Concept-Based Clinical Nursing Skills

FUNDAMENTAL TO ADVANCED

Concept-Based Clinical Nursing Skills

FUNDAMENTAL TO ADVANCED

LOREN NELL MELTON STEIN
MSN, RNC-NIC
Clinical Assistant Professor
Fran and Earl Ziegler College of Nursing
Adjunct Assistant Professor
College of Allied Health
University of Oklahoma Health Sciences Center
Oklahoma City, Oklahoma

CONNIE J. HOLLEN
RN, MS
Adjunct Assistant Professor
College of Allied Health
OUCN Volunteer Adjunct Faculty
Fran and Earl Ziegler College of Nursing
University of Oklahoma Health Sciences Center
Oklahoma City, Oklahoma

ELSEVIER

Elsevier
3251 Riverport Lane
St. Louis, Missouri 63043

Notices

Knowledge and best practice in this field are constantly changing. As new research and experience broaden our understanding, changes in research methods, professional practices, or medical treatment may become necessary.

Practitioners and researchers must always rely on their own experience and knowledge in evaluating and using any information, methods, compounds, or experiments described herein. In using such information or methods they should be mindful of their own safety and the safety of others, including parties for whom they have a professional responsibility.

With respect to any drug or pharmaceutical products identified, readers are advised to check the most current information provided (i) on procedures featured or (ii) by the manufacturer of each product to be administered, to verify the recommended dose or formula, the method and duration of administration, and contraindications. It is the responsibility of practitioners, relying on their own experience and knowledge of their patients, to make diagnoses, to determine dosages and the best treatment for each individual patient, and to take all appropriate safety precautions.

To the fullest extent of the law, neither the Publisher nor the authors, contributors, or editors, assume any liability for any injury and/or damage to persons or property as a matter of products liability, negligence or otherwise, or from any use or operation of any methods, products, instructions, or ideas contained in the material herein.

International Standard Book Number: 978-0-323-62557-9

Senior Content Strategist: Jamie Blum
Senior Content Development Manager: Lisa Newton
Senior Content Development Specialist: Danielle M. Frazier
Publishing Services Manager: Julie Eddy
Book Production Specialist: Clay S. Broeker
Design Direction: Brian Salisbury

Printed in Canada

Last digit is the print number: 9 8 7 6 5 4 3 2 1

Working together
to grow libraries in
developing countries

www.elsevier.com • www.bookaid.org

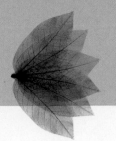

Loren Nell Melton Stein, MSN, RNC-NIC, received her BSN from Duke University in Durham, North Carolina, and her MSN from Marymount University in Arlington, Virginia. She began her clinical experience at Duke University Medical Center in the Neonatal Step-Down and Pediatric Intensive Care Units. She continued her neonatal clinical experience with years in nursing management at Arlington Hospital, now named Virginal Hospital Center. A move to Maryland and completion of her MSN resulted in a faculty position at Salisbury State University and an expansion of her clinical skills to include postpartum and mother/baby care. Upon moving to Oklahoma, she began teaching clinical skills at the College of Nursing, where she first met her co-author. A few years later, she and Connie developed and coordinated a patient care clinical skills class at the College of Allied Health. In Oklahoma, her clinical focus shifted to disaster nursing, and she has served as a Unit Coordinator and statewide Education Coordinator for the Oklahoma Medical Reserve Corps. She has developed a nursing student externship in emergency preparedness and response and was part of a national task force that developed the Core Competencies for Medical Reserve Corps Volunteers. For the last decade, she has been a Clinical Assistant Professor at the Fran and Earl Ziegler College of Nursing, where she coordinates the professional practice lab for the traditional BSN students in Oklahoma City. She has over 2 decades of experience teaching clinical skills to undergraduate students and has contributed to clinical skills and pediatric textbooks.

Loren would like to recognize the unwavering support of her husband and family. She would like to thank her co-author for persevering with this project for many years. In addition, Loren would like to recognize two nurses who inspired her long journey as a nursing educator and as an author to write and continue writing this book: Dean Ruby Wilson, EdD, MSN, RN, FAAN, and Donna Wong, PhD, RN CPN, FAAN. Dean Ruby Wilson was the Dean during her years at Duke and set a wonderfully warm, bright example of a leader and educator. Donna Wong was a fellow Oklahoman who spoke about how writing a book changed her life and who gave so much to the profession of nursing.

Connie J. Hollen, RN, MS, has over 20 years of experience in a variety of areas, including medical/surgical units, the emergency department, post-anesthesia recovery, and critical care. She began her career at University Hospital in Oklahoma City, where she also worked as a charge nurse in the CICU and as a nursing house supervisor. She received her BSN and MS from the University of Oklahoma College of Nursing, where she completed a research thesis and received academic and research awards. After completing her MS, Connie began teaching as an adjunct clinical instructor at the University of Oklahoma College of Nursing and taught junior nursing students in the clinical skills and assessment lab. She has also taught and coordinated a patient care class with her co-author at the University of Oklahoma College of Allied Health. Currently, she is teaching as an adjunct volunteer faculty member in the clinical skills lab at the Fran and Earl Ziegler College of Nursing and as an adjunct assistant professor at the College of Allied Health. Connie is also a volunteer Red Cross instructor and has been a volunteer instructor for the Medical Reserve Corps. In addition, she has been a contributing author and reviewer for several nursing textbooks. Connie has in-depth knowledge about clients who experience terminal and life-threatening illnesses and the strategies and challenges to maintain their quality of life.

Connie would like to recognize the amazing faculty, mentors, colleagues, and clinical nurses at the bedside who continue to be an inspiration. In particular, she would like to thank her friend and co-author who she has taught with for many years. She would also like to thank all of the students who inspired her to keep learning and to keep teaching. Finally, Connie would like to thank her compassionate and brilliant husband, with his gift for humor, who encouraged her to write and continue writing this wonderful book. She would also like to thank her daughter Tori, her son Chris and his wife Kathy, and her sister Ginger for their support.

ACKNOWLEDGEMENTS

This book has involved a tremendous amount of teamwork. We would like to thank the many current and former students, practicing nurses, family members, and friends who served as models and volunteers for the photo shoot and KJ Productions for our wonderful photographs. We appreciate the support of the staff at Elsevier, particularly Anna, Clay, Danielle, and Jamie.

Special thanks go to Cohen Grant and Kim Grant; The Children's Rehabilitation Center; Callie Rinehart, Nurse Educator; and Kyle Leemaster, Director of Nursing, for sharing tracheostomy and gastrostomy tube care with nursing students.

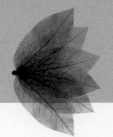

Jean S. Bernard, PhD, MSN, RN
Director of Undergraduate Programs
Appalachian State University
Boone, North Carolina

Morag Dahlstrom, MSN, RN
Professor of Nursing
College of Southern Maryland
LaPlata, Maryland

Amber Nicole Erben, APRN-CNS
Inpatient Neurology Clinical Nurse Specialist
Mercy Hospital
Oklahoma City, Oklahoma

Craig Goforth, MSN, RN
Adjunct Clinical Instructor
College of Nursing
University of Oklahoma Health Sciences Center
Administrative Supervisor
Integris Baptist Medical Center
Oklahoma City, Oklahoma

Tammy W. Howard, MSN, RNC-OB, WHNP-BC
Assistant Professor
Whitson-Hester School of Nursing
Tennessee Technological University
Cookeville, Tennessee

Shelia Hurley, PhD, MSN, MBA/HC, RN
Associate Professor
Whitson-Hester School of Nursing
Tennessee Technological University
Cookeville, Tennessee

Kali Johnson, MSN, RN, PCCN
Adjunct Clinical Instructor
College of Nursing
University of Oklahoma Health Sciences Center
Registered Nurse Clinical Educator
Integris Baptist Medical Center
Oklahoma City, Oklahoma

Jenny Maffett, EdS, MSN, RN
Instructor of Nursing
Whitson-Hester School of Nursing
Tennessee Technological University
Cookeville, Tennessee

Susan E. Piras, PhD, RN
Associate Professor
Whitson-Hester School of Nursing
Tennessee Technological University
Cookcville, Tennessee

Bedelia H. Russell, PhD, RN, CPNP-PC, CNE
Associate Professor
Whitson-Hester School of Nursing
Tennessee Technological University
Cookeville, Tennessee

Karen Zulkowski, DNS, RN
Associate Professor (Retired)
Montana State University
Captain Cook, Hawaii

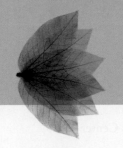

Kali Johnson, MSN, RN, PCCN
Adjunct Clinical Instructor
College of Nursing
University of Oklahoma Health Sciences Center
Registered Nurse Clinical Educator
Integris Baptist Medical Center
Oklahoma City, Oklahoma

Kathleen C. Jones, RN, MSN, CNS
Associate Professor of Nursing
Health Programs
Walters State Community College
Morristown, Tennessee

Lori L. Kelly, RN, EdD, MSN, MBA
Associate Professor of Nursing
South College
Nashville, Tennessee

Patricia T. Ketcham, RN, MSN
Director of Nursing Laboratories
School of Nursing
Oakland University
Rochester, Michigan

Tracy K. Lopez, RN, PhD
Associate Professor and Program Director of Nursing
Doña Ana Community College
New Mexico State University
Las Cruces, New Mexico

Rebecca Otten, RN, EdD
Professor Emeritus of Nursing
California State University—Fullerton
Fullerton, California

Anita K. Reed, RN, MSN
Department Chair of Community Health Practice
St. Elizabeth School of Nursing
Franciscan Health
Lafayette, Indiana

Laura Remy, RN, MPH, BSN
Nurse Researcher and PhD Student
Sinclair School of Nursing
University of Missouri
Columbia, Missouri

Simrit Sandhu, RN, BSN, BSBA RN
Progressive Care Unit
San Antonio Regional Hospital
Upland, California

Susan Parnell Scholtz, RN, PhD
Associate Professor of Nursing
Moravian College
Bethlehem, Pennsylvania

Peter D. Smith, RN, BA, MSN
Instructor and Lead Clinical Educator
Lutheran School of Nursing
Saint Louis, Missouri

Mindy Stayner, RN, PhD, CNE
Professor of Nursing
Capella University
Minneapolis, Minnesota

Lynne Lear Tier, RN, MSN, LNC
Assistant Director of Simulation
Adventist University of Health Sciences
Orlando, Florida

Estella Jo Wetzel, MSN, APRN, FNP-C
Family Nurse Practitioner
Premier Physician Enterprise
Dayton, Ohio

Paige Wimberley, RN, PhD, CNS-BC, CNE
Associate Professor of Nursing
Arkansas State University—Jonesboro
Jonesboro, Arkansas

Jean Yockey, RN, PhD, FNP, CNE
Assistant Professor of Nursing
University of South Dakota
Vermillion, South Dakota

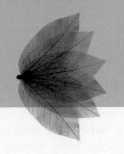

Purpose of the Book

The purpose of this book is to prepare nursing students to provide safe, accurate, client-centered nursing care founded on evidence-based practice. This book takes a unique approach to teaching students nursing skills, as it presents the skills within a framework of critical concepts. The concept-based framework provides students a foundation of seven critical concepts integral to nursing practice on which to develop clinical nursing skills. The concepts allow students to see the patterns and priorities within clinical nursing skills and align well with the competencies of Quality and Safety Education for Nurses (QSEN). The language and concepts often mirror those found in the National Council Licensure Examination-RN (NCLEX-RN). For example, this text uses the term client as the NCLEX-RN does. In addition, the presentation of evidence-based procedures, national standards, and other special features encourages clinical reasoning. This book not only teaches the students "how to" perform a skill but also encourages them to think about "why" they are performing a skill in a certain way. This approach will complement a curriculum that emphasizes clinical judgment and problem-solving skills.

Since the 2003 Institute of Medicine (IOM) report *Health Professions Education: A Bridge to Quality* initiated the appeal for change in nursing education, nursing institutions have been rising to the challenge of developing new ways to teach nursing. Nursing called for new ideas, new tactics in nursing education to meet the urgent need for nurses who are prepared to provide safe, quality nursing care in a rapidly changing environment (Benner, Sutphen, Leonard, & Day, 2010). This text offers a new strategy for teaching clinical nursing skills with a thoughtful, concept-based approach while also acknowledging the importance of the nursing process.

CONCEPT-BASED CLINICAL SKILLS

The purpose of teaching concept-based clinical skills is to facilitate student learning, foster theoretically grounded nursing care, and improve client outcomes. Years of teaching clinical nursing skills culminated in the authors identifying seven nursing concepts that frequently provide the rationales for actions within the clinical skills. We found that presenting and applying these nursing concepts early in nursing students' educational process facilitated student understanding of the nursing concepts and performance of clinical skills.

This text defines each of the critical concepts within the context of performing clinical skills. The definitions provide the rationale and the nursing actions that support the concept. We acknowledge there are other critical concepts;

however, this text is examining the slice of nursing related to performing clinical nursing skills. Sometimes the definition is simple and there is a single statement, such as "Safety measures prevent harm." Sometimes there are multiple ways to operationalize the concept; for example, the concept of infection control includes three possible actions: containing microorganisms, preventing or reducing the transfer of microorganisms, and reducing the number of microorganisms. Communication is one of the broadest concepts, including verbal, nonverbal, written, and electronic communication.

CONCEPT-BASED TEACHING

The authors believe concept-based teaching facilitates student learning and fosters thoughtful, evidence-based nursing care. We believe the method for instructing students should not rely on the memorization of steps in sequence. The application of nursing concepts within the skills improves comprehension and retention of each skill. The noted educator Lynn Erickson (2017) wrote, "The greater the amount of factual information, the greater the need to rise to a higher level of abstraction to organize and process that information." This approach helps students focus less on memorizing the order of steps and more on understanding why they are doing the steps. In this manner, if it becomes necessary to alter the order of the steps in a skill (e.g., as new evidence becomes available, to meet the needs of a client), students will be equipped to make the necessary adaptations without losing sight of the essential concepts that must be done to ensure quality care. For example, if the concept is infection control related to prepping the skin, then whether isopropyl alcohol is applied in a circular scrub or chlorhexidine is applied in a back-and-forth scrub, both are methods of infection control. Teaching within the concept of infection control allows beginning students to apply new evidence and techniques to a foundation of nursing practice concepts without getting stuck in a concrete mode.

Concept-based learning allows students to adapt to new situations and new evidence knowing that the concept has remained the same. As information becomes more complex, conceptual structures are important for sorting information, finding patterns, and processing new information (Erickson, Lanning, & French, 2017). As Giddens (2017) notes in her Preface, "The study of nursing concepts provides the learner with an understanding of essential components associated with nursing practice without becoming saturated and lost in the details for each area of clinical specialty." Concept-based clinical skills and reasoning should facilitate students' ability to adapt to different healthcare settings and client populations with their respective changes in policies and procedures and therefore help bridge the gap between education and practice.

In our experience, nursing faculty and students adapt readily to concept-based teaching. Most nursing faculty readily accept the concepts identified in this text. While concept-based nursing education has been emphasized at different times over the last several decades, it is once again a focus in nursing education. Concepts such as safety and client-centered care permeate nursing and are the backbone of the Quality and Safety Education for Nurses (QSEN) competencies. Furthermore, this text would incorporate beautifully into a concept-based curriculum. For example, Jean F. Giddens' text *Concepts for Nursing Practice* identifies 58 nursing concepts. Three of these concepts are identified as critical concepts within this text. Of Jean Giddens' health and illness concepts, several are components of chapter titles within this text, such as nutrition, elimination, and mobility.

CONTEXT OF THE CLIENT AND FAMILY

Another purpose for teaching clinical skills with a concept-based framework is to foster client-centered care. This concept-based nursing skills text book encourages students to focus on the client and the application of nursing concepts rather than focus primarily on their performance of the skills. When providing nursing care, clinical skills are not a sequential, psychomotor, solo performance. The authors believe that nursing skills are a single component of the full spectrum of nursing care, and nursing care is always in the context of the client and the client's family. We believe providing client-centered care nursing care improves client outcomes.

Critical Concepts

The identification and clarification of the seven critical concepts in this text developed over years of teaching clinical skills. We initially looked at the beginning and ending of skills. Clinical skills begin and end with a predictable sequence of steps. Most skill steps have a rationale, and the rationales fit within broader concepts related to nursing practice. The steps within clinical skills are "the doing," the operationalizing of the nursing concept. For example, "Perform hand hygiene" is a skill step that occurs at the beginning and end of most clinical skills. The larger concept is infection control. The critical concepts also relate to the client's outcome. In this instance, the expected outcome is to prevent client infection. The seven critical concepts identified for performing nursing skills are accuracy, client-centered care, infection control, safety, communication, evaluation, and health maintenance. The critical concept for a skill step is identified in magenta before the step: **ACC, CCC, INF, SAF, COM, HLTH**, and **EVAL**.

ACCURACY

Accuracy is not a concept identified in other skills textbooks, but measurement of blood pressure or placement of a catheter can be correct or incorrect. In this text, we identify variables that impact the accuracy of the skill. There may be subsets of variables that impact accuracy, such as client-related variables, nurse-related variables, and equipment-related variables. For example, when obtaining a manual blood pressure measurement, these three types of variables exist.

Because clinical skills are performed within the context of the client, client-related variables are frequently relevant. A recurring variable is the nurse's assessment of the client, and this text emphasizes the responsibility of the registered nurse to assess the client. For example, accurate assessment of the client's cooperation impacts the performance of the skill and the client outcome. Another frequent, client-related variable is the client's or family's understanding of the procedure. The role of nursing includes explaining the procedure and verifying the client's understanding. For instance, when collecting a urine specimen, the client's understanding of the procedure is paramount for obtaining an uncontaminated clean catch specimen. Likewise, when a client is self-administering pain medication via a patient-controlled analgesia (PCA) pump, it is critical that the client understands the procedure to safely operate the controls to receive adequate pain relief.

An example of a nurse-related variable is the ability to accurately identify anatomical landmarks. The nurse who is placing a urinary catheter in a woman requires knowledge of the anatomy of the pelvic floor and urinary system. The nurse who is giving a viscous intramuscular medication in the ventrogluteal site must be able to accurately identify the anatomical landmarks of the site. Within this text, the accuracy variables provide a list of information that is critical to the accurate performance of the skill. These variables may require a quick review before skill performance. Nursing students' understanding of the identified variables of accuracy is often a prerequisite to skill performance, just as knowledge of anatomy and physiology precede learning nursing skills.

CLIENT-CENTERED CARE

Client-centered care is a recurring concept in healthcare. In this text, client-centered care is based on the concept of respect for the human being. This mirrors the integrated process of caring as defined in the NCLEX-RN test plan that identifies caring as the interaction of the nurse and client in an atmosphere of mutual respect and trust. In this text, specific examples of demonstrating client-centered care include promoting autonomy, providing privacy, ensuring comfort, honoring cultural preferences, and advocating for the client and family. Promoting autonomy is manifested by supporting the decision-making of the client, asking about client preferences, and keeping the focus on the client's needs. Respect for the person means ensuring the client and family understand procedures, including arranging for an approved interpreter if needed and answering questions at any time about a procedure. Respect for the person is also demonstrated by respecting the privacy of the person. Nursing is a trusted profession, and nurses are trusted with a person's body and a person's health information, both of which deserve respect. Another means of showing client-centered care is to ensure the comfort of the client. Assessing, intervening in, and evaluating client comfort is central to providing client-centered care. Assessing cultural preferences and honoring those cultural preferences is another aspect of operationalizing client-centered care. Advocating is sometimes the most difficult and meaningful process of keeping nursing care focused on the client and family.

INFECTION CONTROL

Infection control is a prevalent concern in healthcare, and many nursing skills have an element of infection control. In this text, infection control is the concept related to preventing infection. Infection control may be directed toward preventing infection in the client, in the nurse performing the skill, or in other clients and caregivers in the healthcare setting. Nurses apply three strategies to prevent infection: preventing or reducing the transfer of microorganisms, reducing the number of microorganisms, and containing microorganisms.

Preventing the transfer of microorganisms applies to the individual client, the nurse, and others in the healthcare setting. Nurses prevent the transfer of microorganisms from one anatomical area to another in one client by using specific infection control strategies. For example, wiping female clients from front to back prevents the transfer of microorganisms from the perianal region to the urinary meatus where the microorganisms may cause a urinary tract infection. An example of preventing the transfer of microorganisms to the nurse is the use of personal protective equipment when there is the possibility of exposure to body fluids. Other strategies such as hand hygiene prevent the transfer of microorganisms to both the nurse and to others in the healthcare setting. Within this text we strive to identify the key times for the nurse to perform hand hygiene; however, the student must always consider the specific situation and environment to determine when hand hygiene is warranted based on the principles of infection control.

Reducing the number of microorganisms is another strategy to control infection. There are always organisms in the human mouth, but providing oral care reduces the number of organisms and prevents bacterial overgrowth in the mouth. Nurses use additional strategies to contain microorganisms, such removing soiled gloves by turning them inside out. In this text, infection control is considered in the home and community as well as in the healthcare setting.

SAFETY

Safety is another widely accepted concept in healthcare today. Since the 1999 Institute of Medicine report *To Err is Human* (Kohn, Corrigan, & Donaldson, 1999), improving the safety of healthcare is a recurring goal. For this concept, safety measures are identified to prevent harm and provide a safe care environment. Safety measures are directed primarily toward the client, but at times safety of the nurse and caregivers is an equal concern. For example, in safe client handling and movement, the goal is to prevent harm to both the nurse and the client.

Identified within skills, there are steps to prevent harm and ensure the safety of the client. Safety is always a concern when beginning and finishing an interaction with a client. Before providing care, reviewing orders is a frequently identified safety measure. When entering the room, client identification using two identifiers is a key safety measure. When beginning a skill, this text uses the phrase "Set up an ergonomically safe space" to encourage nursing students to manipulate the client care environment, including the client's bed and surrounding furniture to create a space that is safe for the nurse and client. Using the descriptor "ergonomically safe space" mirrors the NCLEX-RN test plan–related activity statement to use ergonomic principles when providing care. When finishing the skill and preparing to leave a client, several safety measures are consistently identified.

Occasionally a step contains elements of more than one critical concept. If, in this instance, one of those concepts is safety, then we have identified safety. For example, most of the time we identify the labeling of an item as COM for communication. The purpose of a label is to communicate information. However, when labeling tubing to prevent misconnections, which is a significant safety concern, we have identified the step with the critical concept of safety.

COMMUNICATION

Communication is the critical concept that encompasses the exchange of information (verbal, nonverbal, written, or electronic) between two or more people, including nurses and clients and nurses and other members of the healthcare team, as well as documentation in a permanent legal record. Documentation is one aspect of interprofessional communication. Today, interprofessional collaboration is necessary for successful healthcare delivery, and to have successful interprofessional collaboration we must have communication. In this text, we view collaboration as a subset of communication. Collaboration may be with the client and the client's family as well as with other healthcare professionals. Delegation is another subset of communication because the registered nurse must effectively communicate the tasks and information to be delegated. Successful teamwork is contingent upon effective communication.

HEALTH MAINTENANCE

The American Nurses Association (ANA) definition of the scope of practice includes the phrase "Nursing is the protection, promotion, and optimization of health and abilities" (ANA, n.d.). In this text, health maintenance refers to the promotion of the client's well-being, including both the physical health of the body and the ability to provide self-care. The NCLEX-RN test plan identifies self-care as related content within health promotion and maintenance. If a client enters the healthcare facility with healthy teeth and the self-care habit of brushing the teeth twice a day, then within this text it is a nursing health maintenance concept to promote the ability to brush teeth and maintain the health of the mouth. When clients cannot provide self-care to maintain health, the nurse provides the care. Skill steps that reflect the actions taken to maintain and promote health and self-care abilities are identified by the critical concept of health maintenance.

EVALUATION

Evaluation is the critical concept of reflecting on the results to determine the client outcome and efficacy of the care provided. For most skills, evaluation is included as a step within the subheading Finishing the Skill. Evaluation includes checking if the expected client outcomes were achieved and if the method selected by the nurse was effective. We believe it is important for nursing students and nurses to ask the following questions each time a skill is performed: "Did this go well for the client?" "Could it have been done in a way that was better for the client or better for the nurse?" Evaluation is also the concept behind monitoring for specific client outcomes following a skill. The step of evaluation is important in the broader context of nursing clinical research and could include identifying the outcome as data in a clinical research study.

Organization of the Text

The selection of nursing skills in this text reflects current practice and includes a unit on advanced nursing skills not often included in skills textbooks. The first unit introduces fundamental skills used in many settings, because many beginning nursing students begin clinical rotations in low-acuity setting and progress to rotations in acute care and critical care. The reality of nursing education is that nursing students enter clinical sites early in the educational process. One goal of a clinical skills lab is to prepare students to safely enter acute care clinical sites armed with basic skills on a platform of critical nursing concepts. In addition, this text provides a resource for students throughout their clinical rotations, including critical care. Each chapter provides sufficient background information, physiology, and disease-related facts for students to see the relationship between each skill and nursing care.

Unit I, Fundamental Nursing Skills, introduces students to basic nursing skills that frequently appear in a wide range of healthcare settings. The setting may be a healthcare agency, a long-term care residence, a home, or hospice. These fundamental skills will continue to be used in acute care and critical care settings. Like the base of a pyramid, these fundamental skills provide a foundation for nursing care, and other levels of nursing care include and build upon this foundation.

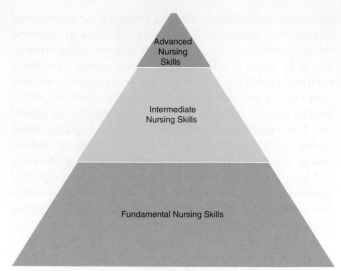

Unit I contains the following chapters, which cover fundamental nursing skills:
- Foundations of Safe Client Care
- Personal Care and Hygiene
- Vital Signs and Vital Measurements
- Performing an Assessment
- Nutrition and Gastrointestinal Tube Therapy
- Supporting Mobility and Immobilization
- Comfort Care
- End-of-Life Care

Building upon the first unit, Unit II, Intermediate Nursing Skills, covers nursing skills typically used in a hospital and prepares students to enter clinical rotations in an acute care facility. This unit contains the following chapters:
- Airway and Breathing
- Sterile Technique
- Medication Administration
- Venous Access
- Central Venous Access
- Bowel Elimination
- Urine Elimination
- Wound Care
- Perioperative Care

In the final unit of the text, Unit III, Advanced Nursing Skills, the chapters cover skills more commonly found in a critical care environment. This unit contains the following chapters:
- Advanced Respiratory Management
- Advanced Cardiovascular Care
- Advanced Neurologic Care

ALIGNING WITH QSEN

This concept-based text acknowledges and responds to the Quality and Safety Education for Nurses (QSEN) competencies (Cronenwett et al., 2007). The critical concepts identified in this text for clinical skills fit well within the quality and safety framework of QSEN. The QSEN competencies encompass all aspects of nursing and are much broader than the seven critical concepts we have identified specific to clinical nursing skills. The Case Study found at the end of each chapter has a QSEN competency–focused question to provide students the opportunity to apply the competencies in a clinical situation. Since the introduction of QSEN competencies, the competencies are increasingly integrated in nursing program curricula. Nursing educators have asked how to best teach and evaluate nursing students using the QSEN paradigm. We believe this text offers a concept-based strategy of how to teach and evaluate the clinical skills of nursing within a framework dedicated to quality and safety.

Safety and Client-Centered Care

Two of the QSEN competencies are also identified in this text as critical concepts for clinical skills, safety and client-centered care. The QSEN definition of safety is "Minimizes risk of harm to patients and providers through both system effectiveness and individual performance" (Cronenwett et al., 2007). One of the identified QSEN skills related to safety is "Demonstrate effective use of strategies to reduce risk of harm to self or others" (Cronenwett et al., 2007). The KSA competencies identified in the QSEN competencies for safety prepare nursing students to perform safety measures to prevent harm. Within this text, the definition of safety is that performing safety measures prevents harm and provides/maintains a safe care environment. The two are totally congruent.

Likewise, the definition of patient-centered care in QSEN is "Recognize the patient or designee as the source of control and full partner in providing compassionate and coordinated care based on respect for patient's preferences, values, and needs" (Cronenwett et al., 2007). Within this text, we identify client-centered care as a critical concept and define it as, "Client-centered care is based on the concept of respect for the human being and is demonstrated through promoting autonomy, providing privacy, ensuring comfort, honoring cultural preferences, and advocating for the client and family." The KSA competencies identified in the QSEN competencies for patient-centered care prepare nursing students to perform client-centered care as identified in this text.

Communication: Informatics, Teamwork, and Collaboration

Within this text, the critical concept of communication is emphasized. Communication is the common element in the QSEN competencies of informatics, teamwork, and collaboration. QSEN competencies within these areas address much broader knowledge, skills, and attitudes than are identified within a clinical skills text.

Quality Improvement

QSEN defines quality improvement as "Use data to monitor the outcomes of care processes and use improvement methods to design and test changes to continuously improve the quality and safety of health care systems" (Cronenwett et al., 2007). In this text, the critical concept of evaluation supports the quality improvement competency. Teaching KSA competencies related to quality improvement strengthens students' ability to evaluate client outcomes and the process

of performing clinical skills. Furthermore, evaluation when finishing a skill is an opportunity to discuss quality improvement and data collection to support evidence-based practice.

Evidence-Based Practice

QSEN defines evidence-based practice as "Integrate best current evidence with clinical expertise and patient/family preferences and values for delivery of optimal health" (Cronenwett et al., 2007). This text emphasizes client-centered care and client preferences in conjunction with evidence-based practice consistent with the QSEN KSA competencies. Throughout this text, emphasis is placed on finding and using evidence-based practice, including identifying areas in which there is a current lack of solid evidence to standardize practice.

Evidence-based practice may direct any and all of the critical concepts. Variables that affect the accuracy of skill performance, such as client assessment, may be impacted through the development of an evidence-based assessment tool. Safety measures may change as evidence supports new processes and new technology to improve client safety. Evidence resulting from research examining improved outcomes with enhanced client autonomy can guide nursing practice related to client-centered care. Infection control practices are frequently changing and evolving as evidence supports new protocols and standards. Evidence supporting improved means of exchanging information and recording information may apply to nurse-client information exchanges, interprofessional team information exchanges, and strategies to document information in the legal health-care record. Health maintenance is a sphere of nursing knowledge and research producing new evidence on how to improve the promotion of client health and self-care abilities. Within this text, the concept of evaluation is present in most skills. Furthermore, evaluation when finishing a skill is an opportunity to discuss quality improvement and data collection to support evidence-based practice.

INTEGRATION OF THE NURSING PROCESS

Although this book uses a concept-based approach, it does not neglect the nursing process. The nursing process is a decision-making model that allows a systematic, cyclic approach to problem-solving. This book seamlessly integrates the nursing process throughout the skills, the sections, and the chapters. At the end of each section, there is a feature titled Application of the Nursing Process that provides an example of a nursing diagnosis, client outcome, and nursing intervention applicable to that section. The objective was not to identify all of the possible nursing diagnoses but rather to give students one or two examples of applicable nursing diagnoses using examples of client outcomes and nursing interventions relevant to the skills within the section.

The authors also support the use of standardized nursing language as a means of improving student understanding and minimizing confusion. Nursing diagnoses and client outcomes are adapted from the International Classification for Nursing Practices (ICNP) (n.d.). The ICNP is used to describe and document the observations (diagnoses) and the interventions of nurses around the world. The ICNP catalogue of Nursing Diagnosis and Outcome Statements is used in many different types of healthcare settings and provides easily understandable terminology for the description of nursing practice. The ICNP is continually updated to reflect changes within the nursing practice, and it has been used extensively in building health information systems. We have found the ICNP diagnoses well organized and comprehensive.

Additionally, at the end of each chapter, an in-depth Case Study and Concept Map provide concrete examples of implementing the nursing process to provide nursing care. Nursing assessment data is always included in the Case Study and identified within the Concept Map. A variety of nursing diagnoses pertinent to the client in the Case Study are identified in the Concept Map. Nursing interventions, often clustered under critical concept headings, are also provided in the Concept Map. The Case Study is structured so that the nursing interventions often require the skills identified within the chapter. In addition, the Case Study analysis encourages clinical judgment and higher-level learning.

Assessment

Nursing assessment is a vital component of performing clinical skills. Often, how a skill is to be performed is dependent upon the nurse's assessment of the cooperation and abilities of the client. Sometimes the skill is an intervention performed as a result of an assessment, such as suctioning a tracheostomy tube based on an assessment of secretions within the tube. Within each skill, the relevant nursing assessment is identified within the procedure. Moreover, within the sections of each chapter, the critical concepts are tailored to the skills within that section. The critical concept for accuracy will identify nursing assessments of specific client traits when those traits impact the accuracy of the skill. For example, assessment of client cooperation, mobility, and level of discomfort impacts the accuracy of several skills.

Nursing Diagnosis

Examples of nursing diagnoses that are appropriate given the skills and nursing care are provided within each section of each chapter. In addition, the concept maps within each chapter integrate key nursing diagnoses related to the Case Study.

Planning and Client Outcomes

Within a concept-based context, expected client outcomes are paramount to developing nursing interventions. If the expected outcome is that the client will not demonstrate any signs of infection, then it follows that the applicable concept is infection control and that the nurse will be implementing measures to prevent infection. Examples of expected client outcomes are given for each section within each chapter.

This text identifies examples of one or more client outcomes within each section throughout the text to give students concrete examples of the expectations.

Interventions

The section Application of the Nursing Process concludes with examples of nursing interventions. These examples are discussed earlier in the text. This helps to reinforce the nursing process.

Evaluation

Evaluation is, of course, the final step in the cycle of the nursing process. It is also a critical concept within this text and often appears as a final step in the skill. We believe that identifying evaluation as an ever-present part of nursing will develop students who value continuous improvement of practice and who question practices that result in suboptimal outcomes. It is important that new nurses develop the skill of evaluation to determine if client outcomes were achieved and to evaluate nursing actions. The evolution of nursing care and the development of new evidence-based practice is dependent upon nurses' ability to evaluate the nursing care given.

SPECIAL FEATURES OF THE TEXT

Literary Quotation

Each chapter begins with a historical, literary, or inspirational quotation. Nursing is an art as well as a science. Literary quotes provide a humanistic approach to nursing practice. The purpose of this feature is to give students a sense of the lives and writings dedicated to nursing, provide a glimpse into the history that preceded our current understanding, or sometimes just to enliven the reading and draw the student into the chapter.

Lessons From the Evidence

These boxes highlight and summarize current research that may contribute to evidence-based clinical practice. They may also identify research studies for which, despite effort and intention, the research lacks sufficient evidence to guide clinical practice. Although some information is featured in boxes, content such as current evidence and lifespan considerations is also found in the narrative text.

Lessons From the Courtroom

These boxes summarize actual court cases related to the skills in the chapter to help students understand legal implications associated with nursing actions and responsibilities. A variety of cases and decisions were selected to reflect the legal consequences of following—or failing to follow—nursing standards.

Lessons From Experience

These boxes use a storytelling format to share the experiences of more seasoned nurses with students. Storytelling is an effective means of sharing clinical experiences and enriching the knowledge of students.

Lifespan Considerations

These boxes present specific considerations for neonatal, pediatric, or geriatric clients, because this text values teaching skills that are applicable to clients across the lifespan. The Essentials of Baccalaureate Education for Professional Nursing Practice (American Association of Colleges of Nursing [AACN], 2008) states that education must include content and experiences across the lifespan. In the United States, approximately 23% of the population is under the age of 18. In addition, while the infant mortality rate has been decreasing, the United States had an infant mortality rate of over 579 per 100,000 live births (Murphy, Xu, Kochanek, & Arias, 2018), which is more than three times that of Finland or Iceland (at 180 deaths per 100,000 births) and more than double that of most European counties (Jacob, 2016).

At the other end of the lifespan are older adults. In the United States, the number of individuals over the age of 65 is expected to more than double by 2060. The population over the age of 85 is the fastest growing demographic in the United States, and while it remains a small percentage of the total population, this demographic is projected to more than triple by 2060 (Mather, Jacobsen, & Pollard, 2015).

As early as 2030, the percentage of the U.S. population under the age of 18 and over the age of 65 could each be about 21%, a total of 42% of the U.S. population. In this text, Lifespan Considerations highlights information related to specialized nursing care of the very young and older adult populations.

Cultural Considerations

These boxes present information related to culture. The United States is an increasingly diverse country. The U.S. Census Bureau (2015) noted that the nation's minority population represents over 37% of the total population. It is a priority of the authors for students to receive information and considerations for minority populations.

Home Care Considerations

These boxes discuss nursing considerations related to home care. While new graduates of nursing programs often initially obtain employment in acute care settings, there has been an overall increase in the number of nurses working in community and home care settings. This text presents skills primarily within the acute care setting, but it provides information and instructions for home care skills as well.

Expect the Unexpected

These boxes use a storytelling format to share unexpected situations have occurred or may occur in nursing practice and to explore appropriate responses in these situations. This feature also helps the student learn how to cope with uncertainty in a challenging healthcare environment.

Case Study

Each chapter will conclude with a Case Study depicting a client with problems that might be experienced in the clinical setting, followed by a series of Case Study questions.

Answers for the Case Study questions are provided on the book's Evolve website.

Concept Map

A Concept Map, based on the subject of the Case Study, provides a visual depiction of the interrelatedness of the client's problems, assessment data, nursing diagnoses, and nursing interventions.

SUMMARY

This textbook offers a unique way of learning skills using a concept-based approach. As noted, the nursing process is also an important element within each of the chapter sections as well as the case studies and concept maps. We believe that the integration of these approaches enhances the student's clinical reasoning and problem-solving skills that will prepare them for the increasingly complex healthcare environment now and in the future.

References

American Association of Colleges of Nursing (AACN). (2008). *The essentials of baccalaureate education for professional nursing practice.* Washington, DC: Author. Retrieved from https://www.aacnnursing.org/Education-Resources/Tool-Kits/Baccalaureate-Essentials-Tool-Kit.

American Nurses Association. (n.d.). *Scope of practice.* Retrieved from https://www.nursingworld.org/practice-policy/scope-of-practice/.

Benner, P., Sutphen, M., Leonard, V., & Day, L. (2010). *Educating nurses: A call for radical transformation* (vol. 15). Stanford, CT: Jossey-Bass.

Cronenwett, L., Sherwood, G., Barnsteiner, J., Disch, J., Johnson, J., Mitchell, P., …, Warren, J. (2007). Quality and safety education for nurses. *Nursing Outlook, 55*(3), 122–131.

Erickson, H. L., Lanning, L.A., & French, R. (2017). *Concept-based curriculum and instruction for the thinking classroom.* Thousand Oaks, CA: Corwin Press.

Giddens, J. F. (2017). *Concepts for nursing practice* (2nd ed.) St. Louis, MO: Elsevier.

Institute of Medicine. (2003). *Health professions education: A bridge to quality.* Washington, DC: National Academies Press.

International Council of Nurses. (n.d.). *About ICNP.* Retrieved from https://www.icn.ch/what-we-do/projects/ehealth-icnp/about-icnp.

Jacob, J. A. (2016). US infant mortality rate declines but still exceeds other developed countries. *Journal of the American Medical Association, 315*(5), 451–452.

Kohn, L. T., Corrigan, J. M., & Donaldson, M. S. (1999). *To err is human: Building a safer health system.* Committee on Health Care in America, Institute of Medicine. Retrieved from https://www.ncbi.nlm.nih.gov/pubmed/25077248.

Mather, M., Jacobsen, L. A., & Pollard, K. M. (2015). Aging in the United States. *Population Bulletin, 70*(2). Retrieved from https://assets.prb.org/pdf16/aging-us-population-bulletin.pdf.

Murphy, S. L,, Xu, J. Q., Kochanek, K. D., & Arias, E. (2018). *Mortality in the United States.* [NCHS data brief, no. 328]. Hyattsville, MD: National Center for Health Statistics.

U.S. Census Bureau. (2015). *U.S. Census Bureau projections show a slower growing, older, more diverse nation a half century from now.* Retrieved from http://www.census.gov/newsroom/releases/archives/population/cb12-243.html.

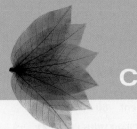

CONTENTS

UNIT 2 Intermediate Nursing Skills

UNIT 3 Advanced Nursing Skills

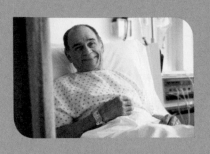

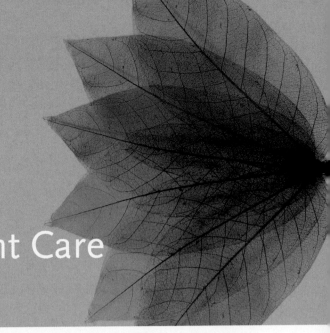

CHAPTER 1

Foundations of Safe Client Care

"It may seem a strange principle to enunciate as the very first requirement in a hospital that it should do the sick no harm." | **Florence Nightingale, 1859**

LEARNING OBJECTIVES

By the end of this chapter, the reader will be able to:

1   Identify a client with two identifiers.
2   Perform hand hygiene with an alcohol-based agent.
3   Perform hand hygiene with soap and water.
4   Apply and remove clean gloves.

5   Apply and remove personal protective equipment: gown, gloves, mask, goggles or face shield, respirator.
6   Apply infection control principles to the environment.
7   Position a client in bed.
8   Move a client up in bed.
9   Transfer a client from a bed to a chair/wheelchair.
10   Move a client with a sling lift.
11   Move a client with a sit-to-stand lift.
12   Transfer a client laterally from a bed to a stretcher.
13   Move clients who have special precautions (logrolling).
14   Apply and remove a vest restraint, limb restraint, elbow restraint, and belt restraint.
15   Apply a mummy restraint.

TERMINOLOGY

Alcohol-based handrub An alcohol-containing preparation designed for application to the hands for reducing the number of viable microorganisms on the hands.

Antimicrobial soap Soap that contains an antiseptic agent.

Antiseptic agent An antimicrobial substance applied to the skin to reduce the number of microbial flora. Examples include alcohols, chlorhexidine, and iodine.

Antiseptic handrub Procedure involving applying an antiseptic handrub product to all surfaces of the hands to reduce the number of microorganisms present.

Antiseptic handwash Procedure involving washing hands with water and soap or other detergents containing an antiseptic agent.

Disinfectant An antimicrobial substance applied to inanimate objects to reduce the number of microorganisms. Examples include bleach solutions and isopropyl alcohol.

Disinfection Process that eliminates many or all pathogenic microorganisms, except bacterial spores, on inanimate objects.

Dorsiflexion Flexion in a dorsal direction; for the foot, flexing upward.

Ergonomic The science of how to fit work to a person's anatomical, physiological, and psychological features in a manner that will enhance well-being.

Hand antisepsis Procedure for antiseptic handwash or antiseptic handrub.

Hand hygiene General term that includes handwashing, antiseptic handwash, antiseptic handrub, or hand antisepsis.

Handwashing Procedure involving washing hands with nonantimicrobial soap and water.

Healthcare-associated infection (HAI) Infection associated with healthcare delivery in any setting (hospitals, long-term care facilities, ambulatory settings, home care).

Nosocomial infection Infection acquired in a hospital.

Sterilization Free from all living microorganisms.

ACRONYMS

AIIR Airborne infection isolation room
APIC Association for Professionals in Infection Control and Epidemiology, Inc.
C-DIFF *Clostridium difficile*
eMAR Electronic medication administration record
HAI Healthcare-associated infection
HEPA High-efficiency particulate air (filtration)
HICPAC Healthcare Infection Control Practices Advisory Committee
IOM Institute of Medicine
MAR Medication administration record
MRSA Methicillin-resistant *Staphylococcus aureus*
NIOSH National Institute for Occupational Safety and Health
PPE Personal protective equipment

Ensuring safety and preventing errors are critical concerns in healthcare. Today, the goals in healthcare include creating a culture of safety and setting the target for zero harm. As we have seen in past reports, healthcare errors cause serious harm, suffering, and even death. In 1999, the Institute of Medicine (IOM), now renamed the National Academy of Medicine, published a shocking report on the safety record of American healthcare facilities. The report, *To Err Is Human: Building a Safer Health System,* stated that "as many as 98,000 people die in hospitals each year as a result of medical errors that could have been prevented." The report also outlined a strategy by which government agencies, healthcare providers, healthcare organizations, and consumers can work together to reduce preventable medical errors. One of the central conclusions of the report is that the majority of medical errors are not due to the actions of individuals but are caused by faulty systems, processes, and conditions. Nurses are in a unique position to identify faulty systems, processes, and conditions and to creatively develop alternatives in which the safety of the client, the client's family, and the healthcare team is paramount. Each section of this chapter identifies an aspect of care related to safety.

Many nongovernmental organizations also address healthcare safety. One of the most important of these is The Joint Commission, an independent accrediting body for healthcare organizations. In order to achieve and maintain accreditation, healthcare facilities must meet specific Joint Commission standards, many of which directly address safety. Today, the standards of an accredited healthcare organization include demonstrating to The Joint Commission that the healthcare facility is building a safety culture (The Joint Commission, 2018).

SECTION 1 Identifying the Client

One of the most critical tasks in delivering safe care is identifying the client for whom the care is intended, including diagnostic procedures, medications, and other treatments. Unfortunately, wrong-client errors continue to happen in all stages of care. To reduce such errors, the first goal of The Joint Commission's National Patient Safety Goals is to improve the accuracy of client identification and to match care to that client (The Joint Commission, 2018). The Joint Commission developed the standard of consistently using two client identifiers every time a client is identified. Acceptable identifiers must be "person specific" and may include name, date of birth, account number, or even telephone number. The client's room number is not an acceptable identifier because it is not person specific. In a hospital setting, clients typically have a wristband that includes several identifiers. The Joint Commission standards stipulate that the two identifiers may be in the same place, such as on the person's wristband. Furthermore, the use of electronic identification technology coding, such as bar coding, meets the two-identifier requirements if there are two or more person-specific identifiers included in the bar code. See Box 1.1 for evidence on whether bar-coding technology reduces medication errors.

In an outpatient setting, where clients do not have a wristband, the Joint Commission standards still require two identifiers. They may be name, date of birth, Social Security number, home address, or phone number. In a behavioral health setting, the clinical record may also include a photograph of the client, which can serve as one of the identifiers. In a home setting, two identifiers are a requirement on the first encounter. After initial contact, a home address or facial recognition may be one of the identifiers. Once the client is identified, then the care is matched to that client.

In all settings, active client involvement in the identification process, when possible, is considered best practice. Nurses ask a client his or her name when first meeting a client, confirm with a client that the information on the wristband is correct, and include a client in eliciting the two person-specific identifiers prior to each diagnostic procedure, medication administration, or other treatment.

APPLICATION OF THE NURSING PROCESS

Examples of Related International Classification for Nursing Practice (ICNP) Nursing Diagnoses, Expected Client Outcomes, and Nursing Interventions:

Nursing Diagnosis: Risk for injury
Supporting Data: Potential for wrong client error

Expected Client Outcome: The client will remain free from injury associated with wrong client errors while in the healthcare setting.
Nursing Intervention Example: Prevent iatrogenic injury by following National Patient Safety Goals of two identifiers.
Reference: International Classification for Nursing Practice. (n.d.). *eHealth & ICNP*. Retrieved from https://www.icn.ch/what-we-do/projects/ehealth-icnp.

CRITICAL CONCEPTS
Identifying the Client

Accuracy (ACC)

Client identification is established through the use of two person-specific identifiers, such as:
- client name
- client date of birth
- client account number.

BOX 1.1 Lessons From the Evidence: Can Bar-Code Technology Decrease Wrong-Client Errors?

A two-part research study conducted in Nebraska used direct observation to collect information about medication administration. In the first part of the study, 9 hospitals participated, and in the second part of the study, 8 hospitals participated; of those 8 hospitals, 5 had been in the first study, so nurses at 12 different hospitals were observed administering medication. One aspect of the study was to determine if a nurse-to-nurse double-check of a medication or the use of bar-code medication administration technology was more effective at preventing a medication administration error. The results showed that bar-code medication administration identified 66.7% of errors prior to administration, whereas nurse-to-nurse double-checking identified only 10%.

In an article that synthesized the findings of 16 systematic reviews of studies regarding safety interventions designed to reduce medication administration errors, the authors found 8 reviews that identified bar-code technology. In general, the authors found that the use of bar-code technology decreases error in medication administration. However, they noted that it also introduces the possibilities of error and interruption in the form of scanning issues and computer malfunction. They concluded that a multifaceted approach that includes the use of bar-code technology is effective in decreasing medication errors. Both articles noted the cost of initiating and sustaining bar-code technology in acute care settings.

References: Cochran, Barrett, & Horn, 2016; Lapkin, Levett-Jones, Chenoweth, & Johnson, 2016.

Client-Centered Care (CCC)

When identifying the client, respect for the client is demonstrated through:
- active client involvement in the identification process
- advocating for the client and family.

Infection Control (INF)

When identifying the client, healthcare-associated infection is prevented by:
- reducing the transfer and number of microorganisms, primarily through hand hygiene.

Safety (SAF)

When identifying the client, safety measures prevent harm and provide a safe care environment.

The use of bar-code technology meets the two person-specific identifiers and enhances client safety.

Communication (COM)

- Communication exchanges information (oral, written, nonverbal, or electronic) between two or more people.
- Collaboration with the client facilitates consistent client identification.

Evaluation (EVAL)

When identifying the client, evaluation of outcomes enables the nurse to determine the efficacy of the care provided.

■ SKILL 1.1 Identifying a Client

EQUIPMENT

Medical record
Medical orders
Medication administration record (MAR) or electronic medication administration record (eMAR)

BEGINNING THE SKILL

1. **INF** Perform hand hygiene.

PROCEDURE

2. **CCC** Introduce yourself to the client and family.
3. **COM** Ask the client to state his or her full name.
4. **ACC** Examine the name on the wristband if present.
   WARNING: Avoid workarounds. If the client's wristband has fallen off or is missing, ensure that it is replaced so that proper identification can occur.

5. **ACC** Examine a second identifier: date of birth, account number.
6. **SAF** Compare identifiers with the medical record, order, MAR, or eMAR depending on your reason for identifying the client.

FINISHING THE SKILL

7. **EVAL** Evaluate your identification of the client. *Are you confident you have correctly identified the client?*

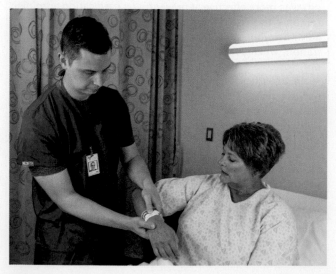

STEP 4 Examine the client wristband.

The goal of infection control practices is to prevent healthcare-associated infections (HAIs). The impact of HAIs includes prolonged hospitals stays, higher medical costs, increased resistance of microorganisms, increased long-term disability, and even death.

One of the well-known risk factors for HAI is the presence of an invasive device. Therefore, clients in healthcare settings with higher acuity and more invasive devices, such as an intensive care unit, are at a greater risk for acquiring an infection. However, greater risk does not automatically mean a greater number of infections. For example, nurses have reduced central line–related bloodstream infections by effectively implementing evidence-based infection control strategies. Healthcare professionals have been less successful in reducing the incidence of catheter-associated urinary tract infections. Today, half of all HAIs occur in non–intensive care settings (Centers for Disease Control and Prevention [CDC], 2018c).

CHAIN OF INFECTION

To prevent infection, one has to understand the transmission of infection, which has specific requirements in a specific sequence, called the chain of infection. The chain of infection is made up of six links: (1) the microorganism or etiologic agent, such as bacteria, viruses, fungi, and parasites; (2) the reservoir—or source—of the microorganism; (3) a portal of exit from the reservoir; (4) a mode of transmission; (5) a portal of entry into the host; and finally (6) a susceptible host. Fig. 1.1 illustrates these six links. For example, a nurse comes to work while in the early stages of influenza. The influenza virus is the microorganism, and the nurse is the reservoir. The nurse sneezes into her hand; the sneeze is the portal of exit for the microorganism. Her hand is the mode of transmission as she then takes a client's pulse and transfers

the microorganism to the client's hand. The client then rubs his eyes and nose, introducing the virus to his mucous membranes. The client's illness and hospitalization have left him susceptible to infection, and 3 days later, he also comes down with influenza.

Breaking the chain of infection that can result in an HAI is one of the foundations of providing safe client care. Although the chain has six links, three are critical for HAI: (1) the reservoir—or source, (2) a mode of transmission for the agent, and (3) a susceptible host. An understanding of the interrelationship of these three elements is necessary if nurses are to prevent the transmission of infectious agents and thereby prevent HAI.

The sources of infectious agents are most often human beings. Clients, family members, visitors, and healthcare personnel contribute to the potential pool of infectious agents. Infectious agents are not always easily identified; whereas some manifest through an active infection, others may be incubating and asymptomatic. Sometimes people are unknowingly colonized with an infectious agent; this can occur, for example, with methicillin-resistant *Staphylococcus aureus* (MRSA). The source may also be the endogenous flora of the gastrointestinal tract or respiratory tract, such as when *Escherichia coli* from the gastrointestinal tract causes an infection in the urinary tract. Occasionally, inanimate objects, such as contaminated faucets or wash basins, are a source of an infectious agent.

Most strategies to prevent the transmission of infectious agents and potential HAI target blocking the mode of transmission. Different types of organisms have different modes of transmission, and some organisms can be transmitted by more than one. Modes of transmission include either direct or indirect contact; droplet transmission, in which respiratory droplets travel by coughing or sneezing; airborne transmission, in which smaller microorganisms can remain airborne; and blood-borne transmission.

One of the most common modes of transmission is contact transmission, specifically, indirect-contact transmission. The difference between indirect- and direct-contact transmission can be clarified with two examples. The herpes simplex virus (HSV) can be transmitted by direct contact. For example, if a healthcare worker did not wear gloves and provided oral care to a client with active oral lesions, a direct-contact transmission could occur, resulting in a herpetic whitlow on the healthcare worker's finger. Indirect-contact transmission happens when the organisms are transferred by an intermediate object or person, for example, through the sharing of a straw or drinking glass. Many years of research confirms that healthcare providers' contaminated hands are a significant source of indirect-contact transmission (Siegel, Rhinehart, Jackson, Chiarello, & Healthcare Infection Control Practices Advisory Committee, 2019). Studies demonstrate that healthcare workers' hands become increasingly

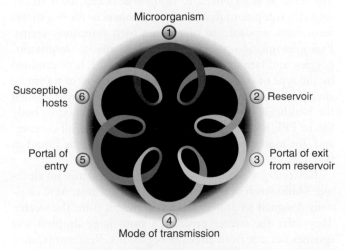

Microorganism
①
② Reservoir
③ Portal of exit from reservoir
④ Mode of transmission
⑤ Portal of entry
⑥ Susceptible hosts

FIG. 1.1 The six chains of infection.

contaminated over time as they provide direct care. The time providing care and the type of care provided affect hand contamination, but hand contamination is very similar for ungloved and gloved hands. The glove surface becomes contaminated, and the gloved hands become a vehicle for indirect-contact transmission. In addition, any device that is shared between clients, such as a thermometer or stethoscope, can serve as a mode of indirect-contact transmission if it is not disinfected between clients.

Many clients within the healthcare system are susceptible hosts because their immune status is compromised by their underlying disease, such as diabetes, or their age. Malignancy and transplants increase susceptibility; some medications change the endogenous flora and increase susceptibility to opportunistic organisms. In healthy individuals, intact skin is the first line of defense against many infectious agents, but surgical procedures and radiation therapy impair this defense. Indwelling devices also promote susceptibility by creating a route along which microorganisms can travel and thus bypass the normal lines of defense.

PREVENTING THE TRANSMISSION OF INFECTION

The CDC developed *Guidelines for Isolation Precautions* in 1996 in order to prevent the transmission of infections. The 2007 version expanded on and updated those first guidelines. Since that time, the CDC has continued to electronically expand on and update the 2007 guidelines. The guidelines identify two tiers of precautions: Standard Precautions and Transmission-Based Precautions.

Standard Precautions

Using Standard Precautions for all clients in all settings, regardless of the suspected or confirmed presence of an infectious agent, is the primary strategy to prevent the transmission of infectious agents in healthcare settings. Standard Precautions are founded on the theory that all blood, body fluids, secretions (except sweat), nonintact skin, and mucous membranes may contain transmissible infectious agents. The specific practices that make up Standard Precautions include:
- hand hygiene
- the use of personal protective equipment (PPE), including gloves, gown, mask, eye protection, or a face shield, depending on the risk of exposure.

Standard Precautions are for the protection of the members of the healthcare team. There are three new elements of Standard Precautions that are in place for the protection of the clients. The three new elements include:
a. specific safe-injection practices (which are discussed in Chapter 11)
b. respiratory hygiene/cough etiquette
c. use of masks for the insertion of catheters or the injection of material into spinal or epidural spaces via lumbar puncture.

Nurses determine which infection prevention practice to use based on the type of client–nurse interaction and the possibility of exposure to blood, other body fluids, or pathogens. Whenever exposure may occur, it is critical to apply infection prevention measures (CDC, 2016b). Review Table 1.1 for recommendations for the application of Standard Precautions for the care of all clients in all healthcare settings.

Hand Hygiene

Hand hygiene has been a critical strategy to prevent the transmission of microorganisms since the mid-1800s, when studies by Ignaz Semmelweis and Oliver Wendell Holmes determined that it could reduce the rate of HAIs. In the 1980s, the United States published the first national hand-hygiene guidelines. Later, in 1995 and 1996, the CDC and Healthcare Infection Control Practices Advisory Committee (HICPAC) recommended hand hygiene when leaving the room of an individual infected with a multidrug-resistant pathogen using either an antimicrobial soap or a waterless antiseptic. In 2002, the HICPAC published hand-hygiene guidelines that represent the most extensive review of the literature to date. The literature showed that alcohol-based handrubs remove organisms more effectively, take less time, and are less irritating to the skin than handwashing with soap and water. In addition, having readily available alcohol-based handrubs increased the total number of times healthcare professionals performed hand hygiene. The CDC and the World Health Organization (WHO) recommend alcohol-based handrubbing as the preferred means and the gold standard of care for hand-hygiene practices in healthcare settings (Siegel et al., 2019; WHO, 2009).

Nevertheless, there are instances when handwashing with soap and water is recommended:
- when hands are visibly dirty or soiled with blood or body fluids
- after using the toilet
- if exposed to spore-forming microorganisms, such as *Clostridium difficile* (C-DIFF) (Siegel et al., 2019).

Review Box 1.2 to identify each time you must perform hand hygiene.

Personal Protective Equipment

The term *personal protective equipment (PPE)* refers to the wearable equipment that protects members of the healthcare team from exposure to or contact with infectious agents. Examples include gloves, gowns, face masks, respirators, goggles, and face shields. The selection of PPE is determined by the type of infectious agent, the mechanism of transmission, the care being delivered, and the varying ways in which the healthcare provider might be exposed to blood or body fluids: PPE is only fully effective if it provides full coverage and, for masks, fits well. A PPE summary can be found in Box 1.3.

Isolation gowns are designed to prevent splatter on clothing. Masks, such as those worn in a surgical area, were originally designed to protect the environment from the wearer. They offer the wearer protection from large droplets and splashes but not from airborne organisms. Respirators, such as the N95 respirator, are designed to protect the wearer

TABLE 1.1 Recommendations for Application of Standard Precautions for the Care of All Clients in All Healthcare Settings

Component	Recommendations
Hand hygiene	After touching blood, body fluids, secretions, excretions, contaminated items; immediately after removing gloves; between client contacts
Personal Protective Equipment (PPE)	
Gloves	For touching blood, body fluids, secretions, excretions, contaminated items; for touching mucous membranes and nonintact skin
Gown	During procedures and client-care activities when contact of clothing/exposed skin with blood/body fluids, secretions, and excretions is anticipated
Mask, eye protection (goggles), face shield[a]	During procedures and client-care activities likely to generate splashes or sprays of blood, body fluids, secretions, especially suctioning, endotracheal intubation
Soiled client-care equipment	Handle in a manner that prevents the transfer of microorganisms to others and to the environment; wear gloves if visibly contaminated; perform hand hygiene.
Environmental control	Develop procedures for routine care, cleaning, and disinfection of environmental surfaces, especially frequently touched surfaces in client-care areas.
Textiles and laundry	Handle in a manner that prevents the transfer of microorganisms to others and to the environment.
Needles and other sharps	Do not recap, bend, break, or hand-manipulate used needles; if recapping is required, use a one-handed scoop technique only; use safety features when available; place used sharps in puncture-resistant container.
Client resuscitation	Use mouthpiece, resuscitation bag, and other ventilation devices to prevent contact with mouth and oral secretions.
Client placement	Prioritize for single-client room if client is at increased risk of transmission, is likely to contaminate the environment, does not maintain appropriate hygiene, or is at increased risk of acquiring infection or developing adverse outcome following infection.
Respiratory hygiene/cough etiquette (source containment of infectious respiratory secretions in symptomatic clients, beginning at initial point of encounter, e.g., triage and reception areas in emergency departments and authorized healthcare provider offices)	Instruct symptomatic persons to cover mouth/nose when sneezing/coughing; use tissues and dispose in no-touch receptacle; observe hand hygiene after soiling of hands with respiratory secretions; wear surgical mask if tolerated or maintain spatial separation, >3 feet if possible.

[a]During aerosol-generating procedures on clients with suspected or proven infections transmitted by respiratory aerosols (e.g., severe acute respiratory syndrome [SARS]), wear a fit-tested N95 or higher respirator in addition to gloves, gown, and face/eye protection.
Refrerence: Centers for Disease Control and Prevention, 2016b.

BOX 1.2 Performing Hand Hygiene

Perform hand hygiene:
- before you touch clients
- before handling an invasive device, regardless of gloving
- after you have contact with blood, body fluids, mucous membranes, nonintact skin, or wound dressings
- after contact with client's intact skin
- before you touch a clean body site after touching a contaminated body site
- after contact with inanimate objects near clients
- after removing your gloves
- before handling medications or food.

Reference: Centers for Disease Control and Prevention, 2018d.

from the inhalation of airborne contaminants. Respirators are made with effective filtering material but must be fit-tested to ensure that the respirator seals well around the face. Face shields and goggles are designed to prevent splashes from reaching the wearer's eyes.

Disposable clean gloves are a critical component of PPE: wearing them protects healthcare personnel from the direct transfer of infection from blood-borne pathogens. Therefore, nurses wear gloves whenever there is the possibility of contact with blood, body fluids, mucous membranes, or nonintact skin. However, gloves can also serve as a means of transferring microorganisms. To prevent this, nurses remove gloves, perform hand hygiene, and reapply fresh gloves whenever they move from handling a contaminated body site to a cleaner body site, and whenever they finish caring for a client, and prior to beginning care for a new client. Using gloves never replaces the need for hand hygiene; nurses always perform hand hygiene before applying new gloves. Gloves are never reused.

Disposable medical gloves are available in a variety of sizes, from extra-small to extra-large, as well as a variety of materials, including latex, polyvinyl chloride (PVC), nitrile, and polyurethane. They also are available powdered and nonpowdered. There has been an increase in the number of people with latex allergies, resulting in increased use of nonlatex gloves.

BOX 1.3 Key Recommendations for Using PPE

Key recommendations for the use of personal protective equipment (PPE) in healthcare settings include:
- Facilities should ensure that sufficient and appropriate PPE is available and readily accessible to members of the healthcare team.
- Educate all members of the healthcare team on proper selection and use of PPE.
- Remove and discard PPE before leaving the client's room or area.
- Wear gloves for potential contact with blood, body fluids, mucous membranes, nonintact skin, or contaminated equipment.
  - Do not wear the same pair of gloves for the care of more than one client.
  - Do not wash gloves for the purpose of reuse.
  - Perform hand hygiene immediately after removing gloves.
- Wear a gown to protect skin and clothing during procedures or activities where contact with blood or body fluids is anticipated.
  - Do not wear the same gown for the care of more than one client.
- Wear mouth, nose, and eye protection during procedures that are likely to generate splashes or sprays of blood or other body fluids.
- Wear a surgical mask when placing a catheter or injecting material into the spinal canal or subdural space.

Reference: Siegel, Rhinehart, Jackson, Chiarello, & the Healthcare Infection Control Practices Advisory Committee, 2019.

Transmission-Based Precautions

The second tier of infection prevention precautions is Transmission-Based Precautions. These do not replace Standard Precautions but are additional measures used whenever Standard Precautions alone may not be sufficient to block the transmission of an infectious agent. When Transmission-Based Precautions are implemented, specific PPE is recommended based on the category of transmission.

Transmission-Based Precautions are often initiated when a client begins to manifest signs and symptoms of infectious disease. Sometimes they are discontinued after the known length of time has passed in which the infectious agent makes the client contagious to others. In other cases, they remain in place until the laboratory tests confirm the agent is no longer infectious.

Transmission-Based Precautions are grouped into three categories: Contact Precautions, Droplet Precautions, and Airborne Precautions. Some diseases can be spread by several modes of transmission; in such cases, prevention of infection may require implementation of more than one category of Transmission-Based Precautions. Implementing Transmission-Based Precautions often means isolating that client in a private room or cohorting clients with the same infection together; this results in the use of the term *isolation precautions* or putting someone on isolation. An example

BOX 1.4 Lessons From the Evidence: Can Use of a Safe Zone Maintain Client Care Without Compromising Infection Control?

Clients in isolation sometimes feel isolated. They have less contact and communication with nurses and other members of the healthcare team. One strategy that has emerged to remove the communication barrier of transmission precautions is the use of a safe zone.

Clients are often placed on transmission precautions because they have a history of a multidrug-resistant infection, even though they do not currently have an active infection. Hospitals in the Trinity Regional Health System in Illinois tested the efficiency of a safe zone in the room of a client with this type of transmission precautions. The safe zone is a 3-foot-square box marked with red duct tape indicating the area just inside the door of the room where healthcare personnel can stand without applying gown or gloves to communicate with and assess the client. The marked area is referred to as the red box. If healthcare personnel enter further than the red box, they must apply personal protective equipment (PPE).

The Trinity study tracked the time saved by nursing staff during 2 full years of use of the red box and extrapolated the cost savings. Without compromising infection control, the time saved represented one full-time staff nurse for 1 year. Other findings included that 8 out of 10 nurses stated that the red box reduced communication barriers and increased client communication and assessment.

Reference: Yi, 2011.

of this is the recommendation to isolate clients who have a history of infection with a multidrug-resistant organism but have no current infection. See Box 1.4 to examine a strategy that is effective in preventing the spread of infection and also saves time and money.

Contact Precautions

Contact Precautions are used to prevent the transmission of infectious agents spread by direct or indirect contact. Contact Precautions are used when there is excessive wound drainage, fecal incontinence, or other bodily discharges that increase the likelihood of environmental contamination and thereby increase the risk of transmission. When Contact Precautions are implemented, a single-person room is preferred. Based on Contact Precautions, the appropriate PPE is, at a minimum, gloves and gown to protect your skin and clothing. If it is possible you could be splashed with blood or body fluids, then a mask and eye protection (goggles or face shield) are also recommended. Standard Precautions always apply; transmission precautions are in addition to the Standard Precautions. Moreover, all members of the healthcare team wear a gown and gloves for all interactions with the client, not just when they suspect exposure may occur.

Droplet Precautions

Droplet Precautions are used to prevent the transmission of infectious agents spread by droplets from respiratory secretions. These agents are not infectious over long distances.

Transmission occurs when respiratory secretions come in contact with another person's mucous membranes or respiratory tract, for example, when an infected person sneezes in close proximity to another person. When Droplet Precautions are implemented, a single-person room is preferred. All members of the healthcare team wear a mask, applied upon entry into the room, for close contact with the infected person. If a client on Droplet Precautions is transported outside of the room, the client should wear a mask. Remember that Standard Precautions apply to all clients and are based on the risk of exposure.

Airborne Precautions

Airborne Precautions are used to prevent the transmission of infectious agents that are suspended in the air and remain infectious even over long distances. When Airborne Precautions are implemented, an airborne-infection isolation room (AIIR) is preferred. An AIIR is a single-person room with special air-handling and ventilation capacity that includes negative air pressure, frequent air exchanges, and air exhausted directly to the outside or through high-efficiency particulate air (HEPA) filtration. All members of the healthcare team wear either a mask or a respirator (depending on the disease), which they apply before entering the room. In addition, when the client has a vaccine-preventable airborne disease, such as measles or chickenpox, only members of the healthcare team who have immunity should provide care. In addition, Standard Precautions apply whenever your care exposes you to blood or body fluids; apply the appropriate PPE, including eye protection.

Disposing of Waste

Hospitals must follow federal and state regulations regarding the management of solid waste. The CDC guidelines state that no additional precautions are needed for non-medical solid waste that is removed from hospital rooms of individuals on Transmission-Based Precautions. Dispose of medical waste without contaminating the outside of the biohazard bag. A biohazard bag is a red waste-disposal bag that meets federal and state requirements for tear resistance. One sturdy, leak-resistant biohazard bag is sufficient. If the bag is punctured, then place it in a second biohazard bag.

Linens

The CDC (2015a) recommends the following strategies to manage soiled linens:
- Contain soiled linens in a laundry bag or designated container.
- Do not handle linens in any way that can make infectious agents airborne; for example, do not shake soiled linens.
- Do not allow soiled linens to touch your person or clothing.

Sharps

Place all sharp items that could break the skin, including needles and syringes, glass tubes and slides, and any other sharp item, in a puncture-resistant biohazard container at the point of use.

Blood and Body Fluids

Check your agency policy to determine the amounts of blood and body fluids that can safely be poured down the sink or flushed down the toilet. Your state may have regulations on the maximum volume that can be poured into the sewer system. Liquid from suction canisters and body fluids from wound-drainage systems are examples of fluids that can typically be disposed of in a toilet. Each state determines if this method of disposal is acceptable and determines if the local sewage treatment system meets the necessary requirements (CDC, 2015b).

Managing the Environment

Preventing infection is a team affair. Nurses represent a critical part of the healthcare team and are invested in establishing a safe and clean care environment. One aspect of preventing the transfer of microorganisms is to ensure that surfaces and objects touched by clients are routinely cleaned and disinfected. These include surfaces around the client, such as the tray table, handrails, doorknobs, and light switches. Also included is medical equipment that touches the client's skin, such as stethoscopes and blood pressure cuffs. Cleaning refers to the removal of any visible contamination, usually by scrubbing with water and detergent. It is an important first step before disinfection, which is the use of disinfectant agents to eliminate many or all microorganisms on inanimate objects. The CDC (2018b) recommends that medical equipment surfaces and environmental surfaces should be disinfected with a low- or intermediate-level disinfectant that is registered with the Environmental Protection Agency (EPA). Medical equipment that comes in contact with mucous membranes, such as an endoscope, requires high-level disinfection or sterilization to prevent the transmission of infective microorganisms.

One issue related to disinfectants is the necessary contact time to eliminate all microorganisms. Some products require several minutes of contact time to be effective (CDC, 2018b). Nurses can advocate for products with shortened contact time and help ensure that label instructions for EPA-registered products are followed. Nurses may not have the primary responsibility to clean or disinfect surfaces within the healthcare environment; however, to reduce the transmission of infective microorganisms, nurses need a clear understanding of the use of disinfectants, issues associated with products, and the PPE required for healthcare environment disinfectants (Table 1.2). Not only are nurses active in managing the healthcare environment, but nurses also instruct families on strategies to reduce the transmission of infective microorganisms at home, as discussed in Box 1.5.

APPLICATION OF THE NURSING PROCESS

Examples of Related ICNP Nursing Diagnoses, Expected Client Outcomes, and Nursing Interventions:

Nursing Diagnosis: Risk for infection

Supporting Data: Increased environmental exposure to pathogens.

Expected Client Outcome: The client will remain free from symptoms of infection while in the healthcare setting, as

TABLE 1.2 Using Disinfectants

Type of Disinfectant	Uses	Examples	Personal Protective Equipment (PPE)
Low-level disinfectants	General disinfecting	Quaternary ammonium compounds	Gloves
	Client room cleaning	Accelerated hydrogen peroxide compound Oxivir®	Gloves
	Cleaning stethoscopes, blood pressure cuffs, tabletops	Ethyl or isopropyl alcohol (70%–90%)	Gloves
Intermediate-level disinfectants	Disinfecting client rooms, isolation rooms, visible blood spills	Diluted bleach 1:50 dilution 1:10 dilution sometimes used	Safety glasses or goggles, gloves, gowns to protect clothing
High-level disinfectants	Disinfecting equipment that comes into contact with mucous membranes (e.g., endoscopes)	Ortho-phthalaldehydes (Cidex®)	Eye protection, gloves, gowns

Reference: Centers for Disease Control and Prevention, 2016b.

demonstrated by temperature and vital signs within established parameters.

Nursing Intervention Example: Use Standard Precautions and perform hand hygiene upon entering and before leaving the client's room.

Reference: International Classification for Nursing Practice. (n.d.). *eHealth & ICNP*. Retrieved from https://www.icn.ch/what-we-do/projects/ehealth-icnp.

CRITICAL CONCEPTS
Preventing Infection

Accuracy (ACC)

When using Standard Precautions, the accuracy of Standard Precautions is subject to the following variables:

Nurse-Related Factors
- Direction, amount of friction, and duration of hand rubbing
- Proper procedures for applying and removing PPE (gowns, gloves, etc.)
- Adherence to infection control policies and guidelines (e.g., CDC, WHO)

Equipment-Related Factors
- Fit and coverage of the protective equipment

Infection Control (INF)

When using Standard Precautions, healthcare-associated infection is prevented by:
- ensuring the containment of microorganisms
- preventing and reducing the transfer of microorganisms
- reducing the number of microorganisms

Communication (COM)

Communication exchanges information (oral, written, nonverbal, or electronic) between two or more people.

Evaluation (EVAL)

When using Standard Precautions, the evaluation of outcomes enables the nurse to determine the efficacy of the care provided.

BOX 1.5 Home Care Considerations: Disinfecting in the Home

Many people are being cared for in the home, including clients with invasive devices such as central lines, immunocompromising conditions, or communicable diseases. Nurses apply the principles of infection control in the home as well as in acute care settings. Information and demonstrations of proper hand hygiene may be needed by families providing home care.

Nurses should also explain how to disinfect objects and surfaces in the home to reduce the number and transfer of microorganisms. Bleach, isopropyl alcohol, and hydrogen peroxide are products recommended by the Centers for Disease Control and Prevention (CDC) for home disinfection of reusable objects. The Association for Professionals in Infection Control and Epidemiology (APIC) recommends that reusable objects that come in contact with mucous membranes, such as a tracheostomy tube, be disinfected by using one of the following methods:
- immersing the object in 70% isopropyl alcohol for 5 minutes
- immersing the object in 3% hydrogen peroxide for 30 minutes
- immersing the object in a 1:50 dilution of household bleach for 5 minutes.

Household cleaning agents that are considered environmentally safe are not registered with the Environmental Protection Agency (EPA) and may not be effective against problematic microorganisms. For example, baking soda, borax, and liquid detergent are not effective disinfectants. Undiluted vinegar and ammonia are effective against *Escherichia coli* and *Salmonella typhi*; however, they are not effective against *Staphylococcus aureus*. Nurses can assist families in identifying situations and sites in their homes where disinfection of surfaces and objects will decrease the risk for the transmission of pathogens.

Reference: Centers for Disease Control and Prevention, 2018a.

■ SKILL 1.2 Performing Hand Hygiene With an Alcohol-Based Agent

EQUIPMENT

Alcohol-based handrub

BEGINNING THE SKILL

1. **INF** Keep fingernails trimmed short, approximately 2 mm in length. Do not wear artificial nails or nail extensions. Follow your healthcare organization's policy regarding the wearing of nail polish.
2. **INF** Remove rings, watches, and jewelry.

PROCEDURE

3. **INF** Apply a palmful of the alcohol-based handrub in a cupped hand. *A palmful of handrub should be sufficient to cover both hands.*

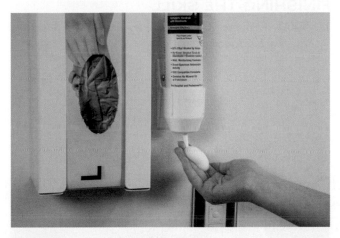

STEP 3 Apply a palmful of the handrub.

4. **ACC** Rub palm against palm with a rotating motion.

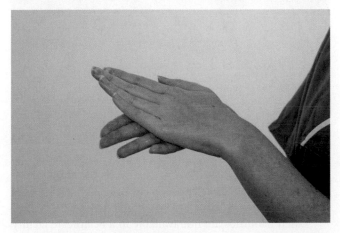

STEP 4 Rub palm against palm.

5. **ACC** Rub between the fingers of both hands by placing your right palm over the back of the left hand and then the left palm over the back of the right hand.

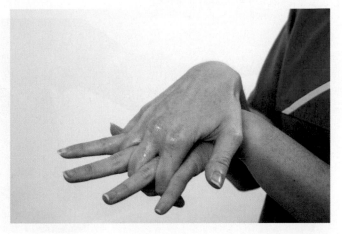

STEP 5 Rub palms over the backs of each hand.

6. **ACC** Rub your palms together, interlacing the fingers.

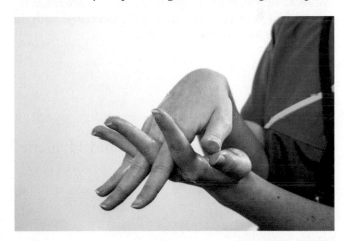

STEP 6 Rub your palms together.

7. **ACC** Rub the backs of your fingers with your opposite palm by curling the fingers around the fingers of the opposite hand and rubbing vertically.

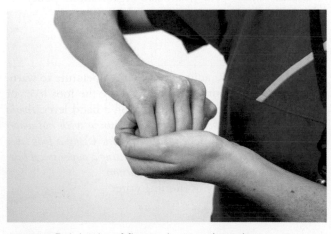

STEP 7 Rub backs of fingers in opposite palm.

8. **ACC** Rub the thumb of one hand by rotating it in the clasped palm of your opposite hand, and then repeat with the opposite thumb.

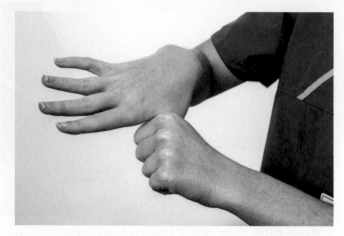

STEP 8 Rub the thumb.

9. **ACC** Rub your fingertips backward and forward in the palm of your opposite hand, and then repeat with the opposite hand in the other palm.

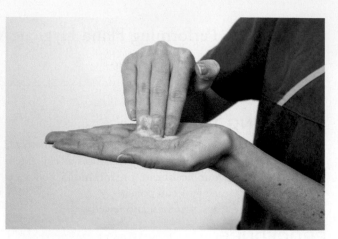

STEP 9 Rub your fingertips.

10. Let your hands completely dry.

FINISHING THE SKILL

11. **EVAL** Evaluate your technique. *Are you confident you washed all surfaces of your hands?*

■ SKILL 1.3 Performing Hand Hygiene With Soap and Water

EQUIPMENT

Nonmedicated soap
Running water
Paper towel

BEGINNING THE SKILL

1. **INF** Keep fingernails trimmed short, approximately 2 mm in length. Do not wear artificial nails or nail extensions. Follow your healthcare organization's policy regarding the wearing of nail polish.
2. **INF** Remove rings, watches, and jewelry.

PROCEDURE

3. **INF** At the sink, adjust the water temperature to warm and water pressure to medium using the foot lever or using a paper towel as a barrier on a hand lever. *Avoid using hot water because frequent washing with hot water may increase the risk of skin irritation. Using a foot lever prevents hand contamination, and using a paper towel barrier decreases the risk of contamination.*
4. Wet your hands with running water.

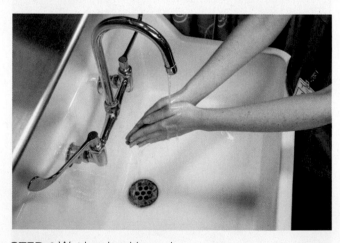

STEP 4 Wet hands with running water.

5. **INF** Dispense sufficient soap covering all hand surfaces. Nonmedicated soaps are recommended when alcohol-based handrubs are not available in a healthcare facility.
6. **ACC** Rub hands for 40 to 60 seconds in the following sequence. Rub palm against palm with a rotating motion.

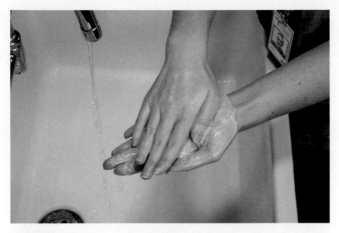

STEP 6 Rub palm against palm.

7. **ACC** Rub between the fingers of both hands by placing your right palm over the back of the left hand and then the left palm over the back of the right hand.

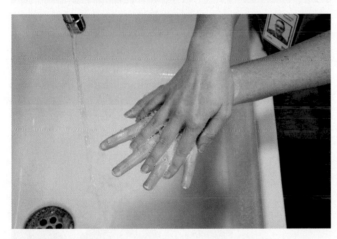

STEP 7 Rub palms over the backs of each hand.

8. **ACC** Rub your palms together, interlacing the fingers.
9. **ACC** Rub the backs of your fingers with your opposite palm by curling the fingers around the fingers of the opposite hand and rubbing vertically.
10. **ACC** Rub the thumb of one hand by rotating it in the clasped palm of your opposite hand, and then repeat with the other thumb.
11. **ACC** Rub your fingertips backward and forward in the palm of your opposite hand, and then repeat with the opposite hand in the other palm.
12. **ACC** Rinse hands with water.

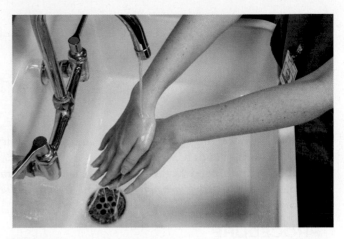

STEP 12 Rinse hands with water.

13. **INF** Dry hands thoroughly with a single-use towel. *A single-use towel reduces the risk of recontamination.*
14. **INF** Use a dry towel to turn off faucet. *Using the towel reduces the risk of recontamination from the sink faucet.*

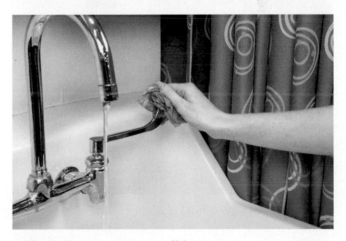

STEP 14 Use towel to turn off faucet.

FINISHING THE SKILL

15. **EVAL** Evaluate your technique. *Are you confident you washed all surfaces of your hands?*

■ SKILL 1.4 Applying and Removing Clean Gloves

EQUIPMENT

Clean gloves

BEGINNING THE SKILL

1. **INF** Remove rings, bracelets, and any other jewelry worn on the hands or wrists.
2. **INF** Perform hand hygiene, ensuring hands are completely dry. *If hands are damp, they will not easily slide into gloves.*

PROCEDURE

Applying Clean Gloves

3. **INF** Remove glove from glove box touching only the outer cuff of the glove.

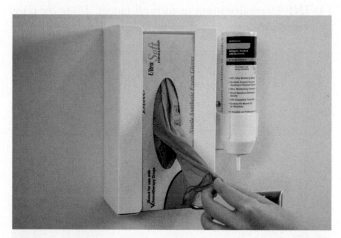

STEP 3 Remove glove from glove box.

4. Put on the glove.

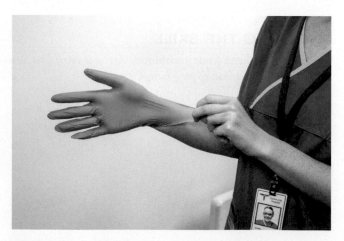

STEP 4 Put on the glove.

5. **INF** Remove another glove from the box with your ungloved hand, touching only the outer cuff of the glove.

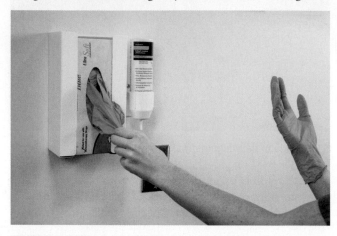

STEP 5 Remove another glove from the box.

6. **INF** Scoop the gloved fingers of your gloved hand under the cuff of the second glove and put on the glove without touching the skin of your hand or forearm. *To keep the gloves uncontaminated, the gloved hand touches only the clean outside surface of the second glove.*

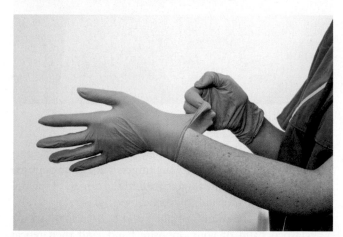

STEP 6 Put on the second glove.

7. **INF** Once gloved, do not touch anything that is not required to be touched to complete the task for which you are gloving. *Gloves are contaminated just as easily as hands are contaminated.*

Removing Soiled Gloves

8. **INF** With your dominant hand, grasp the glove on your nondominant hand near the cuff. Do not touch your skin with the soiled glove. *Dirty only touches dirty.*

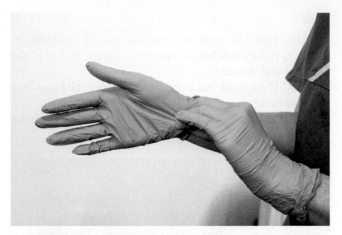

STEP 8 Grasp the glove near the cuff.

9. **INF** Pull the glove off your nondominant hand. The glove will turn inside out as you pull it off.

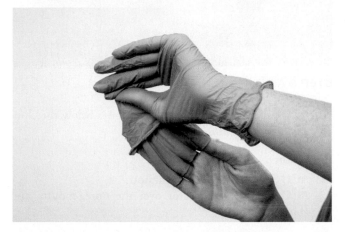

STEP 9 Pull the glove off.

10. **INF** Bunch up the soiled glove in your gloved hand.
11. **INF** With the bare fingers of your nondominant hand, slip two fingers under the cuff of the glove on your dominant hand. *Clean only touches clean.*

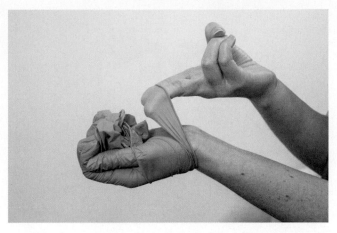

STEP 11 Slip two bare fingers under the cuff.

12. **INF** Pull the glove off your dominant hand. The glove will turn inside out, and the glove from the nondominant hand will be contained within it. *Turning the gloves inside-out contains the microorganisms on the soiled gloves.*

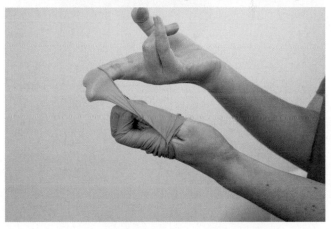

STEP 12 Pull the glove off.

13. Dispose of the gloves in an appropriate receptacle.

FINISHING THE SKILL

14. **INF** Perform hand hygiene.

■ SKILL 1.5 Applying and Removing Personal Protective Equipment

EQUIPMENT

Gown
Mask or respirator
Goggles or face shield
Clean gloves

BEGINNING THE SKILL

1. **INF** Perform hand hygiene.

2. Select appropriate type and size of gown. Gowns should be large enough to close in the back, completely covering clothing.

PROCEDURE
Applying PPE
Gown

3. **ACC** Put on the gown with the ties in the back, and secure the ties at the back of the neck.

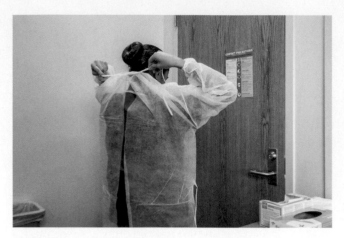

STEP 3 Secure ties at the back of the neck.

4. **ACC** Secure ties at the waist in a bow. *Tying in a bow allows the ties to be easily untied.*

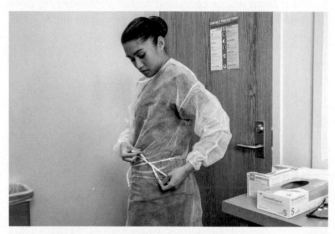

STEP 4 Secure ties at the waist.

5. **INF** Prior to entering the client's room, ensure the gown crosses over itself to completely cover your clothing. (Note: If there is not a gown available that is large enough to cover, use two gowns. Put the first gown on with the ties in the front, and then put on the second gown on with the ties in the back.)

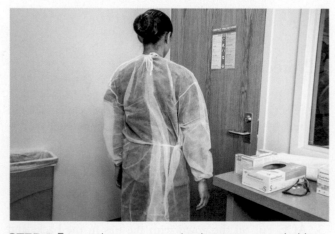

STEP 5 Ensure the gown completely covers your clothing.

Mask

6. **ACC** Place the mask over the nose, mouth, and chin.
7. **ACC** If the mask has ties, secure ties at the middle of the head and the neck.
8. **ACC** If the mask has elastic loops, secure the loops over your ears.
9. **ACC** Squeeze the nosepiece over the bridge of the nose. *Adjusting the nosepiece provides a better fit.*

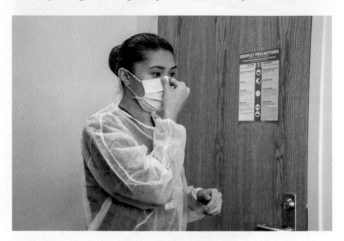

STEP 9 Adjust the nosepiece.

10. **ACC** Adjust mask so that lower edge is below the chin. *A secure fit contains microorganisms.*

Respirator

11. **ACC** Select a fit-tested respirator.
12. **ACC** Place the respirator over the nose, mouth, and chin.

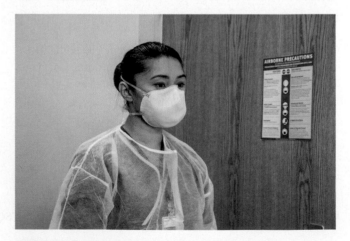

STEP 12 Ensure that the respirator has a snug fit.

13. **ACC** Squeeze the nosepiece over the bridge of the nose. *Adjusting the nosepiece provides a better fit.*
14. **ACC** If the respirator has ties, tie them. If the respirator has elastic loops, secure the loops over your ears.
15. **ACC** Adjust the respirator so that it fits snugly to your face. *A secure fit contains microorganisms.*
16. **ACC** Perform the following fit test. When you inhale, the respirator collapses, and when you exhale, check for air leakage around the face.

Goggles or Face Shield

17. **ACC** To apply goggles, position the goggles over the eyes and secure to the head using the earpieces or headband. *Goggles protect the eyes.* (Note: Personal glasses do not provide adequate protection and cannot be a substitute for goggles. Goggles should fit snuggly over and around the eyes.)

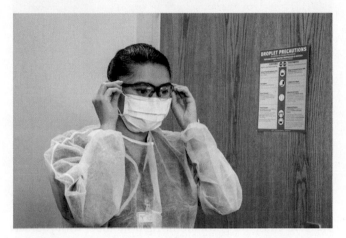

STEP 17 Position goggles over the eyes.

18. **ACC** To apply a face shield, position the face shield over the face and secure it on your brow with a headband. *Face shields protect the face, nose, mouth, and eyes. Face shields should cover your forehead, extend below your chin, and wrap around the sides of your face.*

Clean Gloves

19. **INF** Remove glove from glove box, touching only the outer cuff of the glove, and put on the glove.
20. **INF** Remove another glove from the box with your ungloved hand, touching only the outer cuff of the glove.
21. **INF** Scoop the gloved fingers of your gloved hand under the cuff of the second glove and put on the glove without touching the skin of your hand or forearm. *To keep the clean gloves uncontaminated, the gloved hand touches only the clean outside surface of the second glove.*
22. **INF** Ensure that the gloves cover the gown cuffs.

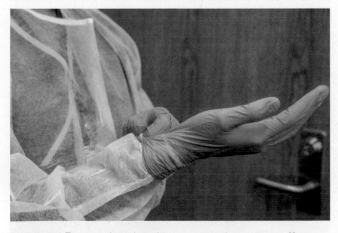

STEP 22 Ensure that the gloves cover the gown cuffs.

23. **INF** Enter the client's room and close the door behind you.
24. **COM** Explain Standard Precautions and Transmission-Based Precautions to the client and client's family. Allow the family to ask questions. Provide client care as needed.
25. **INF** Exit the client's room and close the door behind you.

Removing PPE
Clean Gloves

26. **INF** With your dominant hand, grasp the glove on your nondominant hand near the cuff. Do not touch your skin with the soiled glove. *Dirty only touches dirty.*
27. **INF** Pull the glove off your nondominant hand. The glove will turn inside out as you pull it off.

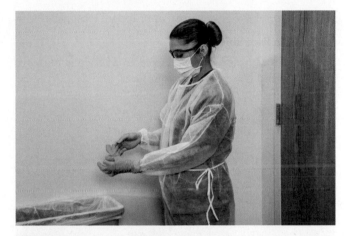

STEP 27 The glove turns inside out as you pull the glove off.

28. **INF** Bunch up the soiled glove in your gloved hand.
29. **INF** Slip two bare fingers or thumb under the cuff of the glove on your dominant hand. *Clean only touches clean.*

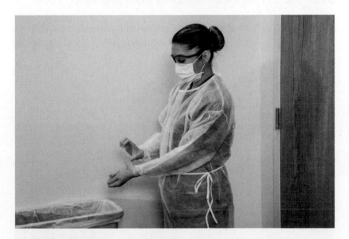

STEP 29 Touch under the cuff to remove the glove.

30. **INF** Pull the glove off your dominant hand. The glove will turn inside out, and the glove from the nondominant hand will be contained within it. *Turning the gloves inside out contains the microorganisms on the soiled gloves.*

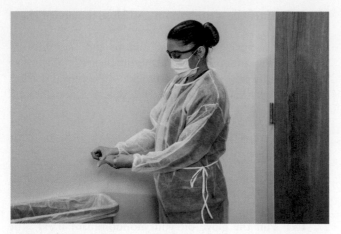

STEP 30 Pull the glove off and dispose of it appropriately.

31. Dispose of the gloves in an appropriate receptacle.

Goggles or Face Shield

32. **INF** Hold headpieces or earpieces with your ungloved hands and lift away from your face.

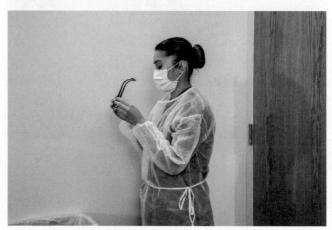

STEP 32 Lift the earpieces away from your face.

33. **INF** Place in appropriate container. *Agencies will designate a specific receptacle for reprocessing or disposing of the equipment.*

Gown

34. Unfasten neck ties.

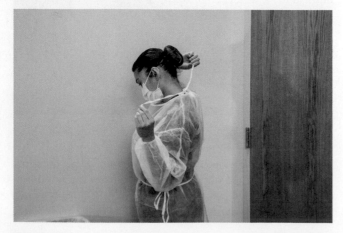

STEP 34 Unfasten neck ties.

35. Unfasten waist ties.

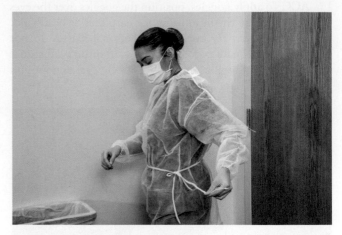

STEP 35 Unfasten waist ties.

36. **INF** Lean forward so that the gown falls away from your body. *Leaning forward prevents the gown from touching you. Gown front and sleeves are contaminated.*
37. **INF** Grasp the gown on the right shoulder with your left hand and the left shoulder with your right hand, then peel the gown away from the neck and shoulder.

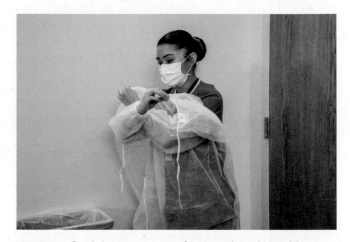

STEP 37 Peel the gown away from neck and shoulder.

38. **INF** Turn contaminated outside of the gown toward the inside.

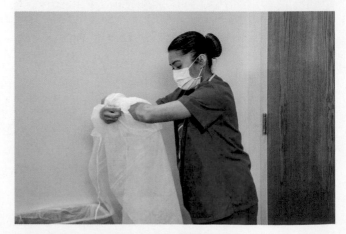

STEP 38 Turn the outside of the gown toward the inside.

39. **INF** Fold or roll gown into a bundle.

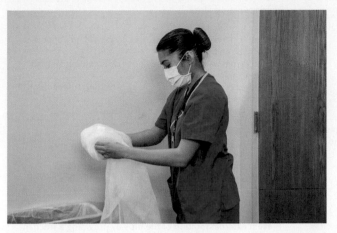

STEP 39 Fold or roll into a bundle.

40. **INF** Place in appropriate container. *Agencies will designate a specific receptacle for reprocessing or disposing of the equipment.*

Mask

41. **INF** Remove mask from face, touching only the loops. *The front of the mask is contaminated.*

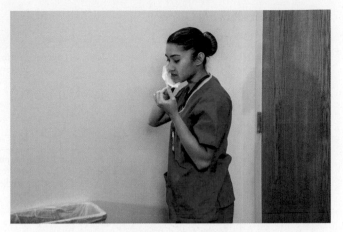

STEP 41 Remove mask from face, touching only the loops.

42. **INF** If the mask has ties, untie the bottom and then untie the top tie. *The front of the mask is contaminated. If the top ties were untied first, then the front of the contaminated mask could flop down onto your clothing*

43. **INF** Place in appropriate container. *Agencies will designate a specific receptacle for reprocessing or disposing of the equipment.*

Respirator

44. **INF** Lift the bottom elastic loop over your head, and then lift off the top one. Touch only the elastic loop. *The front of the respirator is contaminated.*

45. **INF** Place in an appropriate container. *Agencies will designate a specific receptacle for reprocessing or disposing of the equipment.*

FINISHING THE SKILL

46. **INF** Perform hand hygiene.

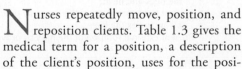

SECTION 3 Moving Clients Safely

Nurses repeatedly move, position, and reposition clients. Table 1.3 gives the medical term for a position, a description of the client's position, uses for the position, and common nursing considerations. In addition, an image of each position is found in Skill 1.6. However, moving clients safely is a two-sided issue: the benefits for and safety of the client must be considered, as well as the health and safety of the nurse or nurses performing the skill.

BENEFITS OF PROPER CLIENT POSITIONING AND REPOSITIONING

When clients have a compromised ability to move purposefully to reposition themselves in the bed, nurses reposition

the client. The first skill in this section describes positioning clients in bed. Effective positioning and frequent repositioning help clients to maintain or recover health in a variety of ways, including the following:

- enhances effective respirations and drainage of oral secretions
- improves oxygenation in respiratory diseases such as asthma and chronic obstructive pulmonary disease
- reduces the risk for atelectasis
- prevents skin breakdown, the development of pressure injury, and contractures
- promotes skin healing
- facilitates childbirth
- provides comfort and decreases discomfort.

TABLE 1.3 Positioning Clients

Position	Client Position	Uses	Nursing Considerations
Supine or dorsal recumbent	Client is on his or her back, facing up, and the bed is level.	Following abdominal or chest surgery	Provide lumbar support. Prevent hyperextension of the neck by providing support of the neck and head. Prevent hyperextension of the knees by providing a small pillow to flex the knees. Prevent external rotation of hips by providing trochanter roll. Prevent heel pressure. Provide foot support to prevent foot drop.
Fowler's High-Fowler's Semi-Fowler's	Client is on his or her back, facing up, and the head of the bed is elevated. Low-Fowler's: 15 degrees Semi-Fowler's: 15–45 degrees (often considered 30 degrees) Fowler's: 45 degrees High-Fowler's: 60–90 degrees	Indicated for nasogastric tube insertion and nasogastric feedings	Provide lumbar support. Prevent hyperextension of the neck by providing support of the neck and head. Provide support for the forearms to prevent shoulder muscle strain, dependent edema of the hands, and flexion contracture of the wrists. Prevent hyperextension of the knees by providing a small pillow to flex the knees. Prevent external rotation of the hips by providing a trochanter roll. Prevent heel pressure. Provide foot support to prevent foot drop.
Lateral	Client is on his or her side with both arms in front of the body; hips and knees are comfortably flexed.	Alternative to supine and removes pressure from scapula, sacrum, and heels	Provide pillow support to keep the head and neck in alignment. Provide pillow to support the upper leg, and prevent internal rotation. Provide pillow to support the upper arm and prevent internal rotation.
Prone	Client is on his or her abdomen with the head turned to one side, and the bed is level.		Provide pillow support for the head, and prevent hyperextension of the neck. Provide support for the lower legs or allow the feet to hang over the end of the bed to prevent foot drop. Provide small pillow or roll under the upper abdomen to prevent hyperextension of the lumbar curvature.
Sim's	Client is on his or her side but rolled almost prone. The lower arm is behind the client, and the hips and knees are flexed, with the upper leg more acutely flexed.	Indicated position for receiving an enema or perineal cleaning	Provide pillow support to keep the head and neck in alignment. Provide pillow to support the upper leg and prevent internal rotation. Provide pillow to support the upper arm and prevent internal rotation. Provide foot support to prevent foot drop.
Trendelenburg's	Client is supine and the bed is level, with the head lower than the feet.	Not commonly used because it causes increased intracranial pressure May be used briefly for chest physiotherapy or central line placement	Provide lumbar support. Prevent hyperextension of the neck by providing support of the neck and head. Prevent hyperextension of the knees by providing a small pillow to flex the knees. Prevent external rotation of the hips by providing a trochanter roll.
Reverse Trendelenburg's	Client is supine and the bed is level, with the feet lower than the head	Indicated to prevent gastroesophageal reflux	Provide lumbar support. Prevent hyperextension of the neck by providing support of the neck and head. Prevent hyperextension of the knees by providing a small pillow to flex the knees. Prevent external rotation of the hips by providing a trochanter roll.

For example, the nurse caring for a premature infant will need to frequently reposition the infant. Box 1.6 describes the physiologic influences of a premature infant's position.

One of the time-honored standards of care is to reposition clients every 2 hours. In fact, some hospitals even play overhead music every 2 hours to remind healthcare workers to reposition clients. Songs like "Turn, Turn, Turn" and "Roll Over, Beethoven" have been used as repositioning reminders.

Hazards of Client Handling

Considering the benefits and frequency of client positioning, the proper technique is critical for nurses, who are at risk for injury from a single incident and for a musculoskeletal disorder from years of wear and tear. Analysis of data from the Bureau of Labor Statistics (2017) shows that the healthcare occupation has the highest rate of injury of all industries in the United States. The most common event leading to injury was found to be overexertion from lifting or moving clients.

BOX 1.6 Lifespan Considerations: Positioning Premature Infants

Very premature infants are not able to reposition themselves. Their inadequate muscular strength and coordination makes them very vulnerable and dependent on the nurses to position them in a manner that supports healthy growth and development. Positioning preterm infants is an important part of nursing care. Research shows that premature infants' positioning influences many physiologic events:

- The right lateral position decreases the incidence of gastroesophageal reflux and aspiration (Mittinty, 2018).
- Midline positioning and bed elevation of 30 degrees may be a potentially better practice to reduce the incidence of intraventricular hemorrhage (Malusky & Donze, 2011).
- Neonates and infants improve ventilation and oxygenation in the prone position, at least for the short term (Mittinty, 2018).
- Positioning in a car seat or sling for an extended period may result in oxygen desaturation, apnea, and/or bradycardia (Khanh-Dao Le, 2017).
- Postural deformities develop without preventive positioning (Khanh-Dao Le, 2017).

BOX 1.7 Body Mechanics Principles

The four principles are as follows:
1. Maintain a wide, stable base with your feet.
2. Put the bed at the correct height (waist level when providing care; hip level when moving a client).
3. Keep the work directly in front of you to avoid rotating the spine.
4. Keep the client as close to your body as possible to minimize reaching.

The most common type of injury was sprains, strains, and/or tears, and the most common body part injured was the trunk, with the back making up the majority of the injuries (Dresser, 2017). Manual lifting, moving, and repositioning of clients is the single greatest risk factor for an overexertion injury (National Institute for Occupational Safety and Health [NIOSH], 2017).

Many factors make moving human beings challenging: Bodies are an awkward size and shape. People may shift abruptly while being moved. Clients often need to be supported in positions for feeding and toileting that strain the nurse. In addition, more and more clients are overweight or obese. At the same time, the age of the nursing workforce in America is increasing. Traditionally, nursing students have been taught only lifting techniques using body mechanics. However, to move people safely, nursing students need an understanding of the broad field of healthcare ergonomics. You will need to know how to use decision-making algorithms and when to use assistive lifting technology to move clients.

ERGONOMICS AND BODY MECHANICS

Ergonomics includes the scientific study of people and their work environments. Ergonomic principles stress fitting the task to the person and the environment. The goal of an ergonomic workspace is to reduce physical stressors and prevent injuries. Nurses need training in ergonomic assessment—that is, in how to examine characteristics of the person, task, and environment. For example, how do the nurse's and the client's size, age, physical abilities, and limitations compare? What unique risk factors are present in the work environment, and what are the unique characteristics of this precise move, transfer, or repositioning? In addition, nurses need training in the steps they can take to alter the work environment and reduce the risk of injury. Such steps can be as simple as raising the bed to an ergonomically appropriate height or moving the wheelchair to the other side of the bed. Throughout this text, *an ergonomically safe space* means the work environment is adjusted to the size and ability of the caregiver and client.

Body mechanics (also known as biomechanics) is a field within ergonomics that applies the laws of mechanics and physics to human movement. It studies physical principles such as load, resistance, and friction within the human body. Research into body mechanics has led to the identification of a group of principles for safe moving and lifting. Principles of body mechanics are identified in Box 1.7. They may be applied when moving a client who can assist with transfer as well as when using assistive lifting equipment. Be aware, however, that an understanding of the principles of body mechanics alone cannot prevent injury. Early research determined weight limits for preventing back injuries while lifting objects, but these objects were not people. Because repositioning and transferring clients often includes unexpected movements, the equation results in a recommended 16-kg (35-lb)maximum weight limit (NIOSH, 2017).

Equipment and Algorithms for Moving Clients Safely

A growing number of research studies indicate that the use of assistive lifting equipment can prevent musculoskeletal injuries and is safer for clients as well. The NIOSH, Veterans Health Administration (VHA), and American Nurses Association (ANA) developed both an assessment tool and algorithms to assist nurses in determining a strategy to safely transfer, reposition, and move clients (NIOSH, VHA, & ANA, 2009).

Determining the best method to move a client requires an accurate assessment of the client's level of assistance, upper-extremity strength, weight-bearing capability, weight, height, level of cooperation, and comprehension of the move. In addition, the nurse assesses for any other conditions likely to impact the move, such as the client's activity level, cognitive function, degree of mobility, and discomfort. After completing the assessment, the nurse follows the appropriate algorithm. Following the algorithm will determine whether

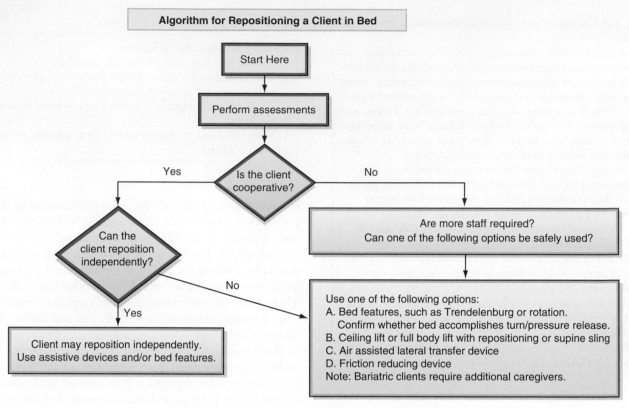

Algorithm for Repositioning a Client in Bed

Start Here

↓

Perform assessments

↓

Is the client cooperative?

— Yes →   Can the client reposition independently?
— No →   Are more staff required? Can one of the following options be safely used?

Can the client reposition independently?
— Yes → Client may reposition independently. Use assistive devices and/or bed features.
— No →

Use one of the following options:
A. Bed features, such as Trendelenburg or rotation. Confirm whether bed accomplishes turn/pressure release.
B. Ceiling lift or full body lift with repositioning or supine sling
C. Air assisted lateral transfer device
D. Friction reducing device
Note: Bariatric clients require additional caregivers.

FIG. 1.2 Algorithm for Repositioning a Client in Bed.

caregiver assistance is not needed or whether assistive lifting equipment or two or more caregivers will be required.

- Skill 1.6 and Skill 1.7 use the Algorithm for Repositioning a Client in Bed shown in Fig. 1.2.
- Skills 1.8 to Skill 1.10 use the Algorithm for Transfer to or From a Seated Position shown in Fig. 1.3.
- Skill 1.11 on transferring clients laterally uses the Algorithm for Lateral Transfer shown in Fig. 1.4.

Review the algorithms to see if the client can partially bear weight and is cooperative; if so, then perhaps transfer without equipment (Skill 1.8) or sit-to-stand lift is indicated (Skill 1.10), depending on the strength and balance of the client. For example, if a client cannot bear weight, is not cooperative, and/or does not have upper-extremity strength, assistive lifting equipment and two caregivers are indicated (Skill 1.9).

Clearly, to move clients safely, nurses must be familiar with the equipment involved. Equipment may be as simple as a transfer belt and as sophisticated as a ceiling-mounted lift. One of the most commonly used items is a draw sheet. A draw sheet is a sheet of heavier fabric that is placed across the bed from the client's shoulders to knees to facilitate moving the client. It is not as efficient as a friction-reducing surface (also called a sliding sheet), but it is found on almost every hospital bed. Table 1.4 summarizes assistive equipment.

Advocacy for Safe Client Handling

Over the last two decades, the ANA has supported legislation and regulations to help prevent nurse injuries and musculoskeletal disorders. For example, the ANA's Safe Patient Handling campaign encourages institutional policies that would reduce or eliminate manual client handling. As of 2016, 11 states had enacted legislation or adopted regulations to protect nurses through the use of assistive lifting equipment. The ANA counters the argument that lifting equipment is too expensive with data showing that when hospitals implement safe client handling equipment, they achieve savings by reducing lost work days and reducing worker compensation costs that meet or exceed the cost of the equipment (ANA, n.d.).

SUMMARY

In summary, moving clients safely involves excellent judgment as well as teamwork and collaboration between the nurse and other healthcare providers and/or between the nurse and the client. The critical concept of accuracy is applied in several ways. Before moving any client, an accurate assessment of the client's abilities must be performed. Accurate selection and use of the safe handling equipment is required and accurate client positioning. Safety is also an important concept. Adherence to established safe client handling algorithms will keep the nurses

Algorithm for Transfer to or From a Seated Position

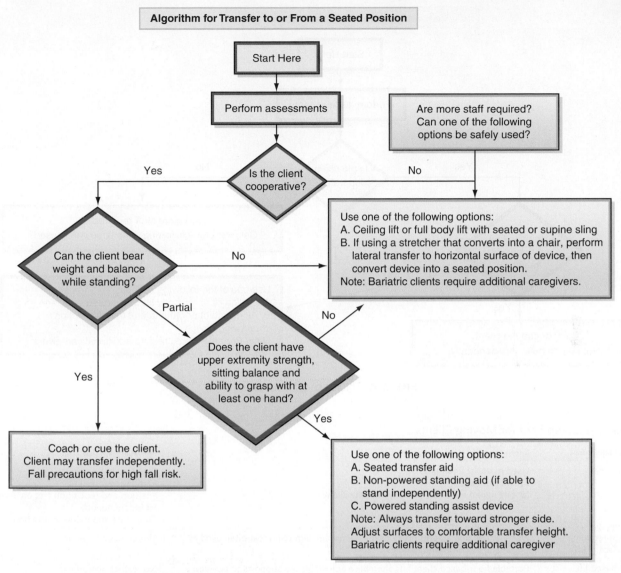

FIG. 1.3 Algorithm for Transfer to or From a Seated Position.

and client safe. Even with the use of safe client handling equipment sound body mechanics are prudent safety measures to keep nurses safe. This section on moving the client includes positioning the client to maintain musculoskeletal alignment and maximize circulation. Finally, effective communication during transfers enhances teamwork and safety.

APPLICATION OF THE NURSING PROCESS

Examples of Related ICNP Nursing Diagnoses, Expected Client Outcomes, and Nursing Interventions:

Nursing Diagnosis: Impaired mobility in bed

Supporting Data: Client is unable to adequately reposition self in bed.

Expected Client Outcome: The client will demonstrate optimal positioning in proper body alignment in bed while in the healthcare setting.

Nursing Intervention Example: Assist client to position in proper body alignment.

Reference: International Classification for Nursing Practice. (n.d.). *eHealth & ICNP.* Retrieved from https://www.iscn.ch/what-we-do/projects/ehealth-icnp.

CRITICAL CONCEPTS
Moving the Client Safely

Accuracy (ACC)

Moving the client is subject to the following variables:
- assessment of client, including abilities and limitations for movement, need for supportive devices, cooperation, strength, mobility, level of discomfort, and activity intolerance
- proper positioning of the client

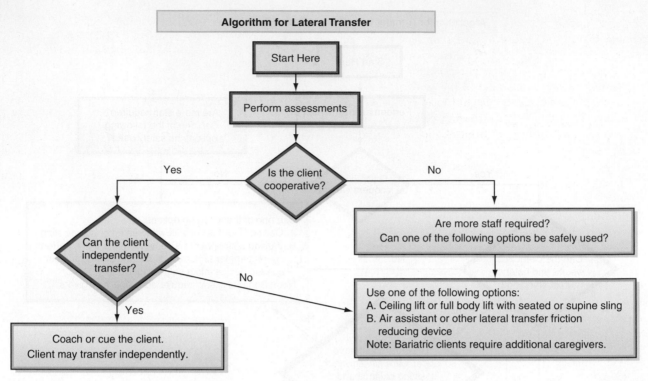

FIG. 1.4 Algorithm for Lateral Transfer.

TABLE 1.4 Equipment for Moving Clients

Type of Equipment	Information About the Equipment	Indications for Use
Transfer belt	Used to assist and guide Provides a handle Not designed for lifting the weight of the client	Client must be able to: Partially bear weight Position and reposition feet on floor Sit independently Cooperate and follow instructions
Friction-reducing surface (FRS)	Flat sheet sliding system provides low-friction movement; most often used in pairs; may come with handles	No restrictions on use
Floor-based lift	Portable floor-based client lift, often have adjustable leg supports to position around chairs, beds	No restrictions on use
Ceiling-mounted lift	Ceiling-mounted client lift; runs along tracks in the ceiling	No restrictions on use
Slings	Fabric device that attaches to lifting equipment; may be disposable or reusable; may be mesh for bathing	No restrictions on use
Sit-to-stand lift	Mobile lift Client is attached to the lift with a sling or belt and is assisted to a standing position from a sitting position.	Client must be able to: Partially bear weight Sit independently Have no hip instability Cooperate and follow instructions
Sliding board	A sliding board may be made of plastic or wood and provides stability when moving from one surface to another. Shapes available to aid in wheelchair transfers and bed-to-stretcher transfers.	Client must: Be unable to bear weight Have no hip instability Cooperate and follow instructions

- selection and use of equipment
- understanding of procedure by client.

Client-Centered Care (CCC)

When moving clients, respect for the client is demonstrated through:
- promoting autonomy
- providing privacy and ensuring comfort

- answering questions and providing an interpreter, if needed
- advocating for the client and family.

Infection Control (INF)

When moving clients, healthcare-associated infection is prevented by:
- reducing the transfer and number of microorganisms, primarily through hand hygiene and cleaning of the transfer belt.

Safety (SAF)

When moving clients, safety measures prevent harm and maintain a safe care environment for the client and nurse by:

- following four principles of body mechanics:
  - Maintain a wide, stable base with your feet.
  - Put the bed at the correct height (waist level when providing care; hip level when moving a client).
  - Keep the work directly in front of you to avoid rotating the spine.
  - Keep the client as close to your body as possible to minimize reaching.

Communication (COM)

- Communication exchanges information (oral, written, nonverbal, or electronic) between two or more people.

- Collaboration with the client and other healthcare providers is essential to achieve safe client handling and movement.
- Documentation records information in a permanent legal record.

Health Maintenance (HLTH)

When moving clients, nursing is dedicated to the promotion of health and abilities, including:

- positioning the client to promote venous return and musculoskeletal alignment
- regaining strength and mobility and supporting health-seeking behaviors.

Evaluation (EVAL)

When moving clients, the evaluation of outcomes enables the nurse to determine the efficacy of the care provided.

■ SKILL 1.6 Positioning a Client in Bed

EQUIPMENT

Trapeze bar
Friction-reducing surface
Pillows
Clean gloves
Assistive devices, as needed
Assistive lifting equipment, as needed

BEGINNING THE SKILL

1. **INF** Perform hand hygiene.
2. **INF** Apply gloves if there is a risk of exposure to body fluids.
3. **CCC** Introduce yourself to the client and family and explain the procedure.
4. **SAF** Identify the client using two identifiers.
5. **CCC** Provide privacy. Close the door; pull the curtain.

PROCEDURE

6. **ACC** Assess the client's activity level, cognitive function, degree of mobility, and discomfort. Premedicate client if indicated. *Your assessment is to determine the extent to which the client can assist with the repositioning.*
7. **SAF** Assess for the presence of intravenous lines and other equipment that might be an impediment to movement, such as Foley catheter, ventilator tubing, or electrocardiogram (ECG) wires.
8. **ACC** Assess the client's weight and ability to assist with the move to determine the need for assistive lifting equipment, such as ceiling- or floor-based lifts or friction-reducing equipment, and the appropriate number of caregivers needed for the move. Follow the Algorithm for Repositioning a Client in Bed (see Fig. 1.2). (Note: Some clients will be able to move without physical assistance but need verbal cueing.) *Assistive equipment is necessary*

whenever a nurse is lifting more than approximately 16 kg (35 lb). Implementing safe handling and movement standards prevents injury to the nurse and client.

9. **ACC** Assess the client's need for supportive devices, such as footboards, hand rolls, or an abduction pillow. *Supportive devices are used to maintain alignment and posture when individuals need assistance to maintain their existing level of muscle and joint health.*
10. **SAF** Lock the wheels of the bed.
11. **SAF** Raise the bed to a comfortable working height. If working alone, raise the side rail on the opposite side. *Setting up an ergonomically safe space prevents injury to the nurse and client. Raising the side rail prevents the client from falling out of the bed.*
12. **Position the client in Fowler's.**

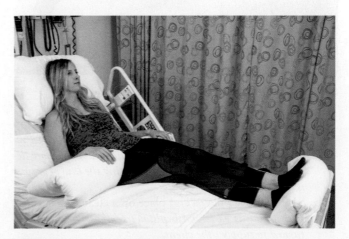

STEP 12 A client in Fowler's.

a. **ACC** Position the client's hips at the break in the bed such that when the head of bed rises, the client's back and head elevate and the hips remain level.

b. **ACC** Elevate the head of the bed to the appropriate position: Low-Fowler's is considered 15 degrees; semi-Fowler's is between 15 and 45 degrees (often considered 30 degrees); Fowler's is typically considered 45 degrees; and high-Fowler's is typically between 60 and 90 degrees (see Table 1.3).

c. **HLTH** Maintain dorsiflexion of feet. Insert a footboard to maintain dorsiflexion of the feet and prevent foot drop, if needed.

d. **HLTH** Maintain alignment of the legs without external rotation of the hips or hyperextension of knees. Position a trochanter roll to maintain alignment of the legs, if needed. Place a small pillow under the knees to provide flexion of the knees, if needed.

e. **HLTH** Maintain the natural curve of the spine. Position a small pillow at the lumbar portion of the back to support the lumbar curvature, if needed.

f. **HLTH** Maintain a neutral position of the neck and head. Position pillows to support the head, neck, and upper back without hyperextending the neck.

g. **HLTH** Support forearms, preventing shoulder strain. Position pillows under the forearms to prevent shoulder strain and to promote venous return of the hands.

h. **HLTH** Maintain wrist and finger position, preventing contractures. Place a handroll in the palm of the hand, if indicated.

13. **Position the client in the lateral position from Fowler's.**

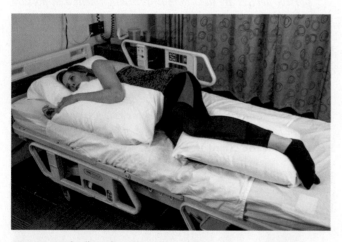

STEP 13 A client in a lateral position.

a. **SAF** Lower the head of the bed to the lowest position tolerated by the client. *Lowering the head of the bed reduces the force needed to move the client and therefore decreases the risk of nurse injury. Fighting the law of gravity is a losing battle.*

b. **SAF** Remove pillows and place on a clean, dry surface. *Positioning is easier with pillows removed and then returned to support the client.*

c. **ACC** Position the client on a friction-reducing surface, as needed. *Friction-reducing surfaces greatly reduce the force needed to move clients.*

d. **ACC** Position the client's hips on the side of the bed closest to you. *Beginning to roll on one side of the bed allows room to turn and position the arms and legs.*

e. **ACC** Position the client's arm nearest you across the client's chest. *Positioning the arm in the direction the client will roll facilitates the roll.*

f. **ACC** Position the client's far arm abducted from the client's body with the client's hand up at head level. *This is the direction the client will roll; therefore, abducting the arm and raising the hand prevents the client from rolling on top of the arm and hand.*

g. **ACC** Position the client's leg nearest you over the other leg. *Positioning the leg in the direction the client will roll facilitates the roll.*

If You Are Alone

h. **SAF** Raise the side rail on the near side where the client's hips are closest to the edge of the bed.

i. Walk around the bed to the far side.

j. **ACC** Place one hand on the client's far shoulder and far hip to roll the client. *Holding the hip and shoulder gives control over the client's torso.*

If You Are Working With a Colleague

k. **ACC** The nurse on the far side places one hand on the client's far shoulder and far hip. *Holding the hip and shoulder gives control over movement of the client's torso.*

l. **SAF** The nurse on the near side assists the client to lift the head and, if the client has long hair, protects the hair. *Lifting the head reduces friction, and moving the hair prevents pulling.*

m. **SAF** Place one foot under the edge of the bed and the other foot behind with a broad stance.

n. **SAF** Flex your knees and hips with your weight over the foot closest to the bed. *Flexing your knees and hips engages the gluteal and quadriceps muscles and reduces stress on your back.*

o. **COM** Coordinate the move with your colleague. Typically, nurses count to three, then move. *Coordinating movement maximizes your efforts and reduces the risk of injury.*

p. **SAF** Tighten your core muscles and transfer your weight to the back foot. Keep your arms in close to your body. *Working close to the body prevents hyperextension and reduces the risk of injury.*

q. **ACC** Roll the client into a lateral position.

r. **HLTH** Position pillows under the client's head to support the head and neck and maintain a neutral position without lateral flexion of the neck.

s. **HLTH** Position pillows under the upper arm to support the shoulder and arm in alignment and to prevent internal rotation.

t. **HLTH** Position pillows under the upper leg to support the leg and hip in alignment and to prevent internal rotation.

14. **Position the client in the Sim's position from Fowler's.**

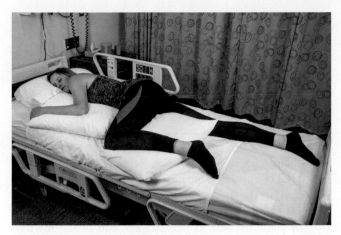

STEP 14 A client in Sim's position.

a. **ACC** Lower the head of the bed to the lowest position tolerated by the client. *Lowering the head of the bed reduces the force needed to move the client and therefore decreases the risk of nurse injury. Fighting the law of gravity is a losing battle.*

b. **SAF** Remove pillows and place one against the headboard and any others on a clean, dry surface. *Positioning is easier with pillows removed and then repositioned to support the client.*

c. **ACC** Position the client on a friction-reducing surface, as needed. *Friction-reducing surfaces greatly reduce the force needed to move clients.*

d. **ACC** Position the client's hips on the side of the bed closest to you. *Beginning to roll on one side of the bed allows room to turn and position the arms and legs.*

e. **ACC** Position the client's arm nearest you across the client's chest. *Positioning the arm in the direction the client will roll facilitates the roll.*

f. **ACC** Position the client's dependent arm close to the client's body. This is the direction the client will roll. *Keeping the arm close to the body allows the client to roll over the arm.*

g. **ACC** Position the client's leg nearest you over the other leg. *Positioning the leg in the direction the client will roll facilitates the roll.*

If You Are Alone

h. **SAF** Raise the side rail on the near side where the client's hips are closest to the edge of the bed.

i. Walk around the bed to the far side.

j. **ACC** Place one hand on the client's far shoulder and far hip. *Holding the hip and shoulder gives control over the client's torso.*

If You Are Working With a Colleague

k. **ACC** The nurse on the far side places one hand on the client's far shoulder and far hip. *Holding the hip and shoulder gives control over movement of the client's torso.*

l. **SAF** The nurse on the near side assists the client to lift the head and, if the client has long hair, protects the hair. *Lifting the head reduces friction, and moving the hair prevents pulling.*

m. **SAF** Place one foot under the edge of the bed and the other foot behind with a broad stance.

n. **SAF** Flex your knees and hips with your weight over the foot closest to the bed. *Flexing your knees and hips engages the gluteal and quadriceps muscles and reduces stress on your back.*

o. **COM** Coordinate the move with your colleague. Typically, nurses count to three, then move. *Coordinating movement maximizes your efforts and reduces the risk of injury.*

p. **SAF** Tighten your core muscles and transfer your weight to the back foot. Keep your arms in close to your body. *Working close to the body prevents hyperextension and reduces the risk of injury.*

q. **ACC** Roll the client into a position halfway between a lateral and prone position.

r. **HLTH** Position pillows under the client's head to support the head and neck and maintain a neutral position without lateral flexion of the neck.

s. **HLTH** Position the upper leg flexed at the hip and knee, and position pillows under the upper leg to support the leg and hip in alignment and to prevent internal rotation.

t. **HLTH** Position a small pillow or sandbag against the plantar surface of the foot to support dorsiflexion and prevent plantar flexion (foot drop).

15. **Position the client prone from Fowler's.**

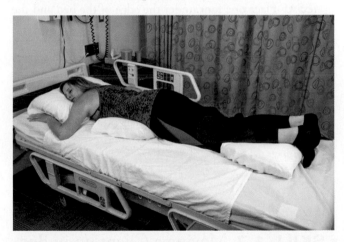

STEP 15 A client in a prone position.

a. **ACC** Lower the head of the bed to the lowest position tolerated by the client. *Lowering the head of the bed reduces the force needed to move the client and therefore decreases the risk of nurse injury. Fighting the law of gravity is a losing battle.*

b. **SAF** Remove pillows and place them on a clean, dry surface. *Positioning is easier with pillows removed and then repositioned to support the client.*

c. **ACC** Position the client on a friction-reducing surface, as needed. *Friction-reducing surfaces greatly reduce the force needed to move clients.*

d. **ACC** Position the client's hips on the side of the bed closest to you. *Beginning to roll on one side of the bed allows room to turn and position the arms and legs.*

e. **ACC** Position the client's arm nearest you across the client's chest. *Positioning the arm in the direction the client will roll facilitates the roll.*

f. **ACC** Position the client's dependent arm close to the client's body. This is the direction the client will roll. *Keeping the arm close to the body allows the client to roll over the arm.*

g. **ACC** Position the client's leg nearest you over the other leg. *Positioning the leg in the direction the client will roll facilitates the roll.*

If You Are Alone

h. **SAF** Raise the side rail on the near side where the client's hips are closest to the edge of the bed.

i. Walk around the bed to the far side.

j. **ACC** Place one hand on the client's far shoulder and far hip. *Holding the hip and shoulder gives control over the client's torso.*

If You Are Working With a Colleague

k. **ACC** The nurse on the far side places one hand on the client's far shoulder and far hip. *Holding the hip and shoulder gives control over movement of the client's torso.*

l. **SAF** The nurse on the near side assists the client to lift the head and, if the client has long hair, protects the hair. *Lifting the head reduces friction, and moving the hair prevents pulling.*

m. **SAF** Place one foot under the edge of the bed and the other foot behind with a broad stance.

n. **SAF** Flex your knees and hips with your weight over the foot closest to the bed. *Flexing your knees and hips engages the gluteal and quadriceps muscles and reduces stress on your back.*

o. **COM** Coordinate the move with your colleague. Typically, nurses count to three, then move. *Coordinating movement maximizes your efforts and reduces the risk of injury.*

p. **SAF** Tighten your core muscles and transfer your weight to the back foot. Keep your arms in close to your body. *Working close to the body prevents hyperextension and reduces the risk of injury.*

q. **ACC** Roll the client into a prone position.

r. **ACC** Position the client's head turned to one side. If a pillow is used, it must be a very flat one to prevent hyperflexion of the neck.

s. **CCC** The arms may be comfortably positioned at the client's side or up at the head level.

t. **HLTH** Position a small pillow under the abdomen to support the lumbar curvature.

u. **HLTH** Position a small pillow under the lower legs or allow the feet to fall over the end of the mattress to allow dorsiflexion and prevent plantar flexion (foot drop).

FINISHING THE SKILL

16. **CCC** Remove friction-reducing surface, if used.

17. **CCC** Provide comfort. Assist the client with positioning, replace the pillows, and rearrange bedding.

18. **SAF** Secure all medical equipment attached to the client and check for patency, such as intravenous lines and Foley catheters. *Equipment can become kinked or disconnected with client movement.*

19. **SAF** Ensure client safety. Place bed in the lowest position and verify that the client can identify and reach the nurse call system. *These safety measures reduce the risk of falls.*

20. **EVAL** Evaluate outcomes. Your evaluation includes how the client tolerated the procedure and the amount of assistance the client required to reposition.

21. **INF** Remove gloves, if used.

22. **INF** Perform hand hygiene.

23. **COM** Document assessment findings, care given, and outcomes in the legal healthcare record.

▪ SKILL 1.7 Moving a Client up in Bed

EQUIPMENT

Trapeze bar
Friction-reducing surface or draw sheet
Clean gloves

BEGINNING THE SKILL

1. **INF** Perform hand hygiene.

2. **INF** Apply gloves if there is a risk of exposure to body fluids.

3. **CCC** Introduce yourself to the client and explain the procedure.

4. **SAF** Identify the client using two identifiers.

5. **CCC** Provide privacy. Close the door; pull the curtain.

PROCEDURE

6. **ACC** Assess the client's activity level, cognitive function, degree of mobility, and discomfort. Premedicate client if indicated. *Your assessment is to determine the extent to which the client can assist with the repositioning.*

7. **SAF** Assess for the presence of intravenous lines and other equipment that might be an impediment to movement, such as Foley catheter, ventilator tubing, or ECG wires.

8. **ACC** Assess the client's weight and ability to assist with the move to determine the need for assistive lifting equipment, such as ceiling- or floor-based lifts or friction-reducing equipment, and the appropriate number of caregivers needed for the move. Follow the Algorithm for Repositioning a Client in Bed (see Fig. 1.2). Some clients will be able to move without physical assistance but need verbal cueing. *Assistive equipment is necessary whenever a nurse is lifting more than approximately 16 kg (35 lb). Implementing safe handling and movement standards prevents injury to the nurse and client.*

Client Cannot Assist

9. **ACC** If a client cannot provide assistance to reduce friction and add force to the movement toward the head of the bed and if the client's weight represents more than approximately 16 kg (35 lb) per nurse, use assistive lifting equipment. See Skill 1.9.

Client Able to Reposition

10. **ACC** If the client has sufficient upper-extremity strength to use a trapeze bar or the side rails to support his or her weight and push with the feet, then:
    a. **COM** Instruct the client to bend the knees and place the feet flat on the mattress.
    b. **COM** Instruct the client to tuck the chin to chest and push into the heels, extending the legs.
    This should move the client up in the bed. If successful, repeat until the client is in the desired position.

Client Able to Assist and Friction-Reducing Device Available

11. **ACC** If the client can partially assist, find the appropriate number of caregivers with whom to complete this activity. Follow the Algorithm for Repositioning a Client in Bed (see Fig. 1.2). If caregivers are not available, use assistive lifting equipment.
12. **SAF** Raise the bed to a comfortable working height. *Setting up an ergonomically safe space prevents injury to the nurse and client.*
13. **SAF** Lower the head of the bed to the lowest position tolerated by the client. *Lowering the head of the bed reduces the force needed to move the client and therefore decreases the risk of nurse injury. Fighting the law of gravity is a losing battle.*
14. **SAF** Remove pillows and place one against the headboard and any others on a clean, dry surface. *Moving is easier with pillows removed. It requires less force and therefore decreases the risk of nurse injury. Placement of one pillow against the headboard creates a soft bumper should the client bump his or her head while moving up in the bed.*
15. **ACC** Position the client on a friction-reducing surface or draw sheet. Ensure the client's head, shoulders, hips, and most of the legs are on the draw sheet or friction-reducing surface. *A friction-reducing surface greatly reduces the force needed to move clients.*

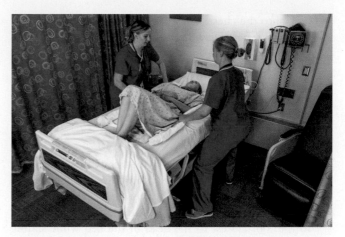

STEP 15 Position the client on a draw sheet.

16. Nurses position themselves on each side of the bed. *Moving clients up in bed is best performed with two or more individuals and a friction-reducing surface, even when clients can provide some assistance. All caregivers should not lift more than approximately 16 kg (35 lb).*
17. **SAF** Position your feet shoulder-width apart. *This gives a broad base of support.*
18. **SAF** Turn slightly toward the head of the bed, and point your foot closest to the client's head in the direction of the head of the bed. *Facing in the direction of movement facilitates body alignment and prevents twisting.*
19. **ACC** Position the client's feet firmly on the bed surface with knees bent. *Having the legs off the sheet reduces friction, and the client can push with the legs to assist in moving up in the bed.*

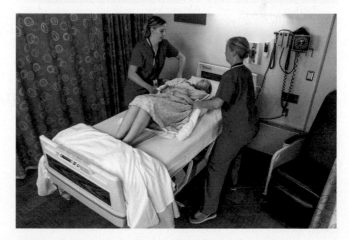

STEP 19 Position the client's feet firmly on the bed.

20. **ACC** If the client has a trapeze bar and the upper-body strength, ask the client to grasp the trapeze bar.
21. **ACC** If the client does not have a trapeze bar, ask the client to cross the arms over the chest. *Clients reduce friction by having their arms off the sheet. They reduce load weight by pulling up with a trapeze bar. Both assist in moving up in the bed.*
22. **COM** Ask the client to lift the head up, tucking the chin to the chest. If the client has long hair, bring the

hair onto the chest. *Lifting the head reduces friction, and moving the hair prevents pulling.*

23. **SAF** Tightly grasp the straps or rolled edge of the friction-reducing surface or draw sheet with your hands at the client's hip and shoulder.

24. **SAF** Flex your knees and hips with your weight over the foot closest to the foot of the bed. *Flexing your knees and hips engages the gluteal and quadriceps muscles and reduces stress on your back.*

25. **COM** Coordinate the move with your colleague. Typically, nurses count to three, then move. *Coordinating movement maximizes your efforts and reduces the risk of injury.*

26. **SAF** Tighten your core muscles and transfer your weight to the foot closest to the head of the bed while sliding the client toward the head of the bed. Keep your arms in close to your body. *Working close to the body prevents hyperextension and reduces the risk of injury.*

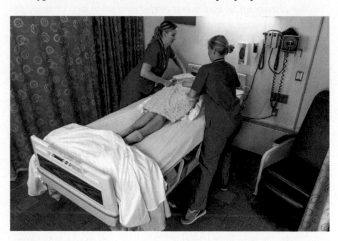

STEP 26 Transfer your weight while sliding the client.

27. **SAF** If the client is not in a good position, adjust your feet and move the client again.

FINISHING THE SKILL

28. **CCC** Remove the friction-reducing surface, if used. (Note: A draw sheet remains beneath the client.)

29. **CCC** Provide comfort. Assist the client with positioning, replace the pillows, and rearrange bedding.

30. **SAF** Secure all medical equipment attached to the client and check for patency, such as intravenous lines and Foley catheters. *Equipment can become kinked or disconnected with client movement.*

31. **SAF** Ensure client safety. Place bed in the lowest position and verify that the client can identify and reach the nurse call system. *These safety measures reduce the risk of falls.*

32. **EVAL** Evaluate outcomes. Your evaluation includes how the client tolerated the procedure, the amount of assistance the client required, and your use of appropriate safe handling equipment.

33. **INF** Remove gloves, if used.

34. **INF** Perform hand hygiene.

35. **COM** Document assessment findings, care given, and outcomes in the legal healthcare record.

▪ SKILL 1.8 Transferring a Client From Bed to Chair

EQUIPMENT

Transfer belt
Trapeze bar
Friction-reducing surface
Bath blanket or sheet
Clean gloves

BEGINNING THE SKILL

1. **INF** Perform hand hygiene.
2. **INF** Apply gloves if there is a risk of exposure to body fluids.
3. **CCC** Introduce yourself to the client and explain the procedure.
4. **SAF** Identify the client using two identifiers.
5. **CCC** Provide privacy. Close the door; pull the curtain. Have a bath blanket or sheet available for additional coverage after the transfer.

PROCEDURE

6. **ACC** Assess the client's activity level, cognitive function, degree of mobility, and discomfort. Premedicate client if indicated. *Your assessment is to determine the extent to which the client can assist with the repositioning.*

7. **SAF** Assess for the presence of intravenous lines and other equipment that might be an impediment to movement, such as a Foley catheter or ECG wires.

8. **ACC** Assess the client's ability to bear weight and cooperate in order to determine the need for assistive lifting equipment. Follow the Algorithm for Transfer to or From a Seated Position (see Fig. 1.3). *The client must be able to stand and pivot and be cooperative to successfully transfer using only a transfer belt. Assistive equipment is necessary whenever a nurse is lifting more than approximately 16 kg (35 lb). Implementing safe handling and movement standards prevents injury to nurse and client.*

Client Cannot Assist

9. **ACC** If client cannot bear weight, follow the Algorithm for Transfer to or From a Seated Position (see Fig. 1.3) and use assistive lifting equipment. See Skill 1.9.

Client Able to Reposition

10. **COM** If the client has the ability and balance to come to a standing position, give the client verbal instructions for the transfer.
    a. Instruct the client to stand. Rocking may help give the client momentum to come to his or her feet.
    b. Instruct the client to reach for the far arm of the chair and use the arm of the chair for support as he or she moves until the chair/wheelchair is behind him or her.
    c. Instruct the client to reach back to the arms of the chair and to lower down to sitting on the chair.

Client Able to Assist

11. **SAF** Lock the wheels of the bed.
12. **SAF** Lower the bed to the lowest position.
13. Move the client into a sitting position (with legs dangling).
    a. **ACC** Position the client in a lateral position, facing you with the legs close to the edge of the bed.
    b. **SAF** Stand at the client's hips. Place your foot nearest the head of bed at the edge of the bed and the other foot behind with a broad stance.
    c. **ACC** Raise the head of the bed.
    d. **ACC** With your hand nearest the head of the bed, grasp forearm to forearm with the client. Place your other arm over the client's ankles or shins (depending on the length of the client's legs).
    e. **SAF** Flex your knees and hips with your weight over the foot closest to the bed. *Flexing your knees and hips engages the gluteal and quadriceps muscles and reduces stress on your back.*
    f. **COM** Instruct the client to push off the mattress or side rail to assist reaching a sitting position. Coordinate the move with your client. Typically, nurses count to three, then move. *Coordinating movement maximizes your efforts and reduces the risk of injury.*
    g. **SAF** Tighten your core muscles and transfer your weight to the back foot while smoothly pulling the client's feet off the bed with one arm and pulling the client's forearm to assist the client to a sitting position. (Note: Gravity will help lower the client's legs, and the momentum helps to pivot the client into position.) *Transferring your weight prevents twisting of the spine and reduces the risk for injury.*
    h. **SAF** Observe the client's color and make eye contact. Ask how the client feels. Remain standing in front of the client. *Clients may experience orthostatic hypotension and may faint.*

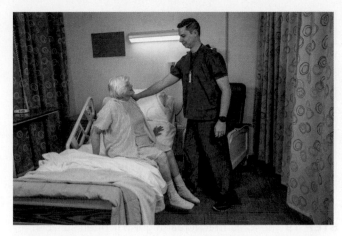

STEP 13H Observe the client's color. Make eye contact.

14. **SAF** Secure a transfer belt around the client's waist. *Using a transfer belt allows a safer hold while guiding a client from one position to another.*
15. **SAF** Assist the client to put on nonslip shoes or slippers. Ensure client can place both feet firmly on the floor with a wide base of support.
16. **SAF** Position the chair or wheelchair at the head of the bed, turned toward the bed on the client's stronger side.
17. **SAF** Lock the wheels if using a wheelchair.
18. **SAF** Stand facing the client and shoulder to shoulder on the client's weak side. Place your foot between the client's feet. Feel where you could connect with the client's knee or shin on the client's weaker side.

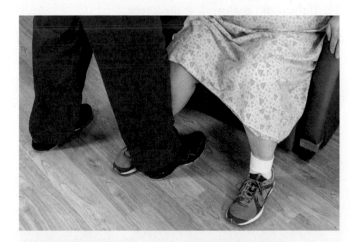

STEP 18 Place your foot between the client's feet.

19. **SAF** Grasp the transfer belt with one hand. You may support the client at the elbow or shoulder with the other hand as needed. The forearm-to-forearm grasp is often suitable. **WARNING:** Do not allow the client to hold on to your neck or shoulders. *This transfers pressure down your spine.*

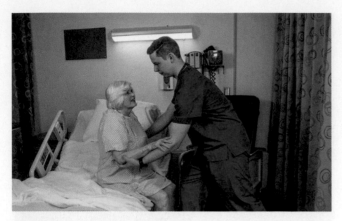

STEP 19 The forearm-to-forearm grasp is often suitable.

20. **COM** Instruct the client to lean forward at the hips and to push to a stand at your command. The client may also use his or her fists to push off the bed.
21. **COM** Coordinate the move with your client. (Note: Typically, nurses count to three and then move or say, "ready, steady, stand.") *Coordinating movement maximizes your efforts and reduces the risk of injury.*
22. **SAF** Flex your knees and hips, and with your weight evenly distributed, come straight up along with the client. *Flexing your knees and hips engages the gluteal and quadriceps muscles and reduces stress on your back*
23. **SAF** Observe the client's color and make eye contact. Ask how the client feels. Remain standing, facing the client and shoulder to shoulder. *Clients may experience orthostatic hypotension and may faint.*
24. If the client goes weak at the knees:
    a. Make contact with the client's knee/shin.
    b. **ACC** Push with your knee, and at the same time, push on the transfer belt or the client's hip bone.

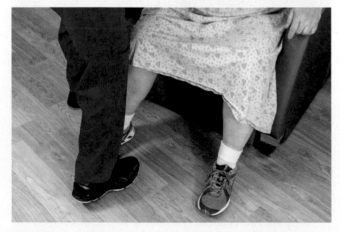

STEP 24B If the client goes weak at the knees, push with your knee.

    c. **ACC** Sit the client back down on the bed.
    d. **ACC** Put your hand on the client's shoulder, and push the client's shoulder to the head of the bed. *This prevents the client from going backward across the bed.*
    e. **CCC** Allow the client to rest.

From Standing to the Wheelchair

25. **COM** Instruct the client to pivot and step back until the chair/wheelchair is behind the client.
26. **COM** Instruct the client to reach back to the arms of the chair.
27. **COM** Instruct the client to lower down slowly to sitting on the chair on your command. Continue grasping the transfer belt with one hand, and support the client's shoulder with the other. You may need to switch hands.
28. **SAF** Plan where your knees and feet will go. You may place one of your knees between the client's knees, or you may place your feet and knees on either side of the client's knees. *Flexing your knees and hips engages the gluteal and quadriceps muscles and reduces stress on your back.*
29. **COM** Instruct the client to sit down slowly. Flex your knees and hips. *Flexing your knees and hips saves you from bending over the client and keeps your back straight.*

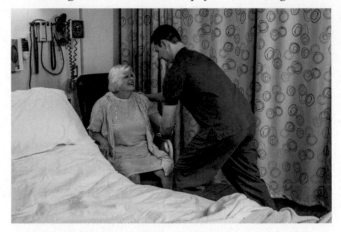

STEP 29 As the client sits, flex your knees and hips.

30. **INF** Remove the transfer belt. Clean the transfer belt if it is used for multiple clients.

FINISHING THE SKILL

31. **CCC** Provide comfort. Ask the client if he or she would like a sheet or bath blanket lap cover.
32. **SAF** Secure all medical equipment attached to the client and check for patency, such as intravenous lines and Foley catheters. *Equipment can become kinked or disconnected with client movement.*
33. **SAF** Ensure client safety. Verify that the client can identify and reach the nurse call system. *These safety measures reduce the risk of falls.*
34. **EVAL** Evaluate outcomes. Your evaluation includes how the client tolerated the procedure and the amount of assistance the client required. Was your communication effective? Was the transfer safely accomplished?
35. **INF** Remove gloves, if used.
36. **INF** Perform hand hygiene.
37. **COM** Document assessment findings, care given, and client transfer outcomes in the legal healthcare record.

■ SKILL 1.9 Using a Sling Lift to Move a Client

EQUIPMENT
Floor-based lift
Ceiling-mounted lift
Appropriate-size sling
Clean gloves

BEGINNING THE SKILL
1. **INF** Perform hand hygiene.
2. **INF** Apply gloves if there is a risk of exposure to body fluids.
3. **CCC** Introduce yourself to the client and explain the procedure.
4. **SAF** Identify the client using two identifiers.
5. **CCC** Provide privacy. Close the door; pull the curtain.

PROCEDURE
6. **ACC** Assess the client's activity level, cognitive function, degree of mobility, and discomfort. Premedicate the client if indicated. *Your assessment is to determine the extent to which the client can assist with or tolerate moving.*
7. **SAF** Assess for the presence of intravenous lines and other equipment that might be an impediment to movement, such as a Foley catheter or ECG wires.
8. **ACC** Assess client's weight, ability to bear weight, ability to cooperate, and upper-extremity strength. Follow the Algorithm for Transfer to or From a Seated Position (see Fig. 1.3). *Your assessment is to determine the appropriate safe handling equipment.*
   If the client is unable to bear weight, cooperate, and/or use upper-extremity strength, then use a sling lift and two caregivers.
9. **ACC** Determine the appropriate sling to use considering the client's size, the client's medical condition, and the purpose of the transfer.
10. **SAF** Find a colleague with whom to complete this activity, as needed.
11. **SAF** Raise the bed to a comfortable working height. *Setting up an ergonomically safe space prevents injury to the nurse and client.*
12. **SAF** Lock the bed wheels.
13. **SAF** Lower the head of the bed to the lowest position tolerated by the client. *Lowering the head of the bed reduces the force needed to move the client and therefore decreases the risk of nurse injury. Fighting the law of gravity is a losing battle.*
14. **SAF** Remove pillows and place on a clean, dry surface. *Positioning in the sling is easier with pillows removed. It requires less force and therefore decreases the risk of nurse injury.*
15. **ACC** Follow the manufacturer's directions for positioning the client in the sling. Many slings are placed in position by rolling the client from side to side. If the

manufacturer recommends rolling, roll the client away from you first.
16. **ACC** Position the fabric sling under the client with the widest part under the client's thighs and the narrower part behind the client's shoulders.
17. **ACC** Position the lift over the client and lower the lift until the attachment bar is in position to attach the sling to the bar without pulling or lifting the client.

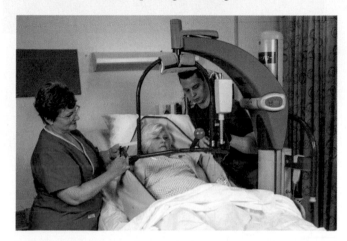

STEP 17 Attach the sling to the bar.

18. **ACC** Determine if the client will be lifted in a sitting position, supine position, or in between, and position the sling accordingly.
19. **SAF** Instruct the client to cross his or her arms. *Crossing the arms ensure they remain inside the sling.*
20. **ACC** Use the lift to raise the client's head.
21. **ACC** Use the lift to raise the client off the bed.

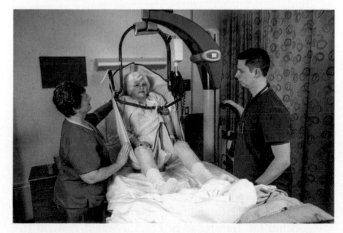

STEP 21 Use the lift to raise the client off the bed.

22. **CCC** Ensure the client is safe and comfortable.
23. **ACC** Transfer the client. Clients can be moved in the bed or to another bed, a chair, a wheelchair, or the toilet.

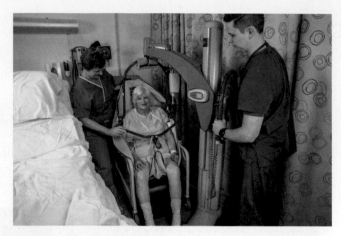

STEP 23 Transfer the client.

24. **SAF** Ensure the brakes are locked on the receiving bed/chair/wheelchair.
25. **ACC** Use the lift to lower the client.
26. Remove the sling.

FINISHING THE SKILL

27. **CCC** Provide comfort. Assist the client with positioning, and ask the client if he or she would like a sheet or bath blanket lap cover.
28. **SAF** Secure all medical equipment attached to the client and check for patency, such as intravenous lines and Foley catheters. *Equipment can become kinked or disconnected with client movement.*
29. **SAF** Ensure client safety. Verify that the client can identify and reach the nurse call system. *These safety measures reduce the risk of falls.*
30. **EVAL** Evaluate outcomes. Your evaluation includes how the client tolerated the procedure and the amount of assistance the client required. Was the transfer safely accomplished? Was the sling the best selection for the transfer?
31. **INF** Remove gloves, if used.
32. **INF** Perform hand hygiene.
33. **COM** Document assessment findings, care given, and outcomes in the legal healthcare record.

■ SKILL 1.10 Using a Sit-to-Stand Lift

EQUIPMENT

Sit-to-stand lift
Appropriate-size sling or belt
Clean gloves

BEGINNING THE SKILL

1. **INF** Perform hand hygiene.
2. **INF** Apply gloves if there is a risk of exposure to body fluids.
3. **CCC** Introduce yourself to the client and explain the procedure.
4. **SAF** Identify the client using two identifiers.
5. **CCC** Provide privacy. Close the door; pull the curtain.

PROCEDURE

6. **ACC** Assess the client's activity level, cognitive function, degree of mobility, and discomfort. Premedicate the client if indicated. *Your assessment is to determine the extent to which the client can assist with the repositioning.*
7. **SAF** Assess the client's ability to bear weight, ability to cooperate, and upper-extremity strength to determine the need for assistive lifting equipment. Follow the Algorithm for Transfer to or From a Seated Position (see Fig. 1.3). *The client must be able to bear weight, have hip stability, and be cooperative to successfully use a sit-to-stand lift. Assistive equipment is necessary whenever a nurse is lifting more than approximately 16 kg (35 lb). Implementing safe handling and movement standards prevents injury to the nurse and client.*

8. **SAF** Assess for the presence of intravenous lines and other equipment that might be an impediment to movement, such as a Foley catheter or ECG wires.
9. **SAF** Determine the appropriate belt to use considering the client's size.
10. **SAF** Lock the wheels of the bed.
11. **SAF** Lower the bed to the lowest position.
12. Move the client into a sitting position.
    a. **ACC** Position the client in a lateral position, facing you with the knees bent and the legs close to the edge of the bed.
    b. **SAF** Stand at the client's hips. Place your foot nearest the head of the bed under the edge of the bed and the other foot behind with a broad stance.
    c. **ACC** Raise the head of the bed.
    d. **ACC** Place your hand nearest the head of the bed under the client's shoulder and your other arm over the client's thighs.
    e. **SAF** Flex your knees and hips with your weight over the foot closest to the bed. *Flexing your knees and hips engages the gluteal and quadriceps muscles and reduces stress on your back.*
    f. **COM** Instruct the client to push off the mattress or side rail to assist in reaching a sitting position. Coordinate the move with your client. Typically, nurses count to three, then move. *Coordinating movement maximizes your efforts and reduces the risk of injury.*
    g. **SAF** Tighten your core muscles and transfer your weight to the back foot while smoothly pulling the client's knees and feet off the bed with one arm and

pushing the client's shoulder to assist the client to a sitting position. *Transferring your weight prevents twisting of the spine and reduces the risk for injury.*

h. **SAF** Observe the client's color and make eye contact. Ask how the client feels. Remain standing in front of the client. *Clients may experience orthostatic hypotension and may faint.*

13. **SAF** Assist the client to put on nonslip shoes or slippers. Ensure the client can place both feet firmly on the floor.

14. **ACC** Position the lift in front of the client close enough that the client can place his or her feet on the footplate.

15. **SAF** Adjust the lift legs on either side of the seated client with a broad base of support. Lock the lift.

16. **SAF** Secure the correct-size belt around the client and attach to the lift.

17. **ACC** Position the client's feet on the footplate of the lift and adjust the shin support to just below the client's patella. The client's shins should touch the shin support. *The shin support provides support for the client's legs when standing.*

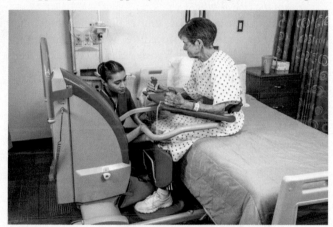

STEP 17 Position the client's feet on the footplate and adjust the shin support.

18. **ACC** Position the client's hands and forearms on the lift. Encourage the client to grip the handlebars. *The client uses upper-extremity strength to assist in standing.*

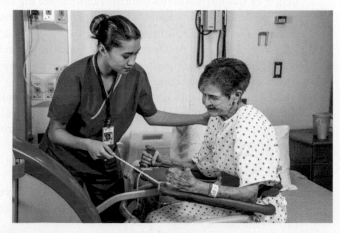

STEP 18 Position the client's hands and forearms on the lift.

19. **COM** Instruct the client to look up and lean back slightly.

20. **COM** Tell the client the lift is starting. *Communication exchange helps to ensure successful movement and reduces the risk of injury.*

21. **ACC** Use the lift to raise the client to a standing position.

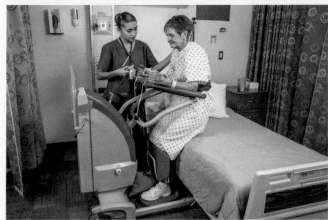

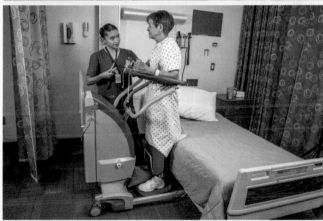

STEP 21 Use the lift to raise the client to a standing position.

22. **CCC** Ensure the client is stable and comfortable.

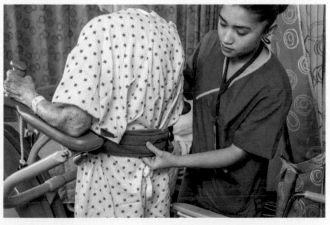

STEP 22 Ensure the client is stable and comfortable.

23. **SAF** Unlock the lift and adjust the lift legs to parallel. *The lift moves more easily if the legs are parallel.*

24. **ACC** Transfer the client to the desired location.

25. **SAF** Ensure the receiving seat is locked, if applicable.

26. **ACC** Use the lift to lower the client to a seated position. Ensure the client is stable.

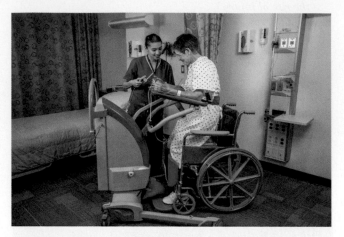

STEP 26 Lower the client to a seated position.

27. Remove belt.

FINISHING THE SKILL

28. **CCC** Provide comfort. Assist the client with positioning and ask the client if he or she would like a sheet or bath blanket lap cover.
29. **SAF** Secure all medical equipment attached to the client and check for patency, such as intravenous lines and Foley catheters. *Equipment can become kinked or disconnected with client movement.*

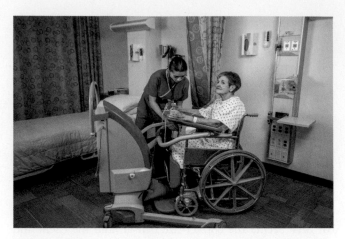

STEP 29 Secure all medical equipment and check for patency.

30. **SAF** Ensure client safety. Verify that the client can identify and reach the nurse call system. *These safety measures reduce the risk of falls.*
31. **EVAL** Evaluate outcomes. Your evaluation includes how the client tolerated the procedure. Was your communication effective? Was the transfer safely accomplished?
32. **INF** Remove gloves, if used.
33. **INF** Perform hand hygiene.
34. **COM** Document assessment findings, care given, and outcomes in the legal healthcare record.

■ SKILL 1.11 Transferring Clients Laterally (From Bed to Stretcher)

EQUIPMENT

Friction-reducing surface
Lateral transfer board
Bath blanket or sheet
Clean gloves
Assistive lifting equipment, as needed

BEGINNING THE SKILL

1. **INF** Perform hand hygiene.
2. **INF** Apply gloves if there is a risk of exposure to body fluids.
3. **CCC** Introduce yourself to the client and explain the procedure.
4. **SAF** Identify the client using two identifiers.
5. **CCC** Provide privacy. Close the door, pull the curtain, and cover the client with a gown. Have a bath blanket or sheet available for additional coverage after the transfer.

PROCEDURE

6. **ACC** Assess the client's activity level, cognitive function, degree of mobility, and discomfort. Premedicate the client if indicated. *Your assessment is to determine the extent to which the client can assist with moving.*
7. **SAF** Assess for the presence of intravenous lines and other equipment that might be an impediment to movement, such as a Foley catheter or ECG wires.
8. **ACC** Assess the client's weight and ability to assist. Follow the Algorithm for Lateral Transfer (see Fig. 1.4). *Your assessment is to determine the appropriate safe handling equipment.*

Client Cannot Assist

9. **ACC** If a client cannot provide assistance and weighs over 90 kg (200 lb), use a lift with a sling and three caregivers. See Skill 1.8.

Client Able to Assist

10. **ACC** If a client can provide assistance and weighs less than 90 kg (200 lb), use a friction-reducing device and two to four caregivers, depending on the client's condition and medical equipment.
11. **SAF** Lock the wheels of the bed.
12. **SAF** Raise the bed to a comfortable working height. *Setting up an ergonomically safe space prevents injury to the nurse and client.*
13. **SAF** Lower the head of the bed to the lowest position tolerated by the client. *Lowering the head of the bed reduces the force needed to move the client and therefore decreases the risk of nurse injury. Fighting the law of gravity is a losing battle.*
14. **SAF** Remove pillows and place on a clean, dry surface. *Moving is easier with pillows removed. It requires less force and therefore decreases the risk of nurse injury.*
15. **ACC** Position the client on a friction-reducing surface, usually by rolling from side to side. *Friction-reducing surfaces greatly reduce the force needed to move clients.*
16. **SAF** Position the stretcher parallel to the bed and at the same height or slightly lower. *A lower-height surface reduces the force needed to move the client.*
17. **SAF** Nurses position themselves on each side of the bed. Position your feet shoulder-width apart with one foot closer to the bed. *This gives a broad base of support.*

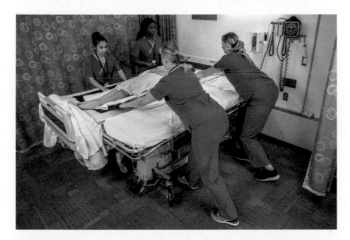

STEP 17 Position feet shoulder-width apart, one foot closer to the bed.

18. **ACC** Ask the client to cross the arms over the chest and lift the head up, tucking the chin to the chest. If the client has long hair, bring the hair onto the chest. *Crossing the arms and lifting the head reduce friction, and moving the hair prevents pulling.*
19. Grasp the straps or rolled edges of the friction-reducing device.
20. **SAF** Flex your knees and hips with your weight over the foot closest to the foot of the bed. *Flexing your knees and hips engages the gluteal and quadriceps muscles and reduces stress on your back.*

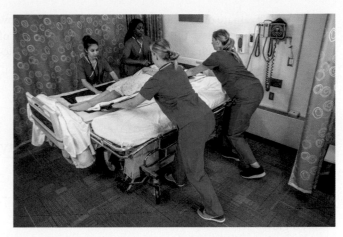

STEP 20 Flex knees and hips, with weight over the foot closest to the foot of the bed.

21. **COM** Coordinate the move with caregivers and client. Typically, nurses count to three, then move. *Coordinating movement maximizes your efforts and reduces the risk of injury.*
22. **SAF** To transfer the client, the nurses on the bed side tighten core muscles, push forward, and transfer weight to the front foot. The nurses on the stretcher side tighten core muscles, pull, and transfer weight to the rear foot. *Working close to the body prevents hyperextension and reduces the risk of injury.*

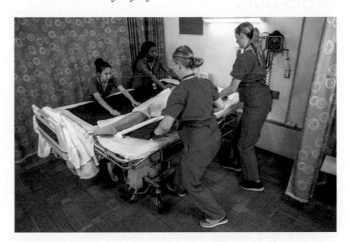

STEP 22 Pull and transfer weight to the rear foot.

FINISHING THE SKILL

23. **ACC** Determine if the friction-reducing device will be needed again or should be removed. Remove if indicated.
24. **CCC** Provide comfort. Assist the client with positioning, replace the pillows if possible, and cover the client with a sheet or bath blanket.
25. **SAF** Secure all medical equipment attached to the client and check for patency, such as intravenous lines and Foley catheters. *Equipment can become kinked or disconnected with client movement.*

26. **EVAL** Evaluate outcomes. Your evaluation includes how the client tolerated the procedure and the amount of assistance the client required. Was the transfer safely accomplished?

27. **INF** Remove gloves, if used.
28. **INF** Perform hand hygiene.
29. **COM** Document assessment findings, care given, and outcomes in the legal healthcare record.

■ SKILL 1.12 Moving Clients Who Have Special Precautions (Logrolling)

EQUIPMENT

Pillow
Clean gloves
Assistive devices, as needed
Assistive lifting equipment, as needed

BEGINNING THE SKILL

1. **INF** Perform hand hygiene.
2. **INF** Apply gloves if there is a risk of exposure to body fluids.
3. **CCC** Introduce yourself to the client and explain the procedure.
4. **SAF** Identify the client using two identifiers.
5. **CCC** Provide privacy. Close the door, pull the curtain, and cover the client with a gown or bath blanket.

PROCEDURE

6. **SAF** Check the order for special precautions and the client's limitations. *Special precautions may be ordered for the hip, knee, shoulder, or spine. Clients with possible cervical injury may have an order to keep the head immobilized.*
7. **ACC** Assess the client's activity level, cognitive function, degree of mobility, and discomfort. Premedicate the client if indicated. *Your assessment is to determine the extent to which the client will be cooperative during the repositioning. Unexpected movement increases the risk of injury.*
8. **SAF** Assess for the presence of intravenous lines and other equipment that might be an impediment to movement, such as Foley catheter or ECG wires.
9. **ACC** Assess the client's weight, degree of cooperation, and ability to assist. Follow the Algorithm for Lateral Transfer (see Fig. 1.4). *Your assessment is to determine the appropriate safe handling equipment and caregivers needed.*

Client Cannot Assist

10. **ACC** If a client is not cooperative or cannot provide assistance, or if the client's weight represents more than approximately 16 kg (35 lb) per nurse, use assistive lifting equipment and at least two caregivers. See Skill 1.8. (Note: Orthopedic units may have additional assistive lifting technology available, such as turning clips or turning straps that attach to the bed or bed sheet and are used with a ceiling or floor lift.)

Client Able to Assist

11. **ACC** If a client can provide assistance and weighs less than 90 kg (200 lb), use a friction-reducing surface and two to four caregivers depending on the client's condition and medical equipment. One caregiver may be needed to ensure neck alignment.
12. **SAF** Lock the wheels of the bed.
13. **SAF** Raise the bed to a comfortable working height. *Setting up an ergonomically safe space prevents injury to the nurse and client.*
14. **ACC** Position the client on a friction-reducing surface, as needed. *Friction-reducing surfaces greatly reduce the force needed to move clients.*
15. **COM** Coordinate the move with caregivers and client. Determine who is responsible for maintaining any special precautions, such as neck alignment or hip abduction. *Coordinating movement maximizes your efforts and reduces the risk of injury.*
16. **ACC** Pull the friction-reducing surface to bring the client's hips to one side of the bed. *Beginning to roll on one side of the bed allows room to turn and position the arms and legs.*
17. **ACC** Position the client's arms across his or her chest. *Positioning the arms across the chest prevents trapping an arm under the client.*
18. **ACC** Place a pillow between the client's knees. *Placing a pillow prevents adduction of the hip when turned.*
19. **ACC** The nurse on the far side places one hand on the client's far shoulder and far hip. *Holding the hip and shoulder gives control over movement of the client's torso.*
20. **SAF** The nurse on the near side assists the client to lift the head and, if the client has long hair, protects the hair. *Lifting the head reduces friction, and moving the hair prevents pulling.*
21. **SAF** Place one foot under the edge of the bed and the other foot behind with a broad stance.
22. **SAF** Flex your knees and hips, with your weight over the foot closest to the bed. *Flexing your knees and hips engages the gluteal and quadriceps muscles and reduces stress on your back.*
23. **COM** Coordinate the move with your colleagues. Typically, nurses count to three, then move. *Coordinating movement maximizes your efforts and reduces the risk of injury.*
24. **SAF** Tighten your core muscles and transfer your weight to the back foot. Keep your arms in close to your body. *Working close to the body prevents hyperextension and reduces the risk of injury.*

25. **ACC** Roll the client as a unit.

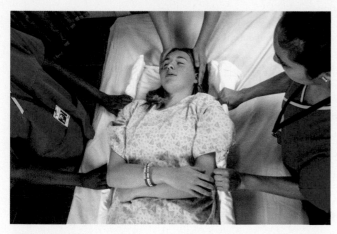

STEP 25 Roll the client as a unit.

26. **CCC** Remove friction-reducing surface, if used.
27. **CCC** Provide comfort. Assist the client with positioning, replace the pillows, and rearrange bedding.
28. **SAF** Secure all medical equipment attached to the client and check for patency, such as intravenous lines and Foley catheters. *Equipment can become kinked or disconnected with client movement.*
29. **SAF** Ensure client safety. Place bed in the lowest position and verify that client can identify and reach the nurse call system. *These safety measures reduce the risk of falls.*
30. **EVAL** Evaluate outcomes. How did the client tolerate the procedure? Was the transfer safely accomplished?
31. **INF** Remove gloves, if used.
32. **INF** Perform hand hygiene.
33. **COM** Document assessment findings, care given, and outcomes in the legal healthcare record.

SECTION 4 Using Restraints

The use of restraints in healthcare settings requires significantly more than knowing how to use them. Restraint use is complex and is the subject of significant regulation. Before restraints are used, there must be a complete assessment to determine the least restrictive intervention to effectively protect the client. Alternatives to restraints must be used and documented. There must be an order for restraints, and the restraint must be the least restrictive intervention that still protects the client's safety. The misuse of restraints can result in physical and emotional harm. Thus, restraints should only be used as a last resort. This section defines restraints, then explains their appropriate safe use and strategies for reducing their use.

DEFINING RESTRAINTS

The definition of physical restraints given by the Centers for Medicare and Medicaid Services (CMS) is "any manual method, physical or mechanical device, material, or equipment that immobilizes or reduces the ability of a patient to move his or her arms, legs, body, or head freely" (CMS, 2017, p. 123). The CMS further stipulates that this definition applies to all uses of restraints in all hospital settings. In some cases, an object or device not primarily designed as a restraint can be used in a manner that makes it a restraint. For example, if full-length side rails are up on both sides of a bed and the individual is not able to get out of the bed, then the side rails are acting as a restraint. If, however, a partial side rail is up to assist a client with getting in and out of bed, then the side rail is not a restraint. Table 1.5 describes restraints, their uses, and whether they are commonly used with adults or pediatric populations.

In addition to physical restraints, medications can in some circumstances be considered a chemical restraint. The CMS definition for chemical restraints is "a drug or medication when it is used as a restriction to manage the patient's behavior or restrict the patient's freedom of movement and is not a standard treatment or dosage for the patient's condition" (CMS, 2017, p. 124).

USE OF SECURING DEVICES

During surgery and recovery from anesthesia, securing devices for client safety are necessary. The CMS explains that "a medically necessary positioning or securing device used to maintain the position, limit mobility, or temporarily immobilize the patient during medical, dental, diagnostic, or surgical procedures is not considered a restraint" (CMS, 2017, p. 128). Furthermore, the restraint used while a client is recovering from anesthesia is considered a part of the surgical procedure. For young children, developmentally appropriate protective safety interventions, such as high-chair lap belts, raised crib rails, or stroller safety belts, that would be used outside a healthcare setting by safety-conscious adults to protect an infant, toddler, or preschool-aged child would not be considered restraint (CMS, 2017). Nurses are to use their judgment when a seatbelt is a safety device and not a restraint.

REGULATIONS GOVERNING USE OF RESTRAINTS

Today, the use of restraints has come under intense scrutiny. Restraints have been implicated in immobility-related

TABLE 1.5 Types of Restraints

Types of Restraints	Uses	Population
Limb restraints—a wide cushioned strap placed around the wrist or ankle with straps to secure it to the bed	To immobilize a limb, often for therapeutic reasons	Adults, children
Belt restraints—strap placed around the waist	To confine persons to a bed or chair	Adults
Vest restraints—a sleeveless vest with straps that can be tied to a bed or wheelchair	To confine a person to a bed or wheelchair	Adults
Mitt restraints—like a mitten without the thumb	To prevent the use of fingers to pick, scratch or pull	Adults, children
Elbow restraint	Prevents flexion of the elbow	Primarily children
Mummy restraint—blanket or sheet used to swaddle a child and prevent movement	Prevents flailing, kicking, and thrashing	Primarily infants and young children

problems such as pressure injury, contractures, and bone loss; in emotional and psychological issues such as confusion and loss of dignity; and in accidental deaths as a result of strangulation and suffocation. Moreover, many of the alleged benefits of restraints have not been supported by research evidence. For example, although it was once thought that restraints helped to prevent falls, numerous studies have shown that the premise is not valid. In fact, the use of restraints may increase the risk of falls and serious injury and increase the length of hospital stay (Khanh-Dao Le, 2018). The current Joint Commission standard, which is applicable to all hospitals, includes the following:

- All clients have the right to be free from physical or mental abuse and corporal punishment.
- All clients have the right to be free from restraint or seclusion, of any form, imposed as a means of coercion, discipline, convenience, or retaliation by staff.
- "Restraint or seclusion may only be imposed to ensure the immediate physical safety of the patient, a staff member, or others and must be discontinued at the earliest possible time" (CMS, 2017, pp. 117–118).
- The decision to use a restraint is not driven by the client's diagnosis but by a comprehensive individual client assessment.

Restraint Use in Acute Care Settings

Historically, healthcare providers have used restraints in medical-surgical areas to prevent clients from disturbing invasive devices, such as intravenous lines. This is particularly the case in intensive care units where clients have many invasive devices. However, as with falls, although the intent was to prevent injury, studies have shown that restraint use does not prevent unplanned extubation and may even cause greater harm (Chang, Wang, & Chao, 2008). Intensive care units have reduced the use of restraints with a variety of alternative strategies, including the following:

- The use of hand mitts that are not pinned
- Offering frequent orientation for the client
- Securing the equipment out of the client's sight
- Giving the client something else to hold
- Ensuring client comfort
- Treating pain and anxiety
- Allowing clients to touch and explore their tubes. (Hurlock-Chorostecki & Kielb, 2006)

Restraint Use in Residential Care Settings

Restraints use was once quite prevalent in long-term care facilities but now is quite rare. In 1987, the U.S. Congress passed the Nursing Home Act, which states that every nursing home must protect and promote the rights of each resident. Among these rights is "the right to be free from … any physical or chemical restraints imposed for purposes of discipline or convenience and not required to treat the resident's medical symptoms." Restraint use has dramatically decreased. In 1991, the percentage of nursing home residents restrained daily was approximately 21%, and by 2015, that number had decreased to 1.0% (CMS, 2008, 2015). The CMS states that the use of physical restraints in nursing homes is an indicator of the quality of care and may be considered a quality-of-life measure as well.

Reducing the Use of Restraints

Today, healthcare facilities are reducing restraint use through increased individual assessment and unit-based strategies such as the use of restraint alternatives. For example, a large study found that the most common type of physical restraint in acute care settings is the wrist restraint; however, some units dedicated to minimal restraint have now replaced wrist restraints with mittens (Minnick, Mion, Johnson, Catrambone, & Leipzig, 2007). Nurses can benefit from training in the use of such alternatives. Moreover, nurses who have used restraints for many years may need education about the risks of restraint use. Nurses may use restraints out of fear of litigation should an unrestrained client be injured. The use of restraints may not be necessary to prevent a lawsuit, provided standards of care are maintained and documented. In fact, healthcare facilities may be held liable for the misuse of restraints rather than for not using them (Salmon & Di Leonardi, 2013). See Box 1.8 for information about lawsuits and an example of a legal case involving the use of restraints.

APPLICATION OF THE NURSING PROCESS

Examples of Related ICNP Nursing Diagnoses, Expected Client Outcomes, and Nursing Interventions:
Nursing Diagnosis: Risk for trauma

Supporting Data: Potential for misuse of restraints and struggling with restraints

Expected Client Outcome: Client will be free from trauma while in the healthcare setting.

Nursing Intervention Example: Appropriate use of unpinned mitt restraint

Reference: International Classification for Nursing Practice. (n.d.). *eHealth & ICNP*. Retrieved from https://www.icn.ch/what-we-do/projects/ehealth-icnp.

BOX 1.8 Lessons From the Courtroom: Understanding the Courtroom and Lawsuit Against Nursing Home Dismissed

To bring a malpractice lawsuit forward, four things usually must be in place. First, there must be a legal duty to provide care. This is the case whenever a client is in the hospital and nurses provide care. Second, there must be a failure to provide reasonable care, or a breach of duty. Third, a client must have sustained an actual injury. Finally, it must be proven that the actual injury was the result of the breach of duty.

If there is a question regarding the care given, the court typically defers to expert testimony about the standard for that care. The plaintiff (person bringing forward the lawsuit) is typically required to submit expert testimony stating that the care provider failed to comply with professional or statutory standards of care. This testimony can be rebutted by expert testimony provided by the defendant. If the hospital or nursing staff did not deviate from the standard of care—for example, if they followed the hospital's policies and procedures—they most likely will not be found guilty of medical malpractice.

It is important for nurses to know when and how they will be held accountable for their judgment. Each state has a nurse practice act that defines the legal scope of practice for nurses within that state. Additionally, there are national professionally acceptable standards, and there may also be statutorily imposed standards for certain medical procedures.

The following case illustrates that following the physician's orders and standard of care resulted in the dismissal of the lawsuit despite the fact that restraints were not used and the client did sustain a fall.

In Tennessee, an 88-year-old woman with Alzheimer's disease was admitted to a skilled nursing facility, where she was identified as at high risk for falls. Her physician did not order restraints because restraints have significant risks. The physician ordered the bed to be placed against the wall on one side and kept in the lowest position with a half side rail elevated. The facility implemented and documented bedside checks every 2 hours. The elderly woman did fall but sustained only minor facial bruising and a cut of one eye. After she died of events unrelated to the fall, her son sued the facility for negligence based on the premise that a fall was in fact evidence of negligence. The physician testified that restraints were not appropriate for this person and that without an order, the nurses could not restrain the client. All facility policies were followed and standards met. The court dismissed the case (Patient not restrained, falls from bed: Lawsuit against nursing home dismissed, 2009).

CRITICAL CONCEPTS
Using Restraints

Accuracy (ACC)

When using restraints, accuracy is subject to the following variables:

Nurse-Related Factors
- Assessment of client and choice of type of restraint use needed
- Adherence to facility policy and regulations of restraint use
- Adherence to manufacturer guidelines regarding restraint use
- Technique used to apply and maintain restraints

Equipment-Related Factors
- Condition of restraints (i.e., ties intact, no fraying)

Client-Centered Care (CCC)

When using restraints, respect for the client is demonstrated through:
- promoting autonomy
- protecting dignity
- providing privacy and ensuring comfort
- answering questions and providing an interpreter, if needed
- advocating for the client and family.

Infection Control (INF)

When using restraints, healthcare-associated infection is prevented by:
- reducing the transfer and number of microorganisms, primarily through hand hygiene.

Safety (SAF)

When using restraints, safety measures prevent harm and maintain a safe care environment for the client and nurse.

Communication (COM)
- Communication exchanges information (oral, written, nonverbal, or electronic) between two or more people.
- Collaboration with other healthcare providers is essential when using and monitoring restraints to provide best practice.
- Documentation records information in a permanent legal record.

Health Maintenance (HLTH)

When using restraints, nursing is dedicated to the promotion of health and abilities, including maintaining skin integrity and mobility.

Evaluation (EVAL)

When using restraints, evaluation of outcomes enables the nurse to determine the efficacy of the care provided.

■ SKILL 1.13 Applying and Removing Restraints

EQUIPMENT

Restraints

BEGINNING THE SKILL

1. **SAF** Perform a thorough, individualized assessment to determine the least restrictive intervention that will effectively protect the client from harm. *A thorough assessment is required by the CMS.*
2. **SAF** Implement and document the use of alternatives to restraints used before the implementation of restraints. *Alternatives are a requirement of the CMS.*
3. **SAF** Determine if the restraint intervention proposed is the least restrictive intervention that protects the client's safety. *This is a requirement of the CMS.*
4. **SAF** Obtain an order for restraints. If restraints must be applied to protect the client or staff prior to an order being obtained, then a written or verbal order must be obtained within 1 hour of applying restraints. *An order is a requirement of the CMS.*
5. **CCC** Notify the individual's family of the initiation of restraints, if indicated.
6. **INF** Perform hand hygiene.

PROCEDURE

7. **SAF** Follow manufacturer's instructions for applying the restraint.
8. **ACC Applying Elbow Restraints**
   a. Release the adjustment straps.
   b. Wrap the elbow restraint around the arm, centering it over the elbow.

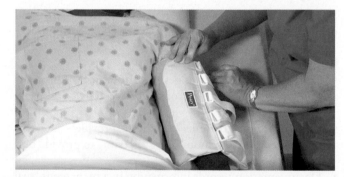

STEP 8B Center the elbow restraint over the elbow.

   c. Secure the hook fastener to the quilted material.
   d. **HLTH** Leave enough room to easily insert two fingers between the restraint and the person's arm to maintain adequate circulation.
9. **ACC Applying Limb Restraints**
   a. **HLTH** Ensure the limb restraint has sufficient padding to prevent skin breakdown.
   b. Apply the limb restraint around the ankle or wrist.

   c. **HLTH** Ensure that two fingers can be inserted between the restraint and the ankle or wrist.

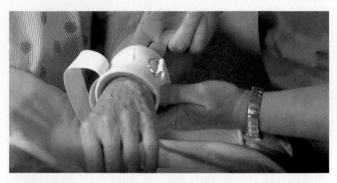

STEP 9C Ensure that the limb restraint is not too tight.

10. **ACC** Applying a Belt Restraint
    a. Inspect the belt. If the belt has Velcro, ensure it will hold securely. Determine the length of the two ties.

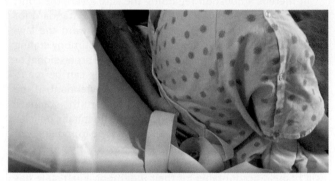

STEP 10A Ensure the belt restraint is smooth in back.

    b. Apply the belt restraint to the client.
    c. **HLTH** Ensure that two fingers can be inserted between the restraint and the client.
11. **ACC Applying a Mitt Restraint**
    a. Apply a thumbless mitt restraint to the hand.

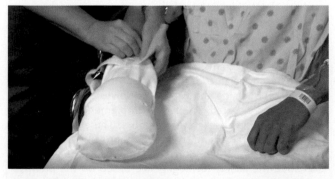

STEP 11A Ensure that the thumbless mitt restraint is secure.

    b. Follow the manufacturer's instructions for securing the mitt restraint.

c. Determine if the client's mitt can remain unpinned or if the restraint is to be secured.

12. **ACC** If restraint is to be secured to the bed frame in a quick release half bow:

a. Insert the ties through a secure section of the bed frame. Bring the end of the ties back across the ties to form a loop.

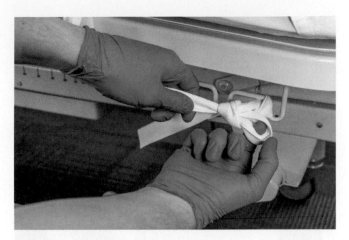

STEP 12C Pull tight.

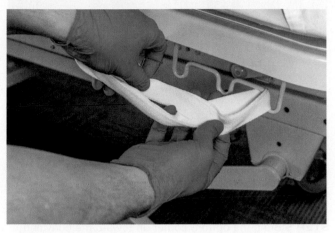

STEP 12A Insert the ties through the bed frame and form a loop.

b. Push a section of the distal end of the tie back through the loop of the ties.

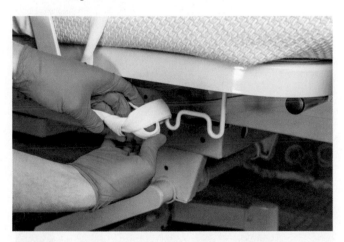

STEP 12B Push a section of the tie through the loop.

c. Pull tight. Note: Pulling the tab should result in a quick release of the knot. If the client pulls on the tie, the knot tightens.

FINISHING THE SKILL

13. **EVAL** Evaluate your actions. *Are you confident the restraint applied was the least restrictive intervention that protects the client?*
14. **INF** Perform hand hygiene.
15. **COM** Document in the client's chart:
    a. the events that resulted in the use of restraints
    b. the restraint alternatives implemented before the use of restraints
    c. the type of restraint selected and the rationale for the selection
    d. the time and the individual ordering the use of restraints
    e. each monitoring of the client, including time, and assessment of the client. *Specific documentation is required by the CMS each time restraints are applied.*
16. **SAF** Monitor the client at least every 2 hours to assess the emotional and physical well-being of the client, the ongoing need for restraint use, and any changes in the client's status, including if the restraint is to be removed. *Monitoring a minimum of every 2 hours is required by the CMS.*
17. **HLTH** Monitor the client's skin under the restraint for any signs of skin irritation or injury. Monitor the client for changes in joint range of motion. *Restraints have been implicated in the development of pressure injury and contractures.*

■ SKILL 1.14 Applying a Mummy Restraint

EQUIPMENT

Blanket or sheet (length equal to two times the length of the infant)
Clean gloves

BEGINNING THE SKILL

1. **INF** Perform hand hygiene.
2. **INF** Apply gloves if there is a risk of exposure to body fluids.

PROCEDURE

3. **INF** Place the blanket on a clean, dry surface and fold down one corner of the blanket.
4. **ACC** Place the infant on the blanket in a supine position with the infant's shoulders below the crease of the folded corner.

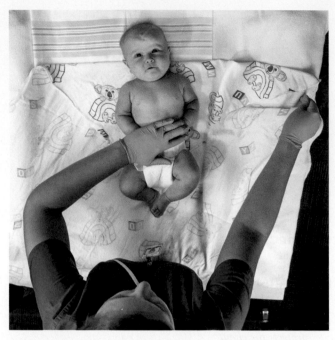

STEP 3 Place the infant's shoulders below the crease of the folded corner.

5. **SAF** Maintain one hand on the infant at all times while applying the mummy restraint.
6. **ACC** Fold the left corner of the blanket over the infant's body, securing the left arm in a relaxed position at the infant's side.

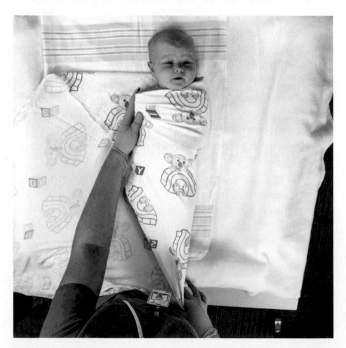

STEP 4 Fold the left corner of the blanket over the infant's body, securing the left arm.

7. **ACC** Roll the infant slightly onto his or her right side and secure the corner of the blanket under the infant's hips.
8. **ACC** Bring the corner of the blanket at the infant's feet up toward the body and secure the corner under the infant's hips or back depending on the length of the blanket.

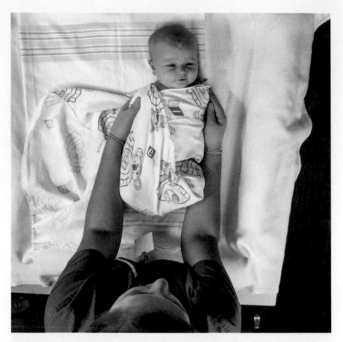

STEP 5 Bring the bottom corner up toward the body and secure.

9. **ACC** Fold the right corner over the infant's body, securing the right arm in a relaxed position at the infant's side.

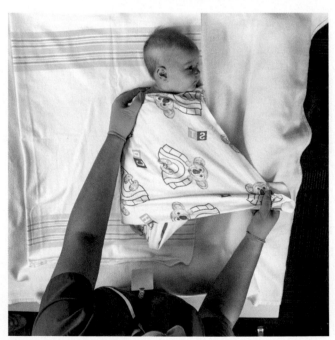

STEP 7 Fold the right corner over the infant's body, securing the right arm.

FINISHING THE SKILL

10. **CCC** Provide comfort, such as rocking or offering a pacifier.

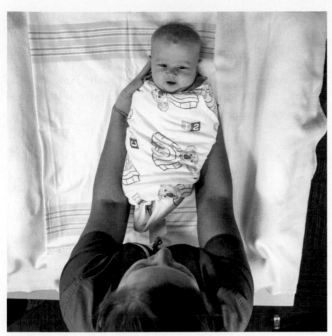

STEP 10 Provide comfort.

11. **SAF** Ensure client safety. Place the infant in a safe environment, such as a crib or bassinet.

12. **EVAL** Evaluate outcomes.
    a. Did the mummy restraint facilitate the performance of another procedure?
    b. How did the infant tolerate the restraint and the procedure?
13. **INF** Remove gloves, if used.
14. **INF** Perform hand hygiene.
15. **COM** Document the care given and client outcomes in the legal healthcare record.

■ **CASE STUDY**

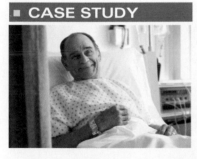

Frank Matousek is an 84-year-old male recently admitted to the Veterans Administration (VA) hospital following a motor vehicle accident in which he sustained a right ankle tibia/fibula fracture and fracture of his right ulna and radius. Surgeons performed an open reduction and internal fixation of the right ankle and placed a lightweight fiberglass cast on his right wrist. He had been living in an assisted-living facility for a year since the death of his wife, Barbara. He has type 2 diabetes and poor circulation in his lower extremities, and he admits to some confusion and forgetfulness. His wife had been ill with cancer for several years before her death in hospice care.

Upon admission to the VA hospital, Frank was tested for methicillin-resistant *S. aureus* (MRSA) with a nasal swab, which came back positive. Although many people in the community are colonized with MRSA, it is speculated that he may have become colonized during his many visits to his wife in hospice care. He is currently receiving antibiotics even though his wounds do not appear to be infected with MRSA. He is in a single room, and he is placed on Contact Precautions.

Since admission, Frank's confusion has increased. He is particularly confused in the evening and at night. He calls the night nurses "Barbara," which is the name of his deceased wife. When awakened, he does not remember that he is in the VA hospital until he is reminded.

Frank is having difficulty positioning himself in the bed. He is unable to use his right hand because the cast is on that wrist. His fingers become swollen if his hand remains down at his side for several hours. The greatest problem is his right ankle. The incision is not red or swollen, but the ankle and foot are swollen. The color of his foot is more pale and gray than his other foot. He complains of pain in the right leg and foot. The surgeon has ordered weight bearing as tolerated, but Frank requires assistance to transfer to a chair.

The nursing student is planning care around several safety concerns: identifying the client, preventing the transfer of infective microorganisms, and positioning the client.

Case Study Questions

1. When Frank is aroused from sleep or sedation, he is disoriented for several minutes. At 8:00 p.m. when the student enters the room, Frank appears asleep. How can the student verify the client's identification?
2. **Application of QSEN Competencies:** One of the Quality and Safety Education for Nurses (QSEN) skills for Safety is to demonstrate effective use of technology and standardized practices that support safety and

quality (Cronenwett et al., 2007). Describe the use of technology to support the National Patient Safety Goal of identifying the patient correctly.

3. Frank has dependent edema in his right hand and in his right foot. He requires assistance with repositioning. What positions might be comfortable and help Frank's venous return?

4. Frank has an order to bear weight as tolerated, but he requires assistance moving to the recliner in his room. How can the nursing student assist Frank in safe bed-to-chair transfers?

5. Frank has a positive MRSA nasal swab. How can the nursing student help to prevent the transfer of the organism to Frank's wounds?

■ CONCEPT MAP

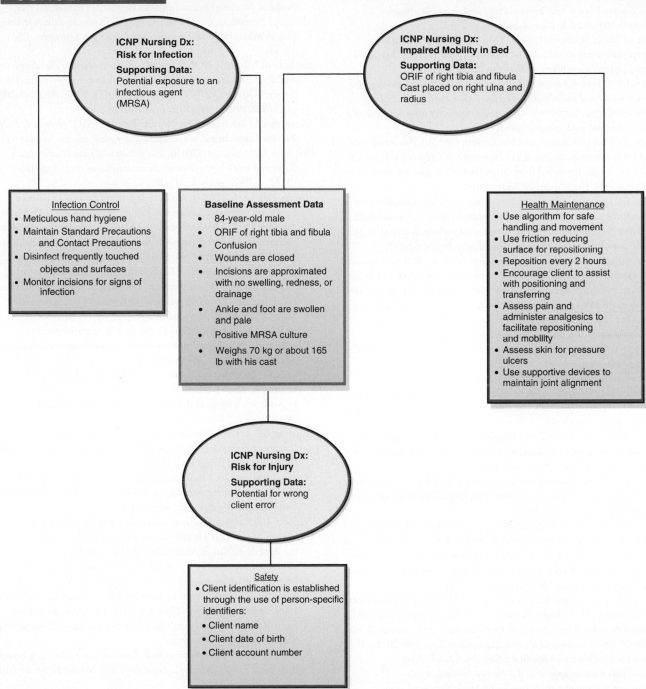

ICNP Nursing Dx:
Risk for Infection

Supporting Data:
Potential exposure to an
infectious agent
(MRSA)

ICNP Nursing Dx:
Impaired Mobility in Bed

Supporting Data:
ORIF of right tibia and fibula
Cast placed on right ulna and
radius

Infection Control
- Meticulous hand hygiene
- Maintain Standard Precautions
  and Contact Precautions
- Disinfect frequently touched
  objects and surfaces
- Monitor incisions for signs of
  infection

Baseline Assessment Data
- 84-year-old male
- ORIF of right tibia and fibula
- Confusion
- Wounds are closed
- Incisions are approximated
  with no swelling, redness, or
  drainage
- Ankle and foot are swollen
  and pale
- Positive MRSA culture
- Weighs 70 kg or about 165
  lb with his cast

Health Maintenance
- Use algorithm for safe
  handling and movement
- Use friction reducing
  surface for repositioning
- Reposition every 2 hours
- Encourage client to assist
  with positioning and
  transferring
- Assess pain and
  administer analgesics to
  facilitate repositioning
  and mobility
- Assess skin for pressure
  ulcers
- Use supportive devices to
  maintain joint alignment

ICNP Nursing Dx:
Risk for Injury

Supporting Data:
Potential for wrong
client error

Safety
- Client identification is established
  through the use of person-specific
  identifiers:
- Client name
- Client date of birth
- Client account number

References

American Nurses Association. (n.d). *Handle with care*. Retrieved from https://www.nursingworld.org/practice-policy/work-environment/health-safety/handle-with-care/.

Bureau of Labor Statistics. (2017). *Injuries, illnesses and fatalities: Frequently asked questions*. Last modified June 9, 2017. Retrieved from https://www.bls.gov/iif/oshfaq1.htm.

Centers for Disease Control and Prevention. (2015a). *Environmental infection control guidelines. Background G. Laundry and bedding*. Retrieved from https://www.cdc.gov/infectioncontrol/guidelines/environmental/background/laundry.html.

Centers for Disease Control and Prevention. (2015b). *Environmental infection control guidelines. I.IV. Treatment and disposal of regulated medical wastes*. Retrieved from https://www.cdc.gov/infectioncontrol/guidelines/environmental/index.html.

Centers for Disease Control and Prevention. (2016a). *Guidelines for disinfection and sterilization in healthcare facilities. Chemical disinfectants*. Retrieved from https://www.cdc.gov/infectioncontrol/guidelines/disinfection/disinfection-methods/chemical.html.

Centers for Disease Control and Prevention. (2016b). *Recommendations for application of standard precautions for the care of all patients in all healthcare settings*. Retrieved from https://www.cdc.gov/infectioncontrol/guidelines/isolation/appendix/standard-precautions.html.

Centers for Disease Control and Prevention. (2018a). *Disinfection in ambulatory care, home care, and the home*. Retrieved from https://www.cdc.gov/infectioncontrol/guidelines/disinfection/healthcare-equipment.html.

Centers for Disease Control and Prevention. (2018b). *Guidelines for disinfection and sterilization in healthcare facilities*. Retrieved from https://www.cdc.gov/infectioncontrol/guidelines/disinfection/healthcare-equipment.html.

Centers for Disease Control and Prevention. (2018c). *Healthcare associated infections: HAI data and statistics*. Retrieved from https://www.cdc.gov/hai/surveillance/index.html.

Centers for Disease Control and Prevention. (2018d). *When and how to perform hand hygiene*. Retrieved from https://www.cdc.gov/handhygiene/providers/index.html.

Centers for Medicare and Medicaid Services. (2008). *Release of report: Freedom from unnecessary physical restraints: Two decades of national progress in nursing home care*. Retrieved from https://www.cms.gov/Medicare/Provider-Enrollment-and-Certification/SurveyCertificationGenInfo/Downloads/SCLetter09-11.pdf.

Centers for Medicare and Medicaid Services. (2015). *Nursing home data compendium 2015 edition*. Retrieved from https://www.cms.gov/Medicare/Provider-Enrollment-and-Certification/CertificationandComplianc/Downloads/nursinghomedatacompendium_508-2015.pdf.

Centers for Medicare and Medicaid Services. (2017). *State operations manual appendix A—Survey protocol, regulations and interpretive guidelines for hospitals*. Retrieved from https://www.cms.gov/Regulations-and-Guidance/Guidance/Manuals/downloads/som107ap_a_hospitals.pdf.

Chang, L., Wang, K. K., & Chao, Y. (2008). Influence of physical restraint on unplanned extubation of adult intensive care patients: A case-control study. *American Journal of Critical Care, 17*(5), 408–416.

Cochran, G. L., Barrett, R. S., & Horn, S. D. (2016). Comparison of medication safety systems in critical access hospital: Combined analysis of two studies. *American Journal of Health-System Pharmacy, 73*, 1167–1173.

Cronenwett, L., Sherwood, G., Barnsteiner, J., Disch, J., Johnson, J., Mitchell, P., ... Warren, J. (2007). Quality and safety education for nurses. *Nursing Outlook, 55*(3), 122–131. Retrieved from http://qsen.org/competencies/pre-licensure-ksas/.

Dresser, M. A. (2017). Hospital workers: An assessment of occupational injuries and illnesses. Monthly Labor Review, U.S. Bureau of Labor Statistics. Retrieved from https://doi.org/10.21916/mlr.2017.17.

Hurlock-Chorostecki, C., & Keilb, C. (2006). Knot-So-Fast: A learning plan to minimize patient restraint in critical care. *Dynamics, 17*(3), 12–18.

Institute of Medicine (IOM). (1999). *To err is human: Building a safer health system*. Retrieved from http://www.iom.edu/~/media/Files/Report%20Files/1999/To-Err-is-Human/To%20Err%20is%20Human%201999%20%20report%20brief.pdf.

International Classification for Nursing Practice. (n.d.). *eHealth & ICNP.* Retrieved from https//www.icn.ch/wht-wedo/projects/eheealth-icnp.

The Joint Commission. (2018). *2018 National patient safety goals*. Retrieved from https://www.jointcommission.org/assets/1/6/2018_HAP_NPSG_goals_final.pdf.

Khanh-Dao Le, L. (2017). *Positioning preterm infants*. [Evidence Summary]. Retrieved from the Joanna Briggs Institute Database.

Khanh-Dao Le, L. (2018). *Restraint: Clinician information*. [Evidence Summary]. Retrieved from the Joanna Briggs Institute EBP Database, BJE@Ovid. JBI3701. Database.

Lapkin, S., Levett-Jones, T., Chenoweth, L., & Johnson, L. (2016). The effectiveness of interventions designed to reduce medication administration errors: A synthesis of findings from systematic reviews. *Journal of Nursing Management, 24*(7), 845–858.

Malusky, S., & Donze, A. (2011). Neutral head positioning in premature infants for intraventricular hemorrhage prevention: An evidence-based review. *Neonatal Network, 30*(6), 381–389.

Minnick, A. F., Mion, L. C., Johnson, M. E., Catrambone, C., & Leipzig, R. (2007). Prevalence and variation of physical restraint use in acute care settings in the US. *Journal of Nursing Scholarship, 39*(1), 30–37.

Mittinty, M. (2018). *Neonates: Mechanical ventilation (positioning)*. [Evidence Summary]. Retrieved from the Joanna Briggs Institute EBP Database, JBI@Obic. JBI971.

National Institute for Occupational Safety and Health (NIOSH). (2017). *Safe patient handling and mobility*. Retrieved from https://www.cdc.gov/niosh/topics/safepatient/.

National Institute for Occupational Safety and Health (NIOSH), & Veterans Health Administration (VHA), and the American Nurses Association (ANA). (2009). *Safe patient handling training for schools of nursing*. Retrieved from http://www.cdc.gov/niosh/docs/2009-127/pdfs/2009-127.pdf.

Nightingale, F. (1860). *Notes on nursing: What it is and what it is not*. [First American edition]. New York, NY: D. Appleton & Company. Retrieved from http://digital.library.upenn.edu/women/nightingale/nursing/nursing.html.

Patient not restrained, falls from bed: Lawsuit against nursing home dismissed. (2009, January). *Legal Eagle Eye Newsletter for the Nursing Profession 17*(1), 7.

Salmon, N., & Di Leonardi, B. C. (2013). *Restraints: The last resort*. RN.com. Retrieved from https://lms.rn.com/getpdf.php/1897.pdf.

Siegel, J. D., Rhinehart, E., Jackson, M., Chiarello, L., & the Healthcare Infection Control Practices Advisory Committee. (2019). *2007 Guideline for isolation precautions: Preventing transmission of infectious agents in healthcare settings*. Retrieved from https://www.cdc.gov/infectioncontrol/pdf/guidelines/isolation-guidelines-H.pdf.

World Health Organization. (2009). *WHO guidelines on hand hygiene in healthcare*. Retrieved from http://whqlibdoc.who.int/publications/2009/9789241597906_eng.pdf.

Yi, S. (2011). Duct tape cuts time and costs related to contact precautions. *Medscape Medical News*. Retrieved from http://www.medscape.com/viewarticle/745502.

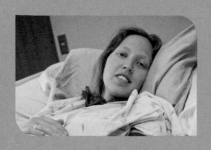

CHAPTER 2
Personal Care and Hygiene

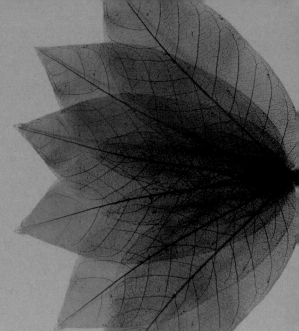

"For cleanliness of body was ever esteemed to proceed from a due reverence to God, to society, and to ourselves."

Francis Bacon, Creator of the Scientific Method (1562-1626)

LEARNING OBJECTIVES

By the end of this chapter, the reader will be able to:

1 Discuss the effect of personal care and hygiene on a client's physical health and sense of well-being.
2 Assist an ambulatory client with bathing.
3 Change the gown for a client who has an IV line.
4 Bathe an adult client in bed.
5 Provide foot care.
6 Provide nail care to the hands and feet.
7 Bathe and diaper an infant.
8 Provide oropharyngeal suctioning.
9 Provide oral hygiene for a conscious client, including brushing and flossing teeth.
10 Provide oral hygiene for an unconscious client.
11 Remove, clean, and insert a client's dentures.
12 Shampoo a nonambulatory client's hair.

13 Shave a client.
14 Discuss the care for a client with lice.
15 Provide eye care for an unconscious client.
16 Remove and clean contact lens.
17 Remove and clean an artificial eye.
18 Assist a client using a bedside commode.
19 Assist a client using a urinal.
20 Assist a client using a bedpan.
21 Apply a condom catheter.
22 Demonstrate mitering a bedsheet corner.
23 Demonstrate changing a pillowcase.
24 Make an occupied bed, make an unoccupied bed, and prepare a surgical bed.

TERMINOLOGY

Abrasion An injury to the top layer of skin or mucous membrane.
Blanching Whitening of the skin.
Decubitus A pressure injury or bedsore.
Dermis Layer of skin below the epidermis layer.
Diaphoresis Sweating.
Epidermis The outermost layer of skin.
Erythema Redness of the skin.
Fan fold Pleated fold used during bed making; sometimes called an accordion fold.
Hygiene An activity conducive to preserve health.
Iatrogenic Resulting from the medical treatment.
Ischemia Diminished blood flow.
Maceration Softening of the skin by soaking in a liquid.
Mitered corners The angled folds made when tucking sheets at the corners of a bed.
Mucosa Mucous membranes lining the nose and mouth.
Necrosis Cellular death.

Nosocomial Acquired during an acute-care hospital stay; an older term.
Pediculosis An infestation of lice.
Perineal Relating to the area between the rectum and the reproductive organs; also used more generally to describe the portion of the body between the legs, including the urogenital passages and the rectum.
Prosthesis/prosthetic An artificial body part, such as an artificial eye.
Purpura Discolored reddish-purple area.
Shearing The distortion of body tissue that may result in injury and occurs when force is applied in opposite but parallel directions, such as sliding skin and subcutaneous tissue away from the musculature beneath.

ACRONYMS

IV Intravenous
MRSA Methicillin-resistant *Staphylococcus aureus*

Personal care and hygiene were emphasized in early nursing history. Even before an understanding of germ theory, Florence Nightingale noted that cleanliness is an effective means of promoting health. In her book *Notes on Nursing*, Nightingale writes, "It cannot be necessary to tell a nurse that she should be clean, or that her patient should be clean seeing that the greater part of nursing consists of preserving cleanliness" (Nightingale, 1860).

Today, cleanliness and infection control continue to be of concern as healthcare facilities face new challenges. The prevalence of infections with antibiotic-resistant organisms, such as methicillin-resistant *Staphylococcus aureus* (MRSA), and of healthcare-associated infections has prompted nurses and nursing researchers to reexamine the role of hygiene protocols in decreasing such infections. Therefore, infection control is a critical concept that applies to personal care and hygiene. The purpose of infection control related to personal hygiene is twofold. The first is to prevent the transfer of microorganisms from one area to another, for example, by wiping front to back on the female perineum. The second aspect of infection control related to personal hygiene is to prevent an overgrowth of microorganisms, for example, by brushing teeth.

Client-centered care is a concept that is central to personal care and hygiene. Maintaining the cleanliness of a client and the client's immediate environment reflects respect for that client. Facilities and individual healthcare providers create an atmosphere of concern and value when they rigorously maintain personal and environmental cleanliness. In fact, healthcare consumers may select their healthcare facility based on this value of cleanliness. Allowing clients control over their personal hygiene choices is another means of demonstrating respect for the client. Several of the personal care skills within this chapter, such as hair care, have many possible variations based on preferences or culture. Honoring cultural and personal preferences, as well as promoting autonomy, are desirable when providing nursing care in most of these skills.

Providing privacy is another way to show respect for the client. Maintaining privacy when providing personal care and assistance with hygiene is an essential aspect of client-centered care. Privacy is best achieved by creating concentric rings or layers of privacy, starting with the client and continuing out into the room (Fig. 2.1). Keeping the client covered and unexposed provides the first layer of privacy. Using a room divider and/or pulling shut the client's privacy curtain creates the next layer of privacy. Another layer of privacy is completed by closing the door, and still another layer is completed by placing signage on the door to indicate the need for privacy.

Health maintenance is another critical concept that applies to many personal care and hygiene skills. Nursing promotes the health of the whole body. The condition of the skin, hair, and nails often indicates the health status of the entire person. Maintaining the hygiene of one part of the body can have a profound effect on the client's general health. For example, providing oral care and maintaining a healthy mouth can prevent pneumonia and systemic infection. Nursing also teaches and encourages clients to manage

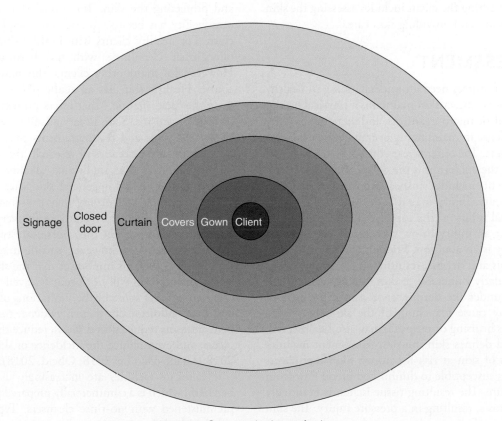

FIG. 2.1 Concentric rings of privacy.

their own hygiene whenever possible with health maintenance behaviors such as washing their face or brushing their teeth. The term *health maintenance* in this chapter refers to both promoting the client's abilities to provide self-care and maintaining the physical health of the person or a specific body part, such as the skin.

Personal care and hygiene are foundations of nursing care; however, these activities are sometimes delegated to assitive personnel. Effective delegation includes clear communication of the critical concepts and nursing interventions to assistants as well as communication back to the registered nurse from the assistants about the physical findings and the client's response to the activity. The registered nurse is always responsible for the client assessment and supervises the outcomes of delegated tasks. In this chapter, many of the variables that affect the accuracy of the skill are related to the assessment of the client. Delegation requires the use of verbal and written communication to ensure the clear transmission of information between members of the healthcare team.

SECTION 1 Bathing a Client

Personal hygiene offers several benefits to the client: an enhanced sense of well-being, cleanliness, and skin care. Each of us recognizes that a bath, shampooed hair, and clean teeth help us feel better. Clients consistently report that they, too, feel better when clean. Bathing provides a refreshed and comforted feeling. Bathing washes away perspiration, body oils, dirt, and odors, as well as microorganisms (Khanh-Dao Le, 2018). One goal of bathing, hair care, oral care, and perineal care is to prevent an overgrowth of microorganisms, whether bacterial, viral, or fungal. Clients who take antibiotics are particularly susceptible to an iatrogenic infection from opportunistic organisms. In addition to providing comfort and cleanliness, bathing the client includes assessing the skin for damage or injury and providing skin care.

SKIN ASSESSMENT

To assess the skin, nurses need an understanding of healthy skin and skin injury. Intact skin maintains a physical barrier against opportunistic microorganisms, and therefore, healthy skin is a vital defense in maintaining overall health. The skin is made up of layers. The outer layer is the epidermis, and the next layer below the epidermis is the dermis (Fig. 2.2).

Skin assessment includes inspecting for possible and potential skin injury. Injury may manifest in several forms, including external injury to the top layer of skin, an injury to the dermis, or an injury below the dermis. An example of external injury is an abrasion. Friction and shearing may tear the epidermis and dermis, resulting in skin tears. Older adults are particularly vulnerable to skin tears (Obeid, 2018). Signs of injury under the dermis, such as the presence of fluid, which may cause blanching of the skin, or pooled blood that causes bruising or purpura, may also be observed. Box 2.1 lists and defines skin injuries. Assessment includes identifying areas of skin at risk for injury. Skin that covers pressure points is susceptible to diminished blood flow from unrelieved pressure. The resulting tissue ischemia eventually may lead to necrosis, resulting in a pressure injury. The skin under a therapeutic device, such as a nasal cannula, is at risk for breakdown, and skin that remains moist, such as in skinfolds or the perianal area, is at risk for moisture-associated skin damage. Many facilities use a standardized risk assessment tool (e.g., the Braden Scale) to assess the risk of skin breakdown. The Braden Scale identifies risk in six categories: sensory perception, moisture, activity, mobility, nutrition, and friction and shear.

SKIN CARE

The goal of skin care is the protection of vulnerable skin, the prevention of skin breakdown, and the restoration of skin integrity. Caring for skin includes cleansing, moisturizing, and protecting the skin. Traditional skin care in a healthcare facility has been soap and water applied with a washcloth. For healthy clients with healthy skin, this technique offers basic cleanliness with few harmful consequences. However, for many other clients, this may not be the best course. Healthy skin has an acidic pH, sometimes referred to as the "acid mantle," that offers protection from opportunistic organisms. Soap is very alkaline, which changes the pH of the skin, and has ingredients that can be irritating to the skin. After decades of research, the best-practice recommendation is that traditional alkaline soap and water should not be used for general skin care (Craven, 2018). Vigorous wiping and drying may cause shearing and tearing in delicate skin, particularly in the very young and old populations. To prevent this, nurses are typically taught to pat delicate skin dry; however, patting may not thoroughly dry the skin, and it is important that the skin be fully dried so that maceration will not occur (Craven, 2018). No-rinse cleansers address some of the limitations of traditional soap and water. Additionally, there is evidence that no-rinse emollient cleansers reduce skin dryness, reduce the risk of pressure ulcers, and even reduce the incidence of skin tears (Haesler, 2018; Khanh-Dao Le, 2018; Obeid, 2018).

Healthcare facilities are increasingly using a disposable bed bath, which is a commercially prepared package of cloths premoistened with no-rinse cleansers. Typically, a disposable bed bath has 8 to 10 cloths moistened with a no-rinse

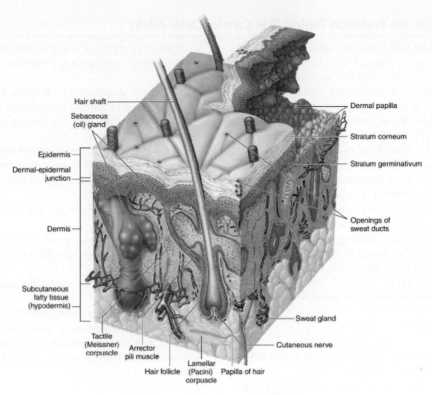

Hair shaft
Sebaceous (oil) gland
Epidermis
Dermal-epidermal junction
Dermis
Subcutaneous fatty tissue (hypodermis)
Tactile (Meissner) corpuscle
Arrector pili muscle
Hair follicle
Lamellar (Pacini) corpuscle
Papilla of hair
Dermal papilla
Stratum corneum
Stratum germinativum
Openings of sweat ducts
Sweat gland
Cutaneous nerve

FIG. 2.2 Cross section of skin and underlying structures.

BOX 2.1 Skin Injuries

- Abrasion: An injury to the top layer of skin or mucous membrane; a scrape or scratch.
- Blanching: Whitening of the skin.
- Erythema: Redness of the skin.
- Ischemia: Diminished blood flow to the skin; may result in discoloration, mottling, or cyanosis.
- Moisture-associated skin damage (MASD): Skin erosion or inflammation caused by prolonged exposure to moisture.
- Necrosis: Cellular death of the skin; may result in black discoloration and eventually decay, causing a sore.
- Skin tear: Traumatic wound that occurs principally on the extremities of older adults, caused by friction or shearing forces that separate the epidermis or both the epidermis and dermis from underlying structures.
- Shearing: The distortion of body tissue that occurs when force is applied in opposite but parallel directions, such as sliding skin and subcutaneous tissue away from the musculature beneath.

cleanser that may also contain aloe, moisturizers, or vitamin E. Packages may be warmed in a designated microwave or stored in a warming device. One package provides a full-body cleansing; one cloth is used to wipe each body part and then is discarded. Although clients may not be familiar with the product, disposable bed baths are effective in terms of time and cost, and they prevent the possibility of bacterial colonization in bath basins. Since a landmark systematic review of the existing literature in 2007 (Hodgkinson, Nay,

& Wilson, 2007), evidence continues to support the finding that no rinse cleansers are preferred to soap and water for older clients (Khanh-Dao Le, 2018). For more information on skin care recommendations, see Box 2.2.

In addition to cleansing the skin, moisturizing the skin helps to maintain the moisture in the outer layers of the skin and mitigates problems with dryness and loss of skin integrity. Moisturizers can be ointments, creams, or lotions. To maintain skin hydration, apply moisturizers at least twice a day and immediately after bathing. Apply moisturizers directly to the skin and gently rub downward in the direction of hair growth to prevent blockage of the hair follicles (Wounds UK, 2012).

Barrier products differ from cleansers and moisturizers in that they create a thin film over the surface of the skin and protect the skin from irritants. Traditional skin barriers include standard zinc-oxide pastes and petroleum jelly. Newer products include those with a water-repellent silicone-based ingredient to form a protective film and those that contain a bioadhesive to adhere to damaged skin (Bradbury, Price, Gaffing, & Yoro, 2017). Although they are expensive, there are also products that cleanse, moisturize, and provide a skin barrier. Currently, nursing research studies are examining skin-care protocols to determine optimal methods of maintaining skin integrity.

BATHING AN ADULT

Methods for bathing an ambulatory adult client are varied and depend on what is available in the facility. Possible methods may include a tub bath, showering while standing,

BOX 2.2 Lessons From the Evidence: Topical Skin Care for Older Adults

The Joanna Briggs Institute (JBI) is an international not-for-profit research and development organization. It is located within the Faculty of Health Sciences at the University of Adelaide, Australia, and collaborates internationally with over 70 other entities that have agreed on definitions of evidence, methodologies, and methods regarding the synthesis of nursing evidence. The JBI promotes and supports the synthesis, transfer, and utilization of evidence through identifying feasible, appropriate, meaningful, and effective healthcare practices. The JBI is involved in the development and dissemination of a number of publications that inform health professionals about clinical practice and specifically what constitutes best practice in healthcare. JBI regularly publishes Evidence Summaries fulfilling the role of translation of research evidence into practice.

In 2018, the JBI published Evidence Summaries on several topics related to skin care:
- Skin care to reduce the incidence of pressure ulcers (Haesler, 2018)
- Skin tears (Obeid, 2018)
- Skin cleansing in older adults (Craven, 2018)
  Systematic reviews of the evidence have led to the following best-practice recommendations for skin care:
- The use of traditional alkaline soaps is not recommended for general skin care.

- A no-rinse cleanser is better than soap and water for cleaning skin to prevent incontinence-associated dermatitis.
- The use of disposable bath wipes and nondetergent, non-rinse-off cleanser reduces the risk of dry skin and reduces skin-tear incidence compared with standard soap and water.
- Use warm water rather than hot water for bathing to decrease the risk of dehydrating the skin.
- Apply hypoallergenic moisturizers or emollients to keep the skin hydrated.
- Ensure adequate nutrition and hydration to prevent fragile, dry skin.
- Avoid using adhesive products on fragile skin.
- Avoid skin massage in order to decrease the risk of skin damage.
- Protect the skin from moisture, such as urine, to prevent skin damage.
  A commonsense skin regimen that takes into account the personal preferences of the client and combines the best practice recommendations on cleaning, moisturizing, and protection from moisture promotes the best clinical outcomes.

References: Craven, 2018; Haesler, 2018; Obeid, 2018.

showering while sitting in a shower chair, a partial bath at a sink, and a complete or partial bed bath. The appropriate type of bath may depend on the client's condition but may also vary from day to day. For example, a client may have an assisted shower one day but only a partial bath while seated near the sink the next day.

Nurses and clients should collaboratively determine the best choice considering the client's ability to provide self-care, condition, preferences, and usual practices. Considerations affecting the ability to provide self-care include activity intolerance, cognitive function, musculoskeletal function, and level of discomfort. In addition, the client's condition may dictate the bathing method. For instance, if there is debris on the skin, a shower would be preferable to a bath because a shower rinses away debris, whereas a tub bath does not.

Hands and feet warrant additional attention. A client's hands require cleaning to prevent them from transferring microorganisms. Assess the client's hands, and determine what activities the client is performing. Provide the client with frequent access to hand hygiene, especially if the client assisting with his or her own toileting needs and before meals. Additionally, bathing the feet may offer physiologic benefits (Box 2.3).

When bathing an adult client on bedrest, the degree to which the client is able to assist with the bath will vary. If a client is unconscious or sedated and unable to assist in any way, it is preferable to have two nurses perform the bath, one on each side of the bed. If only one nurse is available and the client cannot assist, the nurse should move from one side of the bed to the other to prevent poor body mechanics and

potential harm. Other clients, however, may have an order for bedrest but still be able to wash their own face and hands, as well as lift their arms and legs to assist with the bath. In such cases, the nurse may stay on one side of the bed and bathe the farther arm and leg before the nearer extremities. Because the nurse is not supporting the weight of the extremity, there is less potential for harm from poor body mechanics.

The order of the bath is given from cleanest area to dirtiest area, usually starting with the face, followed by the extremities, and finishing with the torso. As discussed previously, a no-rinse cleanser is preferable to soap; however, if soap is used, it should be used sparingly and rinsed thoroughly. If a washcloth becomes soiled, obtain a fresh washcloth. Change the water in the basin whenever it becomes cold or dirty. The water is usually changed after washing the axilla and under the breasts and is always changed after cleaning the genitalia. The skin must be thoroughly dried after bathing to prevent maceration. If the assessment of the skin indicates dry skin, apply a moisturizer. If areas of skin need protection, apply a skin barrier.

BATHING AN INFANT

Although the critical concepts remain the same, the skill of bathing an infant differs from the skill of bathing an adult (Box 2.4). Nurses bathe sick, hospitalized infants and healthy newborns and are responsible for teaching new parents how to bathe an infant at home. Although procedures may differ slightly for these different types of infant baths, the three desired outcomes remain the same.

BOX 2.3 Lessons From the Evidence: Effects of Foot Bathing (a.k.a., Why Do We Love a Pedicure?)

There have been almost two decades of international research studies on the physiological effects of foot bathing. It is a noninvasive, low-cost, low-risk complementary therapy that has been shown to improve sleep in poor sleepers and provide comfort and relaxation after surgery. Foot bathing has been known to be relaxing and is now thought to decrease the sympathetic activity and increase the parasympathetic activity of the nervous system. The following research studies examined the effects of foot bathing:

- Aydin et al. (2016) examined the effect of foot-bathing therapy on heart-rate variability (HRV) parameters in a healthy population. The results were that almost all HRV parameters increased, and heart (pulse) rate and low-frequency/high-frequency activity decreased, after foot-bathing therapy compared with before foot-bathing therapy. The researchers concluded that foot bathing might induce a state of balance between the sympathetic and parasympathetic systems and might be helpful to prevent possible cardiac arrhythmias.
- Cal, Cakiroglu, Kurt, Hartiningsih, and Suryani (2016) examined vital signs and pain scores in mothers after cesarean section to measure the impact of hand- and feet-bathing therapy. The results demonstrated a statistically significant decrease in pain score, systolic and diastolic blood pressure, heart rate, and respiratory rate. The conclusion was that hand and foot bathing is a complementary therapy to decrease anxiety and stress.
- Kim, Lee, and Sohng (2016) examined the effects of foot-bathing therapy using two different water temperatures on the quality of sleep of older adults living in nurs-

ing homes. The results demonstrated improved sleep, especially for the poor sleepers; found 40°C to be a more effective temperature; and determined that sleep benefits waned after 3 weeks.
- Liao et al. (2013) explored warm foot baths as a means to enhance sleep in older adults. The findings demonstrated increased foot temperatures and distal–proximal skin temperature gradients but not a change in perceived quality of sleep after a footbath of 40°C water temperature for 20 minutes.
- Yamamoto, Aso, Nagata, Kasugai, and Maeda (2008) demonstrated increased relaxation, as measured by a significant increase in parasympathetic activity and a significant decrease in sympathetic activity, following a warm wrapped foot bath.
- Saeki, Nagai, and Hishinuma (2007) demonstrated both increased parasympathetic and decreased sympathetic activity and enhanced immune function as measured by significant increases in white blood cell (WBC) count and natural killer (NK) cell cytotoxicity following footbaths at 42°C for 10 minutes.
- Liao, Chiu, and Landis (2008) examined the effect of a 40-minute foot bath at 41°C on sleep, and the results showed that the amount of wakefulness was decreased in the second non–rapid eye movement (NREM) period on the night of the foot bath.

In summary, preliminary findings suggest that foot bathing may be an easily implemented intervention to improve cardiovascular and immune function and promote relaxation and sleep.

First and most importantly, during the bath, the infant should not be cold stressed, a precursor to hypothermia. The combination of water and exposed skin increases heat loss through evaporation, conduction, and radiation. Infants are much more susceptible to heat loss than are adults; cold stress can initiate a physiological cascade of events that includes hypoglycemia and acidosis. A newborn's first bath may be safely given when the newborn has an axillary temperature of 98.2°F (36.9°C) or higher (Lund & Durand, 2016).

The second desired outcome is that the infant not be physiologically or emotionally stressed by the bath. Critically ill infants are cleaned as needed and may not tolerate a full bath. Although healthy infants are physiologically stable, they can become emotionally stressed and cold stressed by a bath. Parents of newborns should be counseled that it is more important for their infant to stay calm and learn to enjoy a bath than to scrub every inch of their new baby. To that end, immersion bathing is recommended for infants, even for newborns and preterm infants. Immersion bathing is placing an infant into warm water (38°C) with only the head and neck above the water (Lund & Durand, 2016). Bathing is recommended no more than every other day. The third and final desired outcome is that the infant is cleaner than before the bath.

An infant's skin is thin, delicate, and susceptible to a variety of rashes, such as diaper rash and prickly heat. Maintaining the acidity of an infant's skin supports the acid mantle that helps to protect the infant from skin infections. Any cleansing product used on an infant should be pH neutral or slightly acidic so as to not disrupt the acid mantle. Protecting an infant's skin from urine and stool is also a priority.

APPLICATION OF THE NURSING PROCESS

Examples of Related International Classification for Nursing Practice (ICNP) Nursing Diagnoses, Expected Client Outcomes, and Nursing Interventions:

Nursing Diagnosis: Self-care deficit, impaired ability to perform hygiene

Expected Client Outcome: Client will participate in own personal cleanliness and hygiene to the extent possible without changes in vital signs or pain level.

Nursing Intervention Example: Allow the client to bathe independently, washing all areas within the client's reach.

Reference: International Classification for Nursing Practice. (n.d.). *eHealth & ICNP*. Retrieved from https://www.icn.ch/what-we-do/projects/ehealth-icnp.

BOX 2.4 Lifespan Considerations: Neonatal Considerations for Bathing

The Association of Women's Health, Obstetric and Neonatal Nurses (AWHONN) recommends the following in its evidence-based reference book *Neonatal Skin Care: Evidence-Based Clinical Practice Guidelines* (2018):

- Bathe neonates every few days with warm tap water; if the infant is greater than 32 weeks' gestation, mild, pH-neutral cleansers can be used.
- Preterm infants can be safely bathed every 4 days without increasing the risk of infection.
- Immersion bathing is the most relaxing method for stable preterm infants and normal newborns.
- Immersion bathing is beneficial as a newborn's first bath.
- Tub baths are not contraindicated for normal newborns or stable preterm infants with umbilical cords because there is no increase in the infection rate or healing time.
- After bathing, provide opportunities for infant recovery, including skin-to-skin contact, swaddling, and dressing in clothing.
- Products with chlorhexidine gluconate should be used with caution on infants less than 2 months of age.
- If chlorhexidine gluconate is used prior to a procedure, it should be washed off with sterile water or saline after the procedure.
- Leave the umbilical cord open to dry without antimicrobial topical agents.

Reference: Association of Women's Health, Obstetric and Neonatal Nurses, 2018.

CRITICAL CONCEPTS
Bathing the Client

Accuracy (ACC)

Bathing the client is subject to the following variables:
- assessment of the client, including mobility, level of discomfort, cooperation, and activity intolerance, and monitoring output
- identification of anatomical landmarks

- identification of accurate musculoskeletal movement
- understanding of procedure by client and family.

Client-Centered Care (CCC)

When bathing, respect for the client is demonstrated through:
- promoting autonomy
- providing privacy
- ensuring comfort
- honoring cultural preferences
- arranging for an interpreter, as needed
- advocating for the client and family.

Infection Control (INF)

When bathing the client, healthcare-associated and client infection is prevented by:
- containment of microorganisms
- preventing and reducing the transfer of microorganisms
- reducing the number of microorganisms.

Safety (SAF)

When bathing the client, safety measures prevent harm and maintain a safe care environment.

Communication (COM)

- Communication exchanges information (oral, written, nonverbal or electronic) between two or more people.
- Collaboration with the client and other healthcare providers is essential when bathing the client to maintain client autonomy and implement a plan of skin care.
- Documentation records information in a permanent legal record.

Health Maintenance (HLTH)

Nursing is dedicated to the promotion of health and abilities related to personal hygiene.

Evaluation (EVAL)

When bathing the client, evaluation of outcomes enables the nurse to determine the efficacy of the care provided.

■ SKILL 2.1 Assisting an Ambulatory Client With Bathing

EQUIPMENT

Washcloth or disposable wipes
Two towels
Clean gown, robe, and nonskid slippers
Clean gloves
Cleanser or soap
Moisturizer
Safe handling equipment, as needed
Linen hamper
Personal items: deodorant, toothbrush and toothpaste, moisturizers, powder, and so forth

BEGINNING THE SKILL

1. **INF** Perform hand hygiene.
2. **INF** Apply gloves.
3. **CCC** Introduce yourself to the client and family and explain the procedure.
4. **SAF** Identify the client using two identifiers.
5. **SAF** Determine if the client has any pertinent allergies.
6. **CCC** Provide privacy; close the door and pull the curtain.

PROCEDURE

7. **ACC** Assess the client's degree of mobility, discomfort, cooperation, and recent activity intolerance. *Your assessment is to determine the extent to which the client can provide independent self-care or assist with the bath.*

8. **SAF** Assess the safe client-handling needs, such as a hoist or wheelchair. *Your assessment is to determine the appropriate safe handling equipment.*

9. **CCC** Assess the preferences of the client, including type of bath, such as shower or bed bath; time of day for the bath; and choice of skin care products.

10. **CCC** Assess for hearing aids, glasses, or watches to be removed before the bath.

11. **SAF** Assist the client with transfer if equipment is needed, and transport the client and equipment to the bath or shower room. See "Moving Clients Safely" in Chapter 1.

12. **SAF** Ensure fall-prevention safety measures are in place: antiskid matt, shower chair.

13. **COM** Instruct the client to use safety measures, and show the client the location of the emergency call system.

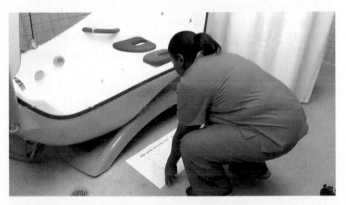

STEP 12 Ensure safety measures are in place.

14. **CCC** Ensure privacy by closing the door and placing signage on the door to identify the bathroom as occupied.

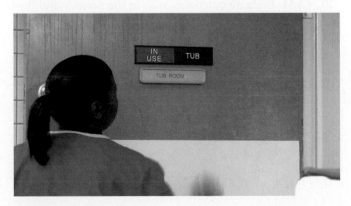

STEP 14 Ensure privacy.

15. **CCC** Assist the client to remove his or her gown, and keep the client covered with a bath blanket for privacy and warmth.

16. **SAF** Assist the client into the shower or tub. If the client is competent to bathe alone, tell the client when you will return.

17. If you will remain with the client and assist with the bath:
    a. **CCC** Keep the client covered with the gown or bath blanket until the water is running in a shower or the client is submerged in a tub.
    b. **HLTH** Allow the client to bathe independently, washing all areas within the client's reach.
    c. **CCC** Assist the client with any areas not within reach, for example, the back or lower extremities.

18. **SAF** Assist the client out of the tub or shower.

19. **HLTH** Use the opportunity to inspect the skin, especially any bony prominences.

20. **HLTH** Assess the skin-care needs of the client, such as the need for a moisturizer or a barrier cream.

21. **CCC** Assist the client to dry thoroughly and put on a clean gown, robe, and slippers.

22. **CCC** Gather all personal items belonging to the client.

23. **SAF** Transport client back to the room and assist the client in transferring into the bed or a chair.

FINISHING THE SKILL

24. **CCC** Provide comfort. Assist the client with positioning and rearranging the bedding.

25. **SAF** Ensure client safety. Place the bed in the lowest position. Verify that the client can identify and reach the nurse call system. *These safety measures reduce the risk of falls.*

26. **INF** Return to the bath/shower room and clean and disinfect the area.

27. **COM** Change the signage on the door to unoccupied.

28. **INF** Remove gloves and perform hand hygiene.

29. **EVAL** Evaluate outcomes, such as the extent to which the client required assistance with the bath and the use of assistive handling equipment.

30. **COM** Document skin assessment findings, care given, and client outcomes in the legal healthcare record.

■ SKILL 2.2 Changing the Gown of a Client With an IV Line

EQUIPMENT

Clean gown
Clean gloves

BEGINNING THE SKILL

1. **INF** Perform hand hygiene.
2. **INF** Apply gloves.
3. **CCC** Introduce yourself to the client and family and explain the procedure.
4. **SAF** Identify the client using two identifiers.
5. **CCC** Provide privacy; close the door and pull the curtain.

PROCEDURE

6. **CCC** Untie the soiled gown and remove the gown from the client's arm with the IV line. Maintain the client's privacy by keeping the soiled gown covering the client.
7. **SAF** Remove the IV bag from the IV pole. If the IV line is on a pump, clamp the tubing and remove the tubing from the pump.
8. **ACC** Thread the bag through the soiled gown sleeve from the end of the sleeve toward the neck of the gown.

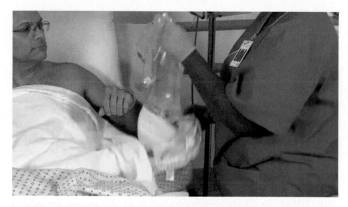

STEP 8 Thread the IV bag through the gown sleeve.

9. **ACC** Pick up the clean gown and thread the IV bag through the sleeve of the gown, as you would put on the gown.
10. **CCC** Cover the client loosely with the clean gown to provide privacy before removing the soiled gown.
11. **INF** Remove the soiled gown from the remaining arm and pull the soiled gown out from under the clean gown. Make a bundle of the soiled gown, and avoid allowing the soiled gown to touch clean items or your own clothing.
12. **INF** Place the soiled gown directly into the linen hamper. Do not place the soiled gown on a chair or on the floor, and do not allow the soiled linens to touch your own clothing.

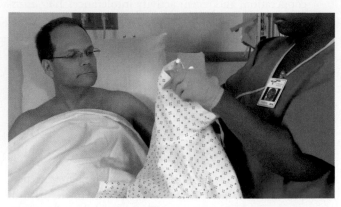

STEP 9 Thread the IV bag through the clean gown sleeve.

13. **ACC** Instruct the client to put his or her arm through the first sleeve of the clean gown, then the second sleeve of the clean gown.
14. Adjust and fasten the clean gown.
15. **SAF** Re-hang the IV bag on the IV pole. If the IV is on a pump, replace the tubing within the pump and unclamp the tubing.
16. **EVAL** Evaluate the patency of the system and the connections. Take the opportunity to assess the IV insertion site.

FINISHING THE SKILL

17. **INF** Remove gloves and perform hand hygiene.
18. **CCC** Provide comfort. Assist the client with positioning and rearranging the bedding.
19. **SAF** Ensure client safety. Ensure that the bed is in the lowest position. Verify that the client can identify and reach the nurse call system. *These safety measures reduce the risk of falls.*
20. **EVAL** Evaluate outcomes, such as the patency and flow of the IV line.
21. **COM** Document assessment findings, care given, and outcomes in the legal healthcare record.

■ SKILL 2.3 Bathing an Adult Client in Bed

EQUIPMENT

Prepackaged bath cloths

Moisturizer

Personal items: deodorant, moisturizers, and powder

Clean gown

Disposable wipes or washcloth, two towels, cleanser or soap, and basin, if prepackaged bath cloths are not available

Clean gloves, if there is a risk of exposure to body fluids

Linen hamper

Safe handling equipment, as needed

BEGINNING THE SKILL

1. **INF** Perform hand hygiene.
2. **INF** Apply gloves if there is a risk of exposure to body fluids.
3. **CCC** Introduce yourself to the client and family and explain the procedure.
4. **SAF** Identify the client using two identifiers.
5. **SAF** Determine if the client has any pertinent allergies.
6. **CCC** Provide privacy; close the door and pull the curtain.

PROCEDURE

7. **SAF** Set up an ergonomically safe space. Raise the bed to a comfortable working height. Raise one side rail. *Setting up an ergonomically safe space prevents injury to the nurse and client.*
8. **ACC** Assess the client's degree of mobility in bed, discomfort, cooperation, and recent activity intolerance. *Your assessment is to determine the extent to which the client can assist with the bath and the client's ability to tolerate the turning and handling associated with bathing.*
9. **SAF** Assess the safe client handling needs, such as a hoist or sliding sheets. Obtain any identified safe handling equipment. *Your assessment is to determine the appropriate safe handling equipment.*
10. **CCC** Assess the preferences of the client, including the timing of the bath and the use of skin-care products.
11. **INF** Place clean gown, linens, and skin-care products on a clean surface.
12. Prepare a clean work surface, such as the over-the-bedside table.
13. **CCC** Warm prepackaged bath cloths and/or fill the basin with warm water.

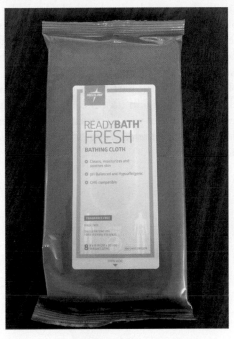

STEP 14 Warmed prepackaged bath cloths.

14. **SAF** Assess the client's medical equipment to determine the risk of electrical shock.
15. **SAF** Adjust all medical lines to ensure sufficient slack to roll the client.
16. **CCC** Assess for hearing aids, glasses, contact lens, or watches that should be removed before the bath.
17. **INF** Fold bedspread and/or blankets from the edges toward the center of the bed if they are to be placed back on the made bed. Remove them and place them on a clean surface. *Clean only touches clean.*
18. **CCC** Keep the client covered with a bath blanket, removing the top sheet. *Covering the client provides privacy and prevents chilling.*
19. Remove the client's gown. If the client has an IV line, follow Skill 2.2, steps 6 to 16.

Face

20. **CCC** Place a towel over the client's chest. *A towel will provide warmth and privacy and catch any drips while wiping the face.*
21. **HLTH** Determine whether the client is able to wash the face independently. If so, encourage the client to do this. *Nursing encourages clients to maintain their own health behaviors.*
22. **CCC** Determine whether the client prefers a prepackaged bath cloth or a washcloth wet with warm water. Provide the client the with an appropriate face cloth. If you will be washing the client's face using a washcloth, make a washcloth mitt.

Making a washcloth mitt:

a. Lay the washcloth on a clean surface.

b. Place your dominant hand palm up on the washcloth with the bottom edge level with the knuckles.

c. Fold the right edge of the washcloth to the center; fold the left edge of the washcloth to the center. The washcloth should now be folded in thirds with the fingers inside.

d. Fold the uppermost part of the cloth down toward the palm of the hand and tuck the edge under the cloth to create a multilayer wiping surface. *The mitt retains heat and water better than a single layer and does not drip as much.*

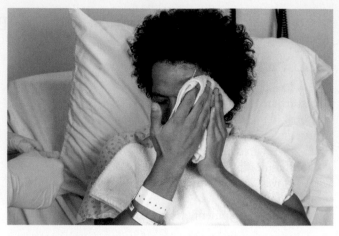

STEP 22 Encourage the client to wash his or her face.

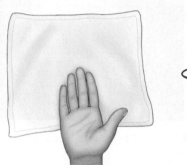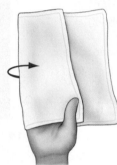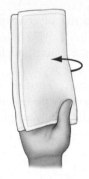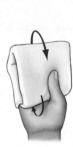

STEP 17C Fold the washcloth into thirds and tuck in the end.

e. Two wash mitts are easier to use, one that is lightly soaped and one for rinsing. By using two, time is not spent rinsing all the cleanser or soap out of one of the washcloths.

23. **INF** Using water only, wipe one eye in one direction from the nose to the ear. *This cleans substances away from the opening of the lacrimal duct.* Use a different section of the cloth for the other eye. *A different section prevents cross-contamination of eye organisms.*

24. **INF** With or without soap/cleanser, according to client preference, gently wash the forehead, cheeks, nose, around the mouth, and neck. Gently clean the outside of the ears.

25. **HLTH** If soap is used, use the second washcloth to rinse all soap residue from the face.

26. **HLTH** Dry gently and thoroughly.

27. **HLTH** Return glasses and hearing aids as appropriate.

Hands

28. **HLTH** Determine whether the client can wash the hands independently. If so, encourage the client to do this. Hands may be placed in the wash basin to soak. *Nursing encourages clients to maintain their own health behaviors.*

29. **INF** Wash the hands and rinse in the basin. Nail care may be given now or after the bath is completed (see Skill 2.6, Providing Nail Care).

30. **INF** If the client's hands were soiled, change the water in the basin.

Upper Body

31. **SAF** Position yourself where you can easily work at waist height without straining your back. If you are supporting the client's extremities, move from one side of the bed to the other in order to prevent straining your back.

32. **INF** Place a towel under the arm to be washed. Wipe with a disposable bath cloth or lightly soap the washcloth mitt and wash the client's arm from hand to axilla using long, smooth strokes.

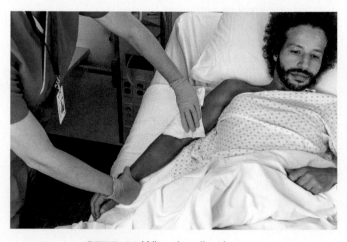

STEP 33 Wipe the client's arm.

33. **INF** Wash the axilla. Discard the disposable bath cloth or rinse out the washcloth.
34. **HLTH** If using soap, rinse carefully using the second washcloth mitt to rinse from the hand, up the arm to the axilla. Rinse the axilla.
35. **HLTH** Dry thoroughly. Apply moisturizer, if indicated.
36. **HLTH** Inspect the skin, especially bony prominences, such as the elbow.
37. **INF** Move the towel and place it under the other arm. Wash, rinse, and dry the other extremity and axilla. If using a disposable bath cloth, discard after use.
38. **CCC** Apply deodorant, as the client desires.
39. **INF** Move the towel to cover the chest and keep the client covered except for the area being bathed. Wash, rinse, and dry the upper chest. Some women may request that powder be applied under their breasts after bathing. *Avoid excessive use of powder, which may cause caking or may be inhaled if suspended in the air.* (Note: Critical care units may prohibit the use of powder.)
40. **INF** Wash, rinse, and dry the abdomen.
41. **INF** Change the water in the basin and rinse the washcloths.

Lower Body

42. **CCC** Place a dry towel under the client's leg. Drape the bath blanket to cover the client's genitalia.
43. **INF** Wipe with a disposable bath cloth or lightly soap the washcloth mitt and wash the client's leg from ankle to groin using long, smooth strokes. If using a disposable bath cloth, discard after use. If using a washcloth, use the second wash mitt to rinse from foot to groin. Dry the leg thoroughly.

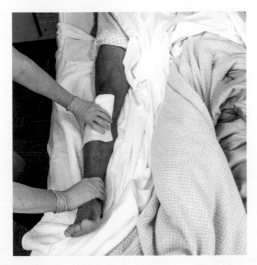

STEP 44 Wipe the client's leg.

44. **INF** Move the towel to the other leg and repeat the bathing sequence.
45. **INF** Place the towel under the feet and wash, rinse, and dry the feet and toes.
46. **HLTH** Inspect the skin, especially bony prominences, such as the heels.
47. **HLTH** Apply moisturizer, if indicated.
48. **INF** Remove the towel. Change the water in the bath basin.

Back

49. **SAF** Ensure all medical lines are secure and with enough slack to reposition the client.
50. **SAF** Assist the client into a side-lying position using appropriate assistive devices, support the client's head with a pillow, and raise the side rail on the side the client is facing.
51. **INF** Place the towel under the client's back. Wipe with a disposable bath cloth or lightly soap the washcloth mitt and wash the client's back from shoulder to buttocks using long, smooth strokes.

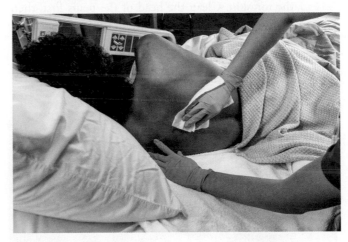

STEP 52 Wipe the client's back.

52. **INF** If using a disposable bath cloth, discard after use. If using a washcloth, use the second wash mitt to rinse from shoulders to buttocks.
53. **HLTH** Dry the back thoroughly.
54. **HLTH** Inspect the skin, especially bony prominences, such as the shoulder blades, spine, and sacrum.
55. **HLTH** Apply moisturizer and/or skin barrier, if indicated. Remove the towel.

Perirectal/Genitals

56. **INF** If not already wearing gloves, apply clean gloves.
For a woman:
   a. **CCC** Place a towel under the buttocks.
   b. **INF** Use a disposable peri-wipe if available.
   c. **CCC** Position the top leg forward into a Sims position to expose the labia and rectum. *Women can seldom reach between their legs to effectively clean between labial folds. Thus, genital self-care is usually not effective for a woman in bed.*

d. **INF** Wash from front to back, cleaning between the labia. Use a different section of the washcloth for each stroke. Wipe the rectal area last. *Clean from the cleanest to the dirtiest area.*

e. **HLTH** If using soap, rinse carefully.

f. **HLTH** Dry thoroughly in all skinfolds. Remove the towel. *Drying thoroughly in skinfolds prevents maceration.*

For a man:

a. **CCC** To clean the peri-rectal area: Place a towel under the buttocks. Use a disposable wipe if available.

b. **CCC** Position the top leg forward into a Sims position to expose the rectum.

c. Wipe over the rectum. Remove the towel.

d. To clean the genitals: Position the client supine and place a towel over his thighs.

e. **HLTH** Determine if the male client can wash his own genitals. If he is able, elevate the head of the bed to facilitate his self-care. *Nursing encourages clients to maintain their own health behaviors.*

f. **INF** If the client is unable to wash himself, determine if the client is circumcised. If uncircumcised, retract the foreskin. Clean the head of the penis first, then clean down the shaft and wipe around and under the scrotum. Return the foreskin to its original position.

g. **INF** If circumcised, clean the head of the penis first, then clean down the shaft, then wipe around and under the scrotum.

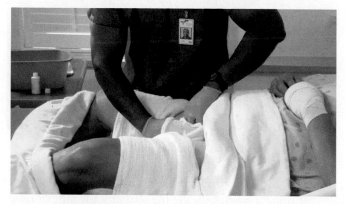

STEP 57G For a man, clean down the shaft, and wipe around the scrotum.

h. Remove the towel from between his legs.

57. **INF** Place a clean gown on the client. Remove the towel on his or her chest. If the client has an IV, follow Skill 2.2, steps 6 to 8.

58. **INF** Empty and disinfect the bath basin. *Bath basins are a potential reservoir for microorganisms.*

59. **INF** Bed linens are usually changed following a bed bath. *Linens may become damp after a bath. Changing the bed linens enhances cleanliness and reduces the number of microorganisms.* See Skill 2.25.

60. **INF** Remove the soiled linens from the room.

FINISHING THE SKILL

61. **INF** Remove gloves and perform hand hygiene.

62. **SAF** Ensure client safety. Place the bed in the lowest position. Verify that the client can identify and reach the nurse call system. *These safety measures reduce the risk of falls.*

63. **CCC** Provide comfort. Assist the client with positioning and rearranging the bedding.

64. **EVAL** Evaluate outcomes, such as the client's tolerance of the activity and use of handling equipment.

65. **COM** Document skin assessment findings, care given, and outcomes in the legal healthcare record.

66. If safe handling equipment was used, return it to the storage area.

■ SKILL 2.4 Providing Alternate Perineal Care

This procedure may be of benefit at times when additional perineal care is needed, such as prior to urinary catheter insertion or when the client is incontinent. This procedure may be used to provide perineal care after childbirth.

EQUIPMENT

Bedpan, commode chair, or toilet
Warm water
Mild soap
Peri-bottle, spray bottle, or pitcher

Absorbent pad
Clean gloves

BEGINNING THE SKILL

1. **INF** Perform hand hygiene.

2. **INF** Apply gloves.

3. **CCC** Introduce yourself to the client and family and explain the procedure.

4. **SAF** Identify the client using two identifiers.

5. **SAF** Determine if the client has any pertinent allergies.

6. **CCC** Provide privacy; close the door and pull the curtain.

PROCEDURE

7. **SAF** Set up an ergonomically safe space. Raise the bed to a comfortable working height. Raise one side rail. *Setting up an ergonomically safe space prevents injury to the nurse and client.*
8. **CCC** Position the client on the bedpan, commode chair, or toilet. If using a bedpan, place an absorbent pad under the client's hips before positioning the bedpan.
9. **INF** Mix mild soap with warm water in the peri-bottle, spray bottle, or pitcher.
10. **INF** Pour or spray warm, soapy water over the perineum.

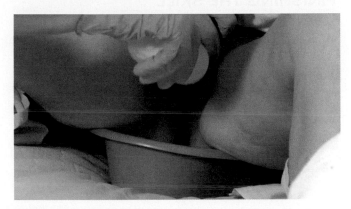

STEP 10 For a woman, pour warm soapy water over the perineum.

11. Refill the bottle or pitcher with warm water.
12. **INF** Rinse off the soap by pouring or spraying water over the perineum.
13. **HLTH** Pat dry with toilet paper or a disposable wipe. *Drying thoroughly in skinfolds prevents maceration.*
14. Assist the client off the bedpan, commode chair, or toilet.
15. **INF** If using a bedpan, empty, rinse, and dry the bedpan.

FINISHING THE SKILL

16. **INF** Remove gloves and perform hand hygiene.
17. **CCC** Provide comfort. Assist the client with positioning and rearranging the bedding.
18. **SAF** Ensure client safety. Place the bed in the lowest position. Verify that the client can identify and reach the nurse call system. *These safety measures reduce the risk of falls.*
19. **EVAL** Evaluate outcomes.
20. **COM** Document assessment findings, care given, and outcomes in the legal healthcare record.

■ SKILL 2.5 Providing Foot Care

EQUIPMENT

Clean gloves, if there is a risk of exposure to body fluids
Basin of warm water
Two towels
Absorbent pad
Disposable wipes or washcloth
Cleanser or soap

BEGINNING THE SKILL

1. **INF** Perform hand hygiene.
2. **INF** Apply gloves if there is a risk of exposure to body fluids.
3. **CCC** Introduce yourself to the client and family and explain the procedure.
4. **SAF** Identify the client using two identifiers.
5. **CCC** Provide privacy; close the door and pull the curtain.

PROCEDURE

6. **SAF** Assist the client to a chair that allows the client's feet to rest firmly on the ground.
7. **HLTH** Inspect the client's feet to assess circulation; skin integrity or irritation; condition of toenails; and presence of a fungal infection, calluses, corns, or warts.
8. **HLTH** Assess the skin care needs of the client, such as the need for a moisturizer or a barrier cream.
9. **SAF** Place the absorbent pad on the floor and place the basin on the absorbent pad.
10. Fill the bath basin with warm water.
11. Assist the client in placing the feet in the basin.
12. **HLTH** Allow the feet to soak for about 10 minutes. **WARNING:** If clients have diabetes mellitus, peripheral neuropathy, or peripheral vascular disease, do not soak the feet.
13. **INF** Apply cleanser or soap on a disposable cloth or washcloth and wash the feet. Wash carefully between the toes. *Microorganisms are reduced by cleaning.*

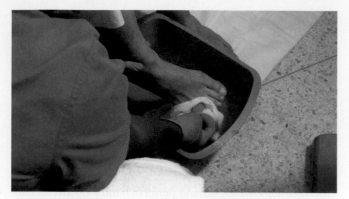

STEP 13 Wash between the toes.

14. Determine if nail care is needed or allowed. *Many facilities prohibit nurses from cutting toenails and sometimes fingernails. Some facilities permit only a podiatrist to cut toenails.*
15. **HLTH** Dry the feet thoroughly, including between the toes. *Drying thoroughly in skinfolds prevents maceration.*
16. **HLTH** Apply moisturizer, if indicated.

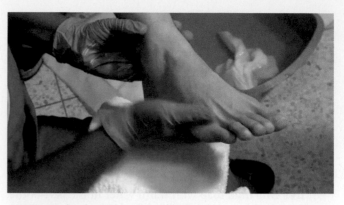

STEP 16 Apply moisturizer, if indicated.

FINISHING THE SKILL

17. **INF** Remove gloves, if used, and perform hand hygiene.
18. **CCC** Provide comfort. Assist the client with positioning and rearranging the bedding.
19. **SAF** Ensure client safety. Place the bed in the lowest position. Verify that the client can identify and reach the nurse call system. *These safety measures reduce the risk of falls.*
20. **EVAL** Evaluate outcomes.
22. **COM** Document foot assessment findings, care given, and outcomes in the legal healthcare record.

■ SKILL 2.6 Providing Nail Care

EQUIPMENT

Scissors or nail clippers
Basin of warm water
Towel
Nail file or emery board
Orangewood stick or plastic nail cleaner
Clean gloves, if there is a risk of exposure to body fluids

BEGINNING THE SKILL

1. **INF** Perform hand hygiene.
2. **INF** Apply gloves if there is a risk of exposure to body fluids.
3. **CCC** Introduce yourself to the client and family and explain the procedure. Ensure that the client consents to the procedure.
4. **SAF** Identify the client using two identifiers.
5. **CCC** Provide privacy; close the door and pull the curtain.
6. **SAF** Determine if nurses may cut nails in your facility. *Many facilities prohibit nurses from cutting toenails and sometimes fingernails. Some facilities permit only podiatrists to cut toenails.*

PROCEDURE

7. Fill the bath basin with warm water.
8. **HLTH** Place the basin of warm water in a position comfortable for the client to soak either the fingernails or the toenails.

9. **HLTH** Soak the nails in warm water for approximately 5 minutes.
10. **INF** Clean under the nails with a plastic nail stick or an orangewood stick.

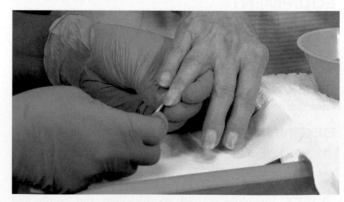

STEP 10 Clean under the nails.

11. **HLTH** Dry fingers and/or toes. *Drying thoroughly in skinfolds prevents maceration.*
12. **HLTH** Cut the nails straight across with clippers or nail scissors to fingertip length. Avoid cutting the nail into a curved shape. *Cutting the nail straight across can help prevent an ingrown nail.*

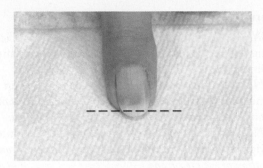

STEP 12 Cut the nails straight across to fingertip length.

13. **CCC** File the nails smooth with a nail file or emery board.

FINISHING THE SKILL

14. **INF** Remove gloves, if used, and perform hand hygiene.

15. **CCC** Provide comfort. Assist the client with positioning and rearranging the bedding.
16. **SAF** Ensure client safety. Place the bed in the lowest position. Verify that the client can identify and reach the nurse call system. *These safety measures reduce the risk of falls.*
17. **EVAL** Evaluate outcomes.
18. **COM** Document assessment findings, care given, and outcomes in the legal healthcare record.

▪ SKILL 2.7 Bathing an Infant

EQUIPMENT

Two receiving blankets or towels
pH-neutral cleanser
Soft nail brush
Clean gloves, if there is a risk of exposure to body fluids
Disposable wipes or washcloth
Cotton balls

BEGINNING THE SKILL

1. **INF** Perform hand hygiene.
2. **INF** Apply gloves if there is a risk of exposure to body fluids. *Prior to the first bath, a newborn will have maternal blood on its body, even if it is not visible. Gloves are worn until the first bath is complete.*
3. **CCC** Introduce yourself and explain the procedure to family members present.
4. **SAF** Identify the client using two identifiers.

PROCEDURE

5. **SAF** Set up an ergonomically safe space to prevent injury to the nurse and client. Determine an appropriate environment and surface for a bath/shampoo. *Bathe the infant in an environment that is warm and free of drafts to prevent cold stressing the infant. In an acute-care facility, infants are bathed within an isolette or under a radiant warmer.*
6. **SAF** Assess the infant's ability to tolerate the turning, handling, and cold stress associated with bathing. This includes noting the infant's current temperature. *A newborn must reach and maintain a given temperature before the first bath is given.*
7. **SAF** Assess the infant's medical equipment to determine the risk of electrical shock and the need to secure medical lines.

Infant Shampoo

If the infant is to have a shampoo and a bath, then give the shampoo first. Dry the hair completely before proceeding to give the bath in order to minimize heat loss.

8. **SAF** Adjust the temperature of the water to be used to wet and rinse the infant's head. (Note: In the hospital, this may be water running in a sink; in the home, it could also be water in a pitcher.)
9. **CCC** Swaddle the infant in a receiving blanket with the hands on the chest. Swaddling prevents the infant from grabbing and enhances the infant's sense of security.
10. **SAF** Tuck the infant securely in a football hold using your nondominant hand.

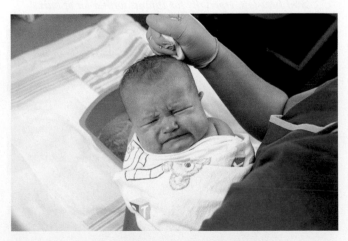

STEP 10 Use a football hold to shampoo a swaddled infant.

11. **SAF** Check the water temperature. The water should not be too hot; the desired range is 98°F to 99°F (36.7–37.2°C). If wearing gloves, check the water temperature with your forearm to ensure it does not feel hot to the touch. *Infants have thin skin and are at greater risk for burns.*

12. **CCC** Using your dominant hand, wet the infant's hair, preventing water from running into the infant's eyes and face.

13. **INF** Apply a mild cleanser and gently clean in a circular motion. *If this is the newborn's first bath, the desired outcome is to remove all maternal blood from the infant's hair.* (Note: Many newborn nurseries use the brush portion of a surgical scrub brush to gently loosen all foreign material from the newborn's scalp.)

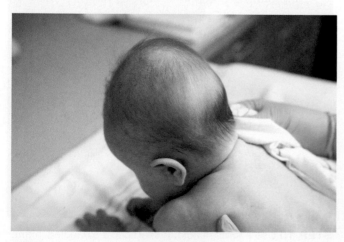

STEP 13 Gently clean the scalp in a circular motion.

14. **SAF** Recheck the water temperature and rinse the infant's scalp thoroughly.

15. **HLTH** Dry the hair thoroughly with a receiving blanket or towel and discard the wet blanket. Comb through the infant's hair to hasten drying. *Wet hair can cause significant heat loss, especially for infants with a lot of hair.*

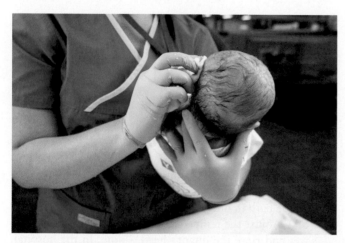

STEP 15 Dry infant's hair thoroughly.

Infant Bath

16. **SAF** Return the infant to the selected safe surface and unswaddle the infant. Keep one hand on the infant at all times.

17. **INF** Wipe one eye from nose to ear, using plain water and a cotton ball or soft disposable wipe. *This cleans substances away from the opening of the lacrimal duct.*

18. **INF** Wipe the other eye with a different section of the wipe or another cotton ball. *This prevents cross-contamination of eye organisms.*

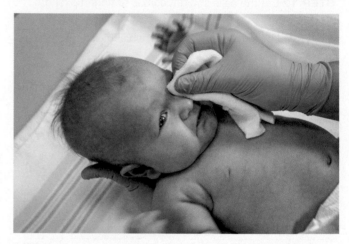

STEP 18 Use a different section of the wipe to prevent cross-contamination.

19. **INF** Gently wash the forehead, cheeks, nose, around the mouth, and neck. Gently clean behind the ears. *Infants' ears have very soft cartilage, which allows their ears to lay flat against their head, forming a hidden crease.*

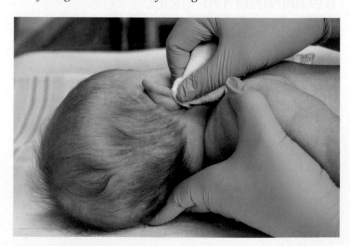

STEP 19 Clean gently behind the ears.

20. **HLTH** Dry face and neck gently and thoroughly. *Drying thoroughly in skinfolds prevents maceration.*

21. **INF** Remove T-shirt, if present. Place a scant amount of pH-neutral cleanser on a disposable wipe or washcloth and wipe the chest, abdomen, and arms. *Unlike adults, infant axillae do not need special attention because newborns do not have any active sweat ducts in their axillae.*

22. **INF** Wet a clean disposable wipe or washcloth and rinse off the cleanser.
23. **INF** Examine the hands and fingers for small particles; then wipe clean. *Newborns' palmar grasp reflex causes them to close their fists around anything they feel, potentially capturing small particles.*

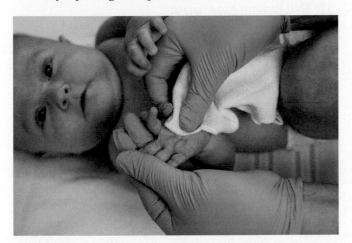

STEP 23 Clean the infant's hands and fingers.

24. **HLTH** Dry the neck, abdomen, arms, and hands gently and thoroughly. Put a clean T-shirt on the infant, which can be prewarmed if the infant is at risk for cold stress.
25. **INF** Examine the feet and between the toes carefully; then apply a scant amount of pH-neutral cleanser on a disposable wipe or washcloth and clean the feet and between the toes. *Newborns plantar grasp reflex causes them to curl their toes in response to sensation on the soles of their feet, potentially capturing small particles between their toes.*

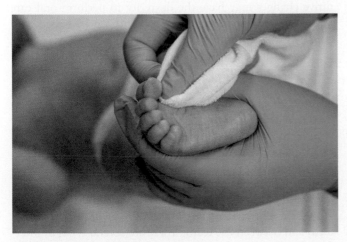

STEP 25 Clean infant's feet and toes.

26. **INF** Wet a clean disposable wipe or washcloth and rinse the cleanser from the legs and feet.
27. **HLTH** Dry the legs and feet.

Diaper Change

28. **ACC** Unfasten the diaper. Be prepared to catch the urine stream, particularly if the infant is on intake and output. *A common reaction of little boys, in particular, is to void in response to the cold air on their genitalia.*
28. **INF** Clean the genitalia gently with a cotton ball or disposable wipe. Wipe creases on the thighs.

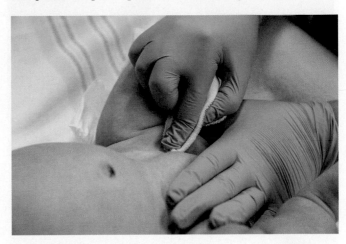

STEP 28 Wipe creases on the thighs

Infant girls: Wipe girls from front to back between the labial folds. Newborn girls may have thick vaginal discharge, and occasionally a newborn girl will have bloody vaginal discharge as a result of the dramatic decrease in maternal hormones. *Wiping from the front to the back prevents the transfer of microorganisms toward the urethra.*
Infant boys: Wipe boys' penis and around and under each testicle. Do not retract the penis on an uncircumcised infant. Do not use soap on freshly circumcised boy's penis. *Male infants' testicles are enlarged because of maternal hormones.*

29. **INF** Turn the infant over and inspect and clean the buttocks, including the sacral dimples.

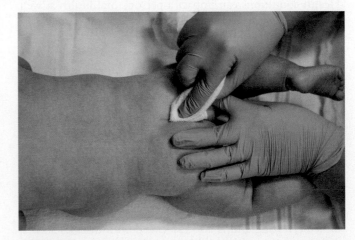

STEP 29 Inspect and clean sacral dimples.

30. **HLTH** Dry thoroughly and gently, especially in skinfolds. *Drying thoroughly in skinfolds prevents maceration.*
31. Position and fasten a clean diaper. (Note: If the umbilical cord is present, fasten the diaper tucked below the umbilicus.)

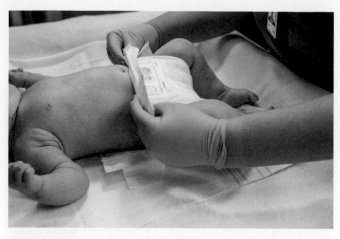

STEP 31 Fasten the diaper folded below the umbilicus.

32. **INF** If the umbilical cord is present, follow facility policy for cord care.
33. **EVAL** Monitor the infant's temperature.

FINISHING THE SKILL

34. **INF** Remove gloves, if used.
35. **INF** Perform hand hygiene.
36. **SAF** Ensure client safety.
37. **CCC** Provide comfort, such as swaddling, nesting, or nonnutritive sucking (pacifier or infant's fingers).
38. **EVAL** Evaluate outcomes.
39. **COM** Document assessment findings, such as urine output and stool characteristics; care given; and outcomes in the legal healthcare record.

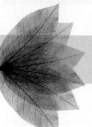

SECTION 2 Oral Hygiene

The mouth is the portal to the human body, an opening to the respiratory and gastrointestinal systems. Consistent, quality oral hygiene is critical to health maintenance and the prevention of infection. Oral health has social implications as well because it impacts speech, facial expressions, and tasting and eating food. Oral health is one of the topics and objectives for *Healthy People 2020*. In the United States, significant disparities in the access to preventative dental care exist that are associated with race/ethnicity, education level, and income. Health conditions can impact a person's oral health as well, such as diabetes (Office of Disease Prevention and Health Promotion [ODPHP], 2018).

Oral care contributes to health in every setting. Oral hygiene decreases not only periodontal infections but also respiratory infections, including pneumonia. In long-term care and acute-care facilities, a landmark review of hundreds of studies concluded that there is solid evidence that oral hygiene reduces the incidence of respiratory diseases (Sjogren, Nilsson, Forsell, Johansson, & Hoogstraate, 2008). In long-term residential settings, maintaining a healthy mouth has the benefit of improving communication, appetite, and the ability to obtain adequate nutrition. On the other hand, problematic oral health may result in pain and difficulty eating and is also associated with diseases such as diabetes, pneumonia, and endocarditis (Jayasekara, 2017). Several nursing studies examined the impact of collaboration with a dental hygienist in residential settings and found positive results. Given the strong relationship between systemic health and oral health and the increasing numbers of older adults, this is an area for continued growth (Mohammadi, Franks, & Hines, 2015).

Most children and adults can provide their own oral care. In such cases, the role of the nurse is to promote the client's self-care capabilities and support healthy behaviors, such as regular flossing and brushing, by providing the appropriate supplies and reminding clients about oral hygiene after each meal and at bedtime. Nurses recognize that clients with cognitive changes may have the dexterity to perform oral care but may need reminders about when to do it. In fact, clients with dementia may develop dental diseases as a result of the loss of awareness of the importance of and need for oral hygiene. Clients with a variety of healthcare concerns, including arthritis, osteoporosis, diabetes, and immune suppression from chemotherapy or radiation therapy, are at increased risk for developing oral complications and may require nursing assistance with oral hygiene. Nurses typically follow the recommendations of the American Dental Association (ADA) for routine brushing and flossing, including brushing with a soft-bristle toothbrush over all of the tooth surface using short, gentle strokes a minimum of twice a day. The objective of flossing is to remove plaque on the teeth and between the teeth. There are several types of interdental cleaners, such as floss heads or interdental sticks, that may require less manual dexterity than dental floss or are easier to use on a client. Electric toothbrushes also require less manual dexterity and remove more plaque. When clients are not able to provide their own oral hygiene, the nurse may assist or provide oral care, including brushing, flossing, and caring for dentures.

DENTURES

Clients who wear dentures will need specific care related to the cleaning, wearing, and storing of dentures. Dentures are very expensive items and require vigilance to ensure that they are not broken or lost during a stay in a healthcare facility. Dentures should be cleaned daily with a denture cleaner or mild dish soap and not be cleaned with whitening or abrasive toothpaste. Products endorsed with the ADA Seal of Acceptance have been evaluated for safety and effectiveness (ADA, 2016). When dentures are not worn, they are always kept in water or a denture-cleaning solution. Dentures may warp if they are allowed to dry out. However, if stored in a cleansing agent, they are to be washed off before the dentures are placed in the client's mouth. Denture storage containers are to be clearly labeled with the client's name and cleaned regularly. Nurses encourage clients who have dentures to remove them at night and to wear them during the day to improve clarity of speech, facilitate eating, and enhance the sense of well-being.

ORAL CARE IN THE ACUTE CARE SETTING

Clients in an intensive care setting on mechanical ventilation require more than the ADA recommended oral care to prevent ventilation associated pneumonia (VAP). In an intensive care setting, research shows a relationship between providing oral hygiene and a subsequent decrease in the incidence of pneumonia in mechanically ventilated adults. Currently, best practice is to provide oral care with chlorhexidine gluconate for all clients on mechanical ventilation (Swe, 2017) (Fig. 2.3). What is not yet established is which concentration of chlorhexidine gluconate and what frequency of providing oral care yield the best results (Hua et al., 2016). For more information, see Box 2.5.

Although more studies on effective oral hygiene practices and protocols are needed, the current best practice recommendations include the following:

- A small, soft-bristle toothbrush used with toothpaste is much more effective at removing plaque, the reservoir for microorganisms, than sponge toothettes (Khanh-Dao Le, 2017).
- Sponge toothettes pose a risk of tearing and leaving a piece of sponge in the mouth or airway. However, for clients with a bleeding risk, they are an alternative (Khanh-Dao Le, 2017).
- Glycerin and lemon swabs are not recommended because they dry the oral mucosa, decalcify teeth, and decrease the pH, thereby increasing the risk of bacterial and fungal infections (Chen, 2015).
- Hydrogen peroxide and sodium bicarbonate (unless properly diluted) are also not recommended for daily use

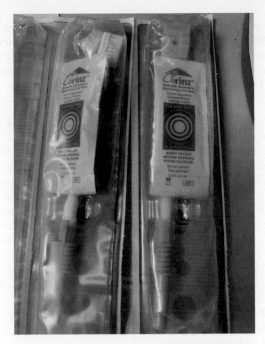

FIG. 2.3 Disposable oral hygiene kits.

because they can cause superficial burns and alter the pH (Chen, 2015).

- Oral chlorhexidine rinses have shown promise in decreasing nosocomial infections in adults in critical care settings, provide effective plaque control, and have antibacterial and fungicidal properties (Slade, 2017).
- Oral fluid intake should be encouraged in order to maintain the hydration of oral mucous membranes, or a saliva substitute should be used (Slade, 2017).

In the acute care setting, suction may be set up to help clear secretions. One device that is commonly used for oropharyngeal suctioning is a Yankauer. It is a rigid, clear plastic catheter with a smooth rounded end, and it is angled to facilitate suctioning in the mouth. It is only used in the mouth and is used when clients have difficulty expelling secretions in the mouth. It is useful when providing oral care.

Oral care needs to be consistently recognized and prioritized within the acute care setting, both to achieve the benefits of good oral care and to avoid the potential complications of neglecting oral care. Progress has been made in developing assessment tools and protocols at individual healthcare facilities however, there is a continued need for a recognized standard of care because even the definition of *oral care* varies between facilities (Hua et al., 2016). Oral care benefits from multidisciplinary collaboration to improve and achieve optimal oral health. Nurses have a key role in the implementation of oral hygiene assessment tools, oral hygiene protocols, and the availability of evidence-based supplies in order to consistently provide quality oral healthcare.

Reference: International Classification for Nursing Practice. (n.d.). *eHealth & ICNP.* Retrieved from https://www.icn.ch/what-we-do/projects/ehealth-icnp.

BOX 2.5 Lessons From the Evidence : What Are the Effects of Oral Hygiene Care on the Incidence of Ventilator-Associated Pneumonia in Critically Ill Clients Receiving Mechanical Ventilation in Intensive Care Units?

A Cochrane Review analyzed 38 studies to identify the best evidence-based care.

It is known that the use of mechanical ventilation for more than 48 hours puts clients at risk for developing ventilator-associated pneumonia (VAP). It is also known that other factors, such as client sedation, positioning, and the use of endotracheal tubes with subglottic secretion drainage ports, also impact the incidence of VAP (Klompas et al., 2014). However, it has also been shown that oral care can reduce the incidence of VAP.

The review grouped the studies into four clusters:
1. Chlorhexidine antiseptic mouth rinse or gel compared to placebo (treatment without the active ingredient chlorhexidine) or usual care (with or without tooth brushing)
2. Tooth brushing compared with no tooth brushing (with or without antiseptics)
3. Powered compared with manual tooth brushing
4. Oral-care solutions with other solutions

The strength of the evidence was limited by the quality of the studies. The authors reported that only 13% were well conducted. The strongest conclusion was that chlorhexidine reduces the risk of VAP whether applied as a mouth rinse or gel. However, the change in VAP did not translate into a change in death rate, days on mechanical ventilation, or days in the intensive care unit.

The other oral-care comparison studies provided limited or weak evidence. There was not enough evidence to determine if any of the interventions studied had unwanted side effects (Hua et al., 2016).

APPLICATION OF THE NURSING PROCESS

Examples of Related ICNP Nursing Diagnoses, Expected Client Outcomes, and Nursing Interventions:

Nursing Diagnosis: Impaired ability to perform oral hygiene

Supporting Data: Client's clinical condition prevents self-care.

Expected Client Outcome: Client will participate as much as possible in oral hygiene. The client's teeth, gums, tongue, palate, mucosa, and odor remain clean.

Nursing Intervention Example: Assist the client with oral hygiene after meals using a soft-bristle toothbrush and interdental cleaning devices, such as dental floss.

Nursing Diagnosis: Lack of knowledge of oral hygiene

Expected Client Outcome: The client will verbalize and demonstrate brushing and flossing using the ADA recommendations for oral care.

Nursing Intervention Example: Instruct and/or demonstrate brushing and flossing using the ADA recommendations for oral care.

CRITICAL CONCEPTS
Providing Oral Care

Accuracy (ACC)

Providing oral care is subject to the following variables:

Nurse-Related Factors
- Assessment of client, including fine motor abilities, level of discomfort, risk for aspiration, and cooperation
- Assessment of the oral cavity, including teeth, gums, tongue, palate, mucosa, and odor
- Identification of anatomical structures
- Angle, pressure, and direction of brushing
- Understanding of procedure by client and family.

Equipment-Related Factors
- Functioning of suction equipment.

Client-Centered Care (CCC)

When providing oral care, respect for the client is demonstrated through:
- promoting autonomy
- providing privacy
- ensuring comfort
- honoring cultural preferences
- arranging for an interpreter, as needed
- advocating for the client and family.

Infection Control (INF)

When providing oral care, healthcare-associated infection and client infection are prevented by:
- reducing the number of microorganisms by regular oral care
- containment of microorganisms
- preventing and reducing the transfer of microorganisms.

Safety (SAF)

When providing oral care, safety measures prevent harm and maintain a safe care environment.

Communication (COM)
- Communication exchanges information (oral, written, nonverbal or electronic) between two or more people.
- Collaboration with the client and other healthcare professionals improves oral care.
- Documentation records information in a permanent legal record.

Health Maintenance (HLTH)

Nursing is dedicated to the promotion of health and abilities related to personal hygiene.

Evaluation (EVAL)

When providing oral care, evaluation of outcomes enables the nurse to determine the efficacy of the care provided.

■ SKILL 2.8 Providing Oropharyngeal Suctioning With a Round-Tip Suction Catheter (Yankauer)

EQUIPMENT

Round-tipped suction catheter (Yankauer)
Wall suction
Connecting tubing
Water
Cup
Emesis basin
Clean gloves

BEGINNING THE SKILL

1. **INF** Perform hand hygiene.
2. **INF** Apply gloves.
3. **CCC** Introduce yourself to the client and family and explain the procedure.
4. **SAF** Identify the client using two identifiers.
5. **CCC** Provide privacy; close the door and pull the curtain.

PROCEDURE

6. **ACC** Assess the client's ability to clear oral secretions, level of discomfort, cooperation, risk for aspiration, and degree of mobility. *Your assessment is to determine if the client requires oropharyngeal suctioning or if the client can remove fluid or secretions without assistance.*
7. **SAF** Position the client with the head of the bed up and the head turned to the side. If sitting up is contraindicated, turn the client on his or her side. *Sitting up and side-lying positions decrease the risk of aspiration.*
8. **ACC** Connect the Yankauer to the distal end of the suction tubing. Ensure the suction tubing is connected to the suction canister. *Loose connections will not provide sufficient suction.*
9. **ACC** Turn wall suction to continuous suction at moderate suction (80–120 mm Hg).
10. **CCC** Pour a small amount (approximately 120 mL [4 oz]) of water into a clean cup or emesis basin. Dip the end of the round-tip catheter or Yankauer into the water. *Lubricating the tip of the Yankauer makes it easier to insert.*
11. **CCC** Place a disposable absorbent pad or towel across the client's chest to catch secretions.
12. **ACC** Place the Yankauer in the client's mouth along the gum line if sitting up right or buccal pocket if client is on his or her side. *Gravity will result in secretions pooling on the dependent side.*

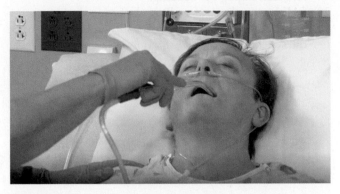

STEP 12 Place the Yankauer in the client's mouth along the gum line.

13. **ACC** Withdraw the Yankauer from the mouth. Assess secretions, and dip the end of the tip into water to flush the secretions into the canister. (Note: Assess secretions for amount, consistency, and color.)

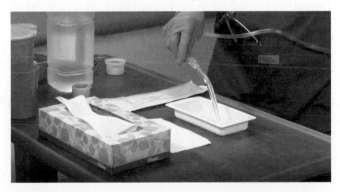

STEP 13 Assess secretions and flush secretions into canister.

14. **ACC** If additional suctioning is needed, place the Yankauer in the client's mouth. Begin on the dependent side, slide it under the tongue, and suction along the other cheek.
15. **EVAL** Reassess secretions. Place the tip of the Yankauer into water to flush the secretions into the canister. *Flushing the secretions into the canister clears the inner lumen of the Yankauer and prevents the secretions from drying and blocking the catheter.*
16. Turn off suction.
17. **INF** Place the Yankauer in a clean container. The packaging it came in is sometimes kept to provide a cover. Remove disposable absorbent pad or towel from his or her chest.

FINISHING THE SKILL

18. **INF** Remove gloves and perform hand hygiene.
19. **CCC** Provide comfort. Assist the client with positioning and rearranging the bedding.
20. **SAF** Ensure client safety. Place the bed in the lowest position. Verify that the client can identify and reach the nurse call system. *These safety measures reduce the risk of falls.*

21. **EVAL** Evaluate outcomes.
22. **COM** Document secretion assessment findings, such as care given, and outcomes in the legal healthcare record.

■ SKILL 2.9 Providing Oral Hygiene for a Conscious Client

EQUIPMENT

Soft-bristle toothbrush
Toothpaste
Water
Emesis basin
Clean gloves
Towel or washcloth
Dental floss, approximately 45-cm (18-inch) section, or alternative interdental cleaner

BEGINNING THE SKILL

1. **INF** Perform hand hygiene.
2. **INF** Apply gloves.
3. **CCC** Introduce yourself to the client and family and explain the procedure.
4. **SAF** Identify the client using two identifiers.
5. **CCC** Provide privacy; close the door and pull the curtain.

PROCEDURE

6. **ACC** Assess the client's fine motor abilities, level of discomfort, cooperation, risk for aspiration, and degree of mobility. *Your assessment is to determine the best position for the client and the extent to which the client can assist with brushing and flossing of the teeth.*
7. **SAF** Position the client sitting up, if he or she able; otherwise, position the client on his or her side. *Sitting up and side-lying positions decrease the risk of aspiration.*
8. **CCC** Assess the client's oral hygiene product requirements and preferences. For example, does the client have dentures or a bridge that requires a specific type of cleanser?
9. **ACC** Assess the client's mouth, including the teeth, gums, tongue, palate, mucosa, and odor.
10. **SAF** Check laboratory results to determine if the client has a bleeding disorder. *Clients with bleeding disorders require additional care with oral hygiene in order to not to cause bleeding.*

Brushing Teeth: Instruct the Client or Perform the Following:

11. **CCC** Place a towel on the client's chest.
12. **CCC** Moisten the toothbrush to soften the bristles, and apply toothpaste.

13. **ACC** Place the toothbrush at a 45-degree angle against the gums.

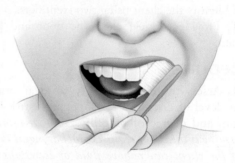

STEP 13 Place the brush against the gums.

14. **ACC** Move the brush back and forth gently in short strokes.
15. **ACC** Move the brush systematically from one area of the teeth to the next, brushing the outer tooth surfaces, inner tooth surfaces, and the chewing surfaces of the teeth on both the upper and lower teeth (ADA, n.d.).
16. **ACC** Use the front end of the toothbrush to clean the inside surfaces of the front teeth, using a gentle up-and-down stroke. *Using the front end of the toothbrush allows the toothbrush bristles to reach these surfaces.*
17. **ACC** Brush the tongue. *This helps to remove bacteria and decrease odor.*
18. **CCC** Encourage the client to spit into the emesis basin as needed.
19. **CCC** Offer water to the client and encourage the client to rinse the toothpaste from his or her mouth and then spit into the emesis basin.
20. **INF** Rinse the toothbrush and empty, rinse, and disinfect the emesis basin.
21. **INF** Store the toothbrush in a clean container.

Flossing Teeth

22. **ACC** Wrap the dental floss around the index fingers on both of your hands. (Note: Alternative interdental cleaners such as tiny brushes or floss heads are also effective to clean between the teeth.)

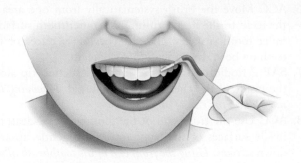

STEP 22 Clean between teeth.

23. **ACC** Guide the floss between the client's teeth, rubbing the floss against the teeth.
24. **ACC** At the gum line, guide the floss along one tooth and gently slide it between the gum and the tooth.
25. **ACC** Rub the tooth, moving away from the gum by curving the floss around the edge of the tooth.
26. **ACC** Repeat with every tooth, including the back side of the last tooth, using a fresh section of the floss for each tooth.

27. **CCC** Offer water and emesis basin to the client and encourage the client to rinse and spit into the basin.

FINISHING THE SKILL

28. **INF** Remove gloves and perform hand hygiene.
29. **CCC** Provide comfort. Assist the client with positioning and rearranging the bedding.
30. **SAF** Ensure client safety. Place the bed in the lowest position. Verify that the client can identify and reach the nurse call system. *These safety measures reduce the risk of falls.*
31. **EVAL** Evaluate outcomes.
32. **COM** Document assessment findings, care given, and outcomes in the legal healthcare record, including:
    * oral assessment of the mouth, including teeth, gums, tongue, palate, mucosa, and odor
    * assessment of client's self-care abilities and deficits
    * client's reported knowledge of oral hygiene
    * client education provided
    * how the client tolerated the procedure.
33. **COM** Refer any dental problems assessed to a dental professional.

■ SKILL 2.10 Providing Oral Hygiene for an Unconscious Client

EQUIPMENT

Round-tipped suction catheter (Yankauer)
Wall suction
Soft-bristle toothbrush
Toothpaste
Water
Emesis basin
Clean gloves
Towel or washcloth
Water-filled syringe
Bite block

BEGINNING THE SKILL

1. **INF** Perform hand hygiene.
2. **INF** Apply gloves.
3. **CCC** Introduce yourself and explain the procedure to family members present.
4. **SAF** Identify the client using two identifiers.
5. **CCC** Provide privacy; close the door and pull the curtain.

PROCEDURE

6. **SAF** Determine if the client has a bleeding disorder. Clients with bleeding disorders require additional care with oral hygiene in order to not cause bleeding.
7. **SAF** Set up an ergonomically safe space. Raise the bed to a comfortable working height. Raise one side rail. *Setting up an ergonomically safe space prevents injury to the nurse and client.*

8. **ACC** Use a tongue depressor to hold back the lips and cheeks, exposing the teeth. Assess the client's mouth, including teeth, gums, tongue, palate, mucosa, and odor.

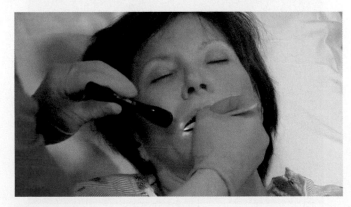

STEP 8 Assess the client's mouth.

9. **SAF** Roll the client into a side-lying position, with the head of the bed elevated if possible. This position allows liquid to drain out of the mouth and prevents aspiration.
10. **CCC** Place a towel or absorbent pad under the client's face. The pad prevents accidentally soiling the sheets.
11. **CCC** Turn on the wall suction and set a Yankauer suction tip at hand in order to catch liquid from the client's mouth.

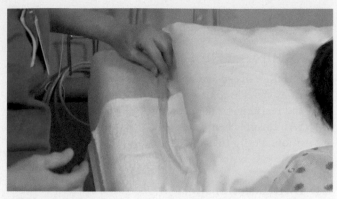

STEP 11 Have a rounded tip Yankauer suction at hand.

12. **SAF** Using a bite block, gently open the client's mouth. **WARNING:** Do not place your fingers in the client's mouth. The *client may bite your fingers.*
13. **CCC** Moisten the toothbrush to soften the bristles, and apply a small amount of toothpaste.
14. **ACC** Place the toothbrush at a 45-degree angle against the gums.
15. **ACC** Move the brush back and forth gently in short strokes.

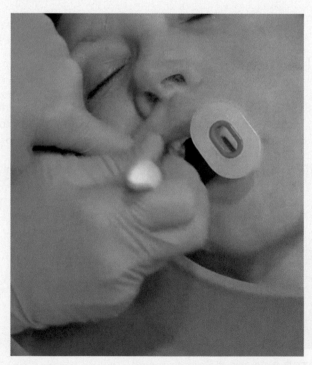

STEP 15 Brush teeth with the bite block in place.

16. **ACC** Move the brush systematically from one area of the teeth to the next, brushing the outer tooth surfaces, inner tooth surfaces, and the chewing surfaces of the teeth on both the upper and lower teeth.
17. **SAF** Periodically insert the Yankauer suction tip along the inside of the cheek to remove liquid. *Removing liquid reduces the risk of aspiration.*
18. **ACC** Use the front end of the toothbrush to clean the inside surfaces of the front teeth with gentle up-and-down strokes. *Using the front end of the toothbrush allows the toothbrush bristles to reach these surfaces.*
19. **ACC** Brush the tongue. Brushing the tongue helps to remove bacteria and decrease odor.
20. **CCC** Rinse the client's mouth with a small amount of water in a syringe and then suction.
21. Remove bite block.
22. **HLTH** Apply moisturizer to the client's lips.
23. **INF** Rinse the toothbrush and store in a clean container.
24. **INF** Place the tip of the Yankauer into water to flush the sections into the canister. *Flushing the secretions into the canister clears the inner lumen of the Yankauer and prevents the secretions from drying and blocking the catheter.*

FINISHING THE SKILL

25. **INF** Remove gloves and perform hand hygiene.
26. **CCC** Provide comfort. Assist the client with positioning and rearranging bedding.
27. **SAF** Ensure client safety. Place the bed in the lowest position. Verify that the client can identify and reach the nurse call system. *These safety measures reduce the risk of falls.*
28. **EVAL** Evaluate outcomes.
29. **COM** Document assessment findings, including teeth, gums, tongue, palate, mucosa, and odor; care given; and outcomes in the legal healthcare
30. **COM** Refer any dental problems assessed to a dental professional.

■ SKILL 2.11 Removing, Cleaning, and Inserting Dentures

EQUIPMENT

Clean gloves
Denture toothbrush
Denture cup
Emesis basin
Denture cleansing agent or dish soap

BEGINNING THE SKILL

1. **INF** Perform hand hygiene.
2. **INF** Apply gloves.
3. **CCC** Introduce yourself to the client and family and explain the procedure.
4. **SAF** Identify the client using two identifiers.
5. **CCC** Provide privacy; close the door and pull the curtain.

PROCEDURE

6. **ACC** Assess the client's fine motor abilities, level of discomfort, cooperation, risk for aspiration, and degree of mobility. *Your assessment is to determine the extent to which the client can assist with removing, cleaning, and inserting dentures.*
7. **ACC** Assess the client's mouth, including the gums, tongue, palate, mucosa, and odor. Ask the client about the fit of the dentures.
8. **SAF** Ask the client to remove the dentures. If the client is unable to do this, grasp the lower denture and lift it out. Grasp the front edge of the top denture to break the seal at the roof of the mouth and lift the upper denture out. *Removing the bottom denture first reduces the bite risk for the caregiver (Jablonski, 2012).*

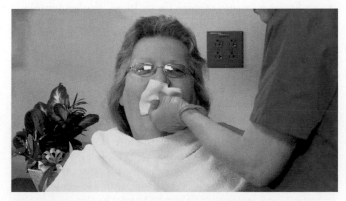

STEP 8 Grasp the edge of the dentures and remove.

9. **SAF** If the client is unable to brush the dentures, place the dentures in an emesis basin to brush them. Brushing dentures in the sink is not recommended. *Dentures can break if they accidentally fall into the sink.*
10. **SAF** If the client is able to brush the dentures independently and prefers to do it over a sink, place a washcloth

or towel in the sink to protect dentures from breaking if they accidentally fall into the sink. *Dentures can break if they accidentally fall into the sink.*

11. **HLTH** Brush the dentures with a toothbrush or denture brush using denture cleanser in the same manner teeth are brushed.
12. **SAF** Rinse the dentures in lukewarm water, never hot water. *Excessively hot water can warp dentures.*
13. **HLTH** If dentures are to be reinserted into the client's mouth, encourage the client to brush the gums and tongue with a toothbrush and toothpaste or rinse with mouthwash before inserting dentures. Denture wearers should practice good dental hygiene by brushing the gums, tongue, and roof of the mouth before inserting dentures to stimulate tissue circulation and to remove plaque.
14. **CCC** Apply denture adhesive to the dentures if the client is accustomed to using it.
15. **CCC** Assist the client to insert the dentures.
16. **INF** Rinse out the denture cup and emesis basin, if used, storing in a secure place within the client's reach.
17. **SAF** If the dentures are to remain out of the client's mouth, place them in a clearly labeled, unbreakable container filled with lukewarm water or lukewarm water with an effervescent cleaning tablet.

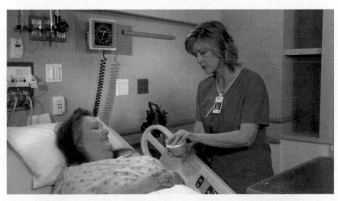

STEP 17 Place dentures in an unbreakable container filled with lukewarm water.

18. **SAF** Place container in a safe place within the client's reach.

FINISHING THE SKILL

19. **INF** Remove gloves and perform hand hygiene.
20. **CCC** Ensure client safety and comfort. Place the call light in reach.
21. **EVAL** Evaluate outcomes.
22. **COM** Document assessment findings, care given, and outcomes in the legal healthcare record.
23. **COM** Refer any problems with how the dentures fit to a dental professional.

SECTION 3   Providing Hair Care

Providing hair care offers an enhanced sense of well-being and cleanliness to the client. In this chapter, hair care encompasses shampooing hair, braiding hair, shaving facial hair, and caring for the client with lice. There are numerous methods of shampooing. Ambulatory clients may be provided with hair care while seated in the shower. For nonambulatory clients, several assistive devices are available. Some facilities may require an authorized healthcare provider's order to provide a shampoo. Considerations that will impact the best method of shampooing the client include activity intolerance, cognitive function, musculoskeletal function, and level of discomfort.

Various shampoo assistive devices are available, including those that allow the nurse to shampoo from a wheelchair or gurney. If the client can be moved to a sink, a molded plastic shampooing device that extends from under the client's head into a sink allows the water to run into the sink. Shampooing at a sink simplifies the process slightly because the sink provides a convenient source of running water and a drain.

If the client cannot be moved to the sink, there are also many different assistive devices available to shampoo the client in bed, including molded trays and inflatable rings. These types of assistive devices usually have a drain long enough to reach near the floor. Select a receptacle large enough to hold all the water. Position the receptacle on the floor away from your feet. In addition to traditional water and shampoo, there are dry shampoos and no-rinse shampoos available in a bag or shower cap (Fig. 2.4).

Different types of hair (e.g., curly, straight, coarse, fine) require different kinds of care, and the nurse should be familiar with culturally appropriate hair-care techniques. Box 2.6 explains the care of African American hair. Caring for hair also encompasses protecting it from damage between shampoos. In healthcare facilities, hair can be braided or wrapped in a scarf to reduce tangles and hair breakage. If braided, the braids must not pull tightly from the scalp. When significant tension is put on hair, there is an inflammatory reaction around the hair bulb, and the hair is released. As a result, tight braids can result in hair breakage and the loss of hair. Even loose braids should be released regularly and culturally appropriate hair care provided.

SHAVING

Clients are usually shaved only upon request. Men may be accustomed to shaving every day, and a daily shave is important to their sense of well-being. Some men are accustomed to shaving with a safety razor, and others use an electric razor. Clients who are at risk for prolonged bleeding times due to anticoagulant therapy should be counseled to use an electric razor to decrease the risk of bleeding from cuts and nicks. Check the facility's policy on the use of electric razors. Many facilities require a safety check of electrical equipment brought from home, and some facilities do not permit their use.

LICE

The term for an infestation of lice is *pediculosis* (Fig. 2.5). There are three different types of lice (singular: louse):
- *Pediculus humanus capitis* (head louse)
- *Pediculus humanus corporis* (body louse, clothes louse)
- *Pthirus pubis* ("crab" louse, pubic louse).

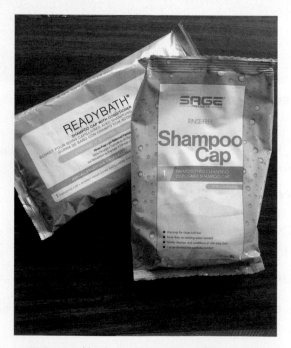

FIG. 2.4 No-rinse shampoo in a bag or cap.

BOX 2.6 Cultural Considerations: African American Hair Care

African American hair differs in structure from Caucasian hair. The dry outer cuticle may be twice as thick. In addition, each hair has more turns, making it more fragile and prone to breakage. It is also drier, with a lower water content, and requires moisture to keep it healthy.

Recommended hair care:
- Wash hair about once a week.
- Follow each shampoo with a leave-in conditioner.
- Using a wide-tooth comb or pick to avoid breaking the hair, comb the conditioner through the hair to the ends.
- Use a natural oil such as shea butter or coconut oil.
- Do not use mineral oil or petroleum jelly. These products are not absorbed.

Adapted from Dellinger, 2017; Bosley & Daveluy, 2015.

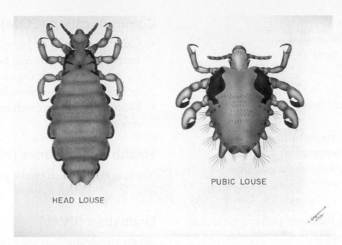

HEAD LOUSE   PUBIC LOUSE

FIG. 2.5 Two types of lice. Note the claws used to grasp onto individual hairs.

All three types of lice are spread by close person-to-person contact and feed on human blood (Centers for Disease Control and Prevention [CDC], 2013). Head lice are common among children and are often a problem in schools or camps, as discussed in Boxe 2.7. Body lice, the only type of lice known to spread disease, are usually found only in individuals with poor hygiene. Infestation can be treated with a bath and change of clothes. Pubic lice are usually only found on adults and may be found in coarse hair in other areas of the body. Pubic lice are spread through sexual contact.

Both over-the-counter and prescription medications are available for the treatment of lice infestations. These medications are insecticides. They are safe and effective when the package instructions are precisely followed; however, overuse or misuse can be dangerous. Note that many products do not kill the eggs, which are called nits. A second treatment is generally recommended within 7 to 9 days in order to kill any surviving hatched lice before they produce new eggs. Some products are not approved for children under the age of 2.

APPLICATION OF THE NURSING PROCESS

Examples of Related ICNP Nursing Diagnoses, Expected Client Outcomes, and Nursing Interventions:

Nursing Diagnosis: Lack of knowledge of treatment regime

Expected Client Outcome: Client (or parent if client is a child) will participate in the learning process and treatment regime, verbalize understanding of therapeutic treatment and measures to prevent lice infestation, perform necessary procedures correctly, and explain reasons for the actions.

Nursing Intervention Examples: Teach the family the therapeutic treatment. Ask the family to explain back to you how to use the prescription medication for lice.

Reference: International Classification for Nursing Practice. (n.d.). *eHealth & ICNP.* Retrieved from https://www.icn.ch/what-we-do/projects/ehealth-icnp.

BOX 2.7 Lifespan Considerations: Facts About Head Lice in Children

- In the United States, approximately 6 to 12 million children between the ages of 3 and 11 become infested with head lice every year.
- Head lice infestation is not related to the cleanliness of the child or the child's home environment.
- Head lice are spread by direct head-to-head contact with a person who already has head lice. This contact frequently occurs when children, especially girls, play together. Such contact is common among children during play at home, school, day care, or camp.
- Lice are occasionally spread through the sharing of hats and scarves, combs and brushes, and pillows and bedding.
- Head lice infestation is much less common among African Americans than other ethnicities. The head louse in the United States may have claws that are not suited to grasping African American hair shafts.

Reference: Centers for Disease Control and Prevention, 2015.

CRITICAL CONCEPTS
Providing Hair Care

Accuracy (ACC)

Providing hair care to the client is subject to the following variables:
- assessment of client, including mobility, level of discomfort, cooperation, and activity intolerance
- assessment of client's hair and scalp
- identification of anatomical landmarks
- time
- accurate musculoskeletal movement
- understanding of procedure by client and family.

Client-Centered Care (CCC)

When providing hair care, respect for the client is demonstrated through:
- promoting autonomy
- providing privacy
- ensuring comfort

- honoring cultural preferences
- arranging for an interpreter, as needed
- advocating for the client and family.

Infection Control (INF)

When providing hair care, client infection and healthcare infestation are prevented by
- containment of microorganisms and lice
- reducing the transfer of microorganisms and lice
- reducing the number of microorganisms and lice.

Safety (SAF)

When providing hair care, safety measures prevent harm and maintain a safe care environment by:
- reducing risk though adherence to specific product or facility instructions.

Communication (COM)

- Communication exchanges information (oral, written, or nonverbal or electronic) between two or more people.
- Collaboration with the client, the client's family, and other healthcare professionals improves care.
- Documentation records information in a permanent legal record.

Health Maintenance (HLTH)

Nursing is dedicated to the promotion of health and abilities related to personal hygiene.

Evaluation (EVAL)

When providing hair care, evaluation of outcomes enables the nurse to determine the efficacy of the care provided.

■ SKILL 2.12 Shampooing a Nonambulatory Client's Hair

EQUIPMENT

Two towels
Warm water
Pitcher to pour water or spray nozzle
Receptacle for drainage water, if needed
Shampoo
Conditioner, according to client's preference or need
Client's hair-care products
Comb and/or brush
Clean gloves, if there is a risk of exposure to body fluids

BEGINNING THE SKILL

1. **INF** Perform hand hygiene.
2. **INF** Apply gloves if there is a risk of exposure to body fluids.
3. **CCC** Introduce yourself to the client and family and explain the procedure.
4. **SAF** Identify the client using two identifiers.
5. **CCC** Provide privacy; close the door and pull the curtain.

PROCEDURE

6. **SAF** Set up an ergonomically safe space. Raise the bed to a comfortable working height. Raise one side rail. *Setting up an ergonomically safe space prevents injury to the nurse and client.*
7. **ACC** Assess the client's degree of mobility, level of discomfort, cooperation, and activity intolerance. *Your assessment is to determine the extent to which the client can assist with hair care.*
8. **CCC** Assess for hearing aids or glasses that should be removed before the shampoo.
9. **CCC** Assess the preferences of the client, including the timing of shampoo and the type of hair-care products.

10. **HLTH** Assess the hair-care needs of the client in order to maintain healthy hair, such as the need for conditioner.
11. **SAF** Assess for the presence of blood or debris in the client's hair that would require special care.
12. **SAF** Assess the need for handling equipment, such as a hoist or sliding sheets. *Implementing safe handling and movement standards prevents injury to the nurse and client.*
13. **SAF** Assess the client's medical equipment to determine the risk of electrical shock.
14. **SAF** Determine the best location for the client's shampoo: gurney, wheelchair, or bed.
15. **CCC** Place disposable pads on the gurney, wheelchair, or bed to prevent them from getting wet.
16. **SAF** If shampooing on a gurney or wheelchair:
    a. Transfer the client to the gurney or wheelchair, using safe handling equipment if needed.
    b. **SAF** Position the wheelchair or gurney at the sink, and then lock all wheels. *Locking the wheels prevents inadvertent movement and falls.*
17. **CCC** Place a towel around the client's neck and shoulders. *The towel prevents the clothing or gown from getting wet.*
18. **CCC** Place the shampoo assistive device under the client's head and adjust the neck for comfort and to prevent water from leaking.
19. **SAF** If shampooing in bed, position a drainage receptacle away from your feet but so that it collects the water. Pour or spray a small amount of water into the molded shelf. *This tests the drainage and ensures the water drains into the sink or drainage receptacle.*
20. **CCC** Fold a washcloth and lay it on the client's forehead. *This helps to prevent water and shampoo from getting into the client's eyes.*
21. **ACC** Pour or spray water along the client's hairline from ear to ear, rinsing the hair.

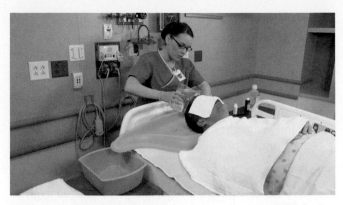

STEP 21 Rinse the hair.

22. **ACC** Place shampoo in your hands and work the shampoo into your client's hair, distributing the shampoo evenly throughout the hair.

23. **CCC** Gently rub the scalp with your fingertips. *Rubbing the scalp will facilitate cleaning the scalp and hair, increase circulation, and relax the client.*

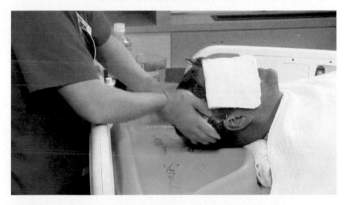

STEP 23 Gently rub the scalp.

24. **ACC** Pour or spray water along the hairline again, from ear to ear, to rinse the shampoo from the hair.

25. **CCC** Ensure the hair is thoroughly rinsed.
26. **CCC** If conditioner is to be used, rub a small amount in the palms of your hands and work it through the hair.
27. **CCC** Rinse the hair thoroughly, or leave the conditioner in and comb it through the hair, depending on the client's needs.
28. If the hair is long enough, squeeze the hair to remove any excess water.
29. **CCC** Wrap a towel around the client's hair, turban style. *Wrapping the hair helps to prevent chilling the client and assists with drying the hair.*
30. Remove the shampoo assistive device and empty the drainage receptacle. Discard the disposable pads.
31. **CCC** Towel dry the client's hair to prevent temperature loss from evaporation. Use a second dry towel to ensure the client is thoroughly dry, if needed.
32. **CCC** Comb through clean hair to remove tangles and help to dry the hair.
33. **SAF** Use a hair dryer if needed and available. *Hair dryers brought from home may not be permitted or may require a safety check prior to use in the facility.*
34. **CCC** Allow the client or client's family to style the client's hair, if possible. If not, the nurse styles the hair as closely as possible to the client's preferences. (Note: For clients who do not have a styling preference, if the client's hair is long enough, a simple loose braid will keep it from tangling.)

FINISHING THE SKILL

35. **INF** Remove gloves and perform hand hygiene.
36. **SAF** Ensure client safety. Place the bed in the lowest position and lower the side rail. Place the call light in reach. *These safety measures reduce the risk of falls.*
37. **CCC** Provide comfort. Assist the client with positioning and rearranging the bedding.
38. **EVAL** Evaluate outcomes.
39. **COM** Document assessment findings, care given, and outcomes in the legal healthcare record.

■ SKILL 2.13 Shampooing a Client With a Dry-Shampoo Cap

EQUIPMENT

Dry-shampoo cap package
Microwave, if recommended by dry-shampoo cap manufacturer
Comb and/or brush
Clean gloves, if there is a risk of exposure to body fluids
Two towels

BEGINNING THE SKILL

1. **INF** Perform hand hygiene.
2. **INF** Apply gloves if there is a risk of exposure to body fluids.
3. **CCC** Introduce yourself to the client and family and explain the procedure.

4. **SAF** Identify the client using two identifiers.
5. **CCC** Provide privacy; close the door and pull the curtain.

PROCEDURE

6. **SAF** Set up an ergonomically safe space to prevent injury to the nurse and client. Position the client sitting up, if possible. *Setting up an ergonomically safe space prevents injury to the nurse and client.*
7. **ACC** Assess the client's degree of mobility, level of discomfort, cooperation, and activity intolerance. *Your assessment is to determine the extent to which the client can assist with hair care.*

8. **CCC** Place a towel around the client's neck and shoulders to prevent the product from getting on the client's gown or clothing.
9. **SAF** Follow the specific directions on the dry-shampoo package. (Note: Some packages are placed in the microwave to warm the contents.)
10. Place the shampoo cap on the client's head.
11. **CCC** Gently rub the scalp with your fingertips through the bag to distribute the dry shampoo evenly in the hair and scalp. *Rubbing the scalp will facilitate cleaning the scalp and hair, increase circulation, and relax the client.*

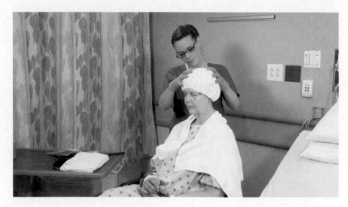

STEP 10 Gently rub the scalp.

12. **ACC** Wait the prescribed amount of time.
13. Remove and discard the shampoo cap.
14. **CCC** Comb through clean hair to remove tangles.
15. **CCC** Allow the client or client's family to style the client's hair, if possible. If not, style the hair as closely as possible to the client's preferences. (Note: For clients who do not have a styling preference, if the client's hair is long enough, a simple loose braid will keep it from tangling.)

FINISHING THE SKILL

16. **INF** Remove gloves, if used, and perform hand hygiene.
17. **SAF** Ensure client safety. Place the bed in the lowest position. Verify that the client can identify and reach the nurse call system. *These safety measures reduce the risk of falls.*
18. **CCC** Provide comfort. Assist the client with positioning and rearranging the bedding.
19. **EVAL** Evaluate outcomes.
20. **COM** Document assessment findings, care given, and outcomes in the legal healthcare record.

■ SKILL 2.14 Shaving a Client

EQUIPMENT

Warm, damp towel or washcloth
Shaving cream/gel or shaving soap
Clean gloves, if there is a risk of exposure to body fluids
Safety razor
Basin of warm water
Two towels
Aftershave lotion, according to client's preference

BEGINNING THE SKILL

1. **INF** Perform hand hygiene.
2. **INF** Apply gloves if there is a risk of exposure to body fluids.
3. **CCC** Introduce yourself to the client and family and explain the procedure.
4. **SAF** Identify the client using two identifiers.
5. **CCC** Provide privacy; close the door and pull the curtain.

PROCEDURE

6. **SAF** Determine if the client has a bleeding disorder. *Clients with bleeding disorders require additional care with shaving in order not to cause bleeding.*
7. **SAF** Set up an ergonomically safe space to prevent injury to the nurse and client. Position the client sitting up, if possible. *Setting up an ergonomically safe space prevents injury to the nurse and client.*

8. **SAF** If using an electric razor, check facility policy. *Many facilities require a safety check of electrical equipment brought from home, and some facilities do not permit their use.*
9. **ACC** Assess the client's degree of mobility, level of discomfort, cooperation, and activity intolerance. *Your assessment is to determine the extent to which the client can assist with shaving.*
10. **CCC** Place a clean, dry towel over the client's chest.
11. **CCC** If using a safety razor, place a warm, damp towel on the beard to soften the hair, and then apply shaving cream, gel, or shaving soap generously to the beard area.

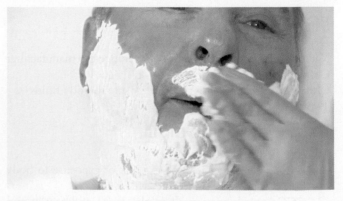

STEP 11 Apply shaving cream to the beard area.

12. **ACC** Hold the skin taut and shave in short strokes in the direction of the hair growth, which is downward on the face. After every few strokes, rinse the razor in the basin of warm water.

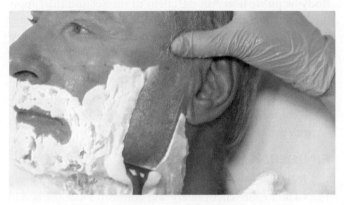

STEP 12 Shave in short strokes.

13. Shaving may be done in a variety of patterns. A suggested pattern is as follows:
    a. Shave on the cheek from beard line to jawline, moving from the area in front of the ear toward the mouth.
    b. Repeat this procedure with the other cheek.
    c. Shave the upper lip and chin area.
    d. To complete the shave, have the client tip his head back to expose his neck. Shave from the jawline down toward the neck to the end of the beard line.
14. **CCC** When finished shaving, wipe any remaining shaving foam from client's face with a damp towel or washcloth.
15. **CCC** If the client wants aftershave lotion, apply a small amount in your hands and pat onto the client's face.
16. Remove the towel on the client's chest.
17. **INF** Rinse and dry the basin; clean and store the razor.

FINISHING THE SKILL

18. **INF** Remove gloves, if used, and perform hand hygiene.
19. **SAF** Ensure client safety. Place the bed in the lowest position and lower the side rail. Place the call light in reach. *These safety measures reduce the risk of falls.*
20. **CCC** Provide comfort. Assist the client with positioning and rearranging the bedding.
21. **EVAL** Evaluate outcomes.
22. **COM** Document assessment findings, care given, and outcomes in the legal healthcare record.

▪ SKILL 2.15 Caring for a Client With Lice

EQUIPMENT

Isolation bags
Clean linen
Change of clothing or gown for client
Treatment shampoo (for head lice infestation)
Treatment lotion or cream (for body or pubic lice infestation)
Clean gloves
Fine-tooth comb or nit comb
Tongue blades
Disinfectant for comb
Towels
Tissues

BEGINNING THE SKILL

1. **INF** Perform hand hygiene.
2. **INF** Apply gloves.
3. **CCC** Introduce yourself to the client and family and explain the procedure.
4. **SAF** Identify the client using two identifiers.
5. **CCC** Provide privacy; close the door and pull the curtain.

PROCEDURE

6. **SAF** Set up an ergonomically safe space to prevent injury to the nurse and client. Position the client sitting up, if possible. *Setting up an ergonomically safe space prevents injury to the nurse and client.*

7. **ACC** Under a bright light, assess the condition of the client's hair and scalp. Tongue blades can be used to lift the hair and examine the scalp and base of the hair shaft. The use of a small magnifying glass may be helpful. *Misdiagnosis of lice infestation is common. Seeing live lice is the best determination.* (Note: Finding nits within 0.6 cm (1/4 inch) of the base of the hair shaft suggests but does not confirm an infestation. Nits are frequently seen behind the ears and near the back of the neck (CDC, 2013).

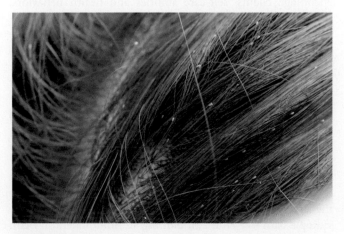

STEP 7 Examine the hair and scalp.

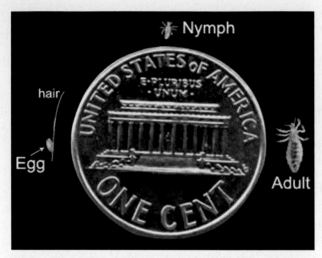

STEP 7 Seeing live lice is the best determination.

8. **INF** If lice are present, remove and bag all clothing and bed linens separately. Provide the client a clean gown.
9. **SAF** Treat the lice.

Head lice: Shampoo according to the package instructions. When using treatment shampoo for lice, follow the package directions precisely because overexposure to treatment shampoo can have toxic effects.

Body or pubic lice: Ask the client to shower and then apply the treatment lotion or cream according to the package instructions. When using treatment lotion for lice, follow the package directions precisely because overexposure to treatment lotion or cream can have toxic effects.

10. **SAF** Rinse thoroughly and towel dry.
11. **ACC** For head lice, comb through the hair with a fine-tooth comb. The shampoo kit may contain a nit comb to remove nits.

FINISHING THE SKILL

12. **INF** Remove gloves and perform hand hygiene.
13. **CCC** Ensure client safety and comfort. Place the bed in the lowest position and lower the side rail. Place the call light in reach. *These safety measures reduce the risk of falls.*
14. **EVAL** Evaluate outcomes.
15. **COM** Document assessment findings, care given, and outcomes in the legal healthcare record.

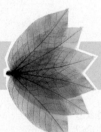

SECTION 4　Eye and Ear Care

Caring for the eyes and ears is vital to maintaining accurate sensory input for clients. Sensory input, such as seeing and hearing clearly, is required for most people in order to maintain optimal communication and their own self-care abilities and health behaviors. Nurses assess clients' activity level, cognitive function, and degree of mobility and discomfort to determine the extent to which clients can perform independent self-care. Additionally, nurses support and encourage clients' self-care abilities and health behaviors, including the ability to provide their own eye and ear care. If a client is able to assist with or perform eye and ear care independently, nurses assess and evaluate the client's knowledge and practice of eye and ear care in order to ensure safe and healthy practices. For example, improper care of contact lenses can result in eye infection or irritation.

In order to promote autonomy, an aspect of client-centered care, clients should be given the supplies needed to care for their own eyes and ears. Clients should be encouraged to make decisions regarding the products and the timing of their eye and ear care. If a client is unable to remove contact lenses or is unconscious, the nurse should remove, clean, and store the lenses. Routine eye and ear cleaning are included in providing a bath (see Skill 2.3, Bathing an Adult Client in Bed). Unconscious, sedated, or medically paralyzed clients may have a diminished or absent blink reflex and therefore require eye care in order to prevent drying.

As our population continues to age, nurses will increasingly have clients who use hearing aids. Hearing aids come in a variety of types and brands, but many have very small components and complicated circuitry. They require careful handling, and maintenance usually requires a hearing aid professional. Here are a few general care recommendations:

- Do not use water, cleaning fluids, solvents, or rubbing alcohol to clean a hearing aid.
- Do not drop a hearing aid on a hard surface. Handle a hearing aid over a soft surface in case it slips through your fingers.
- Avoid heat, including direct sunlight.
- Avoid chemicals, including sprays and body products.
- Protect hearing aids from moisture. Do not store them in a humid bathroom. Do not allow the client to wear them for showering or bathing.
- Keep hearing aids clean with either a soft dry cloth or with a special moist cleansing wipe, designed especially for that hearing aid.
- Keep hearing aids safe within their designated storage compartment.

Like dentures, hearing aids can be very expensive. Just as nurses strive to maintain their clients' health, so, too, do nurses strive to ensure no harm comes to clients' valuable belongings, such as dentures and hearing aids.

APPLICATION OF THE NURSING PROCESS

Examples of Related ICNP Nursing Diagnoses, Expected Client Outcomes, and Nursing Interventions:

Nursing Diagnosis: Impaired ability to perform hygiene

Expected Client Outcome: Client will participate in eye and ear care to the extent possible without changes in vital signs or pain level.

Nursing Intervention Example: Provide the client the supplies needed to care for his or her eyes and ears.

Reference: International Classification for Nursing Practice. (n.d.). *eHealth & ICNP.* Retrieved from https://www.icn.ch/what-we-do/projects/ehealth-icnp.

CRITICAL CONCEPTS
Eye and Ear Care

Accuracy (ACC)

Providing eye and ear care to the client is subject to the following variables:
- assessment of client, including mobility, level of discomfort, cooperation, and activity intolerance
- assessment of client's eyes and ears
- identification of anatomical landmarks
- time
- accurate musculoskeletal movement
- understanding of procedure by client and family.

Client-Centered Care (CCC)

When providing eye and ear care, respect for the client is demonstrated through:
- promoting autonomy

- providing privacy
- ensuring comfort
- honoring cultural preferences
- arranging for an interpreter, as needed
- advocating for the client and family.

Infection Control (INF)

When providing eye and ear care, client infection and healthcare-associated infection are prevented by
- containment of microorganisms
- reducing the transfer of microorganisms
- reducing the number of microorganisms.

Safety (SAF)

When providing eye and ear care, safety measures prevent harm and maintain a safe care environment.

Communication (COM)

- Communication exchanges information (oral, written, nonverbal or electronic) between two or more people.
- Documentation records information in a permanent legal record.

Health Maintenance (HLTH)

Nursing is dedicated to the promotion of health and abilities related to personal hygiene.

Evaluation (EVAL)

When providing eye and ear care, evaluation of outcomes enables the nurse to determine the efficacy of the care provided.

■ SKILL 2.16 Providing Eye Care for an Unconscious Client

EQUIPMENT

Clean gloves
Normal saline
Washcloth or cotton balls
Eye drops or ointment, as ordered

BEGINNING THE SKILL

1. **INF** Perform hand hygiene.
2. **INF** Apply gloves.
3. **CCC** Introduce yourself and explain the procedure to family members present.
4. **SAF** Identify the client using two identifiers.
5. **CCC** Provide privacy; close the door and pull the curtain.

PROCEDURE

6. **SAF** Set up an ergonomically safe space to prevent injury to the nurse and client. Raise the bed to a comfortable working height. *Setting up an ergonomically safe space prevents injury to the nurse and client.*
7. **ACC** Assess for a blink reflex (see Skill 4.5).

8. **ACC** Wipe the eyes from nose to ear using water and a cotton ball or soft disposable wipe. *This cleans substances away from the opening of the lacrimal duct.*

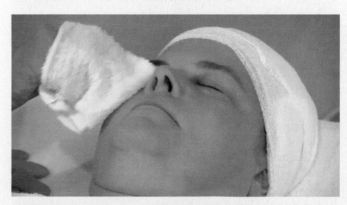

STEP 8 Wipe the eye from nose to ear.

9. **INF** Wipe the other eye with a different section of the wipe or another cotton ball. *This prevents cross-contamination of eye organisms.*

10. **ACC** If there is any dried discharge, place the moist cloth or cotton ball on the discharge until it is softened and will wipe off.
11. If there is an order for eye drops or ointment, apply as ordered (see Chapter 11).

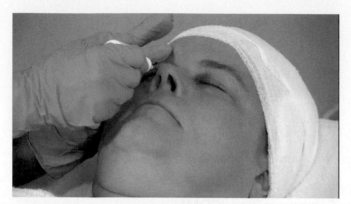

STEP 11 Apply eye drops or ointment.

FINISHING THE SKILL

12. **INF** Remove gloves and perform hand hygiene.

13. **SAF** Ensure client safety. Place the bed in the lowest position. Verify that the client can identify and reach the nurse call system. *These safety measures reduce the risk of falls.*
14. **CCC** Ensure client comfort. Position the client and rearrange the bedding.
15. **EVAL** Evaluate outcomes.
16. **COM** Document assessment findings, care given, and outcomes in the legal healthcare record.

■ SKILL 2.17 Removing and Cleaning Contact Lenses

EQUIPMENT

Clean gloves
Contact lens container
Cleaning and/or disinfecting solution for soft lenses or rigid lenses as appropriate

BEGINNING THE SKILL

1. **INF** Perform hand hygiene.
2. **INF** Apply gloves.
3. **CCC** Introduce yourself and explain the procedure to client and family members present. Determine if the client is able to remove contact lenses. The nurse removes the lenses if the client is unable to do so.
4. **SAF** Identify the client using two identifiers.
5. **CCC** Provide privacy; close the door and pull the curtain.

PROCEDURE

6. **SAF** Set up an ergonomically safe space to prevent injury to the nurse and client. Raise the bed to a comfortable working height. *Setting up an ergonomically safe space prevents injury to the nurse and client.*
7. **ACC** Assess both eyes for contact lenses. *Some individuals wear only one lens.*
8. **ACC** Determine the position of the lens on the eye.
9. Remove the lens from the eye.

For soft contact lenses:
   a. **ACC** Hold the eye open using the nondominant hand by positioning your thumb on the lower lid and forefinger on the upper lid.

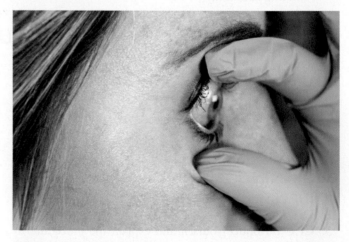

STEP 9A Hold the eye open.

   b. **ACC** Locate the lens on the eye.
   c. **ACC** Using your dominant hand, gently squeeze the lens between your thumb and forefinger.

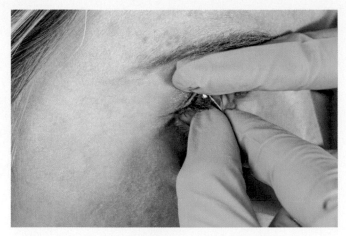

STEP 9C Gently squeeze the lens between thumb and forefinger.

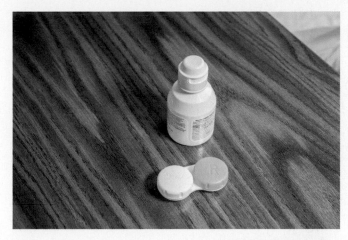

STEP 12 Store lens in the contact lens container with solution.

d. Remove the lens from the eye.

For rigid contact lenses:

    a. **ACC** If the client is able to follow directions, pull laterally on the lateral canthus of the eye and ask the client to blink. Be prepared to catch the contact. The blink should result in dislodging the contact.

10. **INF** To clean the contact lens, follow the instructions on the cleaning solution label.
11. **INF** Rinse with lens cleanser.
12. **SAF** Store lens in the contact lens container with solution. The lens container should have one side marked for the right lens and one marked for the left lens; be sure to place each lens in the correct side of the container.

13. Repeat removal, cleaning, and storage with the other lens.
14. **CCC** If the client has glasses, offer them at this time.

FINISHING THE SKILL

15. **INF** Remove gloves and perform hand hygiene.
16. **SAF** Ensure client safety and comfort. Place the bed in the lowest position and lower the side rail. Place the call light in reach. *These safety measures reduce the risk of falls.*
17. **EVAL** Evaluate outcomes.
18. **COM** Document assessment findings, care given, and outcomes in the legal healthcare record.

■ SKILL 2.18 Removing, Cleaning, and Inserting an Artificial Eye

EQUIPMENT

Clean gloves
Washcloth
Towel
Mild soap
Water or normal saline solution

BEGINNING THE SKILL

1. **INF** Perform hand hygiene.
2. **INF** Apply gloves.
3. **CCC** Introduce yourself and explain the procedure to client and family members present. Determine if the client is able to remove and clean the artificial eye or requires assistance.
4. **SAF** Identify the client using two identifiers.
5. **CCC** Provide privacy; close the door and pull the curtain.

PROCEDURE

6. **SAF** Set up an ergonomically safe space to prevent injury to the nurse and client. Raise the bed to a comfortable working height. *Setting up an ergonomically safe space prevents injury to the nurse and client.*
7. **CCC** Assess the client's accustomed method of cleaning the artificial eye.

8. **CCC** Assess the preferences of the client, including timing and products for eye care.
9. **ACC** Hold the eye open using the thumb and forefinger of your nondominant hand on the upper lid and your dominant hand on the lower lid.
10. **ACC** Depress the lower lid and slide the prosthesis out.

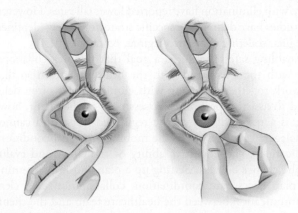

STEPS 9 AND 10 Hold the eye open, depress the lower lid, and slide the prosthesis out.

11. **INF** Wash the prosthesis with water and mild soap. Rinse thoroughly. *Washing and rinsing prosthetic eyes reduces irritation and infection.*
12. **INF** Rinse the empty eye socket with water or normal saline.
13. **HLTH** Assess the tissue within the eye socket for swelling or drainage.
14. **INF** Wipe the eye from nose to ear using water and a cotton ball or soft disposable wipe. *This cleans substances away from the opening of the lacrimal duct.*
15. **INF** Wet the prosthesis with water or normal saline, lift the upper lid, and slide the prosthesis into place.

FINISHING THE SKILL

16. **INF** Remove gloves and perform hand hygiene.
17. **SAF** Ensure client safety and comfort. Place the bed in the lowest position and lower the side rail. Place the call light in reach. *These safety measures reduce the risk of falls.*
18. **EVAL** Evaluate outcomes.
19. **COM** Document assessment findings, care given, and outcomes in the legal healthcare record.

SECTION 5   Assisting With Elimination

Clients may need assistance in elimination in healthcare facilities, long-term care, assisted living, and in their homes. Nurses may provide multidimensional interventions to assist a client with elimination, such as environmental adjustments, changing medications to reduce sedation, and/or promoting mobility through exercise and collaboration with physical therapy (Tzeng & Yin, 2012). When nurses provide assistance with elimination in an acute care setting, key concepts are safety, client-centered care, collaboration, and health maintenance.

APPLYING CONCEPTS OF SAFETY, CLIENT-CENTERED CARE, COLLABORATION, AND HEALTH MAINTENANCE

Safety issues are paramount when assisting with elimination. Studies have shown that about half of the falls in acute-care facilities are elimination-related (Sivapurim, 2018; Tzeng, 2010). Some studies have shown more serious injury with falls related to toileting. Risk factors for elimination-related falls include age and cognitive impairment, including impaired judgment about toileting. Units that implement regular assistance with elimination have reported lower fall rates. However, no studies have defined the specific strategies loosely identified as regular toileting (Barrett, Vizgirda, & Zhou, 2017).

Enabling safe toileting is a goal that requires collaboration with the client and with the healthcare team so that all work together. Assisting with elimination is often delegated to assistive personnel. Assessment of the client, however, is a responsibility of the registered nurse and cannot be delegated. Nurses assess the mobility, medical condition, medications, and cognitive ability of the client and evaluate the client's fall risk. Setting up a plan and implementing the plan necessitate coordination, collaboration, and clear communication between the healthcare team and the client. A study examining the perceptions of registered nurses and patient care technicians revealed the critical need for effective communication, including the sharing impact of the client's medications and medical condition (Barrett et al., 2017).

Providing privacy, an element of client-centered care and maintaining safety is a balancing act. Elimination is a very private act, and protecting dignity is important. Many people are uncomfortable with having a nurse present while they eliminate. However, given the number of falls that occur each year during toileting, many clients should not be left alone when they are on a bedpan or a bedside commode. When staying with clients on a bedpan or bedside commode, you can make them more comfortable by giving them a little space and some noise to cover the sound of eliminating. Running the water at the sink and flushing the toilet in the bathroom are examples of sounds that help promote urination and enhance clients' sense of privacy.

Health maintenance is also a concern in assisting with elimination. Nursing interventions related to maintaining client strength, balance, and mobility have been identified as an element of functional independence, including toileting. Without timely assistance with elimination, clients may have incontinence and accidental soiling, resulting in increased risk for impaired skin integrity and the risk of acquiring a healthcare-associated infection, for example, an *S. aureus* infection in a pressure injury.

BEDSIDE COMMODE, URINALS, BEDPANS, AND CONDOM CATHETERS

There are several methods to assist the client with elimination. The client's mobility is the most significant factor in determining which method is selected. This section includes skills for assisting with elimination using a bedside commode, a urinal, and a bedpan, as well as for applying a condom catheter. For clients who can safely transfer but who are not able to ambulate to and from the toilet, a bedside commode is an option. The bedside commode is a portable chair with a toilet seat and waste receptacle that can be removed

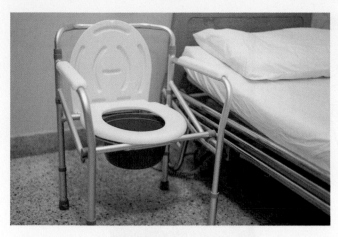

FIG. 2.6 Bedside commode.

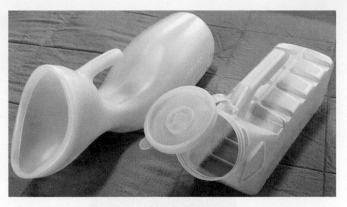

FIG. 2.7 Female urinal (*left*) and male urinal (*right*).

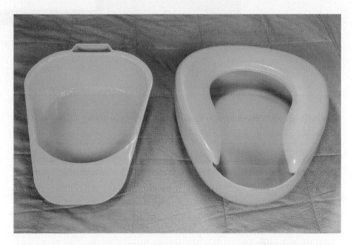

FIG. 2.8 Two types of bedpans. Fracture pan *(left)* and full-size bedpan *(right)*.

and emptied (Fig. 2.6). The advantage of using the bedside commode is that it is most like using a toilet. When clients are restricted to bed or cannot safely transfer, they may use a urinal to urinate (Fig. 2.7). Urinals for women are shaped differently from urinals for men. Use of a urinal for women is fairly new, and so when presented with the option, some women may prefer to use a bedpan. Some men have difficulty voiding while sitting. Assisting male clients into a standing position, even if leaning against the side of the bed and not fully bearing their own weight, may facilitate voiding. Both sexes will need to use a bedpan to pass a bowel movement if they cannot transfer to a bedside commode.

Types of bedpans include a full-size bedpan and a fracture pan. The full-size bedpan is shaped like a toilet seat and is positioned under the client with the closed, rounded end at the client's sacrum. If clients are able to flex their hips, they may use a full-size bedpan. When clients are not permitted to flex their hips or unable to lift their hips, a fracture pan can be used. The low rim on the fracture pan permits easier positioning for clients with restricted hip movement (Fig. 2.8). For incontinent men, a condom catheter is an external device that allows urine management. A condom-like sheath is placed over the penis and attached to drainage tubing and a collection bag (Fig. 2.9). Advantages of the condom catheter include a lower risk of urinary tract infections compared with an indwelling catheter and the prevention of skin breakdown from incontinence. The disadvantages include a risk of skin breakdown on the penis and difficulty keeping the sheath in place, as discussed in Box 2.8. New on the market is an external female catheter that uses low-pressure wall suction combined with an absorbent wicking gauze surface. The external female catheter may remain in position between the labia for eight to 12 hours (Fig. 2.10).

APPLICATION OF THE NURSING PROCESS

Examples of Related ICNP Nursing Diagnoses, Expected Client Outcomes, and Nursing Interventions:

Nursing Diagnosis: Impaired self-toileting

Supporting Data: Client on bedrest

Expected Client Outcome: Client will demonstrate the ability to use adaptive devices to facilitate toileting or will agree to ask for assistance when needed.

Nursing Intervention Example: Collaborate with the client to provide a client-centered toileting regimen.

Reference: International Classification for Nursing Practice. (n.d.). *eHealth & ICNP.* Retrieved from https://www.icn.ch/what-we-do/projects/ehealth-icnp.

CRITICAL CONCEPTS
Assisting With Elimination

Accuracy (ACC)

Assisting the client with elimination is subject to the following variables:

- assessment of client, including cognitive ability, mobility, level of discomfort, cooperation, and activity intolerance
- identification of anatomical landmarks
- identification of accurate musculoskeletal movement
- measurement of urinary output
- understanding of procedure by client and family.

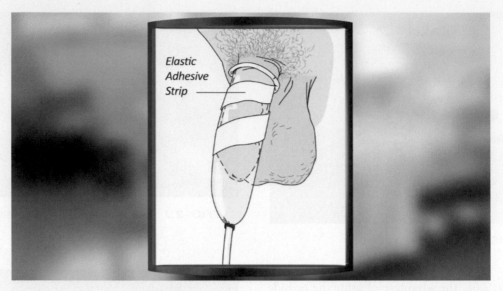

FIG. 2.9 Condom catheter.

BOX 2.8 Lessons From Experience: Evaluating a Condom Catheter

Kelsey was in a clinical rotation on a medical-surgical unit. In the change-of-shift report, she was told that the nurse caring for Mr. Long had secured his condom catheter three times during the night and that at 0600, the catheter was secure. Mr. Long, an 87-year-old, was on his second day post-op for a below-the-knee amputation due to severe peripheral vascular disease secondary to his diabetes.

Kelsey entered Mr. Long's room, introduced herself to him, and began a head-to-toe assessment. To begin her genitourinary assessment, she said, "Mr. Long, I need to check your catheter." She provided privacy, draping the client so that only his genitals were exposed. The condom catheter was secure, but something looked odd. The head of his penis appeared much larger than the shaft.

Kelsey decided to check with her instructor before removing the condom catheter because she knew it had been very difficult to secure. Kelsey and her instructor returned to the client's room, and together they removed the condom catheter and unfastened the wrap. Mr. Long's penis was swollen to about twice its normal size distal to the Velcro wrap. The Velcro had been too tight, and Mr. Long's penis had had insufficient circulation.

Kelsey's nursing instructor said, "Kelsey, it's good that you discovered this. It can be uncomfortable to thoroughly assess the genitourinary system, but it is so important." The condom catheter was discontinued.

Summary: Managing a client's elimination needs requires the evaluation of the outcomes associated with each intervention. A condom catheter offers a lower risk of urinary tract infection compared with an indwelling catheter and prevents skin breakdown from incontinence. Establishing a means to keep the catheter secure without making it too tight can be worth the effort.

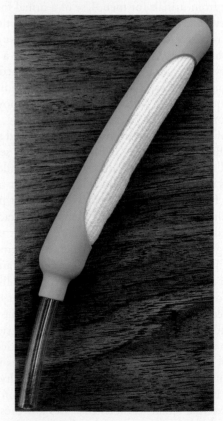

FIG. 2.10 A female external catheter.

Client-Centered Care (CCC)

When assisting with elimination, respect for the client is demonstrated through:

- promoting autonomy
- providing privacy
- ensuring comfort

- protecting dignity
- honoring cultural preferences
- arranging for an interpreter, as needed
- advocating for the client and family.

Infection Control (INF)

When assisting with elimination, client infection and healthcare-associated infection are prevented by:
- containment of microorganisms
- preventing and reducing the transfer of microorganisms
- reducing the number of microorganisms.

Safety (SAF)

When assisting with elimination, safety measures prevent harm and maintain a safe care environment.

Communication (COM)

- Communication exchanges information (oral, written, nonverbal or electronic) between two or more people.
- Collaboration with the client and other healthcare providers is essential to achieve safe toileting.
- Documentation records information in a permanent legal record.

Health Maintenance (HLTH)

Nursing is dedicated to the promotion of health and abilities when assisting with elimination.

Evaluation (EVAL)

When assisting with elimination, evaluation of outcomes enables the nurse to determine the efficacy of the care provided.

■ SKILL 2.19 Assisting a Client Using a Bedside Commode

EQUIPMENT

Bedside commode
Toilet paper
Clean gloves

BEGINNING THE SKILL

1. **INF** Perform hand hygiene.
2. **INF** Apply gloves.
3. **CCC** Introduce yourself to the client and family and explain the procedure.
4. **SAF** Identify the client using two identifiers.
5. **CCC** Provide privacy; close the door and pull the curtain.

PROCEDURE

6. **SAF** Set up an ergonomically safe space to prevent injury to the nurse and client. Position the bedside commode adjacent to the bed. (Note: Be mindful of environmental hazards that may contribute to a fall or prevent the client from toileting independently, including the height of the bed, the use of side rails, and an intravenous line.) *Setting up an ergonomically safe space prevents injury to the nurse and client.*
7. **ACC** Assess the client's orientation to person, time, place, and situation; cognitive function; degree of mobility; medications; and level of discomfort. *Your assessment is to determine the extent to which the client requires assistance with elimination.*
8. **SAF** Use the appropriate safe handling equipment. Have canes and walkers available for clients who are accustomed to using them.
9. **SAF** Position the client on the side of the bed in a sitting position with the bed in the lowest position possible and the feet firmly on the floor.

10. Transfer the client from the bed to the commode chair (see Skill 1.8).
11. **CCC** Provide call light and toilet paper for the client. If the client is not in a gown, assist the client with clothing.
12. **CCC** Provide privacy, but remain close by.
13. **INF** When the client has finished, determine if any assistance with wiping or dressing is required. For female clients, wipe from front to back. *Microorganisms from the perianal region and vaginal outlet may cause an infection if transferred to the urinary meatus.*
14. Transfer the client from the commode chair to the bed or chair (see Skill 1.8).
15. **ACC** Measure and record urine output if the client is on intake and output (I&O).
16. **INF** Empty contents of the commode chair into the toilet and rinse, disinfect, dry, and replace the pan in the commode chair.

FINISHING THE SKILL

17. **INF** Remove gloves and perform hand hygiene.
18. **SAF** Ensure client safety. Ensure that the bed is in the lowest position. Ensure that the client can identify and reach the nurse call system. *These safety measures reduce the risk of falls.*
19. **CCC** Provide comfort. Assist the client with positioning and rearranging the bedding.
20. **EVAL** Evaluate outcomes. Your evaluation includes the amount of assistance the client required and your use of appropriate safe handling equipment.
21. **COM** Document assessment of output, care given, and client outcome in the legal healthcare record.

▪ SKILL 2.20 Assisting a Client Using a Urinal

EQUIPMENT

Urinal
Toilet paper
Clean gloves

BEGINNING THE SKILL

1. **INF** Perform hand hygiene.
2. **INF** Apply gloves.
3. **CCC** Introduce yourself to the client and family and explain the procedure.
4. **SAF** Identify the client using two identifiers.
5. **CCC** Provide privacy; close the door and pull the curtain.

PROCEDURE

6. **SAF** Set up an ergonomically safe space to prevent injury to the nurse and client. Be mindful of environmental hazards that may contribute to a fall or prevent the client from toileting independently, including the height of the bed, the use of side rails, and an IV line. *Setting up an ergonomically safe space prevents injury to the nurse and client.*
7. **ACC** Assess the client's orientation to person, time, place, and situation; cognitive function; degree of mobility; medications; and level of discomfort. *Your assessment is to determine the extent to which the client requires assistance with elimination.*
8. **CCC** Assess the client's preferred position for voiding, and assist the client into a sitting or standing position.
9. **CCC** If sitting, ask the client to bend his knees, press down on his heels, and raise his hips in order to place an absorbent pad under his hips. Once the pad is in place, ask the client to lower his hips again. If the client is unable to lift the hips, the client may turn from side to side to allow positioning of the absorbent pad. *Placing the absorbent pad under the client prevents accidentally wetting the sheets.*
10. Provide the client with the urinal.
11. **ACC** If the client is unfamiliar with the use of a urinal, instruct the client to place the urinal flat between the legs, positioning the penis over the opening of the uri-

nal. Caution the client to watch the angle of the urinal as it fills to prevent urine from spilling onto the bed.
12. **ACC** If the client is unable to assist, place the urinal between his legs and position his penis over the opening of the urinal.

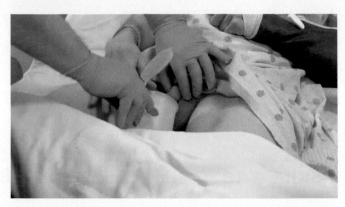

STEP 12 Position penis over urinal opening.

13. **CCC** Provide call light and toilet paper, if desired, for the client.
14. **CCC** Provide privacy, but remain close by.
15. Remove the urinal.
16. **ACC** Measure and record urine output if the client is on I&O. Note the color, clarity, and odor of the urine.
17. **INF** Empty the contents of the urinal into the toilet and rinse, dry, and replace the urinal near the bedside.
18. **INF** Remove and discard any soiled absorbent pads.

FINISHING THE SKILL

19. **INF** Remove gloves and perform hand hygiene. Assist the client to also perform hand hygiene.
20. **SAF** Ensure client safety. Ensure that the bed is in the lowest position. Ensure that the client can identify and reach the nurse call system. *These safety measures reduce the risk of falls.*
21. **CCC** Provide comfort. Assist the client with positioning and rearranging the bedding.
22. **EVAL** Evaluate outcomes. *Your evaluation includes the amount of assistance the client required.*
23. **COM** Document assessment of output, care given, and client outcome in the legal healthcare record.

▪ SKILL 2.21 Assisting a Client Using a Bedpan

EQUIPMENT

Absorbent pad
Full-size bedpan or fracture pan
Toilet paper
Clean gloves
Rolled towel

BEGINNING THE SKILL

1. **INF** Perform hand hygiene.
2. **INF** Apply gloves.
3. **CCC** Introduce yourself to the client and family and explain the procedure.
4. **SAF** Identify the client using two identifiers.

5. **CCC** Provide privacy; close the door and pull the curtain.

PROCEDURE

6. **SAF** Set up an ergonomically safe space to prevent injury to the nurse and client. Be mindful of environmental hazards which may contribute to a fall, including the height of the bed, the use of side rails, and an intravenous line. *Setting up an ergonomically safe space prevents injury to the nurse and client.*

7. **ACC** Assess the client's orientation to person, time, place, and situation; cognitive function, degree of mobility; medications; and level of discomfort. *Your assessment is to determine the extent to which the client requires assistance with elimination.*

8. **ACC** Assess the client's ability to lift and flex the hips. *Your assessment is to determine if a fracture pan or a full-sized bedpan is appropriate. If the client is unable to lift her hips or flex her hips, a fracture pan is indicated.*

9. **SAF** Assess the safe client-handling needs, such as the need for a hoist.

10. **SAF** Raise the side rail on the opposite side of the bed to provide a handrail for the client and prevent falls.

11. Position the head of the bed flat.

12. To position the client who can lift his or her hips:
    a. **CCC** Ask the client to bend the knees, press down on the heels, and raise the hips in order to place an absorbent pad under the hips. Once the pad is in place, ask the client to lower the hips again. *Placing the absorbent pad under the client prevents accidentally wetting the sheets.*
    b. **ACC** Ask the client to raise his or her hips again, and slide the bedpan under the hips. (Note: If using a full-size bedpan, the height of the bedpan creates a sizable gap at the client's lower spine. Slide a tightly rolled small towel into the gap. *Sliding a tightly rolled small towel behind the bedpan may make sitting on the bedpan more comfortable.*)

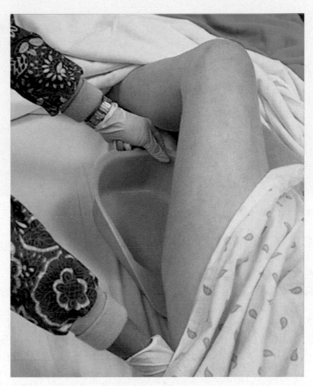

STEP 12A Slide the bedpan under the client's hips.

   c. **ACC** Raise the head of the bed, keeping a firm grip on the bedpan, until the head of the bed reaches a height where the client is sitting comfortably. *Very few people can comfortably eliminate while lying flat on the back. Raising the bed may cause the bedpan to shift, so hold it tightly until the client is in the final position.*

13. To position the client who cannot lift his or her hips:
    a. **ACC** Assist the client to roll to one side.
    b. **CCC** Place an absorbent pad under the hips. *Placing the absorbent pad under the client prevents accidentally wetting the sheets.*
    c. **ACC** Apply the bedpan to the client's buttocks.

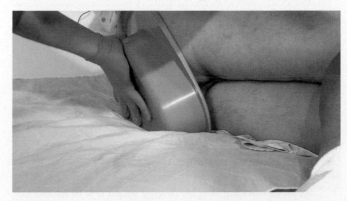

STEP 13C Apply the bedpan to the client's buttocks.

   d. Assist the client to roll onto his or her back again.

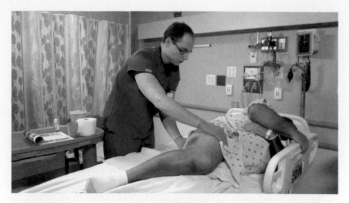

STEP 13D Assist the client onto his or her back.

14. **SAF** Provide call light and toilet paper for the client. Return bed to the lowest position, if raised.
15. **CCC** Cover client with a sheet.
16. **CCC** Remain close by, but allow the client privacy during elimination.
17. **HLTH** Assist with wiping if any assistance is required.
18. **ACC** Lower the head of the bed, keeping a hand on the bedpan, until the client can raise the hips or roll slightly to one side. Push the bedpan down into the mattress to help slide it out smoothly from under the client. *Avoiding jerky movements will help prevent urine from splashing.*

19. **INF** Cover the bedpan with an absorbent pad.
20. **HLTH** Assist with additional perineal clean-up, if needed, by having the client roll into a side-lying position. *Removing stool and urine prevents skin break down.*
21. **INF** Remove and discard any soiled absorbent pads.
22. **ACC** Measure and record urine output if the client is on I&O.
23. **INF** Empty the contents of the bedpan into the toilet and rinse, dry, and replace the bedpan near the bedside.

FINISHING THE SKILL

24. **INF** Remove gloves and perform hand hygiene. Assist the client to also perform hand hygiene.
25. **SAF** Ensure client comfort and safety. Ensure that the bed is in the lowest position. Ensure that the client can identify and reach the nurse call system. *These safety measures reduce the risk of falls.*
26. **EVAL** Evaluate outcomes. *Your evaluation includes the amount of assistance the client required and your use of appropriate safe handling equipment.*
27. **COM** Document assessment of output, care given, and client outcome in the legal healthcare record.

■ SKILL 2.22 Applying a Condom Catheter

EQUIPMENT

Basin of warm water, soap, washcloth, and towel
Condom catheter kit
Scissors
Clean gloves
Absorbent pads
Bath blanket for draping

BEGINNING THE SKILL

1. **INF** Perform hand hygiene.
2. **INF** Apply gloves.
3. **CCC** Introduce yourself and explain the procedure to client and family members present.
4. **SAF** Identify the client using two identifiers.
5. **CCC** Provide privacy; close the door and pull the curtain.

PROCEDURE

6. **SAF** Set up an ergonomically safe space to prevent injury to the nurse and client. Raise the bed to a comfortable working height. *Setting up an ergonomically safe space prevents injury to the nurse and client.*
7. **ACC** Assess the client's orientation to person, time, place, and situation; cognitive function; degree of mobility; medications; and discomfort. *Your assessment is to confirm that a condom catheter is an appropriate elimination choice.*
8. Position client supine, with the legs slightly apart.
9. **HLTH** Determine the client's level of activity. *If the client is ambulatory, a leg collection bag is preferable.*

10. **CCC** Place an absorbent pad under the client's genitalia. *Placing the absorbent pad prevents accidentally wetting the sheets.*
11. **INF** Wash and dry the penis and scrotum (see Skill 2.3, steps 57a–e).
12. **CCC** Trim pubic hair at the base of the penile shaft, if needed.
13. **ACC** Follow the manufacturer's directions in the packaged condom catheter kit.
14. **HLTH** Apply liquid skin protector to the penile shaft, if available in condom catheter kit.
15. **HLTH** Allow liquid skin protector to dry.
16. **ACC** Hold the penis with your nondominant hand. With your dominant hand, place the condom catheter over the head of the penis.

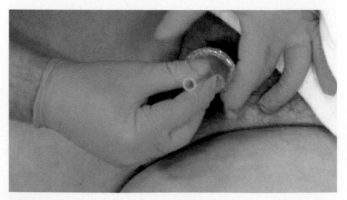

STEP 16 Place the condom catheter over the head of the penis.

17. **ACC** Roll the condom sheath down over the shaft of the penis, leaving 2.5 to 5 cm (1–2 inches) of space between the catheter tip and the head of the penis.

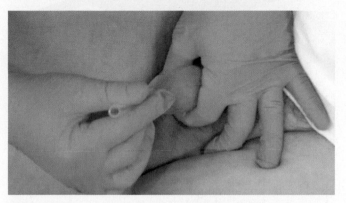

STEP 17 Roll the condom over the penis shaft.

18. **ACC** Secure the catheter according to the manufacturer's directions. Various types are available. One type has a wrap that is wrapped in a spiral on the shaft of the penis. Ensure the wrap is not too tight.

19. **ACC** Attach the funnel end of the condom to the urine collection tubing. Secure the tubing to the client's thigh.
20. **ACC** Attach the urine collection tubing to the urine bag or leg bag.
21. **CCC** Remove the disposable pad and any items from the client's bed. Cover the client with his gown and bedding.
22. **INF** Secure the collection bag below the level of the bladder.

FINISHING THE SKILL

23. **INF** Remove gloves and perform hand hygiene.
24. **SAF** Ensure client comfort and safety. Ensure that the bed is in the lowest position. Ensure that the client can identify and reach the nurse call system. *These safety measures reduce the risk of falls.*
25. **EVAL** Evaluate outcomes. Reassess the penis within 15 to 30 minutes after applying the condom catheter to assess for swelling and client comfort. *Your evaluation includes the method of securing the condom catheter and the use of a leg bag versus a collection bag.* (Note: Perform hand hygiene and apply clean gloves each time you assess the condom catheter.)
26. **COM** Document assessment of output, care given, and client outcome in the legal healthcare record.

SECTION 6 Making Beds

Upon admission to a healthcare facility, clients are routinely assigned a bed, which may be in the emergency department, a preoperative area, or in a hospital room. During their stay, clients spend most of their time in the bed—it becomes their living space. It is the responsibility of the facility and its employees to keep this space clean and free from infectious agents.

TYPES OF BEDS

Hospital beds are twin size, on a metal frame. They have wheels and brakes. Hospital beds can be adjusted to raise the head of the bed, raise the lower section of the bed with a notch for the knees, called the knee gatch, and raise or lower the height of the bed from the floor. Some beds have additional positioning capabilities, including tilting the mattress into a head-down position (Trendelenburg) or a head-up position without flexing the mattress. Some beds may have an integrated bed system rather than a separate frame and mattress. Alternative positioning capabilities allow the healthcare team to position the client for procedures, for comfort, or to promote the client's healing. Control panels for the healthcare providers' use are on the outside of the side rails and at the foot of the bed. These controls usually permit several adjustments at a time, for instance, raising the height of the bed and lowering the head of the bed. Controls for clients to use in order to reposition themselves for comfort are located on the inside of the side rail. Typically, these controls only allow the client to adjust the head of the bed and the knee gatch. Many beds also include controls for the television and the nurse call system on the side rails. Another feature included on many hospital beds is a backboard for cardiopulmonary resuscitation (CPR).

The features of hospital beds vary with different brands; exploring the types of beds at each clinical facility allows nursing students to become familiar with several different brands. Many facilities now have bariatric beds that are designed to assist with the care of the very obese client (Fig. 2.11). These heavy-duty beds accommodate weights up to 1000 lbs. Some beds can convert to a chair. Some have integrated scales that will weigh the client while in the bed.

Hospital beds sometimes have an over-bed frame, such as a Balkan frame, that is securely attached to the bed frame (Fig. 2.12). The over-bed frame allows many types of attachments to be secured, including a traction or suspension system. One common attachment is a trapeze that allows the client to pull up and assist in positioning during activities of daily living, such as bed making and bathing.

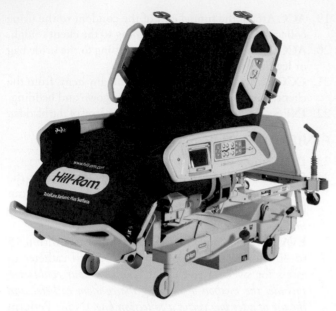

FIG. 2.11 A bariatric bed.

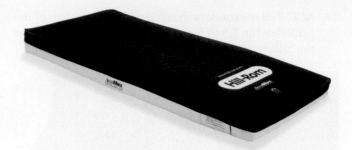

FIG. 2.13 Mattress overlay.

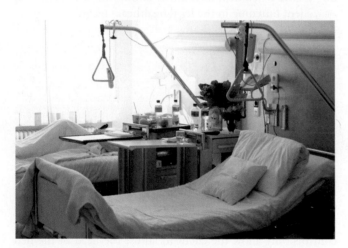

FIG. 2.12 Bed with a Balkan frame.

TYPES OF MATTRESSES

Most hospital mattresses are either inner spring or foam with a waterproof covering to ensure that the mattress does not become soiled. This type of mattress is easy to clean but does not allow air to circulate around the person. This lack of air circulation can promote diaphoresis and increased pressure on points of contact, such as bony areas like the heels. Other types of mattresses, mattress covers, or chair covers are designed to reduce pressure on points of contact.

Pressure-redistribution support surfaces are designed to prevent the formation of pressure injury or promote the healing of pressure injury by reducing the pressure on bony prominences. Most of these support surfaces reduce pressure by conforming to the contours of the body so that pressure is distributed over a larger surface area. Also, numerous types of support-surface overlays can be layered over the mattress (Fig. 2.13). The National Pressure Ulcer Advisory Panel (NPUAP, 2018) defines a support surface as "a specialized device for redistribution designed for management of tissue loads, micro-climate, and/or other therapeutic functions. Support surfaces include, but are not limited to, mattresses, integrated bed systems, mattress replacement, or overlays, or seat cushions, and seat cushion overlays." Table 2.1 describes the functional components of support surfaces as described by the NPUAP. Choosing the most appropriate support surface for the needs of the client can have legal implications, as discussed in Box 2.9.

TYPES OF BEDDING AND BED MAKING

Various items of bedding are used in making beds, as identified in Box 2.10. Unoccupied beds can be prepared in three different ways:

- **Closed bed:** The top sheet, blanket, and bedspread are pulled up at the head of the bed.
- **Open bed:** The top sheet, blanket, and bedspread are turned down at the head of the bed, ready to accept a client. A surgical bed is an example of an open bed.
- **Surgical bed:** The bed for a client who has just had surgery is open and is adjusted to be at the same height as a gurney. A surgical bed is prepared with absorbent pads appropriate for the type of surgery performed and a draw sheet to assist with turning. The surgical bed is prepared to receive a client directly from a surgical department (Fig. 2.14).

Making a bed, either occupied or unoccupied, is most easily accomplished by two people, one on each side of the bed. If a coworker is not available, the nurse makes the bed on one side and then moves to the other side, rather than repeatedly moving back and forth to each side of the bed.

TABLE 2.1 Features of Support Surfaces[a]

Feature	Definition
Air fluidized	A feature of a support surface that provides pressure redistribution by forcing air through a granular medium (e.g. beads) producing a fluid state.
Alternating pressure	A feature of a support surface that provides pressure redistribution via cyclic changes in loading and unloading as characterized by frequency, duration, amplitude, and rate of change parameters.
Lateral rotation	A feature of a support surface that provides rotation about a longitudinal axis as characterized by degree of client turn, duration, and frequency.
Low air loss	A feature of a support surface that provides air flow to assist in managing the heat and humidity (microclimate) of the skin
Multi-zoned surface	A surface in which different segments can have different pressure redistribution capabilities.
Pulsation	A feature of a support surface that provides repeating higher and lower pressures resulting in cyclic changes in stiffness of the surface, typically with shorter duration inflation/deflation, higher frequency, and lower amplitude than alternating pressure.
Reactive support surface	A powered or non-powered support surface with the capability to change its load distribution properties only in response to applied load.

[a]Features can be used alone or in combination.

Reference: National Pressure Ulcer Advisory Panel, 2018.

BOX 2.9 Lessons From the Courtroom: Pressure Ulcers and Litigation

Could Making a Bed Ever Have Legal Implications?

- Pressure ulcers are the second most common legal claim after wrongful death (Agency for Healthcare Research and Quality [AHRQ], 2014).
- Support surfaces are an important tool in the treatment and prevention of pressure ulcers.
- Selection of support surfaces may be a factor in pressure ulcer litigation.
- Documentation of the type of support surface used and any change in support surface is an important aspect of nursing care.

BOX 2.10 Types of Sheets for Bed Making

- Fitted sheet: A sheet with elastic gathered corners, also known as a contour sheet.
- Flat sheet: A sheet without elastic gathered corners that may be used as either a top sheet or a bottom sheet.
- Draw sheet: A sheet of heavier fabric that is placed across the bed from the client's shoulders to knees to facilitate moving the client. A draw sheet is kept tucked in but may be untucked when used to move the client.
- Absorbent pad: Absorbent pads are often disposable and are usually absorbent on one side and waterproof on the other.
- Bath blanket: A soft, absorbent blanket that is placed next to the client's skin and may be used to drape the client for privacy.
- Blanket: A washable blanket placed between the flat sheet and the bedspread.
- Bedspread: Many facilities use a lightweight and easily washed bedspread.

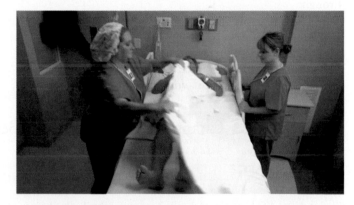

FIG. 2.14 The surgical bed is ready to receive a client directly from a surgical department.

Making an occupied bed is performed in a side-to-side sequence using many of the same steps as in changing an unoccupied bed. Some clients may be able to turn without assistance; however, in many high-acuity settings, clients will need assistance. Assess vital signs, including the level of pain, periodically throughout the procedure to determine the degree to which the client is tolerating bed making. It is strongly recommended to have two nurses available when changing an occupied bed, one on each side of the bed. Prior to beginning the procedure, the nurses clarify their roles, identifying who is primarily focused on client assessment.

APPLICATION OF THE NURSING PROCESS

Examples of Related ICNP Nursing Diagnoses, Expected Client Outcomes, and Nursing Interventions:

Nursing Diagnosis: Risk for impaired skin integrity
Supporting Data: Client is restricted to bed and has impaired bed mobility.

Expected Client Outcome: Client will demonstrate skin integrity and be free of pressure injury with no reddened areas or blisters.

Nursing Intervention Example: Keep linen free of wrinkles and determine if a pressure-redistributing mattress support-surface overlay may be indicated.

Reference: International Classification for Nursing Practice. (n.d.). *eHealth & ICNP.* Retrieved from https://www.icn.ch/what-we-do/projects/ehealth-icnp.

CRITICAL CONCEPTS
Changing a Bed

Accuracy (ACC)

Making beds is subject to the following variables:
* assessment of the client, including mobility, risk for skin breakdown and pressure injury, level of discomfort, and activity intolerance.

Client-Centered Care (CCC)

When making beds, respect for the client is demonstrated through:
* providing privacy
* ensuring comfort
* honoring cultural preferences
* arranging for an interpreter, as needed
* advocating for the client and family.

Infection Control (INF)

When making beds, client infection and healthcare-associated infection are prevented by
* containment of microorganisms
* preventing and reducing the transfer of microorganisms
* reducing the number of microorganisms.

Safety (SAF)

When making beds, safety measures prevent harm and maintain a safe environment.

Communication (COM)

* Communication exchanges information (oral, written, nonverbal or electronic) between two or more people.
* Collaboration with the client and other healthcare professionals facilitates bed making.
* Documentation records information in a permanent legal record.

Health Maintenance (HLTH)

When making beds, nursing is dedicated to the promotion of health and mobility in bed.

Evaluation (EVAL)

Evaluation of outcomes enables the nurse to determine the efficacy of the care provided related to making beds.

▪ SKILL 2.23 Changing an Unoccupied Bed

EQUIPMENT

Bed
Clean gloves, if there is a risk of exposure to body fluids
Linen hamper
Bottom sheet—contour, if available
Top sheet
Draw sheet, if appropriate
Absorbent pad, if appropriate
Blanket
Bedspread
Pillowcases

BEGINNING THE SKILL

1. **INF** Perform hand hygiene.
2. **INF** Apply gloves if there is a risk of exposure to body fluids.
3. **SAF** Identify the client using two identifiers.
4. **CCC** Introduce yourself to the client and family and explain the procedure.
5. **SAF** Set up an ergonomically safe space for client care to prevent injury to the nurse and client.
6. Determine the type of bedding needed.
   a. **CCC** Select the type of bedding needed according to client needs, such as a disposable absorbent pad for drainage or incontinence or a draw sheet and pillow to assist with positioning.
   b. **CCC** Assess the preferences of the client (e.g., more blankets versus fewer blankets).
   c. **HLTH** Evaluate the mattress surface, bedding, and the client's pressure injury risk factors to determine if a pressure-redistributing mattress support-surface overlay may be indicated. *Pressure redistribution is the ability of a support surface to distribute the load over the contact areas of the human body, providing the therapeutic benefit of preventing or managing pressure injury (NPUAP, 2018).*

PROCEDURE

Removing the Soiled Linens

7. **ACC** Assess the client's activity intolerance. *The outcome of the assessment will determine if the client will tolerate moving out of the bed to allow you to make an unoccupied bed.* If the client has a significant risk for activity intolerance, follow Skill 2.25.
8. **SAF** If the client is in bed and needs assistance to transfer, assist the client out of bed to a chair using standards of safe client handling and movement. *Implementing safe handling and movement standards prevents injury to the nurse and client.*
9. Remove any items that should not go into the linen hamper, such as disposable absorbent pads. Dispose of any trash.
10. **SAF** Raise the bed to a comfortable working height and lower the bedrails. *Setting up an ergonomically safe space prevents injury to the nurse and client.*

11. **INF** If the bedspread and/or blankets are to be placed back on the made bed, fold them from the edges toward the center of the bed. Remove them and place them on a clean surface. *Clean only touches clean.*

12. Loosen all the tucked ends of the sheets from under the mattress.

13. **INF** Fold the linens from the outside of the mattress edges toward the center, creating a small bundle of folded, soiled linens. Avoid shaking or flapping soiled linens. Shaking soiled linens disperses microorganism into the air.

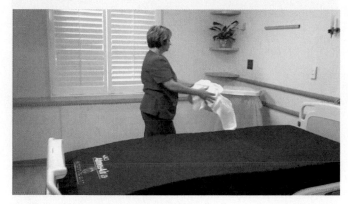

STEP 13 Bundle up the soiled linens.

14. **INF** Place the bundle directly into the linen hamper. Do not place soiled linens on a chair or the floor, and do not allow soiled linens to touch your own clothing.

15. **INF** If the mattress is soiled, clean the mattress according to facility policy.

16. **INF** If using gloves, remove and discard them. Perform hand hygiene before handling clean linens.

Making the First Side of the Bed

17. Place the clean folded bottom fitted sheet in the center of the bed. Unfold the sheet until the sheet is folded in half and fully extended lengthwise from the head of the bed to the foot of the bed. Position the folded edge down the center of the bed with the edges toward the nurse.

18. **HLTH** Secure the bottom sheet to the mattress at the head of the bed. At the head of the bed, bring the contour sheet corner toward the corner of the mattress, but leave the gathered edge inverted. As you face the head of the bed, slide the hand closest to the mattress over the sheet and grasp the corner of the mattress. Use your other hand to pull the gathered edges of the sheet down over the edge of the mattress. Lift the mattress slightly with the hand grasping the corner of the mattress and ensure that the sheet is securely tucked under the mattress.

19. **HLTH** At the foot of the bed, repeat the procedure with the bottom sheet corner. Pull the sheet until it is wrinkle-free. *Smooth bedding protects pressure points from wrinkles that could contribute to pressure ulcers.*

20. Lift the edge of the sheet that will be tucked on the other side of the mattress, and leave it loosely folded down the center of the bed.

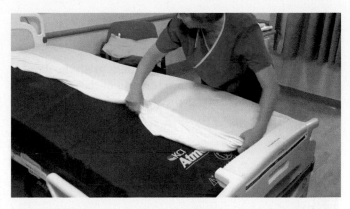

STEP 20 Secure one side of the sheet and place the other loosely folded down the center of the bed.

21. **CCC** If your assessment determined that the client would benefit from a draw sheet to assist with client positioning, place the draw sheet on the bed and unfold the draw sheet until it is folded in half. Place the folded edge of the draw sheet down the center of the bed with the edges toward the nurse. Position the draw sheet on the mattress such that the top border is at the level of the client's shoulders and the bottom border is below the client's hips.

22. Lift the top edge of the draw sheet that will be tucked on the other side of the mattress and loosely fan-fold half of the sheet. Leave the edge easily visible. Tuck the remaining bottom edge of the draw sheet under the mattress securely.

23. **CCC** If an absorbent pad will be used over the draw sheet, place an absorbent pad in the middle of the bed.

24. Place the folded top sheet in the center of the bed. Unfold the sheet until the sheet is folded in half and fully extended lengthwise from the head of the bed to the foot of the bed. Position the folded edge down the center of the bed with the edges toward the nurse. Position the top edge of the sheet so that there will be enough fabric to turn down a cuff over the blanket at the head of the bed and enough fabric at the bottom of the bed to secure the sheet.

25. Lift the top edge of the draw sheet that will cover the other side of the mattress and loosely fan-fold half of the sheet. Leave it loosely folded in the center of the bed.

26. **CCC** If the client has stated a preference for a blanket, place a blanket over the sheet folded in half with the folded edge down the center of the bed and the edges toward the nurse. Position the blanket below the hem of the top sheet at the head of the bed.

27. Lift the top edge of the blanket that will cover the other side of the mattress and fan-fold half of the blanket. Leave it loosely folded in the center of the bed.

28. At the foot of the bed, tuck the bottom edge of the top sheet and blanket under the mattress and miter the corners.

Folding a Mitered Corner

a. Tuck the sheet under the mattress at the foot of the bed.

b. Standing on the side of the mattress, grasp the sheet at the hem about a foot from the end of the mattress.

c. Lift the corner and lay the sheet on the top of the mattress, creating a triangle.

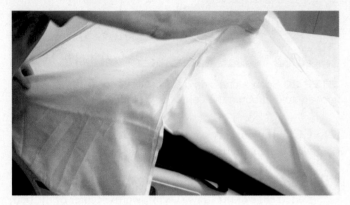

STEP 28C Lift the corner and create a triangle.

d. Tuck the sheet that is not a part of the triangle under the mattress.

e. Pinch a corner of the triangle at the foot of the bed and lower the sheet over the side of the mattress, creating a straight mitered corner.

Making the Second Side of the Bed

29. **HLTH** Walk around the foot of the bed to the other side. Locate the bottom contour sheet and pull it toward you. Facing the foot of the bed, slide the hand closest to the mattress over the sheet and grasp the corner of the mattress. Use the other hand to pull the gathered edges of the sheet down over the edge of the mattress. Lift the mattress slightly with the hand holding the sheet securely on the surface of the bed, and ensure that the sheet is securely tucked under the mattress. Secure the sheet under the mattress, ensuring there are no wrinkles. *Smooth bedding protects pressure points from wrinkles that could contribute to pressure ulcers.*

30. At the head of the bed, repeat the procedure with the bottom contour.

31. **HLTH** Reach to the center of the bed and locate the edge of the draw sheet. Pull the sheet taut and tuck it in under the mattress. *Smooth bedding protects pressure points from wrinkles that could contribute to pressure ulcers.*

32. Locate the absorbent pad and position it in the center of the mattress.

33. Reach to the center of the bed and locate the edge of the top sheet. Pull the sheet taut and adjust the sheet so that the top edge is even across the mattress.

34. **HLTH** Reach to the center of the bed and hold on to the edge of the blanket. Pull the blanket until it is smooth, with no wrinkles or folds.

35. At the head of the bed, fold the top edge of the top sheet into a cuff over the blanket.

36. **HLTH** At the foot of the bed, make a pleat in the top sheet and blanket the width of the foot of the bed. *Having sufficient room for the feet to remain flexed prevents foot drop.*

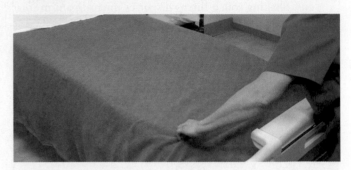

STEP 36 Make a horizontal toe pleat.

37. Tuck the bottom edge of the top sheet and blanket under the mattress and miter the corner. See "Folding a Mitered Corner," steps 28a to 28e earlier in this skill.

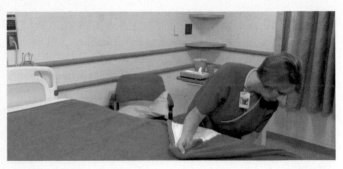

STEP 37 Miter the corners.

Changing a Pillowcase

38. Bunch up the pillowcase from the open end to the closed end.

39. Grasp the outside of the closed end of the pillowcase with one hand, push toward the inside of the pillowcase, and grasp the short edge of the pillow.

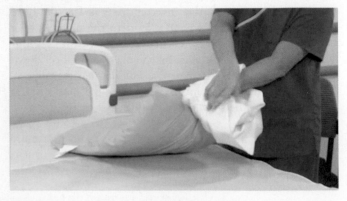

STEP 39 Grasp the short edge of the pillow.

40. Hold firmly to the pillowcase and the edge of the pillow.
41. With the other hand, pull the pillowcase over the pillow.

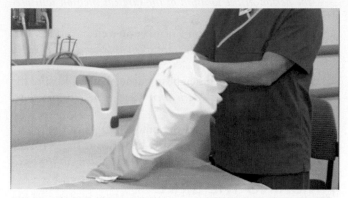

STEP 41 Pull the pillowcase over the pillow.

42. Place the pillow at the head of the bed. Traditionally, nurses place the open end of the pillowcase away from the door. *This position has a neater appearance.*

FINISHING THE SKILL

43. **SAF** Return the bed to the lowest height, and position the side rails to assist the client in entering the bed. *Implementing safe handling and movement standards prevents injury to the nurse and client.*
44. **INF** Perform hand hygiene.
45. **EVAL** Evaluate outcomes, such as how the client tolerated the activity and use of handling equipment.
46. **SAF** Ensure client safety and comfort. Verify that the client can identify and reach the nurse call system. *These safety measures reduce the risk of falls.*
47. **COM** Document assessment findings, if significant; care given; and outcomes in the legal healthcare record.

■ SKILL 2.24 Making a Surgical Bed

EQUIPMENT

Bed
Bottom sheet—contour, if available
Top sheet
Draw sheet, if appropriate
Absorbent pad, if appropriate
Blanket

BEGINNING THE SKILL

1. **INF** Perform hand hygiene.

Removing the Soiled Linens

2. **INF** Apply gloves. Remove and dispose of soiled linens if present following steps 9 to 14 in Skill 2.23, Changing an Unoccupied Bed.
3. **INF** If the mattress is soiled, clean the mattress according to facility policy.
4. **INF** If using gloves, remove and discard them. Perform hand hygiene before handling clean linens.
5. **CCC** Determine the type of bedding needed. Select the type of bedding needed according to client needs, such as a disposable absorbent pad for drainage or incontinence or a draw sheet and pillow to assist with positioning.
6. **ACC** Assess the mattress surface, bedding, and the client's pressure ulcer risk factors to determine if a pressure-redistributing mattress support-surface overlay may be indicated. *Pressure redistribution is the ability of a support surface to distribute the load over the contact areas of the human body, providing the therapeutic benefit of preventing or managing pressure ulcers (NPUAP, 2018).*

PROCEDURE

7. **SAF** Raise the bed to a comfortable working height and lower the bedrails. *Setting up an ergonomically safe space prevents injury to the nurse.*

8. Place the contour sheet, draw sheet, and absorbent pad as needed on the mattress from one side of the bed, following step 17 through step 23 in Skill 2.23, Changing an Unoccupied Bed.
9. Tuck in the contour sheet and draw sheet following step 29 through step 32 in Skill 2.23, Changing an Unoccupied Bed.
10. Place the folded top sheet in the center of the bed. Unfold the sheet until the sheet is folded in half and fully extended lengthwise from the head of the bed to the foot of the bed. Position the folded edge down the center of the bed with the edges toward the nurse. Position the top edge of the sheet along the mattress at the head of the bed.
11. Lift the long edge of the sheet that will be on the other side of the mattress and spread the top sheet flat on the mattress.
12. Make a cuff with the sheet at the head of the bed.
13. Make a larger cuff at the foot of the bed with end of the sheet so that the sheet is the same length as the mattress.
14. Fold in each corner to make a triangle at the head and the foot of the bed

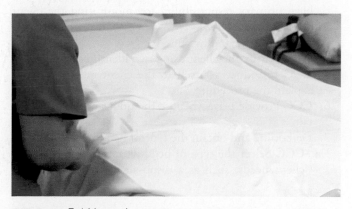

STEP 14 Fold in each corner.

15. Lift the remaining hanging portion of the sheet and fan-fold it on the bed.
16. Walk to the opposite side of the bed, lift the top sheet, and pull it toward you. Place it along the edge of the bed nearest you and fan-fold it in segments approximately 22.30 cm (9–12 inches) in length. Leave the last segment pointed toward the center of the bed.

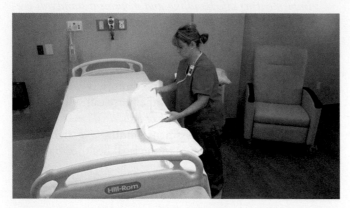

STEP 16 Fan-fold the top sheet.

17. **CCC** Position absorbent pads on the bed as appropriate for the surgical incision. *Absorbent pads positioned under the person at the location of the surgical incision will prevent soiling the sheets.*
18. **CCC** Place an additional blanket on a clean surface. *Clients coming from surgery are often cold and will need a blanket.*
19. **SAF** Adjust the bed height to gurney height. Ensure the bed is locked. *The bed is then ready to receive the client from surgery on a gurney.*
20. Place the pillowcase on the pillow and place the pillow on a clean surface, not on the bed. *Client transfer is accomplished more efficiently without the pillow on the bed.*

FINISHING THE SKILL

21. **INF** Perform hand hygiene.

▪ SKILL 2.25 Changing an Occupied Bed

EQUIPMENT

Bed
Clean gloves, if there is a risk of exposure to body fluids (soiled linens)
Linen hamper
Bottom sheet—fitted, if available
Top sheet
Draw sheet, if appropriate
Absorbent pad, if appropriate
Blanket
Bedspread
Pillowcases

BEGINNING THE SKILL

1. If possible, find a colleague to assist you with this activity and determine whether you or your colleague will have primary responsibility for monitoring the client during this activity.
2. **INF** Perform hand hygiene.
4. **SAF** Identify the client using two identifiers.
5. **CCC** Introduce yourself to the client and family and explain the procedure.
6. **CCC** Provide privacy. Close the door and pull the curtain.
7. Determine and obtain the type of bedding needed.
   a. **CCC** Select the type of bedding needed according to client needs, such as a disposable absorbent pad for drainage or incontinence or a draw sheet and pillow to assist with positioning.
   b. **CCC** Assess preferences of the client (e.g., more blankets vs. fewer blankets).
   c. **ACC** Assess the mattress surface, bedding, and the client's pressure injury risk factors to determine if a pressure-redistributing mattress support-surface overlay may be indicated. *Pressure redistribution is the ability of a support surface to distribute the load over the contact areas of the human body, providing the therapeutic benefit of preventing or managing pressure ulcers (NPUAP, 2018).*
   d. **INF** Place clean linens on a clean surface in the order you will need them.

PROCEDURE

8. **ACC** Assess the client's activity intolerance and the client's ability to lie flat. *The outcome of the assessment will determine if the client will tolerate the turning and handling associated with changing an occupied bed and the client's ability to lie flat. Medical restrictions may require you to keep the client's head elevated.*
9. **SAF** Assess the need for handling equipment, such as a hoist or friction-reducing surfaces, by using the repositioning algorithm in Chapter 1. *Implementing safe handling and movement standards prevents injury to the nurse and client.*

10. **SAF** Set up an ergonomically safe space for you and for the client. Raise the bed to a comfortable working height. Raise one side rail. Lower the head of the bed to the extent tolerated by the client. *Setting up an ergonomically safe space prevents injury to the nurse and client.*

11. **SAF** Apply clean gloves and check intravenous lines and other equipment, such as Foley catheter, ventilator tubing, or electrocardiogram (ECG) wires, to ensure sufficient slack to roll the client.

12. **INF** If the bedspread and/or blankets are to be placed back on the made bed, fold them from the edges toward the center of the bed. Remove them and place them on a clean surface. *Clean only touches clean.*

13. **CCC** Keep the client covered with a sheet or bath blanket. *Covering the client provides privacy and prevents chilling.*

14. **SAF** Assist the client to roll into a side-lying position toward the raised side rail, support the head with a pillow, and have the client hold on to the side rail, if possible. For critically ill clients, one nurse remains on the client's side of the bed, monitoring the client and equipment.

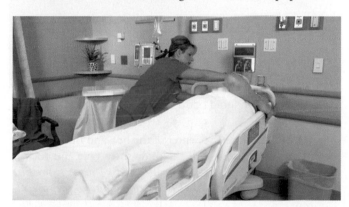

STEP 14 Assist the client into a side-lying position.

Removing the Soiled Linens From the First Side of the Bed

15. On the other side of the bed, lower the bedrails and loosen all the tucked ends of the soiled sheets from under the mattress.

16. **INF** Loosely roll the soiled bottom sheet and draw sheet toward the client's back.

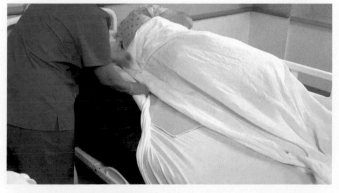

STEP 16 Roll the soiled sheets toward the client's back.

17. **INF** If the mattress is soiled, clean and dry the mattress according to facility policy.

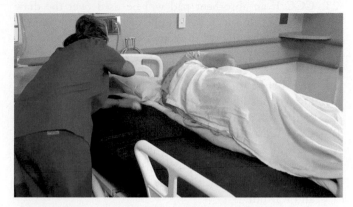

STEP 17 If the mattress is soiled, clean and dry it.

18. **INF** Remove gloves and discard them. Perform hand hygiene before handling clean linens.

Making the First Side of the Bed

19. Place the clean folded bottom sheet in the center of the bed. Extend the sheet to the top and bottom of the bed, folded in half with the center in the middle of the bed and the edges toward the nurse.

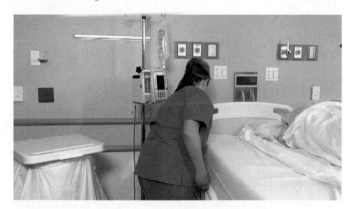

STEP 19 Place a clean bottom sheet on half the bed.

20. Lift the top edge of the sheet and fan-fold it to the middle of the sheet. Leave it folded in the middle of the bed.

21. **HLTH** Tuck the corners of the bottom sheet at the head and foot of the bed if the sheet is contoured. Make mitered corners if it is not a contoured sheet. Smooth the sheet to remove wrinkles. *Smooth bedding protects pressure points from wrinkles that could contribute to pressure ulcers*

22. **CCC** If your assessment determined that the client would benefit from a draw sheet, place the draw sheet on the bed, folded in half with the center in the middle of the bed and the edges toward the nurse. Position the sheet to ensure that the top border is at the level of the client's shoulders and the bottom border is below the client's hips. Lift the far edge of the draw sheet that is parallel to the edge of the mattress and fan-fold it to the center of the sheet. Leave the edge easily visible. Tuck

the remaining edge of the draw sheet under the mattress securely.

23. **CCC** If an absorbent pad will be used over the draw sheet, position it in the middle of the bed and fold the far edge back toward the center of the bed.

Rolling the Client to the Other Side

24. **SAF** Before moving the client, apply gloves and check intravenous lines and other equipment to ensure sufficient slack to roll the client.

25. **CCC** Raise the side rails and assist the client in rolling over the rolled-up soiled linens and the fan-folded clean linens. Assist the client into a side-lying position with the head supported. Keep the client covered for privacy and warmth.

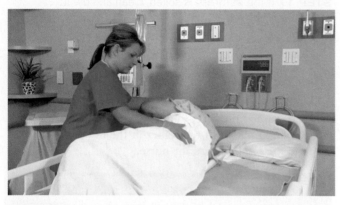

STEP 25 Assist the client to roll over the rolled-up sheets.

26. **SAF** Instruct the client to hold on to the side rail. If the client is unable to assist, one nurse helps the client maintain the side-lying position, and a second nurse changes the linens.

Removing Soiled Linens From the Second Side of the Bed

27. Move to the opposite side of the bed. Lower the side rail.

28. Remove any items that should *not* go into the linen hamper, such as disposable absorbent pads, and dispose of any trash.

29. **INF** Fold the soiled linens from the top and bottom of the mattress toward the center, creating a small bundle of folded, soiled linens.

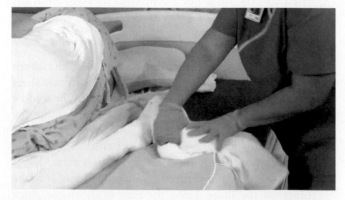

STEP 29 Fold in the soiled linens from the top and bottom.

30. **INF** Place the bundle directly into the linen hamper. Do not place soiled linens on a chair or on the floor, and do not allow the soiled linens to touch your own clothing.

31. **INF** If the mattress is soiled, clean and dry it according to facility policy.

32. **INF** Remove gloves and discard. Perform hand hygiene before handling clean linens.

Making the Second Side of the Bed

33. **HLTH** Reach to the bottom layer of clean sheets and find the fitted bottom sheet. Pull the sheet taut, tucking it securely at the top and bottom of the mattress. *Smooth bedding protects pressure points from wrinkles that could contribute to pressure ulcers.*

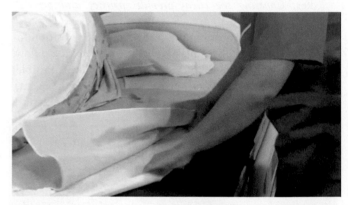

STEP 33 Pull the fitted bottom sheet taut.

34. **HLTH** Reach to the center of the bed and find the edge of the draw sheet. Pull the draw sheet taut and tuck it in under the mattress. *Smooth bedding protects pressure points from wrinkles that could contribute to pressure ulcers.*

35. **HLTH** If an absorbent pad will be used, find the edge of the pad and smooth it flat.

The Top Layers

36. Assist the client to roll back into the middle of the bed.

37. **CCC** Unfold a clean sheet and place it over the client. If the client is able, ask the client to hold on to the clean sheet. Remove the soiled sheet or bath blanket used to cover the client while maintaining privacy with the top sheet.

38. **CCC** Add the blanket to cover the client. Keep the blanket parallel with the sheet and fold the sheet over the blanket.

39. Tuck the end of the top sheet and blanket under the mattress at the foot of the bed to keep them in place. Miter the corners, but allow the sides to hang freely.

40. **HLTH** Make a pleat in the top sheet and blanket at the foot of the bed. *The pleat allows room for the feet to remain flexed and prevents foot drop.*

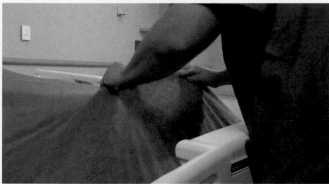

STEP 40. Make a horizontal toe pleat.

41. Change the pillowcases, as described in Skill 2.24.
42. **INF** Place soiled pillowcase directly into the linen hamper. Do not place soiled linens on a chair or on the floor, and do not allow the soiled linens to touch your own clothing.

43. **CCC** Assist the client into a comfortable position. Assist the client with positioning and rearranging the bedding.
44. **SAF** Secure all medical equipment attached to the client and check for patency, such as intravenous lines and Foley catheters.

FINISHING THE SKILL

46. **SAF** Ensure client safety. Place the bed in the lowest position. Verify that the client can identify and reach the nurse call system. *These safety measures reduce the risk of falls.*
47. **CCC** Provide for client comfort.
48. **INF** Remove gloves and perform hand hygiene.
49. **EVAL** Evaluate outcomes, such as the client's tolerance of the activity and use of handling equipment.
50. **COM** Document assessment findings, care given, and outcomes in the legal healthcare record.

■ CASE STUDY

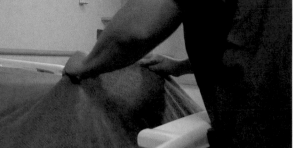

Stephanie Johnston is a 28-year-old female who is 32 weeks pregnant and expecting her first baby. She has been in the antepartum special-care unit for 5 days, on strict bedrest, for preeclampsia. Her authorized healthcare providers plan to medically manage her preeclampsia until she is at least 34 weeks pregnant. At that time, if necessary, they will deliver the baby. She shows signs of mild preeclampsia: elevated blood pressure, edematous lower extremities, and hyperproteinuria. She is not to get out of bed and is to remain positioned either on her left side or supine with her head elevated. Her baseline blood pressure in the supine position is 130/85. When she sits up fully, her blood pressure goes up as well, as high as 150/90.

Stephanie is on medication for her hypertension, and she is also on seizure precautions. She has an IV line in her left forearm. She has an indwelling Foley catheter, and the nurses are monitoring her urine output.

The nurse asks Stephanie if she would like a complete bed bath and shampoo today. Stephanie states, "I would love to get my hair washed. I normally wash it every day, and I just can't stand it dirty like this! I haven't had much of a bath since I got here." She has very sensitive skin and states that her skin reacts to a lot of things." When discussing her bath, Stephanie states, "It itches down there," and she points to her labia. You notice that there is still betadine visible on her perineum.

Stephanie is very nearsighted and normally wears contact lens. She is accustomed to caring for them herself.

Case Study Questions

1. What is the best position for Stephanie's bed bath? How will you clean her back? State your rationale for your answers.
2. **Application of QSEN Competencies:** One of the Quality and Safety Education for Nurses (QSEN) (Cronenwett et al., 2007) concepts is Patient-Centered Care (which we call client-centered care). The definition is to recognize the client as the source of control and the full partner in providing compassionate and coordinated care based on respect for the client's preferences, values, and needs. How can Stephanie's preferences, values, and needs be incorporated into her bath?
3. How would you respond, both verbally and with interventions, to Stephanie's complaint about itching?
4. Are there any vital signs you would measure before continuing with hair care? If so, give your rationale.
5. How would you position Stephanie for her shampoo? How could you position Stephanie to make her bed while complying with her position restrictions?
6. Considering Stephanie's IV line and Foley catheter placement, what precautions do you need to take when changing her bed?
7. What assessments would be appropriate to measure Stephanie's tolerance of the procedure?
8. Identify the factors needed to facilitate the care of Stephanie's contact lenses.
9. What interventions are essential before you leave Stephanie's room?

■**CONCEPT MAP**

ICNP Nursing Dx:
Risk for Injury:

Supporting Data:

Preeclampsia
Seizure precautions

Baseline Assessment Data

- 28-year-old white female
- Pregnant, 32 weeks gestation
- Strict bedrest
- Mild preeclampsia
- History of elevated BP
- Edematous lower extremities
- Proteinuria
- IV in left forearm
- Foley catheter
- Positioning restrictions
- Contact lenses
- Sensitive skin
- Stated concern for baby's well-being

Safety: Seizure Precautions
and Prevention

- Keep soft pillows around the bed
- Keep side rails up and bed in lowest position
- Monitor electrolytes, especially magnesium
- Monitor subjective/objective symptoms
- Protect IV and Foley catheter lines

ICNP Nursing Dx:
Anxiety

Supporting Data:
Loss of independence
Fear for her baby's well being
Restrictions related to Foley catheter and IV
Decreased mobility

ICNP Nursing Dx:
Impaired Ability to Perform Hygiene

Supporting Data:
Activity restrictions secondary to labile hypertension.

Communication

- Use therapeutic communication
- Bathe with assistance of a caregiver without anxiety
- Avoid false reassurance
- Ask open-ended questions

Client-Centered Care

- Verbalize knowledge of skin care
- Perform self-care activities as able, clean and insert contact lenses, and wash face
- Client to choose bath and hair products
- Client to choose the time of day for a bath

References

Agency for Healthcare Research (AHRQ). (2014). *Are we ready for this change?* Retrieved from https://www.ahrq.gov/patient-safety/settings/hospital/resource/pressureulcer/tool/pu1.html.

American Dental Association. (n.d.). *How to brush.* Retrieved from https://www.mouthhealthy.org/en/az-topics/b/brushing-your-teeth.

American Dental Association. (2016). *Oral health topics: Dentures.* Retrieved from http://www.ada.org/en/member-center/oral-health-topics/dentures.

Association of Women's Health, Obstetric and Neonatal Nurses. (2018). *Neonatal skin care: Evidence-based clinical practice guidelines* (4th ed.). Washington, DC: Author.

Aydin, D., Hartiningsih, S. S., Izgi, M. G., Bay, S., Unlu, K., Tatar, M. O., … Dane, S. (2016). Potential beneficial effects of foot bathing on cardiac rhythm. *Clinical & Investigative Medicine*, *39*(6), S48–S51.

Barrett, M. B., Vizgirda, V. M., & Zhou, Y. (2017). Registered nurse and patient care technician perceptions of toileting patients at high fall risk. *Medsurg Nursing*, *26*(5), 317–323.

Bosley, R. E., & Daveluy, S. (2015). A primer to natural hair care practices in black patients. *Cutis*, *95*(2), 78–80, 106.

Bradbury, S., Price, J., Gaffing, J., & Yoro, E. (2017). Evaluating an incontinence cleanser and skin protectant ointment for managing incontinence associated dermatitis. *Wounds UK*, *13*(1), 79–85.

Cal, E., Cakiroglu, B., Kurt, A. N., Hartiningsih, S. S., & Suryani, D. S. (2016). The potential effects of hand and foot bathing on vital signs in women with caesarean section. *Clinical & Investigative Medicine*, *39*(6), S86–S88.

Centers for Disease Control and Prevention. (2019). *Parasites—Lice.* Retrieved from https://www.cdc.gov/parasites/lice/index.html.

Centers for Disease Control and Prevention. (2015). *Head lice: Frequently asked questions.* Retrieved from https://www.cdc.gov/parasites/lice/head/gen_ info/faqs.html.

Chen, Z. (2015). *Mouth care.* [Evidence summary]. Retrieved from The Joanna Briggs Institute EBD Database.

Craven, D. (2018). *Skin cleansing: Older adults.* [Evidence summary]. Retrieved from The Joanna Briggs Institute EBD Database.

Cronenwett, L., Sherwood, G., Barnsteiner, J., Disch, J., Johnson, J., Mitchell, P., … Warren, J. (2007). Quality and safety education for nurses. *Nursing Outlook*, *55*(3), 122–131 Retrieved from http://qsen.org/competencies/pre-licensure-ksas/.

Dellinger, M. (2019). *Caring for your African American or biracial child's hair.* Retrieved from http://adoption.about.com/od/africanamericanhaircare/ss/blackhaircare_2.htm.

Haesler, E. (2018). *Pressure injuries: Skin care to reduce the risk of pressure injuries.* [Evidence summary]. Retrieved from The Joanna Briggs Institute EBD Database.

Hodgkinson, B., Nay, R., & Wilson, J. (2007). A systematic review of topical skin care in aged care facilities. *Journal of Clinical Nursing*, *16*(1), 129–136.

Hua, F., Xie, H., Worthington, H. V., Furness, S., Zhang, Q., & Li, C. (2016). Oral hygiene care for critically ill patients to prevent ventilator-associated pneumonia. *Cochrane Database of Systematic Reviews*, *10*, 10137. https://doi.org/10.1002/14651858.CD008367.pub3.

International Classification for Nursing Practice. (n.d.). *eHealth & ICNP.* Retrieved from https://www.icn.ch/what-we-do/projects/ehealth-icnp.

Jablonski, R. (2012). Oral health and hygiene content in nursing fundamental textbooks. *Nursing Research and Practice*, 1–7. Retrieved from https://doi.org/10.1155/2012/372617.

Jayasekara, R. (2017). *Oral health: Implementation strategies for residential care.* [Evidence summary]. Retrieved from The Joanna Briggs Institute EBD Database.

Khanh-Dao Le, L. (2017). *Oral care: Foam swabs/foam sponges.* [Evidence summary]. Retrieved from The Joanna Briggs Institute EBD Database.

Khanh-Dao Le, L. (2018). *Bathing/showering: Techniques and cleansing solutions.* [Evidence summary]. Retrieved from The Joanna Briggs Institute EBD Database.

Kim, H. J., Lee, Y., & Sohng, K. Y. (2016). The effects of footbath on sleep among the older adults in nursing home: A quasi-experimental study. *Complementary Therapies in Medicine*, *26*, 40–46.

Klompas, M., Branson, R., Eichenwald, R., Greene, L. R., Howell, M. D., … Berenholtz, S. M. (2014). Strategies to prevent ventilator-associated pneumonia in acute care hospitals: 2014 update. *Infection Control and Hospital Epidemiology*, *35*(8), 915–936.

Liao, W. C., Chiu, M. J., & Landis, C. A. (2008). A warm footbath before bedtime and sleep in older Taiwanese with sleep disturbance. *Research in Nursing & Health*, *31*(5), 514–528.

Liao, W. C., Wang, L., Kuo, C. P., Lo, C., Chiu, M. J., & Ting, H. (2013). Effect of a warm footbath before bedtime on body temperature and sleep in older adults with good and poor sleep: An experimental crossover trial. *International Journal of Nursing Studies*, *50*(12), 1607–1616.

Lund, C., & Durand, D. (2016). Skin and skin care. In S. L. Gardner, B. S. Carter, M. E. Hines, & J. E. Hernandez (Eds.), *Merenstein & Gardner's handbook of neonatal intensive care* (8th ed.) (pp. 464–478). St. Louis, MO: Mosby.

Mohammadi, J. J. Y., Franks, K., & Hines, S. (2015). Effectiveness of professional oral healthcare intervention on the oral health of residents with dementia in residential aged care facilities: A systematic review protocol. *The Joanna Briggs Institute Database of Systemic Reviews & Implementation Reports*, *13*(10), 110–122.

National Pressure Ulcer Advisory Panel. (2018). *Terms and definitions related to support surfaces.* Retrieved from https://cdn.ymaws.com/npuap.org/resource/resmgr/s3i_terms-and-defs-feb-5-201.pdf.

Nightingale, F. (1860). *Notes on nursing: What it is and what it is not* (1st American ed.). New York, NY: D. Appleton & Company. Retrieved from http://digital.library.upenn.edu/women/nightingale/nursing/nursing.html

Obeid, S. (2018). *Skin tears: Prevention.* [Evidence summary]. Retrieved from The Joanna Briggs Institute EBD Database.

Office of Disease Prevention and Health Promotion. (2018). *Healthy people 2020: Oral health.* Retrieved from https://www.healthypeople.gov/2020/topics-objectives/topic/oral-health.

Saeki, Y., Nagai, N., & Hishinuma, M. (2007). Effects of footbathing on autonomic nerve and immune function. *Complementary Therapies in Clinical Practice*, *13*(3), 158–165.

Sivapurim, M. S. (2018). *Fall prevention: Toileting.* [Evidence summary]. Retrieved from The Joanna Briggs Institute EBD Database.

Sjogren, P., Nilsson, E., Forsell, M., Johansson, O., & Hoogstraate, J. (2008). A systematic review of the preventive effect of oral hygiene on pneumonia and respiratory tract infection in elderly people in hospitals and nursing homes: Effect estimates and methodological quality of randomized controlled trials. *Journal of the American Geriatrics Society*, *56*(11), 2124–2130.

Slade, S. (2017). *Oral hygiene care: Acute care setting.* [Evidence summary]. Retrieved from The Joanna Briggs Institute EBD Database.

Swe, K. K. (2017). *Ventilator associated pneumonia: Oral hygiene care.* [Evidence summary]. Retrieved from The Joanna Briggs Institute EBD Database.

Tzeng, H. M. (2010). Understanding the prevalence of inpatient falls associated with toileting in adult acute care settings. *Journal of Nursing Care Quality, 22*(1), 22–30.

Tzeng, H. M., & Yin, C. Y. (2012). Toileting-related inpatient falls in adult acute care settings. *Medsurg Nursing, 21*(6), 372–377.

Wounds UK. (2012). *Best practice statement: Care of the older person's skin.* Retrieved from http://www.woundsinternational.com/pdf/content_10608.pdf.

Yamamoto, K., Aso, Y., Nagata, S., Kasugai, K., & Maeda, S. (2008). Autonomic, neuro-immunological and psychological responses to wrapped warm footbaths—A pilot study. *Complementary Therapies in Clinical Practice, 14*(3), 195–203.

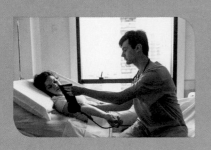

CHAPTER 3
Vital Signs and Vital Measurements

"The most important practical lesson that can be given to nurses is to teach them what to observe." | **Florence Nightingale, 1860**

VITAL SIGNS

VITAL MEASUREMENTS

SECTION 6 Assessing Oxygen Saturation

- **SKILL 3.17**   Obtaining a Pulse Oximeter Measurement

SECTION 7 Assessing Blood Glucose

- **SKILL 3.18**   Obtaining Capillary Blood Glucose Measurements

LEARNING OBJECTIVES

By the end of this chapter, the reader will be able to:

1 Identify factors that affect vital signs.
2 Identify the established parameters of vital signs for various age groups.
3 Discuss febrile and afebrile states.
4 Measure temperature with a digital electronic thermometer.
5 Measure temperature with a tympanic thermometer.
6 Measure temperature with an infrared temporal artery thermometer.
7 Discuss interventions related to regulating temperature.
8 Use a conductive heating or cooling blanket.
9 Use an infant radiant warmer.
10 Explain the physiologic hemodynamics of pulse and blood pressure.
11 Palpate a radial pulse rate.
12 Palpate carotid pulses.
13 Palpate and evaluate peripheral pulses.
14 Use a Doppler ultrasound device to assess peripheral pulses and systolic blood pressure.
15 Assess an apical pulse via palpation and auscultation.
16 Assess respirations.
17 Measure blood pressure through various methods.
18 Measure oxygen saturation with a pulse oximeter.
19 Measure capillary blood glucose with a glucometer.

TERMINOLOGY

Afebrile Characterized by a normal body temperature; without fever.

Amplitude In reference to pulses, the extent of fullness and height with each arterial pulsation.

Apnea Absence of breathing.

Auscultation Assessment through listening, usually through a stethoscope.

Bradycardia Heart rate below the normal acceptable range, less than 60 beats per minute.

Bradypnea Respiratory rate below the acceptable range, usually less than 12 breaths per minute in an adult.

Conduction Method of heat transfer from the human body to objects touching the body (e.g., cold sheets).

Convection Method of heat transfer from the human body to the surrounding air (e.g., a draft).

Core temperature Internal body temperature.

Cyanosis Color change, often a blue or gray tone, associated with decreased oxygenation; most noticeable in the lips, fingers, mucous membranes, or tongue.

Diastolic pressure The blood pressure reading during diastole, the lowest arterial pressure during the cardiac cycle.

Dorsiflex To bend or extend backward.

Dyspnea Labored breathing resulting from air hunger—can be subjective (client reports) or objective (nurse observes).

Evaporation Method of heat transfer due to vaporization of liquid to gas, resulting in cooling (e.g., of the body during sweating).

Febrile Characterized by a temperature above the normal limits; having a fever.

Fossa Anatomical term referring to a shallow depression or groove; used to describe the inside of the elbow (popliteal fossa) and behind the knee (antecubital fossa).

Handoff The transfer of information, primary responsibility, and authority from one or more nurses to other nurses.

Hemodynamics Dynamics of blood flow; mechanisms within the circulatory system that maintain a circulatory equilibrium.

Hypertension State characterized by blood pressure above the normal range.

Hyperthermia State characterized by temperature greatly above the thermoregulatory set-point.

Hypotension State characterized by blood pressure below the normal range.

Hypothermia State characterized by temperature greatly below the thermoregulatory set-point.

Hypovolemia Decreased circulating blood volume in the vascular system.

Korotkoff sounds Vascular sounds with five distinct phases that the body produces during blood pressure measurements.

Mean arterial pressure (MAP) The average arterial pressure of one cardiac cycle.

Orthopnea Difficulty breathing when in a supine position.

Palpation Assessment through touch.

Postural (orthostatic) hypotension Decrease in blood pressure related to a sudden change in position (e.g., from supine to sitting or standing).

Pulse deficit Difference between the apical and radial pulse rate.

Pyrexia State of being febrile.

Radiation Method of heat transfer from a warm body to cooler surroundings.

Sublingual Under the tongue.

Systolic pressure The blood pressure reading during systole, the highest arterial pressure during the cardiac cycle.

Tachycardia Heart rate above the normal acceptable range, greater than 100 beats per minute in an adult.

Tachypnea Respiratory rate above the acceptable range, greater than 20 breaths per minute in an adult.

Total parenteral nutrition An intravenous nutritional support that includes carbohydrate, protein, fat, electrolytes, vitamins, minerals, and fluids.

ACRONYMS

AX Axillary
bpm Beats per minute
PMI Point of maximal impulse
TPN Total parenteral nutrition
TPR Temperature, pulse, respiration

VITAL SIGNS

Vital signs is the term for the collection of measurements that includes temperature, pulse, and respirations (TPR) and blood pressure. Vital signs are a critical assessment because they provide healthcare professionals clues to clients' underlying physiologic health and their response to physiologic and environmental stressors. Subtle changes in a client's baseline vital signs may serve as an early warning sign that the body is initiating a compensatory mechanism. Changes in vital signs may reflect a physiologic change, such as an infection or pain. Vital signs can also be affected by the physical environment and the client's emotional state, activity level, and medications. Vital sign parameters vary according to age and medical history. It is important for the nurse to determine if any of these elements have influenced the client's vital signs.

Although vital signs are a part of many members of the healthcare team's training, measuring vital signs is primarily within the nurse's domain. It is not unusual for a nurse to delegate this skill, but it is the nurse's responsibility to ensure vital signs are completed and reviewed in a timely manner. Accurate measurement of vital signs is a safety concern because inaccurate vital sign measurement may result in potentially dangerous overtreatment or undertreatment.

Vital signs are taken in almost every healthcare setting. The frequency with which nurses assess vital signs varies according to the condition of the client and the setting. For example, in a clinic or healthcare provider's office, vital signs are assessed at each visit, whereas in a critical care setting, vital signs may be assessed as often as every 5 minutes. In any case, vital signs must be taken at least as often as ordered. Even if vital signs are ordered only once per shift, it is the standard of care for a nurse to take vital signs additionally at any time they are warranted. For example, if the nurse gives a medication that is known to decrease respiratory rate and blood pressure but the vital signs are ordered only once per shift and have already been completed, it is the nurse's responsibility to take the vital signs before and after giving

the medication to ensure the client's safety. Nurses must use their own judgment to determine when additional assessment of vital signs is needed.

Communication is a key critical concept when obtaining vital signs, beginning with communication with the client. Vital signs are typically shared with the client. Clients may need to be educated on norms for temperature in Celsius and their pulse, respiratory rate, and blood pressure. They often want to know more about the normal variations and the optimal measurements.

Electronic communication affects vital signs in a couple of ways. Electronic communication of vital signs, such as heart rate and blood pressure, may be monitored electronically from a remote site, which is often called remote patient monitoring. The remote site may be a site within the acute care setting or it may be in a different town. Telehealth is the use of telecommunications tools, including telephones, smart phones, and mobile wireless devices, to assist in the remote provision of healthcare (Dorsey & Topol, 2016). One of the current trends of telehealth is monitoring an individual's vital signs from his or her home. Future advances in physiologic sensors and smart phone technology may facilitate the growth and value of remote monitoring.

In addition, electronic equipment used within an acute care setting may record the vital sign measurements directly into the electronic medical record (EMR), thus documenting the vital signs. In this instance, the nurse is still responsible for knowing the vital signs and determining if they represent a change from the client's baseline. Any significant change in the client's health status must be communicated to the authorized healthcare provider. This is a particular concern when vital sign measurement has been delegated to another member of the healthcare team. Teamwork and clear communication is necessary to ensure that any significant change in health status is communicated to the registered nurse and the authorized healthcare provider for that client.

Nurses measure temperature in order to assess whether a client is afebrile or febrile as a means of detecting infection. Even before the invention of a clinical thermometer, Florence Nightingale (1898) instructed nurses to note "if a patient is feverish" (p. 5). Other reasons to measure temperature include to obtain a baseline measurement and to assess for hyperthermia or hypothermia. At home, some women take their temperature measurement each day to track their basal body temperature to predict ovulation. Accurate temperature measurement is critical because temperature is used to diagnose, inform treatment, and evaluate treatment. There are a variety of instruments and sites for measuring temperature, each with advantages and disadvantages.

How did 98.6°F become the accepted normal temperature? In the 1860s, Dr. Carl Wunderlich studied the results of over 1 million measurements of axillary temperatures taken with early mercury thermometers on about 250,000 people. He concluded from his analysis of the data that 98.6°F (37°C) was the mean temperature (Mackowiak & Worden, 1994). Although such a large study sample has never been replicated, neither have his results. A study performed at the University of Maryland found 98.2°F to be the mean oral temperature (Mackowiak, Wasserman, & Levine, 1992).

However, two of Dr. Wunderlich's conclusions were supported by the University of Maryland study and continue to be substantiated today. The first is the diurnal nature of our body temperature. Body temperature fluctuates throughout the day—it is lower in the morning and higher in the evening. Thus, normal temperature is best expressed as a range. The second is that older adults have lower temperatures than younger adults. Large studies and systematic reviews have consistently found that body temperatures in older adults are lower than those in young adults (Lu, Leasure, & Dai, 2010; Waalen & Buxbaum, 2011). Given the variations within the day and the lower temperatures of older adults, assessing temperature requires carefully identifying a baseline in order to determine a febrile state, particularly for older adults.

SITES AND METHODS OF TEMPERATURE ASSESSMENT

The core temperature is the body's internal temperature. It is the optimal temperature measurement because it is less influenced by the environment than the surface of the body. The body surface reflects both the environment, such as a cold room, and the body's response to the environment, such as sweating in a hot room. However, the core temperature is only assessed by invasive methods. In intensive care settings, temperature probes may be placed in the esophagus or bladder. In other settings, a rectal temperature is an invasive but low-technology method of measuring a core temperature. In most settings, nurses measure temperature using noninvasive methods.

The ideal site for measuring temperature is noninvasive, safe, easily accessed, and culturally acceptable and provides a temperature that is consistent with the core temperature. Sites for measuring temperature include the mouth, the axillae, in the ear (reflecting the temperature of the tympanic membrane), on the forehead by scanning the temporal artery, and lastly, in the rectum. In the mouth and under the tongue near the sublingual artery is a site that is a close measure of core temperature. The mouth is not a safe choice for young children or clients who are uncooperative or have an altered level of consciousness, but it is a frequently used site for cooperative, alert clients. Recent intake of food or drink is a factor that can alter the reading and must be assessed in order to prevent an inaccurate measurement. The axilla is a frequently used site for young children but does not provide as accurate a reflection of the core temperature. The rectum provides a close approximation of the core temperature; however, it is neither easily accessed nor culturally acceptable. It is a very vascular area with safety risks, including rectal perforation, so it is seldom used for adults. The American Academy of Pediatrics (AAP) advice to parents is to take a rectal temperature for children less than 3 years of age (AAP, 2015). However, it is contraindicated for infants less than 1 month of age due to their small size and the risk for rectal perforation (Hockenberry, Rodgers, & Wilson, 2017). Within a healthcare agency, follow the department's policy for selecting the site to measure a temperature.

In addition to the variety of sites that exist for temperature measurement, there are also a variety of types of thermometers. The oldest type of thermometer is a glass mercury thermometer. Because of the safety risks of broken glass and the toxic risk of mercury, these thermometers are no longer found in acute care settings. Electronic digital thermometers are frequently used in healthcare settings and may be used in the mouth, axillae, or rectum. The electronic digital thermometer used in the oral site has been shown to measure as accurately and consistently as the glass mercury thermometer (Dolkar, Kapoor, Singh, & Suri, 2013). A tympanic thermometer and temporal artery thermometer (TAT) are specifically designed for those sites and cannot be used for any other route. Glass thermometers with a nonmercury indicator or a small digital thermometer may be used for a client on isolation precautions. See Fig. 3.1 for two types of thermometers.

The TAT is one of the most recent types of thermometers. The thermometer is swept across the forehead, intersecting the temporal artery, and then touched behind the ear. TATs are noninvasive and easily accepted by clients. However, The Joanna Briggs Institute provided an evidence summary of 10 adult research studies and found consistent evidence that the TAT has low sensitivity and is not accurate enough to replace more invasive temperature measurements (Slade, 2017). An analysis of 11 pediatric research articles reached a similar conclusion. The accuracy and reliability of the TAT are not well

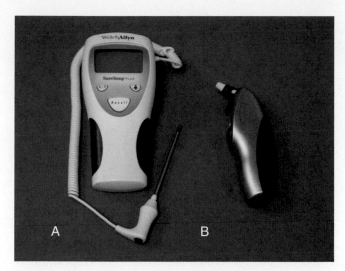

FIG. 3.1 Types of thermometers. **A,** Electronic. **B,** Tympanic.

BOX 3.1 Lifespan Considerations: Obtaining Temperatures in Pediatric Clients

- The oral method is recommended in children 4 to 5 years and older.
- The axillary method can be used to screen for fever in children of all ages. It is the least accurate method of determining fever.
- The rectal method can be used from birth to 3 years of age. Insert the probe 1 to 2.5 cm (½–1 inch) inside the anus and hold loosely.
- The tympanic (infrared) method can be used in children 6 months of age or older; correct positioning of the ear must be ensured.
- Temporal artery thermometers should not be used in infants who are less than 90 days old. Temporal artery thermometry is accurate with clients greater than 3 months of age with or without fever, ill or well.

Reference: American Academy of Pediatrics, 2015.

established, particularly in children with fevers (Khanh-Dao Le, 2017). The conclusion of a systematic review of 30 articles found TAT measurements have an unacceptably low sensitivity to detecting fever in children and are not recommended in this population. Furthermore, fever may still be present after a TAT measurement shows an afebrile measurement (Kiekkas, Aretha, Almpani, & Stefanopoulos, 2019). Studies with neonates have found significant differences when comparing the TAT temperature with axillary temperatures in newborns (Robertson-Smith, McCaffrey, Syers, Williams, & Taylor, 2015).

Tympanic membrane thermometers have been in use for a couple of decades. They are positioned in the ear canal and use an infrared sensor to read the temperature of the tympanic membrane, which reflects a core temperature. They are recommended for infants over the age of 4 weeks up to older adults. The site is easily accessed, and the reading is delivered very quickly. The sensor probe is covered with a probe cover as a means of infection control between clients. The tympanic membrane thermometer is not recommended in clients with ear drainage or eardrum scarring, but readings are accurate in cases of otitis media. When the tympanic thermometer is placed in the ear canal, the nurse straightens the canal by pulling the pinna up and back for an adult and down and back for a child. Tympanic temperature readings have also been researched for accuracy and found to have good reliability (Haugan et al., 2013). All thermometers must be used according to the manufacturer's recommendations to ensure accurate results. Box 3.1 discusses factors that should be taken into consideration when determining what route to use to measure a pediatric client's temperature, and Table 3.1 reports adult temperature ranges for different measurement sites.

APPLICATION OF THE NURSING PROCESS

Examples of Related International Classification for Nursing Practice (ICNP) Nursing Diagnoses, Expected Client Outcomes, and Nursing Interventions:

Nursing Diagnoses: Fever
Supporting Data: Client has symptoms and laboratory data (elevated white blood cell [WBC] count) suggestive of infection.
Expected Client Outcomes: The client will have no evidence of fever:
- temperature within established parameters for client
- client reports a sense of comfort related to temperature.

Nursing Intervention Example: Monitor client's temperature as indicated with appropriate thermometer at an appropriate site.
Reference: International Classification for Nursing Practice. (n.d.). *eHealth & ICNP.* Retrieved from https://www.icn.ch/what-we-do/projects/ehealth-icnp.

CRITICAL CONCEPTS
Assessing Temperature

Accuracy (ACC)

Temperature measurement is sensitive to the following variables:
Client-Related Factors
- Client age and time of day
- Environment (e.g., room temperature)
- Increased skin moisture (if measuring in the axillae)
- Ingestion of hot or cool liquids 30 minutes before measurement
- Recent exercise or exertion

Nurse-Related Factors
- Site selection of the temperature measurement
- Proper measurement technique

Equipment-Related Factors
- Type of equipment

TABLE 3.1 Adult Temperature Ranges From Different Body Sites

Oral	Axillary	Rectal	Tympanic	Temporal
36.0°C–37.6°C	35.5°C–37.0°C	34.4°C–37.8°C	35.6°C–37.4°C	36.1°C–37.3°C
(96.8°F–99.68°F)	(95.9°F–98.6°F)	(93.92°F–100.04°F)	(96.08°F–99.32°F)	(96.98°F–99.14°F)

From Davie, A., & Amoore, J. (2010). Best practice in the measurement of body temperature. *Nursing Standard, 24*(42), 42–49. Reprinted with permission from Yoost and Crawford.

Client-Centered Care (CCC)

When assessing temperature, respect for the client is demonstrated through:
- promoting autonomy
- providing privacy
- ensuring comfort.

Infection Control (INF)

When assessing temperature, healthcare-associated infection is prevented by:
- containment of microorganisms
- preventing and reducing the transfer of microorganisms
- reducing the number of microorganisms.

Safety (SAF)

When assessing temperature, safety measures provide a safe care environment and prevent harm to the client.

Communication (COM)

- Communication exchanges information (oral, written, nonverbal or electronic) between two or more people.
- Collaboration with other healthcare providers to use a consistent measurement technique improves accuracy.
- Documentation records information on temperature assessment in a permanent legal record.

Health Maintenance (HLTH)

When assessing temperature, nursing is dedicated to the promotion of health, including:
- protecting the client's rectal mucosa.

Evaluation (EVAL)

When assessing temperature, the evaluation of outcomes enables the nurse to determine the efficacy of the care provided.

▪ SKILL 3.1 Measuring Temperature With an Electronic Thermometer

EQUIPMENT

Electronic thermometer
Thermometer probe cover
Antiseptic wipes
Clean gloves (may not be needed with the oral site)

BEGINNING THE SKILL

1. **INF** Perform hand hygiene.
2. **INF** Apply gloves.
3. **CCC** Introduce yourself to the client and family and explain the procedure.
4. **SAF** Identify the client using two identifiers.

PROCEDURE

5. **ACC** Assess the client's activity level (including recent bathing) and ingestion of hot/cool liquids within the last 30 minutes.
6. **SAF** Assess for contraindications at the site. For the oral site, assess for client cooperation. For the rectal site, age is the primary consideration because this site is usually only selected for children. Contraindications for the rec-

tal site, if it is indicated, include risk for bleeding, immunosuppression, and recent rectal surgery.
7. **INF** Determine if the correct probe is on the thermometer for the selected site, usually a blue probe for oral sites and a red probe for rectal sites.
8. **INF** Turn on the thermometer and apply the thermometer probe cover by pushing the probe into the cover. (Note: On many models, the thermometer is turned on by simply withdrawing the probe.)
9. **ACC** Place the thermometer in the correct anatomical position.

Oral Site

10. Place the thermometer tip underneath the tongue in the sublingual pocket, ensuring that the client keeps the lips closed around the thermometer. *The temperature in the posterior sublingual pocket reflects the body's core temperature because the sublingual arteries bring blood from the core to the site.*

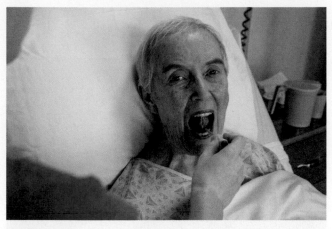

STEP 9 Oral site: Place the thermometer tip underneath the tongue.

Axillary Site

11. Place the thermometer tip in the center of the axilla. Ask the client to cover the probe, ensuring that the probe is in contact with the skin. *If the probe is exposed to the air, it may measure the temperature of the environment rather than the client's temperature, resulting in a false reading.*

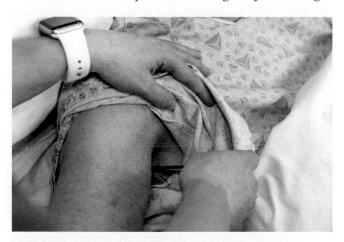

STEP 9 Axillary site: Place the thermometer tip in the center of the axilla.

Rectal Site

12. **For an infant or toddler:**
    a. Place the infant or toddler in a supine or prone position. Place water-soluble lubricant on the probe cover to ease insertion of the probe. Place the probe inside the anus and advance the probe 1 to 2.5 cm (½–1 inch) based on the size of the infant. If resistance is met, stop. Keep your hand cupped around the infant's buttocks.

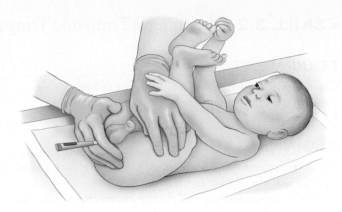

STEP 9. Rectal site: Place the probe inside the anus.

13. **For an adult:**
    a. Provide privacy and position the client in the Sims position, exposing only as much of the body as necessary. *The Sims position makes it anatomically easier to insert the probe into the rectum.*
    b. Lift the top buttock to expose the anus. Have the client take a deep breath and release. *This will relax the sphincter.*
    c. Place water-soluble lubricant on the probe cover to ease the insertion of the probe. Place the probe inside the anus and advance the probe about 2.5 to 3 cm (1–1½ inches), moving in the direction of the umbilicus. **WARNING**: If resistance is met, stop. *This ensures that the probe is within the rectum but does not perforate the colon.*
14. **ACC** Hold the thermometer in place until the auditory signal is heard.
15. **ACC** Note the temperature before turning off the thermometer.
16. **INF** Eject the probe cover into a facility-approved waste container by pushing the button on the back of the probe. If the thermometer is rechargeable, return it to the charger.

FINISHING THE SKILL

17. **INF** Remove gloves.
18. **INF** Perform hand hygiene.
19. **SAF** Ensure client safety and comfort. Ensure that the bed is in the lowest position and verify that the client can identify and reach the nurse call system. *These safety measures reduce the risk of falls.*
20. **EVAL** Evaluate the results for accuracy by comparing them to previous results and observing the client's current condition.
21. **COM** Document temperature assessment findings, noting the site in the legal healthcare record.
22. **COM** Share the results with the client, and if the temperature is outside of the established parameters for the client, notify the authorized healthcare provider.

■ SKILL 3.2 Obtaining a Tympanic Temperature

EQUIPMENT

Clean gloves, if there is a risk of exposure to body fluids
Tympanic thermometer
Probe cover

BEGINNING THE SKILL

1. **INF** Perform hand hygiene. Apply clean gloves if there is a risk of exposure to body fluids.
2. **CCC** Introduce yourself to the client and family and explain the procedure.
3. **SAF** Identify the client using two identifiers.

PROCEDURE

4. **ACC** Assess the client's activity level within the last 30 minutes.
5. **INF** Cover the thermometer probe and turn on the thermometer.
6. **ACC** Position the ear for the best placement of the probe in the ear canal.
   For adults and children older than 3 years: Gently pull the pinna up and back.

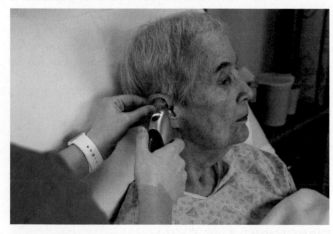

STEP 6 For adults: Gently pull the pinna up and back.

   For children younger than 3 years: Gently pull the pinna down and back.

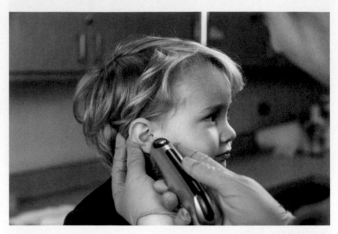

STEP 6 For children younger than 3 years: Gently pull the pinna down and back.

Pulling the pinna straightens the ear canal and helps ensure that the infrared light accesses the tympanic membrane.

7. **ACC** Place the probe firmly inside the ear canal.
8. **ACC** Hold the thermometer in place until the auditory signal is heard, usually within 5 to 30 seconds.
9. Remove the thermometer and read the temperature measurement on the display screen. Eject the probe cover into a facility-approved waste container by pushing the button on the back of the probe.
10. Make sure to make note of the temperature reading before turning off the thermometer. Return the instrument to its charger.

FINISHING THE SKILL

11. **INF** Perform hand hygiene.
12. **SAF** Ensure client safety and comfort. Ensure that the bed is in the lowest position and verify that the client can identify and reach the nurse call system. *These safety measures reduce the risk of falls.*
13. **EVAL** Evaluate the results for accuracy by comparing them to previous results and observing the client's current condition.
14. **COM** Document temperature assessment findings, noting the site, in the legal healthcare record.
15. **COM** Share the results with the client, and if the temperature is outside of the established parameters for the client, notify the authorized healthcare provider.

▪ SKILL 3.3 Obtaining a Temperature Using a Temporal Artery Thermometer

EQUIPMENT

Temporal artery thermometer
Probe cover (may be optional—check facility policy)

BEGINNING THE SKILL

1. **INF** Perform hand hygiene.
2. **CCC** Introduce yourself to the client and family and explain the procedure.
3. **SAF** Identify the client.

PROCEDURE

4. **ACC** Assess the client's activity level within the last 30 minutes.
5. **ACC** Ensure that the skin is dry. If the skin is wet, pat dry.
6. **INF** Cover the thermometer probe, if indicated.
7. **ACC** Place the probe at the center of the forehead, directly onto the skin. Press the "on" button and keep it depressed while measuring the temperature.

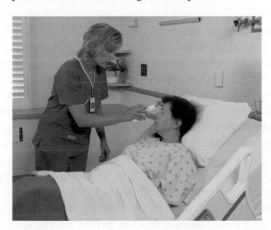

STEP 7 Place the probe at the center of the forehead.

8. **ACC** While continuing to maintain contact with the skin, slowly slide the probe across the forehead to the hairline.

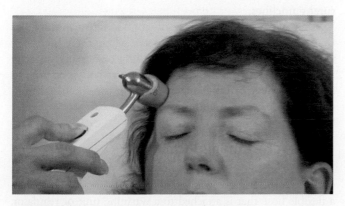

STEP 8 Slide the probe across the forehead.

9. **ACC** While still depressing the "on" button, lift the probe away from the hairline and place it on the skin directly behind the ear. *Measuring the temperature in two places (over the forehead and behind the ear) ensures that heat loss that may occur from the forehead due to evaporation is taken into account. In addition, a temporal artery temperature taken behind the ear is not always accurate on its own because vessel dilatation may not always be present.*

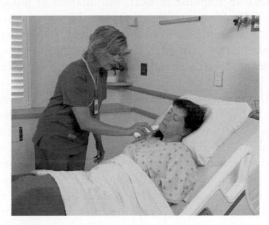

STEP 9 Place the probe behind the ear.

10. Release the "on" button and read the temperature.
11. **INF** Eject the probe cover into a facility-approved waste container by pushing the button on the back of the probe.

FINISHING THE SKILL

12. **INF** Perform hand hygiene.
13. **SAF** Ensure client safety and comfort. Ensure that the bed is in the lowest position and verify that the client can identify and reach the nurse call system. *These safety measures reduce the risk of falls.*
14. **EVAL** Evaluate the results for accuracy by comparing them to previous results and observing the client's current condition.
15. **COM** Document temperature assessment findings, noting the site, in the legal healthcare record.
16. **COM** Share the results with the client, and if the temperature is outside of the established parameters for the client, notify the authorized healthcare provider.

SECTION 2 Regulating Temperature

In the previous section, the range of expected body temperatures and methods of measuring temperature are discussed. As humans, we have a sophisticated system of thermoregulation to keep our body temperature within a certain range. Our body temperature reflects the difference between the heat produced and the amount of heat loss. In response to heat, vasodilation of blood vessels and diaphoresis increase heat loss. In response to cold, vasoconstriction reduces heat loss, and shivering increases heat production. Although temperature may vary slightly, significant deviations from a stable temperature can be fatal.

Serious deviations from a normothermic temperature are hyperthermia and hypothermia. Hyperthermia occurs when the body reaches a dangerous temperature level above the thermoregulatory set-point. It can occur in certain metabolic states in which the body expends a vast amount of energy. One such state is fever, or pyrexia, and another cause of hyperthermia is heat stroke, which occurs when the body is exposed to an environment that is too hot. In both of these examples, the increased body temperature can be fatal if not treated quickly. When the body temperature rises above the thermoregulatory set-point, it is difficult, without intervention, for the body to regain homeostasis. The body may attempt to achieve thermoregulation through sweating, in which fluid released from sweat glands to the skin surface vaporizes into the environment, cooling the body. This method of heat loss, called evaporation, is less effective in a humid environment.

Conversely, hypothermia is a state in which the body temperature decreases below the thermoregulatory set-point. Hypothermia can occur from exposure to a low-temperature environment, such as when a driver becomes stranded in the car during a blizzard. Hypothermia can also occur by design during a medical intervention. For example, in some types of cardiac surgery, temperatures are intentionally lowered in order to decrease metabolic need. Both the very young and the very old are most at risk for hypothermia.

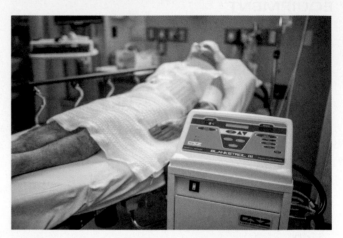

FIG. 3.2 Conductive thermal unit for cooling/heating.

blankets, wraps, or pads that are placed on the client (Fig. 3.2). After the thermal transfer device (e.g., blanket/wrap) is attached to the machine, distilled water (which has been cooled or warmed by the thermal unit) circulates through the thermal transfer device at a prescribed target temperature. Depending on the thermal machine, the target temperature may also be referred to as the set-point (Stryker, 2016). The target temperature or set-point requires an order by the authorized healthcare provider.

The cooling or heating regulation for this type of system can be manual or automatic. If it is set on manual, the nurse monitors the client's temperature and adjusts the temperature of the system according to the order and target temperature. If an automatic mode is used, a temperature probe, supplied by the manufacturer, is placed on the client and then connected by cable to the thermal machine to provide continuous monitoring. This provides a way for the machine to adjust the temperature of the water based on the client's temperature and prescribed set-point. Because there may be variations between thermal machines, check the manufacturer guidelines.

One of the disadvantages of conductive technology is that cooling or heating can only occur where there is contact with the client's skin. Thus, the cooling or heating capacity might be limited, depending on the client's body position. In addition, injury or ischemia can occur if the client has poor circulation or certain conditions, such as Raynaud's disease or diabetes.

Forced-Air Warming Technology

Forced-air warming is a type of convective technology. With this system, temperature-controlled, filtered air is circulated through a flexible hose that is attached to a warming unit or regulator. The hose is also attached to a blanket, vest, or gown that is placed

REGULATING TEMPERATURE

Conductive Cooling/Heating Technology

For clients who need systemic cold or heat therapy to regulate their temperature, conductive technology may be used. This type of technology involves direct cooling or heating by contact with the client's skin. The system usually consists of a thermal unit or machine, connector hoses with clamps, and thermal transfer devices such as full-body

on the client. Some of these systems have specialized high-efficiency particulate air (HEPA) filters and diffusion systems that can prevent the disruption of airflow. The primary indications for forced-air warming are to prevent and treat hypothermia. These systems are often used during perioperative care to help clients maintain a normothermic temperature. To prevent complications, follow the manufacturer guidelines closely. For more information about forced-air warming, see Chapter 17.

Pediatric Considerations

Children, especially neonates, have many risk factors for hypothermia. They have a much higher ratio of surface area to body mass than adults. Newborns cannot shiver. They may have fewer fat reserves and glycogen stores for ready energy to increase their temperature. Nurses caring for newborns and premature infants use isolettes (incubators) and radiant heat warmers to assist with regulating temperature. A radiant heat warmer is designed to warm infants on a mattress below the radiant heater. A probe is attached to the infant to provide feedback to adjust the output of the heater unit. Infants may also be placed inside an isolette, a modern incubator that manages the heat and humidity of the environment.

Safety Considerations

When using heating or cooling technology, be aware of systemic physiologic effects. Because a heating or cooling blanket and/or wraps cover a larger surface area than localized heat/cold, changes in vital signs may occur. To prevent skin damage or burns, keep the area between the client and blanket dry, and follow the manufacturer guidelines regarding time limitations. Before initiating any type of systemic heat or cold therapy, check the order and assess the client carefully to ensure it is the appropriate choice.

APPLICATION OF THE NURSING PROCESS

Examples of Related ICNP Nursing Diagnoses, Expected Client Outcomes, and Nursing Interventions:

Nursing Diagnosis: Impaired thermoregulation
Supporting Data: Potential for hypothermia or hyperthermia
Expected Client Outcomes: The client will exhibit effective thermoregulation:
- temperature within established parameters for client.
Nursing Intervention Examples: Apply thermal units and thermal transfer devices per manufacturer instructions. For an infant, maintain a neutral thermal environment under a radiant warmer.

Nursing Diagnosis: Risk for impaired skin integrity
Supporting Data: Potential for burns or disruptions in the skin from thermal devices
Expected Client Outcomes: The client will have no evidence of redness, skin breakdown, or burn injury.
Nursing Intervention Example: Use burn precautions (e.g., placing a dry barrier between the client's skin and the thermal blanket/wrap, limiting heating or cooling therapy per manufacturer instructions, monitoring skin closely during therapy).
Reference: International Classification for Nursing Practice (n.d.) *eHealth & ICNP*. Retrieved from https://www.icn.ch/what-we-do/projects/ehealth-icnp.

CRITICAL CONCEPTS
Regulating Temperature

Accuracy (ACC)

Accuracy when regulating temperature is sensitive to the following variables:
- temperature of the environment.

Client-Related Factors
- Client history, including allergies, medications, and past procedures
- Client's age, medical history, and indications for heating or cooling therapy
- Presence of impaired circulation or any contraindications, such as Raynaud's disease

Nurse-Related Factors
- Site selection for probe placement
- Selection and use of equipment
- Proper monitoring of client's temperature and effect of therapy

Equipment-Related Factors
- Type of equipment
- Proper functioning of thermal transfer devices (e.g., thermal blankets or wraps)
- Proper functioning of thermal unit or radiant heat warmer

Client-Centered Care (CCC)

When regulating temperature, respect for the client is demonstrated through:
- providing privacy and minimizing client exposure when placing the thermal blankets
- ensuring comfort by proper positioning and ensuring thermal devices are placed properly
- honoring cultural preferences
- advocating for the client and family.

Infection Control (INF)

When regulating temperature, healthcare-associated infection is prevented by:
- preventing and reducing the transfer of microorganisms
- reducing the number of microorganisms.

Safety (SAF)

When regulating temperature, safety measures prevent harm and maintain a safe care environment by:
- ensuring that alarms on thermoregulation equipment are set and remain on at all times
- ensuring that thermoregulation equipment meets medical facility standards.

Communication (COM)

- Communication exchanges information (verbal, nonverbal, or electronic) between two or more people.
- Documentation records temperature regulation in a permanent legal record.
- Collaboration with other healthcare professionals to regulate a client's temperature improves care.

Health Maintenance (HLTH)

When regulating temperature, nursing is dedicated to the promotion of health, including:

- protection of the client's skin integrity and prevention of burns or injury.

Evaluation (EVAL)

When regulating temperature, the evaluation of outcomes enables the nurse to determine the safety and efficacy of the care provided.

■ SKILL 3.4 Using Conductive Cooling or Heating Therapy

EQUIPMENT

Clean gloves, if there is a risk of exposure to body fluids
Washcloth and towels
Blood pressure cuff
Stethoscope
Thermometer
Antiseptic wipes
Equipment for taking temperature manually
Sterile distilled water (if needed)
Temperature probe (supplied by manufacturer)
Disposable protective sheaths for temperature probe
Thermal unit/machine for systemic cooling or heating therapy
Thermal transfer devices (thermal blankets or wraps) for thermal machine

BEGINNING THE SKILL

1. **SAF** Review the order for cooling or heating therapy, including the set-point or target temperature. *When the thermal unit/machine is in automatic mode, the set-point or target temperature is the desired and prescribed temperature for the client; in the manual mode, the set-point is the desired temperature for the water (Stryker, 2016).*
2. **INF** Perform hand hygiene.
3. **CCC** Introduce yourself to the client and family and explain the procedure.
4. **SAF** Identify the client using two identifiers.
5. **CCC** Obtain informed consent.
6. **CCC** Provide privacy.

PROCEDURE

7. **ACC** Assess the following:
   a. Client's level of orientation and ability to follow instructions
   b. Client and family's understanding of cooling or heating therapy
   c. Client's level of pain and discomfort
   d. Client's age, medical history, and indications for cooling or heating therapy
   e. Possible contraindications/precautions (e.g., circulatory disorders, Raynaud's disease, diabetes, skin disorders)
   f. Presence of transdermal medication patches. *A cooling/heating device could affect transdermal medication delivery.*
8. **ACC** Assess vital signs and peripheral pulses. *Systemic cooling or heating therapy covers a larger surface area than localized therapy and may have a more systemic physiologic effect. Assessing vital signs before the procedure establishes a baseline assessment.*
9. **HLTH** Examine skin on client's body where thermal transfer devices (cooling or heating blanket/wraps) will be in contact; assess for any redness, irritation, or breakdown of skin integrity. (Note: Avoid these areas if possible).
10. **SAF** Check the thermal machine and thermal transfer devices (cooling or heating blankets/wraps).
    a. Ensure that outlets, cables, and connectors are intact, without breaks or frays.
    b. Ensure that thermal transfer devices (blankets/wraps) are clean and intact.
    c. Secure wheel locks of the machine by pressing locks down with feet. *Prevents machine from moving or rolling away.*
11. **ACC** Prepare thermal machine and thermal transfer devices.
    a. Check the water level in the thermal machine. If needed, fill reservoir with sterile distilled water per manufacturer guidelines. Do not overfill. *Distilled water prevents damage to the internal components. Overfilling could cause overflow from blanket drainage when the machine is off.*
    b. While the clamps are closed on the connectors, attach connector hoses to the thermal transfer devices

(blankets/wraps) and to the thermal machine per the manufacturer guidelines. Check the connector hoses to ensure there are no kinks.

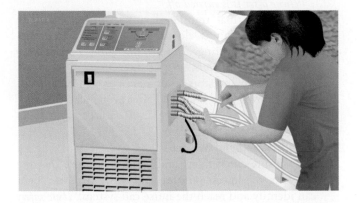

STEP 11B Attaching and checking the connector hoses.

c. Open the clamps on the connector hoses prior to turning the thermal machine on. *Failure to open the clamps before the thermal machine is turned on will prevent water from flowing properly to the blankets/ body wraps (Stryker, 2016).*

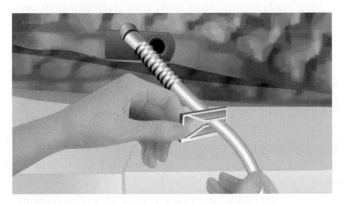

STEP 11C Opening the connector hose clamps.

12. **ACC** Plug the power cord into the grounded receptacle and press the "on" button of the thermal machine.
13. **SAF** Ensure that no leaks are present.
14. **INF** Apply gloves, if there is a risk of exposure to body fluids.
15. **ACC** Assist the client to the appropriate position and adjust the thermal transfer device (blankets or body wraps) as ordered.
16. **SAF** Ensure that there is a sheet or barrier between the client and the thermal transfer devices, and keep areas between the client and thermal transfer devices dry. *Placing a dry absorbent sheet or barrier between the client and the thermal transfer devices will facilitate uniform distribution and prevent burn injury.*

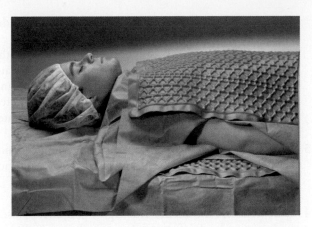

STEP 16 A dry barrier should be between the client and the thermal transfer device.

17. **SAF** Place extra protection and barriers around sensitive areas or genitalia. *Prevents burn injury.*
18. **SAF** Avoid placing any fluids or any other heat source under the client or allowing moisture to get between the client and the thermal transfer devices. *Heating or cooling can increase the toxicity of certain solutions and injure the client's skin.*
19. **SAF** Avoid metal items on bedding or client clothing, such as snaps or pins. *Metal is a conductor of heat, and these items could become hot and uncomfortable.*
20. **SAF** Adjust initial settings on thermal machine per order and manufacturer guidelines. **WARNING:** Ensure that all alarms are on and working properly.
21. **ACC** If using the thermal machine in the manual mode:
    a. Press the button for manual mode.
    b. Adjust the set-point for water temperature on the thermal machine as ordered.
    c. Monitor the client's temperature closely and adjust heating or cooling based on the needs of the client and the order of the authorized healthcare provider.
    d. Follow facility policy and order regarding when to turn the machine off. *Some facilities require that the unit be turned off when the client's temperature is within 0.05 to 0.01 degrees of the desired temperature in order to avoid inadvertent temperature drift.*
22. **ACC** If using the thermal machine in the automatic mode:
    a. **INF** Apply clean gloves. (Note: After the probe is placed, remove gloves and perform hand hygiene before continuing care for the client.)
    b. Prepare and place the temperature probe as directed by the manufacturer. The probe should measure the client's core temperature. (Note: Some facilities use a bladder or esophageal probe to measure core temperature.) **WARNING:** Avoid using a rectal probe in an adult or if the client has contraindications, such as neutropenia (low WBC count), a rectal abscess, or rectal bleeding. *Rectal procedures can cause irritation or trauma of the rectal mucosa and abscesses in clients who are at risk for infections.*

c. Place the cable of the temperature probe into the thermal machine.

d. Adjust the set-point or target temperature on the thermal machine as ordered. (Note: When in automatic mode, the thermal machine monitors and compares the client's temperature with the ordered set-point and then automatically adjusts the water temperature.)

23. **SAF** Ensure that the temperature of the water does not exceed the maximum recommended contact surface temperature (usually no greater than 40°C [104°F]). *This prevents burn injury (Stryker, 2016).*

24. **CCC** Reassess the client's vital signs, peripheral pulses, and comfort level at frequent intervals during cooling or heating therapy as indicated by policy and client needs.

25. **HLTH** Reinspect the client's skin at frequent intervals for any irritation, redness, or other changes.

26. **ACC** Continue to monitor the water level in the thermal machine reservoir. *If the water level becomes too low, mechanisms could overheat and be damaged.* (Note: If the device will not heat or cool, double-check that there is water in the reservoir and ensure that the flow to the pad is not blocked. Check again to make sure there are no kinks in the hoses.)

27. **ACC** Discontinue cooling or heating therapy as ordered. *Some facilities require the thermal machine to be turned off when the client is at certain level or near the desired temperature.*

a. Press the "off" or "standby" button and unplug the thermal machine.

b. Allow the thermal transfer device (blanket/body wrap) to remain on for 5 to 10 minutes before removing. *Allows for water to drain back into the machine after it is turned off.*

c. If the thermal transfer device (e.g., blanket/body wraps) has clamps, close them or pinch them off before disconnecting. *This prevents water from spilling out of the connectors.*

d. **INF** Clean and store equipment per facility policy.

28. **INF** Remove gloves if applied after probe placement.

FINISHING THE SKILL

29. **INF** Perform hand hygiene.

30. **SAF** Ensure client safety and comfort. Ensure that the bed is in the lowest position and verify that the client can identify and reach the nurse call system. *These safety measures reduce the risk of falls.*

31. **EVAL** Evaluate the client outcomes. *Was the cooling or heating therapy effective? Did your client tolerate the procedure?*

32. **COM** Document assessment findings, care given, and outcomes in the legal healthcare record, including:

- set-point or target temperature that was used for cooling or heating therapy
- type of temperature probe used and location (if automatic mode used)
- condition of client's skin before, during, and after application
- client's temperature before, during, and after cooling or heating therapy.

■ SKILL 3.5 Using an Infant Radiant Warmer

EQUIPMENT

Radiant warmer
Heat reflective skin patch
Skin probe

BEGINNING THE SKILL

1. **SAF** Review the authorized healthcare provider's order and hospital policy. *Verifying the plan of care prevents injury to the client.*

2. **INF** Perform hand hygiene.

3. **SAF** Set up an ergonomically safe space. Ensure the wheels are locked. Ensure the bed is the appropriate distance from the warming unit. Ensure the unit is plugged in and working.

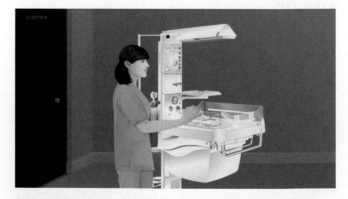

STEP 3 Set up an ergonomically safe space.

4. **SAF** Turn on the warmer and prewarm the unit according to the manufacturer's instructions. Many units are prewarmed in manual mode, then switched to skin or Servo mode when the infant is placed in the warmer.

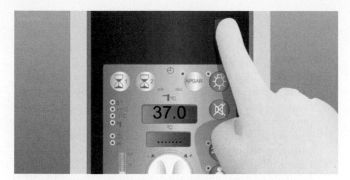

STEP 4 Turn on the warmer and prewarm the unit.

PROCEDURE

5. **INF** Perform hand hygiene.
6. **SAF** Identify the client using two identifiers.
7. **CCC** If family members are present, explain the procedure.
8. **ACC** When the unit is warm, place the infant in the warmer.
9. **ACC** Attach the skin probe metal-side down over the liver area of the infant's abdomen using a heat-reflective patch. The foil side of the patch faces the heater, and the adhesive side secures the patch to the infant. Do not apply over a bony area. Do not allow the infant to lie on the skin probe. *Consistent contact between the probe and the infant's skin is required for accurate warming. The foil is reflective, ensuring the probe measures the infant's temperature and is not directly heated by the warming units.*

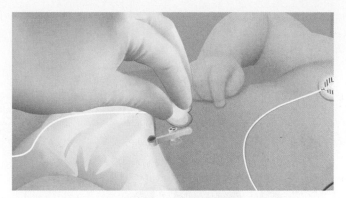

STEP 9 Attach the skin probe.

10. **ACC** Ensure the heater is in the correct mode to read the surface temperature of the infant (Servo vs. manual) and is accurately reading the skin temperature.
11. **ACC** Ensure that the alarms for high and low temperatures are set appropriately for the infant.

FINISHING THE SKILL

12. **INF** Perform hand hygiene.
13. **SAF** Ensure client safety and comfort.
14. **EVAL** Evaluate the contact between the probe and the infant's skin every half hour or per the manufacturer's guidelines. Evaluate the infant's temperature per hospital policy or authorized healthcare provider's orders.
15. **COM** Document temperature assessment findings, such as infant temperature measurements and temperature settings on the warmer; care given; and outcomes in the legal healthcare record.

SECTION 3 Assessing Pulses

The client's pulse reflects left ventricular contraction and the subsequent force of blood flowing through the arteries. The strength (amplitude or volume) or quality of the pulse also indicates the amount of circulating blood and the efficiency of the heart. As with other vital sign parameters, it is important to identify the client's baseline in order to know if interventions are needed.

According to the American Heart Association (2017), the average resting pulse rate for adults is 60 to 100 beats per minute. Pulse rates in children vary depending on the child's age (Table 3.2). When a client's pulse rate is not within established parameters, it is important to look at trends and other factors. For example, how does the client's pulse rate compare to the client's baseline pulse rate on admission? Does the client's pulse feel weak or thready? What is abnormal for one client may not be unusual for another client. Other factors to consider are associated signs and symptoms. Does the client feel light-headed or dizzy? Is the client having palpitations?

LOCATION AND DIFFERENTIATION OF PULSES

Pulses are assessed in several locations: carotid, peripheral (which includes radial, brachial, femoral, popliteal, dorsalis pedis, and posterior tibial), and apical (Fig. 3.3). As part of a head-to-toe physical assessment, it is common for the nurse

TABLE 3.2 Pulse Rate Parameters

Age Group	Normal Resting Pulse Rate (Beats/Minute)
Newborn	80–160
1-year-old	80–140
15-year-old	50–90
Adult	60–100
Older adult	60–100

References: American Heart Association, 2017; Yoost & Crawford, 2016.

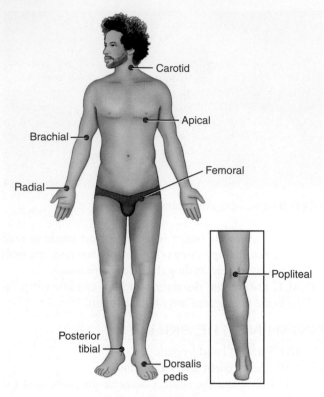

FIG. 3.3 Pulse sites.

to check all of these pulses. The radial pulse is the most commonly used peripheral pulse to count the client's pulse rate. This is recorded as beats per minute (bpm). If the radial pulse is not easily palpated, other pulses, such as the carotid pulse rate, may be used. The carotid pulse is a reflection of arterial blood flow to the brain, and the peripheral pulses reflect circulation to the upper and lower extremities.

APICAL PULSE

In contrast to the other pulses (which are obtained by palpation), the apical pulse is usually obtained by direct auscultation of the heartbeat at the apex of the heart or the point of maximal impulse (PMI). An apical pulse is often used for adults and is preferred for infants and children. (For more information on children, see Box 3.2) The advantage of obtaining an apical pulse is that it facilitates a more accurate count of the client's heart rate while also allowing the nurse to note any irregularities or unusual sounds of the heartbeat. When obtaining an apical pulse rate, a rhythmic, two-beat "lub-dub" sound should be heard, and these two sounds count as one heartbeat when you are counting the apical heart rate. The rate should be counted for 60 seconds.

A discrepancy between the apical and radial pulse rate is called a pulse deficit. When checking for a pulse deficit, auscultate the apical pulse and palpate the radial pulse for a full minute at the same time. This procedure should be done by two different nurses if possible. If the client has a pulse deficit that deviates from the client's baseline, it may be related to decreased perfusion of the extremities. Perform a system-specific (heart and lungs) assessment (see Chapter 4) and notify the authorized healthcare provider as indicated.

BOX 3.2 Lifespan Considerations: Obtaining Heart Rates in Pediatric Clients

- In infants and children younger than 2 years, the pulse rate is obtained by auscultating an apical pulse at the point of maximum impulse (PMI). It is helpful to perform this procedure while the infant/child is resting if possible.
- In older children, the pulse rate may be obtained by palpating either the radial or brachial pulse.
- Count the pulse rate for 1 full minute as a baseline; if frequent readings are required, use shorter times (15–30 seconds).
- If the pulse is irregular, count for 1 full minute to ensure accurate measurement. Sinus arrhythmia (the heart rate increasing with inspiration and decreasing with expiration) may be quite noticeable in infants and children.

BOX 3.3 Tips for Using a Stethoscope

- Turn the ear tips of the stethoscope to follow the path of the ear canal.
- Move your chin toward your chest and determine the position where the earpieces best fit into your ear canals and you do not hear sounds from the room.
- If the stethoscope has a rotating end piece, the side you wish to use (bell or diaphragm) must be turned to the opening ensure the sound travels up the tubing.
- The bell is designed to hear low-pitched tones, and the diaphragm is designed to hear higher-pitched tones.
- Use light pressure when placing the chest piece against the client's skin. Heavy pressure may prevent you from hearing well.
- In order to prevent your stethoscope from becoming a vector and transferring microorganisms from one client to another, clean the end piece with an antiseptic wipe before using it with a client. Clean the earpieces with an antiseptic wipe anytime you place a shared stethoscope in your ears.
- Never submerge the chest piece of a stethoscope in water.
- If your stethoscope tubing is made of polyvinyl chloride (PVC) and you wear it against your skin, the tubing will harden over time. Therefore, keep your stethoscope in your pocket when not in use, and clean the entire stethoscope regularly.

In order to obtain an accurate apical pulse, the nurse must identify the proper landmarks for placement of the stethoscope, and the stethoscope must be used correctly. Tips for using a stethoscope are listed in Box 3.3.

TECHNIQUE FOR ASSESSING PULSES

When palpating pulses, accuracy is one of the most important critical concepts to consider. To ensure accuracy, use the pads of the first two or three fingers, not the fingertips. Note the characteristics of the pulse, such as the overall strength,

TABLE 3.3 Grading Palpated Pulses

Grade	Description
4+	Full and bounding Easily palpated with light pressure Difficult to obliterate May be able to see pulsation
3+	Normal Able to palpate pulse without difficulty using normal pressure
2+	Weak Difficult to palpate but can feel steady pulse
1+	Thready Barely able to palpate May not be able to feel pulse consistently

Note: Grading scale can only be used for palpation (not Doppler pulses).

amplitude, and rhythm, and whether or not the pulses are equal bilaterally. To express the strength (amplitude or volume) of the pulse, use a 4-point palpation grading system ranging from 1+ (thready) to 4+ (bounding; see Table 3.3). The rhythm may be determined by assessing whether the pulse is regular or irregular.

To determine if the peripheral pulses are equal bilaterally, palpate and compare the pulses in both extremities at the same time. When palpating the carotid pulses, avoid pressing too hard. Palpate one side at a time because simultaneous palpation may decrease blood flow to the client's brain.

Palpation of the pulse requires the nurse's nails to be short. Long nails may interfere with finger-pad contact or injure the client when pressure is applied. If the peripheral or carotid pulses are difficult to locate by palpation, a Doppler ultrasound may be used. A Doppler is a small handheld (noninvasive) device that amplifies the sound of the pulse or blood flow. As discussed in Box 3.4, it is important not to assume or document that the client's pulses are absent just because you don't feel them. You may be able to locate the pulses with the Doppler, and this should be properly documented. It is also important to consider other assessment parameters, such as warmth, sensation, and movement. If there is a significant change from the baseline assessment of the client's pulses, notify the authorized healthcare provider, and document the findings accordingly.

ALTERATIONS OF THE CLIENT'S PULSE

If a client has alterations in his or her pulse, such as when the pulse deviates from the expected rate or is irregular, the nurse must attempt to determine the underlying cause. Because the pulse is affected by the autonomic nervous system, factors such as anxiety, fear, pain, or discomfort, as well as stress, can affect the pulse. A variety of substances, such as caffeine, nicotine, certain herbs, and medications, can also affect the pulse rate, as can recent physical activity, room temperature, and even noise. Physiologic changes may also directly affect the pulse rate. For example, a decreased circulating blood volume related to hypovolemia may result in a weak and thready palpated peripheral pulse as well as compensatory tachycardia.

BOX 3.4 **Expect the Unexpected: Unable to Find Peripheral Pulses**

On a medical-surgical unit, Tori, a student nurse, is caring for Mr. Carter, a client who had a femoral catheter placed in his right femoral artery on the previous shift. Mr. Carter has an order for his dorsalis pedis and posterior tibial pulses to be assessed every 2 hours. When checking Mr. Carter's pulses, Tori is unable to feel anything. She notes that on the previous shift, the pulses were graded as 2+ bilaterally. She also observes that Mr. Carter's lower extremities are warm to the touch and pink in color. She documents on her written assessment for her clinical instructor, "Pulses absent bilaterally, grading 0, extremities pink and warm to touch."

The clinical instructor responds, "Tori, I see that you charted that Mr. Carter's lower extremities were pink and warm but that the pulses were absent bilaterally. Generally, if the extremity is pink and warm, there is, in fact, a pulse, even if you were having trouble palpating it. In this situation, it's critical not to assume that the pulse is absent. Remember that your assessment of the client is important and becomes a part of the medical record. If you are having trouble palpating a client's pulses, additional assessment tools, such as the Doppler ultrasound device, and other circulatory assessment parameters, such as measuring capillary refill, can be used to obtain accurate information. It is important not to document "pulses absent" unless you also document additional assessment parameters and interventions that were done. In addition, it is important to document whom you notified about these findings."

After using the Doppler ultrasound device to assist with finding the pulses, Tori correctly documents the following:
Extremities pink and warm; brisk capillary refill
Dorsalis pedis—heard with Doppler bilaterally
Posterior tibial—heard with Doppler bilaterally

Because the pulse reflects the client's underlying heart rhythm, alterations may indicate that more advanced cardiac monitoring is necessary. The nurse might make this determination, for example, when the client's pulse is very irregular or deviates significantly from the client's baseline. If the client is already receiving cardiac monitoring and develops a dysrhythmia, assessment of the pulse will allow the nurse to determine the client's peripheral perfusion (see Chapter 19). When the client's pulse is irregular, obtain the pulse rate for a full minute (60 seconds) to facilitate an accurate assessment and heart rate.

APPLICATION OF THE NURSING PROCESS

Examples of Related ICNP Nursing Diagnoses, Expected Client Outcomes, and Nursing Interventions:

Nursing Diagnosis: Risk for impaired peripheral tissue perfusion

Supporting Data: Peripheral pulses weak and thready, apical-radial pulse deficit

Expected Client Outcomes: The client will demonstrate adequate peripheral tissue perfusion:
- peripheral pulses 2+ bilaterally on palpation
- pulse rate within established parameters for client

- upper and lower extremities warm to touch
- capillary refill time in nailbeds of less than 2 seconds.

Nursing Intervention Examples: Palpate pulses and compare/grade bilaterally. Monitor skin warmth of extremities.

Reference: International Classification for Nursing Practice (n.d.). *eHealth & ICNP.* Retrieved from https://www.icn.ch/what-we-do/projects/ehealth-icnp.

CRITICAL CONCEPTS
Assessing Pulses

Accuracy (ACC)

Pulse measurement is sensitive to the following variables:

Client-Related Factors
- Recent ingestion of nicotine, caffeine, medications, or herbal preparations
- Recent exercise or exertion
- Pain, anxiety, or a full bladder
- Environment (e.g., room temperature, room noise)

Nurse-Related Factors
- Site selection of the pulse
- Proper identification of anatomical landmarks for pulse sites
- Proper technique when palpating pulses
- Auscultation technique for apical pulse

Equipment-Related Factors

Equipment, such as a Doppler machine, must be in good working order and have a battery if needed.

Client-Centered Care (CCC)

When assessing pulses, respect for the client is demonstrated through:
- promoting autonomy
- ensuring comfort
- providing privacy and only exposing what is necessary when assessing peripheral and apical pulses.

Infection Control (INF)

When assessing pulses, healthcare-associated infection is prevented by:
- reducing the transfer and number of microorganisms, primarily through hand hygiene.

Safety (SAF)

When assessing pulses, safety measures provide a safe care environment and prevent harm to the client.

Communication (COM)

- Communication exchanges information (oral, written, non-verbal, electronic) between two or more people.
- Documentation records information on pulse assessment in a permanent legal record.

Evaluation (EVAL)

Evaluation of the outcomes allows the nurse to determine the efficacy of the care provided

---

▪ SKILL 3.6 Obtaining a Radial Pulse Rate

EQUIPMENT

Digital watch or watch with a second hand

BEGINNING THE SKILL

1. **INF** Perform hand hygiene.
2. **CCC** Introduce yourself to client and family and explain the procedure.
3. **SAF** Identify the client using two identifiers.
4. **CCC** Provide privacy.

PROCEDURE

5. **ACC** Assess the client for exercise and nicotine or caffeine intake within the last 30 minutes.
6. **ACC** Seat the client in a quiet, calm environment.
7. **ACC** Expose the client's wrist so that the radial artery is not covered with clothing.

8. **CCC** Support the client's wrist. *Supporting the client's wrist stabilizes the joint and facilitates client comfort.*
9. **ACC** Identify the anatomical landmarks for the radial pulses. The radial pulse is located on the inner wrist, thumb side, medial to the bony prominence of the radial head.
10. **ACC** Using the first two or three finger pads (not fingertips), locate the radial pulse. If it is difficult to locate the radial pulse, assist the client in slightly dorsiflexing (bending back) the wrist. Use sufficient pressure to feel a steady, uninterrupted pulse beat. Do not use the thumb or press so hard as to completely occlude the artery. *Using two or three finger pads increases the surface area and sensitivity for assessment of the pulse. Dorsiflexing brings the artery closer to the surface so that the pulse is easier to palpate. The thumb is not used because the thumb has a pulse that could confound assessment.*

11. **ACC** Observe the time while counting the radial pulse rate and note whether the rhythm is regular or irregular. If the client's pulse is regular, count for 30 seconds and multiply by 2. If the client's pulse is irregular or weak, count the client's pulse for 1 full minute. *The rhythm and regularity of the pulse reflect the client's underlying heart function. Assessment for 1 minute facilitates obtaining an accurate assessment of the pulse when it is irregular.*

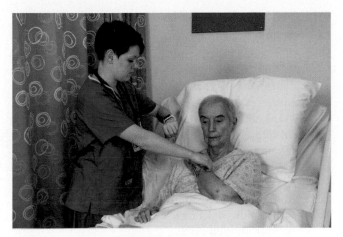

STEP 11 Obtaining the radial pulse rate.

12. **ACC** Palpate both radial pulses at the same time and compare bilaterally. Assess the strength and character of the pulses; grade the force or amplitude by using a grading scale 1+ (thready) to 4+ (bounding; see Table 3.3). *The strength, character, and amplitude of the pulses reflect the circulating blood volume and efficiency of the heart.*

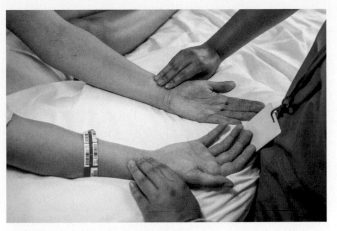

STEP 12 Compare radial pulses bilaterally.

FINISHING THE SKILL

13. **INF** Perform hand hygiene.
14. **SAF** Ensure client safety and comfort. Ensure that the bed is in the lowest position and verify that the client can identify and reach the nurse call system. *These safety measures reduce the risk of falls.*
15. **EVAL** Evaluate the results for accuracy by comparing them to previous results and observing the client's current condition.
16. **COM** Document assessment findings in the legal healthcare record, including:
    - radial pulse rate in beats per minute (bpm)
    - which side (right or left wrist) was used to obtain the radial pulse rate
    - character, quality, and rhythm of radial pulse
    - strength of palpated radial pulse using a 4-point scale (see Table 3.3).
17. **COM** Share the results with the client, and if the radial pulse rate is outside of the established parameters for the client, notify the authorized healthcare provider.

■ SKILL 3.7 Assessing Carotid Pulses

EQUIPMENT

Digital watch or watch with a second hand

BEGINNING THE SKILL

1. **INF** Perform hand hygiene.
2. **CCC** Introduce yourself to client and family and explain the procedure.
3. **SAF** Identify the client using two identifiers.
4. **CCC** Provide privacy.

PROCEDURE

5. **ACC** Assess the client for exercise and nicotine or caffeine intake within the last 30 minutes.

6. **ACC** Seat the client in a quiet, calm environment.
7. **ACC** Identify the anatomical landmarks for the carotid pulses. (Note: The carotid pulse is located in the groove in the neck between the sternocleidomastoid muscle and the trachea.)
8. **ACC** Use the first two or three finger pads (not fingertips) to locate the carotid pulse. Use sufficient pressure to feel a steady, uninterrupted pulse beat. Do not use the thumb or press so hard as to completely occlude the artery. *Using the first two or three finger pads increases the surface area and sensitivity for assessment of the pulse. The thumb is not used because the thumb has a pulse that could confound the assessment.*

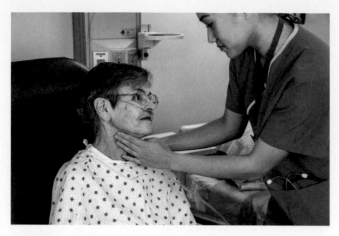

STEP 8 Locating the carotid pulse.

9. **SAF** Palpate the carotid pulses one at a time. **WARNING:** Do not press down on the carotid pulses bilaterally at the same time. *Palpating both carotid arteries at the same time may decrease blood flow to the brain. Compressing the carotid sinus may stimulate the vagus nerve and cause reflex bradycardia.*

10. **ACC** Observe the time while counting the carotid pulse rate and note whether the rhythm is regular or irregular. If the client's pulse is regular, count for 30 seconds and multiply by 2. If the client's pulse is irregular or weak, count the client's pulse for 1 full minute. *This enhances accuracy. The rhythm and regularity of the pulse reflect the client's underlying heart function.*

11. **SAF** Assess the strength of the carotid pulses, and grade the force or amplitude bilaterally (one at a time) by using the palpation technique and a grading scale of 1+ (thready) to 4+ (bounding; see Table 3.3). *The strength and amplitude of the pulses reflect the circulating blood volume and efficiency of the heart. Grading pulses bilaterally facilitates accurate assessment.* **WARNING:** Avoid massaging the client's neck. *Massaging may stimulate the vagus nerve and result in bradycardia.*

FINISHING THE SKILL

12. **INF** Perform hand hygiene.
13. **SAF** Ensure client safety and comfort. Ensure that the bed is in the lowest position and verify that the client can identify and reach the nurse call system. *These safety measures reduce the risk of falls.*
14. **EVAL** Evaluate the results for accuracy by comparing them to previous results and observing the client's current condition.
15. **COM** Document assessment findings in the legal healthcare record, including:
    - carotid pulse rate in beats per minute (bpm)
    - which side (right or left carotid) was used to obtain the carotid pulse rate
    - character, quality, and rhythm of pulse
    - strength of palpated carotid pulse using a 4-point scale (see Table 3.3).
16. **COM** Share the results with the client, and if the carotid pulse findings are outside of the established parameters for the client, notify the authorized healthcare provider.

■ SKILL 3.8 Assessing Peripheral Pulses

EQUIPMENT

Clean gloves for palpating femoral pulses
Pillow
Doppler if needed

BEGINNING THE SKILL

1. **INF** Perform hand hygiene.
2. **CCC** Introduce yourself to the client and family and explain the procedure.
3. **SAF** Identify the client using two identifiers.
4. **CCC** Provide privacy.

PROCEDURE

5. **ACC** Assess the client for exercise and nicotine or caffeine intake within the last 30 minutes.

6. **ACC** Seat the client in a quiet, calm environment.
7. **ACC** Identify the anatomical landmarks for each peripheral pulse. Use the first two or three finger pads (not fingertips) to locate the peripheral pulse. Use sufficient pressure to feel a steady, uninterrupted pulse beat. Do not use the thumb or press so hard as to completely occlude the artery. *Using the first two or three finger pads increases the surface area and sensitivity for assessment of the pulse. The thumb is not used because the thumb has a pulse that could confound the assessment.*
   a. **Palpate the brachial pulses:** The pulse is located on the inner aspect of the arm in the antecubital area medial to the biceps tendon. Ensure that the client's palms are facing up so that the antecubital area is exposed. To facilitate palpation, ask the client to extend the arm and rest it on a pillow. (Note: If a pillow

is not available, support the client's arm behind the elbow with your nondominant hand.) *Extending and supporting the arm brings the artery closer to the surface and facilitates palpation.*

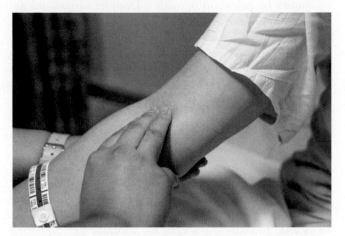

STEP 7A Palpating the brachial pulse.

b. **Palpate the femoral pulses:** The femoral pulse is located midway between the anterior iliac spine and the symphysis pubis. Apply gloves before palpating the femoral pulses, palpate the pulses, and then remove the gloves and perform hand hygiene before palpating other pulses. To facilitate palpation of the femoral pulses, have the client lie flat in bed, if tolerated, and extend the lower extremities. It may also be helpful to place one hand over the other and press more firmly. For obese clients, it may be helpful to assist the client to turn or externally rotate the hip in order to allow more surface area for palpation. *The femoral artery may be fairly deep and, thus, may require deeper compression.*

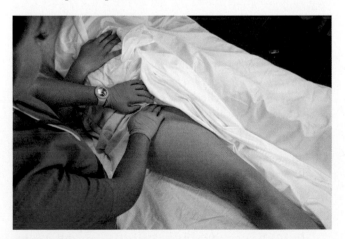

STEP 7B Palpating the femoral pulse.

c. **Palpate the popliteal pulses:** The popliteal pulse is located behind the knee in the popliteal fossa, which is marked by the lower edge of the femur and the upper edge of the tibia. It is often adjacent to the medial tendon. With the client's leg extended, place two or three finger pads into the popliteal fossa and compress the artery against the bone. (Note: It may be helpful to turn the client on his or her side to assess the popliteal pulse and to place a pillow between the client's knees to facilitate proper alignment and extension.) *Extending the leg brings the artery closer to the surface and facilitates palpation.*

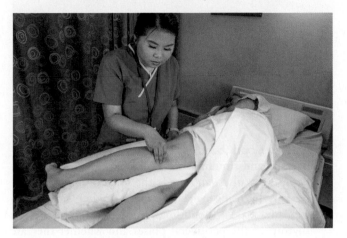

STEP 7C Palpating the popliteal pulse.

d. **Palpate the posterior tibial pulses:** The posterior tibial pulse is located along the inside of the foot around the medial malleolus. If you are having difficulty palpating the posterior tibial pulses, ask the client to dorsiflex the foot so that the toes point toward the knee. *Dorsiflexing the foot brings the artery closer to the surface and facilitates palpation.*

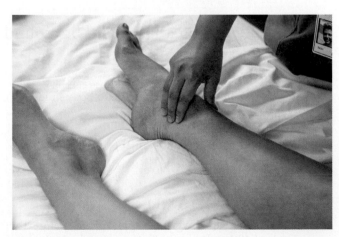

STEP 7D Palpating the posterior tibial pulse.

e. **Palpate the dorsalis pedis pulses:** The dorsalis pedis pulse is located on the dorsum of the foot. Identify the pulse in the groove midway or just distal to the arch of the foot and parallel with the first and second toe. (Note: This location may vary slightly, depending on the client.) *Identifying the groove may allow the pulse to be more easily palpated.*

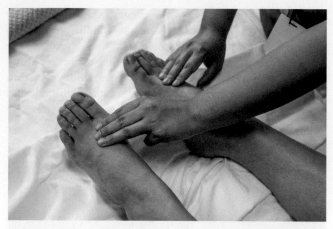

STEP 7E Palpating the dorsalis pedis pulses and comparing bilaterally.

8. **ACC** Use both hands to assess the peripheral pulses bilaterally and simultaneously. Assess the strength of the peripheral pulses, and grade the force or amplitude bilaterally by using palpation and a grading scale of 1+ (thready) to 4+ (bounding; see Table 3.3). Note the rhythm of the peripheral pulses and whether they are regular or irregular. *The strength, amplitude, and rhythm of the pulse reflect the circulating blood volume and efficiency of the heart. Grading pulses bilaterally facilitates accurate assessment and allows comparison of the circulation in the left and right extremities. The rhythm and regularity of the pulses are also a reflection of the client's underlying heart rhythm.*

9. **ACC** If the peripheral pulses are difficult to locate by palpation, use a Doppler ultrasound device to audibly obtain the pulses (see Skill 3.9) and mark their location with a waterproof pen. If you are unable to locate the pulses by palpation or with a Doppler ultrasound device, notify the authorized healthcare provider. *The client's pulse may be present even though it is not palpable. The Doppler ultrasound device detects pulses by amplifying sound waves that are created by the movement of the pulsation through the arteries. Marking pulses that are hard to locate makes them easier to find for follow-up assessments.*

FINISHING THE SKILL

10. **INF** Perform hand hygiene.
11. **SAF** Ensure client safety and comfort. Ensure that the bed is in the lowest position and verify that the client can identify and reach the nurse call system. *These safety measures reduce the risk of falls.*
12. **EVAL** Evaluate the results for accuracy by comparing them to previous results and observing the client's current condition.
13. **COM** Document assessment findings in the legal healthcare record, including:
    * Bilateral strength of pulses (if palpated) using a 4-point scale (see Table 3.3)
    * Character, quality, and rhythm of pulses
14. **COM** Share the results with the client, and if the pulse findings are outside of the established parameters for the client, notify the authorized healthcare provider.

■ SKILL 3.9 Using a Doppler Ultrasound Device to Assess Pulses

EQUIPMENT

Clean gloves, if there is a risk of exposure to body fluids
Doppler ultrasound device with probe
Extra battery if needed
Ultrasonic conductive gel or individual packets of gel
Waterproof pen or marker
Tissue or paper towel

BEGINNING THE SKILL

1. **INF** Perform hand hygiene. Apply gloves before the procedure, if there is a risk of exposure to body fluids.
2. **CCC** Introduce yourself to the client and family and explain the procedure.
3. **SAF** Identify the client using two identifiers.
4. **CCC** Provide privacy.

PROCEDURE

5. **ACC** Turn on the Doppler ultrasound device and check that it is functioning properly. *Identifying technical problems before entering the client's room saves time.*
6. **ACC** Assess the client for exercise and nicotine or caffeine intake within the last 30 minutes.
7. **ACC** Seat the client in a quiet, calm environment.
8. **ACC** Identify the anatomical landmarks for the selected pulse. Place a generous amount of conductive gel directly on the anatomical landmark over the arterial pulsation site. *A sufficient amount of conductive gel facilitates the transfer of sound.*
9. **ACC** Position the entire end of the Doppler probe in the conductive gel, making direct contact with the skin where the pulse site is located. *Increasing the contact area of the end of the probe facilitates identification of the pulse waves.*

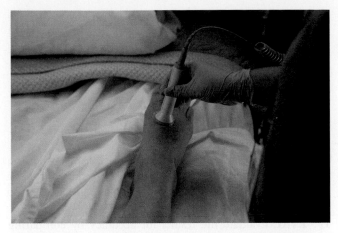

STEP 9 Place the end of the probe in the conductive gel.

10. **ACC** Turn the Doppler ultrasound device to the "on" position after the probe is placed and adjust the volume as needed.

11. **ACC** Move the probe over the anatomical landmark until you hear a "swishing" pulse sound. Apply more conductive gel if needed.

12. **ACC** Assess the audible rhythm of the pulse and note whether it is regular or irregular. If the client's pulse is regular, count for 30 seconds and multiply by 2. If the client's pulse is irregular or weak, count the client's pulse for 1 full minute. *The rhythm and regularity of the pulse is*

a reflection of the client's underlying heart function. Assessment for 1 minute facilitates obtaining an accurate assessment of the pulse.

13. **CCC** Clean the conductive gel from the client's skin.

14. **ACC** If it was difficult to find the pulse, mark the area with a waterproof pen at the site. *This expedites identification and makes it easier to find the pulse for follow-up assessments.*

15. Turn the Doppler ultrasound device off.

16. Clean the probe by wiping off the conductive gel with a tissue.

18. **INF** Disinfect equipment (Doppler and probe) per facility policy.

FINISHING THE SKILL

19. **INF** Remove gloves if worn and perform hand hygiene.

20. **SAF** Ensure client safety and comfort. Ensure that the bed is in the lowest position and verify that the client can identify and reach the nurse call system. *These safety measures reduce the risk of falls.*

21 **EVAL** Evaluate the outcomes.

22. **COM** Document pulse assessment findings in the legal healthcare record, including:
   - location of pulse or pulses obtained by Doppler.

23. **COM** Share the results with the client, and if the pulse findings are outside of the established parameters for the client, notify the authorized healthcare provider.

■ SKILL 3.10 Obtaining an Apical Pulse

EQUIPMENT

Digital watch or watch with a second hand
Stethoscope
Antiseptic wipes

BEGINNING THE SKILL

1. **INF** Perform hand hygiene.
2. **CCC** Introduce yourself to the client and family and explain the procedure.
3. **SAF** Identify the client using two identifiers.
4. **CCC** Provide privacy. Close the door, pull the curtain, and cover the client with a gown or bath blanket.

PROCEDURE

5. **INF** Clean the stethoscope endpiece with an antiseptic wipe before using. Clean the earpieces with an antiseptic wipe if the stethoscope is shared.
6. **CCC** If not contraindicated by facility policy or infection control procedures, warm the stethoscope for a few seconds in your hand. *Warming promotes comfort and prevents startling the client when you place the stethoscope on his or her skin.*
7. **ACC** Assess the client for exercise and nicotine or caffeine intake within the last 30 minutes.
8. **ACC** Seat the client in a quiet, calm environment.

9. **ACC** Locate the apical pulse, also known as the point of maximum impulse (PMI). The PMI is located at the fifth intercostal space (ICS) at the left midclavicular line (MCL).

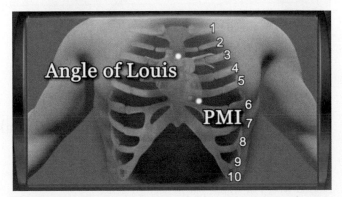

STEP 9 Locating the point of maximum impulse (PMI; apical pulse).

a. Palpate the sternal angle a few centimeters below the suprasternal notch. After placing your finger to the left of the sternal angle, identify the second intercostal space and count downward to the PMI.

b. Attempt to palpate the apical pulse using your first two or three finger pads with enough pressure to feel a consistent beat before auscultating the apical pulse rate. (Note: The apical pulse may not be palpable in some clients. In addition, the location of the apical pulse may vary slightly.)

10. **ACC** Auscultate the apical pulse by placing the bell or diaphragm of the stethoscope directly on the skin where the PMI is located. If you are unable to hear the apical pulse, reposition the stethoscope on the skin and/or ask the client to lie on the left side if tolerated. *Changing the client's position to the left side displaces the heart closer to the chest wall, which may enhance the sound of the apical pulse. Using the bell enhances the auscultation of low-pitched sounds; using the diaphragm enhances the auscultation of high-pitched sounds.* (Note: An alternative way to locate the PMI in a woman is to place, or ask her to place, the stethoscope just underneath her left breast and slide the bell or diaphragm of the stethoscope up as far as is comfortable. If needed, ask the client to lift her breast up. If the client has a pendulous breast, it may help to displace her breast to one side in order to improve access to her PMI.)

11. **ACC** Count the apical pulse rate for 1 full minute. Each lub-dub sound is equivalent to one beat. *Counting for a full minute facilities an accurate assessment.*

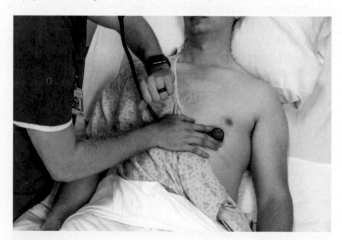

STEP 11 Auscultating the apical pulse rate.

12. **ACC** Assess the character, quality, and rhythm of the apical pulse. Note whether or not the client's apical pulse has murmurs or extra beats and whether the pulse is regular or irregular. *The character and rhythm of the pulse reflect the client's underlying heart function and overall condition.*

FINISHING THE SKILL

13. **INF** Perform hand hygiene.

14. **SAF** Ensure client safety and comfort. Ensure that the bed is in the lowest position and verify that the client can identify and reach the nurse call system. *These safety measures reduce the risk of falls.*

15. **EVAL** Evaluate the results for accuracy by comparing them to previous results and observing the client's current condition.

16. **COM** Document assessment findings in the legal healthcare record, including:
    - apical heart rate (auscultated) in beats per minute (bpm)
    - position used to obtain the apical pulse (e.g., left side, sitting upright)
    - character, quality, and rhythm of the apical pulse; presence of any unusual heart sounds.

17. **COM** Share the results with the client, and if the apical pulse findings are outside the established parameters for the client, notify the authorized healthcare provider.

■ SKILL 3.11 Obtaining an Apical-Radial Pulse

EQUIPMENT

Digital watch or watch with a second hand
Stethoscope
Antiseptic wipes

BEGINNING THE SKILL

1. **ACC** Ensure that there are two nurses available for the procedure. (Note: The second person may be another member of the healthcare team qualified to take vital signs.)

2. **INF** Perform hand hygiene.

3. **CCC** Introduce yourself and the second nurse to the client and family. Explain to the client why two nurses are needed for the procedure.

4. **SAF** Identify the client using two identifiers.

5. **CCC** Provide privacy. Close the door, pull the curtain, and cover the client with a gown or bath blanket.

PROCEDURE

6. **ACC** Assess the client for the following:
   a. Signs and symptoms that could be associated with a possible pulse deficit (e.g., feelings of palpitations

or chest pain, fluttering in chest, cool extremities, edema in lower extremities)

   b. Any shortness of breath or changes in the client's blood pressure or pulse oximetry reading.

7. **COM** Determine which nurse will obtain the apical pulse and which nurse will obtain the radial pulse. *Facilitates collaboration.* (Note: The nurse who will be obtaining the radial pulse will hold the watch. In some facilities, there is a clock on the client's wall that can be used for counting the pulse rates)

8. **SAF** Place the client in a comfortable position at an ergonomically safe working height. *Prevents injury to the nurse.*

9. **ACC** Using the appropriate landmarks, locate the pulse sites for obtaining the apical and radial pulses. Refer to Skill 3.6, Obtaining a Radial Pulse, and Skill 3.10, Obtaining an Apical Pulse.

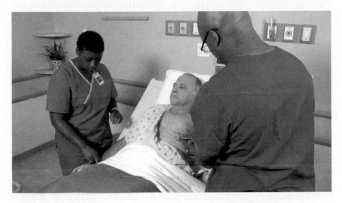

STEP 9 Locating the apical and radial pulse sites.

10. **ACC** After stating "start," simultaneously obtain the radial pulse (first nurse) and apical pulse (second nurse). Ensure that the watch or the clock on the client's wall can be seen by both nurses.

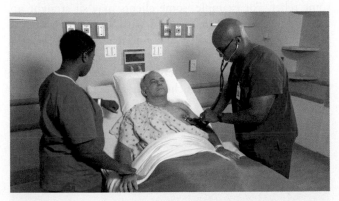

STEP 10 Obtaining the apical-radial pulse rate.

11. **ACC** Count the radial and apical pulse for a full minute (60 seconds). *This facilitates accuracy, particularly if the pulse is irregular.* (Note: At the end of 60 seconds, the nurse who said "start" will say "stop" while both healthcare providers look at the watch or clock.)

12. **ACC** During the procedure, assess the radial and apical pulse for rhythm, quality, and strength. Note if the client's extremities are cool, diaphoretic, or clammy to the touch. *Assessment while obtaining pulses can provide clues about the client's underlying condition.*

13. **ACC** Repeat the procedure if indicated using both left and right radial pulses.

14. **ACC** Compare the results and determine if there is an apical-radial pulse deficit. Subtract the radial rate from the apical rate (if there is a difference) and compare to the client's baseline. Report findings to the authorized healthcare provider if there is an apical-radial pulse deficit or if results are not within established parameters.

FINISHING THE SKILL

15. **INF** Perform hand hygiene.

16. **SAF** Ensure client safety and comfort. Ensure that the bed is in the lowest position and verify that the client can identify and reach the nurse call system. *These safety measures reduce the risk of falls.*

17. **EVAL** Evaluate the results for accuracy by comparing them to previous results and observing the client's current condition.

18. **COM** Document assessment findings in the legal healthcare record, including:
   - apical heart rate (auscultated), radial pulse rate, and apical-radial pulse deficit, if present, in beats per minute (bpm)
   - position used to obtain the apical-radial pulse rate (e.g., left side, sitting upright)
   - character, quality, and rhythm of the apical and radial pulses
   - side used (left or right radial) to obtain peripheral pulse rate
   - additional assessment parameters, such as cool extremities or palpitations.

19. **COM** Share the results with the client, and if the pulse findings are outside of the established parameters for the client or if the client has an apical-radial pulse deficit, notify the authorized healthcare provider.

SECTION 4 Assessing Respirations

The respiratory rate is measured by counting the breaths per minute. A breath includes both inhalation and exhalation. The thoracic diaphragm is the primary muscle responsible for respiration. The contraction of the diaphragm and expansion of the thoracic cavity result in inspiration. Exhalation occurs when the diaphragm relaxes and the thoracic cavity recoils. The respiratory rate is an objective, quantitative measurement and is an important part of a complete respiratory assessment. The established parameters for respirations in an adult are 12 to 20 breaths per minute (Table 3.4). Sleep and rest result in a lower respiratory rate, whereas activity increases respirations. When there is a need for more oxygen, the first compensatory mechanism is to increase the respiratory rate. A respiratory rate above the established parameters (hyperventilation) is termed *tachypnea*. A respiratory rate below the established parameters (hypoventilation) is termed *bradypnea*. Opioids, sedatives, and anesthesia have a side effect of respiratory depression, which may result in bradypnea. The potential for respiratory depression from medications is discussed further in Chapter 7. Apnea is a period of time during which there is an absence of breathing. A respiratory rate above the established parameters is a signal that there is a physiologic demand that has triggered the body's compensatory system. Therefore, when there is a change in a client's respiratory rate, the nurse documents the findings, investigates the reasons, and notifies the authorized healthcare provider in a timely manner.

When you count a respiratory rate, you do not want clients to be aware that you are counting their respirations because they may change their breathing pattern. Typically, nurses place their fingers on the client's radial pulse, perhaps folding the client's arm across his or her chest as well. First count the pulse rate, and then count the respiratory rate. The respiratory rate is primarily an observation, but when the client's arm is across his or her chest, it is supported, and you may feel the movement of the client's arm as he or she breathes and perhaps even hear the client's breath as well (Fig. 3.4). If the client is an adult and the first 30 seconds provides a rate within the established parameters, you may count the respiratory rate for 30 seconds and multiply it by 2 to get the breaths per minute. If the client is a child or infant, or if the respirations

are irregular or outside of the established parameters, then it is best to count the respiratory rate for a full 60 seconds.

In addition to counting the breaths per minute, the nurse notes several characteristics of the client's respirations, including their depth and rhythm. Respiratory depth refers to how shallow or deeply the client is breathing. Shallow breaths have less air movement, and deep breaths take in more air, filling the lungs. In physiologic terms, the depth of respirations reflects the size of the tidal volume. Shallow breaths have a smaller tidal volume, and deep breaths have a greater tidal volume. Rhythm reflects how evenly spaced each breath is within a minute. Adults usually breathe rhythmically, but infants do not. For an infant, irregular respirations are the norm. Infants will take several rapid breaths and then pause.

The nurse also assesses the effort the client is making to breathe, sometimes referred to as the work of breathing. This can be subtle; notice if the client can talk comfortably in full sentences. When people are having difficulty breathing, they use a variety of strategies to help them pull air into their lungs and force air out while keeping the alveoli open (Fig. 3.5). They increase the depth of their respirations and engage accessory muscles. In addition to the diaphragm and the intercostal muscles, the sternocleidomastoid muscles and scalene muscles in the neck will become active. You may see flaring nostrils with inhalation in adults, although this is more often seen in infants. Exhaling through pursed lips is a compensatory mechanism that should be noted. By exhaling through pursed lips, the client is maintaining a minimum air pressure in the alveoli throughout the exhalation. Note the client's position. When clients are having difficulty breathing, they position themselves in the manner that brings them some relief. For example, some clients may sit straight up, and other clients, such as those with chronic obstructive pulmonary disease (COPD), will find relief leaning forward, resting their hands or forearms on a surface. This is referred to as a tripod position, illustrated in Fig. 3.6. Terms used to describe respiratory effort include *dyspnea* (labored breathing)

TABLE 3.4 Respiratory Rate Parameters

Age Group	Range (Breaths/Min)
Newborn	30–60
1-year-old	24–40
6-year-old	15–25
15-year-old	15–20
Adult	12–20
Older adult	15–20

References: Lowdermilk, Perry, Cashion, & Alden, 2016; Yoost & Crawford, 2016.

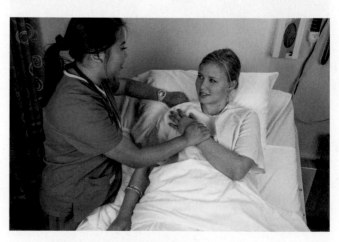

FIG. 3.4 Assess the client's respiratory rate.

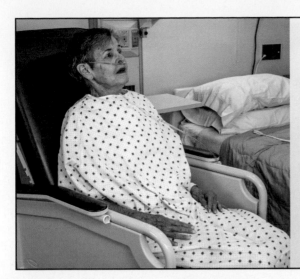

- Straining neck muscles
- Cyanosis: periorbital and/or circumoral
- Pursed lips
- Flaring nostrils
- Adventitious breath sounds
- Altered level of consciousness: confusion, combativeness, anxiety, dizziness,
- Loss of consciousness
- Use of intercostal muscles
- Coughing

FIG. 3.5 Signs of labored breathing.

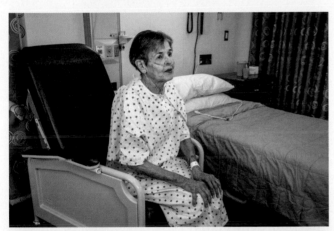

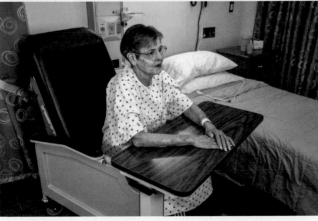

FIG. 3.6 Person in a tripod position.

and *orthopnea* (difficulty breathing when in a supine position). If the client's respiratory pattern is not regular or the effort seems to be greater than normal, ask the client to rate his or her ease of breathing on a scale of 1 to 10, with 10 being very difficult to breathe. An increased respiratory rate is predictive of clinical deterioration (Sharma, 2018). Respiratory patterns that seem unusual or effort greater than expected must be documented and quickly communicated to the authorized healthcare provider.

ASSESSING RESPIRATIONS IN PEDIATRIC CLIENTS

Children and neonates present some challenges when assessing respirations. Their respiratory rates are typically rapid and irregular. They are reactive to stimulation, so obtaining a respiratory rate should be done while the child is quiet and before obtaining other vital signs. Initially, observe and count without touching, particularly for infants. Placing a cold stethoscope on the chest can dramatically increase the respiratory rate. In infants and children, count the respiratory rate for 1 full minute. In children younger than 6 or 7 years of age, look for abdominal movement rather than the chest excursion that you see in adults. Although the initial respiratory rate is simply counted, the quality of breath sounds must also be evaluated as part of your respiratory assessment. Compare the rate to the established range for the infant or child's age. An increased respiratory rate is an early warning sign that there is a change in status. This can be very subtle. If you observe an elevated respiratory rate, check again when the child is at rest.

In adults, the nurse notes depth and rhythm. Infants and children have small tidal volumes, so an increase in depth does not give them much more air movement. Therefore, infants and children primarily compensate by increasing their respiratory rate. The breathing rhythm of infants is irregular: huff, puff, huff, puff, pause. Assess the effort of breathing. Strategies to increase air movement include nasal flaring during inhalation and grunting during exhalation. Retractions may become visible as the work of breathing increases (Fig. 3.7). Retractions are named for where they are anatomically visible: substernal retractions, suprasternal retractions, and intercostal retractions. As in adults, note the presence of anxiety, restlessness, irritability, and position of comfort. Observe the child's color, including central and extremity color. Pediatric clients can deteriorate quickly. Therefore, timely reporting and accurate documentation of alterations in the client's assessment and vital signs are essential.

In summary, adults as well as pediatric clients need accurate assessment and follow-up if they exhibit alterations in

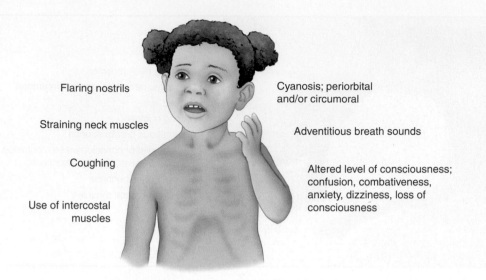

Flaring nostrils

Straining neck muscles

Coughing

Use of intercostal muscles

Cyanosis; periorbital and/or circumoral

Adventitious breath sounds

Altered level of consciousness; confusion, combativeness, anxiety, dizziness, loss of consciousness

FIG. 3.7 Assess the effort of breathing.

their respirations. If compensatory mechanisms are not sufficient for adequate gas exchange, the client may show signs of hypoxia, such as anxiety, confusion, diaphoresis, paleness, and tachycardia. Remember that cyanosis is a very late sign of hypoxia. Whenever a client has an elevated respiratory rate or signs of respiratory distress, including increased respiratory effort, you should also check the client's oxygen saturation and quickly relay your assessments to the authorized healthcare provider because supplemental oxygen may be needed.

APPLICATION OF THE NURSING PROCESS

Examples of Related ICNP Nursing Diagnoses, Expected Client Outcomes, and Nursing Interventions:

Nursing Diagnosis: Impaired breathing
Expected Client Outcome: The client will demonstrate effective breathing:
- respiratory rate within established parameters
- depth and rhythm appropriate for age
- unlabored respirations.

Nursing Intervention Example: Monitor client's respiratory rate, depth, and effort.
Reference: International Classification for Nursing Practice. (n.d.). *eHealth & ICNP.* Retrieved from https://www.icn.ch/what-we-do/projects/ehealth-icnp.

CRITICAL CONCEPTS
Assessing Respirations

Accuracy (ACC)

Respiratory assessment is sensitive to the following variables:
- client age, medical history, and medical condition
- increased client activity

- client awareness of being monitored.

Nurse-Related Factors
- proper assessment of respiratory rate, depth, rhythm, or effort

Client-Centered Care (CCC)

When assessing respirations, respect for the client is demonstrated through:
- promoting autonomy
- ensuring comfort
- providing privacy and only exposing what is necessary.

Infection Control (INF)

When assessing respirations, healthcare-associated infection is prevented by:
- reducing the transfer and number of microorganisms, primarily through hand hygiene.

Safety (SAF)

When assessing respirations, safety measures provide a safe care environment and prevent harm to the client.

Communication (COM)

- Communication exchanges information (oral, written, non-verbal, electronic) between two or more people.
- Documentation records information on respiratory assessment in a permanent legal record.

Evaluation (EVAL)

When obtaining a respiratory assessment, the evaluation of outcomes enables the nurse to determine the efficacy of the care provided.

▪ SKILL 3.12 Obtaining a Respiratory Rate and Respiratory Assessment

EQUIPMENT

Digital watch or watch with a second hand

BEGINNING THE SKILL

1. **INF** Perform hand hygiene.
2. **CCC** Introduce yourself to the client and family and explain the procedure.
3. **SAF** Identify the client using two identifiers.

PROCEDURE

4. **ACC** Assess the client's activity level within the last 30 minutes. If you are obtaining a full set of vital signs, you count a radial pulse first.
5. **ACC** Without removing your fingers from the client's wrist, count the breaths per minute by observing the rise and fall of the client's chest. You may find it helpful to breathe along with the client.

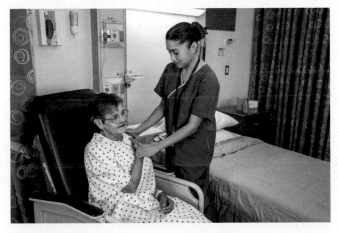

STEP 5 Count the breaths per minute.

a. If the client's respiratory rhythm is regular, count for 30 seconds and multiply by 2.
b. If the client's respiratory rhythm is irregular, count the client's respirations for 1 full minute.
c. Describe the respiratory rate as within established parameters, bradypnea, or tachypnea. *A respiratory rate outside of the established parameters can be a compensatory signal that there is a physiologic change.*

6. **ACC** Assess respiratory depth. *With deep inspirations, adults will use more use of the diaphragm and intercostal muscles. Increases in respiratory depth may be a compensatory signal that there is a physiologic change, and decreases in respiratory depth may be the result of medications, such as opioids.*
7. **ACC** Assess the rhythm of breathing. Rhythm is classified as regular or irregular. *An irregular breathing pattern is abnormal in an adult.*
8. **ACC** Assess for respiratory effort, especially the use of accessory muscles. If increased work of breathing is noted, identify which muscles are active. Are they assisting primarily on inhalation or both inhalation and exhalation? *Your assessment provides a baseline for comparison, as later intervention provides relief. Supplemental oxygen can relieve the work of breathing.*
9. **ACC** Assess the client's position while breathing. *Clients who are having difficulty breathing will seek positions of physical comfort while breathing.*
10. **ACC** Inspect for signs of hypoxia, including anxiety, restlessness, paleness, or even cyanosis in the nailbeds. Obtain an oxygen saturation if any signs of hypoxia are noted. *Cyanosis is a late sign that hypoxia is occurring.*

FINISHING THE SKILL

11. **INF** Perform hand hygiene.
12. **SAF** Ensure client safety and comfort. Ensure that the bed is in the lowest position and verify that the client can identify and reach the nurse call system. *These safety measures reduce the risk of falls.*
13. **EVAL** Evaluate the results for accuracy by comparing them to previous results and observing the client's current condition.
14. **COM** Document assessment findings in the legal healthcare record, including:
    * respiratory rate in breaths per minute (bpm)
    * respiratory depth and rhythm
    * respiratory effort and use of accessory muscles, if present
15. **COM** Share the results with the client, and if the respiratory rate is outside of the established parameters for the client, notify the authorized healthcare provider.

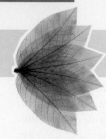

A blood pressure reading measures both the greatest pressure within the arterial walls and the lowest pressure within the arterial walls. The greatest pressure, called the systolic pressure, occurs during systole when the heart ejects blood into the systemic circulation. The systolic pressure is dependent on the stroke volume (the volume of blood ejected with each heartbeat) and the heart rate. The lowest pressure, called the diastolic pressure, occurs during diastole when the heart muscle relaxes. It primarily represents the vascular resistance of the body. Blood pressure is a product of the blood flow out of the heart and the vascular resistance. Blood pressure is measured in millimeters of mercury (mm Hg) and is written as a fraction: systolic pressure over diastolic pressure.

CLASSIFICATION OF HYPERTENSION

The current criteria for categories of hypertension were established by the American College of Cardiology (ACC) and the American Heart Association (AHA) in 2017. Under the new guidelines, the optimal blood pressure for an adult is a systolic pressure of less than 120 and a diastolic pressure of less than 80.

The elevated blood pressure category includes a systolic pressure between 120 and 129 and a diastolic pressure of less than 80.

- Stage 1 hypertension is categorized as 130 to 139 mm Hg systolic or 80 to 89 mm Hg diastolic.
- Stage 2 hypertension is categorized as greater than or equal to 140 mm Hg systolic or greater than 90 mm Hg diastolic.

The new guidelines removed the prehypertension category. Previously, stage 1 hypertension began with a systolic pressure of 140. The revised categories will result in more individuals being identified as hypertensive. Table 3.5 lists these guidelines. Identifying and treating hypertension are critical to improving the health of our population. Hypertension is second only to cigarette smoking as a cause of death. Hypertension is an important risk factor for cardiovascular events, such as stroke, coronary heart disease, and heart failure, as well as end-stage renal disease (Whelton et al., 2017). Many individuals with hypertension monitor their blood pressure at home. See Box 3.5 for a discussion of

the issues and information nurses need to help clients measure their blood pressures at home.

Along with the new adult hypertension classification guidelines in 2017, the hypertension guidelines for children and adolescents were also revised. For children less than 13 years of age, an elevated blood pressure is identified as greater than the 90th percentile for gender, age, and height, and stage 1 hypertension in children less than 13 years of age is identified as a blood pressure that is greater than the 95th percentile for gender, age, and height. In 2017, revised tables for gender, age, and height were published by the American Academy of Pediatrics. For adolescents older than 13 years of age, the classification is very similar to the adult delineations. See the classifications identified in Table 3.6.

As discussed, hypertension is a blood pressure higher than the optimal level. The other end of the spectrum is hypotension, which is a blood pressure lower than that needed to optimally maintain perfusion. There are not classifications of levels of hypotension as there are with hypertension. Hypotension may result from dehydration, bleeding, and other factors. If blood pressure is too low, perfusion is poor, resulting in decreased oxygen to the organs and cellular tissue. The provision of intravascular fluid volume may be required to increase the blood pressure.

FACTORS AFFECTING BLOOD PRESSURE

A variety of physiologic factors can affect blood pressure, most of which are seen in the acute care setting. Blood volume, because of the impact on stroke volume, has a direct effect on blood pressure. An increase in blood volume will increase both the systolic and diastolic blood pressure; a decrease in blood volume will decrease both the systolic and the diastolic blood pressure. The autonomic nervous system affects blood pressure as well. Conditions that stimulate the autonomic system, including pain, anxiety, fear, and exertion, may increase blood pressure. When you measure blood pressure, assess for recent events such as activity, exertion, or pain that would impact the measurement. Body position and the length of time in that position are also variables in blood pressure measurement; however, within a hospital setting, many clients will be supine in bed. The sitting position produces a higher diastolic blood

TABLE 3.5 Classification of Hypertension in Adults

Category	Systolic Blood Pressure Measurement (mm Hg)		Diastolic Blood Pressure Measurement (mm Hg)
Optimal adult blood pressure	<120	and	<80
Elevated blood pressure	120–129	and	<80
Stage 1 hypertension	130–139	or	80–89
Stage 2 hypertension	>140	or	>90

Reference: Whelton et al., 2017.

BOX 3.5 Home Care Considerations: Blood Pressure Monitoring

Increasingly, clients with hypertension are monitoring their blood pressure at home. The primary advantage of home blood pressure monitoring is the ability to identify sustained high blood pressure. Research is demonstrating that home monitoring of blood pressures is more accurate than clinic monitoring for identifying clients at risk for complications of high blood pressure, such as organ damage. Additionally, home blood pressure measurements were found to be better predictors of morbid events, such as stroke, than clinic measurements. Two methods are available for measuring blood pressure at home. Ambulatory blood pressure measurement (APBM) monitoring measures blood pressure every 15 to 30 minutes over a 24-hour period. Home blood pressure (HBP) is an automated oscillometric blood pressure measuring device that may have memory storage and allows individuals to take their blood pressure at home at the same time over several days. Typically, a person's blood pressure is lower at night when sleeping. ABPM has demonstrated that people whose blood pressure does not decrease at night are at increased risk for complications and morbidity associated with high blood pressure (Mancia et al., 2013).

An oscillometric device that records pressure from the brachial artery is most commonly used for home monitoring of blood pressure. One difficulty of home monitoring is ensuring that the results are recorded accurately. Studies in which clients were asked to record their home blood pressure readings, not knowing that their blood pressure monitors recorded and stored the readings, demonstrated that readings were omitted and that some were fabricated (Pickering et al., 2005). Another study demonstrated that cognitively impaired older adults successfully monitored their blood pressure with a home oscillometric device with memory capability that records their blood pressures (Plichart et al., 2013). To help ensure accurate records, the current recommendation is for the use of monitors with memory capability to store the blood pressure readings or systems for sending stored readings over the telephone (Whelton et al., 2017).

To facilitate accurate home monitoring of blood pressure, the nurse teaches the client about factors that affect blood pressure and the accuracy of blood pressure measurements (e.g., caffeine intake, nicotine intake, body position, and arm position) and the importance of accurate record keeping.

pressure than the supine position, often by as much as 5 mm Hg. The standing position results in a very slight decrease in blood pressure; however, after 1 or 2 minutes, the blood pressure increases to a greater pressure than a sitting position would produce. Therefore, when appropriate, blood pressure should be consistently obtained with the client in the same position, preferably seated with the back supported and the feet on the floor (Whelton et al., 2017).

One very common condition that impacts blood pressure is getting older. As we age, our vascular system becomes less compliant, vascular resistance increases, and there is an increased incidence of atherosclerosis. In fact, over half of all Americans over the age of 60 have elevated blood pressure, particularly systolic pressure. When the systolic pressure is elevated but the diastolic is not, it is called isolated systolic hypertension. Two out of three adults over the age of 60 have isolated systolic hypertension (National Heart, Lung, and Blood Institute [NHLBI], 2017). Another blood pressure condition more common in older adults is orthostatic hypotension, also called postural hypotension, which is a transient decrease in blood pressure caused by a change in body position (e.g., from lying down or sitting to a standing position). It is often accompanied by dizziness and is a risk factor for falls. Orthostatic hypotension is defined as a decrease of 20 mm Hg in the systolic pressure and a decrease of 10 mm Hg in the diastolic pressure within 3 minutes of standing (Mancia et al., 2013). Postural hypotension is more frequently found in people with diabetes. Measuring blood pressure at 1 minute after assuming a standing position and again 3 minutes after standing assesses for clients with postural hypertension (Mancia et al., 2013).

MEASURING BLOOD PRESSURE

Blood pressure can be measured in several ways. Arterial blood pressure can be measured directly in an intensive care setting when an arterial line is in place. Without such an invasive device, an indirect measurement of blood pressure can be obtained in any extremity but is most often measured in the upper arm. The skills that follow outline four different techniques for measuring blood pressure. The first and simplest is to palpate the radial artery while inflating the blood pressure cuff. The pressure on the sphygmomanometer gauge when the radial pulse disappears is an estimation of the systolic blood pressure. Remember that systolic pressure is the force with which the heart pushes blood into the

TABLE 3.6 Classification of Hypertension in Children and Adolescents

Category	Children	Adolescents 13 and Older
Optimal blood pressure	Less than the 90th percentile for age, sex, and height	<120/80
Elevated blood pressure	≥90th percentile and <95th percentile for age, sex, and height	120–129/<80
Stage 1 hypertension	≥95th percentile for age, sex, and height to <95th percentile + 12 mm Hg	≥130/80
Stage 2 hypertension	≥95th percentile + 12 mm Hg for age, sex, and height	>140/90

Reference: Flynn & Falkner, 2017.

arteries. How much pressure it takes to cut off that flow should mirror the arterial pressure. The second method is auscultating the systolic and diastolic pressures using a stethoscope, which is used to listen for the emergence and disappearance of Korotkoff sounds while slowly releasing air from a blood pressure cuff (Table 3.7). Korotkoff sounds are created by changing blood flow and turbulence within the artery as the blood pressure cuff compresses and then releases blood flow. The third skill describes how to use an automatic oscillometric blood pressure monitor. This is an electronic automatic blood pressure device that calculates blood pressure by first determining the MAP via changes in the amplitude of arterial wall pulsations, then calculating the systolic and diastolic pressure using an algorithm. The fourth skill uses a Doppler ultrasound device (which is more sensitive than feeling a pulse) to detect a systolic pressure

Steps to Ensure an Accurate Blood Pressure Measurement

Measuring blood pressure accurately is critical. The blood pressure measurement is used to determine a diagnosis; to initiate, evaluate, and terminate treatment; and to evaluate prognosis. Inaccurate blood pressure measurements could result in mismanagement and poor outcomes.

To measure blood pressure accurately with a brachial cuff, several procedural techniques must be followed. Assess the client for factors that will alter the reading, select the proper equipment, and properly position and prepare the client. It is worth emphasizing the importance of determining the correct size of the cuff (Table 3.8); incorrect cuff size has been implicated within nursing research as the most common reason for obtaining an incorrect blood pressure measurement. A cuff that is too large will result in a pressure measurement that is lower than the actual blood pressure, and a cuff that is too small will result in a pressure measurement that is higher than the actual blood pressure (Khanh-Dao Le, 2016). See Box 3.6 for a case study illustrating the potential problems stemming from an incorrect cuff size. Further considerations include the following:

- Assess the client for recent activity and/or caffeine or nicotine consumption.
- Assess whether the client has recently emptied his or her bladder.
- Select the appropriate-size cuff and equipment that has been validated and calibrated.
- When possible, position the client seated, with the back supported and the feet on the floor.
- Position and support the client's arm at the level of the heart.
- Place the cuff on the skin and not over clothing.

TABLE 3.7 Korotkoff Sounds

Phase	Description
I	Pressure level at which the first faint, clear tapping sounds are heard, which increase as the cuff is deflated (reference point for systolic blood pressure)
II	Phase during cuff deflation when a murmur or swishing sounds are heard
III	Period during which sounds are clearer and increase in intensity
IV	Phase where a distinct, abrupt muffling sound is heard
V	Pressure level when the last sound is heard (reference point for diastolic blood pressure)

TABLE 3.8 Recommended Cuff Sizes

Arm Circumference	Cuff Size
22–26 cm	Small adult size: 12–22 cm
27–34 cm	Adult size: 16–30 cm
35–44 cm	Large adult size: 16–36 cm
45–52 cm	Adult thigh size: 16–42 cm

The size of the cuff used should be appropriate to the size of the client's extremity. Using an inappropriately sized cuff will produce inaccurate readings. The cuff should be wide enough to encircle 80% of the upper arm and long enough to be fastened securely.
Reference: Pickering et al., 2005. Reprinted in Whelton et al., 2017.

BOX 3.6 Lessons From Experience: The Importance of Selecting the Correct Cuff Size

On a postpartum unit, a mother who had just had her third baby was preparing to go home. Mrs. Williams was tall and muscular, and her body mass index (BMI) was somewhere between overweight and obese. Mrs. Williams's authorized healthcare provider was reviewing her hospital records before writing the discharge order and noticed that her blood pressure measurements were consistently elevated, often in the range of 135 to 140/85 to 90. In determining whether or not to send Mrs. Williams home on antihypertensive medication, the authorized healthcare provider asked the charge nurse to check Mrs. Williams's blood pressure a couple of times that morning before her discharge.

The charge nurse took the automatic blood pressure machine into Mrs. Williams's room. Upon wrapping the cuff around Mrs. Williams's upper arm, the nurse noted that the circumference of Mrs. Williams's arm exceeded the marked range on the cuff. The nurse asked Mrs. Williams if any other nurse had tried this cuff and then found and used a larger cuff, and Mrs. Williams replied, "No, they used this one." After obtaining a cuff appropriate for Mrs. Williams's arm size, the nurse measured Mrs. Williams's blood pressure, and the measurement was about 10 mm Hg below the previous measurements. Three blood pressure measurements taken with the correct-size cuff on the morning of discharge were below the hypertensive range, and Mrs. Williams was discharged home without antihypertensive medication. In summary, incorrect cuffing is a serious problem recognized by nursing and medical organizations. Incorrect blood pressure measurement leads to incorrect diagnosis and medical treatment.

When the arm is below the level of the heart, the pressure reading is higher; when the arm is above the level of the heart, the pressure is lower (Mancia et al., 2013; Seckel, 2016).

The most accurate method of measuring blood pressure is to first estimate the palpated systolic pressure (Skill 3.13) and then auscultate the systolic and diastolic pressures (Skill 3.14), listening for the emergence and disappearance of Korotkoff sounds. Don't talk to the client, and ask the client not to speak to you, during blood pressure measurement.

Palpating the systolic pressure before auscultating the systolic and diastolic pressure is important for several reasons. First, it prevents the error of missing a hypertensive reading on an individual with an auscultatory gap. An auscultatory gap is the temporary disappearance of phase 2 Korotkoff sounds. If first palpated, the true systolic will be felt. If the nurse only listens, the systolic blood pressure may be underestimated. Second, palpation of the systolic pressure allows the nurse to determine the regularity and rate of the pulse. The rate of the pulse affects the rate with which the nurse releases the cuff pressure. The slower the pulse rate, the slower the release. Third, initial palpation of the systolic pressure allows the nurse to individualize inflation of the cuff based on the client's actual systolic pressure and prevents overinflation of the cuff. When auscultating the systolic/diastolic pressure, the cuff is inflated to 30 mm Hg above the palpated systolic pressure. If the client has a systolic of 90, then the cuff only needs to be inflated to 120 mm Hg. Overinflation of the cuff may result in spasm of the vessels, pain, and a falsely elevated reading. Finally, if an individual is very hypovolemic and the blood pressure cannot be auscultated, the palpatory method may be used as an alternate means of determining systolic pressure. A skilled nurse may first palpate the systolic pressure (Skill 3.13) and then move right into auscultating the systolic and diastolic pressures by continuing to inflate the cuff to 30 mm Hg above the palpated systolic pressure (Skill 3.14). Students should practice these skills separately until they are proficient in each skill separately before combining the two skills.

Authorities recommend measuring a client's blood pressure in both arms when measuring the client's blood pressure for the first time, but in the acute care setting, this may not always be possible (Seckel, 2016; Whelton et al., 2017). Documenting the anatomical location of the blood pressure measurement is critical because the location of the measurement will affect the reading. Blood pressure readings are typically taken in the upper arm, and in fact, blood pressure norms were established with the right arm. However, your client may have conditions that prohibit obtaining a blood pressure measurement in the right arm, such as the presence of a peripherally inserted central catheter (PICC) or an infusing peripheral intravenous line. Do not measure blood pressure in extremities with an arteriovenous fistula, deep vein thrombosis, or any grafts. Other contraindications for blood pressure measurement in an extremity are the presence of lymphedema following a mastectomy or lumpectomy (Seckel, 2016). Sometimes a cuff cannot be found to fit on the upper arm of an obese client, and the blood pressure is measured on the forearm. However, blood pressure measurements obtained by placing a blood pressure cuff on the forearm will not consistently be the same as measurements obtained from the upper arm. The site must be noted because it cannot be compared to an arm blood pressure measurement (Seckel, 2016). At times, it may be necessary to assess blood pressure using a lower extremity (Box 3.7). Like a forearm measurement, the lower extremity measurement cannot be compared to a brachial measurement.

To measure blood pressure accurately, nurses need equipment that measures accurately. For decades, the gold standard for measuring blood pressure was mercury sphygmomanometers. Today, most mercury sphygmomanometers have been replaced, due to concerns about mercury toxicity, with either aneroid sphygmomanometers or automated oscillometric monitors (Fig. 3.8). Neither tool has been shown to be as accurate as the mercury sphygmomanometer (Skirton, Chamberlain, Lawson, Ryan, & Young, 2011). Aneroid sphygmomanometers require regular calibration and additional research to further validate their accuracy. Although automatic oscillometric monitors are popular and eliminate the potential for user error, many studies conclude that these devices deliver inaccurate measurements, particularly in high blood pressure ranges and in clients with irregular heart rates (Skirton et al., 2011). Furthermore, different manufacturers of automatic oscillometric blood pressure monitors use different algorithms, and therefore consistent use of a device made by the same manufacturer is needed to accurately monitor blood pressure over time. When

---

BOX 3.7 Measuring a Lower Extremity Blood Pressure

- If measuring blood pressure in the thigh or calf, use the same guidelines for determining cuff size that are used when measuring blood pressure in the arm—that is, the cuff should have a bladder width that is at least 40% of the leg's circumference and a bladder length that is 80% of the leg's circumference.
- When measuring a thigh blood pressure, place the client in a prone or side-lying position and listen for Korotkoff sounds over the popliteal artery.
- When measuring an ankle blood pressure with the cuff over the calf, place the client supine and listen over the dorsalis pedis or posterior tibial artery.
- Generally, a lower-extremity systolic pressure is 10% to 20% higher than that obtained from the brachial artery. Comparisons of mean and diastolic arm blood pressures with calf measurements are not consistent. In adults, calf blood pressure measurements should only be taken when an upper arm is not available.

Reference: Seckel, 2016.

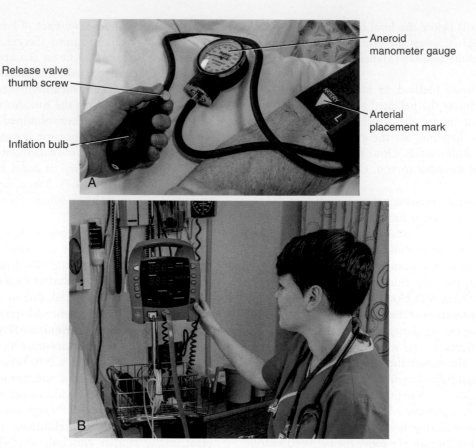

Release valve
thumb screw

Aneroid
manometer gauge

Inflation bulb

Arterial
placement mark

A

B

FIG. 3.8 Blood pressure sphygmomanometers. **A,** Aneroid. **B,** Oscillometric blood pressure monitors.

using an automatic oscillometric monitor for continuous blood pressure monitoring, the precautions identified in Box 3.8 need to be followed. In addition, agencies need to determine that the oscillometric devices purchased meet the Association for the Advancement of Medical Instrumentation standards for accuracy, which will ensure accuracy when compared with the auscultatory method (Seckel, 2016).

APPLICATION OF THE NURSING PROCESS

Examples of Related ICNP Nursing Diagnoses, Expected Client Outcomes, and Nursing Interventions:

Nursing Diagnosis: Altered blood pressure
Expected Client Outcomes: The client will demonstrate:
- blood pressure measurement at client's baseline or within established parameters
- pulse rate and rhythm within established parameters for client.

Nursing Intervention Examples: Monitor blood pressure by auscultating the systolic and diastolic blood pressure using an appropriate-size blood pressure cuff and taking steps to ensure an accurate measurement, including palpating a systolic blood pressure.

Reference: International Classification for Nursing Practice. (n.d.). *eHealth & ICNP.* Retrieved from https://www.icn.ch/what-we-do/projects/ehealth-icnp.

CRITICAL CONCEPTS
Assessing Blood Pressure

Accuracy (ACC)

Blood pressure measurement is sensitive to the following variables:
Client-Related Factors
- Age, medical history, and medical condition
- Recent ingestion of nicotine, caffeine, medications, or herbal preparations
- Recent exercise or exertion
- Past surgeries that change vasculature (mastectomy, lymphadenectomy)
- Conditions that compromise circulation (arteriovenous [AV] shunt, intravenous line)
- Pain, anxiety, or a full bladder
- Environment (e.g., room temperature, room noise)
- Body position: seated, standing, or lying down; legs crossed; back supported or not supported
- Arm position in relation to the heart

BOX 3.8 Precautions for Continuous Blood Pressure Monitoring

- Ensure the accuracy of the blood pressure monitor by first auscultating the blood pressure with a manual device and comparing the measurements.
- Allow at least 1 full minute between cuff inflations because too-frequent blood pressure measurements may result in venous congestion.
- If using an automatic oscillometric blood pressure monitor for continuous monitoring, set high and low alarm limits for the systolic and diastolic pressure before beginning.
- Do not turn off the alarms, and check periodically that others have not turned off the alarms.
- Check the position of the cuff frequently, and remove the cuff regularly to assess the skin condition of the arm.
- Use the least frequent cycle time to meet blood pressure assessment needs and only for the duration required.

Reference: Seckel, 2016.

Equipment-Related Factors
- Blood pressure cuff not the appropriate size
- Type of equipment
- Battery charge and working order of equipment

Nurse-Related Factors
- Proper selection of equipment
- Proper positioning and preparation of the client
- Selection of the appropriate size cuff
- Adherence to procedural techniques, such as palpation of the the systolic pressure prior to measuring an auscultated blood pressure
- Auscultation and interpretation of Korotkoff sounds

Client-Centered Care (CCC)

When assessing blood pressure, respect for the client is demonstrated through
- promoting autonomy
- providing privacy
- ensuring comfort.

Infection Control (INF)

When assessing blood pressure, healthcare-associated infection is prevented by:
- reducing the transfer and number of microorganisms, primarily through hand hygiene.

Safety (SAF)

When assessing blood pressure, safety measures provide a safe care environment and prevent harm to the client.

Communication (COM)

- Communication exchanges information (verbal, nonverbal, or written) between two or more people.
- Documentation records information in a permanent legal record.

Health Maintenance (HLTH)

When measuring blood pressure, nursing is dedicated to the promotion of health, including:
- protecting the client's skin integrity.

Evaluation (EVAL)

When assessing blood pressure, the evaluation of outcomes enables the nurse to determine the efficacy of the assessment provided.

■ SKILL 3.13 Palpating a Systolic Blood Pressure

EQUIPMENT

Sphygmomanometer with blood pressure cuff

BEGINNING THE SKILL

1. **INF** Perform hand hygiene.
2. **CCC** Introduce yourself to client and family and explain the procedure.
3. **SAF** Identify the client using two identifiers.
4. **CCC** Provide privacy if needed.

PROCEDURE

5. **ACC** Assess the client for exercise and nicotine or caffeine intake within the last 30 minutes.
6. **ACC** Assess for factors that can cause compromised circulation, such as AV shunts, previous (past) mastectomy or lymphadenectomy, or the presence of an intravenous line.
7. **ACC** Seat the client in a quiet, calm environment with the legs uncrossed and the back supported; wait 5 minutes while the client is in this position before measuring the blood pressure.
8. **ACC** Expose the client's arm so that the brachial artery is not covered with clothing. Ensure the sleeve is not constricting the upper arm. *A sleeve that constricts the upper arm could act as a tourniquet, affecting the accuracy of the blood pressure measurement (Pickering et al., 2005).*
9. **ACC** Place the client's arm in a supported position at the level of the heart, with the palm facing up and the elbow straight.

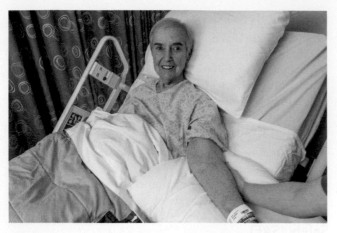

STEP 9 Support the client's arm at heart level.

10. **ACC** Measure the circumference of the bare upper arm at the midpoint between the shoulder and elbow, and select a cuff with a bladder width that is at least 40% of the arm circumference and a bladder length that is 80% of the arm circumference.
11. **ACC** Place the cuff around the client's upper arm 2.5 to 5 cm (1 to 2 inches) above the elbow. Ensure the bladder is centered on the arm. Some cuffs may be marked to indicate this position. The cuff should be snug enough not to slip but not so tight as to be uncomfortable.

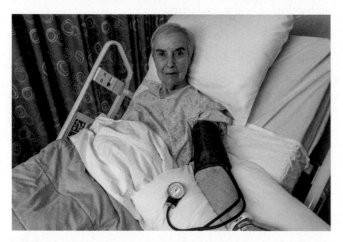

STEP 11 Place the cuff around the client's upper arm.

12. Palpate the radial artery with the finger pads of the non-dominant hand. It is also acceptable to palpate the brachial artery; however, students often find the radial artery is easier to palpate. *The nondominant hand is used to palpate because the dominant hand is used to manipulate the valve of the sphygmomanometer bulb.*

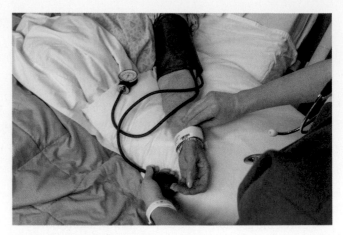

STEP 9 Palpate the radial artery.

13. **ACC** Hold the sphygmomanometer bulb in the dominant hand, close the valve by rolling the thumbscrew gently to the right, and inflate the cuff rapidly at first, then inflate incrementally and more slowly while continuing to palpate the radial or brachial pulse. *Rapid inflation is acceptable within the very low pressures that could not represent a systolic pressure. Inflating more slowly and in smaller increments as you near the low range of a systolic pressure will allow you to pinpoint the pressure at which the pulsations cease.*

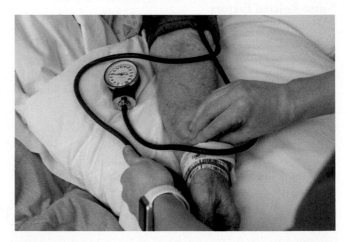

STEP 13 Inflate the cuff while palpating the brachial pulse.

14. **ACC** Note the pressure at which the pulse disappears. This pressure is the palpated systolic pressure and is recorded as one number with the term "palpated." (Note: It is not a fraction. For example, if the pulse is no longer palpable at 130 mm Hg as the cuff is inflated, then the blood pressure is recorded as 130 palpated systolic.)
15. **ACC** Assess the rate and rhythm of the pulse in order to apply the information when obtaining an auscultated blood pressure. *The heart rate impacts the rate of cuff deflation (2 mm Hg per heartbeat is recommended when the heart rate is lower than 60 bpm (Pickering et al., 2005). The rhythm affects the accuracy of the reading. Clients with an irregular heart rhythm have significant variation in*

blood pressure measurement from beat to beat and may require additional assessment.

16. **HLTH** Deflate the cuff by releasing the valve, rolling the thumbscrew to the left. If only a palpated systolic pressure is needed, remove the cuff from the client's arm. If taking an ausculated systolic and diastolic pressure, advance to step 14 in Skill 3.14. *Removing the blood pressure cuff when it is not in use protects the client's skin.*

17. **INF** Wipe off the cuff with a disinfectant if the cuff is shared between clients.

FINISHING THE SKILL

18. **INF** Perform hand hygiene.

19. **SAF** Ensure client safety and comfort. Ensure that the bed is in the lowest position and verify that the client can identify and reach the nurse call system. *These safety measures reduce the risk of falls.*

20. **EVAL** Evaluate the results for accuracy by comparing them to previous results and observing the client's current condition.

21. **COM** Document the assessment findings, noting palpated systolic pressure and whether the right or left arm was used to obtain the measurement, in the legal healthcare record.

22. **COM** Share the results with the client, and if the blood pressure is outside of the established parameters for the client, notify the authorized healthcare provider.

■ SKILL 3.14 Measuring a Systolic and Diastolic Blood Pressure by Auscultation

EQUIPMENT

Stethoscope
Sphygmomanometer with blood pressure cuff
Antiseptic wipes

BEGINNING THE SKILL

1. **INF** Perform hand hygiene.
2. **CCC** Introduce yourself to the client and family and explain the procedure.
3. **SAF** Identify the client using two identifiers.
4. **CCC** Provide privacy if needed.

PROCEDURE

5. **ACC** Assess the client for recent exercise and nicotine or caffeine intake within the last 30 minutes.
6. **ACC** Assess for factors that can compromise circulation, such as AV shunts, previous (past) mastectomy or lymphadenectomy, or the presence of an intravenous line.
7. **ACC** Seat the client in a quiet, calm environment with the legs uncrossed and the back supported; wait 5 minutes while the client is in this position before measuring the blood pressure.
8. **ACC** Expose the client's arm so that the brachial artery is not covered with clothing. Ensure the sleeve is not constricting the upper arm. *Stethoscopes are designed to listen directly on the skin, not over clothing. A sleeve that constricts the upper arm could act as a tourniquet, affecting the accuracy of the blood pressure measurement (Pickering et al., 2005).*
9. **ACC** Place the client's arm in a supported position at the level of the heart, with the palm facing up.
10. **ACC** Assess the circumference of the bare upper arm at the midpoint between the shoulder and elbow and select

a cuff with a bladder width that is at least 40% of the arm circumference and a bladder length that is 80% of the arm circumference.

11. **ACC** Place the cuff around the client's upper arm 2.5 to 5 cm (1–2 inches) above the elbow. Ensure the bladder is centered on the arm. Some cuffs may be marked to indicate this position. *The cuff should be snug enough not to slip but not so tight as to be uncomfortable.*

12. **ACC** Obtain a palpated systolic blood pressure using the steps identified in Skill 3.13. *This prevents a false reading for clients with an auscultatory gap (loss of Korotkoff sounds at pressures higher than the true diastolic), particularly those with hypertension; allows the nurse to individualize inflation of the cuff based on the client's actual systolic pressure; and prevents overinflation of the cuff. Overinflation of the cuff may result in spasm of the vessels, pain, and a falsely elevated reading.*

13. **ACC** Deflate the cuff and wait 1 to 2 minutes to allow the venous congestion to dissipate. *Venous congestion may result in increased venous pressure.*

14. **INF** Clean the stethoscope endpiece with an antiseptic wipe. Clean the earpieces with an antiseptic wipe if the stethoscope is shared.

15. **ACC** Place the stethoscope earpieces in the ear canals. Place the diaphragm of the stethoscope over the brachial artery with your nondominant hand. Ensure that the stethoscope maintains contact with the skin but does not press too hard and does not come into contact with the cuff or the rubber tubing. *Korotkoff sounds may be listened to with either the diaphragm or the bell, but students may initially find it easier to maintain contact when using the diaphragm. Avoiding contact with the cuff or rubber tubing decreases artifact.*

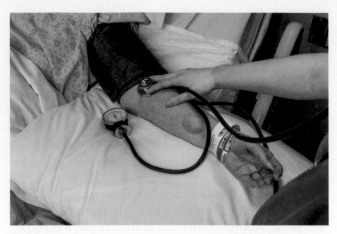

STEP 15 Place the bell over the brachial artery.

16. **ACC** Hold the sphygmomanometer bulb in the dominant hand, close the valve by rolling the thumbscrew gently to the right, and rapidly inflate the cuff to 30 mm Hg above the palpated systolic pressure. *Inflating the cuff 30 mm Hg above the palpated systolic pressure prevents overinflation of the cuff and allows sufficient time to adjust the rate of descent.*

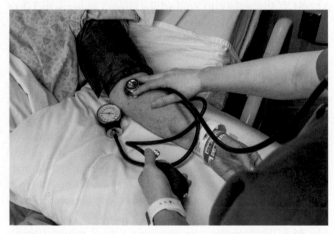

STEP 16 Inflate the cuff.

17. **ACC** Deflate the cuff slowly by gently rolling the thumbscrew to the left; release the pressure at a rate of about 2 mm Hg per second. Listen carefully. Note the pressure at which repetitive sounds first appear (Korotkoff phase 1) to the nearest 2 mm Hg. Do not round off this number. This is the systolic pressure reading. *The heart rate impacts the rate of cuff deflation (2 mm Hg per heartbeat is recommended when the heart rate is lower than 60 bpm [Pickering et al., 2005]). The rhythm affects the accuracy of the reading. Clients with an irregular heart rhythm have significant variation in blood pressure measurement from beat to beat and may require additional assessment.*

18. **ACC** Continue to listen to the Korotkoff sounds. Note any distinct muffling of the sounds (Korotkoff phase IV) and note the pressure. Determine the pressure when the pulsations disappear completely (Korotkoff phase V). This is the diastolic pressure reading.

19. **ACC** Continue to deflate the cuff slowly for at least another 10 mm Hg and then rapidly deflate the cuff. *Cautious deflation of the cuff ensures that no additional sounds are missed.*

20. **ACC** Wait 1 minute and obtain a second reading. *A minimum of two readings should be taken at intervals of at least 1 minute. An average of the two readings may be recorded* (Mancia et al., 2013; Pickering, 2005).

21. **HLTH** Remove the cuff from the client's arm. *Removing the blood pressure cuff when it is not in use protects the client's skin.*

22. **INF** Wipe off the cuff with a disinfectant if the cuff is shared between clients.

FINISHING THE SKILL

23. **INF** Perform hand hygiene.

24. **SAF** Ensure client safety and comfort. Ensure that the bed is in the lowest position and verify that the client can identify and reach the nurse call system. *These safety measures reduce the risk of falls.*

25. **EVAL** Evaluate the results for accuracy by comparing them to previous results and observing the client's current condition.

26. **COM** Document assessment findings, noting palpated systolic pressure and whether the right or left arm was used to obtain the measurement, in the legal healthcare record.

27. **COM** Share the results with the client, and if the blood pressure is outside of the established parameters for the client, notify the authorized healthcare provider.

■ SKILL 3.15 Measuring Blood Pressure With an Automatic Oscillometric Monitor

EQUIPMENT

Blood pressure cuff
Automatic oscillometric blood pressure monitor

BEGINNING THE SKILL

1. **INF** Perform hand hygiene.
2. **CCC** Introduce yourself to client and family and explain the procedure.
3. **SAF** Identify the client using two identifiers.
4. **CCC** Provide privacy if needed.

PROCEDURE

5. **ACC** Assess the client for exercise and nicotine or caffeine intake within the last 30 minutes.
6. **ACC** Assess for any factors that can compromise circulation, such as AV shunts, previous (past) mastectomy or lymphadenectomy, or the presence of an intravenous line.

7. **ACC** Seat the client in a quiet, calm environment with the legs uncrossed and the back supported; wait 5 minutes while the client is in this position before measuring blood pressure.
8. **ACC** Expose the client's arm. *The brachial artery must be free of clothing.*
9. **ACC** Place the client's arm in a supported position at the level of the heart, with the palm facing up.
10. **ACC** Assess the circumference of the bare upper arm at the midpoint between the shoulder and elbow and select a cuff with a bladder width that is at least 40% of the arm circumference and a bladder length that is 80% of the arm circumference.
11. Ensure that the cuff is completely deflated and attached securely to the automatic oscillometric blood pressure monitor.
12. **ACC** Place the cuff around the client's upper arm 2.5 to 5 cm (1 to 2 inches) above the elbow. Ensure the cuff is facing the correct direction and the arrow indicating the artery is placed appropriately. *The cuff should be snug enough not to slip but not so tight as to be uncomfortable.*

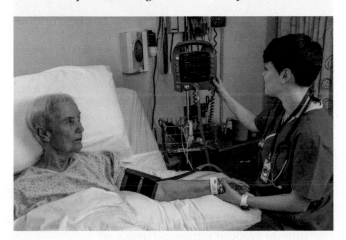

STEP 12 Place the cuff around the client's upper arm.

13. **SAF** Determine if setting the alarm limits for the automatic oscillometric blood pressure monitor is appropriate. *High and low alarm limits are set at readings that reflect the client's baseline and allow for the fluctuations expected with normal activity. The alarm limits function to alert the nurse to any unexpected decrease or increase in the client's blood pressure.*
14. **ACC** Turn on the automatic oscillometric blood pressure monitor. Follow the manufacturer's instructions for obtaining a blood pressure. (Note: Most automatic oscillometric blood pressure monitors display systolic pressure, diastolic pressure, mean arterial blood pressure, and heart rate.)
15. **HLTH** Remove the cuff from the client's arm. *Removing the blood pressure cuff when it is not in use protects the client's skin.*
16. **INF** Wipe off the cuff with a disinfectant if the cuff is shared between clients.

FINISHING THE SKILL

17. **INF** Perform hand hygiene.
18. **SAF** Ensure client safety and comfort. Ensure that the bed is in the lowest position and verify that the client can identify and reach the nurse call system. *These safety measures reduce the risk of falls.*
19. **EVAL** Evaluate the results for accuracy by comparing them to previous results and observing the client's current condition.
20. **COM** Document assessment findings, noting palpated systolic pressure and whether the right or left arm was used to obtain the measurement, in the legal healthcare record.
21. **COM** Share the results with the client, and if the blood pressure is outside of the established parameters for the client, notify the authorized healthcare provider.

■ SKILL 3.16 Using a Doppler Ultrasound Device to Hear Systolic Blood Pressure

EQUIPMENT

Sphygmomanometer with blood pressure cuff
Doppler ultrasound device with probe
Ultrasonic conductive gel, in bottle or individual packets
Tissue or paper towel

BEGINNING THE SKILL

1. **INF** Perform hand hygiene.
2. **CCC** Introduce yourself to the client and family and explain the procedure.
3. **SAF** Identify the client using two identifiers.
4. **CCC** Provide privacy if needed.

PROCEDURE

5. **ACC** Turn on the Doppler ultrasound device and check that it is functioning properly. *Identifying technical problems before entering the client's room saves time.*
6. **ACC** Assess the client for exercise and nicotine or caffeine intake within the last 30 minutes.
7. **ACC** Assess for factors that can compromise circulation, such as AV shunts, previous (past) mastectomy or lymphadenectomy, or the presence of an intravenous line.
8. **ACC** Seat the client in a quiet, calm environment with the legs uncrossed and the back supported; wait 5 minutes while the client is in this position before measuring blood pressure.
9. **ACC** Expose the client's arm so that the brachial artery is not covered with clothing. The conductive gel and Doppler probe will be placed on the skin directly over the

brachial artery. *Ensure the sleeve is not constricting the upper arm because constriction could act as a tourniquet and affect the blood pressure measurement (Pickering et al., 2005).*

10. **ACC** Place the client's arm in a supported position at the level of the heart, with the palm facing up.

11. **ACC** Measure the circumference of the bare upper arm at the midpoint between the shoulder and elbow and select a cuff with a bladder width that is at least 40% of the arm circumference and a bladder length that is 80% of the arm circumference.

12. **ACC** Place the cuff around the client's upper arm 2.5 to 5 cm (1–2 inches) above the elbow. Ensure the bladder is centered on the arm. Some cuffs may be marked to indicate this position. *The cuff should be snug enough not to slip but not so tight as to be uncomfortable.*

13. **ACC** Place a generous amount of conductive gel directly on the client's brachial artery (the radial artery may also be used). *Conductive gel facilitates the transfer of sound.*

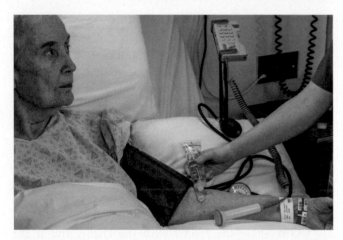

STEP 13 Apply a generous amount of gel over the brachial artery.

14. **ACC** Position the entire end of the Doppler probe in the conductive gel, making direct contact with the skin where the pulse is located. *Increasing the contact area of the end of the probe facilitates identification of the pulse waves.*

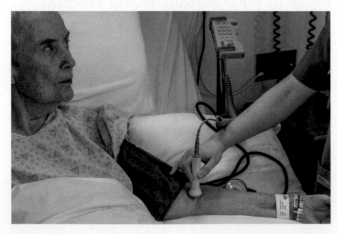

STEP 14 Place the end of the probe in the gel.

15. Turn the Doppler ultrasound device to the "on" position after the probe is placed and adjust the volume as needed.

16. **ACC** Move the probe until you hear a "swishing" pulse sound. Apply more conductive gel if needed. In order to use your dominant hand to manipulate the thumbscrew of the pressure bulb, transfer the Doppler ultrasound device to your nondominant hand.

17. **ACC** When you hear a consistent pulse, hold the sphygmomanometer bulb in the dominant hand, close the valve by rolling the thumbscrew gently to the right, and rapidly inflate the cuff to 30 mm Hg above the palpated systolic pressure. *Inflating the cuff 30 mm Hg above the palpated systolic pressure prevents overinflation of the cuff and allows sufficient time to adjust the rate of descent.*

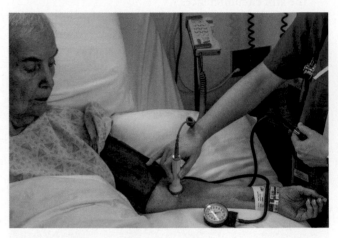

STEP 17 Inflate the cuff.

18. **ACC** Deflate the cuff slowly by gently rolling the thumbscrew to the left, releasing the pressure at a rate of about 2 mm Hg per second. Listen carefully. Note the pressure at which a pulsation is first heard to the nearest 2 mm Hg. Do not round off this number. This is the systolic reading.

19. Turn the Doppler ultrasound device off.

20. **HLTH** Remove the cuff from the client's arm. *Removing the BP cuff when it is not in use protects the client's skin.*

21. **CCC** Clean the conductive gel from the client's skin and from the probe.

22. **INF** Wipe off the cuff with a disinfectant if the cuff is shared between clients.

FINISHING THE SKILL

23. **INF** Perform hand hygiene.

24. **SAF** Ensure client safety and comfort. Ensure that the bed is in the lowest position and verify that the client can identify and reach the nurse call system. *These safety measures reduce the risk of falls.*

25. **EVAL** Evaluate the results for accuracy by comparing them to previous results and observing the client's current condition.

26. **COM** Document assessment findings, noting systolic blood pressure auscultated using a Doppler and whether the right or left arm was used to obtain the measurement, in the legal healthcare record.

27. **COM** Share the results with the client, and if the blood pressure is outside of the established parameters for the client, notify the authorized healthcare provider.

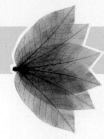

VITAL MEASUREMENTS

In addition to measuring vital signs, there are other quantitative objective assessments that are frequently measured, such as pulse oximeter measurement and capillary blood glucose measurement. The timing of a pulse oximeter measurement will often occur with vital signs; however, blood glucose measurements will coincide more with mealtimes. Both measurements are routine for certain populations, and nursing students will be expected to perform these measurements in the clinical area.

SECTION 6 Assessing Oxygen Saturation

Oxygen saturation (SpO_2) is the amount of oxygen bound to hemoglobin, measured as a percentage of the total possible binding capacity. The established parameter for oxygen saturation is 95% to 100% in healthy individuals not receiving supplemental oxygen. Oxygen saturation is measured with a pulse oximeter. A pulse oximeter measures the oxygen saturation with a probe that emits red and infrared light. Hemoglobin absorbs different wavelengths of light depending on its level of oxygen saturation. The oxygen saturation is then measured based on the light absorption of the saturated hemoglobin and is expressed as a percentage. Nurses measure oxygen saturation either intermittently or continuously, and oxygen saturation is frequently recorded along with vital signs.

For intermittent measurement, portable pulse oximeters are used. They are designed to take readings on a variety of people and usually attach to the client's fingertip with a plastic clip. When a client is receiving oxygen and is more unstable, then continuous monitoring at the bedside occurs. Continuous oximeters may attach with a flexible, bandage-style wrap that is for one individual only. However, different types of clips exist that may be used to attach to a toe or an earlobe or the nose. Bedside pulse oximeters have programmable alarms for high and low oxygen saturations.

The SpO_2 provides an easy, noninvasive, and cost-effective estimate of the oxygen saturation. This is a valuable measurement in a wide variety of settings and situations. SpO_2 measurements can help caregivers to detect hypoxia and can monitor oxygenation when supplemental oxygen is ordered or during sedation or surgeries. However, the SpO_2 does not always provide the full picture. For example, if a person has anemia or blood loss (i.e., insufficient red blood cells), then an SpO_2 of 100% does not ensure adequate organ perfusion and oxygenation. Likewise, if supplemental oxygen is being given, an SpO_2 of 100% does not tell you if too much oxygen is perhaps being administered. The SpO_2 measurement is part of a bigger assessment that includes the clinical assessment and may include an arterial blood gas for a more detailed analysis.

OBTAINING AN SpO₂ READING

When the clip or wrap is applied and turned on, the pulse oximeter will display a pulse rate, an SpO_2 percentage, and sometimes a waveform. In order to determine that the device is reading accurately, check for a correlation between the pulse that you assess and the pulse the device is sensing. Only record the SpO_2 if the device is accurately reading the pulse and there is an uninterrupted waveform. Many factors can cause inaccurate pulse oximetry readings. See Table 3.9 for a list of problems that result in inaccurate readings and for possible solutions.

APPLICATION OF THE NURSING PROCESS

Examples of Related ICNP Nursing Diagnoses, Expected Client Outcomes, and Nursing Interventions:

Nursing Diagnosis: Impaired gas exchange

Supporting Data: Client receiving supplemental oxygen

Expected Client Outcome: Client demonstrates sufficient O_2/CO_2 exchange through:
- unlabored respirations within established parameters (12–20 breaths/minute)
- pulse oximetry results within established parameters for client
- oriented mental status

Nursing Intervention Example: Monitor oxygen saturation.

Reference: International Classification for Nursing Practice. (n.d.). *eHealth & ICNP*. Retrieved from https://www.icn.ch/what-we-do/projects/ehealth-icnp.

CRITICAL CONCEPTS
Assessing Oxygen Saturation

Accuracy (ACC)

Obtaining a pulse oximeter measurement is sensitive to the following variables:

Client-Related Factors
- Client medical history, including recent use of intravascular dyes or exposure to carbon monoxide, cigarette smoking

TABLE 3.9 Problems With Measuring Pulse Oximetry

Problem	Reason	Solution
Carbon monoxide Jaundice Intravascular dyes	Interfere with the light reflected from the hemoglobin (Hgb)	Obtain an arterial blood gas (ABG).
Diabetic neuropathy Peripheral vascular disease (PVD) Hypothermia Cigarette smoking	Impaired circulation to fingertips	Apply the probe on the nose or earlobe.
Light—strong sunlight or artificial light	Interferes with the light sensors	Put the finger and fingertip probe under the bedcovers.
Nonadherence of bandage-wrap-style probe Excessive sweating Poorly positioned sensor Obesity—finger too large to fit into clip	With bandage-wrap-style probes, the light source must align with the light receptor.	Apply the bandage-wrap-style probe with the light source and light receptor in alignment.
Nail polish Acrylic nails Dark skin pigment Unclean skin surface	Interfere with the amount of light received	Remove nail polish or acrylic nails. Reposition probe.
Shivering Excessive movement	In older models, movement can interfere with receiving light consistently.	Warm the client. Swaddle moving infants. Use an ear clip.
Methemoglobinemia	Abnormal Hgb	Obtain an ABG.
Anemia	Not enough red blood cells/Hgb can result in hypoxia even when each cell carries an oxygen.	Blood transfusion Obtain an ABG.

Adapted from WHO, 2011.

- Client medical condition, including peripheral vascular disease, diabetic neuropathy, jaundice, or hypothermia
- Dark pigmentation
- Hypothermia
- Excessive sweating
- Excessive movement, including shivering
- Presence of nail polish or acrylic nails

Blood-Related Factors
- Anemia
- Methemoglobinemia

Nurse-Related Factors
- Site selection for sensor
- Positioning of the sensor

Equipment-Related Factors
- Condition of the sensor
- Capabilities of the model

Environmental Factors
- Strong natural or artificial light

Client-Centered Care (CCC)

When assessing oxygen saturation, respect for the client is demonstrated through:
- promoting autonomy
- providing privacy
- ensuring comfort
- honoring cultural preferences
- advocating for the client and family.

Infection Control (INF)

When assessing oxygen saturation, healthcare-associated infection is prevented by:
- preventing and reducing the transfer of microorganisms
- reducing the number of microorganisms.

Safety (SAF)

When assessing oxygen saturation, safety measures provide a safe care environment and prevent harm to the client.

Communication (COM)

- Communication exchanges information (oral, written, nonverbal or electronic) between two or more people.
- Documentation records information on oxygen saturation in a permanent legal record.

Health Maintenance (HLTH)

When assessing oxygen saturation, nursing is dedicated to the promotion of health, including:
- protecting the client's skin integrity.

Evaluation (EVAL)

When assessing oxygen saturation, the evaluation of outcomes enables the nurse to determine the efficacy of the care provided.

▪ SKILL 3.17 Obtaining a Pulse Oximeter Measurement

EQUIPMENT

Clean gloves, if there is a risk of exposure to body fluids
Antiseptic wipes
Pulse oximeter

BEGINNING THE SKILL

1. **SAF** Review the authorized healthcare provider's order and hospital policy. Determine if intermittent or continuous measurement is ordered. *Verifying the plan of care prevents injury to the client.*
2. **INF** Perform hand hygiene. Apply gloves, if there is a risk of exposure to body fluids.
3. **CCC** Introduce yourself to the client and family and explain the procedure.
4. **SAF** Identify the client using two identifiers.
5. **CCC** Provide privacy. Close the door and pull the curtain.

PROCEDURE

6. **ACC** Check the following by asking the client about:
   - client's allergies, such as allergies to topical antiseptics or latex
   - client's history related to conditions that may interfere with pulse oximetry.
7. **ACC** Turn on the pulse oximeter device and check it is functioning properly. Check that the sensor is clean and dry.
8. **ACC** Select a site that is intact, warm, dry, and adequately perfused for pulse oximetry measurement. *Review Table 3.9 for factors that impede pulse oximetry measurement.*
9. **ACC** Apply the sensor:

If using a clip:
   a. Squeeze the ends of the clip to open it.
   b. Position on the client.
   c. Release the ends of the clip.

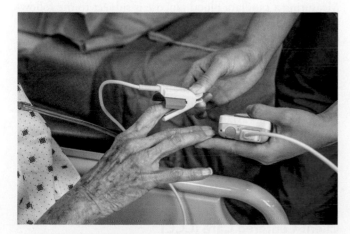

STEP 9A Position the clip on the client.

If using a wrap:
   a. Position the bandage-style sensor around the hand, foot, or digit such that the light source and receptor are aligned.

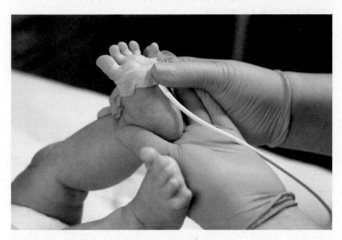

STEP 9A Position the bandage-style sensor.

   b. Secure the bandage-style sensor snugly, but do not restrict blood flow.
10. Turn the pulse oximeter to the "on" position after the sensor is secured. Adjust volume as needed.
11. **ACC** Set the alarm parameters according to the authorized healthcare provider's order and hospital policy.
12. **ACC** Measure the SpO$_2$ and pulse rate.
13. **EVAL** Evaluate the results measured. Compare the pulse rate on the pulse oximeter and the client's radial pulse or heart rate monitor. *If there is no correlation between the pulses, then reposition the sensor and check again.*
14. If obtaining an intermittent measurement, turn the pulse oximeter off.
15. **INF** Clean the probe with an antiseptic wipe.
16. **HLTH** If using a wrap, reposition the wrap as needed to protect the client's skin integrity.

FINISHING THE SKILL

17. **INF** Remove gloves if worn and perform hand hygiene.
18. **SAF** Ensure client safety and comfort. Ensure that the bed is in the lowest position and verify that the client can identify and reach the nurse call system. *These safety measures reduce the risk of falls.*
19. **EVAL** Evaluate the outcomes. Ensure that the client's pulse oximeter measurement is within the prescribed parameters. If it is not, then determine if there are existing orders in the event that the client is not within the prescribed parameters, or contact the authorized healthcare provider promptly.
20. **COM** Document assessment findings, including respiratory assessment; sensor site assessment; supplemental oxygen if present; date, time, and site of SpO$_2$ measurement; client and family education if provided; and client outcomes in the legal healthcare record.

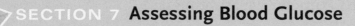

SECTION 7 Assessing Blood Glucose

MEASURING BLOOD GLUCOSE WITH A GLUCOMETER

Blood glucose is the readily available source of energy for cellular and metabolic needs. Blood glucose levels vary throughout the day based on caloric intake. The body maintains a homeostatic range of blood sugar by releasing glucagon and insulin. The established parameters for fasting blood sugar (defined as no caloric intake for at least 8 hours) is between 70 and 110 mg/dL. A level of less than 40 to 50 is considered a critically low level. At this level, there is not sufficient energy for cellular metabolism. Shortly after eating, it is expected to have blood sugar levels greater than 200 mg/dL. The physiologic response to an elevated blood sugar is to produce insulin, and within 2 hours, blood sugar levels should be less than 140 mg/dL for those under 50 years of age, under 150 mg/dL for those between 50 and 60 years of age, and under 160 mg/dL for those over 60 years of age. A reading of over 400 mg/dL is considered a critical value indicative of hyperglycemia.

Several factors can impact blood glucose levels. Diabetes is a disease defined by hyperglycemia and glucose intolerance. Approximately 9.4% of the American population has diabetes; however, a little less than one-quarter of these individuals are undiagnosed (Centers for Disease Control and Prevention [CDC], 2017). In addition, physiologic stressors can increase glucose levels, including trauma, infection, or myocardial infarction. Intravenous fluids containing dextrose will increase blood glucose levels, particularly those solutions with a greater concentration of dextrose, including total parental nutrition (TPN). Many medications will affect glucose levels; some medications will increase the glucose level, and others will decrease the level. Pregnancy and the development of gestational diabetes will result in glucose intolerance during the pregnancy and a subsequent risk of developing diabetes later in life.

Although a blood glucose level is included in a blood chemistry sent via blood sample to the laboratory, nurses also frequently measure blood glucose at the bedside with a glucose meter or glucometer. This is also referred to as a finger-stick blood sugar (FSBS). Typically for clients with diabetes, blood glucose levels are checked before each meal and before bedtime. Clients who are on TPN may have blood glucose measurements ordered with vital signs. Glucometers are small handheld devices that require only a drop of capillary blood to measure the blood glucose. If appropriate, allow the client to select the site for puncture. Nurses may use strategies to increase blood flow to the selected site, such as applying a warm compress or holding it in a dependent position, thus using gravity to aid blood flow.

Glucometers: Present and Future

There are many types and brands of glucometers with a variety of features. As a student, familiarize yourself with the types of strips and meters found at your clinical site. Clients with diabetes have glucometers at home and may be very knowledgeable about the differences between brands. Future innovations may enable noninvasive glucose monitoring, which would change the assessment of blood glucose. Noninvasive glucose monitoring promises improved management of diabetes with the removed discomfort of frequent finger sticks. Individuals with diabetes may use an invasive continuous glucose monitoring system that provides trends and early notification of high and low blood sugars. The FDA has approved a combination continuous glucose monitor and an insulin pump.

APPLICATION OF THE NURSING PROCESS

Examples of Related ICNP Nursing Diagnoses, Expected Client Outcomes, and Nursing Interventions:

Nursing Diagnosis: Nonadherence to diagnostic testing regimen

Supporting Data: Client has diabetes and states that she has not been testing her blood sugar

Expected Client Outcome: Client will check her blood sugar with a glucometer before breakfast each day.

Nursing Intervention Example: Monitor client's blood glucose with a glucometer before each meal and at bedtime.

Reference: International Classification for Nursing Practice. (n.d.). *eHealth & ICNP.* Retrieved from https://www.icn.ch/what-we-do/projects/ehealth-icnp.

CRITICAL CONCEPTS
Assessing Blood Glucose

Accuracy (ACC)

Measuring a capillary blood glucose is subject to the following variables:

Client-Related Variables
- Client medical history, including allergies, medications, and diseases
- Condition of fingers, including scarring and bruising
- Client current medications

Nurse-Related Variables
- Site of lancet insertion
- Selection and use of equipment
- Preparation of equipment

Equipment-Related Variables
- Glucometer and glucometer strips

Client-Centered Care (CCC)

When assessing blood glucose, respect for the client is demonstrated through:
- promoting autonomy
- providing privacy

- ensuring comfort
- honoring cultural preferences
- advocating for the client and family.

Infection Control (INF)

When assessing blood glucose, healthcare-associated infection is prevented by:
- containment of microorganisms
- preventing and reducing the transfer of microorganisms
- reducing the number of microorganisms.

Safety (SAF)

When assessing blood glucose, safety measures provide a safe care environment and prevent harm to the client.

Communication (COM)

- Communication exchanges information (oral, written, nonverbal, or electronic) between two or more people.
- Documentation records information in a permanent legal record.

Health Maintenance (HLTH)

When assessing blood glucose, nursing is dedicated to the promotion of health and self-care abilities, including:
- protecting the client's skin integrity by rotating sites.

Evaluation (EVAL)

When assessing blood glucose, the evaluation of outcomes enables the nurse to determine the efficacy of the care provided.

■ SKILL 3.18 Obtaining Capillary Blood Glucose Measurements

EQUIPMENT

Clean gloves
Antiseptic wipes
Glucometer
Glucometer strips
Lancet
Cotton ball or gauze pad
Bandaid
Control solution and check strip, if performing quality control test

BEGINNING THE SKILL

1. **SAF** Review the authorized healthcare provider's order and hospital policy. Determine the ordered frequency and timing of blood glucose measurements. Determine if orders are present for specific high or low blood glucose measurements. *Verifying the plan of care prevents injury to the client.*
2. **INF** Perform hand hygiene.
3. **CCC** Introduce yourself to the client and family and explain the procedure.
4. **SAF** Identify the client using two identifiers.
5. **CCC** Provide privacy. Close the door and pull the curtain.

PROCEDURE

6. **ACC** Check the following:
   - client's fingertips for bruising, circulation, or repeated use
   - client's medications for anticoagulants
   - client's allergies, such as allergies to topical antiseptics or latex.

7. **ACC** Examine the glucometer and glucometer strips to ensure compatibility. Check the expiration date on the glucometer strips. Check that quality control tests on the glucometer are current.
8. **ACC** Check that the glucometer indicates readiness for blood glucose measurement. Follow the manufacturer's instructions for the specific model. Turn on the glucometer, if appropriate for the model. Enter the client name and appropriate information into the glucometer per agency policy.
9. Remove a glucometer testing strip from the bottle and reseal the bottle. (Note: Some glucometers will instruct you to insert the glucometer strip into the glucometer now.)
10. **HLTH** Select a site for testing, or ask the client to select a site. The lateral sides of the fingertips are the appropriate site for capillary blood sampling in adults. Be sure to consistently rotate sites by selecting a new finger and a different side of the finger selected. *Rotating fingers and sites on the finger will prevent the short-term effect of soreness and prevents the long-term effect of thickened, discolored skin.*

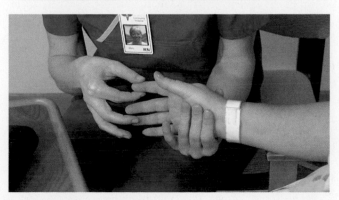

STEP 10 Select a site for testing.

11. **INF** Apply clean gloves. Cleanse the site with an antiseptic wipe. Allow the site to air dry.
12. **ACC** Remove the cover from the lancet. If the lancet is adjustable, select the depth based on the client recommendation and the condition of the skin.
13. **COM** Tell the client there will be a stick.
14. **ACC** Place the lancet on the selected site and pierce the skin. If using a lancing device with a release, push the release.

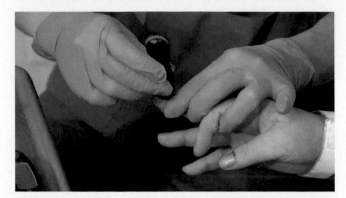

STEP 14 Place the lancet on the selected site.

15. **SAF** Discard lancet into puncture-proof sharps container.
16. **ACC** Wipe the first blood drop if indicated by the manufacturer's recommendation or agency policy. *The first drop may contain alcohol and a greater amount of interstitial fluid.*
17. **ACC** Obtain a second droplet of blood and apply it to the glucometer strip. Note that newer model glucometer strips will "wick" the blood onto the strip, but with older-model glucometers, you must place a blood droplet on the glucometer strip.

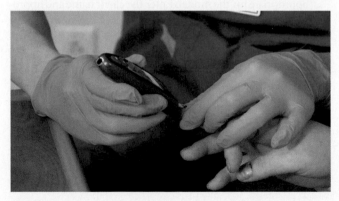

STEP 17 Apply the drop to the glucometer strip.

18. Press the cotton ball over the site where the blood was drawn.

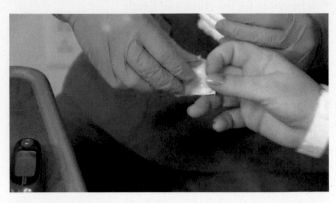

STEP 18 Press the cotton ball over the site.

19. **COM** Watch for a reading on the glucometer. Share the results with the client.
20. **INF** When you have a reading, discard the glucometer strip.

FINISHING THE SKILL

21. **INF** Remove gloves and perform hand hygiene. (Note: Do not touch clean surfaces with dirty gloves.)
22. **SAF** Ensure client safety and comfort. Ensure that the bed is in the lowest position and verify that the client can identify and reach the nurse call system. *These safety measures reduce the risk of falls.*
23. **EVAL** Evaluate the outcomes. Ensure the client's blood glucose level is within the prescribed parameters. If the client is not within the parameters, then act on existing orders or contact the authorized healthcare provider promptly.
24. **COM** Document assessment findings, such as glucose measurement results; date, time, and site of blood glucose measurement; condition of the fingertips; client and family education, if provided; and client outcomes in the legal healthcare record.
25. **HLTH** Encourage the client to participate in capillary blood glucose measurements. Observe the client demonstrate self-care before discharge.

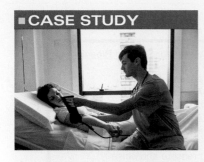

■ CASE STUDY

Ms. Torres is a 29-year-old client who was admitted to the hospital for abdominal surgery for the removal of fibroids. Her current weight is 46 kg (102 pounds), and she is 168 cm (5'6") tall. In the recovery room, her postoperative baseline vital signs were as follows: temperature 37.3°C (99°F) using a temporal artery thermometer (TAT); pulse 89; respirations 16. Her blood pressure was 134/78 mm Hg using a pediatric cuff. She has a dry, intact abdominal dressing and a Foley catheter draining 40 mL/hr of clear, yellow urine. In the recovery room, Ms. Torres rated her pain as a 1 on a 0- to 10-point scale.

Upon admission to the surgical unit, the authorized healthcare provider ordered Ms. Torres's vital signs to be taken every hour for 4 hours and every 4 hours thereafter due to instability during surgery. Her vital signs on admission to the floor were temperature 36.0°C (97°F; axillary); respirations 15; and her radial pulse was 84 with a regular rate and rhythm. Her blood pressure was 106/58 mm Hg in the left arm. However, the blood pressure cuff seemed loose on Ms. Torres.

Several hours later on the night shift (7:00 PM to 7:00 AM shift), another nurse obtains Ms. Torres's vital signs. Her temperature at that time is 37.0°C (98.6°F; oral); respirations 16; and blood pressure 104/58 using a regular adult-size cuff. Her radial pulse rate is 66 bpm but is irregular and somewhat difficult to palpate. Her extremities are warm to touch, and she has no other complaints or symptoms at this time. Although Ms. Torres rated her pain as a 2, her discomfort has stabilized after receiving pain medication.

Case Study Questions

1. Each time a vital sign is obtained, the nurse is responsible for evaluating the results to ensure accurate measurement. Identify the vital signs that deviate from Ms. Torres's baseline when she is initially admitted to the surgical unit from the recovery room.
2. When comparing the blood pressure measurement obtained when Ms. Torres was in the recovery room to the first blood pressure measurement obtained on the surgical unit, there was a significant decrease. How would you explain the difference?
3. The admitting surgical unit nurse obtained a temperature lower than the temperature obtained by the recovery room nurse. Explain some reasons for the change.
4. Explain how the admitting surgical unit nurse could have evaluated Ms. Torres's vital signs when they deviated from baseline. Describe measures the nurse could have taken to evaluate the validity of the vital sign results.
5. Describe the potential impact of the documented vital signs on Ms. Torres's care.
6. During the night shift, Ms. Torres's radial pulse assessment changed from the previous shift. Explain this change. How can the nurse ensure that the measurement and assessment of Ms. Torres's pulse are accurate?
7. **Application of QSEN Competencies:** One of the Quality and Safety Education for Nurses (QSEN) skills for Teamwork and Collaboration is to follow communication practices that minimize the risks associated with handoffs during transitions in care (Cronenwett et al., 2007). How could the nurses improve handoff communication in this situation?

■CONCEPT MAP

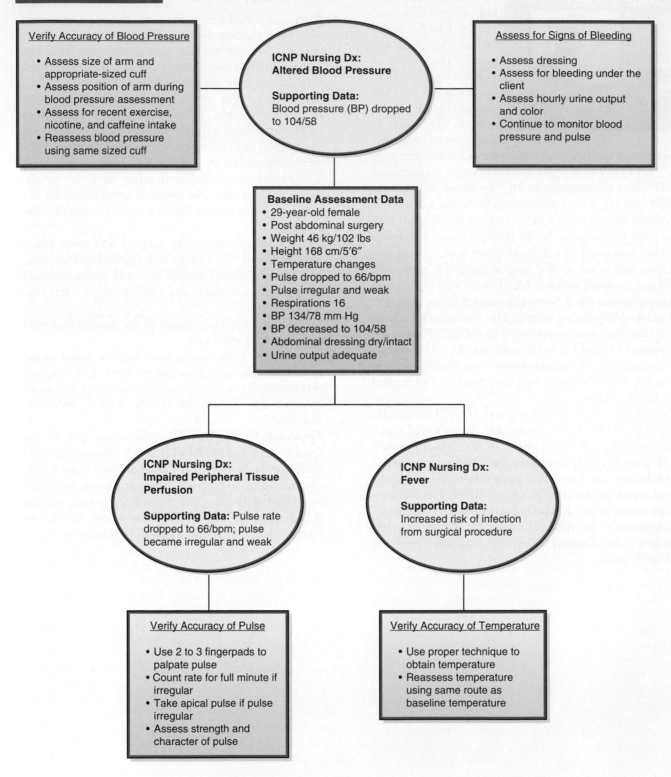

Verify Accuracy of Blood Pressure

- Assess size of arm and appropriate-sized cuff
- Assess position of arm during blood pressure assessment
- Assess for recent exercise, nicotine, and caffeine intake
- Reassess blood pressure using same sized cuff

**ICNP Nursing Dx:
Altered Blood Pressure**

Supporting Data:
Blood pressure (BP) dropped to 104/58

Assess for Signs of Bleeding

- Assess dressing
- Assess for bleeding under the client
- Assess hourly urine output and color
- Continue to monitor blood pressure and pulse

Baseline Assessment Data
- 29-year-old female
- Post abdominal surgery
- Weight 46 kg/102 lbs
- Height 168 cm/5′6″
- Temperature changes
- Pulse dropped to 66/bpm
- Pulse irregular and weak
- Respirations 16
- BP 134/78 mm Hg
- BP decreased to 104/58
- Abdominal dressing dry/intact
- Urine output adequate

**ICNP Nursing Dx:
Impaired Peripheral Tissue Perfusion**

Supporting Data: Pulse rate dropped to 66/bpm; pulse became irregular and weak

**ICNP Nursing Dx:
Fever**

Supporting Data:
Increased risk of infection from surgical procedure

Verify Accuracy of Pulse

- Use 2 to 3 fingerpads to palpate pulse
- Count rate for full minute if irregular
- Take apical pulse if pulse irregular
- Assess strength and character of pulse

Verify Accuracy of Temperature

- Use proper technique to obtain temperature
- Reassess temperature using same route as baseline temperature

References

American Academy of Pediatrics. (2015). *How to take a child's temperature*. Retrieved from https://www.healthychildren.org/English/health-issues/conditions/fever/pages/How-to-Take-a-Childs-Temperature.aspx.

American Heart Association. (2017). *All about heart rate (pulse)*. Retrieved from http://www.heart.org/HEARTORG/Conditions/HighBloodPressure/GettheFactsAboutHighBloodPressure/All-About-Heart-Rate-Pulse_UCM_438850_Article.jsp.

Centers for Disease Control and Prevention. (2017). *National diabetes statistics report: Estimates of diabetes and its burden in the United States, 2017*. Atlanta, GA: U.S. Department of Health and Human Services.

Cronenwett, L., Sherwood, G., Barnsteiner, J., Disch, J., Johnson, J., Mitchell, P., ... & Warren, J. (2007). Quality and safety education for nurses. *Nursing Outlook, 55*(3), 122–131. Retrieved from http://qsen.org/competencies/pre-licensure-ksas/.

Dolkar, R., Kapoor, S., Singh, N. V., & Suri, V. (2013). A comparative study on the recording of temperature by the clinical mercury thermometer and digital thermometer. *Nursing and Midwifery Research Journal, 9*(1), 40–46.

Dorsey, E. R., & Topol, E. J. (2016). State of telehealth. *New England Journal of Medicine, 375*, 154–161.

Flynn, J. T., & Falkner, B. E. (2017). New clinical practice guidelines for the management of high blood pressure in children and adolescents. *Hypertension, 70*(4), 683–686.

Haugan, B., Langerud, A. K., Kalvey, H., Frøslie, K. F., Riise, E., & Kapstad, H. (2013). Can we trust the new generation of infrared tympanic thermometers in clinical practice? *Journal of Clinical Nursing, 22*, 698–709.

Hockenberry, M. J., Rodgers, C. C., & Wilson, D. (2017). *Wong's essentials of pediatric nursing* (10th ed.). St. Louis, MO: Elsevier.

International Classification for Nursing Practice. (n.d.). *eHealth & ICNP*. Retrieved from https://www.icn.ch/what-we-do/projects/ehealth-icnp.

Khanh-Dao Le, L. (2016). *Vital signs: Clinician information*. [Evidence Summary]. Retrieved from The Joanna Briggs Institute EBP Database.

Khanh-Dao Le, L. (2017). *Temperature measurement (pediatrics): Temporal artery thermometers*. [Evidence Summary]. Retrieved from The Joanna Briggs Institute EBP Database.

Kiekkas, P., Aretha, D., Almpani, E., & Stefanopoulos, N. (2019). Temporal artery thermometry in pediatric patients: Systematric review and meta-analysis. *Journal of Pediatric Nursing, 46*, 89–99.

Lowdermilk, D. L., Perry, S. E., Cashion, K., & Rhodes Alden, K. (2016). *Maternity and women's health care* (11th ed.). St. Louis, MO: Elsevier.

Lu, S. H., Leasure, A. R., & Dai, Y. T. (2010). A systemic review of body temperature variations in older people. *Journal of Clinical Nursing, 19*, 4–16.

Mackowiak, P. A., Wasserman, S. S., & Levine, M. M. (1992). A critical appraisal of 98.6 degrees F, the upper limit of the normal body temperature, and other legacies of Carl Reinhold August Wunderlich. *JAMA, 268*(12), 458–467.

Mackowiak, P. A., & Worden, G. (1994). Carl Reinhold August Wunderlich and the evolution of clinical thermometry. *Clinical Infectious Diseases, 18*(3), 458–467.

Mancia, G., Fagard, R., Narkiewicz, K., Redón, J., Zanchetti, A., Böhm, M., & Task Force Members. (2013). 2013 ESH/ESC guidelines for the management of arterial hypertension: The Task Force for the Management of Arterial Hypertension of the European Society of Hypertension (ESH) and of the European Society of Cardiology (ESC). *Journal of Hypertension, 31*(7), 1281–1357.

National Heart, Lung, and Blood Institute. (2017). *High blood pressure*. Retrieved from https://www.nhlbi.nih.gov/health-topics/high-blood-pressure.

Nightingale, F. (1898). *Notes on nursing: What it is, and what it is not*. Retrieved from https://www.fulltextarchive.com/page/Notes-on-Nursing/.

Pickering, T. G., Hall, J. E., Appel, L. J., Falkner, B. E., Graves, J., Hill, M. N., ... Roccella, E. J. (2005). Recommendations for blood pressure measurement in humans and experimental animals: Part 1: Blood pressure measurement in humans: A statement for professionals from the Subcommittee of Professional and Public Education of the American Heart Association Council on High Blood Pressure Research. *Hypertension, 45*(1), 142–161.

Plichart, M., Seux, M. L., Caillard, L., Chaussade, E., Vidal, J. S., Boully, C., & Hanon, O. (2013). Home blood pressure measurement in elderly patients with cognitive impairment: Comparison of agreement between relative-measured blood pressure and automated blood pressure measurement. *Blood Pressure Monitoring, 18*(4), 208.

Robertson-Smith, J., McCaffrey, F. T., Syers, R., Williams, S., & Taylor, B. J. (2015). A comparison of mid-forehead and axillary temperatures in newborn intensive care. *Journal of Perinatology, 35*, 120–122.

Seckel, M. A. (2016). Obtaining noninvasive accurate blood pressure measurements in adults. [AACN Practice Alert]. *Critical Care Nurse, 36*(3), e12–e16.

Sharma, L. (2018). *Vital signs: Clinician information*. [Evidence Summary]. Retrieved from The Joanna Briggs Institute EBP Database.

Skirton, H., Chamberlain, W., Lawson, C., Ryan, H., & Young, E. (2011). A systematic review of variability and reliability of manual and automated blood pressure readings. *Journal of Clinical Nursing, 20*(5–6), 602–614.

Slade, S. (2017). *Temperature measurement (adults): Temporal artery thermometers*. [Evidence Summary]. Retrieved from The Joanna Briggs Institute EBP Database.

Stryker. (2016). *Product brochure and operations manual. Altrix™ precision temperature management system*. Retrieved from https://techweb.stryker.com/Temp_Management/8001/0916/Operations/8001-009-001G.pdf.

Turner, M., Burns, S. M., Chaney, C., Conaway, M., Dame, M., Parks, C., ... Zarzyski, M. (2008). Measuring blood pressure accurately in an ambulatory cardiology clinic setting: Do patient position and timing really matter? *MEDSURG Nursing, 17*(2), 93–98.

Waalen, J., & Buxbaum, J. N. (2011). Is older colder or colder older? The association of age with body temperature in 18,630 individuals. *Journals of Gerontology, Series A, Biological Sciences and Medical Sciences, 66A*, 487–492.

Whelton, P. K., Carey, R. M., Aronow, W. S., Casey, D. E., Collins, K. J., Dennison Himmelfarb, C., ... Wright, Jr., J. T. (2017). 2017 ACC/AHA/AAPA/ABC/ACPM/AGS/APhA/ASH/ASPC/NMA/PCNA guideline for the prevention, detection, evaluation, and management of high blood pressure in adults. *Journal of the American College of Cardiology, 138*(17), e426–e483.

World Health Organization. (2011). *Pulse oximetry training manual*. Retrieved from http://www.who.int/patientsafety/safesurgery/pulse_oximetry/who_ps_pulse_oximetry_training_manual_en.pdf.

Yoost, B. L., & Crawford, L. R. (2016). *Fundamentals of nursing. Active learning for collaborative practice*. St. Louis, MO: Elsevier.

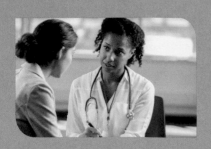

CHAPTER 4

Performing an Assessment

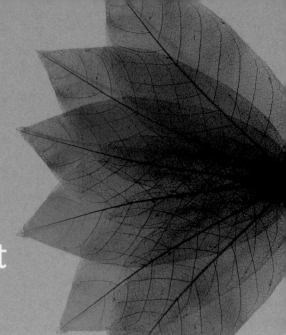

"We see only what we look for, and we look for only what we know." | **Adapted from Johann Wolfgang Goethe (1749–1832), Poet, Playwright, and Natural Philosopher**

LEARNING OBJECTIVES

By the end of this chapter, the reader will be able to:

1 Identify the assessment process.
2 Differentiate between subjective and objective data.
3 Identify components of a complete health history.
4 Describe how to conduct an interview with a client.
5 Discuss how to avoid personal bias when interviewing a client.
6 Identify communication techniques that may be used when interviewing a client.
7 Identify components of a physical exam.
8 Collect objective data through performing inspection, auscultation, percussion, and palpation.

9 Perform a preliminary survey.
10 Perform a rapid head-to-toe bedside assessment.
11 Perform a system-specific assessment:
  a Skin/integumentary system
  b Head (HEENT) and neck
  c Neurologic
  d Thorax (heart and lungs)
  e Abdominal
  f Musculoskeletal
  g Genitourinary

TERMINOLOGY

Abduction Movement or pulling of an extremity (e.g., leg) away from the midline of the body.

Accommodation Focus on a near object, then a far object, with corresponding pupillary constriction noted in eyes bilaterally.

Adduction Movement or pulling of an extremity toward the midline of the body.

Atrophy Decrease in size or shape of a body part that can affect its function.

Bilateral Occurring on both sides of the body as if a mirror image.

Crepitus Crackling, popping, or grating sensation that may be palpated just under the skin or create a faint sound. Crepitus is usually caused by air in the subcutaneous tissues.

Dorsal Anatomical term that refers to the back or upper side of something (e.g., back of hand).

Dorsiflexion Bending backward or flexing back of a part of the body, such as foot or hand.

Edema Excess fluid in interstitial spaces.

Eversion Movement to turn the sole of the foot away from the midline of the body.

Inspection Objective technique for collecting assessment data through observation.

Inversion Movement to turn the sole of the foot toward the body's midline.

Objective data Information obtained through observation and inspection of the client.

Ophthalmoscope Tool used to examine the external and internal structures of the eyes.

Otoscope Tool used to examine the external ear, ear canal, and tympanic membrane.

Palmar Palms or "grasping sides" of the client's hands.

Palpation Objective assessment gathered through touching the client to detect the condition of tissue.

Paresthesia A burning, tickling, or prickling pain sensation verbalized by client.

Percussion Objective assessment elicited when the person examining gently strikes a given point of contact on the client's body.

Peristalsis Physiologic sequential muscular contractions of the gastrointestinal tract.

Phalange Any of the bones of the fingers.

Pitting edema Edema characterized by an indentation of skin and tissue that remains after pressure is applied and released. It is often seen in the lower extremities.

Reflex hammer Small hammer device with a rubber head used to elicit deep tendon reflexes.

Reflexes An involuntary response to a stimulus. In a physical exam, reflexes can be elicited with a reflex hammer to assess central and peripheral nervous system function.

Stereognosis The ability to identify an object by using the "tactile" sense.

Subjective data Information client shares about self.

Tuning fork Two-pronged tool with tines in the shape of the letter "U" that can be used to assess a client's ability to hear sound and feel vibration when the fork is vibrated.

ACRONYMS

CVA Costovertebral angle

DTRs Deep tendon reflexes

HEENT Head, eyes, ears, nose, and throat

HIPAA Health Insurance Portability and Accountability Act

JVD Jugular venous distention

LEP Limited English proficiency

LOC Level of consciousness

PERRLA Pupils equal, round, regular, reactive to light, and accommodation

---

Assessment is an essential nursing skill. The American Nurses Association (ANA) identifies assessment as, "Standard 1. The registered nurse collects pertinent data and information relative to the healthcare consumer's health or the situation." (ANA, 2015, p. 53). The standards of nursing practice, as explained by the ANA (2015), are statements of the duties that all registered nurses are expected to perform competently. There are various types of assessments that nurses use depending upon the client and the situation. Nurses adapt the breadth and depth of the assessment to the situation. Nurses must also prioritize the collection of pertinent data based on the client's immediate needs. For example, a client who receives a certain treatment may require assessment and reassessment to ensure there are no adverse effects of the treatment and to identify the effectiveness of the therapy. Likewise, a client with an acute injury or condition may require ongoing assessment to monitor for complications. Regardless of whether a client's condition is acute or chronic, it is important for nurses to assess and monitor trends and changes, and to provide the appropriate interventions.

The following types of assessments will be described in this chapter. Each of these assessments collects both subjective and objective data.

- Performing a Preliminary Survey
- Performing a Comprehensive Health Assessment (which may also include obtaining a health history)
- Performing a Rapid Head-to-Toe Bedside Assessment
- Performing a System-Specific Assessment

Effective communication and accurate documentation of the information collected during assessment is also identified as an essential competency of the registered nurse (ANA, 2015). Nurses have consistent, personal interactions with the client and the opportunity to observe, communicate, and assess his or her needs. This unique relationship often means that more information is shared between the client and nurse.

The purpose of this chapter is to help students perform assessment in a systematic and logical way. It is not intended to replace a comprehensive assessment text but rather to provide the reader with a quick reference of various types of assessments to use at the bedside. This chapter will also help the reader identify what needs to be assessed in various settings. In most settings, the registered nurse is responsible for initial and ongoing assessment of the client.

THE ASSESSMENT PROCESS

Assessment begins upon entering the client's room. As you introduce yourself, observe the client closely. In what position is the client lying? How does the client respond to the opening door or your voice? Is the client alert and oriented? When you shake your client's hand, how firm is the grip? What is the client's skin temperature? What color is the skin? As you look at the client's armband, can the client tell you his or her name and birthdate correctly? Is the intravenous (IV) site intact? Within minutes, the nurse has already gathered valuable information. It is also important to assess the client's immediate environment. The client's environment must be safe and conducive to healing (see Chapter 7). For example, is the client's room clean and well ventilated with a comfortable temperature? Are there any unnecessary sights, odors, noises or distractions?

Assessment continues in an orderly way using a planned method of progression. For example, a head-to-toe or system-specific assessment (as described in this chapter) may be used. A systematic method ensures that no area is overlooked and that a complete assessment has been performed.

SECTION 1 Collecting Subjective and Objective Data

During the assessment and data collection process, the critical concepts of accuracy, client-centered care, and communication are paramount. Subjective data is information that is shared with the nurse from the client's perspective. Objective data is the information collected by the nurse and/or other healthcare providers by direct observation or examination. This observation will include most of the senses: sight, touch, sound, and smell. Many times, subjective and objective data are collected simultaneously.

COLLECTING SUBJECTIVE DATA

There are several ways to collect subjective data, and one of the most common is to ask the client questions while performing the physical assessment (discussed shortly). Another important part of the subjective assessment is to assess whether the client is having pain. Pain can be a distraction for the client, and it may also affect aspects of the physical assessment. When assessing the client's pain, use a facility-approved tool that is consistent, age appropriate, and culturally sensitive. (For more information on pain assessment, see Chapter 7). Another way of collecting subjective data is by obtaining a health history and conducting an interview.

Obtaining a Health History

The health history allows clients to relate why they are seeking healthcare at this time. Nurses and other healthcare providers may have health history data to collect. Most healthcare organizations will have approved paperwork that can be used as a guide to collect health history data. It is important to not omit information from these forms. The client's legal health record begins with the collection and documentation of this information. Four types of health histories are possible during a client visit (Wilson & Giddens, 2017), as follows:

- **Comprehensive health assessment interview:** This is an interview that allows for better understanding of the client's current health status, general welfare, and personal understanding about ongoing health concerns regarding the treatment plan.
- **Focused, problem-oriented health interview:** This is an interview that allows for more in-depth information to be elicited from the client pertaining to a known healthcare condition needing detailed attention.
- **Follow-up history:** The follow-up history is a variation of the focused, problem-oriented health interview and occurs after a client has been treated and returns for reevaluation. This type of health history will help determine the client's progress since his or her treatment.
- **Emergency history:** The emergency history elicits information regarding the immediate health concern for the client that could be potentially life threatening.

Before the oral interview begins, the client may be asked to complete a written health history. The nurse will utilize this information while conversing with the client. The primary components of the client's health history usually include the following:
- Identifying data and source of the history
- Chief complaint(s)
- History of present illness
- Past medical/surgical history
- Medications/allergies
- Family history/social history
- Review of systems

The chief complaint is the main problem that led to the client seeking care, and it must be documented in the client's own words, preferably in quotes—for example, "I have been feeling more tired lately" or "I haven't been able to do my usual activities."

Conducting an Interview

Client interviewing is a skill that takes time to develop. To facilitate trust and enhance communication, it is important to provide client-centered care during all phases of the interview process. Many facilities have programs for healthcare providers to improve this essential skill. Obtaining as much information as possible from the client's point of view about his or her particular healthcare concerns is the goal (Garlock, 2016). Communication can also be enhanced by avoiding personal bias and using effective interview techniques.

Avoiding Personal Bias

When conducting an interview as part of the assessment, it is important to avoid bias and maintain objectivity. Avoiding bias is a critical aspect of providing client-centered care. For example, emotionally charged topics such as the client's sexual orientation or drug use are to be approached in an unbiased, nonconfrontational way. In addition, the nurse must recognize his or her own personal discomfort during the interview process. The nurse must also avoid making assumptions based on the client's ethnicity, gender, or age. Sometimes the client will make assumptions that can lead to denial, such as "Oh I am way too young to have chest pain!" Unfortunately, false assumptions may affect the accuracy of the assessment and cause serious conditions to be overlooked.

Factors to Consider Before Conducting an Interview

In order to conduct an effective interview, there are several factors to consider. For example, the environment where nurses interview clients is more conducive to conversation if it is private and quiet, with a comfortable temperature. A quiet environment allows for the client's undivided attention, which facilitates the collection of important data. To protect the client's privacy, healthcare facilities are required to recognize the Healthcare Information Portability and Accountability Act (HIPAA). Thus securing and protecting private health information during the interview is essential.

Another factor to consider during an interview is the client's ability to communicate in English. If a client has a different primary language or has significant hearing loss, a certified interpreter would be an essential member of the healthcare team. Cross-cultural communication can create a problem during the collection of subjective information in the healthcare setting. Federal laws require that clients who have limited English proficiency (LEP) must have access to interpretation services (U.S. Department of Health and Human Services, 2013). For a variety of reasons, federal law discourages the use of family or friends as interpreters. Most hospitals have interpretation services (Massachusetts General Hospital, 2018). In addition, electronic interpretation services may be available. When working with an interpreter and a client from another culture, cultural considerations must be addressed. For a list of cultural considerations, see Box 4.1.

BOX 4.1 Cultural Considerations

Factors to consider when working with an interpreter and a client from another culture include the following:
- Talk to the interpreter privately before you begin. Make sure the interpreter understands the information that you will try to convey during the interview.
- Some people from other cultures like to have family present when they are encountering difficult times, such as a health crisis. Find out from your interpreter whom the client prefers to have present during the health interview and assessment.
- If any communication is not understood on either side, restate the communication. Make sure the client also knows to tell the interpreter this.
- Begin by having introductions from everyone present. Explain to the client how the interpreter will work so that the client will understand that the interpreter is accurately relaying what the client is saying.
- Speak directly to the client and not the interpreter.
- Clarify any misunderstandings that may occur during the interview.

References: Garlock, 2016; Kachirskaia, Mate, & Neuwirth, 2018; Wilson & Giddens, 2017.

Techniques for Conducting an Interview

One of the most important techniques when interviewing or speaking to a client is to position yourself at the client's level and make eye contact (Fig. 4.1). In addition to facilitating trust and enhancing communication, this technique sends the message that you care about the client and are concerned about what he or she has to say. Some additional strategies that will facilitate an effective interview between the nurse and client include the following:
- Phrase questions in an open-ended format so that the client can provide as much detail, in his or her own words, as possible. Open-ended questions or statements elicit answers that will be more than one word. Details expressed in the answer to an open-ended question or statement help the nurse learn more about the factors affecting the client. An example of an open-ended question is, "What

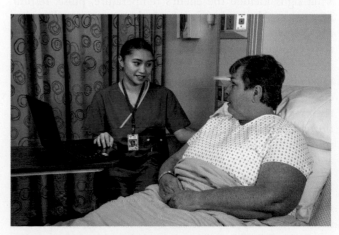

FIG. 4.1 Sitting at eye level with the client enhances communication.

brings you here today?" Asking a broad, open-ended question such as, "Is there anything I have not asked that you are concerned about?" allows the client to verbalize any unspoken concerns.

In contrast to open-ended questions, closed-ended questions will often be answered by the client with just "yes" or "no." An example of a closed-ended question is "Are you having severe pain?" Closed-ended questions or statements often impede the flow of information from the client, hinder self-expression, and limit elaboration on pertinent details. A better option is using an open-ended statement such as "Describe your pain and tell me how it is affecting your activities."

- Avoid using medical jargon, and speak as plainly as possible (Carr, 2017).
- Repeat back information that is shared by the client. This validates the information and also ensures that what you are hearing is correct.
- Speak in a clear and confident tone. This will facilitate trust and enhance communication. It is also helpful to face the client when speaking.
- Promote an atmosphere of safety where the client is comfortable sharing personal information with the nurse without fear of retribution. This demonstrates that the client's health is at the center of the conversation (Carr, 2017).

The client is a vital member of the healthcare team. Effective communication between the nurse and the client will elicit valuable information for ensuring excellent care.

COLLECTING OBJECTIVE DATA

Objective data is what you can see, hear, feel or smell, such as findings from a physical exam or head-to-toe assessment. It is sometimes quantitative data, such as the client's vital signs, pulse oximetry, lab results, or height and weight. An image such as a radiograph is also objective data. The nurse's attention to detail and technique will enhance accuracy when collecting objective data.

Vital Signs

Vital signs include the client's temperature, pulse, respiratory rate, and blood pressure. Vital signs are usually taken routinely at set intervals. Depending on the client's condition, the nurse may have to take the vital signs at more frequent intervals. It is often the nurse's judgment as to when the vital signs must be obtained. When the client's condition changes, the nurse must take vital signs as a part of the client's rapid bedside assessment. Many facilities require routine measurement of pulse oximetry readings when the vital signs are obtained. (For information on obtaining vital signs and pulse oximetry, see Chapter 3.)

Height and Weight

In an inpatient setting, a weight will be collected in the manner most appropriate for the client's age and physical condition. Weight and height are also obtained in outpatient settings and are especially important in tracking the growth and development of infants and children. When using a standing scale, ensure that the scales are zeroed and calibrated according to your facility policy. If the client is going to be weighed every day for monitoring, ensure that the same scale is used, and weigh the client at the same time of day.

If the client is on bedrest, has limited mobility, or is unable to stand, a bed scale may need to be used. Many facilities are now equipped with beds that are able to weigh the client automatically. (For more information on measuring a client's height and weight, as well as measuring other anthropometric data, see Skill 5.1 in Chapter 5.)

Physical Exam

Performing a physical assessment is a critical aspect of nursing care. Many times, the subjective assessment, such as the interview and health history, will help the nurse determine what type of physical exam may be required and how urgently it will need to be done. For example, if the client states that he or she is having some difficulty breathing, then the nurse may need to promptly perform a system-specific respiratory assessment. The four main types of physical examination techniques are inspection, auscultation, percussion, and palpation. These techniques are discussed in the following subsections (Wilson & Giddens, 2017).

Inspection

Inspection is the purposeful observation of a client, including the client's appearance, behavior, and movement. Examples of inspection may include looking at the client's skin as well as the symmetry of his or her facial features. Inspection may also include looking for any lesions, wounds, bruises, or rashes and observing the client's gait and any body movements, such as spasms, tremors, or pulsations. A thorough inspection requires adequate lighting. To respect the client's dignity, inspection of certain areas of the body also requires privacy.

Auscultation

In the technique of auscultation, a stethoscope is used to listen to sounds produced by the heart, lungs, blood vessels, and bowels. Both the bell and diaphragm are used when assessing the heart. The bell is used alone when listening for vascular sounds, such as the carotid arteries. The diaphragm of the stethoscope is often used to assess the lungs and bowel. Using a stethoscope is also important for taking vital signs and obtaining a blood pressure (see Chapter 3).

Percussion

Percussion is a technique that produces sounds that can help determine the state of the underlying tissue or organs. For example, upon palpation, a nurse may find a lump or mass in the client's abdomen. Based on the sounds this area produces through percussion, it can be determined if the lump is more solid (a dull sound) or less dense, like a gas (which would be a more resonant, tympanic, or hollow sound). Not all body systems benefit from using percussion. Three types of percussion that may be used are direct, indirect, and blunt:

- **Direct percussion:** This technique involves tapping the fingertip directly over the area to be examined, as in percussion of the sinuses.
- **Indirect percussion:** This is a technique of tapping the nondominant third finger by the dominant hand's fingertip with two rapid strokes, which produces a sound that may be used to determine the density of the organs below. In order to obtain the best quality of sound, indirect percussion is generated from the flicking action of the examiner's wrist, not the entire hand (Fig. 4.2).
- **Blunt percussion:** This technique is commonly used to assess kidney inflammation. The nurse places the palm of the nondominant hand over the area to be examined and strikes the back of the hand with the dominant fist. Use caution and assess the client carefully for any contraindications before performing this type of percussion (Fig. 4.3).

Palpation

In the palpation technique, pressure is gently applied to the skin by the palmar surface of the fingers and hands using a rotary motion. This technique assesses temperature, tenderness, organ contour, and joint crepitus. Palpation may be light, as used for temperature and tenderness. The deep palpation technique may be used to assess the client's underlying organs. However, if a client is having abdominal pain, use extreme caution. Avoid deep or pointed percussion of the left upper quadrant where the client's spleen is located because vigorous palpation could cause rupture and/or bleeding. Assess the client for any contraindications, such as appendicitis.

The purpose of palpation is to feel, using the fingers and/or hands, for changes in body structure, including organ sizes. In some areas, such as the chin, the fingers are needed to provide shallow or light palpation, which is no greater than 1 cm in depth (Fig. 4.4), whereas in others, such as the abdomen, the fingers and hands are used for deeper palpation. One method that may be used is the bimanual technique (Fig. 4.5), whereby the dominant hand is placed over the nondominant hand. The top hand performs the pressing rotary motion while the bottom hand remains stationary. When palpating a pulse, the pads of two or three fingers are usually used.

When performing a physical exam, it is helpful to ask the client follow-up questions. For example, upon palpation of the lymph nodes in the neck, the nurse finds that there are two enlarged nodes in the left posterior cervical

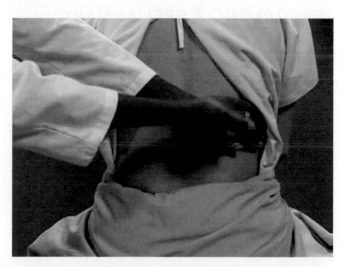

FIG. 4.3 Blunt percussion.

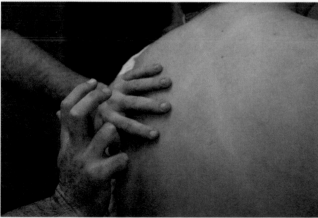

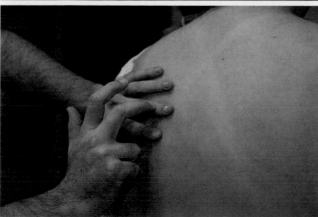

FIG. 4.2 Indirect percussion.

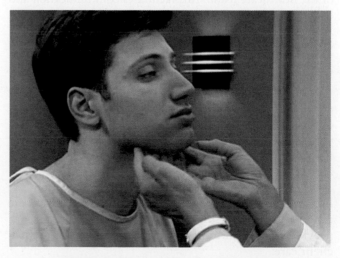

FIG. 4.4 Light palpation of lymph nodes.

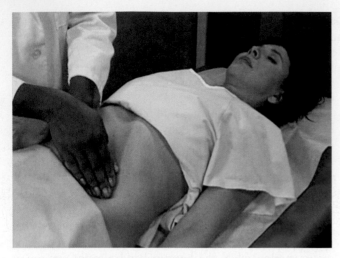

FIG. 4.5 Deep palpation (bimanual technique).

chain. When questioned, the client replies, "I'm getting over an ear infection. It's not as tender as it was last week." These pieces of information help the nurse recognize and analyze cues to complete the client's assessment.

PERFORMING A PRELIMINARY SURVEY

When a client is initially admitted into an inpatient setting or seen in a clinic, the nurse may be required to perform a preliminary assessment. This type of assessment is usually a general survey of the client, and it includes both subjective and objective data collection. During this assessment, the nurse is observing the overall appearance and behavior of the client, as well as the client's mobility and orientation level. The initial interview and collection of the health history (including medical/surgical history, medications, and allergies) are often performed during the preliminary survey. In addition, the preliminary survey can determine the need for a more in-depth head-to-toe system specific assessment. The nurse can also determine if the client requires immediate medical attention or a referral to other members of the healthcare team. This facilitates communication and collaboration.

SUMMARY

When collecting subjective and objective data, three of the most important critical concepts to consider are client-centered care, accuracy, and communication. These critical concepts are also interrelated. For example, providing client-centered care enhances communication with the client and facilitates trust, which in turn also enhances accuracy.

Both subjective and objective data collection are important for the client's overall assessment. They are rarely performed in isolation of each other, and they both provide valuable information that is necessary for optimal client care.

CRITICAL CONCEPTS
Collecting Subjective and Objective Data

Accuracy (ACC)

Subjective and objective data collection may be sensitive to the following variables:

Client-Related Factors
- Age and developmental level
- Level of consciousness and orientation
- Level of pain, discomfort, or emotional distress
- Culture and language
- Vision, hearing, or any disabilities
- Environment (e.g., noise, temperature, distractions)
- Modesty
- History of sexual trauma or posttraumatic stress disorder (PTSD)
- Lack of knowledge/understanding

Nurse-Related Factors
- Technique used to collect subjective data (interview and health history)
- Thoroughness of interview questions and ability to listen to the client
- Position when interviewing client (e.g., sitting at eye level)
- Personal bias or assumptions
- Language barriers
- Observational skills and technique used to collect objective data
- Ability to verify findings and perform further assessment, as needed

Client-Centered Care (CCC)

When collecting subjective and objective data, respect for the client is demonstrated through:
- promoting client autonomy and allowing flexibility during the data collection process
- providing client privacy and comfort when collecting subjective and objective data
- respecting cultural preferences
- speaking with age-appropriate language and arranging an interpreter if necessary
- advocating for the client and family needs.

Infection Control (INF)

When collecting subjective and objective data, healthcare-associated infection is prevented by:
- reducing the transfer and number of microorganisms, primarily through hand hygiene.

Safety (SAF)

When collecting subjective and objective data, safety measures prevent harm by:
- maintaining focus on the client
- maintaining a safe care environment for the client and nurse
- utilizing age-appropriate equipment.

Communication (COM)

- Communication exchanges information (oral, written, nonverbal, or electronic) between two or more people. Maintain HIPAA compliance with all communication.
- Documentation records information in a permanent legal record.
- Communication between the nurse, the client, and other healthcare providers is vital for assessment and data collection.

Evaluation (EVAL)

When collecting subjective and objective data, evaluation of outcomes enables the nurse to determine the efficacy of the assessment process.

- Comparison of current subjective and objective data with previous results facilitates evaluation of trends and changes in the client's clinical status.

■ SKILL 4.1 Performing a Preliminary Survey

EQUIPMENT

Clean gloves, if there is a risk of exposure to body fluids
Scales, if indicated (for weight measurement)
Stethoscope, blood pressure (BP) cuff, watch, and other equipment for obtaining vital signs as needed

BEGINNING THE SKILL

1. **INF** Perform hand hygiene.
2. **CCC** Introduce yourself to the client and family and explain the procedure.
3. **SAF** Identify the client using two identifiers.
4. **ACC** Assess the client's level of consciousness and orientation to person, time, place, and situation. *Provides a baseline assessment for comparison to subsequent assessments.*
5. **CCC** Provide privacy.

PROCEDURE

Collecting Subjective Assessment Data

6. **ACC** Ask the client why he or she is seeking healthcare. *Determines client's chief complaint.*
7. **ACC** Interview the client and obtain the health history. The health history is a chance for the client to relate why he or she is seeking healthcare at this time. (Note: Prior to the interview, ensure that the client is aware of HIPAA rights as required by law.)
   a. **CCC** Establish with the client whom he or she wants to be present for the interview. *The client may or may not want certain family members or individuals present for the interview.*
   b. **CCC** Ensure that environment for the interview is private and has a comfortable temperature and good lighting. *Promotes comfort and facilitates accuracy.*
   c. **ACC** Sit down at the client's eye level, facing the client.
   d. **ACC** Assess the client's primary health concern through open-ended questioning.
   e. **ACC** Assess the characteristics of the health concern, including the severity, potential triggers, and what relieves the primary concern.
   f. **ACC** Ask the client for how long and how often the concern has occurred.
   g. **ACC** Ask whether the concern has occurred before and what was done about it.

8. **CCC** Assess the client's level of pain or discomfort. *Pain can be a distraction.*
9. **CCC** Assess the client for any language barriers. Arrange for an interpreter if necessary. *Addresses cultural considerations and facilitates communication with the client.*
10. **COM** Ask the client whether he or she would like to discuss any other concerns regarding his or her healthcare. *Helps facilitate communication if the client has additional concerns.*

Collecting Objective Assessment Data

11. **ACC** Observe the client's overall appearance, behavior, and general demeanor. Does the client appear to be in any distress that requires immediate attention? Does the client appear clean and well kempt? Does the client have any unusual behaviors or physical movements?
12. **ACC** Observe the client's gait and mobility. Does the client appear to have any difficulty with ambulation? Does the client appear to have balance or posture issues?
13. **ACC** Assess the client's nutritional status. Does the client appear hydrated and well-nourished? Obtain the client's height and weight on calibrated scales.
14. **ACC** Assess the client's vital signs and pulse oximetry value if indicated.
15. **ACC** If indicated, perform a system-specific physical exam on the client. (see Section 2 of this chapter). Apply gloves if there is a risk of exposure to body fluids (Note: The findings from the preliminary survey will help the nurse identify the need for a system-specific exam.)

FINISHING THE SKILL

16. **INF** Remove gloves, if used, and perform hand hygiene.
17. **SAF** Ensure safety and comfort. Ensure that the bed is in the lowest position and verify that the client can identify and reach the nurse call system. *These safety measures reduce the risk of falls.*
18. **EVAL** Evaluate the outcomes. Was the client able to answer questions without difficulty?
19. **COM** Make appropriate referrals to other healthcare professionals as needed. *Referrals to other healthcare professionals as needed facilitates collaboration and improves care.*
20. **COM** Document assessment findings, outcomes, and referrals made based on the preliminary assessment in the legal healthcare record.

A head-to-toe assessment is a physical exam that begins at the client's head and progresses down to the feet. This type of assessment is a purposeful examination that facilitates collection and integration of data. Nurses perform head-to-toe assessments every day in a variety of settings, including outpatient clinics; emergency rooms; and acute care, long-term care, and home care settings. For the purpose of this chapter, the head-to-toe exam will be conducted as though the client is new to the agency or facility. The nurse may also need to perform a system-specific assessment. Moreover, the client may have medical equipment that needs to be addressed, such as a urinary catheter, intravenous catheter, or wound drain.

Nurses care for and assess clients of various ages. Each developmental age offers unique variations in assessment. Most of the information in this chapter is written with the adult client in mind. However, for helpful hints when assessing infants, children, maternal/child, and geriatric clients, refer to the discussion of lifespan considerations in Box 4.2.

As discussed in Box 4.3, the nurse must remain alert and watchful for changes in the client's physical assessment. Any changes that are not expected or deviate from the client's baseline must be reported to the authorized healthcare provider in a timely manner. This is an important aspect of client care. Failure to report changes could result in serious harm to the client.

CRITICAL CONCEPTS WHEN PERFORMING A HEAD-TO-TOE OR SYSTEM-SPECIFIC ASSESSMENT

As with the interview process, accuracy is one of the most important critical concepts to consider when performing a systematic physical assessment. Client-centered care is also important to promote client comfort and facilitate the exam. For example, cultural considerations must be addressed, and an interpreter should be arranged if there is a language barrier. In addition, the client's modesty must be protected during the physical exam to protect the client's dignity and help him or her feel at ease. Moreover, it is helpful to ensure that the room temperature is comfortable. Additional critical concepts such as infection control, evaluation, communication, and collaboration are also important to consider.

PERFORMING A RAPID HEAD-TO-TOE BEDSIDE ASSESSMENT

The rapid head-to-toe bedside assessment is an assessment tool a nurse utilizes to prioritize client acuity when preparing to give care throughout the shift. A nurse may have several clients under his or her care. Performing this type of assessment allows the nurse to understand how to allot time for care to be given safely and efficiently. This assessment also incorporates observations from initial acts of care for the client. In contrast to the preliminary health survey that may involve an in-depth interview and health history, the rapid assessment may only take a few minutes.

During the rapid bedside assessment, it is important to compare findings with the client's baseline assessment upon admission. Any significant changes should be noted and reported to the authorized healthcare provider. Priorities during this assessment include circulation, airway, and breathing; orientation level; and general appearance. Does the client look and act well? Is the client responsive to verbal stimuli? Does the client answer questions and follow simple commands? Inspect the client's skin color, turgor, and other characteristics closely when obtaining vital signs. This is an opportunity to notice any unexpected findings that might not have been previously observed (Box 4.4). Auscultate the client's heart, lungs, and abdomen and note any unusual sounds. Palpate the client's abdomen, and assess the client's strength and range of motion. It is also important to palpate the client's peripheral pulses.

Throughout the assessment, note any IV lines, fluids, dressings, catheters, or drains attached to the client. For clients who have catheters in extremities or the groin area, assess the circulation and pulses distal to those catheters. Assess the safety of the client related to bed and side-rail positions and the proximity of the nurse call system, and note any individuals who are at the bedside. Once the general welfare and safety of one client are ensured, the nurse can assess other assigned clients. This process helps maintain a safe care environment and allows for planning as well as prioritization of care.

PERFORMING A SYSTEM-SPECIFIC ASSESSMENT

A system-specific assessment is useful when your client has a specific health concern or problem within a certain body system. When assuming care for a client, the nurse will usually take report from the previous shift. During this report, primary concerns are communicated between staff. Thus, your first visit with the client may include a quick bedside assessment to follow up and validate concerns raised by previous care providers. Based on the rapid bedside assessment and the client's condition, a system-specific assessment may be performed. For example, a postoperative client who had gastrointestinal surgery with an abdominal incision may need a more detailed abdominal assessment. During this assessment, the client may raise new concerns that will require additional system-specific assessments based on the complaint. For example, this client may complain about soreness on his sacral area, and the nurse may observe that it is reddened, possibly as a result of being immobilized for a long time on a hard surface during surgery.

BOX 4.2 Lifespan Considerations: Assessment Techniques

PEDIATRIC CONSIDERATIONS

The age and developmental stage of a child are essential to know in order to assess the child accurately. The nurse may use this knowledge to incorporate play or a child's curiosity to facilitate the exam (Wilson & Giddens, 2017). The extra time spent allowing the child to explore the equipment or spent demonstrating an exam on a teddy bear may go a long way toward having an environment for a cooperative exam that provides accurate findings. The inclusion of family and knowledge of psychosocial issues surrounding pediatric clients may help the nurse to adjust the evaluation for the individual situation (Wilson & Giddens, 2017). Some specific considerations for clients across the lifespan follow.

Infants

- Assessment of infants is usually best accomplished by seizing the opportunity to listen when the baby is asleep, with warm hands and stethoscope, and may drift away from the standard head-to-toe approach, instead being more opportunistic (Wilson & Giddens, 2017).
- Older infants like to grab and hold things—give the infant a tongue depressor or something to do with their hands to keep them away from equipment.

Toddlers (Ages 1 to 3)

- There is a wide range of development in this group, and characteristics include increased movement, separation anxiety, and curiosity.
- An exam might best be accomplished with the child sitting on a parent's lap rather than on the exam table.
- A curious older toddler may want to listen to his or her own heart.
- Engage the child by having him or her "blow out" the otoscope light.
- Distraction is useful to help focus or refocus a child—for example, singing or looking at a book.

Child (Ages 4 to 9)

- Engage the child more in conversation and explanation of findings.
- Allow the child to handle equipment.
- Acknowledge a child's fears.

Older Child (Ages 10 to 12)

- Engage the child in the exam by talking with and to the child.
- Answer questions.

Teen

- Empower the teen to communicate his or her concerns about the exam.
- Assess the level of knowledge that the teen has about his or her condition.

PREGNANT FEMALE (OBSTETRICS [OB])

- Some pregnant females may be immunocompromised. Assess vaccine history.
- Deep tendon reflexes (DTRs): In pregnant women, assessment of the patellar reflex (usually first choice) or the triceps reflex is often preferred.

POSTPARTUM CLIENTS

- Many times, the client will have slept for a few hours prior to the early morning head-to-toe postpartum exam and may need to get up and void. You can listen to the client's lung sounds and complete the DTR assessment while she is sitting on the side of the bed.
- Reassess postpartum fundus status after the client voids.
- If the postpartum fundus is elevated to the umbilicus or above and/or deviated from the midline position, assess bladder status and bleeding status.
- When palpating the postpartum fundus, use the side of hand instead of the fingertips. This allows you to better palpate and massage the fundus.

GERIATRIC CONSIDERATIONS

Environment

- Allow room for mobility aids, such as a walker.
- Ensure that the environment has a comfortable temperature.
- Avoid extremely low and soft seating surfaces.
- Avoid highly polished and slick surface materials that could create a fall risk for the client.
- Minimize background noise, such as blaring TVs, people talking, and background music.
- Ensure the client is wearing glasses or hearing aids or using other needed assistive aids.
- When using printed items, make sure the type is large enough and can be easily read.
- Ensure that a restroom or portable commode is nearby.

Assessment

- Use proper form of address (don't call by first name unless client asks you to).
- Speak slowly and clearly. Don't shout.
- Avoid slang, especially potentially generational slang.
- Use common language.
- Face the client when speaking, and sit or stand at eye level.
- Allow plenty of time for the assessment and the older client's response. Don't interrupt.
- Conserve the client's energy by grouping assessment items that require position changes.
- Observe the client for fatigue. Allow for rest periods.
- Assist the older client on and off the exam table.

References: National Institutes of Health, National Institute on Aging, 2015; Wilson & Giddens, 2017.

BOX 4.3 Lessons From the Courtroom: Failure to Report Significant Findings of a Physical Assessment

A client was admitted to the hospital with diabetic ketoacidosis (DKA). He had a history of insulin-dependent diabetes and drug abuse. The plan was to rehydrate the client and stabilize his blood sugar. The next morning after he was admitted, the nurse on the day shift performed two head-to-toe assessments during her shift. There were no problems noted other than his DKA, which was beginning to improve.

The night nurse took over care of the client at 7:00 PM. The client's wife reported that his legs were numb and that he had moved one leg off the bed. The nurse stated this was related to his condition. Her head-to-toe assessment about an hour later noted different findings compared to the day nurse. Her abdominal assessment revealed a "firm" abdomen, whereas the day nurse had found a "soft" abdomen. The night nurse also found that the client was weak in his extremities, yet during the day, there had been no weakness. There was no mention of numbness in the chart.

At about 3:40 AM, the client notified the nurse he could no longer move his legs. He also had not urinated since 1:30 PM the day before. The nurse catheterized him and obtained a large amount of dark urine. She notified the charge nurse, who notified the resident. Diagnostic tests eventually revealed an epidural abscess in the thoracic spine, which left the client with irreversible paraplegia. The agency that assigned the night nurse to the hospital was found liable for the $1.4-million-dollar judgment because the nurse had failed to report significant findings in a timely manner (Nursing assessment: Damages awarded for negligence, 2013).

This case demonstrates how important it is to note changes in the client's head-to-toe assessment and to report these changes in a timely manner as they are occurring. In this situation, the night nurse did not notify anyone of changes in the client's condition until 3:40 AM.

Although this case occurred in 2013, malpractice suits against healthcare providers, including nurses, are still on the rise, according to information reported by Healthcare Risk Management. As the case reviewers noted, a leading contributing factor for the rise in healthcare-related lawsuits is inadequate client assessments (More nurses, hospitalists being sued for malpractice, studies say, 2016).

BOX 4.4 Expect the Unexpected: Assessing the Skin: A Critical Observation

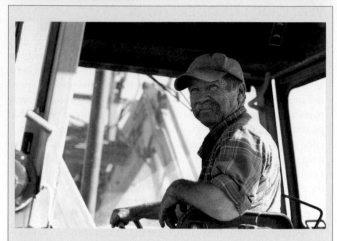

Mr. Green, a 74-year-old retired farmer, is admitted to the surgical unit after an orthopedic procedure. Jamie, a second-year nursing student, is assigned to care for Mr. Green on his second post-op day. As part of her clinical assignment, Jamie performs a rapid head-to-toe assessment on Mr. Green and obtains his vital signs. During the assessment, Jamie inspects Mr. Green's skin and notices that he has numerous flat round age spots on his skin that have well-defined borders and are uniform in color. However, when she obtains his tympanic temperature, Jamie also notices that he has a raised lesion on the posterior side of the pinna of his right ear that is pigmented and slightly ulcerated. When Jamie asks Mr. Green if he was aware of the lesion, he states "Aww…It doesn't bother me. My cap rubs on my ear sometimes, and then it bleeds. I have freckles and moles all over the place—I'm not worried about it!" Nevertheless, Jamie is aware that some of the characteristics of this lesion are different from those of his other skin spots, and the discoloration, ulceration, and irregular edges concern her. She notifies Mr. Green's authorized care provider, who refers him to a dermatologist for a biopsy. The biopsy reveals that Mr. Green has malignant melanoma, a serious type of skin cancer that requires immediate treatment.

This case underscores how important it is to be alert for any unusual findings during a head-to-toe assessment. It also demonstrates that taking vital signs is a great opportunity to observe your client closely. Mr. Green's lesion on his ear was unusual and not related to his history or reason for his hospitalization. However, if left untreated, the lesion could have become fatal. According to the Centers for Disease Control and Prevention (CDC), malignant melanoma has an increased mortality rate. An acronym used to help identify lesions that require further evaluation is ABCDE (CDC, 2019):

A—asymmetrical shape
B—irregular, jagged borders
C—color variation (red, brown, tan, or black)
D—diameter (often >6 mm or larger than the size of a pea)
E—lesion that is evolving or changing

Jamie's assessment and astute observation while caring for Mr. Green facilitated early recognition and treatment of a potentially life-threatening disease.

Different systems are interdependent and influence each other. Thus, it is important to note that even if a system-specific assessment is being performed, the findings must be considered within the context of the overall clinical condition and head-to-toe assessment of the client.

Assessing the Skin/Integumentary System

The skin/integumentary system covers the entire body and is assessed throughout the integrated physical exam using inspection as well as palpation. Physical assessment of any body system requires looking at and/or touching the client's skin. The hair and nails, as well as the sebaceous and sweat glands, are auxiliary components of the client's skin that must also be assessed (Wilson & Giddens, 2017).

When providing care for a client, there are many opportunities for the nurse to perform a system-specific assessment of the integumentary system. During this assessment, the skin, hair, and nails of the client must be visible. It is also important to create an environment that is comfortable for the client and will facilitate an accurate exam. In addition, optimum lighting is necessary in order to visualize nuances regarding the skin's color and condition.

Direct contact between the examiner's fingers and the client's skin with palpation yields the most concrete assessment data. For example, how does the client's skin feel to the touch? Is it warm and dry, or does it feel cool and clammy? Are the client's extremities cool in comparison to the rest of the body? Examination of the client while he or she is dressed in a medical gown and the use of a drape when viewing areas of the body maintains modesty and decreases the loss of heat.

Positioning the client so that all surfaces of the skin may be viewed is also necessary. Enlist the client's assistance in self-positioning when able, making sure to maintain safety from falls. For clients who are unable to follow commands to reposition themselves, the nurse, utilizing proper body mechanics and enlisting the help of peers when needed, can accomplish this task.

When examining the client's skin, it is important to assess whether the client has edema. Using the pad (not tip) of your forefinger, press and release the edematous areas and note if there is pitting (Fig. 4.6). Many facilities use a 4-point scale to grade for pitting edema, as shown in Fig. 4.7. Assess the client's skin turgor. The expected finding is that the skin will have immediate recoil when the turgor is checked. Turgor recoil that does not "bounce-back" or is not immediate may be an indication of volume depletion (Wilson & Giddens, 2017).

In addition to the client's skin assessment, the risk for pressure injury must be considered as part of the systematic physical assessment. There are a variety of scales that may be used to measure the client's level of risk. Some of the variables assessed to measure risk include sensory perception, skin moisture, activity level, mobility, nutritional status, and skin sheer/friction. The Centers for Medicare and Medicaid Services (CMS) requires that hospitalized clients receive a risk assessment using a valid and reliable tool. (For more information, see Chapter 16).

Assessing the Head (HEENT) and Neck and the Neurologic System

The assessment of the head and neck area includes the client's head, eyes, ears, nose, and throat (HEENT). This exam may also involve the client's skin and the neurologic, musculoskeletal, respiratory, cardiovascular, and psychologic systems. These systems work together harmoniously. For example, the nose and mouth, as well as the trachea located in the neck area, are the beginning of the client's respiratory system. An assessment of the head and neck area helps to ensure that the client is maintaining adequate airflow and oxygenation and that the client's airway is intact.

The neurologic system innervates every system of the body and can be assessed as the client interacts with the environment. The brain is housed in the skull, and the spinal cord runs down the spine, with nerves extending into each extremity and organ of the body. The client's response to stimuli is examined

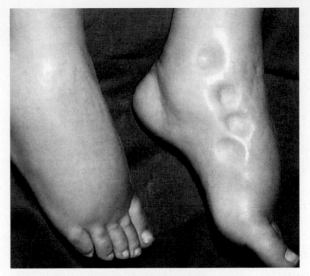

FIG. 4.6 Pitting edema.

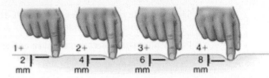

Scale	Description
1+	Barely perceptible pit
2+	Deeper pit, rebounds in a few seconds
3+	Deep pit, rebounds in 10-20 seconds
4+	Deeper pit, rebounds in >30 seconds

FIG. 4.7 Grading scale for pitting edema.

to ensure that the neurologic system and cranial nerve function are intact. For a list of cranial nerves, see Table 4.1.

There are many opportunities for the nurse to assess the head and neck and neurologic system during the general care of the client. For example, conversations between the client and nurse allow the nurse to hear the client's voice and observe the symmetry of the client's facial features at rest and with movement. The nurse can also assess the client's hearing by noting if the client is able to comprehend and answer questions. An assessment of these systems may occur during routine procedures such as taking the client's temperature, cleaning the client's teeth, washing the client's hair, placing a nasogastric tube, or adjusting a nasal cannula. Activities of daily living (e.g., eating and other activities) allow the nurse to assess the client's hand–eye coordination and cranial nerve function when the client is bringing food to the mouth, chewing, swallowing, and using eating utensils.

It is important to note that changes in a client's neurologic status or increased confusion may actually be related to hearing loss, vision, or other changes in the client's daily routine. When performing an assessment, ensure that the client has his or her hearing and visual aids in place, and verify that these devices are working properly (Box 4.5).

TABLE 4.1 List of Cranial Nerves and Function

Cranial Nerve	Function
Olfactory (I)	Sensory: Smell reception and interpretation
Optic (II)	Sensory: Visual acuity and visual fields
Oculomotor (III)	Motor: Raise eyelids, most extraocular movements
	Parasympathetic: Pupillary constriction, change lens shape
Trochlear (IV)	Motor: Downward, inward eye movement
Trigeminal (V)	Motor: Jaw opening and clenching, chewing and mastication
	Sensory: Sensation to cornea, iris, lacrimal glands, conjunctiva, eyelids, forehead, nose, nasal and mouth mucosa, teeth, tongue, ear, facial skin
Abducens (VI)	Motor: Lateral eye movement
Facial (VII)	Motor: Movement of facial expression muscles except jaw, close eyes, labial speech sounds (*b, m, w*, and rounded vowels)
	Sensory: Taste on the anterior two-thirds of tongue, sensation to pharynx
	Parasympathetic: Secretion of saliva and tears
Acoustic or vestibulocochlear (VIII)	Sensory: Hearing and equilibrium
Glossopharyngeal (IX)	Motor: Voluntary muscles for swallowing and phonation
	Sensory: Sensation of nasopharynx, gag reflex, taste on the posterior one-third of tongue
	Parasympathetic: Secretion of salivary glands, carotid reflex
Vagus (X)	Motor: Voluntary muscles of phonation (guttural speech sounds) and swallowing
	Sensory: Sensation behind ear and part of external ear canal
	Parasympathetic: Secretion of digestive enzymes; peristalsis; carotid reflex; involuntary action of heart, lungs, and digestive tract
Spinal accessory (XI)	Motor: Turn head, shrug shoulders, some actions for phonation
Hypoglossal (XII)	Motor: Tongue movement for speech sound articulation (*l, t, n*) and swallowing

From: Wilson & Giddens, 2017.

Assessing the Thorax (Heart and Lungs)

The heart and lungs work together to provide effective gas exchange and perfusion in order to deliver oxygen to organs and cells though out the body and remove carbon dioxide.

Direct assessment of the client using a stethoscope to auscultate the heart tones and lung sounds occurs on a routine basis during the clinical day. Before proceeding with this assessment, the nurse must first be able to identify the primary landmarks and reference lines of the client's thorax (anterior, lateral, and posterior views), as shown in Fig. 4.8. This is important for accurate placement of the stethoscope as well as other aspects of the physical exam.

BOX 4.5 Lessons From Experience: Confusion or Hearing Loss?

Daniel was a first-year nursing student in a clinical rotation at a rehabilitation facility. At preclinical, Daniel introduced himself to Mr. Webber, who was oriented and speaking clearly. Mr. Webber had experienced a stroke 4 weeks earlier and had lost significant muscle control on his left side. He wore glasses and had a hearing aid due to long-term hearing loss. On the day of clinical, Daniel entered Mr. Webber's room and reintroduced himself. When Daniel asked, "How are you doing Mr. Webber?" Mr. Webber answered loudly, "What? There aren't any cows in here!" Daniel paused and said, "Excuse me?" Mr. Webber said angrily, "What are you talking about?" Daniel reported this to Mr. Webber's nurse and told her that the client was talking about cows and seemed confused and agitated. The nurse suggested that they visit Mr. Webber together and start a head-to-toe assessment. When they entered the room, the nurse noticed Mr. Webber fiddling with his hearing aid. She asked, "Sir, please tell me your full name." Mr. Webber did not answer. The nurse moved closer and asked again. This time Mr. Webber shouted, "What are you doing in here?" Daniel then touched his arm and pointed to his own ear. "Mr. Webber, is your hearing aid turned on?" Daniel asked. Mr. Webber took out his hearing aid and said, "Oh, I don't think this thing is working." The nurse and Daniel then replaced the battery in the hearing aid. When they returned the hearing aid to Mr. Webber, he slipped it into his ear and smiled. "Hi, Daniel! No wonder I didn't know what you were talking about!"

When clients have a change in their sensory acuity, including hearing or vision, they may appear to be confused. The nurse and the student realized that Mr. Webber was not confused but, instead, his hearing aid was not functioning properly, and he was having difficulty hearing. This case demonstrates why it is important to consider these factors as part of the overall physical assessment. Nurses validate that their clients are hearing and seeing well.

As part of the cardiac assessment, it is also important to assess the client's circulation by checking the carotid and peripheral pulses bilaterally and rating the quality and strength. Checking the client's capillary refill and vital signs is also important. In addition, the nurse can observe the client's skin tone and feel the warmth of the skin during routine care, which helps to evaluate overall heart and lung health as well as adequate circulation and perfusion.

A client's ability to tolerate activities of daily living offers functional assessment opportunities of the heart and lungs. For example, does the client become tired walking across the room? Because certain cardiovascular conditions may deteriorate quickly, it is important to report unexpected findings to the authorized healthcare provider in a timely manner.

Assessing the Abdomen

The abdomen is a large cavity that includes the digestive, urinary, and reproductive systems. Because there are many organs lying within the abdominal cavity, it is helpful to visualize where various abdominal organs are located beneath the skin's surface (Box 4.6). Utilizing landmarks such as the iliac crest, the lower edge of the rib cage, or the umbilicus can facilitate an accurate assessment.

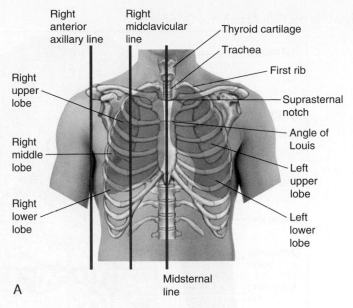

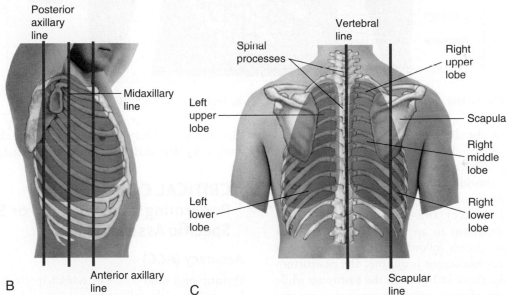

FIG. 4.8 Reference lines for assessment of thorax. **A,** Anterior view; **B,** lateral view; **C,** posterior view.

For the purposes of assessment, the abdomen is usually divided into four quadrants (the right upper and lower quadrant and the left upper and lower quadrant). When assessing the abdomen, nurses usually begin with inspection and auscultation before palpation and percussion. This is because manipulation of the bowels by palpation and/or percussion can actually produce peristalsis, which causes bowel sounds. Sounds should be heard in every quadrant. If no bowel sounds are heard, listen for at least 5 minutes. Sometimes after surgery, bowel peristalsis may be less active due to anesthesia. However, if bowel sounds are never heard or if there are unexpected findings with the exam, notify the authorized healthcare provider.

Assessing the Musculoskeletal System

The musculoskeletal system is the framework of the body and facilitates movement. Muscles are innervated by nerves that receive impulses from the neurologic system in order to initiate movement.

When assessing the musculoskeletal system, the nurse must assess portions of the neurologic system because they work closely together to produce movement. The nurse should also be aware that significant blood and lymphatic vessels closely follow along the skeletal framework, and thus pulses may be evaluated during the musculoskeletal assessment.

During the musculoskeletal system assessment, the nurse will want to ensure the safety of the client against falls or injury. Ensure that the environment is well lit and free from tripping hazards. Wearing nonslip shoes will also help prevent client falls. In addition, the bed or exam table should be in its lowest position, with a chair provided to sit on or hold for stability.

Assessing the Genitourinary System

When assessing the genitourinary system, the nurse recognizes that this is a private area for the client and requires professionalism and sensitivity. It is important to listen to the client for any vocalized concerns about this private area of the body. It is

BOX 4.6 Organs in the Four Abdominal Quadrants

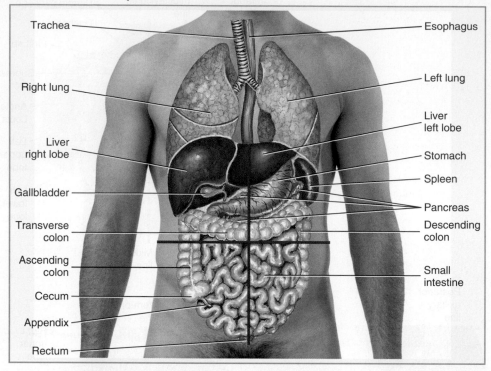

Trachea — Esophagus — Right lung — Left lung — Liver left lobe — Liver right lobe — Stomach — Spleen — Gallbladder — Pancreas — Transverse colon — Descending colon — Ascending colon — Small intestine — Cecum — Appendix — Rectum

From Wilson, S., & Giddens, J. (2017). *Health assessment for nursing practice* (6th ed.). St. Louis, MO: Elsevier, p. 246.

also critical to honor the client's cultural preferences and any requests regarding the gender of the examiner. For example, some cultures only allow a female client to be examined by a female healthcare provider. You will be held responsible for following your facility's policy. See Chapter 15 for further discussion of the legal aspects of same-sex assignments.

With some populations in an acute care setting, such as with postpartum clients following a vaginal delivery, a genitourinary system assessment is routine. The postpartum nurse may assess the client in bed or in the bathroom while on the toilet. Nurses often complete the genitourinary system assessment while assisting the client with elimination. This provides a very natural opportunity to observe the client's genitalia and ask questions, such as "Do you feel like you are completely emptying your bladder when you void?" or "Do you have any difficulty initiating a stream of urine?"

SUMMARY

To summarize, the critical concepts of accuracy, client-centered care, infection control, communication, and evaluation are all essential when performing a head-to-toe or system-specific assessment. In addition, a head-to-toe physical assessment must be performed in a systematic and logical manner. The nurse's decision as to what type of assessment to perform will depend on the clinical setting as well as the status or condition of the client.

Regardless of the type of assessment, the nurse must consider the whole person and integrate the information. The nurse must also consider the findings within the overall context of the client's history and previous exams (Jarvis, 2016).

This strategy will help the nurse identify the client's needs and analyze the data to develop an individualized plan of care.

CRITICAL CONCEPTS
Performing a Head-to-Toe or System-Specific Assessment

Accuracy (ACC)

Performing a head-to-toe or system-specific assessment may be sensitive to the following variables:

Client-Related Factors
- Age and developmental level
- Level of consciousness and orientation
- Level of pain, discomfort, or emotional distress
- Culture and language
- Vision, hearing, or any disabilities
- Environment (e.g., noise, temperature, distractions)
- Modesty
- History of sexual trauma or PTSD
- Lack of knowledge/understanding

Nurse-Related Factors
- Proper technique and sequence used to perform physical exam using inspection, auscultation, percussion, and palpation
- Proper use of equipment (stethoscope, otoscope, ophthalmoscope, tuning fork, reflex hammer, etc.) to perform physical exam
- Correct technique for identifying anatomical landmarks
- Decision making regarding type of physical assessment needed

Equipment-Related Factors

- Proper functioning of equipment used for physical assessment, with batteries and bulbs intact (e.g., otoscope and ophthalmoscope)

Client-Centered Care (CCC)

When performing a head-to-toe or system-specific assessment, respect for the client is demonstrated through:

- promoting client autonomy and allowing flexibility of when the exam is performed
- providing comfort and privacy, and protecting the client's dignity during the assessment
- respecting the client's cultural preferences
- honoring requests regarding gender preferences for the physical exam
- speaking with age-appropriate language and arranging an interpreter if necessary
- avoiding personal bias when performing the assessment and interpreting the results.

Infection Control (INF)

When performing a head-to-toe or system-specific assessment, healthcare-associated infection is prevented by:

- reducing the transfer and number of microorganisms, primarily through handwashing
- ensuring that equipment for physical assessment is properly cleaned.

Safety (SAF)

When performing a head-to-toe or system-specific assessment, safety measures prevent harm by:

- maintaining a safe care environment for client and nurse
- utilizing age-appropriate equipment
- using equipment (e.g., otoscope, ophthalmoscope) properly.

Communication (COM)

- Communication exchanges information (oral, written, nonverbal, or electronic) between two or more people. Maintain HIPAA compliance with all communication.
- Documentation records information in a permanent legal record.
- Communication between the nurse, the client, and other healthcare providers when performing a head-to-toe or system-specific assessment improves data collection and client care.

Evaluation (EVAL)

When performing a head-to-toe or system-specific assessment, evaluation of outcomes enables the nurse to determine the efficacy of the care provided.

- Comparison of current systematic head-to-toe physical assessment data with previous results facilitates evaluation of trends and changes in the client's clinical status.

■ SKILL 4.2 Performing a Rapid Head-to-Toe Bedside Assessment

EQUIPMENT

Clean gloves, if there is a risk of exposure to body fluids
Stethoscope, BP cuff, watch, and other equipment for obtaining vital signs as needed
Pulse oximetry device (if needed)
Equipment for physical exam (if needed)

BEGINNING THE SKILL

1. **INF** Perform hand hygiene.
2. **CCC** Introduce yourself to the client and family and explain the procedure.
3. **SAF** Identify the client using two identifiers.
4. **CCC** Provide privacy.
5. **INF** Apply gloves if there is a risk of exposure to body fluids.

PROCEDURE

6. **ACC** Observe the client from a standing position near the head of the bed or the area where he or she is resting. *This allows for a full view of the client's body and immediate surroundings.*
7. **CCC** Assess the client's environment. Determine if there are any other individuals in the room and whether or not the client wants them to remain in the room during the quick bedside assessment.

8. **ACC** Assess the client's level of consciousness (LOC) and orientation to person, time, place, and situation, and compare to the client's baseline. *Any change in LOC could be significant.*
9. **ACC** Ask the client how he or she is feeling. *Determines client's chief complaint. This also allows the nurse to assess the client's responsiveness and ability to communicate appropriately.*
10. **ACC** Observe the client's overall appearance, behavior, and demeanor. Does the client appear to be in distress that requires immediate attention? Is the client having any difficulty breathing? If the client has any signs of distress, notify the authorized healthcare provider. *Any difficulty with airway, breathing, and circulation must be addressed immediately.*
11. **ACC** Note any tubes or special equipment the client has and ensure the equipment is intact and working properly. *Any disruption of tubes or equipment requires rapid attention.*
12. **CCC** Assess the client's level of pain or discomfort using a culturally appropriate, facility-approved scale. If the client is having uncontrolled pain, intervene appropriately (see Chapter 7).
13. **ACC** Ask the client if he or she is having any difficulty toileting (voiding or defecating), taking note of whether a bedpan, bedside commode, or restroom toilet is utilized (see Chapter 2).

14. **ACC** Assess client's skin and mucous membranes:
    a. Note if skin is pink, warm, and dry, without disruptions, noting any alterations such as intravenous or arterial lines, wounds, dressings, and drains. Ensure that dressings and drains are clean, dry, and intact, without signs of excessive drainage or bleeding.
    b. Note if mucous membranes are pink and moist.
    c. Assess skin turgor for elasticity and immediate recoil (see Skill 4.3).
15. **ACC** Observe the client's gait and mobility as applicable to the current situation. Does the client appear to have any difficulty with movement when asked to do simple tasks such as lifting the arm while the blood pressure cuff is applied or turning to the side so that the back may be inspected and auscultated? Does the client appear to have balance or posture issues? How are the client's strength and range of motion?
    a. Assess hand grip for strength and equality bilaterally (see Skill 4.8).
    b. Assess foot presses for strength and equality bilaterally (see Skill 4.8).
16. **ACC** Obtain vital signs: temperature, pulse, respirations, BP, and oxygen saturation if indicated. Obtain apical pulse if indicated (see Chapter 3).
17. **ACC** Auscultate heart tones and identify S1 and S2. Note any unusual heart sounds, including murmurs, gallops, or rubs (see Skill 4.6). If telemetry is in use, ensure that the leads are intact and note the client's cardiac rhythm on the monitor (see Chapter 19).
18. **ACC** Palpate radial and pedal peripheral pulses bilaterally, noting any edema.
19. **ACC** Press nailbed and check capillary refill, measuring in seconds (see Skill 4.3).
20. **ACC** Auscultate posterior, lateral, and anterior breath sounds in all lobes, taking note of the quality of respirations (see Skill 4.6). Note the presence of any pleural or mediastinal tubes.
21. **ACC** Inspect abdomen for contour with the client in a supine position (see Skill 4.7).
22. **ACC** Auscultate for abdominal sounds in all four abdominal quadrants (see Skill 4.7).
23. **ACC** Check genitourinary status, noting urine output for color and amount. Note external or indwelling catheter. Ensure that it is intact and positioned properly (see Chapter 15).

FINISHING THE SKILL

24. **INF** Remove gloves, if used, and perform hand hygiene.
25. **SAF** Ensure safety and comfort. Ensure that the bed is in the lowest position and verify that the client can identify and reach the nurse call system. *These safety measures reduce the risk of falls.*
26. **EVAL** Evaluate the outcomes. Did the client tolerate the rapid assessment without difficulty? Are there any trends or changes in the client's assessment from the previous exam?
27. **COM** If the findings of the rapid assessment are outside of the established parameters for the client, notify the authorized healthcare provider.
28. **COM** Document assessment findings, care given, and outcomes in the legal healthcare record, including:
    • any variation or change in the client's condition, action taken, and who was notified
    • position and condition of intravenous lines and extremities of placement
    • position of any tubes, drains, or dressings and on which side they are present.

▪ SKILL 4.3 Assessing the Skin/Integumentary System

EQUIPMENT

Clean gloves, if there is a risk of exposure to body fluids
Additional lighting source
Measuring tape
Wound measuring bullseye
Cotton-tipped applicator
Nail polish remover
Drape for modesty

BEGINNING THE SKILL

1. **ACC** Review the client's history for any skin disorders, reactions, or allergies.
2. **INF** Perform hand hygiene.
3. **CCC** Introduce yourself to the client and family and explain the procedure.
4. **SAF** Identify the client using two identifiers.
5. **CCC** Provide privacy. Keep the client covered with a drape or gown.
6. **CCC** Ensure that room has good lighting and a comfortable temperature.
7. **INF** Apply gloves if there is a risk of exposure to body fluids.

PROCEDURE

8. **ACC** Assess the client for any subjective symptoms the client may have related to his or her skin, hair, or nails. If the client voices concerns, ask questions regarding onset, location, duration, associated manifestations, relieving or exacerbating factors, and treatment (Wilson & Giddens, 2017).
9. **ACC** Examine the client's skin surface both anteriorly and posteriorly from head to toe. (Note: This may require repositioning the client to view needed areas.)
10. **ACC** Inspect the client's skin appearance with an initial general survey.
    a. Assess for symmetry between the skin on the left and right sides of the body at rest and with client movement.

b. Note whether mucous membranes are pink and moist.

c. Assess color of skin, paying attention to any pigmentation, lack of pigmentation, cyanosis or pallor, jaundice, or other changes in skin color.

d. Note excessive dryness in the form of cracking or flaking, sweating, or oiliness, taking care to inspect skinfolds. *Skinfolds could conceal skin breakdown and irritation.*

e. Assess for the presence of edema.

f. Assess scars and lesions of the skin, noting their location, patterns and shapes, type, color, and elevation.

11. **ACC** Inspect the client's hair.

a. Note general grooming.

b. Note texture.

c. Note distribution and amount.

d. Visualize the client's scalp utilizing a cotton-tipped applicator to lift the hair on the head in several areas. Observe the scalp condition, texture of hair, distribution of hair, and any infestations or debris present.

12. **ACC** Inspect the client's nails. Remove nail polish so that the natural nail may be assessed.

a. Note general grooming and condition of nail.

b. Note color of nailbed and nail surfaces.

c. Note contour, shape, and thickness of nails.

d. Assess the angle between the nail base and nail. If the angle is >180 degrees, the client may have clubbed nails. (Note: Clubbing may occur when the client has an underlying systemic alteration such as cardiac or pulmonary disease.)

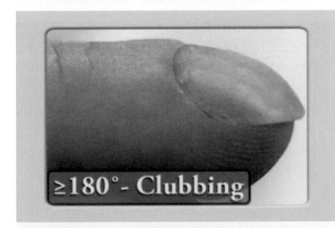

STEP 12(D) Assessing for clubbed nails.

13. **ACC** Palpate the skin.

a. Note any moisture or oiliness to the touch.

b. Use the back of the hand to assess temperature.

c. Note if skin is rough or smooth with light palpation using the fingerpads during palpation. *The fingerpads have a greater ability to discern differences in texture.*

d. Note location, size, shape, and texture of any mass palpable beneath the skin's surface. Report any new or unusual mass to the authorized healthcare provider.

e. Palpate for edema by pressing your finger pad into the skin, using moderate pressure. (Note: If client has pitting edema, note the grade; see Figs. 4.6 and 4.7.)

14. **ACC** Assess the client's skin turgor for elasticity and immediate recoil when grasped between the thumb and in-

dex finger. (Note: The expected finding is recoil of skin. If the skin stays elevated, this is called "tenting," which may be a sign of dehydration or volume depletion.)

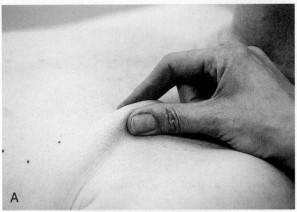

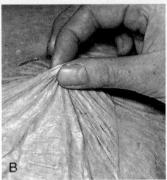

STEP 14 Skin turgor assessment. **A,** Elastic skin turgor. **B,** Poor skin turgor.

15. **ACC** Check the mobility of the skin by lifting a fold of skin between the your thumb and forefinger noting the ease of movement as it is lifted up.

16. **ACC** Palpate the hair, noting the texture.

17. **ACC** Palpate the nails.

a. Note if the nail is firmly attached to the nailbed.

b. Press the nailbed and note time it takes for capillary refill. (Note: The expected finding is that there will be brisk capillary refill of <2 seconds.)

FINISHING THE SKILL

18. **INF** Remove gloves if used and perform hand hygiene.

19. **SAF** Ensure safety and comfort. Ensure that the bed is in the lowest position and verify that the client can identify and reach the nurse call system. *These safety measures reduce the risk of falls.*

20. **EVAL** Evaluate the outcomes. Compare current findings with previous results.

21. **COM** If the findings of the skin/integumentary assessment are outside of the established parameters for the client, notify the authorized healthcare provider.

22. **COM** Document assessment findings, care given, and outcomes in the legal healthcare record, including any change in the client's skin assessment, any action taken, and who was notified.

▪ SKILL 4.4 Assessing the Head (HEENT) and Neck

EQUIPMENT

Clean gloves
Examination light and/or penlight
Measuring tape
Wound-measuring bull's eye
Stethoscope
Ophthalmoscope (for eyes)
Otoscope (for ears)
Vision charts—near, far, color
Opaque cover for use during eye exam
Tuning fork
Two tongue blades with straight edges
Sweet and salty taste samples—sugar and salt
Sour and bitter taste samples—lemon juice and cream of tartar
Two different scent vials—peppermint and cinnamon
Cotton-tipped applicators

BEGINNING THE SKILL

1. **ACC** Review client's medical and surgical history.
2. **INF** Perform hand hygiene.
3. **CCC** Introduce yourself to the client and family and explain the procedure.
4. **SAF** Identify the client using two identifiers.
5. **CCC** Provide privacy. Keep the client covered with a drape or gown.
6. **CCC** Ensure that room has good lighting and a comfortable temperature.
7. **ACC** Ensure that the bed or exam table has the ability to incline 45 degrees.
8. **ACC** Obtain all needed assessment tools for use at the bedside.
9. **INF** Apply gloves if there is a risk of exposure to body fluids and as directed within skill.

PROCEDURE

10. **ACC** Assess the client for any subjective symptoms he or she may have related to the eyes, ears, nose, mouth, head, or neck area. If the client voices concerns, ask questions regarding onset, location, duration, associated manifestations, relieving or exacerbating factors, and treatment.
11. **ACC** Inspect the shape, contour, and symmetry of head and neck anteriorly, posteriorly, and laterally. *Inspecting the client from different angles will facilitate accuracy.*

Assessing the Client's Neck and Jaw Area

12. **ACC** Visualize the position and movement of the client's trachea.
    a. Ask the client to swallow. (Note: Offer the client a glass of water if needed.)
    b. Observe, as client swallows, if the trachea is midline, with freedom of movement.
13. **ACC** Visualize for carotid pulsations on either side of the neck.

14. **ACC** Visualize the left and right neck for jugular venous distention (JVD). Look between the sternal and clavicular heads of the sternocleidomastoid muscle with the client sitting and inclined at a 45-degree angle.

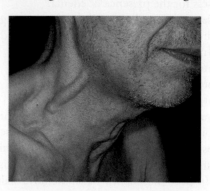

STEP 14 Jugular venous distention (JVD).

15. **ACC** Auscultate both carotid arteries (one at a time) using the bell and/or diaphragm of the stethoscope.
16. **ACC** Palpate the movement and position of the thyroid tissue as well as for the trachea. Use the palmar surface of the fingers resting lightly on each side of the client's neck while the client swallows. (Note: Palpation can occur from in front of the client or from behind the client while you are reaching forward to access the tracheal area.)

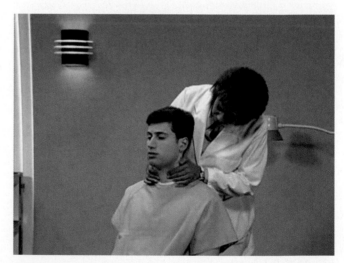

STEP 16 Thyroid and trachea palpation (from behind).

17. **ACC** Using the pads of the index and middle fingers, lightly palpate the client's carotid arteries one side at a time. **WARNING:** The carotid arteries must be palpated one at a time so that bilateral occlusion and compromised blood flow does not occur.
18. **ACC** Assess the client's neck strength (cranial nerve [CN] XI).
    a. Rest the palm of your hand against the client's left cheek.
    b. Ask the client to rotate the head to the left, as if looking over his or her shoulder.
    c. Offer gentle resistance against the client's head rotation.

d. Repeat steps 18a through 18c on the client's right side.
19. **ACC** Ask the client to shrug shoulders upward (CN XI) as you apply gentle resistance with the palms of your hands, taking note of shoulder strength bilaterally.
20. **ACC** Palpate the cheeks bilaterally for any masses or tenderness that may be associated with the salivary glands.
21. **ACC** Ask the client to clench the jaw (CN V) while you attempt to unclench the jaw by placing your thumbs (exerting moderate pressure) to the left and right of the anterior portion of the mandible (or chin).
22. **ACC** Palpate for lymph nodes to the left and right sides of the neck, one side at a time. *This prevents bilateral occlusion of the carotid artery.*
23. **ACC** Using the pads of the index and middle fingers, palpate the superficial lymph nodes of the head and neck.

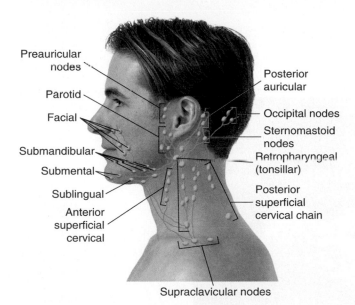

STEP 23 Head and neck lymph nodes.

a. Palpate in front of the ears (preauricular nodes).
b. Palpate behind the ears (postauricular nodes).
c. Palpate at the base of the posterior skull (occipital nodes).
d. Palpate at the base of the mandible beneath the ears (submandibular nodes).
e. Continue forward and palpate from the angle of the mandible anteriorly to the center front (submental nodes).
f. Move the tips of your fingers down either side of the trachea in an alternating pattern toward the sternal notch (cervical nodes).
g. Continue laterally toward the midclavicular line above the clavicle (supraclavicular nodes), then dropping the fingertips below the clavicular line (infraclavicular nodes). (Note: Healthy nodes should *not* be palpable. Take note of any palpable nodes, including their position, size, and texture, and note whether the client complains of discomfort when the nodes are palpated.)

Assessing the Client's Eyes

24. **ACC** Inspect the eyes for symmetry, color, lid position, eyelashes, and eyebrows. Observe the size of the pupils bilaterally. (Note: An expected finding is that the pupils should be equal in size bilaterally.)
25. **ACC** Inspect the conjunctiva and sclera of eyes bilaterally.
26. **ACC** Inspect the conjunctival sac while gently retracting the lower eyelid using the pads of the thumbs bilaterally. Note ease of movement, color, moistness, and ease of retraction when the lower eyelid is released.

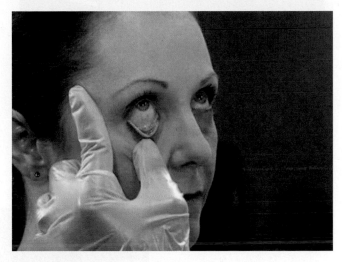

STEP 26 Inspection of conjunctiva and conjunctival sac.

27. **ACC** Assess corneal light reflex (CN III, IV, VI). (Perform exam in a dimly lit area.)
a. Ask the client to visualize an object in the distance with both eyes. The pupils should dilate.
b. Ask the client to look at your finger within 15 cm (6 inches) from the nose with both eyes. The pupils should constrict.
c. Shine the light toward the bridge of nose as the client looks at an object in the distance. Note if the light reflects in the same place in both eyes, symmetrically.
d. If a discrepancy is found, then perform the cover/uncover test.
28. **ACC** Perform the cover/uncover test if indicated.
a. Ask the client to cover one eye and look toward an object in the distance with both eyes.
b. Then uncover the eye and note if both eyes are looking toward the object or if there is a deviation. (Note: The expected finding is that there is no deviation.)
29. **ACC** Assess the client's pupillary response to light. (Perform exam in a dimly lit area.)
a. Ask the client to visualize an object in the distance with both eyes.
b. Using a penlight, direct the light from the side toward the center of the eye, briefly shining light at the pupil. Assess the pupillary response of the eye that the light is shining on. Then glance to the opposite eye and note the response. (Note: The pupillary response in

the illuminated eye and opposite [nonilluminated] eye should be constriction. This is a consensual response.)

c. Repeat steps 29a and 29b on the other eye. (Both pupils should be equal, round, regular, and reactive to light and accommodation [PERRLA].)

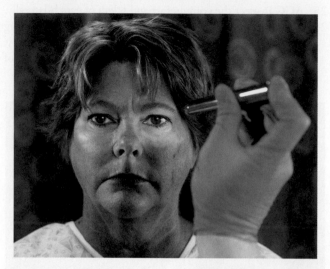

STEP 29 Assessing pupillary response to light.

30. **ACC** Assess visual fields of gaze (CN III, IV, VI). Ask the client to hold the head still and track the movement of an object about 2/3 meter (2 feet) in front of the client through six planes, as follows:

a. Visualize the client's head as a clock, with the nose at the center position.

b. Move an object horizontally from the left ear (3 o'clock), passing through the nose, to the right ear (9 o'clock) and then back.

c. Move an object from the left mid-eyebrow (1 o'clock) diagonally downward through the nose to the opposite right side's shoulder (7 o'clock), then back.

d. Move an object from the right mid-eyebrow (11 o'clock) diagonally downward through the nose to the opposite left side's shoulder (5 o'clock), then back.

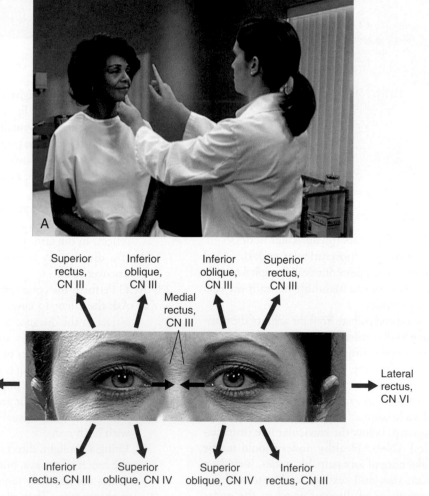

STEP 30 A, Assessment of visual fields. **B,** Visual fields and cranial nerves that innervate the extraocular muscles.

31. **ACC** Assess the visual acuity of the client.
    a. Ask the client to stand at a distance of 20 feet (CN II) in front of the eye chart.
    b. Then ask the client to cover one eye at a time with an opaque cover.
    c. Ask the client to read the letters starting from the top and reading down the chart. The last row in which the client is able to read the majority of letters should be recorded. (Note: A visual acuity of 20/20 is the expected finding [Jarvis, 2016].)
32. **ACC** Assess color vision as mandated by the specific test used (CN II).
33. **ACC** Assess peripheral vision (CN II) using a confrontation test.
    a. Stand face to face with the client, about ⅔ meter (2 feet) between you.
    b. Ask the client to alternately cover the left, then the right eye using the opaque cover.
    c. Cover your eye opposite the client's eye using an opaque cover so that the covered eyes of both the client and yourself are directly across from each other.
    d. Proceeding from a central position midway between yourself and the client, bring your extended arm with pointed index finger toward midline until the client visualizes your fingertip. (Note: The client and the nurse should both visualize the fingertips at the same time for a test of normal peripheral vision.)
34. **ACC** Assess for the red reflex. (Note: The presence of a red reflex, which is caused by light illuminating the retina, is the expected finding.)
    a. Stand about ⅔ meter (2 feet) in front of the client.
    b. Hold the ophthalmoscope in the hand corresponding to the client's eye that is to be examined (e.g., your right hand across from client's right eye).
    c. Ask the client to look at a fixed point in the distance.
    d. Lean toward the client while directing the beam of light into the eye being examined. While holding the ophthalmoscope close, look through the lens with your same eye that is being examined on the client (e.g., your left eye to examine client's left eye).
    e. Assess if the red reflex is present. (Note: If you are performing a more detailed exam of the internal structures of the eye, move toward the client's eye as closely as possible with the ophthalmoscope while also maintaining the position of the ophthalmoscope close to your eye.)

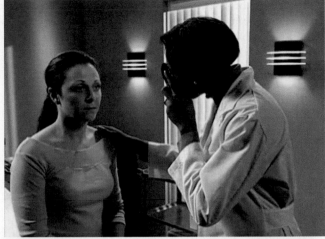

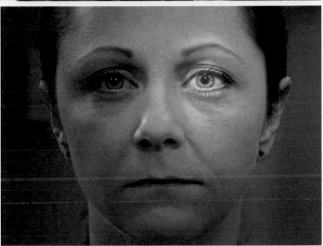

STEP 34 Assessment of red reflex.

Assessing the Client's Facial Movement and Characteristics

35. **ACC** Inspect the client's face during conversation and at rest for symmetry of features.
36. **ACC** Ask the client to follow commands while inspecting the symmetry of the client's facial features (CN VII):
    a. Raise eyebrows.
    b. Frown.
    c. Smile without showing teeth.
    d. Smile showing upper and lower teeth.
    e. Purse lips and puff out cheeks while gently pressing the cheeks with the palms of his or her hands, trying to express air.

f. Have the client close his or her eyes tightly while you are facing the client and placing your thumbs beneath the client's eyes. Place your forefingers beneath the client's eyebrows and try to gently open the client's eyes against resistance.

Assessing the Client's Ears

37. **ACC** Inspect the ears for symmetry, shape, and size, noting the condition of the skin.

38. **ACC** Using a penlight or otoscope, visualize the client's external ear canals bilaterally. Assess for any blockage, foreign body, or discharge in the ear. (Note: If a blockage is visualized, use caution not to push the foreign body, wax, or any other object farther into the client's ear.)

39. **ACC** Palpate the auricles and mastoid areas, touching the tragus of ear bilaterally, noting if any discomfort is elicited.

40. **ACC** Assess the client's hearing (CN VIII).
   a. Stand behind the client.
   b. Ask the client to occlude an ear with his or her finger as directed by you.
   c. Lean toward the open ear and whisper a two-syllable word (e.g., *baseball*).
   d. Alternate steps 40b and 40c. on the other ear.
   e. Take care to use the same volume for both ears.
   f. Raise the volume of your voice equally bilaterally as needed until the client hears your spoken word in each ear.
   g. Assess if the spoken word was heard by the client at an equal volume in each ear. (Note: The expected finding is that your spoken word is heard at the same volume in both ears by the client.)

41. **ACC** If indicated, perform Rinne or Weber test (see Skill 4.5).

Assessing the Nose

42. **INF** Perform hand hygiene.
43. **INF** Apply clean gloves.
44. **ACC** Inspect the external nasal area for symmetry of nares or any observed drainage.
45. **ACC** Visualize both nares using a penlight. Ensure the following:
   • Nares are free from obstruction.
   • Nasal septum is midline.
   • Turbinates are pink and moist.
46. **ACC** Assess CN I (olfactory nerve):
   a. Occlude one nostril while the client inspires. Check for patency of the open nostril.
   b. Ask the client to close his or her eyes and continue occluding the present nostril.
   c. Present a fragrance beneath the open nostril.
   d. Ask the client to identify the fragrance.
   e. Repeat steps 46b through 46d using a different fragrance to test smell. (Note: The expected finding is proper identification by the client of each fragrance presented.)

47. **INF** Remove gloves.
48. **INF** Perform hand hygiene.

Assessing the Mouth

49. **INF** Apply gloves.
50. **ACC** Inspect the mouth area, including the condition of the lips and any scars, lesions, or drainage.
51. **ACC** Assess CNs IX and X and examine the oral pharynx:
   a. Ask the client to open his or her mouth and say "Ahh."
   b. Assess the oropharynx. Use the penlight and tongue blade to visualize the entire oral cavity.
   c. Assess the color and condition of the oral tissue.
   d. Assess the appearance and movement of the soft palate and uvula. *The expected finding is that the movements of the soft palate should be symmetrical, with the uvula staying midline.*
   e. Observe for the symmetry of features, with the tongue being midline. Assess the tonsils for size, color, and presence of exudate. Inspect the condition of the teeth, gums, and tongue.
   f. Palpate the area between the teeth and gums, as well as beneath the tongue, using the index finger of your gloved, dominant hand. Note any nodules, masses, or discomfort.
   g. Elicit a gag reflex by sliding the tongue blade toward the back of the tongue. (Note: Warn the client first and use caution because of the concern for choking or aspiration potential.)
52. **ACC** Assess the movement of the client's tongue in the following ways (CN XII):
   a. Ask the client to protrude the tongue midline, then upward and down.
   b. Ask the client to push the tongue against the inside of the cheek as your hand rests against the outside of the cheek, offering gentle resistance. (Note: The tongue should have good range of motion, and strength should be equal bilaterally.)
53. **ACC** Ask the client to say "light, tight, dynamite" (Jarvis, 2016, p. 646); listen for clarity of speech quality as the words using the letters *l, t, d,* and *n* are spoken.
54. **ACC** Explain to the client that four tastes will be introduced into the mouth one at a time while their eyes are closed so that identification of tastes may take place.
55. **ACC** Ask the client to identify tastes introduced into the mouth from the damp end of a cotton-tipped applicator. Alternate between sweet and salty on the anterior portion of the tongue (CN VII), then sour and bitter on the posterior portion of the tongue (CN IX and CN X). Use a different swab for each test. This will prevent confusion between taste tests.
56. **INF** Remove gloves.

FINISHING THE SKILL

57. **INF** Perform hand hygiene.
58. **SAF** Ensure safety and comfort. Ensure that the bed is in the lowest position and verify that the client can identify and reach the nurse call system. *These safety measures reduce the risk of falls.*
59. **EVAL** Evaluate the outcomes. Compare current findings with previous results. Was the client able to follow directives in the head (HEENT) and neck exam?

60. **COM** If the findings of the head (HEENT) and neck assessment are outside of the established parameters for the client, notify the authorized healthcare provider.
61. **COM** Document findings, care given, and outcomes in the legal healthcare record, including any change in the client's head (HEENT) and neck assessment, any action taken, and who was notified.

■ SKILL 4.5 Assessing the Neurologic System

EQUIPMENT

Clean gloves, if there is a risk of exposure to body fluids
Examination light and/or penlight
Measuring tape
Wound-measuring bull's eye
Stethoscope
Ophthalmoscope
Vision charts—near, far, color
Opaque cover for use during eye exam
Tuning fork
Reflex hammer
Three tongue blades with straight edges
Two cotton balls
Cotton-tipped applicators
Sweet and salty taste samples—sugar and salt
Sour and bitter taste samples—lemon juice and cream of tartar
Two different scent vials—peppermint and cinnamon
Two test tubes
Objects to feel: paper clip, ink pen, coin

BEGINNING THE SKILL

1. **ACC** Review client's medical and surgical history.
2. **INF** Perform hand hygiene.
3. **CCC** Introduce yourself to the client and family and explain the procedure.
4. **SAF** Identify the client using two identifiers.
5. **CCC** Provide privacy. Keep the client covered with a drape or gown.
6. **CCC** Ensure that room has good lighting and a comfortable temperature.
7. **ACC** Ensure that the bed or exam table has the ability to incline 45 degrees.
8. **ACC** Obtain all needed assessment tools for use at the bedside.
9. **INF** Apply gloves if there is a risk of exposure to body fluids and as directed within skill.

PROCEDURE

10. **ACC** Ask the client questions to assess orientation.
    a. Person: "What is your full name?"
    b. Place: "Where are you right now?"
    c. Time: "What is today's date?" or "What year is it?"
    d. Situation: "Why are you here today?"
11. **ACC** Assess client for any subjective symptoms he or she is experiencing, such as changes in vision, balance, hearing, gait, or cognition. If the client voices concerns, ask questions regarding onset, location, duration, associated manifestations, relieving or exacerbating factors, and treatment.

Assessing Cranial Nerve I

12. **ACC** Assess client's sense of smell. (See Skill 4.4.)

Assessing Cranial Nerve II

13. **ACC** Assess the visual acuity of the client. (See Skill 4.4.)
14. **ACC** Assess for the red reflex of the optic disc. (See Skill 4.4.)

Assessing Cranial Nerves III, IV, and VI

15. **ACC** Assess visual fields of gaze. (See Skill 4.4.)

Assessing Cranial Nerve V

16. **ACC** Assess the corneal reflex using the twisted end of a cotton ball as follows:
    a. Direct the client's focus to an object on the opposite side of the room.
    b. Avoid the client's line of vision while drawing the twisted end of the cotton ball lightly across the cornea of the eye closest to you.
    c. Repeat steps 16a and 16b on the opposite side. (Note: The normal finding is that the client blinks when the cornea is touched.)
17. **ACC** Assess the client's recognition of soft and sharp sensation using the twisted end of a cotton ball (soft) and the broken, pointed end of a tongue depressor (sharp) in the following manner:
    a. Demonstrate the two sensations to the client on the anterior surface of the client's hand, stating "soft" when touching the client with the cotton ball twist and stating "sharp" when touching with the pointed end of the tongue depressor.

b. Ask the client to close the eyes, reiterating that the client must say "soft" or "sharp" when the particular sensation is felt.

c. Ask the client to identify sharp and soft sensations while alternately touching the left and right forehead, cheek, and jaw areas with the soft and sharp objects. (Note: The expected finding is that the client identifies both sharp and dull sensations in the three identified areas of the face bilaterally. If there is a discrepancy, test hot and cold sensation by filling one test tube with hot water and one with cold water. Ask the client to discern between these bilaterally in the three identified areas—forehead, cheek, and jaw.)

18. **ACC** Ask the client to clench the jaw.

19. **ACC** Place your thumbs to the left and right center of the client's chin while exerting moderate pressure and attempting to unclench the jaw passively.

Assessing Cranial Nerve VII

20. **ACC** Inspect the client's face during conversation and at rest for symmetry of features.

21. **ACC** Ask the client to follow simple commands while inspecting for facial symmetry. (See Skill 4.4.)

22. **ACC** Ask the client to identify the taste of sweet and salty using different swabs for each test.

Assessing Cranial Nerve VIII

23. **ACC** Visualize the external ear canals bilaterally for blockage, foreign body, or discharge using a penlight. (See Skill 4.4.)

24. **ACC** Assess the client's hearing. (See Skill 4.4.)

25. **ACC** Assess for lateralization of sound using the Weber test.
   a. Hold the tuning fork at the base.
   b. Strike the tuning fork tines against the side of your palm to create a vibration.
   c. Place the base of the tuning fork on top of the client's head midline between both ears.
   d. Ask the client where the sound is heard best: on the left, right, or both ears equally.
   (Note: The expected finding is to hear the sound in both ears equally.)

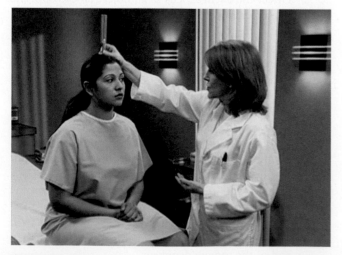

STEP 25 Weber test.

26. **ACC** Assess for bone versus air conduction of sound using the Rinne test.
   a. Strike a tuning fork against the side of your palm to create a vibration.
   b. Place the base of the vibrating tuning fork on the client's mastoid bone behind one ear. *This part of the Rinne test measures bone conduction.*

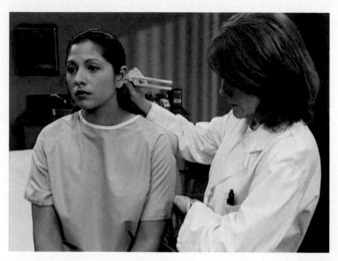

STEP 26B Rinne test (bone).

   c. Ask the client to raise a hand when he or she can no longer hear the sound.
   d. Bring the tuning fork quickly beside the client's ear canal, making sure not to impede the vibration of the tines. *This part of the Rinne test measures air conduction.*

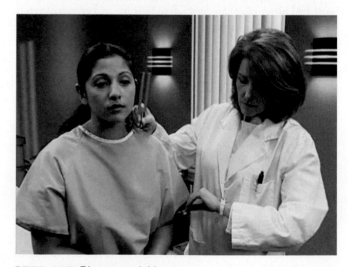

STEP 26D Rinne test (air).

   e. Ask the client if he or she still hears the sound and to raise a hand when the sound is no longer heard. (Note: The expected finding is that air conduction is greater than bone conduction.)
   f. Repeat steps 26a through 26e on the alternate ear.

Assessing Cranial Nerves IX and X

27. **ACC** Inspect the mouth and oropharynx, looking for symmetry. Use a tongue blade to visualize the entire oral cavity. (Note: Apply gloves if they are not already on.)

28. **ACC** Ask the client to say "Ahhh" while assessing the soft palate and uvula. (Note: The expected finding is that soft palate movements should be symmetrical, with the uvula staying midline.)

29. **ACC** Assess the client's ability to swallow. (See Skill 4.4.)

30. **ACC** Ask the client to identify the taste of sour and bitter, which you alternately introduce into the mouth from the damp end of a cotton-tipped applicator.

31. **ACC** Elicit a gag reflex judiciously with the client, due to concern for aspiration potential, by sliding the tongue blade toward the back of the tongue.

Assessing Cranial Nerve XI

32. **ACC** Assess the client's neck mobility and strength. (See Skill 4.4.)

33. **ACC** Ask the client to shrug shoulders upward while you apply downward pressure on both shoulders. Note the quality and symmetry of shoulder strength bilaterally.

Assessing Cranial Nerve XII

34. **ACC** Assess the client's tongue strength and mobility. (See Skill 4.4.)

35. **ACC** Ask the client to say "light, tight, dynamite" as you listen for vocal quality (focusing on the client's pronunciation of *l, t, d,* and *n*).

Assessing Proprioception and Cerebellar Function

36. **ACC** Ask the client to sequentially touch each finger to thumb in a forward motion then back again with increasing speed.

37. **ACC** Ask the client to alternately touch his or her nose and then your finger (which is moved to different locations), as you stand at arm's length from the client. Assess the accuracy of the client's touches in the following situations:
    a. Client, with eyes open, touches his or her own nose and then your index finger.
    b. Client, with eyes closed, touches his or her own nose and then your index finger with his or her own index finger.

38. **ACC** Ask the client to lie down with his or her eyes open and place his or her heel on the knee of the opposite leg running down the shin to the great toe. Repeat on the other side.

39. **SAF** Perform the Romberg test. Ask the client to stand with the feet slightly apart, arms at the sides, and eyes closed for 30 seconds while you stand close to the client. *This is important for safety in case the client becomes unbalanced and needs assistance.* (Note: The expected finding is that the client will be able to remain balanced for 30 seconds [Wilson & Giddens, 2017].)

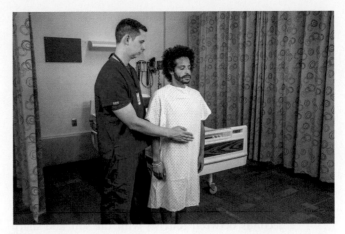

STEP 39 Romberg test.

40. **ACC** Perform the pronator drift test. Ask the client to sit or stand while holding the arms straight forward with the palms facing upward with the eyes closed for 20 to 30 seconds while you observe the client's ability to maintain the arms at the same height. Stand near the client for safety. (Note: An unexpected finding is for one of the client's arms to be lower than the other.)

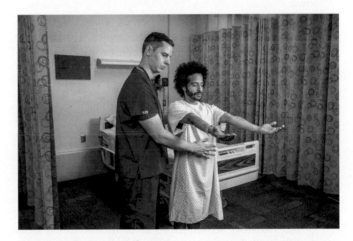

STEP 40 Pronator drift test.

41. **ACC** Ask the client to walk across the room, then turn and come back to the starting point. Observe posture and balance. (Note: The expected finding is coordinated movement and stability. If instability or uncoordinated movements are noted, there may be a motor pathway injury.)

42. **ACC** Ask the client to walk forward on the toes, then on the heels. (Note: The expected finding is the ability to walk on the toes and heels with stable movement. An inability to complete this task reflects altered muscle strength and balance that may require additional testing [Wilson & Giddens, 2017].)

Assessing Sensory Function

43. **ACC** Assess the client's recognition of soft and sharp sensations utilizing the twisted end of a cotton ball

(soft) and the broken, pointed end of a tongue depressor (sharp).

a. Demonstrate the two sensations to the client on the anterior surface of the client's hand, stating "soft" when touching the client with the cotton ball twist and stating "sharp" when touching with the pointed end of a tongue depressor.

b. Ask the client to close his or her eyes, reiterating that the client must say "soft" or "sharp" when the particular sensation is felt.

c. Ask the client to identify sharp and soft sensations while alternately touching the lower arms, hands, abdomen, lower legs, and feet bilaterally, waiting 2 seconds between touches with the soft and sharp objects. (Note: The expected finding is that the client identifies both sharp and soft sensations to all of the identified areas bilaterally [Wilson & Giddens, 2017].)

44. **ACC** Assess the client's recognition of vibratory sensations. Strike the tines of a tuning fork (so that it vibrates) and place the stem of the vibrating tuning fork against the bony prominences of the client's finger and toe joints bilaterally. Continue the procedure as follows:

a. Initially place the stem of the vibrating tuning fork on the anterior surface of the client's hand so that it is felt, and then stop the vibration so that the client understands the difference between vibration and stillness with this exam.

b. Ask the client to close the eyes, reiterating that the client should say which finger or toe joint is being touched with the vibrating tuning fork.

c. Ask the client to identify vibratory sensations while alternately touching the lower arms, hands, abdomen, lower legs, and feet bilaterally, waiting 2 seconds between touches with the vibrating tuning fork. (Note: The expected finding is that the client identifies vibratory sensations to all of the identified areas bilaterally.)

45. **ACC** Ask the client to close his or her eyes and identify a familiar object placed in his or her hand (stereognosis). Repeat with the alternate hand using a new object. (Note: The usual finding is that the client should correctly identify the object within 5 seconds [Wilson & Giddens, 2017].)

Assessing Deep Tendon Reflexes

46. **ACC** Assess the patellar reflex. Ask the client to flex the knee to 45-degree angle while you use a reflex hammer to briskly strike the patellar tendon just below the patellar. (Note: The expected finding is 2+ movement, where 0 is no movement and 4+ is hyperactive [Wilson & Giddens, 2017].)

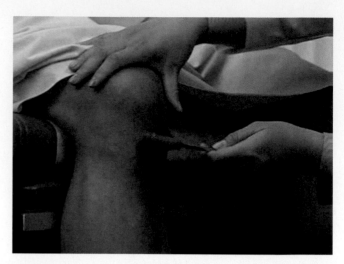

STEP 46 Assessing the patellar reflex.

47. **ACC** Assess the triceps reflex. Ask the client to relax while you support the client's upper arm at the elbow. Using the reflex hammer, directly strike the triceps tendon above the elbow. Observe for contraction of the triceps muscle and extension of the forearm. (Note: The expected finding is 2+ movement, where 0 is no movement and 4+ is hyperactive [Wilson & Giddens, 2017].)

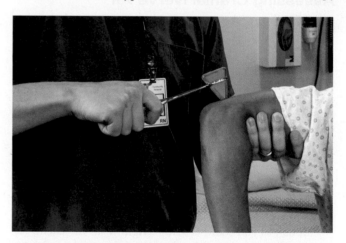

STEP 47 Assessing the triceps reflex.

48. **ACC** Assess the plantar reflex, also known as the Babinski reflex. Stroke the client's heel upward to just below the little toe, then across the ball of the foot toward the great toe, with the rounded end of a reflex hammer handle or other tool. (Note: The expected finding for a client older than 2 years old is plantar flexion of all of the toes and inversion or turning in of the foot. This is known as a negative Babinski reflex. For children from birth to around 18 months, the expected finding is dorsiflexion, or upgoing, of the great toe and fanning of the other toes. However, in adults, this is abnormal and is considered a positive Babinski reflex, which may be related to a defect of an upper motor neuron or other alteration [Jarvis, 2016].)

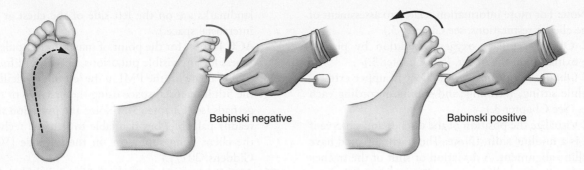

Babinski negative

Babinski positive

STEP 48 Assessing the plantar or Babinski reflex.

FINISHING THE SKILL

49. **INF** Remove gloves if used and perform hand hygiene.
50. **SAF** Ensure safety and comfort. Ensure that the bed is in the lowest position and verify that the client can identify and reach the nurse call system. *These safety measures reduce the risk of falls.*
51. **EVAL** Evaluate the outcomes. Compare current findings with previous results. Did the client remain alert and oriented for the exam? Was the client able to follow directives for the exam?
52. **COM** If the findings of the neurologic assessment are outside of the established parameters for the client, notify the authorized healthcare provider.
53. **COM** Document findings, care given, and outcomes in the legal healthcare record, including any variation or change in the client's neurologic assessment, any action taken, and who was notified.

■ SKILL 4.6 Assessing the Thorax (Heart and Lungs)

EQUIPMENT

Clean gloves, if there is a risk of exposure to body fluids
Stethoscope
Measuring tape
Two tongue blades
Pulse oximeter
Towel to use as drape

BEGINNING THE SKILL

1. **ACC** Review client's medical and surgical history.
2. **INF** Perform hand hygiene.
3. **CCC** Introduce yourself to the client and family and explain the procedure.
4. **SAF** Identify the client using two identifiers.
5. **CCC** Provide privacy. Keep the client covered with a drape or gown.
6. **CCC** Ensure that room has good lighting and a comfortable temperature.
7. **INF** Apply gloves if there is a risk of exposure to body fluids.

PROCEDURE

8. **ACC** Assess the client for any subjective symptoms he or she is experiencing, such as palpitations or difficulty breathing. If the client voices concerns, ask questions regarding onset, location, duration, associated manifestations, relieving or exacerbating factors, and treatment.
9. **ACC** Inspect the neck and thoracic region anteriorly, laterally, and posteriorly. Note skin characteristics, including color, texture, lesion, scars.
10. **ACC** Inspect neck contour for spinal deviations. Note any deviations or abnormalities.
11. **ACC** Inspect chest contour for symmetry bilaterally. Note any deviations or abnormalities such as barrel chest, pectus carinatum (chest wall is pushed outward instead of flush, also known as "pigeon chest"), or pectus excavatum (sunken chest with a concave appearance).
12. **ACC** Observe the anterior–posterior (AP) to lateral thoracic diameter. (Note: The expected finding is normally 1:2 ratio in an adult.)
13. **ACC** Assess the client for ease of breathing.
    a. Listen for even, audible, unlabored respirations during inspiration and expiration.
    b. Visualize chest expansion while examining the anterior, lateral, and posterior chest. Observe the rate, rhythm, and depth of respiration. (Note: Chest movement should be bilaterally symmetrical during the inspiration and expiration phases, without any retractions of the intercostal muscles or accessory muscle use.)
    c. If the client's respiratory rhythm is regular, count for 30 seconds and multiply by 2.
    d. If the client's respiratory rhythm is irregular, count the client's respirations for 1 full minute. *Counting respirations for a full minute if irregular facilitates accuracy.*

(Note: For more information related to assessment of the client's respirations, see Chapter 3.)

14. **ACC** Obtain capillary oxygen saturation by placing pulse oximeter on the finger. (See Chapter 3.)

15. **ACC** Obtain blood pressure of client in upper extremity while sitting, reclining, and supine, recording each value. (See Chapter 3.)

16. **ACC** Visualize the position of the trachea and observe if there is a midline shift. (Note: The trachea should have a midline alignment. A deviation or shift of the trachea from the client's midline may indicate a change in lung volume caused by a pneumothorax, a large pleural effusion, or a significant amount of consolidation [Wilson & Giddens, 2017].)

17. **ACC** Visualize either side of the neck for carotid pulsations to the left and right of the tracheal area. (Note: The character of the carotid pulse may be altered by aortic stenosis.)

18. **ACC** Assess for JVD. (See Skill 4.4.)

19. **ACC** Auscultate the carotid arteries bilaterally using the bell of the stethoscope placed over the medial end of the clavicle and sternocleidomastoid muscle. (Note: In addition to the bell, the diaphragm of the stethoscope can also be used to assess the carotid arteries.)

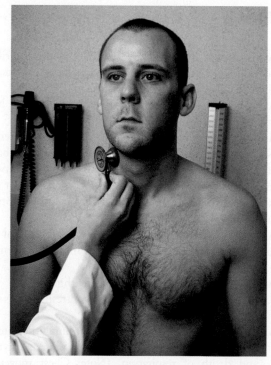

STEP 19 Auscultation of carotid artery.

20. **ACC** Palpate carotid pulsations (one at a time) and compare with the apical pulse to see if rates coincide. (Note: The expected finding is that they are the same rate.)

21. **ACC** Inspect the chest and observe for apical pulsations at eye level. (Note: The apical pulse anatomical landmarks are on the left side of the chest at the fifth intercostal space.)

22. **ACC** Inspect for the point of maximum impulse (PMI). Assess for any visible pulsations, heaves, or lifts.

23. **ACC** Palpate for the PMI in the left midclavicular line at the 5th intercostal space using the first two or three fingerpads (see Chapter 3). (Note: The pulsation should be readily palpable, but if unable to palpate, recheck with the client lying supine or on the left side [Wilson & Giddens, 2017].)

24. **ACC** Palpate with the palms of hands held lightly on the client's skin in the following areas:
    - apex of the heart along the inferior left sternal border
    - left sternal border of the heart
    - base of the heart.

(Note: Unexpected findings would be a heave or lift signified by a palpable impulse that is vigorous upon palpation. Another abnormal finding would be a thrill, which is a fine, palpable, rushing vibration that indicates turbulence of blood flow [Wilson & Giddens, 2017].)

Auscultate Cardiac Areas

25. **ACC** Auscultate the five cardiac points with both the diaphragm and bell of the stethoscope, first with the client sitting up and then supine. It may also help to roll the client to the left side. (Note: The cardiac points represent the auscultatory areas where the heart sounds, which radiate from the valves, are likely to be heard.) Auscultate in the following sequence:
    a. second right intercostal space at the right sternal border (aortic valve area)
    b. second left intercostal space at the left sternal border (pulmonic valve area)
    c. third left intercostal space at the left sternal border (Erb's point area)
    d. fourth left intercostal space at the left sternal border (tricuspid valve area)
    e. fifth left intercostal space in the left midclavicular line (mitral valve area).

26. **ACC** Identify S1 and S2 and note the client's heart rhythm. Is it regular? Assess the pitch, intensity, duration, and timing. Note any unusual sounds, including murmurs, clicks, gallops, or rubs.

27. **ACC** During auscultation, instruct the client to breathe normally and then hold his or her breath in expiration while you listen for 10 to 15 seconds. *This may facilitate the identification of heart sounds.*

Assess Thoracic Expansion

28. **ACC** Place the palms of your hands, with the fingers spread and thumbs touching, on client's posterior chest at the 10th rib bilaterally.

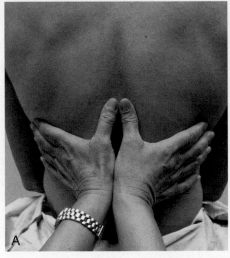
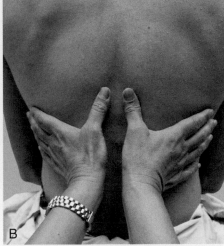

STEP 28 Thoracic expansion assessment (posterior). **A,** Place hands in the correct location. **B,** Observe for expansion during inspiration.

a. Ask the client to take a deep breath.

b. Observe for bilateral and symmetrical expansion of the rib cage as your thumbs move farther apart during the client's inspiration. If indicated, repeat the process on the anterior side of the chest.

Palpate for Thoracic Tactile Fremitus

29. **ACC** Place your palms on the posterior chest bilaterally at the apex of the lungs, moving down the midclavicular line to the mid-scapular, the base of scapula, then to the lateral chest.

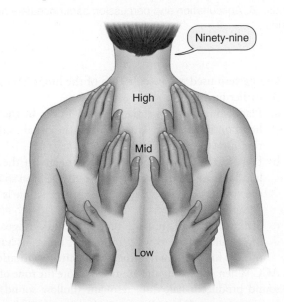

STEP 29 Posterior fremitus assessment.

a. Ask the client to speak the number "99" in a firm, loud voice.

b. Palpate for tactile fremitus during client's vocalization of "99."

c. Palpate for symmetric areas of fremitus as the client repeats "99" in a low, firm voice.

d. Repeat this process on the anterior side at the second and fifth intercostal spaces. (Note: The absence of tactile fremitus is an unexpected finding that may be caused by lung consolidation.)

Auscultation of the Lungs

30. **ACC** Auscultate throughout the lung fields using the diaphragm of the stethoscope. Use a systematic method from one side to the other in sequence while maintaining the same horizontal plane posteriorly, laterally, and anteriorly. (Note: In addition to auscultation, this suggested sequence can also be used for systematic percussion of the lungs.)

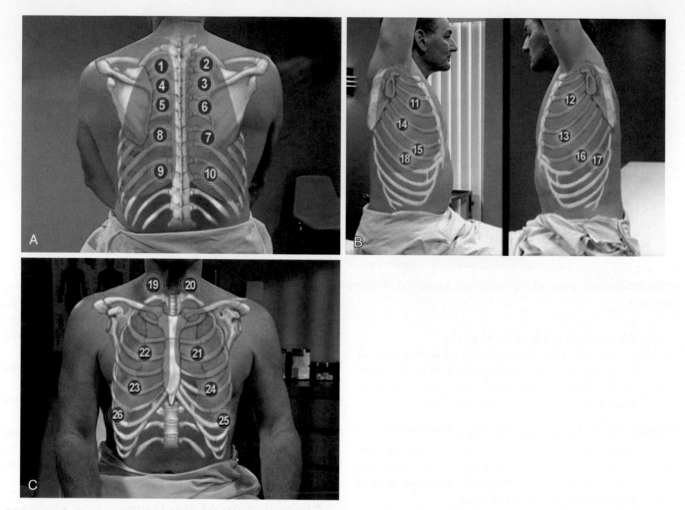

STEP 30 A, Auscultation and percussion sequence (posterior lung fields). **B,** Auscultation and percussion sequence (lateral lung fields). **C,** Auscultation and percussion sequence (anterior lung fields).

31. **ACC** As you auscultate, compare breath sounds bilaterally and assess for amplitude, pitch, and quality. Expected breath sounds will vary depending on the location (Jarvis, 2016).
    a. Bronchial (tracheal): high-pitched, loud, hollow, or tubular sounds
    b. Bronchovesicular: moderate pitch and amplitude, heard posteriorly between scapula
    c. Vesicular: softer, blowing sound; usually heard throughout lung fields

(Note: Abnormal or adventitious breath sounds may include fine or coarse crackles, wheezes, and rhonchi. If any are heard, ask the client to cough and try to clear airway, and then listen again.)

32. **ACC** During auscultation, ask the client to breathe deeply through an open mouth.
    (Note: Be alert for any client discomfort or feeling of faintness, and allow for rest as needed.)

Percussion of the Lungs

33. **ACC** Percuss the lung fields (using indirect percussion method shown in Fig. 4-2). Follow the same sequence and pattern used for auscultation of the lungs. (See step 30 earlier in this skill.)
    a. Place your hyperextended middle finger of the left hand on the client's skin and press the distal joint of that finger down firmly.
    b. Hyperextend or spread all other fingers on the left hand, lifting them away from the client's skin so that the sound produced with indirect percussion is not dampened.
    c. Strike the distal joint of the left middle finger using a quick forward wrist motion of the right hand's middle finger like a hammer, transmitting vibrations.

34. **ACC** When percussing the lung fields, note the tone of the sound produced: flat, dull, resonant (hollow sound), or hyperresonance. (Note: Resonance is the expected tone.)

35. **ACC** Percuss for diaphragmatic excursion.
    a. Ask the client to exhale fully and hold his or her breath.
    b. Percuss the posterior, left back along the midclavicular line starting at the mid-thoracic region moving downward until the sound changes from resonant to dull.

c. Mark this point with a small ink mark.

d. Ask the client to inhale fully and hold his or her breath.

e. Continue to percuss downward from the marked point and again listen for a change in sound from resonant to dull.

f. When dullness is heard, mark this point with a small ink mark.

g. Repeat percussion steps 35a through 35f on the right posterior back along the midclavicular line.

h. Measure the distance between the two marks to determine the client's diaphragmatic excursion. The measurements on the client's right side are usually higher than those on the left side due to the presence of the liver.

(Note: Diaphragmatic excursion is usually 3 to 5 cm in a healthy adult or greater if the client is athletic [Jarvis, 2016].)

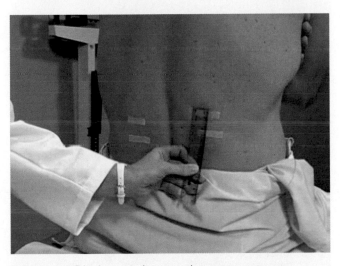

STEP 35H Diaphragmatic excursion measurement.

FINISHING THE SKILL

36. **INF** Remove gloves, if used, and perform hand hygiene.

37. **SAF** Ensure safety and comfort. Ensure that the bed is in the lowest position and verify that the client can identify and reach the nurse call system. *These safety measures reduce the risk of falls.*

38. **EVAL** Evaluate the outcomes. Compare current findings with previous results. Did the client tolerate the exam? Did the client have any shortness of breath during the exam?

39. **COM** If the findings of the heart and lung assessment are outside of the established parameters for the client, notify the authorized healthcare provider.

40. **COM** Document findings, care given, and outcomes in the legal healthcare record, including any variation or change in the client's heart and lung assessment, any action taken, and who was notified.

■ SKILL 4.7 Assessing the Abdomen

EQUIPMENT

Clean gloves, if there is a risk of exposure to body fluids
Stethoscope
Measuring tape
Ink pen

BEGINNING THE SKILL

1. **ACC** Review client's medical and surgical history.
2. **INF** Perform hand hygiene.
3. **CCC** Introduce yourself to the client and family and explain the procedure.
4. **SAF** Identify the client using two identifiers.
5. **CCC** Provide privacy. Keep the client covered with a drape or gown.

6. **CCC** Ensure that room has good lighting and a comfortable temperature.
7. **INF** Apply gloves if there is a risk of exposure to body fluids.

PROCEDURE

8. **ACC** Assess the client for any subjective symptoms he or she is experiencing, such as abdominal pain, bloating, or nausea. If the client voices concerns, ask questions regarding onset, location, duration, associated manifestations, relieving or exacerbating factors, and treatment.

Inspection of the Client's Abdomen

9. **ACC** Inspect the client's abdomen noting:
   - general appearance and symmetry

- skin's surface for any lesions, scars, or striae and tautness
- presence of surface motion
- venous patterns.

10. **ACC** Note the contour of the abdomen at eye level, noting if flat, scaphoid, rounded, or protuberant.

11. **ACC** Inspect for abdominal hernia or separation of the abdominal muscles. (Note: This can be assessed by asking the client to raise the shoulders and head off of the bed surface from a supine position.)

Auscultation of the Client's Abdomen

12. **ACC** Auscultate the client's abdomen using the diaphragm of the stethoscope. (Note: The diaphragm of the stethoscope is used to detect higher-pitch sounds.)
    a. Listen to the client's abdomen for up to 5 minutes if needed to validate if bowel sounds are present.
    b. Listen in each of the abdomen's four quadrants, noting:
       - frequency of activity (hypoactive, active, and hyperactive)
       - character (low/high pitch) in all four quadrants.

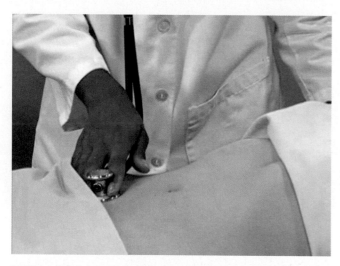

STEP 12B Auscultating bowel sounds.

13. **ACC** Auscultate the abdomen using the bell of the stethoscope. (Note: The bell of the stethoscope is used to detect lower-pitch sounds or bruits.)
    a. Place the stethoscope midway between the xyphoid and umbilicus, slightly to the left of midline. Note if a bruit is present.
    b. Auscultate in all four quadrants, noting if a bruit is present.

Percussion of the Client's Abdomen

14. **ACC** Percuss using the indirect method (see step 33 of Skill 4.6), across the abdomen in a zigzag pattern. Note the tone of the sound produced by percussion. (Note: The expected tone in the abdomen is mostly tympanic, which is a clear, hollow sound. However, dullness may

be elicited over the liver or scattered areas over feces [Wilson & Giddens, 2017].)

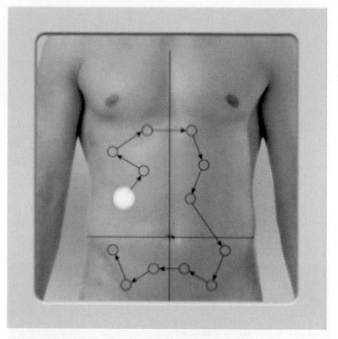

STEP 14 Abdominal percussion sites.

15. **ACC** Percuss for liver span. (Note: Ensure that client is in the supine position.)

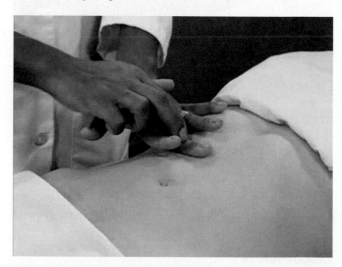

STEP 15 Liver span percussion.

    a. Discern lower border by starting at the midclavicular line over an area of intestinal tympany. Percuss upward on the abdomen until you hear dullness.
    b. Mark this point with a small ink mark.
    c. Discern the upper border of the liver by starting at the midclavicular line over lung resonance and percussing downward until you hear dullness, which may begin in the fifth to the seventh intercostal space (Wilson & Giddens, 2017).
    d. Mark this point with a small ink mark.

e. Measure the distance between these two marks and record this measurement.

Palpation of the Client's Abdomen

16. **ACC** Ask the client to relax the abdominal musculature while supine by bending the knees, with feet resting on the examination table.
17. **ACC** Palpate lightly using the palmar surface of extended fingers.
    a. Depress the abdominal wall to a 1-cm depth along a zigzag pattern using a circular motion.
    b. Palpate three points per each of the four abdominal quadrants.
    c. Note any irregularities or elicited pain.
18. **ACC** Palpate deeply using the palmar surface of the extended fingers. **WARNING:** Do not use deep palpation if the client has contraindications, such as a possible abdominal aortic aneurysm or enlarged spleen, or if the client exhibits pain responses, such as muscle guarding.
    a. Depress the abdominal wall deeply to a 4- to 6-cm depth (unless contraindicated) in the four abdominal quadrants.
    b. Note any irregularities or elicited pain.

Deep Palpation of the Client's Specific Abdominal Organs

19. **ACC** Palpate deeply to a 4- to 6-cm depth (if not contraindicated) for specific organ areas, noting any irregularities or elicited pain (Wilson & Giddens, 2017). **WARNING:** Use caution when using deep palpation and check for contraindications.
    a. **Liver:** Elevate the right flank with the left hand while standing on the client's right side, at the 11th to 12th rib posteriorly. Ask the client to take a deep breath and blow out while you are palpating for the liver's edge in the right midclavicular line. Using the palmar surface of your fingers and your right hand, feel for the edge of the client's liver. Avoid jabbing the client with your fingertips. (Note: The expected finding is that the liver edge is usually not easily palpable. If the liver is palpable, note firmness, nodularity, or any tenderness.)

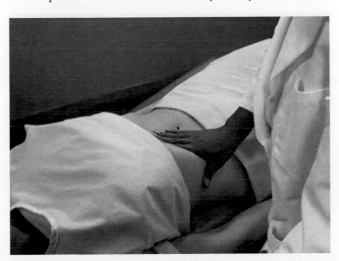

STEP 19A Palpation of liver edge.

b. **Kidneys:** Elevate the left flank by reaching across the client, placing the left hand's palm beneath the client's flank, lifting upward. Ask the client to take a deep breath and hold. Using the palmar surface of the extended fingers on the right hand, depress inward, feeling for a displaced kidney. Repeat on the opposite side to assess the client's right flank area. (Note: The expected finding is that the kidneys are not palpable, although the right kidney, which is about 1 cm lower than the left kidney, may sometimes be palpable.)

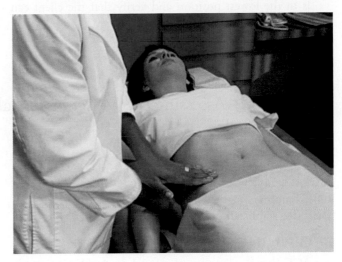

STEP 19B Palpation of the kidneys.

c. **Aorta:** Deep palpation just to the left of midline, near the umbilicus, will allow the nurse to feel aortic pulsations. (Note: The expected finding is that midline palpation of pulsations on either side of the umbilicus for an adult is 2.5 to 4 cm wide.)
d. **Spleen:** Ask the client to lie on his or her right side. Press upward with the left hand at the client's left costovertebral angle while palpating for the spleen with the palmar surface of the extended fingers on the right hand below the left costal margin. (Note: The expected finding is that the spleen is not palpable.) **WARNING:** Use caution when palpating the spleen area, particularly if the spleen is enlarged or if the client has clotting/bleeding disorders.
e. **Gallbladder:** Palpate below the liver margin at the lateral border of the rectus abdominal muscle with the palmar surface of the extended fingers on the right hand. (Note: The expected finding is that the gallbladder is normally not palpable.)
f. **Bladder:** Palpate just above the symphysis pubis with the palmar surface of your right hand. (Note: The expected finding is that the bladder is not palpable unless the bladder is distended with urine; then it may be palpable.)
20. **ACC** Check costovertebral angle (CVA) tenderness. *Helps evaluate kidney function.*
    a. Stand directly behind the client while placing your open, nondominant hand over the client's left costovertebral angle.

b. Using the blunt percussion technique, tap the surface of the nondominant hand with a fist from the dominant hand (see Fig. 4.3).

c. Repeat percussion technique on the opposite side.

d. Note if the client complains of discomfort. (Note: The expected finding is no discomfort.)

FINISHING THE SKILL

21. **INF** Remove gloves and perform hand hygiene. .

22. **SAF** Ensure safety and comfort. Ensure that the bed is in the lowest position and verify that the client can identify and reach the nurse call system. *These safety measures reduce the risk of falls.*

23. **EVAL** Evaluate the outcomes. Compare current findings with previous results. Did the client tolerate the positioning required for the abdominal exam?

24. **COM** If the findings of the abdominal assessment are outside of the established parameters for the client, notify the authorized healthcare provider.

25. **COM** Document findings, care given, and outcomes in the legal healthcare record, including any variation or change in client's abdominal assessment, any action taken, and who was notified.

■ SKILL 4.8 Assessing the Musculoskeletal System

EQUIPMENT

Clean gloves, if there is a risk of exposure to body fluids
Measuring tape
Reflex hammer
Chair (for stabilization)

BEGINNING THE SKILL

1. **ACC** Review client's medical and surgical history.
2. **INF** Perform hand hygiene.
3. **CCC** Introduce yourself to the client and family and explain the procedure.
4. **SAF** Identify the client using two identifiers.
5. **CCC** Provide privacy. Keep the client covered with a drape or gown.
6. **CCC** Ensure that room has good lighting and a comfortable temperature.
7. **CCC** Provide a safe environment for client movement.
8. **CCC** Ensure that there is an exam table or chair for the client to hold for stability as needed.
9. **INF** Apply gloves if there is a risk of exposure to body fluids.

PROCEDURE

10. **ACC** Assess the client for any subjective symptoms he or she is experiencing, such as difficulty with mobility, gait, or activity level. If the client voices concerns, ask questions regarding onset, location, duration, associated manifestations, relieving or exacerbating factors, and treatment.
11. **ACC** Inspect the client's general posture from head to toe from all sides, noting any asymmetry or exaggerated curvature.
12. **ACC** Inspect the client for symmetry of muscle mass and movement throughout.
13. **ACC** Inspect the client's head. Note if there are any disruptions in the symmetry of the skull.
14. **ACC** Ask the client to open, close, protrude, and retract the lower jaw. Observe for the temporomandibular joint's ease of movement, and assess for any pain.

15. **ACC** Palpate for displacement or crepitus of the temporomandibular joint with the fingertips resting just in front of the tragus bilaterally as the client opens and closes the mouth.
16. **ACC** Observe the alignment and curvature of spinous processes from the nape of the neck to the gluteal cleft as the client sits or stands. (Note: The client's back should be straight, without deviations.)
17. **ACC** Palpate on either side of each spinous process using the tips of the fingers and thumbs in a walking motion down either side of the spine from the nape of the client's neck to the gluteal cleft. Assess for asymmetry, masses, bulges, or tenderness. (Note: An abnormality could indicate a bulging disc.)
18. **ACC** Observe the movement of the neck when the client turns the head from left to right as if looking over his or her shoulder. Note range of motion and if the client has any pain.
19. **ACC** Assess the strength of the client's sternocleidomastoid muscle. Using your open palm, gently apply resistance to either side of the client's jaw as the head rotates left and right. Note if strength is equal bilaterally.

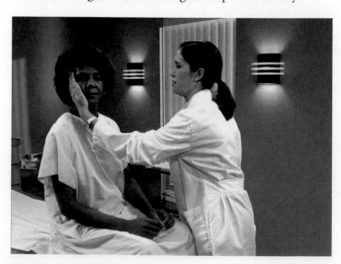

STEP 19 Sternocleidomastoid muscle resistance assessment.

20. **ACC** Observe for hyperextension (ask client to look up), flexion (ask client to touch chin to chest), and lateral bending (ask client to touch ear toward shoulder, to the left and the right).
21. **ACC** Assess for possible scoliosis.
    a. Stand behind the client so that his or her back is directly in front of you.
    b. While the client remains in a standing position, observe for lateral curvature of the spine, and observe for asymmetry and/or elevation of the shoulder or hip (left or right).
    c. Ask the client to bend forward from the waist as if touching the toes.
    d. While the client is bending directly forward, observe for asymmetry and/or elevation of the left or right shoulder, for lateral curvature of the spine, and for asymmetry and/or elevation of the left or right hip.

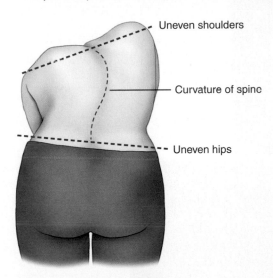

Uneven shoulders

Curvature of spine

Uneven hips

STEP 21D Assessment for scoliosis.

22. **ACC** Instruct the client to stand and twist at the waist to the left and then to the right as if turning to look behind him- or herself, and observe for asymmetry. Ask the client to bend at the waist laterally to the left and then to the right while allowing the hands to slide down the lateral aspect of each leg during each bending motion. Observe for asymmetry and range of motion.
23. **ACC** Ask the client to shrug the shoulders up and down. Observe symmetry and range of motion.
24. **ACC** Ask the client to move the arms from a starting position at the sides, laterally with the dorsal surface of hands forward, through forward flexion, hyperextension, abduction, adduction, internal rotation (hands behind back), and external rotation (hands behind neck). Observe for coordination and the extent of the client's range of motion, which should be symmetrical between the left and right sides.
25. **ACC** Palpate the shoulder with your hand cupped over the client's acromioclavicular and glenohumeral joints

while the client moves the joints one at a time. Note any pops or clicks.
26. **ACC** Ask the client to hold both arms out to the side while your hands are gently pressing down on each shoulder/upper arm. Note if strength is equal bilaterally.

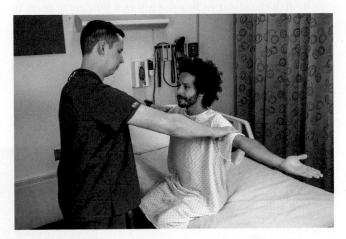

STEP 26 Shoulder strength assessment.

27. **ACC** Inspect, then palpate the olecranon process (elbow) and each side of medial and lateral epicondyles for abnormalities.
28. **ACC** Inspect, then palpate the elbow as the client flexes and extends each elbow, noting any abnormality or limitations in range of motion bilaterally.
29. **ACC** Inspect, then palpate the elbow and wrist as the client pronates (palms down) and supinates (palms up) the hands, noting any abnormality, difference in symmetry, or difference in range of motion bilaterally.
30. **ACC** Inspect, then palpate each joint of the wrists and hands using a gentle massaging motion with the tips of the fingers and thumbs. Note any abnormality or lack of symmetry bilaterally.
31. **ACC** Assess the client's grip strength. Ask the client to grip your crossed middle and index fingers. While attempting to pull your fingers from the client's grasp, assess whether or not the strength of the client's grip is bilaterally symmetric.

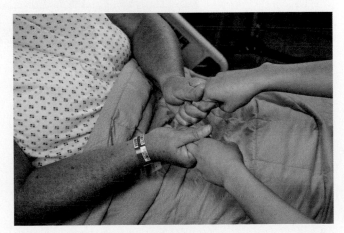

STEP 31 Grip strength assessment.

32. **ACC** Inspect, then palpate the client's hip joint bilaterally.
33. **ACC** Observe the range of motion of the hip and knee joint as follows:
    a. Ask the client to flex the knee 90 degrees.
    b. Ask the client to flex the hip at a 90-degree angle to the chest.
    c. Ask the client to externally rotate (knee directed laterally), then internally rotate (knee across midline) the hip.
    d. Ask the client to extend and adduct the leg toward midline.
    e. Assess for any abnormality or decrease in range of motion bilaterally.

    f. Ask the client to repeat steps 33a through 33e on the opposite leg.
34. **ACC** Inspect, then palpate the knee joint as the client flexes and extends each knee. Note any abnormalities or limitations in range of motion bilaterally.
35. **ACC** Inspect, then palpate the ankle and each joint of the toes as the client flexes and extends the foot.
36. **ACC** Observe the range of motion of ankles and feet as the client performs (A) plantarflexion and dorsiflexion, (B) eversion and inversion, and (C) abduction and adduction.

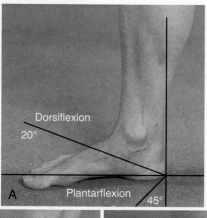

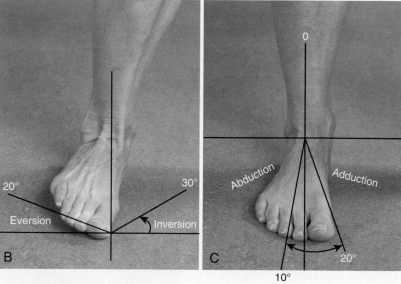

STEP 36 Assessment of ankle/foot range of motion.

37. **ACC** Assess the strength of the ankles and feet.
    a. Use a flexion maneuver. While providing resistance, place the palmar surfaces of your hands on top of the client's feet and ask the client to flex both feet up "as if pulling AWAY from a gas pedal" *(see the red arrow).*

    b. Use an extension maneuver. While providing resistance, ask the client to press the sole of each foot against your hands "as if pushing DOWN on a gas pedal" *(see the blue arrow).*
    c. Note if strength is equal in both feet.

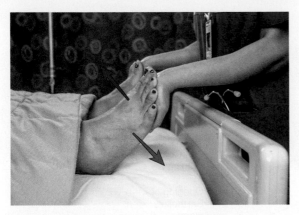

STEP 37 Assessment of ankle/foot strength

38. **ACC** Measure the calf size at the same spot on each leg, and measure the length of each leg from the iliac crest to the medial malleolus, noting if the distance is symmetrical bilaterally.

FINISHING THE SKILL

39. **INF** Remove gloves if used and perform hand hygiene.
40. **SAF** Ensure safety and comfort. Ensure that the bed is in the lowest position and verify that the client can identify and reach the nurse call system. *These safety measures reduce the risk of falls.*
41. **EVAL** Evaluate the outcomes. Compare current findings with previous results. Did the client tolerate the movements required for the musculoskeletal exam?
42. **COM** If the findings of the musculoskeletal assessment are outside of the established parameters for the client, notify the authorized healthcare provider.
43. **COM** Document findings, care given, and outcomes in the legal healthcare record, including any variation or change in client's musculoskeletal assessment, any action taken, and who was notified.

■ SKILL 4.9 Assessing the Genitourinary System

EQUIPMENT

Clean gloves
Additional lighting source (e.g. Gooseneck lamp, flashlight)

BEGINNING THE SKILL

1. **ACC** Review client's medical and surgical history.
2. **INF** Perform hand hygiene.
3. **CCC** Introduce yourself to the client and family and explain the procedure.
4. **SAF** Identify the client using two identifiers.
5. **CCC** Provide privacy. Close the door and pull the curtain. Keep the client covered with a drape or gown.
6. **CCC** Ensure that room has good lighting and a comfortable temperature.
7. **CCC** Provide a pillow for comfort and head support.
8. **CCC** Ensure that another provider is present during examination of this personal area.

PROCEDURE

9. **ACC** Assess the client for any subjective symptoms he or she is experiencing related to the genitourinary system. If the client voices concerns, ask questions regarding onset, location, duration, associated manifestations, relieving or exacerbating factors, and treatment.
10. **CCC** Ask the client to empty the bladder prior to examination. *Emptying the bladder facilitates examination of the genitourinary system and promotes comfort.*

Examining Female

11. **INF** Perform hand hygiene again and apply gloves.

12. **CCC** Inform the client that you will be inspecting and touching the client's genitalia during this examination. Obtain verbal consent. *Promotes respect and client autonomy.*
13. **ACC** Position the client in the lithotomy position, taking care to drape for modesty. If the client is on an examination table, ensure that the client's hips are on edge of the table. *Positioning client so the hips are on the end or edge of the table facilitates access and visibility of genitalia.*
14. **ACC** Inspect the mons pubis area for skin color and hair distribution. Note the presence of nits or lice.
15. **ACC** Inspect the labia majora for symmetry, color, and the presence of lesions.
16. **ACC** Inspect the general perineal area and rectum, noting symmetry, skin color, and the presence of any lesions.
17. **ACC** Separate the labia majora with the gloved nondominant hand using the forefinger and thumb.
18. **ACC** Inspect the labia minora, clitoris, urethral meatus, vaginal opening, and rectum for symmetry and skin color and the presence of any lesions, nodules, scars, or breaks in the skin. During inspection, be aware of odor or discharge. (Note: Expected findings are a lack of discharge and a lack of foul-smelling odor.)

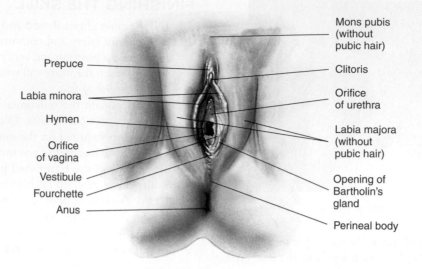

Mons pubis (without pubic hair)

Prepuce

Clitoris

Labia minora

Orifice of urethra

Hymen

Labia majora (without pubic hair)

Orifice of vagina

Vestibule

Fourchette

Opening of Bartholin's gland

Anus

Perineal body

STEP 18 Assessment of female genitalia.

19. **ACC** Ask the client to take a deep breath and bear down while observing for any bulging of perineal tissue or escape of urine from the urethra.
20. **ACC** Lightly palpate the general perineal area using the pads of fingers on the dominant hand, noting any nodules or elicitation of discomfort.
21. **INF** Remove gloves and perform hand hygiene

Examining Male

22. **INF** Perform hand hygiene and apply gloves.
23. **ACC** Verbalize that you will be inspecting and touching the client's genitalia as part of the exam. Use a deliberate (not stroking) motion (Jarvis, 2016). (Note: If an erection response occurs, tell the client that this is a normal physiological response and finish the exam in a professional manner.)
24. **ACC** Position the client in a supine position with the knees slightly bent.
25. **ACC** Inspect the general pubic area for color and hair distribution. Note any nits or lice.
26. **ACC** Inspect the general perineal area—penis, scrotum, urinary meatus, and rectum—for symmetry and skin color and the presence of any lesions, nodules, scars, or breaks in the skin.

27. **ACC** Inspect the penile shaft and determine if it is midline and if the dorsal vein is visible. Note the color of the client's skin and whether or not there are any scars or lesions.
28. **ACC** Inspect the glans penis for symmetry and centrally located urethral meatus. If the client is uncircumcised, gently retract (with gloved hand) the foreskin to view the glans penis and then carefully slide the foreskin to the original position. Note any lesions, discharge, or elicited discomfort.
29. **ACC** Ask client to lift his penis out of way so that you may inspect the dorsal and posterior surface of the penis and scrotum. Observe for swelling, lesions, nodules, or breaks in the skin. (Note: The expected finding is asymmetry of the scrotum, whereby the left scrotal half is usually lower than the right [Jarvis, 2016].)
30. **ACC** Palpate each scrotal sac between the fingertips and thumb of your gloved dominant hand. Note if the scrotal contents and testes slide easily. Note any masses or tenderness.

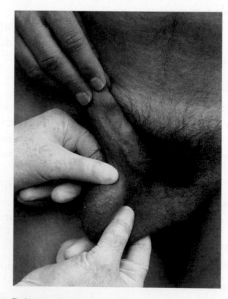

STEP 30 Palpate the scrotal sacs.

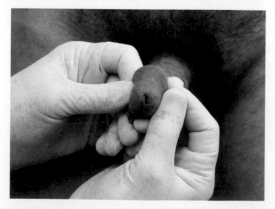

STEP 26 Assessment of male genitalia.

31. **ACC** Ask the client to stand, taking care to stabilize himself by holding to the exam table or the locked bed. Then ask the client to take a deep breath while bearing down. While the client is bearing down, inspect for any bulges or hernias in the abdominal, inguinal, or scrotal areas.

32. **INF** Remove gloves and perform hand hygiene.

FINISHING THE SKILL

33. **SAF** Ensure safety and comfort. Ensure that the bed is in the lowest position and verify that the client can identify and reach the nurse call system. *These safety measures reduce the risk of falls.*

34. **EVAL** Evaluate the outcomes. Compare current findings with previous results. Did the client tolerate the exam? Was the client's modesty and dignity protected during the exam?

35. **COM** If the findings of the genitourinary assessment are outside of the established parameters for the client, notify the authorized healthcare provider.

36. **COM** Document findings, care given, and outcomes in the legal healthcare record, including any variation or change in the client's genitourinary assessment, any action taken, and who was notified.

References

American Nurses Association (ANA). (2015). *Nursing: Scope and standards of practice* (3rd ed.). Silver Spring, Maryland.

Carr, D. D. (2017). Motivational interviewing supports patient centered-care and communication. *Journal of the New York State Nurses Association, 45*(1), 39–43.

Centers for Disease Control and Prevention. (2019). *What are the symptoms of skin cancer?* Retrieved from https://www.cdc.gov/cancer/skin/basic_info/symptoms.htm.

Garlock, A. (2016). Professional interpretation services in health care. *Radiologic Technology, 88*(2), 201–204.

Jarvis, C. (2016). *Physical examination and health assessment* (7th ed.). St. Louis, MO: Elsevier.

Kachirskaia, I., Mate, K. S., & Neuwirth, F. (2018). Human-centered design and performance improvement: Better together. *NEJM Catalyst.* Retrieved from http://www.ihi.org/resources/Pages/Publications/Human-Centered-Design-and-Performance-Improvement.aspx.

Nursing assessment: Damages awarded for negligence. (January, 2013). *Legal Eagle Eye Newsletter for the Nursing Profession.* Retrieved from http://www.nursinglaw.com/assessment5.htm.

Massachusetts General Hospital. (2018). *Working with an interpreter.* Retrieved from https://www.massgeneral.org/interpreters/working/.

More nurses, hospitalists being sued for malpractice, studies say. (2016). [Serial online]. *Healthcare Risk Management, 36*(4), 47. Retrieved from https://www.reliasmedia.com/articles/137567-more-nurses-hospitalists-being-sued-for-malpractice-studies-say.

National Institutes of Health, National Institute on Aging. (2015). *Talking with your older patient: A clinician's handbook.* Retrieved from https://www.nia.nih.gov/health/publication/talking-your-older-patient/understanding-older-patients.

U.S. Department of Health and Human Services. (2013). *Summary of the HIPAA rule.* Retrieved from http://www.hhs.gov/ocr/privacy/hipaa/understanding/summary/.

Wilson, S., & Giddens, J. (2017). *Health assessment for nursing practice* (6th ed.). St. Louis, MO: Elsevier.

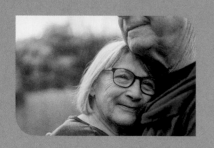

CHAPTER 5

Nutrition and Gastrointestinal Tube Therapy

"A patient's stomach must be its own chemist." | **Florence Nightingale (*Notes on Nursing: What It Is, and What It Is Not*, 1860)**

LEARNING OBJECTIVES

By the end of this chapter, the reader will be able to:

1 Identify different types of nutrients and methods of assimilation of nutrients.

2 Identify disorders that cause or contribute to malnutrition.

3 Identify dysphagia, risk of aspiration, and silent aspiration.

4 Identify standardized nutritional guidelines and nutritional assessment parameters.

5 Perform a basic nutritional screening or assessment on a client.
6 Discuss oral nutrition and different types of diets.
7 Prepare a client to receive a meal.
8 Provide assistance with eating for a client who has a physical or cognitive impairment.
9 Provide assistance with eating for a client who has dysphagia or risk for aspiration.
10 Discuss large-bore gastric tube intubation and gastric tube therapy.
11 Insert a large-bore nasogastric (NG) sump tube.
12 Demonstrate the critical elements of caring for a client with a large-bore NG sump tube.
13 Perform gastric suction/decompression using a large-bore NG sump tube.

14 Irrigate a large-bore NG sump tube.
15 Remove a large-bore NG sump tube.
16 Discuss different routes and types of enteral nutrition (EN).
17 Discuss the preparation, administration, and potential complications of EN.
18 Place and/or care for a client with a nasally inserted small-bore feeding tube.
19 Provide care for a client with a gastrostomy, PEG tube, or jejunostomy tube.
20 Perform an intermittent or a continuous enteral tube feeding.
21 Demonstrate the use of a kangaroo style feeding pump.

TERMINOLOGY

Absorption Process by which digested nutrients are transferred through the alimentary canal and intestinal mucosa into the client's circulatory system.

Anthropometric Refers to measurements used to assess the size, shape, and physical properties of the body (e.g., height and weight, skinfold thickness).

Aspiration (pulmonary) Inadvertent entry or reflux of substances from the client's oropharynx or gastrointestinal system into the lungs or tracheobronchial area.

Assimilation The biological use of substances and nutrients that have been consumed.

Body mass index Refers to a measurement or value that is obtained by calculating a person's weight in kilograms divided by the square of their height in meters.

Decompression To relieve excessive pressure or bloating caused by excess air or fluid.

Digestion The mechanical and chemical processes for breaking down and converting food into nutrients simple enough to be absorbed by the body.

Dysphagia Difficulty swallowing.

Enteral nutrition (EN) Refers to feeding directly into the stomach or small intestine via a feeding tube.

Hydration Status of fluid balance that impacts circulatory volume.

Irrigation Process of using fluid for the flushing, rinsing, or cleaning of a body cavity or tube.

Lavage Washing or cleaning out a body organ (usually done with a tube), such as in gastric irrigation.

Metabolism Sum total of chemical and physical changes that take place in an organism utilizing cellular energy for the assimilation of nutrients.

Nutrients Substances found in food or supplements that nourish the body.

Nutrition Process that involves ingestion, digestion, absorption, assimilation, and metabolism of food and that facilitates growth, repair, and maintenance of the body.

Pyloric Opening between the stomach and duodenum; post-pyloric enteral feedings are given directly into the small intestine (duodenum or jejunum) as opposed to the stomach.

Reflux Backward or nonphysiologic flow of a fluid, as in gastroesophageal reflux.

ACRONYMS

BMI Body mass index
EN Enteral nutrition
GI Gastrointestinal
ND Nasoduodenal
NG Nasogastric
NI Nasointestinal
NJ Nasojejunal
OG Orogastric
PEG Percutaneous endoscopic gastrostomy
USDA U.S. Department of Agriculture

Throughout history, the interconnection between food and a person's health has been recognized. As far back as the 4th century BC, Hippocrates described the relationship of certain foods with the presence of disease patterns in people. However, as nurses realize, health is not merely the absence of disease. From a holistic point of view, food helps the "mind and soul" as well as the body, and it can have a significant impact on a person's social, psychological, and physical well-being (Dudek, 2018).

As professionals at the bedside, nurses are invaluable with respect to assisting clients with individualized nutritional care. Depending on the setting, the nurse's role may include screening for nutritional disorders and making referrals as necessary; intervening on behalf of clients who have difficulty eating; monitoring the client's intake, response, and tolerance for food; and providing care for clients who need more advanced therapy or gastrointestinal tube management. To promote clients' nutritional health, an understanding of nutrients and nutrition-related alterations is essential.

ESSENTIAL AND NONESSENTIAL NUTRIENTS

Nutrients are components of foods and beverages that have been recognized as necessary for human health and functioning. Nutrients are also important for healing. The U.S. Department of Agriculture (USDA) and other nutritional experts note that individuals must have specific nutrients in their diet every day in order to achieve optimal nutritional balance. Two of the major categories of nutrients are *essential* and *nonessential* nutrients. Essential nutrients cannot be manufactured by the body and must be obtained in the food we eat. Nonessential nutrients are usually synthesized without food, although these may also be present in the client's daily intake (Mazur & Litch, 2019).

MACRONUTRIENTS AND MICRONUTRIENTS

Other categories of nutrients that are critical for health are macronutrients and micronutrients. *Macronutrients* are the "energy-packed" nutrients that make up most of the client's intake and are required in large amounts. Macronutrients also supply the majority of the *essential nutrients* to the body. These include fats, carbohydrates, proteins, fiber, essential amino acids, macrominerals, and water (USDA, 2016).

Micronutrients are components of physiologic reactions that facilitate the production of substances important for growth and development (World Health Organization [WHO], 2017). They include water-soluble vitamins such as vitamin C and B complex, biotin, folate, niacin, thiamine (vitamin B_1), pantothenic acid, riboflavin (vitamin B_2), vitamin B_6 (pyridoxine), and B_{12} (cobalamin). Micronutrients also include fat-soluble vitamins (A, D, E, K) and trace minerals such as iron and iodine, which may be toxic at too-high levels. Although micronutrients are only needed in small amounts, deficiencies can cause severe nutritional problems. For example, scurvy is caused by an insufficient amount of the micronutrient vitamin C. Another example of a condition caused by a micronutrient deficiency is iron deficiency anemia.

DIGESTION AND ASSIMILATION OF NUTRIENTS

If a client has difficulty eating or has a particular nutritional disorder, the digestion and assimilation of nutrients may be affected. Digestion is a process by which food is broken down by mechanical and chemical actions. Under normal conditions, digestion begins with chewing, an activity that breaks food apart and mixes it with saliva, which contains digestive enzymes. The food is further broken down in the stomach and small intestine, which also is the site where

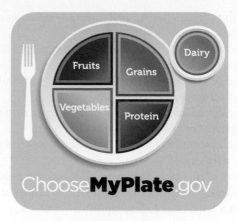

FIG. 5.1 The Choose MyPlate initiative.

many nutrients are absorbed into the client's circulatory system. The nutrients are then carried to the cells of the body, where they are used to build, maintain, and repair structures and to generate energy.

NUTRITIONAL GUIDELINES

To provide consistent information, various entities publish standardized nutrition guidelines. For example, the USDA, in conjunction with the National Academy of Sciences National Research Council, issues the Dietary Reference Intakes (DRIs) that identify the nutrient recommendations for various populations by age and gender. The USDA and Department of Health and Human Services (DHHS) also release the Dietary Guidelines for Americans every 5 years. The goal of these evidence-based guidelines is to promote health and wellness and reduce the risk of chronic disease.

In conjunction with these guidelines, ChooseMyPlate.gov (USDA, 2017) is an interactive website that offers personalized diet and activity recommendations to the public. The MyPlate graphic is a familiar dinner plate and it illustrates the relative proportions of the five food groups recommended at each meal. For example, notice that half of the plate on the MyPlate graphic is fruits and vegetables (Fig. 5.1).

In many facilities, the *Nutrition Care Manual* (NCM) of the Academy of Nutrition and Dietetics (2019) is used as a primary online reference. These guidelines mirror the USDA standards and offer updated nutritional information as well as recommendations for modified or therapeutic diets that may be prescribed for clients with certain conditions. These guidelines also offer educational materials and can be useful in acute care or other settings (Academy of Nutrition and Dietetics, 2019). Regardless of the setting, nurses can collaborate with other healthcare professionals to ensure the client maintains a proper intake of nutrients.

ALTERATIONS THAT CAN CAUSE NUTRITIONAL DEFICIENCIES

When a client's intake of nutrients does not meet the body's requirements, it can create an imbalance in the client's nutritional status. Nutritional deficiencies may also be caused by alterations in the processing of nutrients. This can lead to illness or exacerbate an existing condition. The stress of daily life and hospitalization can aggravate this further. Some disorders may be overlooked, particularly among vulnerable populations such as older adults and the very young or clients who have chronic conditions (Mazur & Litch, 2019).

Malnutrition

Malnutrition occurs when a client receives too much or too few of one or more nutrients in his or her diet. *Overnutrition* can occur when a client's intake exceeds energy requirements and may contribute to chronic diseases such as obesity, hypertension, heart disease, or diabetes mellitus. *Undernutrition,* particularly of proteins and calories, is caused by an inadequate intake of nutrients that may be related to altered metabolism, increased demands due to cancer or systemic infection, or malabsorption. Social deprivation, isolation, poverty, or food insecurities and lack of resources may also lead to undernutrition (Morley, 2018).

Additional causes of inadequate intake and undernutrition may be related to mechanical problems with chewing due to dentition problems or missing teeth. Oral pain and other oral conditions such as xerostomia (dry mouth) may cause problems with chewing and swallowing due to lack of salivary enzymes. When a client has had treatment for cancer or has a medical condition that causes a compromised immune system, the client may develop mucositis or other painful lesions and breakdown of the oral mucosa. If the pain associated with severe mucositis is not controlled, clients with this condition may be at extremely high risk for inadequate intake and undernutrition.

Depending on the cause, malnutrition may develop gradually. Unfortunately, the signs and symptoms of malnutrition may not be obvious until after it has become advanced (Morley, 2018). One distinct warning sign of malnutrition is unintentional weight loss. Additional warning signs of malnutrition are listed in Box 5.1. Worldwide, malnutrition continues to be a serious problem, particularly among older adults and other vulnerable populations (WHO, 2017). Nurses play a critical role in recognizing and preventing malnutrition in many different settings.

Dysphagia and Pulmonary Aspiration Risk

One condition that can lead to undernutrition is dysphagia. Dysphagia comes from the Greek word meaning "disordered eating" and can be caused by problems with oral, pharyngeal, or esophageal phases of swallowing (Paik, 2017). In addition to malnutrition, dysphagia can lead to life-threatening disorders such as dehydration, volume depletion, airway obstruction, and pulmonary aspiration. Aspiration pneumonia can occur if food accidentally enters the pharynx and passes into the client's lung, causing irritation and bacterial infection. Many clients understand this as "food going down

BOX 5.1 Signs and Symptoms of Malnutrition

- Hair that is dull, brittle, dry, or falls out easily
- Dry or rough skin; thin skin with lack of subcutaneous fat
- Poor or delayed wound healing; pressure sores
- Muscle wasting; weakened hand grip
- Generalized edema, especially of the lower extremities
- Depressed mood; altered balance and coordination
- Abnormal heart rate or rhythm or low blood pressure
- Enlarged liver or spleen; swollen lymph nodes

References: Dudek, 2018; Morley, 2018.

BOX 5.2 Possible Warning Signs of Dysphagia or Pulmonary Aspiration

- Does the client cough, choke, or gag when attempting to eat or drink?
- Does the client appear to have nasal regurgitation or reflux when eating?
- Does the client appear to have drooling or poor tongue control?
- Does the client complain of pain or wince/grimace when swallowing?
- Does the client appear to have throat clearing or "tearing up" while eating?
- Does the client appear to be "cheeking" or pocketing food in the cheek?
- Does the client complain of feeling as if food is "stuck in the throat"?
- Does the client appear to have poor tongue control and closure of the lips?
- Does it require multiple swallowing attempts for the client to swallow food?
- Does the client have a "gurgly" voice, hoarseness, or complete voice loss?
- Does the client have an increased respiratory rate or other changes in vital signs?

References: Metheny, 2018; Nestlé, 2017.

the wrong pipe," which causes choking and breathing problems. Clients who have a decreased cough or gag reflex are at high risk for aspiration. Although signs of aspiration may be obvious (e.g., coughing or gagging), they may also be "silent" or subtle. For example, some clients who have aspirated may complain of a sore throat, acute hoarseness, or voice loss.

There are several conditions that may cause dysphagia or pulmonary aspiration, including clients who have an altered level of consciousness or those with neurological conditions such as stroke, traumatic brain injury, or motor disorders. Clients who have certain types of cancer, such as tumors of the head and neck, may also be at risk. It is important to identify early warning signs and prevent complications (Mazur & Litch, 2019; Paik, 2017). For a list of possible warning signs of dysphagia and signs or symptoms of aspiration, see Box 5.2.

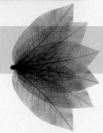

One of the best ways to assess a client's nutritional needs or determine if a client is at risk for a nutritional disorder is to perform a screening. This allows the nurse to look for areas of concern that may indicate the need for a more in-depth nutritional assessment and/or a referral to a registered dietician (Box 5.3).

The Joint Commission stipulates that a nutritional screening should be performed within 24 hours after admission, using a tool developed by the facility. The Joint Commission also recommends that the facility assess and reassess the client's nutritional needs throughout the client's hospital stay. As part of the screening, it is helpful to assess the client's personal preferences, including "comfort foods" normally eaten at home (Dudek, 2018).

The process of nutritional screening and assessment involves more than just filling out paperwork or a required form at the time of the client's admission. It is an ongoing evaluation of the client's intake and ability to eat, how the client is tolerating food, and whether the client likes the meals he or she is receiving. Clients with significant wounds or other medical conditions that place them at risk for malnutrition may need to be assessed more often (Dudek, 2018).

CRITERIA USED FOR A NUTRITIONAL SCREENING OR ASSESSMENT

The criteria for a nutritional screening or assessment usually includes anthropometric data (e.g., height, weight), laboratory data (e.g., albumin, pre-albumin), a physical exam (e.g., condition of skin, hair, and nails), and objective/subjective assessment data (see Chapter 4). Assessing a client's food allergies and evaluating intake of herbs, medications, or certain foods that place the client at risk for medication–food interactions are also crucial (Academy of Nutrition and Dietetics, 2019). It is important to remember that no one parameter is specific for assessment of nutritional status. Nevertheless, a number of tests within the usual laboratory values may be helpful indicators for nutritional disorders, including total protein, albumin, pre-albumin, white blood cell (WBC) count, total lymphocyte count, and hemoglobin. However, some parameters may be misleading and should not be considered alone. For example, a client's low albumin, low WBC count, or low hemoglobin level may be related to overhydration, trauma, or infection rather than malnutrition.

When evaluating nutritional screening criteria, be alert for changes in the client's weight, such as unintentional weight loss of more than 5% over a short period of time (e.g., 3 months). Significant unintended weight loss may be an indication of a serious nutritional disorder.

ASSESSING AND MONITORING A CLIENT'S FOOD AND FLUID INTAKE

During a nutritional screening, it is helpful to assess what the client has been eating at home in order to get a baseline understanding of what the client's needs may be in the acute care setting. For example, asking the client "How many meals do you usually eat in a 24-hour period?" may help determine whether or not the client tends to "skip" meals or might need additional snacks throughout the day. A client's 24-hour recall can also help determine the type of food the client prefers and how the client likes his or her food prepared. However, a more accurate method may be a 4-hour recall because it may be difficult for clients to remember what they ate over the past 24 hours. Observation of the client eating several meals is also helpful (Academy of Nutrition and Dietetics, 2019).

When monitoring clients' intake in the acute care setting, ask them how much they are eating in the hospital compared to home and how they like the food they are receiving in the hospital. This can help identify potential problems with their meals or if any changes need to be made. Document the percentage and the type of food eaten and observe the client's appetite, nonverbal behavior, and facial expressions before

---

BOX 5.3 Major Indicators That Client May Need a Nutritional Referral

ALTERATIONS IN INTAKE OF FOOD
- Altered or reduced appetite
- Need for a restricted or modified diet
- Difficulty or pain when chewing or swallowing
- Dentition problems such as missing teeth or dentures

ALTERATIONS IN BIOCHEMICAL TESTS AND LABORATORY DATA
- Albumin level <3.5
- Prealbumin level <15

ALTERATIONS IN WEIGHT OR OTHER CONDITIONS
- Unexplained weight loss that was not intentional
- Loss of lean body mass or signs of malnutrition (see Box 5.1)
- Body mass index (BMI) that is not within expected parameters for the client (e.g., <18, >30)
- Food allergies or risk for food–medication interactions
- Nausea, vomiting, abdominal pain, or history of abdominal problems
- Chronic conditions such as diabetes, heart disease, or chronic obstructive pulmonary disease (COPD)
- Healing wounds, burns, or risk for pressure injury (Mazur & Litch, 2019)

References: Academy of Nutrition and Dietetics, 2019; Mazur & Litch, 2019.

and during meals (Dudek, 2018). It may also be helpful to monitor the client's calorie count, particularly if the client is at risk for malnutrition.

In addition to food intake, it is important to monitor the client's fluid intake, which is a parameter for assessing the client's hydration status. In the acute care setting, fluid intake is recorded in mL For example, 1 ounce is equivalent to 30 mL, and an 8-oz glass of fluid is 240 mL. Additional ways to evaluate hydration status include assessing the client for any edema in the extremities and assessing the client's skin turgor (see Skill 5.1 and also Chapter 4).

Monitoring Carbohydrate, Fat, and Protein Intake

If a client has diabetes or another metabolic disorder, it may be necessary to monitor (or teach the client to monitor) the client's carbohydrate intake. Some insulin pumps (see Chapter 11) can be programmed to adjust doses based on the client's total intake or projected intake of these nutrients. Initially, this procedure may require consultation with a specialist such as a diabetic nurse educator or a registered dietitian. These professionals help develop a meal plan and a target range for the total grams of carbohydrates the client may have with each meal. Based on the unique needs and characteristics of the client, the pre-meal insulin dosages are determined on an individual basis. Although carbohydrates have the most *immediate* effect on the client's glucose level, the consumption of a large amount of fat or protein can also contribute to higher glucose levels. Thus, the amount of fat and protein the client consumes must also be considered (De Alaiz, 2018).

As part of discharge planning and follow-up, the nurse can help reinforce client and family teaching. Electronic resources are also available for clients, such as the online nutrient database from the USDA that provides a nutrient calculator and information on thousands of foods (USDA, 2016). Several apps are available on most smartphones and other devices. As with other interventions, the collaboration between the nurse, the client, and other healthcare professionals is invaluable.

SUMMARY

When performing a nutritional assessment, accuracy, client-centered care, and communication are key critical concepts. For example, accuracy is important when collecting subjective and objective data, as well as anthropometric data such as the client's height and weight. Client-centered care is provided by protecting the client's privacy and ensuring that an interpreter is present if needed during the screening and assessment process. Communication regarding proper recording of the client's intake and making referrals as necessary are also important.

The initial nutritional screening and ongoing assessment of clients is usually performed by the registered nurse. However, monitoring and recording of food/fluid intake can be delegated to assistive personnel as needed. To reduce the risk for impaired nutritional status, collaboration between the nurse, the client, and other members of the healthcare team is essential.

APPLICATION OF THE NURSING PROCESS

Examples of Related International Classification for Nursing Practice (ICNP) Nursing Diagnoses, Expected Client Outcomes, and Nursing Assessment:

Nursing Diagnosis: Risk for impaired nutritional status

Supporting Data: Client has >5% weight loss over 3 months and a decreased appetite.

Expected Client Outcomes: Client will have no evidence of impaired nutritional status, as seen by:
- body weight within established parameters for the client
- no physical signs of malnutrition (e.g., muscle wasting; dry, brittle nails)
- lab values (hemoglobin [Hgb], albumin, prealbumin) within established parameters
- food intake of at least 80% of meals.

Nursing Assessment Example: Perform a nutritional assessment using a facility-approved tool.

Reference: International Classification for Nursing Practice. (n.d.) *eHealth & ICNP*. Retrieved from https://www.icn.ch/what we do/projects/ehealth-icnp.

CRITICAL CONCEPTS
Nutritional Assessment

Accuracy (ACC)

Accuracy when providing a nutritional assessment is affected by the following variables:
- the client's level of consciousness (LOC) and orientation level
- the client's medical history and level of pain or discomfort
- the client's nutritional history, including intake of herbs and supplements
- the client's social history and socioeconomic history
- screening tool used for collecting objective and subjective data
- the client's language and culture and ability to understand questions
- technique for collecting anthropometric data (e.g., height, weight)
- equipment used for measuring anthropometric data (e.g., calibrated scales).

Client-Centered Care (CCC)

Respect for the client when providing a nutritional assessment is demonstrated by:
- promoting autonomy by obtaining consent before the nutritional screening and allowing the client to participate in monitoring his or her food and fluid intake

- providing privacy and ensuring comfort during the assessment or screening
- honoring cultural preferences by exploring the client's food preferences and restrictions
- advocating for the client and family.

Infection Control (INF)

Healthcare-associated infection when providing a nutritional assessment is prevented by reducing the number and transfer of microorganisms, primarily through hand hygiene.

Safety (SAF)

Safety measures when providing a nutritional assessment prevent harm and provide a safe care environment by checking for food allergies and ensuring that the client is not at risk for food interactions.

Communication (COM)

- Communication exchanges information (oral, written, nonverbal, and electronic) between two or more people.
- Communication between the client and the nurse ensures that the client's food intake and food preferences are acknowledged.
- Collaboration with other healthcare professionals and making referrals when needed enhances the nutritional assessment and improves client care.
- Documentation records information in a permanent legal record.

Evaluation (EVAL)

Evaluation of the outcomes allows the nurse to determine the effectiveness of the screening tool.

■ SKILL 5.1 Performing a Nutritional Screening

EQUIPMENT

Clean gloves, if there is a risk of exposure to body fluids
Screening assessment tool
Scales (for height and weight measurement)
Measuring tape if needed

BEGINNING THE SKILL

1. **INF** Perform hand hygiene.
2. **CCC** Introduce yourself to the client and family and explain the procedure.
3. **SAF** Identify the client using two identifiers.
4. **CCC** Provide privacy.
5. **CCC** Obtain consent before the nutritional screening. *Promotes autonomy.*
6. **INF** Apply gloves if there is a risk of exposure to body fluids.

PROCEDURE

7. **ACC** Assess the client's LOC and orientation to person, time, place, and situation. *A baseline assessment of the client's LOC and orientation must be done to determine if an accurate nutritional screening of subjective data can be obtained.*
8. **ACC** Assess the client for any language barriers. Arrange for an interpreter if necessary. *Language barriers can interfere with the accuracy of the nutritional screening.*
9. **CCC** Assess the client's level of pain or discomfort. If the client is having discomfort, intervene accordingly (see Chapter 7). *Pain can be a distraction during screening.*
10. **SAF** Assess the client for food allergies. *Prevents allergic reactions and complications.*

Obtain Subjective Data Related to Client's Nutritional Status

11. **CCC** Assess the client's nutritional preferences for the following:
    - time of day the client prefers to eat meals
    - types of food the client prefers to eat, including "comfort foods"
    - any foods the client likes to avoid
    - availability of between-meal snacks or supplements
    - cultural/ethnic or religious preferences or restrictions regarding food choices and preparation (e.g., Does the client need kosher or vegetarian meals?).
12. **COM** Ask the client about his or her usual food intake, including number of meals eaten each day, approximate portion sizes, time interval between meals, and tolerance of meals.
13. **ACC** Assess the client's medical history and review medications the client is taking, including herbs and vitamins. *Helps determine potential medication and food interactions.*
14. **ACC** Assess the client for nausea and vomiting or any other complaints related to gastrointestinal issues. Ask the client "Are you able to keep your food down okay?" or "Have you lost weight without trying?" *These parameters may help screen for nutritional disorders.*
15. **ACC** Assess the client's bowel function. Is the client having regular stools? Is the client experiencing diarrhea or anything unusual? *Helps determine tolerance and digestion of food.*
16. **ACC** Assess the client's social history. Ask the client if he or she prefers to eat with others or usually eats alone. *Helps determine the type of setting where the client prefers to eat.*

Obtain Objective Data Related to Client's Nutritional Status

17. **ACC** Review the client's laboratory data (e,g., albumin). Although never considered in isolation, laboratory data can help provide clues about a client's nutritional status.
18. **ACC** Collect anthropometric data:
    a. Obtain the client's weight by using a calibrated scale. Record in kilograms (kg).

b. Use the same scale for each subsequent weight measurement if possible. *This enhances accuracy.*

c. Note if the client has a significant change in his or her weight from baseline. *If the client has significant, unintended weight loss (>5%), it could be an indication of a disorder.*

d. Obtain the client's height by measuring from the back of the heel to the top of the head. Ask the client to look straight ahead and maintain good posture and alignment, and remind the client not to tilt the head back or forward. If the client is standing, ensure that the back of the client's heels are close together and are flush with the wall. Measure the client's height to the nearest 0.1 cm (Academy of Nutrition and Dietetics, 2019).

e. If indicated, calculate and record the client's body mass index (BMI). (Note: BMI is calculated by dividing a client's weight in kilograms by the client's height squared in meters.)

19. **ACC** Perform a head-to-toe or system-specific assessment of the client (see Chapter 4).

a. Observe the overall appearance of the client. Does the client appear frail or emaciated or exhibit muscle wasting? Does the client have brittle nails or hair? *Indicates malnutrition.*

b. Inspect the client's skin. How is the skin tone? Does the client's skin look hydrated and supple? Does the client's skin have brisk recoil? *Brisk recoil is an indication of hydration.*

c. Ask the client to open his or her mouth. Inspect for mucositis, lesions, dentition problems, or dentures. *Dentition problems could interfere with eating.* (Note: If you are going to be checking the client's mouth manually, perform hand hygiene and apply gloves, then remove gloves and perform hand hygiene again after examination of the client's mouth.)

d. Assess the client's ability to take in food. Is the client able to chew and swallow without difficulty? Does client grimace when swallowing? *This could indicate dysphagia.*

e. Assess the client's mobility. Is the client able to sit up in a chair? Is the client able to hold eating utensils? Is the client able to open packages or wrappers?

20. **ACC** Assess the client's abdomen and observe (look) for distention. Auscultate (listen) for bowel sounds in all four quadrants, and palpate (feel) the abdomen and note whether it is soft or firm. *A baseline abdominal assessment can help screen for existing problems.*

21. **COM** Ask the client if he or she would like to discuss any other concerns related to food and nutrition. *Helps facilitate communication if the client has additional fears or concerns.*

22. **COM** Make appropriate referrals to other healthcare professionals such as a registered dietitian as needed. *Promotes collaborative care and communication.*

FINISHING THE SKILL

23. **INF** Remove gloves if used and perform hand hygiene.

24. **SAF** Ensure safety and comfort. Ensure that the bed is in the lowest position and verify that the client can identify and reach the nurse call system. *These safety measures reduce the risk of falls.*

25. **EVAL** Evaluate the outcomes. Did the client tolerate the nutritional screening?

26. **COM** Document assessment findings, care given, referrals made, and outcomes in the legal healthcare record.

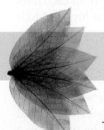

SECTION 2 Assisting Clients With Oral Nutrition

After the client's nutritional screening or assessment the authorized healthcare provider determines what type of diet the client will receive. Most facilities require a specific diet order for every client admitted. Ideally, the client should have as much independence and control as possible regarding meals. This facilitates client centered care. Some facilities have menus, allowing the client to have a variety of choices within parameters. Most facilities honor client requests and adhere to cultural and religious needs by offering food that requires special preparation, such as vegetarian or kosher meals. The nurse can determine any requests or restrictions the client has during the screening process (see Section 1 of this chapter).

TYPES OF DIETS

Depending on his or her needs, a client may be placed on a regular, texture-modified consistency, or therapeutic diet.

When clients are on a *regular diet,* they usually have no restrictions, although most facilities ensure the meals are age-appropriate. Clients who are being prepared for surgery or a procedure and clients who are critically ill may be on NPO (nothing to eat or drink by mouth) status. Some clients who have abdominal distention, nausea/vomiting, or other problems may be temporarily restricted to clear liquids. Clear liquids are defined as "anything you can see through" and include ice chips, gelatins, and different types of broth.

A full liquid diet is similar to a clear liquid diet with the addition of milk products and small amounts of fiber (e.g., puddings, cereal). Because liquid diets lack adequate nutrients (particularly clear liquids), they should only be used for the short term. To enhance recovery after surgery, the goal is for the client to be placed on a regular diet as soon as possible. Oral supplements may be ordered based on the client's individual needs (Academy of Nutrition and Dietetics, 2019).

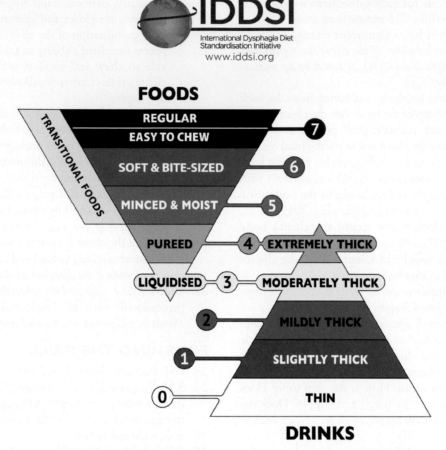

FIG. 5.2 International Dysphagia Diet Standardization Initiative (IDDSI) Framework.

Texture-Modified Diets

For clients who have dysphagia or difficulty chewing, a *texture-modified diet* may be ordered. Traditionally, the National Dysphagia Diet (NDD) has been used, which includes three primary levels: level I (pureed), level II (mechanically altered soft), and level III (advanced mechanical soft). A pureed diet usually has a pudding consistency that can be swallowed without chewing. Foods that are chunky, sticky, or chewy should be avoided. A mechanically altered soft or advanced mechanical soft diet consists of foods that are moist, softly textured, and can be easily formed into a bolus for swallowing (Academy of Nutrition and Dietetics, 2019).

More recently, the International Dysphagia Diet Standardization Initiative (IDDSI) has been implemented to promote culturally neutral terminology and to improve communication across all settings. As shown in Fig. 5.2, this framework has 8 levels (0–7) that identify drinks (levels 0–4) and foods (levels 3–7). These levels are based on characteristics such as liquid thickness, moisture (e.g., hardness, dryness), texture (e.g., tenderness, mashability), and sizes and shapes of food pieces. For example, in level 5 of the framework, minced and moist includes foods that must have a particle or lump width of 4 mm or less (for adult clients), and 2 mm or less (for pediatric clients). This size facilitates chewing and makes the food easier to swallow (Academy of

Nutrition and Dietetics, 2019). For more information on the IDDSI framework, including requirements for each level and testing methods, see the IDDSI website at http://iddsi.org/resources/framework/.

Therapeutic Diets

Therapeutic diets may be ordered for clients who have specific needs or disorders. For example, clients who have diabetes may be placed on a consistent carbohydrate diet, and clients who have cardiovascular disease may be placed on a heart healthy cardiac diet. Clients who have healing wounds, pressure injuries, or burns may have specific dietary requirements and need more calories from certain nutrients, and some clients may require frequent meals or between-meal snacks (Academy of Nutrition and Dietetics, 2019). Assess the client closely and make appropriate referrals as needed. For more information regarding different types of diets, consult with the registered dietitian in your facility.

PREPARING A CLIENT TO RECEIVE A MEAL

When clients are in a hospital or away from home, they may have a great deal of stress and a decreased appetite. One of the best ways to facilitate a client's appetite is to

BOX 5.4 Lifespan Considerations: Assisting an Older Adult With Nutritional Needs

Mrs. Hoang is an 84-year-old Vietnamese American client who has been admitted for dehydration and low blood pressure. She also has a history of arthritis and weakness. Her husband has recently passed away, and her children live in another state. Although Mrs. Hoang's vital signs have now stabilized, her intake record indicates she has been eating less than 50% of her meals. One morning, the nurse notices that Mrs. Hoang has eaten very little of her food, and she has thrown her eating utensils across the bed. Realizing that Mrs. Hoang may be frustrated, the nurse offers to assist with cutting up her meat, opening her milk cartons, or anything else she may need. The nurse also tends to Mrs. Hoang's cultural needs by asking her if she has any special needs or requests.

As part of the normal aging process, many older clients may have a decreased appetite and less tolerance for larger quantities of food. In addition, some older clients, like Mrs. Hoang, may have limited mobility. Offering frequent small meals as well as foods that are easy to pick up (e.g., finger foods, bite-size fruits and veggies, and sandwiches cut in halves or quarters) may help facilitate intake. In addition, providing plate stabilizers and cups with easy-to-hold handles may help (Academy of Nutrition and Dietetics, 2019).

If an older client has decreased visual acuity, providing natural light and ensuring the client knows where everything is on the plate can also be helpful. Because Mrs. Hoang lost her husband, she may be experiencing feelings of social isolation and loneliness (which is common among older clients). It may be helpful to encourage her to eat with others. Sitting and talking with Mrs. Hoang may also facilitate her appetite. An older person's condition can change quickly. Observe the client closely, and make referrals as necessary.

BOX 5.5 Reducing the Risk of Choking and Aspiration During Meals

- Encourage the client to eat slowly and chew the food thoroughly.
- Encourage the client to sit upright in a chair (that has a back) while eating.
- Encourage the client to remain upright for at least 1 to 2 hours after eating.
- Encourage the client to completely swallow food between each bite or sip.
- Assist the client to remove loose dentures if needed.
- Avoid distractions and loud noises during the meal.
- Encourage the client to take small bites or only half a teaspoon at a time.
- Provide meticulous oral care before and after meals and at regular intervals.
- Assist the client with managing oral/pharyngeal secretions if necessary.

References: Metheny, 2018; Nestlé, 2017.

ASSISTING A CLIENT WHO HAS DIFFICULTY EATING

Clients who have disabilities may require assistance with eating. For example, a client who has a visual impairment may need help setting up the meal. Inform the client which side the utensils, napkins, and other items are on. Tell the client what is on the plate by using the clock method (see Skill 5.3). If the client is partially impaired, use contrasting backgrounds, such as white plates with dark placemats. If the client has a cognitive impairment, use plate guards, high-lipped plates, and safe utensils. Avoid rushing clients, and allow them to have as much control and independence as possible (Chang & Roberts, 2011).

Clients who have dysphagia or difficulty swallowing may be at high risk for aspiration. Ensure that the client's head of the bed (HOB) is elevated and that the client is sitting upright. It is also important to cut food into smaller bites and follow the client's texture-modified diet as ordered, and allow plenty of time for the client to chew and swallow the food. Assess the client during the meal by observing verbal and nonverbal clues to ensure the client is not having difficulty. For a summary of ways to reduce the risk of choking and aspiration, see Box 5.5.

APPLICATION OF THE NURSING PROCESS

Examples of Related ICNP Nursing Diagnoses, Expected Client Outcomes, and Nursing Interventions:

Nursing Diagnosis: Impaired swallowing

Supporting Data: The client has verbalized difficulty swallowing at times during meals.

Expected Client Outcomes: Client will exhibit minimal difficulty when swallowing, as seen by:

- absence of coughing, gagging, hoarseness, or choking or signs of aspiration

enhance the client's environment (Dudek, 2018). This can be done by simple measures such as opening curtains to allow natural light to flow in and screening the client from unpleasant odors. As previously discussed, it is important to allow the client to have as much control as possible in order to provide client-centered care. For additional ways to encourage the client to eat, see Skill 5.2.

When preparing a client for a meal, assist the client with opening wrappers, opening cartons, and arranging utensils as needed. Attend to cultural needs by allowing the client to use utensils that are familiar to the client. During the meal, assess the client for any difficulty with chewing or swallowing and determine the need for further assistance. If the client is not eating well, look for subtle clues and ask yourself, "Is the client getting his or her comfort foods? Is the client experiencing discomfort?" (Dudek, 2018). Ask the client if he or she is enjoying the meal or would like substitute foods. In particular, older adults may have special needs associated with the aging process, as discussed in Box 5.4.

- vital signs within established parameters, including respiratory rate
- absence of excessive drooling or "pocketing" of food in cheek during eating
- absence of "wincing" or "grimacing" when swallowing food.

Nursing Intervention Examples: Elevate the client's head of the bed (HOB). Encourage client to chew food thoroughly before swallowing. Implement aspiration precautions.

Reference: International Classification for Nursing Practice. (n.d.) *eHealth & ICNP.* Retrieved from https://www.icn.ch/what-we-do/projects/ehealth-icnp.

CRITICAL CONCEPTS
Assisting Clients With Oral Nutrition

Accuracy (ACC)

Accuracy when assisting clients with oral nutrition is affected by the following variables:

- assessment of the client, including gastrointestinal function, LOC, and orientation level
- client's medical history and any physical or cognitive impairment
- client's motor skills and ability to use eating utensils
- techniques used for facilitating communication with client
- techniques and tools used for assisting client with eating.

Client-Centered Care (CCC)

Respect for the client when assisting clients with oral nutrition is demonstrated through:

- promoting autonomy by allowing client choices regarding types of meals and timing of meals

- protecting the client's dignity by allowing as much independence as possible during meals
- providing privacy and ensuring comfort during mealtime
- honoring cultural preferences by respecting client's food restrictions/choices
- advocating for the client and family regarding food preferences.

Infection Control (INF)

When assisting clients with oral nutrition, infection is prevented by reducing the number and transfer of microorganisms, primarily through hand hygiene.

Safety (SAF)

When assisting clients with oral nutrition, safety measures prevent harm and create a safe care environment, including:
- Following the client's texture-modified diet plan and orders to prevent choking and assessing for any allergies.

Communication (COM)

- Communication exchanges information (oral, written, nonverbal, or electronic) between two or more people.
- Collaboration with the client and other members of the healthcare team facilitates honoring client preferences and enhances nutritional care.
- Documentation records information in a permanent legal record.

Evaluation (EVAL)

Evaluation of the outcomes with oral nutrition allows the nurse to determine the safety and efficacy of the care provided.

▪ SKILL 5.2 Preparing a Client to Receive a Meal

EQUIPMENT

Cloth protectors, napkins, towels, washcloths
Oral care supplies

BEGINNING THE SKILL

1. **INF** Perform hand hygiene.
2. **CCC** Introduce yourself to the client and family.
3. **SAF** Identify the client using two identifiers.

PROCEDURE

4. **SAF** Review the client's diet order with the client and ensure that the client has received the correct tray. *Reviewing the order and tray with the client reduces risk and enhances safety.*

5. **SAF** Assess the client for food allergies. *Assessing for allergies prevents complications.*
6. **ACC** Assess the client's LOC and orientation to person, time, place, and situation. *Helps determine if the client is alert enough to eat without the risk of aspiration.*
7. **ACC** Assess the client for any alteration in gastrointestinal function (complaints of nausea, abdominal distention, etc.) and listen for bowel sounds in all four quadrants. If the client has signs or symptoms of impaired gastrointestinal function, perform a system-specific assessment (see Chapter 4) and notify the authorized healthcare provider. *Alterations in the client's gastrointestinal function could affect the client's ability to eat and properly digest food.*

8. **CCC** Assess the client's level of pain or discomfort. If the client is having pain or discomfort, intervene accordingly (see Chapter 7). *Pain can be a distraction and affect appetite.*

9. **ACC** Assess the client's motor skills and ability to hold and use eating utensils. *Assessing the client's motor skills helps determines if the client may need more assistance with eating.*

10. **CCC** Prepare the client's environment for eating a meal. *A pleasant environment enhances appetite.*
    a. Open curtains and let natural light into the room.
    b. Remove bedpans or any other unpleasant sights or odors in the room.
    c. Reduce unnecessary noise in the room (TVs, outside chatter, etc.).
    d. Ensure that the temperature in the room is pleasant for the client.
    e. Provide music preferred by the client if desired.
    f. Provide extra seating for family and friends if desired.

11. **CCC** Assist the client to empty the bladder prior to the meal if needed. *This promotes comfort.*

12. **SAF** Assist the client to sit up in a chair or sit up on the side of the bed if possible, and ensure that client does not become dizzy or light-headed. *Ensures the client can tolerate sitting up.*

13. **CCC** Assist the client with hand hygiene and any other needs the client may have. Ensure that the client's glasses, dentures, hearing aids, or other personal devices are in place as needed. *Assistive devices will facilitate the client's ability to eat.*

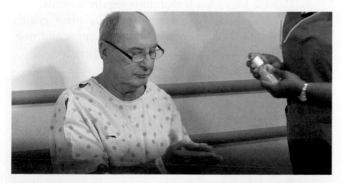

STEP 13 Offer hand hygiene before a meal.

14. **CCC** Assist with oral care if indicated and desired by the client.

15. **CCC** Position the overhead table for the meal tray at a comfortable height for the client.

16. **CCC** Ensure that food is at a proper temperature for the client.

17. **CCC** Ask the client if he or she needs assistance with opening packages, cartons, or other items, and ensure the client has seasonings and anything else the client may need.

18. **SAF** Assist the client with cutting up food into small bites, and provide assistance with other preparation as desired by the client. *Ensures safety and prevents aspiration.*

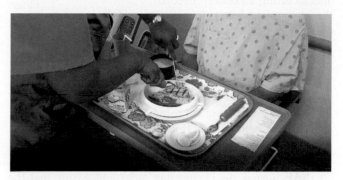

STEP 18 Help the client with food preparation if needed.

19. **CCC** Allow the client to give thanks if desired. *Adheres to the client's cultural needs.*

20. **SAF** Observe the client during eating and ensure that the client is not having difficulty. *This is a safety measure.*

21. **CCC** Sit down at eye level and talk with your client if desired. Allow flexible visiting hours (if allowed by policy) and encourage the client to eat with others. *Meals are often a social time, and interacting with others may enhance the client's mood and appetite.*

22. **SAF** Leave the client's HOB elevated for at least 1 hour after the meal. *Leaving the HOB elevated will prevent aspiration of food into the client's lungs.*

23. **COM** Ask the client how he or she is tolerating the food or if he or she has any additional requests or preferences.

24. **ACC** Measure the client's intake and record the type of foods and percentage of food eaten.

25. **CCC** Provide post-meal oral care or assist the client with hand hygiene as desired.

FINISHING THE SKILL

26. **INF** Perform hand hygiene.

27. **SAF** Ensure safety and comfort. Ensure that the bed is in the lowest position and verify that the client can identify and reach the nurse call system. *These safety measures reduce the risk of falls.*

28. **EVAL** Evaluate the outcomes. Did the client eat at least 80% of the meal? Did the client tolerate the meal?

29. **COM** Document assessment findings, care given, and outcomes in the legal healthcare record. Record the percentage of food eaten and the amount of fluid consumed in mL.

■ SKILL 5.3 Assisting Clients With a Physical or Cognitive Impairment

EQUIPMENT

Cloth protectors, napkins, towels, washcloths
Special eating utensils (if needed)
Plate guards, high-lipped plates (if needed)
Oral care supplies

BEGINNING THE SKILL

1. **INF** Perform hand hygiene.
2. **CCC** Introduce yourself to client and family.
3. **SAF** Identify the client using two identifiers.
4. **CCC** Provide privacy if needed.

PROCEDURE

5. **SAF** Review the client's diet order and ensure that the client has received the correct tray.
6. **SAF** Assess the client for food allergies. *Prevents allergic reaction and complications.*
7. **ACC** Assess the client's LOC and orientation to person, time, place, and situation. *Helps determine if the client is alert enough to eat without risk of aspiration.*
8. **CCC** Assess the client for any pain or discomfort, and prepare the client (and the client's environment) for receiving a meal (see Skill 5.2). *Providing a calm and pleasant environment will help minimize distractions during the meal.*
9. **ACC** Assess the client's motor skills and level of impairment (e.g., Does the client have visual, physical, or cognitive impairments? Is the client partially or totally blind? Can the client safely use eating utensils? Can the client safely sit up in a chair?) *Assessing the client's motor skills and level of impairment helps determine the level of assistance and any special devices needed.*
10. **CCC** Ensure that the client has any assistive devices available during the meal, such as hearing aids, glasses, or other personal devices. *Facilitates independence and autonomy.*
11. **CCC** Provide cloth protectors, napkins, or towels as needed and desired by the client.
12. **SAF** Elevate the client's HOB to 90 degrees if possible. *Elevating the impaired client's HOB will prevent choking and aspiration during eating (Metheny, 2018).*
13. **CCC** Position the bedside table for the meal tray at a comfortable height for the client.
14. **CCC** Assist the client with opening packages and cartons, buttering bread, cutting up meat into smaller pieces, and so forth as needed. *Prevents injury and risk of aspiration.*
15. **CCC** Sit down with the client at eye level, face the client, and speak slowly. *Sitting at eye level, speaking slowly, and facing the client facilitate communication.*
16. **CCC** Place the plate on the table with the main dish closest to the client.

17. **ACC** If the client is visually impaired:
    a. Tell the client what is on the plate.
    b. Describe to the client where seasonings and other items are located.
    c. Describe where each item is on the plate by using the clock method (e.g., meat at 12:00, potatoes at 9:00, peas at 3:00, and fruit at 6:00)

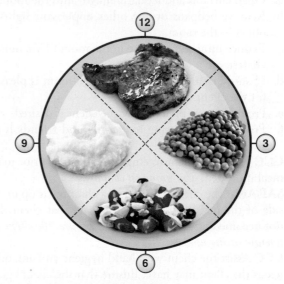

STEP 17C Use the clock method.

18. **ACC** If the client has a motor impairment:
    a. Provide finger foods that don't require utensils.
    b. Provide special equipment, such as plate guards, high-lipped plates, and two-handle cups, and non-sharp utensils with special handles as needed.

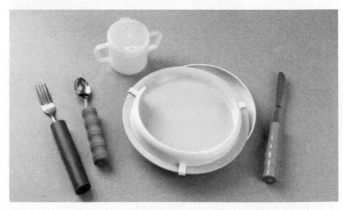

STEP 18B Special mealtime equipment.

19. **ACC** If the client is cognitively impaired:
    a. **SAF** Provide spoons whenever possible, and avoid sharp utensils. *Sharp utensils could injure a cognitively impaired client.*
    b. Provide finger foods that don't require utensils.

c. Provide verbal prompts during the meal, such as touching the client's hand or saying, "Try some of your potatoes now" (Chang & Roberts, 2011).

d. **CCC** Minimize distractions as much as possible during the meal (e.g., play soft music, avoid loud noises, reduce outside chatter, lower television volume).

20. **CCC** If the client cannot feed him- or herself, ask the client what food he or she would like to start with. Alternate solid food and liquids (e.g., sips of water).

21. **CCC** Give food in the order of the client's preference, and give the client as much control as possible during the meal. *This facilitates the client's dignity during the meal.*

22. **SAF** Give the client small bites and allow time to chew and swallow the food. *This reduces the risk of choking.*

23. **CCC** Talk to the client and ask questions during the meal (e.g., "Would you like some water now?" or "What food would you like next?"). *Shows respect and meets social needs.*

24. **SAF** If the client can only use one side of the mouth because of partial paralysis or another disorder, place food and drinking straw on the side the client can use (Metheny, 2018). *This is a safety measure and prevents choking.*

25. **SAF** During feeding, fill spoon only half-full, warn the client if foods are hot, and tell the client what you are feeding with each bite (Nestlé, 2017).

26. **CCC** If the client can partially feed him- or herself, guide the client's hand to his or her mouth. (Note: Allow the client as much independence as possible.)

27. **SAF** During the meal, observe the client and ensure that the client is not having difficulty with chewing or swallowing the food. *This could indicate that the client has a risk of aspiration.*

28. **EVAL** Monitor the client's nonverbal behavior, body language, and gestures during the meal, such as wincing, turning the head away, grimacing, and so forth. *Indicates difficulty with swallowing.*

29. **SAF** Leave the client's HOB elevated for at least 1 to 2 hours after the meal. *Leaving the HOB elevated will prevent aspiration of food into the client's lungs.*

30. **COM** Ask the client how he or she is tolerating the food or if he or she has any additional requests or preferences.

31. **ACC** Measure the client's intake and record the type of foods and percentage of food eaten.

32. **CCC** Provide post-meal oral care or assist the client with hand hygiene as desired.

FINISHING THE SKILL

34. **INF** Perform hand hygiene.

35. **SAF** Ensure safety and comfort. Ensure that the bed is in the lowest position and verify that the client can identify and reach the nurse call system. *These safety measures reduce the risk of falls.*

36. **EVAL** Evaluate the outcomes. Was the client able to eat the meal without difficulty? Did the client tolerate the meal? Was the client able to use special tools without difficulty?

37. **COM** Document assessment findings, care given, and outcomes in the legal healthcare record. Record the percentage of food eaten and the amount of fluid consumed in mL.

■ SKILL 5.4 Assisting Clients With Dysphagia or Aspiration Risk

EQUIPMENT

Cloth protectors, napkins, towels, washcloths
Oral care supplies
Special mealtime equipment if needed

BEGINNING THE SKILL

1. **INF** Perform hand hygiene.
2. **CCC** Introduce yourself to the client and family.
3. **SAF** Identify the client using two identifiers.
4. **CCC** Provide privacy if needed.

PROCEDURE

5. **SAF** Review the client's diet order with the client. Assess the viscosity (thickness) of the food on the tray and ensure that it is appropriate for the client. (Note: Some clients may have orders to thicken food in order to facilitate swallowing. This will vary depending on the facility.)

6. **SAF** Assess the client for food allergies. *Prevents allergic reaction and complications.*

7. **ACC** Assess the client's LOC and orientation to person, time, place, and situation. *Helps determine if the client is alert enough to eat without risk of aspiration.*

8. **CCC** Assess the client for any pain or discomfort and prepare the client (and client's environment) for receiving a meal (see Skill 5.2). *Providing a calm and pleasant environment and attending to the client's physical, social, and cultural needs will help minimize distractions during the meal.*

9. **CCC** Ensure that the client has assistive devices available during the meal, such as hearing aids, glasses, or other personal devices if needed.

10. **ACC** Assess the client's level of swallowing impairment and gag reflex per facility policy. *Helps determine the client's aspiration risk and the level of assistance the client will need.*

11. **CCC** Provide oral care before the meal and ensure that dentures are in place if needed by the client. *Enhances swallowing and reduces risk of aspiration. Oral care also decreases bacterial proliferation in the oropharynx, which reduces the risk of aspiration pneumonia.*
12. **CCC** Allow the client to rest for at least 30 minutes prior to the meal. *Swallowing disorders can cause fatigue during meals. Adequate rest reduces the client's risk of aspiration (Metheny, 2018).*
13. **CCC** Provide cloth protectors, napkins, or towels as needed and desired by the client.
14. **SAF** Elevate the client's HOB fully upright if possible. If not contraindicated, position the client with the body slightly leaning forward. *Elevating the impaired client's HOB will help prevent choking and aspiration. Positioning the client in a slightly forward position may facilitate swallowing,*
15. **CCC** Position the bedside table for the meal tray at a comfortable height for the client.
16. **CCC** Assist the client with opening packages and cartons, buttering bread, cutting up meat into smaller pieces, and so forth as needed. *Prevents injury and reduces the risk of aspiration.*
17. **CCC** Place the plate on the table with the main dish closest to the client.
18. **CCC** Give food in the order of the client's preference, and give the client as much control as possible during the meal. *This will help preserve the client's dignity during the meal.*
19. **SAF** Give small bites and allow the client time to chew and swallow the food. *This reduces the risk of choking.*
20. **SAF** Give the client at least 5 to 10 seconds between each bite or sips of water and adjust rate of feeding depending on the client's tolerance (Metheny, 2018).
21. **SAF** Ensure that the client's mouth is empty before and after each bite and ensure that food is completely chewed between each bite.
22. **SAF** When using a spoon, fill half of the spoon with food at a time. *Small volumes are easier for the client to swallow and will cause less choking (Nestlé, 2017).*
23. **SAF** Place food in the client's mouth on the side that is less impaired. If the client has right-sided weakness, place food on the left side. *Reduces the risk of choking and aspiration.*
24. **SAF** Ask the client to open his or her mouth; carefully inspect the client's mouth to ensure that he or she is not unconsciously "pocketing" food inside the buccal cavity. If this occurs, use your gloved hand to gently remove the food with one finger. *Prevents accumulation of food and reduces the risk of choking (Metheny, 2018).*

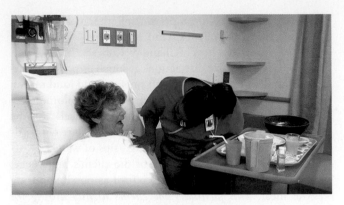

STEP 24 Check for "pocketing" of food.

25. **SAF** During the meal, observe the client closely and ensure that the client is not having any difficulty or displaying signs of choking or aspiration (see Box 5.2).
26. **EVAL** Monitor the client's nonverbal behavior, body language, and gestures during the meal, such as wincing, turning the head away, grimacing, grabbing throat, and so forth.
27. **SAF** Leave the client's HOB elevated for at least 1 to 2 hours after the meal. *Leaving the HOB elevated helps prevent aspiration of food into the client's lungs.*
28. **COM** Ask the client how he or she is tolerating the food or if he or she has any additional requests or preferences. (Note: If the client is not tolerating the food, make referrals to other healthcare professionals as needed.) *Collaboration enhances client care.*
29. **ACC** Measure the client's intake and record the type of foods and percentage of food eaten.
30. **CCC** Provide post-meal oral care and assist the client with hand hygiene as desired.

FINISHING THE SKILL

31. **INF** Perform hand hygiene.
32. **SAF** Ensure safety and comfort. Ensure that the bed is in the lowest position and verify that the client can identify and reach the nurse call system. *These safety measures reduce the risk of falls.*
33. **EVAL** Evaluate the outcomes. Did the client tolerate the meal without difficulty swallowing food? Did the client show any signs of coughing, gagging, or aspirating food during the meal?
34. **COM** Document assessment findings, care given, and outcomes in the legal healthcare record. Record percentage of food eaten and amount of fluid consumed in mL.
35. **EVAL** Provide follow-up monitoring after the meal. Ensure that the client has no signs of silent aspiration, such as voice hoarseness or a change in vital signs.

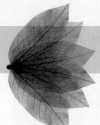

Gastric tube therapy may be used for three primary reasons-to empty the stomach (gastric decompression), to administer a feeding or medication into the stomach, or to irrigate the client's stomach (also called gastric lavage). Large-bore gastric tubes may be used for any of these reasons and are typically only used short term in acute care settings. Depending on the needs of the client, these tubes may be placed orally (orogastric) or nasally (nasogastric), and they require an order by the authorized healthcare provider. For adults, nasogastric (NG) tubes are usually preferred rather than orogastric (OG) tubes because of client discomfort, as well as difficulty with the placement and stabilization of OG tubes in the oral cavity. However, pediatric clients who are obligate nose breathers (such as infants or neonates) or clients who have had recent nasal or sinus surgery or other nasal and sinus complications may not be good candidates for NG tubes. For a list of indications and contraindications for large-bore NG tubes, see Box 5.6.

NASOGASTRIC SUMP TUBE

One of the most common types of large-bore gastric tubes used in the clinical setting is the NG sump tube. These tubes come in a variety of sizes (10, 12, 14, 16, and 18 Fr). The adult-size NG tube is usually 14 to 18 Fr, whereas the pediatric-size NG tube will vary with the size of the child. The larger the number of the tube size, the larger the diameter of the lumen (C. R. Bard, 2017). An example of the NG sump tube is seen in Fig. 5.3, *A,* and the components of the tube are illustrated in Fig. 5.3, *B.*

One of the distinct features of the NG sump tube is that it has two lumens. The main lumen (suction drainage lumen) is used for suction, aspirating gastric contents, or instillation of medications or short-term feedings. This is often done by using a three-way valve to provide a closed system (e.g. Lopez valve) on the end of the main lumen (see Fig. 5.3, *A*). The second smaller lumen is an air vent with an external blue "pigtail". The air vent prevents the mucosal lining of the stomach from being traumatized or suctioned against drainage holes when suction is applied. Some manufacturers have antireflux filters that fit at the end of the blue pigtail and provide two-way airflow. This filter allows the air vent to neutralize vacuum pressure in the stomach. It also allows gases to exit the vent if it becomes clogged while also allowing the nurse to see gastric secretion reflux that may need to be cleared. Although air may be used to clear the blue "dry" air vent of gastric contents, fluid should *never* be injected into the dry air vent (C. R. Bard, 2017).

A primary indication for the NG sump tube is decompression and suctioning to relieve distention if the client has excess air or gastric contents in the stomach. NG sump tubes may also be used for various diagnostic and therapeutic reasons, including short-term enteral tube feedings (discussed in the next section). In addition, NG tubes may be used

after surgery to rest the gastrointestinal tract or to prevent complications. In emergency situations (e.g., if a client is in cardiac arrest), an NG sump tube may be used to prevent aspiration of gastric contents into the client's lungs caused by abdominal distention or emesis. Because of the potentially life-saving purposes of NG sump tubes, it is important to ensure that these tubes and the equipment for gastric suctioning are readily available at the client's bedside.

LEVIN TUBES AND GASTRIC LAVAGE TUBES

One type of large-bore gastric tube that may be less commonly used than the NG sump tube is the Levin tube. These tubes may be used for aspiration of gastric drainage as well as intestinal contents and are usually 12 to 14 Fr (Fig. 5.4). Similar to NG sump tubes, Levin tubes may be used for the short-term administration of tube feedings or medications. The main difference between the Levin tubes and the NG sump tubes is that the NG sump tube has a double lumen, whereas the Levin tube has a single lumen.

Another large-bore gastric tube is the gastric lavage tube. These tubes are usually placed *orally* because their diameter is much too large (22–32 Fr) to be safely inserted nasally (C. R. Bard, 2017). The primary indication for the gastric lavage tube is lavage procedures such as charcoal therapy to remove toxic substances or for gastric ice lavage to control

---

BOX 5.6 Major Indications/Contraindications for Nasogastric Sump Tubes

INDICATIONS
- Diagnostic purposes
  - Aspiration and evaluation of gastric fluid content
  - Administration of contrast for visualization
  - Identification of stomach and esophagus by radiograph
- Therapeutic purposes
  - Gastric decompression and suctioning
  - Irrigation of stomach or gastrointestinal tract
  - Medication administration
  - Short-term feedings

CONTRAINDICATIONS
- Mid-facial or nasal trauma
- Recent maxillofacial, nasal, or sinus surgery
- Basilar skull fracture
- Tumors of the head and neck
- Esophageal or bleeding disorders
- Esophageal tumors or strictures

References: C.R. Bard, 2017; Shlamovitz & Kulkarni, 2018.

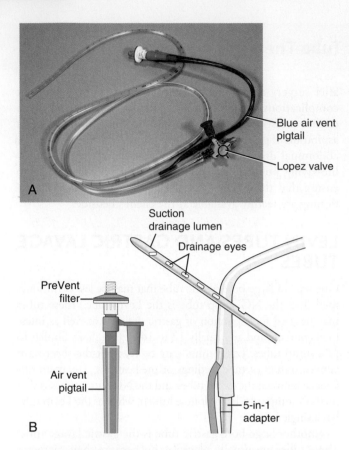

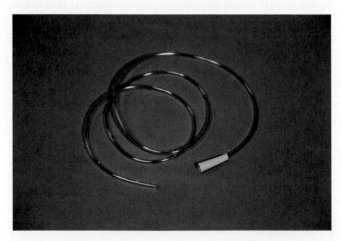

FIG. 5.3 **A,** Example of a nasogastric (NG) sump tube with attached Lopez valve. **B,** Components of a nasogastric (NG) sump tube.

FIG. 5.4 Levin tube with graduated markers.

gastric bleeding. However, these tubes must be used with caution because there may be an increased risk of oropharynx trauma due to their larger diameter.

PLACEMENT AND CARE OF A NASOGASTRIC SUMP TUBE

Before inserting an NG sump tube, review the order and the client's medical/surgical history and make sure there are no contraindications (see Box 5.6). Use extreme caution for clients who have had anatomically altering procedures such as bariatric surgery. Some facilities do not allow nurses to place

BOX 5.7 Lessons From the Evidence: Estimating Length of Insertion for Nasogastric Tubes

According to several studies, the traditional nose–earlobe–xiphoid process (NEX) method may not always give an accurate prediction of the estimated length needed for insertion into the gastric pool. For example, in one study, researchers used an electromagnetic (EM) trace of the tube path to study the accuracy of the NEX method or the opposite xiphoid–earlobe–nose (XEN) method on 71 critically ill clients. According to the authors, the findings suggested that external measurement cannot reliably predict the length of tube required to reach the gastric area and that the NEX and XEN approaches both come up too short to ensure gastric placement. They recommended adding 10 cm (4 inches) to the estimate for greater accuracy. However, the researchers also cautioned that only direct visualization or an EM trace can guarantee accurate placement (Taylor, Allan, McWilliam, & Deirdre, 2014).

A study by Santos, Woith, Freitas, and Zeferino (2016) found similar results. Using an integrative review design, the authors found that the NEX method was not as reliable as other methods. This finding was based on the review of 20 studies that met the inclusion criteria. The authors recommended using a method based on gender and weight, and measuring from the nose to the umbilicus while the client is lying flat to determine a more accurate estimate. More research is needed to compare different methods with various populations.

NG tubes in these clients without special training and supervision. The approximate NG tube insertion length must also be estimated. Traditionally, the NEX (nose-earlobe-xiphoid process) approach has been used to estimate the NG tube depth in adults. However, as discussed in Box 5.7, evidence suggests that the NEX method alone is not reliable and that the estimate may fall short of the gastric pool. A better method may be the NEX + 10 (cm) approach (Taylor, 2014). For pediatric clients, the NEMU (**N**ose-**E**arlobe-**M**idway between the xiphoid and **U**mbilicus) approach is preferred (Brown, 2017; Irving et al., 2018). As shown in Fig. 5.5, the NEMU estimate starts at the tip of the client's nose to the earlobe and then to the midpoint or halfway between the end of the xiphoid process and the umbilicus (Brown, 2017). The NEMU method may also provide an accurate estimate for some adult clients, particularly those who have a long torso.

If you are inserting the NG sump tube for intermittent gastric suctioning, check ahead of time and ensure that the suction regulator and suction canister are set up and working properly. During insertion, observe the client closely for signs of respiratory distress, coughing, or other problems. If there is any indication that the NG tube has been inadvertently placed in the client's airway, withdraw the tube immediately and allow the client to recover before attempting the insertion procedure again.

Checking Placement

After the insertion of an NG sump tube or any type of gastrointestinal tube, the placement should be checked using a combination of methods (American Association of Critical Care

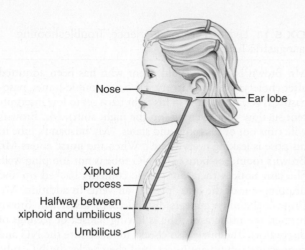

FIG. 5.5 Method for estimating nasogastric (NG) tube insertion length in children: NEMU (**N**ose-**E**arlobe-**M**idway between the xiphoid and **U**mbilicus).

Nose — Ear lobe
Xiphoid process
Halfway between xiphoid and umbilicus
Umbilicus

Nurse [AACN], 2016a). A summary of these methods and evidence-supported recommendations are provided in Box 5.8. An evidence-based review (Metheny et al., 2019) found a general consensus that x-ray verification, (when performed properly) is the most accurate and reliable method for checking tube placement. Regarding nonradiologic methods, checking the pH of gastric contents is most favored, although the authors noted limitations of this method if the client is taking antacids or other medications that could affect gastric pH. The least favored methods include the auscultatory method, the appearance of aspirate, and signs of respiratory distress. These findings are consistent with other guidelines. In particular, there is consensus that the auscultatory method or "swoosh" test is NOT a reliable method for checking placement.

To ensure the tube remains securely in place, check the pre-identified mark at the naris, and measure and record the external length of the tube upon insertion and at regular intervals (at least every 4 hours) thereafter. Even though placement may be initially confirmed by x-ray, follow-up monitoring is essential because the tube can migrate and become displaced later (Boullata et al. 2017). If there is any doubt, check with the authorized healthcare provider and obtain another x-ray if necessary and ordered. Serious errors, fatalities, and legal consequences have occurred as a result of misplaced or displaced NG tubes (Box 5.9).

In addition to using a variety of methods for checking placement, monitor the odor, consistency, texture, and color of the gastric contents (which should be a grassy-green color). Any unusual drainage or signs of bleeding (e.g., bright red blood, coffee-ground emesis) should be immediately reported to the authorized healthcare provider. For a list of potential complications of NG tubes, see Box 5.10.

Using the Nasogastric Sump Tube for Decompression

When NG tubes are used for decompression, the main lumen is connected to low intermittent suction using an

BOX 5.8 Lessons From the Evidence: Verification of Placement for Gastric and Enteral Tubes

Research regarding checking placement for nasogastric (NG), orogastric (OG), and other types of enteral tubes is ongoing. The consensus of best-practice information is that listening over the client's epigastrium and using the auscultatory or "swoosh test" method for checking placement is *not* reliable. A summary of other recommendations is as follows:

- Use a combination of methods (not just one) to determine placement. They all have some limitations. (AACN, 2016a)
- X-ray confirmation of placement is the gold standard. Obtain x-ray confirmation of tube placement *before* initiating irrigation, feedings, or medication administration. However, x-rays must be used with caution for pediatric clients due to concerns regarding radiation exposure and variations in imaging technique. (Irving et al, 2018; Lyman et al. 2016)
- Use pH testing. The pH aspirate of gastric contents should be ≤5. Respiratory secretions usually have a pH of >6. Secretions from the small intestine will usually have a pH value that is higher than that of gastric contents. However, enteral nutrition (EN) formula and acid-suppressing drugs can affect these values. (AACN, 2016a). If the client is on EN, follow your facility policy.
- Monitor for changes in the external length of the tube. Measure from the exit site (or marked portion of tube) at the nose for NG tubes or the corner of the mouth for OG tubes to the end of the lumen of the tube and compare to previous measurements. At the time of the initial x-ray, the exit site of the tube should be marked in centimeters and documented for subsequent measurements.
- Observe the appearance of the aspirate. Gastric contents should be grassy or yellow green. It should basically look like vomit. Aspirate of small intestine contents is often bile-stained. However, the appearance of gastric content aspirate alone is not a reliable indicator of differentiating gastric secretions from respiratory secretions.
- Use capnography (carbon dioxide sensor) or colorimetric capnometry if available. Although this technology can determine that the tube is not in the lungs, it cannot ensure it is in the stomach (AACN, 2016a). In addition, this method may not be available in every setting.
- Verify placement of the tube at least every 4 hours for clients receiving EN (see Section 4 of this chapter). Placement should be rechecked at least every 4 hours and prior to *every* feeding, irrigation, or medication administration. Placement should also be checked if there has been movement in the external length or appearance of the tube or if the tape, commercial stat-lock device, or nasal bridle has moved.

References: AACN, 2016a; Irving et al. 2018; Lyman, Yaworski, Duesing, & Moore, 2016.

BOX 5.9 Lesson From the Courtroom: Nasogastric Tube Misplacement Causes Client's Death

In a lawsuit filed in Jefferson County, Texas *(Thomas v. Baptist Hospital),* a jury awarded more than $2 million to the family of a client who died after nasogastric (NG) tube misplacement. The client, a 64-year-old male who had surgery for a benign tumor, had a nasogastric tube accidentally inserted into his lungs (instead of his stomach) by his physicians. However, the error wasn't discovered until 3 days later. By that time, the client had already received fluid and nutrients through the tube. According to the jury, the fluid instillation into the client's lungs caused pneumonia, coughing, and wound dehiscence (caused by the coughing), and the client eventually died. Although the physicians and their groups paid settlements, the hospital was held 60% liable for negligence on the part of the client's nurses. The jury noted in this case that the nurses had a responsibility to verify the correct placement of the NG tube before administering anything into it because the consequences of misplacement are so severe.

Reference: Nasogastric Tube Misplaced, 2008.

BOX 5.10 Examples of Potential Complications of Nasogastric Tubes

- Misplacement or migration of tube into client's lungs or esophagus
- Aspiration pneumonia caused by tube displacement or reflux of stomach contents
- Inadvertent esophageal perforation or bleeding
- Inadvertent entry of tube into brain during placement, leading to cerebral hemorrhage
- Skin irritation and breakdown (especially around nares)
- Mucosal irritation or development of retropharyngeal abscess

References: C.R. Bard, 2017; Shlamovitz & Kulkarni, 2018.

adapter (such as a 5-in-1 connector) to connect to suction tubing which then attaches to the suction drainage canister (see Skill 5.6). Intermittent suction requires an order, and it is important to use the lowest setting possible. Monitor the client closely to ensure that the blue "pigtail" air vent stays above the level of the stomach and remains clear of gastric fluid. If gastric contents appears in the air vent, this may be an indication of an obstruction in the main lumen. The blue pigtail may need to be cleared using a syringe and a small amount of air per facility policy. As noted, the blue air vent pigtail may only be cleared with air, *not* fluid (C. R. Bard, 2017).

Irrigation of the Nasogastric Sump Tube

In order to maintain the patency of an NG tube, the nurse must irrigate the tube at regular intervals (after verifying placement) as recommended by the manufacturer and facility policy. Irrigation may also be needed if the tube is not

BOX 5.11 Lessons From Experience: Troubleshooting Nasogastric Tubes

Mr. Brown is a 34-year-old client who has been admitted after cholecystectomy surgery. He has a double-lumen nasogastric (NG) sump tube in his right naris set to low intermittent suction. One evening (on the night shift), Mr. Brown's wife runs out of his room and states, "My husband's tube in his nose is leaking everywhere!" When the nurse enters Mr. Brown's room, she notices his NG tube is not sumping well. She also notices there are gastric contents backed up and dripping out of the blue "pigtail" air vent. In addition, Mr. Brown's abdomen appears distended. To assess Mr. Brown further, the nurse asks if he is having nausea or feelings of discomfort. The nurse also checks to make sure the NG and connecting tubing are intact, and she checks the NG tube for placement. In addition, the nurse measures the external length of the tubing to ensure it has not changed from baseline. Realizing the blue air vent should be dry and clear of gastric contents to sump properly, the nurse injects a small amount of air into the blue port to clear the gastric contents per guidelines. In addition, she gently irrigates the main lumen of the NG tube with 30 mL fluid per order (after placement checked). Before the nurse leaves, she also ensures the blue pigtail air vent is above the level of the stomach.

In this situation, Mr. Brown's NG tube was obstructed, causing a backflow of gastric contents into the blue air vent. In an NG sump tube, the blue air vent helps the tube work properly, and it prevents trauma to the mucosal lining of the stomach. The nurse assessed the client and intervened appropriately. If the nurse had experienced difficulty irrigating the NG tube, she could also reposition or turn the client (in order to move the tube off of his stomach wall). In addition, the nurse should monitor Mr. Brown and ensure his abdominal distention has improved.

sumping properly. The amount and type of irrigation are ordered by the authorized healthcare provider. For clients receiving enteral feedings (see Section 4 of this chapter), irrigation may need to be done more often. During irrigation, use gentle pressure, and never *force* fluid in. If difficulty is encountered, use problem-solving and troubleshooting skills (Box 5.11).

Care of Clients With Nasogastric Sump Tubes

When the client has an NG sump tube, it is essential to ensure the tube is working properly and that the tube remains taped securely in place so that it doesn't move around. Meticulous skin care is essential. Inspect the client's nares and make sure they are not becoming dry or irritated and that skin breakdown is not occurring. It is also important to ensure that the client's comfort needs are met. NG tubes can be uncomfortable. Clients with a large-bore NG tube are usually not eating. Therefore, it is important to provide frequent oral care, and if allowed, offer the client ice chips or mouth sponges to prevent the mucous membranes from getting dry and cracked.

SUMMARY

Gastric tube placement and gastric tube therapy must be performed by the licensed nurse. However, the monitoring and recording of fluid intake and gastric output/drainage can be performed by assistive personnel as needed. Delegation to assistive personnel will vary, depending on the state's nurse practice act. When providing care to clients who are receiving gastric therapy, safety is one of the most important critical concepts to consider in order to avoid complications. Because an NG tube can be uncomfortable and cause physical irritation during and after insertion, the client's comfort needs and client-centered care must also be addressed.

APPLICATION OF THE NURSING PROCESS

Examples of Related ICNP Nursing Diagnoses, Expected
    Client Outcomes, and Nursing Interventions:
Nursing Diagnosis: Impaired comfort
Supporting Data: Client is restless and states NG tube is
    "uncomfortable."
Expected Client Outcomes: Client will have decreased discomfort, as seen by:
  - no complaints of pain at NG sump tube insertion/exit site
  - absence of nonverbal signs of discomfort (e.g., picking at NG tube, rubbing nose at NG tube exit site, grimacing, agitation, restlessness).
Nursing Intervention Example: Stabilize NG tube to minimize movement.
Nursing Diagnosis: Risk for impaired skin integrity
Supporting Data: Client verbalizes that skin feels irritated at
    NG sump tube exit site.
Expected Client Outcomes: Client will have no evidence of impaired skin integrity, redness, or skin breakdown at the NG tube exit site or around the naris.
Nursing Intervention Example: Keep naris and NG tube exit site clean and dry.
Reference: International Classification for Nursing Practice. (n.d.) *eHealth & ICNP*. Retrieved from https://www.icn.ch/what-we-do/projects/ehealth-icnp.

CRITICAL CONCEPTS
Providing Gastric Tube Therapy

Accuracy (ACC)

Accuracy when providing gastric tube therapy is affected by the following variables:
  - assessment of the client, including LOC and orientation level, history, nutritional status, and gastrointestinal function
  - identification and selection of appropriate site (naris) for inserting the gastric tube

  - identification and selection of appropriate landmarks for measuring distance of the gastric tube insertion
  - technique used for the gastric tube placement and placement checks
  - technique used for checking and maintaining patency of the gastric tube
  - proper setup of equipment and settings used for suction (if using a gastric sump tube for decompression).

Client-Centered Care (CCC)

Respect for the client when providing gastric tube therapy is demonstrated through:
  - promoting autonomy and obtaining consent before inserting the tube
  - providing privacy and ensuring comfort during and after the procedure
  - honoring cultural preferences and using an interpreter if needed when explaining procedure and providing instructions
  - advocating for the client and family during and after the procedure.

Infection Control (INF)

Healthcare-associated infection when providing gastric tube therapy is prevented by:
  - preventing and reducing the transfer of microorganisms
  - reducing the number of microorganisms.

Safety (SAF)

Safety measures when providing gastric tube therapy prevent harm and create a safe care environment by reducing the risk of injury and ensuring that the gastric tube is placed correctly and remains securely taped in place.

Communication (COM)

  - Communication exchanges information (oral, written, nonverbal, or electronic) between two or more people.
  - Documentation records information in a permanent legal record.
  - Communication between the nurse and other healthcare providers and measurement of the length of exposed tubing ensures that the client's gastric tube remains securely in place and has not migrated.

Health Maintenance (HLTH)

Nursing is dedicated to the promotion of health during gastric tube therapy by:
  - preventing skin breakdown during gastric tube therapy
  - providing oral care and skin care during gastric tube therapy.

Evaluation (EVAL)

Evaluation of the outcomes with gastric tube therapy allows the nurse to determine the safety and efficacy of the care provided.

■ SKILL 5.5 Placement and Care of a Nasogastric (NG) Sump Tube

EQUIPMENT

NG sump tube (large bore), size 14 to 18 Fr (adults) or 10 to 14 Fr (pediatric clients)

Suction regulator, 5-in-1 connector, and connecting tubing if indicated

Yankauer suction catheter, if indicated

Topical anesthetic (if ordered)

Water-soluble lubricant

50- to 60-mL Piston/Toomey syringe

Irrigation fluid (if indicated)

Measuring tape, stethoscope, and pH paper

Clean gloves

Glass of water

Disposable absorbent pads

Towels and washcloths

Tissues and emesis basin (if needed)

Oral care supplies

Chlorhexidine mouth wash if indicated (and ordered)

Cotton-tipped applicators and normal saline

Hypoallergenic tape, commercial stat device, or nasal bridle

BEGINNING THE SKILL

1. **SAF** Review the order and review the client's medical/surgical history for contraindications (e.g., nasal or sinus surgery, nasal septum defects, basilar skull fracture) (see Box 5.6).
2. **INF** Perform hand hygiene.
3. **CCC** Introduce yourself to the client and family and explain the procedure.
4. **SAF** Identify the client using two identifiers.
5. **CCC** Provide privacy.
6. **ACC** Assess the client's orientation to person, time, place, and situation. *A baseline assessment of the client's LOC and orientation must be done in order to determine if the client can tolerate the placement of an NG sump tube and comprehend instructions.*
7. **CCC** Assess comfort needs. If the client is having pain, intervene accordingly before the procedure, and provide comfort measures (see Chapter 7). *Pain increases anxiety.*
8. **CCC** Ensure client consent has been obtained for the procedure. *Facilitates client autonomy.*

PROCEDURE

9. **INF** Apply clean gloves.
10. **SAF** Set up an ergonomically safe space. Raise the bed to a comfortable working height. Raise one side rail. *Setting up an ergonomically safe space prevents injury to the nurse and client.* (Note: After the procedure, return the bed to the lowest position to reduce the risk of falls.)
11. **ACC** Assess the client for nausea and/or vomiting, and assess the client's abdomen (all four quadrants) for bowel sounds. Note any distention or other problems. *An abdominal assessment is important to help establish a baseline for future comparison during gastric tube therapy.*
12. **HLTH** Assess the client's nares for obstructions, deviations, or skin breakdown, and inspect mucous membranes at the back of the throat for mucositis or any lesions.
13. **ACC** Assess one naris at a time for patency. Ask the client to place his or her finger on the side of each naris while breathing through the other. Select the naris that is more patent for tube placement. *This ensures that the correct naris is selected for the NG tube.*
14. **ACC** Prepare the environment for the procedure:
    a. Get a temporary piece of tape ready and tab the ends of the tape.
    b. If the client will be on intermittent suction for decompression, set up canisters and connecting tubing ahead of time and make sure the suction is working.
    c. **SAF** If the client is at high risk for aspiration, set up Yankauer-tip suction.
15. **ACC** Prepare the client for the procedure:
    a. Elevate the client's HOB to the high-Fowler's position if not contraindicated. *Facilitates placement of the tube.*
    b. **CCC** Place towels or disposable absorbent pads over the client's chest.
    c. **CCC** Provide tissues and emesis basin for the client.
    d. **CCC** If ordered, spray topical anesthesia as needed for comfort.
16. **ACC** Estimate the length of tubing that will be inserted by using the NEX + 10 (cm) approach. Measure from the tip of the nose to the earlobe, and from the earlobe to the xiphoid process (NEX), then add 10 cm. Place a piece of tape at this point or use a marker to mark the tube. *The NEX method alone may not provide an accurate estimate. Adding an additional 10 cm to the NEX estimate or using an alternative method may help ensure that the NG tube will reach the client's gastric pool (Taylor, 2014) (see Box 5.7)*

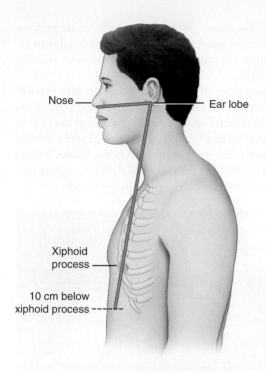

STEP 16 Estimate length of tubing for insertion.

17. **SAF** Lubricate the tube generously with a water-soluble lubricant along the full length that will be inserted, or follow the manufacturer recommendations (C. R. Bard, 2017). *Generous lubrication prevents damage to the client's mucous membranes.* **WARNING:** Avoid the use of petroleum-based products on the tube. Petroleum-based products can harm the client's respiratory tract if there is an inadvertent insertion into the lungs.

18. **ACC** Ask the client to lean forward slightly. Ensure that the client's head is neutral or flexed down slightly if not contraindicated. *This helps avoid insertion of the tube into the airway* (C. R. Bard, 2017).

19. **SAF** Ask the client to raise a hand or finger and alert you if he or she experiences any distress or significant discomfort during the procedure. *Prevents harm to the client.*

20. **ACC** While the client is leaning forward slightly, insert the NG tube into the selected naris. Gently advance the tube back toward the nasopharynx. If needed, rotate the tip of the tube gently to help the tube advance through the selected naris. **WARNING:** Do NOT angle the tube up into the nose. (Note: When you reach the crest of the nasopharynx, you may feel a slight resistance as the pathway turns down.)

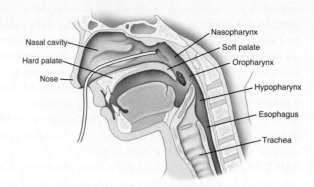

STEP 20 Insert NG tube and advance it toward nasopharynx.

21. **ACC** Once you reach the nasopharynx, guide the tube down by placing your thumb under the tube to achieve an arc. Instruct the client to tuck his or her chin toward the chest and flex the neck forward slightly while looking down. *This angle will close the epiglottis and facilitate passage of the tube through the oropharynx and into the esophagus.*

22. **ACC** As you continue to advance the tube, ask the client to take sips of water and swallow while keeping the neck flexed down. (Note: Be prepared for the tube to advance when the client swallows. Do not prevent the tube from moving with swallowing.)

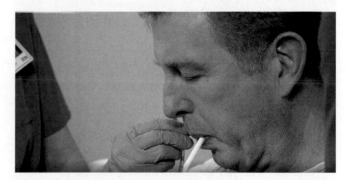

STEP 22 Instruct the client to swallow as you advance the tube.

23. **SAF** If you feel significant resistance, inspect inside the oral cavity (with a penlight if necessary) and check to see if the tube has coiled or kinked. **WARNING:** Never force the tube into the client. *Forcing the NG tube could damage the client's mucosa and cause injury* (McGinnis, 2017).

24. **SAF** If you are having difficulty advancing the tube, reposition the client, unkink the tube if necessary by pulling back enough to straighten the tube, and try again. Encourage the client to swallow. *Client swallowing facilitates moving the tube past the epiglottis into the esophagus.*

25. **SAF** During insertion, continuously monitor the client for signs of respiratory distress (e.g., coughing, inability to speak). If the client experiences these symptoms or

any other problems, such as significant bleeding or severe pain, stop the procedure, immediately withdraw the tube, and allow the client to recover. *Coughing, gagging, and/or an inability to speak are signs the tube may have inadvertently entered the lungs and must be removed immediately.*

26. **SAF** If the tube has to be withdrawn and reinserted, use a different naris if possible. *This is a safety measure.*
27. **ACC** If the client is tolerating the procedure without distress, continue to advance the tube to the identified mark or tape, and hold the tube in place.
28. **SAF** While continuing to hold the tube in place, tape the tube securely with the temporary tape while you check the placement. *Prevents the tube from becoming displaced.*
29. **ACC** Aspirate (draw back) the NG tube contents and note the odor, color, consistency, and texture. Gastric aspirate is usually grassy green or yellow. If there is significant bleeding, notify the authorized provider. *Assessing aspirate alerts the nurse of proper placement and certain disorders.* (Note: Bright red blood or coffee-ground emesis should be reported immediately because it could indicate bleeding or other disorders.)

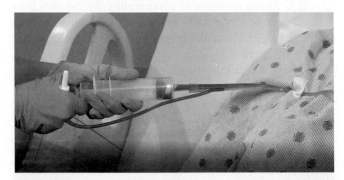

STEP 29 Assess gastric aspirate.

30. **ACC** Verify the placement of the NG tube by using a variety of methods, including checking the pH of the aspirate. The pH of gastric aspirate should be ≤5 (see Box 5.8). **WARNING:** The "swoosh test" alone is *not* a valid or reliable check for NG tube placement.

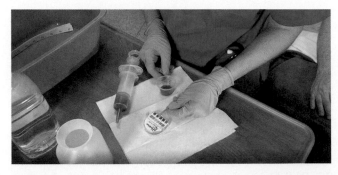

STEP 30 Check gastric pH.

31. **SAF** Before irrigation, tube feedings, or medication administration, NG tube placement must be verified by an x-ray per policy. *An x-ray is the gold standard and most accurate method for checking NG tube placement* (AACN, 2016a).
32. **SAF** After NG tube placement is verified, prep skin and secure tape or commercial stat-lock device in place.

Prevents dislodgement. (Note: Many facilities are now using commercial stat-lock devices or nasal bridles to secure NG tubes because they may provide more stability [Mann, 2016].)

33. **ACC** If using tape: (A) Split half of the tape into two different tails and secure the un-split part of the tape on the bridge of the client's nose vertically. (B) Wrap each of the split pieces (one at a time) in a downward spiral around the NG sump tube in opposite directions. (Note: If there is a risk of exposure to the client's body fluids, ensure that clean gloves are worn during the taping procedure.)

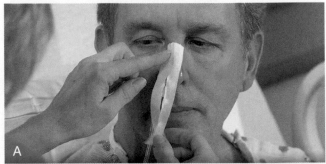

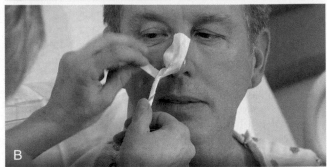

STEP 33 Prepare and secure tape.

34. **SAF** If using a commercial stat-lock device or nasal bridle, ensure that it is placed securely on the nose and NG tube.

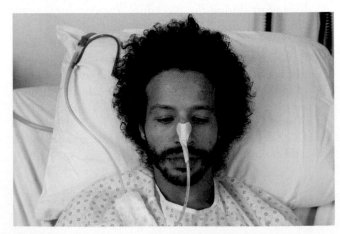

STEP 34 Client with a commercial stat-lock device.

35. **ACC** If the client will be on gastric suction, connect the NG tube securely to the connecting tubing (see Skill 5.6).

36. **ACC** Ensure that the blue pigtail air vent of the NG sump tube is above the level of the stomach and that the NG sump tube is working properly. *Prevents reflux into the NG sump tube and helps the tube sump properly.*

37. **ACC** If the NG sump tube will be capped or there will be a delay in initiating feedings, flush the main lumen of the NG tube with 30 mL of irrigation fluid as required by facility policy, AFTER placement is confirmed. *Flushing prevents clogging of the NG tube*

38. **ACC WARNING:** Do *not* inject fluid into the blue pigtail air vent or antireflux filter. (Note: The purpose of the air vent is to allow air in while fluid is being drawn out of the stomach.) *The blue pigtail air vent is designed for air only, not fluid (C. R. Bard, 2017).*

39. **SAF** Mark the tube at the naris exit site with indelible marker and measure the length of the exposed tube from where it is taped at the nose to the end of the main lumen of the NG tube. Record the length of the exposed tube in centimeters. *This is an important safety measure that provides information to help verify placement.*

40. **CCC** Secure the NG sump tube securely to the client's gown with tape if needed. Avoid using safety pins. *Securing the NG tube provides stability and prevents dislodgement.*

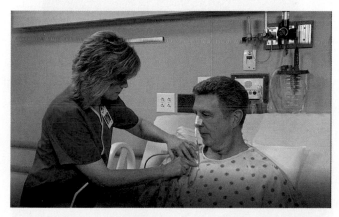

STEP 40 Secure the nasogastric tube to the gown.

41. **CCC** Provide comfort care to the client by providing washcloths and offering oral care.
42. **INF** Dispose of equipment according to facility policy.

FINISHING THE SKILL

43. **INF** Remove gloves and perform hand hygiene.
44. **SAF** Ensure safety and comfort. Ensure that the bed is in the lowest position and verify that the client can identify and reach the nurse call system. *These safety measures reduce the risk of falls.*
45. **EVAL** Evaluate the outcomes. Did the client tolerate the procedure? If the client was placed on NG tube gastric suction, is the NG tube secure and sumping properly?

46. **COM** Document assessment findings, care given, and outcomes in the legal healthcare record:
    • type, size, and purpose of NG tube
    • naris chosen for NG sump tube insertion
    • verification of placement and methods used
    • length of exposed tubing recorded in centimeters

Providing Follow-up Care After Placement of an NG Sump Tube

(Note: Perform hand hygiene and apply clean gloves for all follow-up steps as indicated)

47. **EVAL** Continue to monitor and verify placement of the NG tube at regular intervals.
48. **SAF** Measure and record (in centimeters) the exposed length of the NG tubing from the exit site at the nose to the end of the main lumen of the NG tube and compare it to previous measurements at regular intervals. *Helps ensure that the NG tube has not migrated.*
49. **EVAL** If the client is on NG sump tube suction, continue to monitor the color of the gastric aspirate and ensure that the NG tube is sumping properly (see Skill 5.6).
50. **ACC** If the client is not on NG sump tube suction, flush or irrigate the tube (after placement is verified) at regular intervals per facility policy (see Skill 5.7).
51. **INF** Clean the entire length of exposed NG sump tube as needed with a washcloth and soap and water. *Prevents crust buildup on the tube and promotes hygiene.*
52. **HLTH** Inspect the naris for skin irritation, inflammation, or breakdown. If the nares are dry and irritated, use cotton-tipped applicators and apply water-soluble lubricant as indicated.
53. **HLTH** Clean the area around the naris as needed using warm water and/or saline and cotton-tipped applicators. *Cleaning prevents the buildup of debris that could cause irritation.*
54. **CCC** Provide oral care at regular intervals and as needed. *Clients with NG tubes can easily get dry mouth, and they need meticulous oral care to prevent irritation and lesions.*
    a. Inspect oral cavity for dryness, irritation, or lesions.
    b. Use saline swabs if indicated and clean the buccal cavity and under the tongue.
    c. Use chlorhexidine mouthwash if indicated and ordered. (Note: This may be recommended for clients who have a high risk of aspiration pneumonia.)
    d. Lubricate lips with water or water-soluble lubricant as needed.

■ **SKILL 5.6** Initiating and Managing Nasogastric (NG) Sump Tube Suction

EQUIPMENT

Wall or portable suction regulator
Connecting tubing (2 sets)
Adapter or 5-in-1 connector
Suction canisters
Measuring tape, stethoscope, and pH paper
60-mL Piston/Toomey syringe
Irrigation fluid (if indicated)
Clean gloves
Disposable absorbent pads
Oral care supplies

BEGINNING THE SKILL

1. **ACC** Review order for:
   - purpose of suction (e.g., decompression)
   - type of suction (usually low intermittent)
   - amount of suction (e.g., mm Hg). (Note: Use the lowest suction setting that will allow gastric decompression. For wall suction, set at low—30–40 mm Hg [C. R. Bard, 2017])
2. **INF** Perform hand hygiene.
3. **CCC** Introduce yourself to the client and family and explain the procedure.
4. **SAF** Identify the client using two identifiers.
5. **CCC** Provide privacy.

PROCEDURE

6. **SAF** Prepare equipment for the procedure:
   a. Set up and secure suction regulator (portable or wall) per order and ensure that it is working properly.

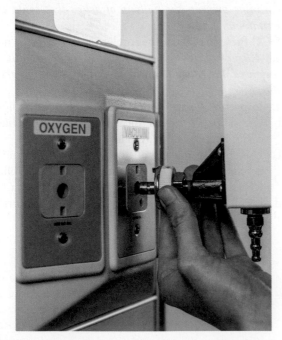

STEP 6A Secure the suction regulator.

b. Attach connecting tubing to regulator.

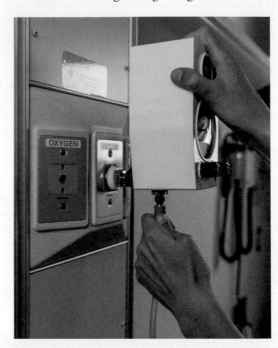

STEP 6B Attaching connecting tubing to regulator.

c. Attach connecting tubings to canisters.

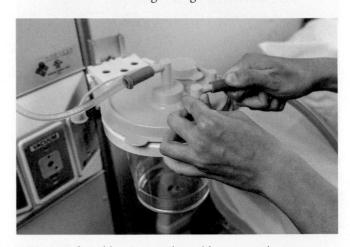

STEP 6C Attaching connecting tubings to canisters.

d. Turn on gastric low intermittent suction. Ensure that suction is working and does not exceed the maximum recommended mm Hg by placing your thumb over the distal end of the suction tubing. (Note: When the end of the suction tubing is occluded, the reading on the suction regulator will increase). *Setting the suction regulator to the appropriate range includes determining the greatest amount of suction incurred when the end is occluded because this could potentially be the amount of suction if the catheter becomes lodged against the mucosa.*

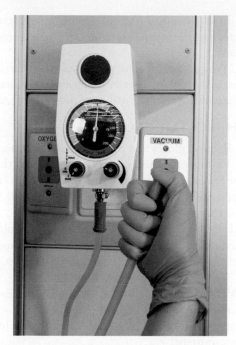

STEP 6D Check to ensure the suction is working.

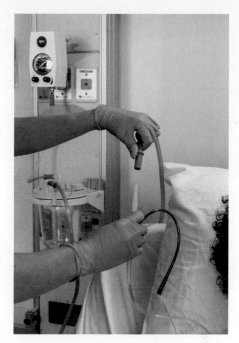

STEP 12 Attach the connecting tubing to the nasogastric tube.

7. **INF** Apply clean gloves (if not already on).
8. **ACC** Assess the client for nausea and/or vomiting, and assess the client's abdomen (all four quadrants) for bowel sounds. Note any distention or other problems. *A baseline abdominal assessment is important for monitoring improvements or future problems.*
9. **CCC** Place disposable absorbent pads or towels under the client's NG sump tube. *Promotes comfort and prevents the client from becoming soiled by gastric contents.*
10. **SAF** Check the placement of the NG sump tube (see Box 5.8) and ensure that the client's tube is taped securely. *Placement must be confirmed before fluids can be instilled into the NG tube.*
11. **SAF** Measure the exposed length of tubing and compare it to length on insertion in centimeters. *Helps ensure that the NG sump tube has not migrated or become displaced.*
12. **SAF** Attach the connecting tubing from the suction canister to the main lumen of the client's NG tube and ensure that these connections are secure. Use a 5-in-1 adapter if necessary.

13. **SAF** Increase intermittent suction gradually and use the lowest suction possible per order that will decompress the stomach. *This procedure will reduce trauma to the mucosal lining of the stomach.*
14. **ACC** Observe tubing until gastric contents begin suctioning and flowing into the receptacles. *This ensures that gastric suction is working properly.*
15. **ACC** Assess gastric contents being suctioned and note the odor, color, consistency, and texture. If there is unusual or excessive bleeding, notify the appropriate healthcare provider. *Assessing gastric contents alerts the nurse of proper placement. Gastric contents should be grassy green. Significant bright red bleeding or coffee-ground emesis should be reported.*
16. **ACC** If the NG tube does not appear to be sumping or allowing suctioning to occur, reposition the client and reassess sumping. If the NG tube is still not sumping properly, irrigate the tube with 5 to 10 mL fluid per order (after placement check; see Skill 5.7). *Repositioning may allow the end of the NG tube to dislodge and suction properly.*
17. **ACC** Ensure that the blue pigtail air vent is above the level of the stomach and that the NG tube is working properly. *Facilitates efficiency and prevents reflux of gastric contents into the air vent.*
18. **SAF** If gastric contents are noted in the blue pigtail air vent, inject a small amount of air into the antireflux valve or the air vent per the manufacturer recommendations. **WARNING:** Never inject fluid into the blue pigtail air vent. It is only designed for air injections. *The blue pigtail prevents reflux into the NG tube. Keeping the blue pigtail dry and clear of gastric contents facilitates proper sumping of the NG tube.*

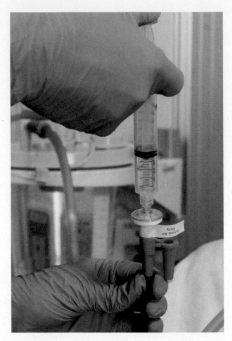

STEP 18 Clear the air vent, if needed, with air only (not fluid).

19. **EVAL** Continue to monitor the client for proper sumping and suctioning of the NG tube.
20. **EVAL** Evaluate the client's abdomen and compare to baseline assessment. Note if the client's abdomen is soft and if the distention is decreasing. *It is important to ensure that gastric suctioning is properly decompressing the stomach.*
21. **CCC** Provide oral care and moist oral swabs for the client as needed. *Provides moisture and prevents dryness, irritation, and skin breakdown of mucosa from lack of oral intake.*

FINISHING THE SKILL

22. **INF** Remove gloves and perform hand hygiene.
23. **SAF** Ensure safety and comfort. Ensure that the bed is in the lowest position and verify that the client can identify and reach the nurse call system. *These safety measures reduce the risk of falls.*
24. **EVAL** Evaluate the outcomes. Did the client tolerate the procedure? Is the NG sump tube sumping properly? Is the client's abdominal distention or discomfort improving?
25. **COM** Document assessment findings, care given, and outcomes in the legal healthcare record:
    - type and amount of gastric suction used (e.g., low intermittent)
    - exposed length of external tubing recorded in centimeters
    - placement verification
    - odor, color, consistency, and texture of gastric contents.

■ SKILL 5.7 Irrigating a Nasogastric (NG) Sump Tube

EQUIPMENT

Sterile water (room temperature)
Irrigation kit (if available)
50- to 60-mL Piston/Toomey syringe
Measuring tape and pH paper
Clean gloves
Disposable absorbent pads
Towels and washcloths
Oral care supplies

BEGINNING THE SKILL

1. **ACC** Review order for type and amount of irrigation fluid.
2. **INF** Perform hand hygiene.
3. **CCC** Introduce yourself to the client and family and explain the procedure.
4. **SAF** Identify the client using two identifiers.
5. **CCC** Provide privacy.

PROCEDURE

6. **INF** Apply clean gloves.
7. **CCC** Place disposable absorbent pads or towels on the client's chest and/or under the client's NG sump tube.

Prevents the client from becoming soiled from gastric contents and irrigation fluid.

8. **SAF** Check the placement of the NG sump tube (see Box 5.8) and ensure that the client's tube is taped securely. *Placement must be confirmed before fluids can be instilled into the NG tube.*
9. **SAF** Measure the exposed length of tubing and compare it to the length on insertion in centimeters. *Helps ensure that the NG sump tube has not migrated or become displaced.*
10. **SAF** Evaluate the patency of the NG sump tube.
    a. If the client is on gastric suction, observe gastric contents and observe the odor, color, consistency, and character of NG sump tube aspirate.
    b. If the client's NG sump tube is capped, aspirate a small amount of gastric contents.
    c. Observe the blue pigtail air vent for the presence of gastric contents. *Gastric contents within the blue air vent could be an indication of an obstruction.*
11. **ACC** Draw up 30 to 50 mL (or whatever is ordered) of irrigation fluid. Ensure the fluid is at room temperature. *Irrigation fluid that is cold could cause cramping or spasms.*

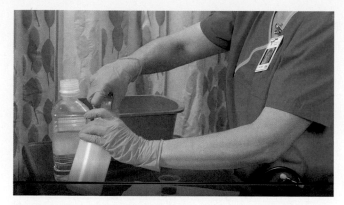
STEP 11 Draw up irrigation fluid.

12. **ACC** If the client is on gastric suction, turn the suction off, fold over or pinch the end of the tube, and disconnect the NG sump tube from the connecting tubing. *Folding over the tube before disconnecting from the connecting tubing prevents excess air from inadvertently entering the client's stomach.*

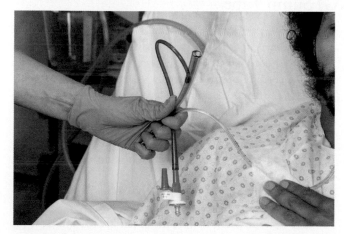
STEP 12 Fold over or clamp the nasogastric tubing.

13. **ACC** Place piston syringe in the main clear lumen of the NG sump tube.

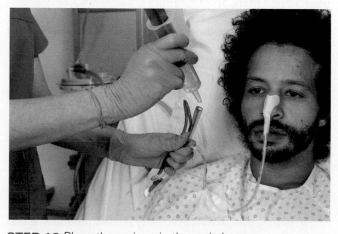
STEP 13 Place the syringe in the main lumen.

14. **SAF** Release tubing and gently instill irrigation fluid. **WARNING:** Do *not* irrigate blue pigtail air vent. *Only the*

main clear lumen of the NG tube may have fluids instilled. The blue air vent is not designed for fluid instillation.

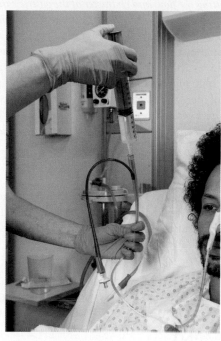
STEP 14 Instill irrigation fluid after releasing or unclamping the tube.

15. **ACC If irrigating by the gravity method:**
    a. Remove the plunger from barrel of the piston/Toomey syringe.
    b. Pinch, clamp, or fold over the tubing of the NG sump tube. *Prevents air from entering the client's stomach before the piston syringe barrel is placed on the tube.*
    c. Place the syringe barrel on the main (clear) port of the NG tube.
    d. Hold the syringe barrel and tube securely as a unit to prevent slipping. *Holding the syringe/tube securely prevents disconnection and loss of fluid.*
    e. While the NG sump tubing remains clamped, pour irrigation fluid into barrel of syringe. Then un-clamp or release the tubing and allow fluid to slowly flow in by gravity. (Note: The amount of irrigation fluid used may vary, depending on the order.)
    f. During irrigation, elevate the syringe barrel above level of client's stomach no more than 45 centimeters (18 inches). *The height of the syringe affects the gravity flow. The higher the syringe, the faster the flow. If the syringe is lowered, the rate will slow down.*

16. **ACC** If the irrigation fluid won't go in or resistance is met, reposition the client, wait a few minutes, and try again. If irrigation fluid still will not go in, gently aspirate the tube back and forth in a "milking" pattern. **WARNING:** Do not force irrigation. *Repositioning the client may help release the end of the NG tube if it is up against the wall of the stomach. Forcing irrigation may damage and disrupt the integrity of the tube.*

17. **ACC** When irrigation is complete, pinch end or fold over NG sump tubing, remove piston/Toomey syringe, and reconnect the tube to suction or cap tube per order.

18. **EVAL** If the NG sump tube is connected to suction, evaluate the flow and character of the gastric contents. *Evaluating the flow and character of the gastric contents after irrigation helps determine the effectiveness of the procedure.*

19. **ACC** Ensure that the blue pigtail air vent is above the level of the stomach and that there are no gastric contents in the blue air vent. If gastric contents are noted in the blue pigtail, inject a small amount of air into the air vent per manufacturer recommendations. *The blue pigtail prevents reflux into the NG tube. Keeping the pigtail dry and clear of gastric contents facilitates the functioning of the tube.*

FINISHING THE SKILL

20. **INF** Remove gloves and perform hand hygiene.
21. **SAF** Ensure safety and comfort. Ensure that the bed is in the lowest position and verify that the client can iden-tify and reach the nurse call system. *These safety measures reduce the risk of falls.*

22. **EVAL** Evaluate the outcomes. Did the client tolerate the procedure? Did irrigation fluid go in without any dif-ficulty? If the client is on suction, is the tube sumping properly after irrigation? Is the gastric aspirate flowing into the canister without any difficulty?

23. **COM** Document assessment findings, care given, and outcomes in the legal healthcare record:
    - type and amount of irrigation fluid used
    - tube placement verification
    - exposed length of external tubing recorded in centi-meters
    - odor, color, consistency, and texture of gastric con-tents.

■ SKILL 5.8 Discontinuing a Nasogastric (NG) Sump Tube

EQUIPMENT

Clean gloves
50- to 60-mL Piston/Toomey syringe, sterile water (if needed)
Airway suction apparatus (if needed)
Disposable absorbent pads
Towels and washcloths
Tissues and emesis basin (if needed)
Oral care supplies

BEGINNING THE SKILL

1. **SAF** Review order.
2. **INF** Perform hand hygiene.
3. **CCC** Introduce yourself to the client and family and explain the procedure.
4. **SAF** Identify the client using two identifiers.
5. **CCC** Provide privacy.

PROCEDURE

6. **ACC** Assess the client for nausea/vomiting, and assess the client's abdomen (all four quadrants) for any disten-tion. If the client is having emesis or any other signs of gastrointestinal distress, notify the authorized healthcare provider before discontinuing the NG sump tube.

7. **INF** Apply clean gloves.
8. **SAF** Prepare the client for the procedure:
    a. Elevate the client's HOB at least 45 degrees.
    b. Place towels or disposable absorbant over the client's chest.
    c. Provide tissues and emesis basin for the client.
    d. Set up airway suction or Yankauer-tip suction if needed.
9. **SAF** Prepare the NG tube for removal:

a. If the client is on gastric suction, turn off suction and use a small amount of air to clear the NG tube according to facility policy. *(McGinnis, 2017)*

b. If the client is on tube feeding, turn off the pump and clear the tube before removal. *Prevents aspira-tion of gastric tube contents during removal (McGinnis, 2017).*

10. **HLTH** Remove tape gently from the nose. Use adhesive remover if necessary.

11. **SAF** Clamp or fold over the NG tube. *Prevents aspira-tion of residual contents from the tube.*

12. **SAF** Ask the client to hold his or her breath and close his or her eyes while you carefully remove the tube. *This may prevent aspiration by closing off the client's airway during removal. Closing the eyes during removal may prevent gas-tric contents from spraying into the client's eyes.*

13. **ACC** Measure the NG sump tube gastric aspirate/drain-age in the suction canister and record before disposal. *Provides proper documentation of amount and character of drainage.*

14. **INF** Dispose of equipment according to facility policy.

15. **CCC** Clean the client's face and mouth as needed. *Pro-vides moisture and prevents dryness, irritation, and skin breakdown of mucosa from lack of oral intake.*

16. **HLTH** Provide skin care around the naris where the tape was attached and around the client's other naris if needed. *Skin care promotes comfort and prevents skin breakdown.*

17. **CCC** Provide oral care and use moist oral swabs for the client as needed. *Provides moisture and prevents dryness, irritation, and skin breakdown of mucosa from lack of oral intake.*

FINISHING THE SKILL

18. **INF** Remove gloves and perform hand hygiene.
19. **SAF** Ensure safety and comfort. Ensure that the bed is in the lowest position and verify that the client can identify and reach the nurse call system. *These safety measures reduce the risk of falls.*
20. **EVAL** Evaluate the outcomes. Did the client tolerate the procedure? Was the NG tube intact upon removal?

21. **COM** Document assessment findings, care given, and outcomes in the legal healthcare record:
    - color and character of gastric aspirate/drainage in canister before disposal
    - appearance of NG tube, including tip, upon removal (e.g., Is it intact?).
22. **EVAL** Provide follow-up monitoring by ensuring that the client is tolerating removal of the tube and has no signs of abdominal distention or nausea and vomiting.

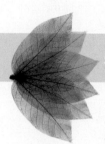

SECTION 4 Providing Enteral Nutrition

Ideally, taking in food orally is the best way to receive nutrients as chewing and saliva initiate digestion. However, when a client is unable to meet his or her nutritional requirements orally, the client may require enteral nutrition (EN). EN is the direct administration of nutrients into the stomach, duodenum, or jejunum by way of a feeding tube, catheter, or stoma, and it usually requires an order by the authorized healthcare provider. EN may be temporary or long term, and it may be needed for clients who are having difficulty chewing or swallowing or for those who have altered digestion in the upper gastrointestinal tract. It may also be indicated for clients who cannot eat because they are comatose or those who have a decreased LOC.

ROUTES OF ENTERAL FEEDING

Depending on the needs of your client, a variety of different routes may be selected. The placement and choice of a feeding route are usually determined by the client's medical and social history, the duration for which the client may need enteral therapy, and the client's risk of aspiration (Dudek, 2018). Feeding tubes are classified as to where they are inserted and where the distal tip ends up (e.g., stomach, duodenum, jejunum). For example, the tubes may be placed through the nose and into the stomach (e.g., nasogastric) or the small intestine (e.g., nasoduodenal [ND], nasojejunal [NJ]). As an alternative, the tubes may be inserted percutaneously or through an adapter into a surgically made stoma such as a gastrostomy or jejunostomy (Mazur & Litch, 2019). An illustration of these routes is seen in Fig. 5.6. The advantages, disadvantages, and various routes are discussed shortly.

Enteral Tubes

In the acute care setting, most of the tubes that are inserted nasally, such as NG, ND, and NJ tubes, are usually for short-term use (<4–6 weeks). In particular, a large-bore NG sump tube (see Section 3 of this chapter) is only appropriate for very short-term feeding because of irritation to the nasal tissues and the discomfort caused by the larger diameter of the tube. Small-bore feeding tubes come in a variety of sizes and are preferred for feeding over large-bore tubes to reduce the risk of esophageal trauma, sinusitis, and tissue necrosis (Dudek, 2018). Examples of various small-bore feeding tubes are seen in Fig. 5.7.

Occasionally, feeding tubes are inserted orally; however, the orogastric (OG) route is primarily used with premature infants prior to the development of a gag reflex. When a premature infant begins to take some feedings orally but continues to receive tube feedings, then the route is usually NG (Brown et al., 2016). For more information on enteral feeding of neonates and infants, see Box 5.12 and Fig. 5.8.

One of the disadvantages of a small-bore feeding tube is that it may become easily obstructed or it may be difficult to aspirate through the tube. Some facilities discourage aspirating through a small-bore tube because of the risk of tube collapse, resulting in damage to the tube.

It is important to note that nasally inserted small-bore feeding tubes are single-lumen tubes, and they are *not* designed for suctioning of gastric contents or decompression. If your client develops severe nausea and/or vomiting, a large-bore NG sump tube may be indicated for suction or decompression (see Section 3 of this chapter).

Nasally Inserted Tubes That Use Electromagnetic Technology

One option available to some clients is a nasally inserted feeding tube that uses electromagnetic technology to guide placement. With this system, the tip of the feeding tube stylet contains an electromagnetic transmitter that generates a signal that is tracked by a receiver that is placed at the client's xiphoid process as the tube is placed in the client. By using a computer screen that displays a graphic representation (both anterior and cross-sectional), placement of the feeding tube can be validated by showing the location of the tip of the tube as it is advanced. Other emerging technologies involve integrated systems whereby a camera is embedded in the feeding tube to allow the nurse or other provider to identify anatomical markers during placement.

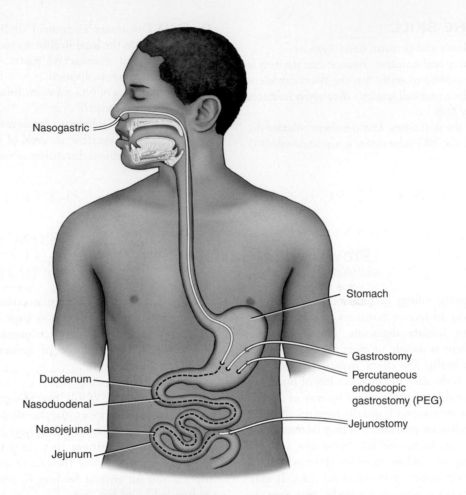

FIG. 5.6 Examples of routes for feeding tubes.

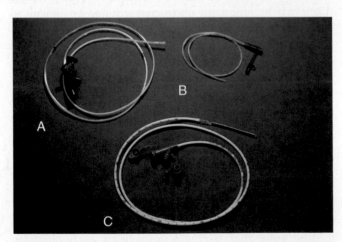

FIG. 5.7 Examples of small-bore feeding tubes. **A,** Feeding tube with non-weighted tip. **B,** Premature infant/neonatal feeding tube. **C,** Feeding tube with weighted tip.

Placement of Nasally Inserted Small-Bore Feeding Tubes

When placing a small-bore feeding tube, the procedure is similar to placing a large-bore NG sump tube (see Section 3 of this chapter). However, small-bore tubes are usually softer and more flexible, and they may be weighted in order to facilitate insertion into the stomach or small intestine. Some feeding tubes may also have a guidewire that facilitates insertion and a special coating that self-lubricates when placed in water. If using a guidewire, never place it back into the tube once the tube has been placed because this could cause a serious injury. Check your facility policy. Some facilities do not allow nurses to place feeding tubes that require a guidewire because of potential complications.

Once the feeding tube is in place, check the placement according to policy using a variety of methods (see Box 5.8). In most facilities, the placement of a feeding tube must first be verified by x-ray prior to feedings or irrigation, then rechecked at regular intervals thereafter. To maintain patency, flush the client's feeding tube on a regular basis (Box 5.13), and provide meticulous oral care even if the client is not eating.

Gastrostomy and PEG Tubes

For clients who need long-term feedings, a gastrostomy (G-tube) may be indicated. G-tubes (usually large bore) are placed directly into the stomach through a surgically created opening (stoma) in the abdominal wall. G-tubes are commonly used to deliver feedings or hydration, although they can also be used to vent air and drainage from the stomach.

A variation of a surgical gastrostomy is a percutaneous endoscopic gastrostomy (PEG) tube, which is placed by

BOX 5.12 Lifespan Considerations: Caring for Pediatric Clients Receiving Enteral Nutrition

An infant or a child receiving enteral nutrition (EN) may have specific needs, depending on their age, size, and developmental level. Infants or children may receive enteral nutrition when requiring respiratory support that prevent oral feedings. Premature infants may also receive a combination of oral and enteral feedings when they are not strong enough to take all of their feedings orally. Orogastric placement is preferred for premature infants with high oxygen needs and without a gag reflex. Nasogastric placement is preferred in infants who are also breastfeeding or other oral feedings and/or who show a gag reflex. (Brown et al., 2016)

Additional considerations regarding pediatric EN include the following:

- For gastric intubation, the NEMU (**N**ose-**E**arlobe-**M**idway between the xiphoid and **U**mbilicus) approach is preferred for estimating the length of insertion (Brown, 2017) (see Fig. 5.5). For additional information related to gastric tube therapy, see Section 3 of this chapter.
- If the client is a child >2 weeks old, specific age-related, height-based methods may need to be used for predicting the length of the enteral tube. However, this method can only help predict the length of the initial placement of the tube, not the location (Lyman et al. 2016).
- The formula chosen for infants and children will depend on the client's clinical and medical condition as well as the client's specific nutrient requirements.
- Infants and children <1 year of age will receive breast milk if available.
- Infants receiving enteral feeding may benefit from non-nutritive sucking (NNS).
- After insertion, check the tube for placement according to best practice (see Box 5.8) and facility policy. As with adult clients, tube placement must be monitored before *each* feeding, irrigation, or medication administration and at regular intervals.
- When administering intermittent feedings, allow the feeding to go in slowly by gravity. (Note: 30 minutes is appropriate for a premature infant.) (Brown et al., 2016)
- When aspirating the tube to check gastric contents, pull back *gently* to avoid traumatizing the child's gastric mucosa.
- When flushing an enteral tube on a pediatric client, use the lowest volume necessary to clear the tube. For example, neonates may need less than 1 to 2 mL and infants may only require 2 to 3 mL to clear the tube (Brown et al., 2016; Boullata, 2017).
- If child has NG or OG tube, ensure that tube is secured to the face in a manner that does not cause an adhesive-related skin injury (see Fig. 5.8).
- Provide emotional support and family teaching as needed.

References: Boullata et al. 2017; Brown, 2017; Brown et al, 2016; Lyman et al. 2016.

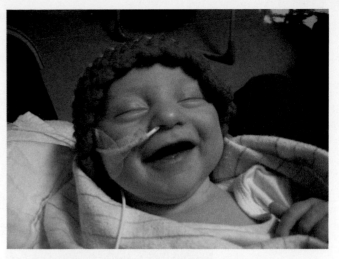

FIG. 5.8 A child with a feeding tube securely taped in place.

BOX 5.13 Recommendations for Flushing Enteral Tubes

To maintain patency of enteral tubes, regular flushing is recommended. The type and amount of flush used will vary depending on the order and the manufacturer recommendations. The client's age, medical status, and type of tube must be considered. For example, a client who is immunosuppressed, a neonate or pediatric client, or a client who has a jejunostomy may require sterile water for flushes. If the client is at risk for volume overload, keep track of the volume of flushes he or she is receiving. Carefully check the placement of the tube *before* flushing or irrigation (see Box 5.8). Depending on policy, flushing should be done at the following times:

- Before and after every feeding
- Each time a feeding is discontinued
- Each time a feeding set is discontinued
- Each time a feeding is stopped or interrupted
- Every 4 hours during continuous feedings or between bolus/intermittent feedings
- Before and after medication administration
- After Gastric Residual Volume (GRV) checks

References: Boullata et al., 2017; Covidien, n.d.

using an endoscope. With this procedure, the authorized healthcare provider places a flexible tube directly into the stomach through a small incision in the abdominal wall. Both the surgical G-tube and the PEG tube are made of special materials to prevent long-term damage to the tube by digestive acids. As seen in Fig. 5.9A, the PEG tube may have a mushroom catheter tip that is held in place by a collapsible internal bumper. An external bumper or flange also helps stabilize the PEG tube. Depending on the style of the appliance and the manufacturer, the internal and external bumpers may vary in appearance and name (e.g., retention disk, crossbar). As an alternative, the PEG tube may be held in place by a retention balloon (see Fig. 5.9B). For both styles of PEG tubes, an adapter is usually attached to the distal or

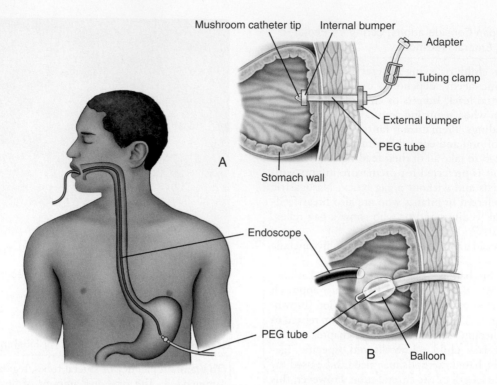

FIG. 5.9 A, PEG tube with mushroom catheter tip. **B,** PEG tube with retention balloon.

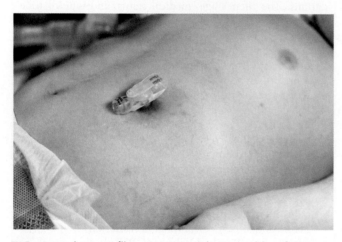

FIG. 5.10 Low-profile gastrostomy button with safety cap in place.

external end of the tube to allow administration of feedings, fluids, or medications (Ecklund, 2017).

Another option that is becoming increasingly common is a low-profile gastrostomy feeding button (e.g., MIC-KEY style button). These devices are held in place by a mushroom-shaped dome that is level with the client's skin (Fig. 5.10). Feedings are given through the button into the stomach using an adapter. Between feedings, the button is flushed and stays in place. It is also capped by an attached safety plug. Gastrostomy buttons are often the first choice for pediatric clients or clients who have an active lifestyle.

Jejunostomy Tubes

If a client is at high risk for aspiration or has had a gastrectomy (partial or total removal of the stomach), then the client may receive feedings into the jejunum. There are several options for delivering feedings into the jejunum. The client may require a jejunostomy or a percutaneous endoscopic jejunostomy (PEJ), which allows feedings directly into the small intestine (see Fig. 5.6). Because the acidic fluids of the stomach are bypassed, strict infection control is required, and sterile water is recommended when flushing the jejunostomy tube (Mann, 2016). One of the disadvantages of a jejunostomy is that the tube is much *smaller* than a gastrostomy tube, and it may be more prone to clogging. Some jejunostomies have dual ports that allow decompression as well as feeding. Another option is a gastric-jejunostomy tube (G-J tube), which enters into the stomach and has longer tubing that descends into the jejunum and allows the feedings to be delivered into the jejunum. An example of a G-J tube (as well as examples of other types of G-tubes) is provided in Fig. 5.11. Many of the newer enteral devices have the EN-Fit features that meet international standards for safe enteral connections. An example of a G-tube with safe enteral connections is seen in Fig. 5.12.

DAILY CARE FOR CLIENTS WITH GASTROSTOMY, PEG, AND JEJUNOSTOMY TUBES

One complication of gastrostomy tubes is increased granulation tissue at the insertion site caused by chronic irritation. Therefore health maintenance and infection control are two of the most important critical concepts. Meticulous skin care and minimizing movement and tension on the

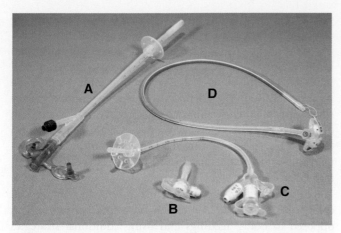

FIG. 5.11 Examples of various enteral tubes. **A and C,** Examples of gastrostomy tubes. **B,** Low-profile gastrostomy feeding button. **D,** Low-profile gastric-jejunal enteral feeding tube.

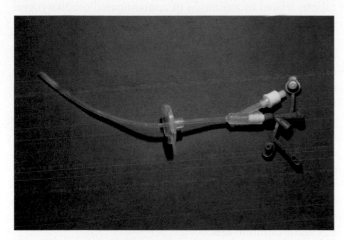

FIG. 5.12 Example of a gastrostomy tube with safe enteral connections. *Top to bottom (right side):* balloon port (top white port), feeding port (middle purple port), and medication port (lower purple port).

tubes are essential. Care at the insertion/exit site is also important to maintain the client's skin integrity. If the client has any signs and symptoms of infection such as redness, warmth, pain at the insertion site or drainage, notify the authorized healthcare provider (Ecklund, 2017). For gastrostomy and PEG tubes, keep the area under the external bumper clean and dry, and rotate the bumper every day (if ordered) to prevent skin breakdown. In order to prevent damage to the client's skin and underlying tissues, it is important to ensure that the bumper is not too tight. In other words, the bumper should rest gently against the skin without leaving an imprint.

DELIVERY METHODS FOR ENTERAL NUTRITION

The major types of delivery methods for EN are intermittent and continuous feeding. The type of formula and method chosen require an order and are based on

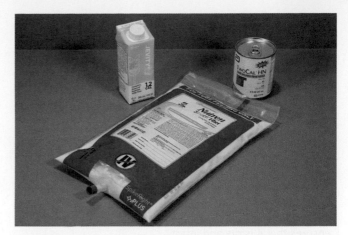

FIG. 5.13 Various types of enteral nutrition (EN) formula.

the client's nutritional needs. The EN formula may be available in ready-to-use cans or cartons (for open systems) or pre-prepared bags/containers for closed feeding systems (Fig. 5.13). Because of the risks associated with EN, the American Society for Parenteral and Enteral Nutrition (ASPEN) has specific recommendations and guidelines regarding the preparation and delivery of EN, as well as precautions for EN. The nurse's primary role is to ensure proper delivery, monitor the client's tolerance and response to EN, and intervene appropriately if there are complications.

Bolus/Intermittent Tube Feedings

Bolus or intermittent feedings involve giving the client a volume of formula within a certain amount of time at designated intervals. These feedings may be given by the syringe method or bag/tubing set method. The disadvantage of bolus feedings is that they may increase the risk of pulmonary aspiration and therefore are not usually recommended for these clients. Bolus feedings can also cause abdominal discomfort and cramping. To reduce the risk of these complications, allow the formula to go in *slowly* by gravity and ensure that the formula is at room temperature. It is also important for the client to sit upright for at least 2 hours after a bolus feeding (Mazur & Litch, 2019). Because soft, flexible feeding tubes could rupture, avoid forcing the feeding into the tube (Dudek, 2018).

Continuous Tube Feedings

Continuous feedings are given over 16 to 24 hours (usually by infusion pumps with steady flow rates) in order to maximize absorption. This is often the preferred method of enteral feeding, particularly for clients at risk for aspiration. Continuous feedings may also be better tolerated than bolus feedings by many clients. Many times, continuous infusions are started at a slower rate and then increased gradually to give the client time to adjust to the feeding (Mazur & Litch 2019). When providing continuous feedings, flush the tube at least every 4 hours per guidelines and facility policy (Boullata et al., 2017) (see Box 5.13).

BOX 5.14 Expect the Unexpected: Feeding Tube Issues

Jennifer, a junior nursing student, is caring for Torie, a 14-year-old female who was admitted for multiple injuries after a motor vehicle accident (MVA). Although Torie's vital signs have stabilized, she is still having difficulty eating on her own. The authorized healthcare providers decide to place a small-bore feeding nasogastric (NG) tube for intermittent tube feedings. One morning during Torie's morning care, she begins to pick at the tape on her nose and states, "This tube is bugging me—it really itches! When do I get it out?" Torie's registered nurse (RN) discusses the importance of the tube with her and provides naris care. She also cleans the visible portion of the NG tube, changes the tape, and ensures that it is dry and intact.

Later that day, Jennifer (the nursing student) notices there are small remnants of adhesive some distance below Torie's NG tube exit site. Realizing this is a "red flag," Jennifer measures the external length of the tube and discovers it is 16 cm longer than what had been recorded after initial insertion. Although Torie's NG tube was still taped at the naris, Jennifer was concerned the feeding tube might have become displaced, so she alerted Torie's RN. When the placement was rechecked, it was discovered that Torie's feeding tube had migrated back into her esophagus! After further assessment, Torie confessed to the nursing student and RN that her tube "accidentally came out" and she had moved the tape back to her nose because she was afraid of "getting in trouble."

This case is a good example of why the placement of feeding tubes has to be carefully checked before each feeding or flushing and rechecked on a regular basis. Even though Torie's tube had initially been verified to be correctly in place after insertion, it became displaced and migrated later into her esophagus. In this situation, the astute observation and reporting from the nursing student, Jennifer, prevented possible complications.

REDUCING RISKS OF ENTERAL NUTRITION

There are many potential risks related to EN that can be reduced with excellent nursing care and adherence to safety measures. One of the most life-threatening complications is pulmonary aspiration of a feeding caused by a misplaced or a displaced tube that has migrated into the client's lungs or esophagus after insertion (Box 5.14). A client who has an altered level of consciousness or a neurological disorder is particularly vulnerable.

One of the simplest ways to prevent aspiration is to elevate the client's HOB at least 30 to 45 degrees during and after feedings. Accurate placement checks also prevent aspiration. Placement must be initially validated by x-ray and then rechecked at least every 4 hours (AACN, 2016b). (see Box 5.8). Placement must also be checked before feedings and medications. It is also important to monitor the client's tolerance of the feedings. Is the client's abdomen distended or firm? Does the client have a feeling of fullness? Some facilities require gastric residual volume (GRV) checks before each feeding and at regular intervals. If a client's GRV is greater than facility policy allows (e.g., >250–500 mL), notify the authorized healthcare provider. In addition, consider the client's clinical status and individual needs. For critically ill adult clients in the ICU, current ASPEN guidelines do not advise routinely interrupting continuous feedings to check GRV unless required by facility policy or unless the client has signs and symptoms (e.g., nausea, cramping, firm distended abdomen, large residual volume) that indicate the client is not tolerating the feedings (McClave et al., 2016).

For clients who are at risk for pulmonary aspiration, evidence based guidelines emphasize using continuous, as opposed to bolus, feedings and using additional strategies such as minimizing sedation as much as possible (AACN, 2016b). Recent guidelines also recommend meticulous oral care twice a day with chlorhexidine mouthwash (if ordered by the authorized healthcare provider) to prevent complications related to aspiration of contaminated oropharyngeal secretions (McClave et al., 2016).

Another serious complication of enteral feeding is misconnection errors. Feeding tubes have been inadvertently connected to intravenous (IV) lines, dialysis catheters, or other lines and tubes. As noted previously, some manufacturers have developed ENFit products that meet the criteria of the International Standards Organization (ISO) for safe enteral connections. These products do not accept the Luer lock connections found on IV lines and other types of nonenteral tubing. Other safety strategies to prevent misconnections include placing tubes or catheters with different purposes in different locations; tracing tubing back to its origin; and providing clear, bold labeling on the EN bag and EN administration sets.

One complication that can lead to infections, diarrhea, or other problems is contamination of the tube feeding formula. Many facilities require the use of closed feeding systems and three-way valves for EN. Most facilities also have strict infection control guidelines as to how long formula can be hung at room temperature. In addition, tubing and administration sets for continuous feedings (including feeding adapters, three-way valves, and other equipment) are usually changed at regular intervals. For a summary of EN risk reduction strategies, see Box 5.15.

HOME CARE CONSIDERATIONS

If the client will continue to receive EN after discharge, provide client and family teaching and follow-up care in order to prevent complications related to storage and administration, as discussed in Box 5.16. If needed, refer the client to other members of the healthcare team, and encourage the client and family to ask questions.

Home care considerations may be particularly important for pediatric clients who will continue to receive EN after discharge. The family may feel anxious and concerned

BOX 5.15 Summary of Risk Reduction Strategies for Enteral Nutrition

REDUCING THE RISK OF ASPIRATION AND TUBE MISPLACEMENT/DISPLACEMENT
- Keep the client's head of the bed (HOB) elevated during and after enteral feedings.
- Use a combination of methods to check enteral tube placement (see Box 5.8).
- Check and recheck tube placement after initial insertion, *before* every feeding, *before* irrigation or medication, and every 4 to 8 hours per policy.
- Investigate "red flags" that could be a sign of tube displacement, such as changes in the visible external length of the tubing. Document the external length of the tube in cm after initial placement and compare to subsequent measurements.
- Provide close observation and monitoring of your client. Ensure that the client is tolerating enteral nutrition (EN) without any nausea, abdominal distention, or distress.
- Provide meticulous oral care on a regular basis to reduce oral pathogens.

REDUCING THE RISK OF COMPLICATIONS RELATED TO MISCONNECTION ERRORS
- Trace tubes back to their origin and ensure they are secure.
- Retrace tubes and recheck all connections during shift change.
- Ensure there is complete handoff communication at the time of transfer of care.

- Identify/confirm the location of all feedings and infusions at shift change.
- Don't force connections if the device doesn't easily fit the tubing.
- Place tubes and catheters with different purposes in different locations.
- Don't confuse bags intended for intravenous use with bags intended for EN use.
- Place bold, bright labels on tubing and bags for EN that state "WARNING! FOR TUBE FEEDING ONLY" or "NOT FOR IV USE!"

REDUCING THE RISK OF COMPLICATIONS RELATED TO CONTAMINATION
- Wear gloves and use closed feeding systems or three-way valves if possible.
- Change EN administration sets, tubing, bag, 3 three-way valves (e.g. Lopez valve), and catheter tip syringe or piston/Toomey used for flushing per facility policy.
- Limit "hang time" of formula per manufacturer recommendations.
- Avoid "topping off" or adding new formula to old formula in the bag.
- Check formula closely for foul odor, mold, or anything unusual.
- If using ready-to-use formula, check the expiration date and wipe off the top of the can with an antiseptic wipe or washcloth prior to opening.

References: Boullata et al., 2017; McClave et al., 2016.

about complications and whether or not they are administering the feedings correctly to their child. Return demonstrations before discharge will help family members feel more comfortable with the procedure. In addition, there are a number of resources, such as the Feeding Tube Awareness Foundation, that offer information and support. The nurse can also encourage the family to include the child in activities and provide as normal of a lifestyle as possible. For more information related to pediatric considerations and EN, see Box 5.12.

PROVIDING CLIENT-CENTERED CARE DURING ENTERAL NUTRITION

Imagine how it must feel to miss out on all of the social and cultural experiences of eating orally. The emotional issues that clients experience when they are receiving EN are often overlooked. Eating is a social event. Many of these clients (particularly those who are on EN long term), feel socially isolated. When caring for clients on EN, use strategies to try and make the feedings feel like a normal mealtime as much as possible. For example, during an intermittent feeding, you can interact and chat with the client, make eye contact, and offer emotional support.

SUMMARY

The initiation of EN and ongoing assessment must be performed by the licensed nurse. However, monitoring of intake and output and assisting the client with oral hygiene can be performed by assistive personnel. Delegation to assistive personnel will vary depending on the state's nurse practice act. As with gastric tube therapy (see Section 3), safety and client-centered care are two of the most important critical concepts when administering EN. In particular, risk reduction strategies such as prevention of pulmonary aspiration are imperative.

APPLICATION OF THE NURSING PROCESS

Examples of Related ICNP Nursing Diagnoses, Expected Client Outcomes, and Nursing Interventions:
Nursing Diagnosis: Risk for aspiration
Supporting Data: Potential for tube displacement
Expected Client Outcomes: Client will have no evidence of aspiration, as seen by:
- respirations, temperature, and vital signs within expected parameters
- absence of dyspnea, gurgling, crackling, wheezing, or abnormal breath sounds

BOX 5.16 Home Care Considerations: Reducing the Risk of Contamination

Ms. Lowe is a 66-year-old client who has been discharged to home after a partial gastrectomy. She has a percutaneous endoscopic gastrostomy (PEG) tube placed for her feedings and received instructions related to her feedings before discharge from the hospital. Several days after her discharge, a tornado hit the city and left Ms. Lowe without power for approximately 36 hours. She also has low water pressure. One afternoon Ms. Lowe contacts the nursing staff at the hospital and reports, "My tube feeding smells different." On further questioning, Ms. Lowe relates that she had stored her extra formula (that was delivered in a pre-mixed bag) in an "ice chest" when her electricity went off because the refrigerator didn't work. She also tells the nurse that she did not want to throw away or "waste" her formula because it is so expensive.

In this situation, the portable ice chest Ms. Lowe used was not adequate. The feedings likely spoiled, causing the foul odor. To prevent contamination-related complications, these feedings should be discarded. After natural disasters, such as tornados, hurricanes, or other disasters, public health officials often advise, "When in doubt, throw it out." Additional ways that Ms. Lowe can prevent contamination at home is to carefully check expiration dates (for ready-to-use or premade formula), label any leftover feedings with the date and time, and discard them after the recommended amount of time. In addition, she should be taught to carefully wash her hands before handling feedings and to thoroughly wash any reusable components of her feeding setup at least once a day using hot water. Ms. Lowe should also be taught not to "top off" or add new formula to any existing formula in the bag. Because Ms. Lowe's water pressure is low, she may have to use distilled or purified water or obtain ready-to-use formula. For additional ways to reduce the risks associated with enteral nutrition, see Box 5.15.

- breath sounds (by auscultation) clear and equal bilaterally
- absence of signs and symptoms of "silent aspiration," such as voice hoarseness.

Nursing Intervention Examples: Implement aspiration precautions. Monitor the client's tolerance of the feedings and elevate the client's HOB at least 30 to 45 degrees during and after the feedings.

Reference: International Classification for Nursing Practice. (n.d.) *eHealth & ICNP*. Retrieved from https://www.icn.ch/what-we-do/projects/ehealth-icnp.

CRITICAL CONCEPTS
Providing Enteral Nutrition

Accuracy (ACC)

Accuracy when providing EN is affected by the following variables:
- assessment of the client, including LOC and orientation level, history, nutritional status, and gastrointestinal function (e.g., presence of bowel sounds and abdominal assessment)
- technique and measurements used for placing small-bore feeding tube

- technique for managing gastrostomy, jejunostomy, and PEG feeding tubes
- adherence to standardized guidelines, such as the ASPEN EN recommendations
- preparation and labeling of tubing, equipment, and formula used for EN
- frequency and timing of checking placement of feeding tubes
- frequency and timing of flushing feeding tubes.

Client-Centered Care (CCC)

Respect of the client when providing EN is demonstrated through:
- promoting autonomy by obtaining consent for EN
- providing privacy and ensuring comfort during EN
- honoring cultural preferences
- advocating for the client and family.

Infection Control (INF)

When providing EN, infection is prevented by:
- preventing and reducing the transfer of microorganisms
- reducing the number of microorganisms
- ensuring that EN guidelines are followed for proper storage, labeling, and administration.

Safety (SAF)

Safety measures when providing EN prevent harm and provide a safe care environment, including:
- using risk reduction strategies to prevent injury as well as pulmonary aspiration and misconnection errors.

Communication (COM)

- Communication exchanges information (oral, written, nonverbal, or electronic) between two or more people.
- Documentation records information in a permanent legal record.
- Communication between the nurse and other members of the healthcare team enhances the safety and effectiveness of EN, including using risk reduction strategies such as measuring and documenting the exposed external length of the tube.

Health Maintenance (HLTH)

Nursing is dedicated to the promotion of health and abilities when providing EN by:
- preventing skin breakdown with nasally inserted feeding tubes
- preventing skin breakdown, redness, and irritation around exit sites of gastrostomy, jejunostomy, and PEG tubes
- preventing skin breakdown and excess granulation tissue around the stomas of gastrostomies and jejunostomies.

Evaluation (EVAL)

Evaluation of the outcomes with EN allows the nurse to determine the safety and efficacy of the care provided.

■ SKILL 5.9 Placement and Care of a Nasally Inserted Small-Bore Feeding Tube

EQUIPMENT

Small-bore flexible feeding tube
Topical anesthetic (if ordered)
Water-soluble lubricant (if needed)
Hypoallergenic tape, stat-lock device, or nasal bridle
50- to 60-mL non-Luer syringe and irrigation fluid (if indicated)
Measuring tape, stethoscope, and pH paper
Clean gloves
Glass of water
Disposable absorbent pads
Towels and washcloths
Airway suction equipment (if needed)
Tissues and emesis basin (if needed)
Oral care supplies
Chlorhexidine mouthwash if indicated and ordered

BEGINNING THE SKILL

1. **SAF** Review the order and review the client's medical/surgical history for contraindications (e.g., nasal or sinus surgery, nasal septum defects, basilar skull fracture; see Box 5.6).
2. **INF** Perform hand hygiene.
3. **CCC** Introduce yourself to the client and family and explain the procedure.
4. **SAF** Identify the client using two identifiers.
5. **CCC** Provide privacy.
6. **ACC** Assess the client's orientation to person, time, place, and situation. *A baseline assessment of the client's LOC and orientation must be done in order to determine if the client can tolerate the placement of a feeding tube and comprehend instructions.*
7. **CCC** Ensure client consent has been obtained for the feeding tube. *Facilitates client autonomy.*
8. **CCC** Assess comfort needs. If the client is having pain, intervene accordingly before the procedure, and provide comfort measures (see Chapter 7). *Pain increases anxiety.*

PROCEDURE

9. **INF** Apply clean gloves.
10. **SAF** Set up an ergonomically safe space. Raise the bed to a comfortable working height. Raise one side rail. *Setting up an ergonomically safe space prevents injury to the nurse and client.* (Note: After the procedure, return the bed to the lowest position to reduce the risk of falls.)
11. **ACC** Assess the client for nausea and/or vomiting, and assess the client's abdomen (all four quadrants) for bowel sounds. Note any abdominal distention. *A baseline abdominal assessment is important to ensure the client can tolerate the procedure.*
12. **HLTH** Assess the client's nares for obstructions, deviations, or skin breakdown, and inspect the mucous membranes at the back of the throat for mucositis or any lesions.

13. **ACC** Assess one naris at a time for patency. Ask the client to place his or her finger on the side of each naris while breathing through the other. Select the naris that is more patent for tube placement. *This ensures that the correct naris is selected for the NG tube.*
14. Prepare the environment for the procedure:
    a. **ACC** Get a temporary piece of tape ready and tab the ends of the tape.
    b. **SAF** If the client is at high risk for aspiration, set up airway or Yankauer-tip suction.
15. Prepare small-bore feeding tube before placement:
    a. **SAF** Inspect tube and stylet for any defects.

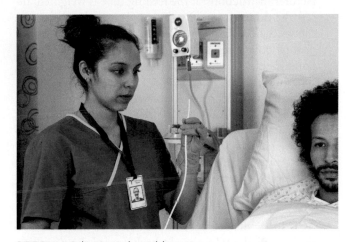

STEP 15A Inspect the tubing.

    b. **SAF** Cap the side port of the feeding tube (if there is one).
    c. **ACC** If using a stylet, test it by inserting it into the tube and ensuring it is working.
    WARNING: Do not allow the stylet to go through the side port or the end of the tube.
16. Prepare the client for the procedure:
    a. **ACC** Elevate the client's HOB to at least 45 degrees.
    b. **CCC** Place towels or absorbent pads over the client's chest.
    c. **CCC** Provide tissues and emesis basin for the client.
    d. **CCC** If ordered, spray topical anesthesia as needed for comfort.
17. **ACC** If the feeding tube will be placed into the gastric pool, estimate the length of tubing that will be inserted by using the NEX + 10 (cm) approach. Measure from the tip of the nose to the earlobe, and from the earlobe to the xiphoid process (NEX), then add 10 cm. Place a piece of tape at this point or use a marker to mark the tube. *The NEX method alone may not provide an accurate estimate. Adding an additional 10 cm to the NEX estimate or using an alternative method may help ensure that the tube will reach the gastric pool (Taylor, 2014)* (see Box 5.7 and Skill 5.5). (Note: For pediatric clients, the NEMU method is recommended. [Brown, 2017] [see Fig. 5.5]).

18. **ACC** If the goal is for the tube to advance into the small intestine (i.e., the duodenum), add approximately 25.4 cm (10 inches) to the estimate per the manufacturer guidelines (Covidien, n.d.). *Postpyloric placement into the small intestine requires a greater length of tubing.*

19. **SAF** Lubricate the tube generously with a water-soluble lubricant along the full length that will be inserted. *Prevents damage to the client's mucous membranes.* **WARNING:** Avoid the use of petroleum-based products on the tube. These products can harm the client's respiratory tract if there is inadvertent insertion into the lungs (C. R. Bard, 2017).

20. **SAF** If using a self-lubricating tube with stylet, inject 10 mL into the feeding tube according to policy and manufacturer instructions; if the feeding tube is weighted, insert the tip into water for 5 seconds in order to activate the special coating (Covidien, n.d.). (Note: Check your facility policy regarding the use of stylet guidewires. Some facilities do not authorize nurses to place feeding tubes that involve guidewires.)

21. **ACC** Ask the client to lean forward slightly. Ensure that the client's head is neutral or flexed down slightly , if not contraindicated. *This helps prevent insertion of the NG feeding tube into the airway.*

22. **SAF** Ask the client to raise his or her hand or finger and alert you if he or she experiences any distress or significant discomfort during the procedure. *Prevents harm to the client.*

23. **ACC** Insert the NG tube into the selected naris and gently advance the tube straight back toward the nasopharynx. If needed, rotate the tip of the tube gently to help the tube advance through the selected naris. **WARNING:** Do *not* angle the tube up into the client's nose. (Note: When you reach the crest of the nasopharynx, you will feel a slight resistance.)

24. **ACC** Once you reach the nasopharynynx, guide the tube down by placing your thumb under the tube to achieve an arc. Instruct the client to tuck his or her chin toward the chest and flex the neck forward while looking down. *This angle will close the epiglottis and facilitate passage of the tube through the oropharynx and esophagus and prevent airway insertion.*

25. **ACC** As you continue to advance the tube, ask the client to take sips of water and swallow while keeping their neck flexed down. (Note: Be prepared for the tube to advance when the client swallows. Do not prevent the tube from moving with swallowing.)

26. **SAF** If you feel significant resistance, or you cannot advance the tube, inspect inside the oral cavity (with a penlight if necessary) and check to see if the tube has coiled or kinked. **WARNING:** Never force the tube into the client. *Forcing the tube into the client could damage the mucosa and cause injury.*

27. **SAF** If you are having difficulty advancing the tube, reposition the client, un-kink the tube if necessary by pulling back enough to straighten the tube, and try again. Encourage the client to swallow. *Client swallowing facilitates moving the tube past the epiglottis into the esophagus.*

28. **SAF** During insertion, assess the client for signs of respiratory distress (e.g., coughing or inability to speak). If the client is experiencing these symptoms or any other problems, such as bleeding or severe pain, stop the procedure, immediately withdraw the tube, and allow the client to recover. *Coughing, gagging, and/or inability to speak are signs the tube may have inadvertently entered the lungs and must be removed.*

29. **SAF** If the tube has to be withdrawn and reinserted, use a different naris if possible.

30. **ACC** If the client is tolerating the procedure without distress, continue to advance the tube to the identified mark or tape, and hold the tube in place. *This helps ensure accurate placement.*

31. **SAF** While continuing to hold the tube in place, tape the tube securely with the temporary tape while you check the placement. *Prevents the tube from becoming displaced.*

32. **ACC** Verify the placement of the nasally inserted feeding tube per facility policy. (see Box 5.8 and Skill 5.5)

33. **SAF WARNING:** Before irrigation, tube feedings, or medication administration, feeding tube placement must be verified initially by x-ray per facility policy. *An x-ray is the gold standard and most accurate method for checking NG tube placement.*

34. **SAF** After feeding tube placement has been confirmed by x-ray:
    a. Prep skin per facility policy and secure tape or commercial device in place.
    b. Mark the exit site of the feeding tube at the naris with a permanent marker.

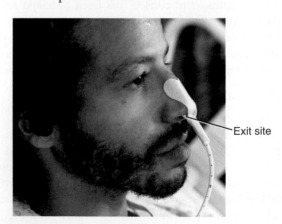

STEP 34B Mark the exit site.

   c. If using tape, place one piece on the bridge of the nose vertically and wrap each of the split pieces around the tube, and then reinforce with a horizontal piece of tape (see Skill 5.5, Step 33).

d. If a stylet was used, *carefully* remove it while holding the tube securely in place at the nose. **WARNING:** Never reinsert the stylet back into the feeding tube after the tube has been placed in the client. *This could cause severe damage and injury to the client's mucosa.*

35. **ACC** If the goal is for the feeding tube to advance to the small intestine (duodenum), then turn the client to the right side per facility policy (Covidien, n.d.).

36. **SAF** If there will be a delay in initiating feedings, flush the tube with irrigation fluid according to facility policy (after tube placement verification) and securely cap as recommended by the manufacturer. *Flushing prevents clogging of the enteral tube.*

37. **SAF** Measure the length of the exposed tube from where it is taped at the nose to the end of the main feeding tube port and record the measurement. Record the number in centimeters as the exposed visible length. *This is an important safety measure that provides information to help verify placement.*

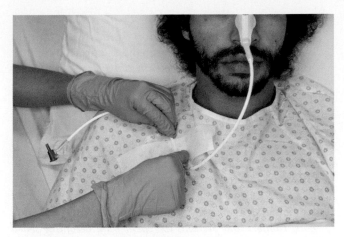

STEP 38 Tape excess tubing to the gown.

39. **CCC** Provide comfort care to the client by providing washcloths and offering oral care.
40. **INF** Dispose of equipment.

FINISHING THE SKILL

41. **INF** Remove gloves and perform hand hygiene.
42. **SAF** Ensure safety and comfort. Ensure that the bed is in the lowest position and verify that the client can identify and reach the nurse call system. *These safety measures reduce the risk of falls.*
43. **EVAL** Evaluate the outcomes. Did the client tolerate the procedure? Is the feeding tube securely in place? Does the x-ray show that the feeding tube is positioned properly?
44. **COM** Document assessment findings, care given, and outcomes in the legal healthcare record:
    * type, size, and location of small-bore feeding tube
    * naris chosen for small-bore feeding tube insertion
    * placement check of the feeding tube and time of x-ray verification
    * length of exposed tubing (from exit site at naris to end of tube) recorded in centimeters.

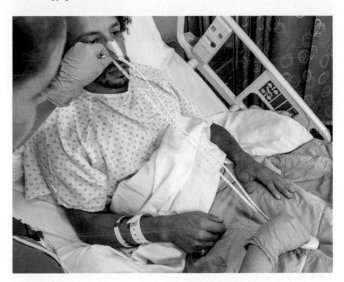

STEP 37 Measure the exposed tubing and record in cm.

38. **CCC** Tape excess feeding tube securely to the client's cheek or gown as needed. *This prevents pulling and tension on the feeding tube.*

■ SKILL 5.10 Providing Care for a Client With a Gastrostomy, PEG Tube, or Jejunostomy

EQUIPMENT

Cotton-tipped applicators
Sterile water
Protective skin barrier product (if ordered)
Hypoallergenic tape
Non-Luer syringes and irrigation fluid (if indicated)
Measuring tape, stethoscope, and pH paper
Clean gloves
Oral care supplies

Chlorhexidine mouthwash if indicated and ordered
Disposable absorbent pads
Towels and washcloths

BEGINNING THE SKILL

1. **INF** Perform hand hygiene.
2. **CCC** Introduce yourself to the client and family and explain the procedure.
3. **SAF** Identify the client using two identifiers.

4. **CCC** Provide privacy.
5. **CCC** Assess the client's comfort needs. If the client is having pain, intervene accordingly, and provide comfort measures (see Chapter 7). *Pain can increase the client's anxiety.*

PROCEDURE

6. **INF** Apply clean gloves.
7. **ACC** Assess the client's abdomen (all four quadrants) for distention or other symptoms. *A baseline assessment is important for monitoring improvement or future problems.*
8. **CCC** Place disposable absorbent pads or towels around the stoma area and the exit site of the enteral tube. *Promotes comfort and prevents the client from becoming soiled during care.*

Monitoring the Appearance and Placement of the Enteral Tube

9. **ACC** Assess the appearance of the client's enteral tube (e.g., gastrostomy, PEG tube, jejunostomy, low-profile feeding button). Note if there is a dressing around the stoma and note if the dressing is dry and intact. *Helps ensure the enteral device is secure, patent, and the tube has not migrated or become displaced since the initial insertion.*
10. **ACC** Validate the placement of the enteral tube by using a combination of methods (e.g., pH checks; see Box 5.8). Recheck every 4 hours or according to facility policy, and check placement before feedings, medication administration, and irrigation. *Even though the tube was initially validated, it can migrate later and become displaced.*
11. **SAF WARNING**: If the enteral tube has accidentally been removed or if there is significant bleeding or leaking around exit sites or the stoma, notify the authorized healthcare provider immediately. *An enteral tube site can close within a few hours unless a new tube is inserted into the tract. Excessive bleeding or drainage requires immediate attention.*
12. **ACC** Inspect the stoma and the skin around the stoma and under the bumper (if present) for redness, irritation, erosion, unusual or excessive drainage, or any sign of excess granulation tissue. If present, report the finding to the authorized healthcare provider. *These signs are an indication of excessive skin irritation that could lead to pressure injury or infection.*
13. **ACC** Measure the length of exposed tubing (from the stoma to the end of the tube) or check the external markings in centimeters on the enteral tube and compare to the length on insertion. *Helps ensure enteral tube has not migrated or become displaced since the initial insertion.*
14. **ACC** For gastrostomy and PEG tubes, assess the position of the external bumper (if present). (Note: The external bumper should rest gently on the client's skin

and keep the tube secure. *Excess pressure can cause tissue damage and excess movement can increase the development of granulation tissue due to chronic irritation.*
15. **ACC** Ensure that the client's skin next to the gastrostomy or PEG bumper (if present) is dry and intact and ensure that the bumper is not too tight or pressing into the client's skin. *Moisture under the bumper and tightness can erode skin and lead to skin breakdown.*

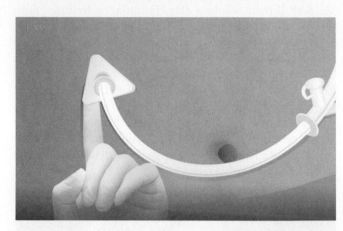

STEP 15 Check the client's skin and position of the bumper.

16. **ACC If the client has a low-profile gastrostomy feeding button:** Ensure that the feeding button is level with the client's skin. *Helps ensure that the feeding button is intact and not displaced.*
17. **INF** Ensure that the skin around the feeding button is dry and intact, without signs of redness, irritation, or leaking. *These measures prevent infection and complications.*
18. **SAF** Ensure that the protective cap on the feeding button is closed securely.

Cleaning and Caring for the Enteral Tube

19. **ACC** If client has a Gastrostomy, PEG tube, or jejunostomy
    a. Inspect sutures (if present) for redness or irritation.
    b. For gastrostomy and PEG tubes, minimize movement of the external bumper (if present) for the first 48 hours. *Minimizing movement provides stability and decreases irritation.*
    c. Gently clean site with cotton-tipped applicators or gauze dipped in saline or other solution (if ordered). If the gastrostomy or PEG tube has an external bumper, clean under and around the bumper. Remove any accumulated drainage and allow the skin to air dry.
    d. Use a split hydrogel or split gauze dressing above the bumper, not below, to avoid significant tension on the enteral tube insertion site.

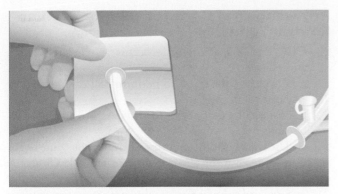

STEP 19D Use a pre-split hydrogel dressing if needed.

   e. For established gastrostomy or PEG tubes without sutures, rotate the external bumper every day (if ordered). *This procedure may prevent pressure injury.*
   f. If the client has a gastrostomy or PEG tube with a retention balloon, deflate the balloon at regular intervals (if ordered) to relieve pressure per order and manufacturer instructions.
   g. Use a protective skin barrier product as needed (if ordered).
20. **ACC** If the client has a low-profile gastrostomy feeding button:
   a. Ensure that the area around the button is dry and intact.
   b. If ordered, rotate the button once per day to relieve pressure.

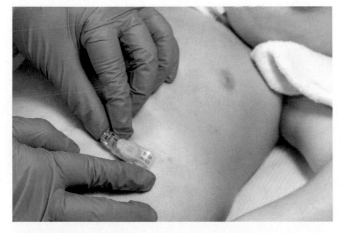

STEP 20B Rotate low-profile gastrostomy button.

   c. Clean the area around and under the low-profile button with moistened cotton-tip applicators as ordered. *Prevents crust buildup and debris.*

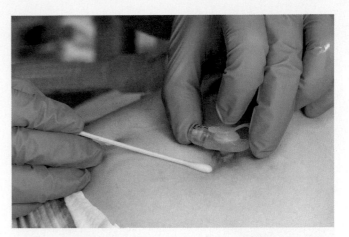

STEP 20C Clean under and around the button.

Maintaining Patency and Flushing the Enteral Tube

21. **ACC** Maintain patency by flushing the enteral tube (e.g., Gastrostomy, PEG, Jejunostomy, and low-profile feeding button) at regular intervals per order and policy. (Note: The volume and type of flushing depend on the type and size of the enteral tube. Some enteral tubes, like jejunostomies, require sterile water for flushing.)
   a. If the client is receiving tube feedings, flush the enteral tube every 4 hours and before and after feedings (see Skill 5.11 and Box 5.13).
   b. If the client is receiving enteral medications, flush before and after medications and between each medication (see Chapter 11).
22. **ACC** If the client has a low-profile feeding button (e.g., MIC-Key), attach an extension set (that has been primed) and flush according to manufacturer instructions or as follows:
   a. Insert the "nose" of the extension set into the feeding port by matching and aligning the black line on the connector with the black line on the feeding port. *Alignment of the black lines ensures that the extension set is secure.*

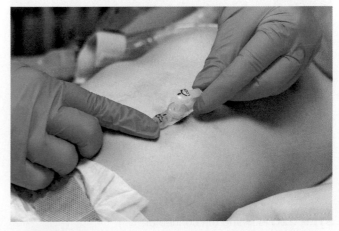

STEP 22A Insert primed extension set into the feeding port.

b. Turn the extension set connector clockwise and lock securely in place. **WARNING.** Do not turn connector past stop point.

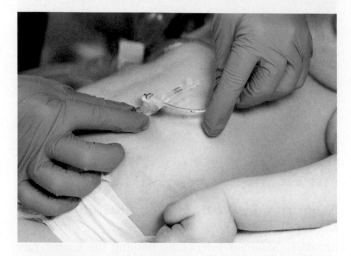

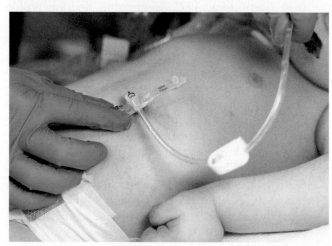

STEP 22B Turning the extension set connector clockwise.

c. After verifying placement, flush with ordered amount of fluid.

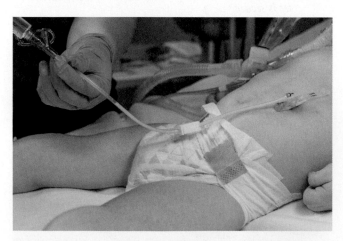

STEP 22C Flushing the connector.

Providing Oral Care for Clients With an Enteral Tube

23. **CCC** Ensure that oral care occurs at regular intervals and as needed:
    a. Encourage the client to perform oral care himself or herself if desired.
    b. Inspect the oral cavity for dryness, irritation, or lesions.
    c. Use chlorhexidine mouthwash and/or or saline swabs as ordered if the client is at increased risk. Clean the buccal cavity and under the tongue. *The client is at increased risk of infection when not eating and drinking as the mouth is not lubricated in the same way.*
    d. Lubricate the client's lips with water or a water-soluble lubricant as needed. *The client's lips are at an increased risk of blistering when not lubricated by eating and drinking.*
24. **INF** Dispose of equipment.

FINISHING THE SKILL

25. **INF** Remove gloves and perform hand hygiene.
26. **SAF** Ensure safety and comfort. Ensure that the bed is in the lowest position and verify that the client can identify and reach the nurse call system. *These safety measures reduce the risk of falls.*
27. **EVAL** Evaluate the outcomes. Did the client tolerate the procedure? Does the stoma site or exit site look clean, without signs of irritation, redness, or excess granulation tissue?
28. **COM** Document assessment findings, care given, and outcomes in the legal healthcare record:
    • appearance of exit sites and/or stoma of the enteral device
    • appearance and character of any drainage
    • placement check and length of exposed tubing
    • amount and type of flushing and cleaning product used.

▪ SKILL 5.11 Administering a Tube Feeding (Intermittent or Continuous)

EQUIPMENT

EN formula for open or closed system feedings (room temperature)

Appropriate catheter-tipped syringe or piston Toomey (usually 50–60 mL)

Oral syringes (10 mL) for smaller enteral tubes (gastrostomy button or jejunostomy)

Irrigation fluid (usually sterile water)

Tube feeding set or feeding bag and pole (if needed)

Labels for feeding bags and containers

Feeding pump (if needed)

Measuring tape, stethoscope, and pH paper

Disposable absorbent pads

Towels and washcloths

Clean gloves

Lopez valve or three-way valve (if needed)

Connecting tubing or feeding adapter (if needed)

BEGINNING THE SKILL

1. **SAF** Review order for the following:
   a. Type of enteral feeding (intermittent or continuous)
   b. Open or closed type of feeding
   c. Route of enteral administration (e.g., nasally inserted tube, gastrostomy, PEG)
   d. Product or generic name of formula
   e. Rate of administration and time intervals of feedings.
2. **SAF** Review the client's medical/surgical history. If the client has been receiving feedings, determine if the client has had any difficulty. *Helps determine the client's risk for aspiration.*
3. **SAF** Verify with authorized healthcare provider that tube placement has been checked by x-ray. *X-ray verification of feeding tube placement is the gold standard prior to feeding.*
4. **INF** Perform hand hygiene.
5. **CCC** Introduce yourself to the client and family and explain the procedure.
6. **SAF** Identify the client using two identifiers.
7. **CCC** Provide privacy.
8. **ACC** Assess the client's orientation to person, time, place, and situation. *A baseline assessment or orientation must be done to determine the client's risk of aspiration.*
9. **SAF** Assess the client for any food or formula allergies.
10. **CCC** Ensure that client consent has been obtained for EN. *Promotes autonomy and client centered care.*

PROCEDURE

11. **INF** Apply clean gloves.
12. **ACC** Assess the client for nausea (if client is verbal) and vomiting; observe (look) at client's abdomen for distention, auscultate (listen) for bowel sounds in all four quadrants, and palpate (feel) the abdomen and note whether it is soft. *A baseline abdominal assessment can help determine if the client can tolerate enteral feedings.*

Preparing for the Intermittent or Continuous Tube Feeding

13. Prepare the client for the procedure:
    a. **SAF** Elevate the client's HOB to at least 45 degrees. *Prevents reflux or aspiration.*
    b. **CCC** Place towels or disposable absorbent around the enteral site.
14. Prepare enteral feedings or formula for the procedure.
    a. **INF** Clean bedside table with antiseptic solution.
    b. **INF** If using ready-to-use canned formula (for open system), check expiration dates and shake cans before using.
    c. **INF** Wipe off the top of the cans with an antiseptic wipe. *Reduces pathogens.*
    d. **ACC** If using reconstituted or diluted powder formula, mix only with sterile or purified water and use immediately after mixing.
    e. **ACC** If using pre-prepared feeding and enteral tubing set (for closed system), check for unusual consistency or odor. If present, discard and do not use.
    f. **CCC** Ensure that formula is room temperature. *Formula that is too cold could cause cramping and poor tolerance, especially among older adults (Dudek, 2018).*

Preparing the Client's Feeding Tube or Enteral Access Device

15. **SAF WARNING:** Prior to initiating flushing or feeding, verify the placement of the feeding tube by using a variety of methods (e.g., checking pH; see Box 5.8). *Because an enteral tube can migrate, the placement must be validated before each feeding, even if the placement was initially confirmed by x-ray.*
16. **SAF** If feedings are being given to the client for the first time or if there is any question about the placement of the tube, placement must be validated by x-ray per policy. *This is an important safety measure (AACN, 2016a).*
17. **ACC** If required by the facility policy, check the GRV before the feeding by gently aspirating the tube with an appropriate-size syringe. If the GRV is greater than your facility policy or the order allows, notify the authorized healthcare provider. (Note: If you are having difficulty aspirating gastric contents, it may help to instill a small amount of air first, or turn the client side to side [AACN, 2016b]. For pediatric clients, it may be helpful to flush the tube with 2 to 3 mL of air, reposition the client to the left side and wait 10 to 15 minutes [Irving et al., 2018].) *Turning the client side to side or injecting the feeding tube with air may help move the distal end of*

the tube away from the gastric wall to facilitate aspiration of gastric contents.

18. **If the client has a nasally inserted tube (nasogastric or nasointestinal):**
    a. **SAF** Ensure that tape is dry and intact and securely in place on the nose. If the tape on the nose has moved, the tube may have migrated or become displaced.
    b. **ACC** Measure the length of exposed tubing from the base of the nose to the end of the main port of the clear tube and compare it to the length on insertion. *Ensures tube has not migrated or become displaced since initial insertion.*

19. **If the client has a gastrostomy, jejunostomy, or PEG tube:**
    a. **SAF** Ensure that stoma and external bumpers (if present) are intact and that the dressing around the stoma (if present) is dry and intact. *Helps ensure the device is secure.*
    b. **ACC** Measure the length of exposed tubing or check external markings from stoma or exit site to the end of the main port of the tube, and compare to the length on insertion. *This helps to ensure the tube has not migrated or become displaced.*
    c. **SAF WARNING:** If the exit site on the enteral device has signs of significant bleeding, drainage, or leakage around the stoma, notify the authorized healthcare provider, and do not administer feedings in the enteral tube.
    d. **ACC** Prime the feeding adapter or extension set with sterile water as ordered or recommended by the manufacturer. (Note: If the client has a jejunostomy or a PEG tube, the client may receive continuous as opposed to bolus/intermittent feedings to facilitate the proper absorption and tolerance of feedings [Dudek, 2018].)

20. **ACC If the client has a low-profile gastrostomy feeding button:**
    a. Ensure that feeding button is dry and intact and level with the client's skin.
    b. Prime the bolus extension set or continuous extension set for the gastrostomy feeding button according to the manufacturer instructions.
    c. When attaching the primed extension set to the feeding button, insert the extension set into the feeding port by matching and aligning the black line on the extension set connector with the black line on the feeding port. Turn the extension set connector clockwise and lock it securely into place (see Skill 5.10).

Administering a Bolus or Intermittent Tube Feeding

21. **ACC If using the syringe/gravity method:**
    a. Remove the plunger from the barrel of the piston/Toomey syringe. (Note: The size of the syringe depends on the age of the client, type of appliance, and the volume to be administered. For example, if the client has a gastrostomy feeding button or a jejunos-

tomy, a smaller oral syringe may be used as opposed to a larger syringe.)
    b. Pinch, clamp, or fold over the enteral tubing, feeding adapter, or extension set. *Prevents air from entering the client's stomach before the syringe barrel is placed.*
    c. Place the syringe barrel on the main port or feeding adapter of the enteral tube.
    d. Hold the syringe barrel and tube securely as a unit to prevent slipping. *Holding the syringe/tube securely prevents disconnection and loss of fluid and feeding.*
    e. While the tubing remains clamped, pour irrigation fluid into the barrel of the syringe. Then un-clamp the tubing and allow fluid to slowly flush the tube. *Flushing the tube prior to feeding maintains the patency of the tube.* (Note: The amount of irrigation fluid used may vary, depending on the type of enteral tube the client has. Gastrostomy and jejunostomy tubes will require less volume than nasogastric tubes.)
    f. During irrigation, elevate the syringe barrel above the level of the client's stomach (no more than 45 cm [18 inches]). *The height of the syringe affects gravity flow. The higher the syringe, the faster the flow. If the syringe is lowered, the rate will slow down.*
    g. After irrigation, clamp the tubing first and then pour the prescribed formula into the syringe barrel. *Clamping the tube first prevents air from entering the client.*

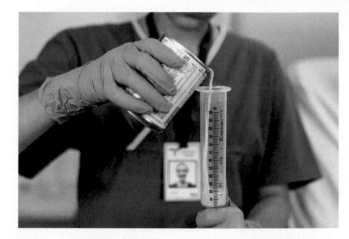

STEP 21G While tubing is clamped, pour formula into the syringe.

    h. Un-clamp the tubing and allow feeding to slowly go in by gravity. If the feeding is going in too fast, lower the syringe. *Slow gravity feeding reduces the risk of nausea or cramping.*
    i. Repeat as necessary until feeding is complete. Ensure that the client is tolerating the feedings. Refill the barrel of syringe before it is empty. *Avoids air entering the tube.*
    J. **WARNING:** Do not force a feeding into the tube. *Forcing a feeding into the enteral tube, especially a small-bore tube, could rupture the tube.*
    k. After the feeding is complete, flush the tube again per policy or order.

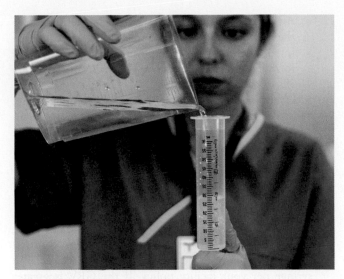

STEP 21K Flush tubing after feeding.

WARNING: Do not allow the barrel of the syringe to run completely dry or allow air to enter the tube. *Excess air in the client's stomach could cause distention.* (Note: Before or after feedings, some clients may require decompression or venting of the enteral tube. Check specific manufacturer recommendations.)

22. **ACC If using the bag/tubing set method for intermittent feeding:**
    a. Prepare feeding bag/tubing set according to the manufacturer instructions. If using an open feeding system, close the clamp on the feeding bag tubing, and then pour formula into the feeding bag using aseptic technique.

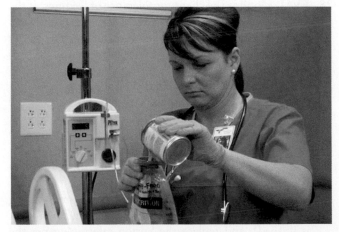

STEP 22A While the tubing is clamped, pour formula into the bag.

    b. If using a closed tube feeding system, remove the protective cover from the closed container, and spike the closed feeding tube set into the container.
    c. Hang the feeding bag on a pole at the recommended height (usually approximately 25–45 centimeters [10–18 inches]). Open the clamp and *slowly* prime the tubing with formula to remove air. After the

tubing is primed, close the clamp. *Slow priming at a lower velocity of flow reduces air.* (Note: If using an infusion pump for the feeding, see Skill 5.12.)
    d. Connect the distal end of the feeding bag tubing to the proximal end of the client's enteral tube or feeding adapter. Use a push-and-twist motion. **WARNING:** Before you attach the tube feeding to the client and open the clamp, trace the client's tube to its point of origin. *Tracing tubes to their origin prevents misconnection errors.* (Note: Some facilities are using special safety adapters such as ENFit connectors that only allow enteral connections.)

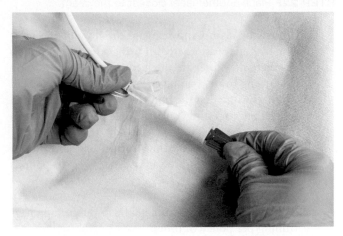

STEP 22D Trace the tubing to the point of origin, then connect the feeding adapter.

    e. **SAF** Remove gloves and perform hand hygiene. Place a label on the feeding bag tubing that states **"TUBE FEEDING ONLY"** and **"NOT FOR IV USE"** and ensure that the label on the bag matches the client identification and contains correct information (e.g., type, strength, and amount of feeding; date, time, and initials of the healthcare provider who hung the bag). *Proper labeling prevents misconnection errors.* (Note: If required by your facility, place the labels on the tubing BEFORE connecting the feeding to the client)

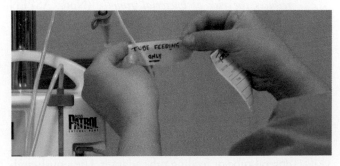

STEP 22E Label the bag and tubing.

    f. **SAF** Place another label on the feeding tube or enteral adapter closest to the source (client). *Additional safety buffers and labels prevent misconnection errors.*

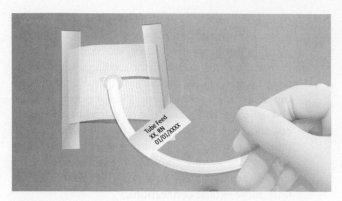

STEP 22F Place another label closest to the client.

g. Open the clamp and regulate the flow of the feeding by gravity as ordered. If using a feeding pump to regulate flow, prepare the feeding administration set according to the manufacturer instructions (see Skill 5.12). Ensure that the pump is working properly and adjust pump settings and rate of feeding according to order.

h. **SAF** Do not allow feedings to run dry, and do not use a pump with a pressure that exceeds 40 pounds per square inch (psi). *Excess pressure could rupture the tube.*

i. After the feeding is complete, flush the feeding bag/tubing per policy or order.

Administering a Continuous Tube Feeding

23. **ACC** Prepare and initiate a continuous tube feeding.
    a. Perform hand hygiene and apply clean gloves.
    b. Prepare the feeding pump and feeding administration set according to the manufacturer instructions. (If using a kangaroo pump, see Skill 5.12.)
    c. Prepare the feeding. If the feeding bag and set are not already pre-prepared, prime the tubing in the pump and follow steps 22a through 22c. Initiate only enough feeding for 4 to 8 hours of "hang time" per facility policy or manufacturer recommendations. *Limiting how long continuous tube feedings are hung reduces the risk of bacterial growth.* (Note: ASPEN guidelines state that closed feedings are preferred. In the acute care setting, infusion times for closed feedings are limited to 24 to 48 hours per the manufacturer. If an open feeding system is used, the infusion time should be limited to 4 to 8 hours. [Boullata et al. 2017])
    d. After placement is checked and other preliminary procedures are done, connect the distal end of the feeding bag tubing to the proximal end of the client's enteral tube or feeding tube adapter. Use a push-and-twist motion. **WARNING:** Before you attach tube feeding to the client and open the clamp, trace the tube to its point of origin. (Note: Many facilities are now using special safety adapters, such as ENFit connectors, that only allow safe enteral connections.)

e. After the primed tubing or adapter is connected to the client, open the clamp and adjust the rate of feeding on the pump according to order. Ensure that the formula is infusing properly. *Monitoring is essential to ensure the pump is working.*

24. **SAF** During the continuous feeding, flush the feeding tube at regular intervals (according to order and policy), and monitor the client's infusion closely. **WARNING:** Do NOT rely on the pump rate and volume alone to determine if feeding is infused (Boullata et al. 2017).

25. **SAF** Replace the feeding bag and/or administration set before the tube feeding runs completely dry. *Prevents air from entering the client's gastrointestinal tract.*

26. **SAF** If required by your facility, check the GRV during continuous feedings every 4 to 8 hours (or as required) by gently aspirating the tube with the appropriate-size syringe per your facility policy. If the GRV is greater than your facility allows, notify the authorized healthcare provider. (Note: For critically ill clients in the ICU, current ASPEN guidelines do not advise routinely interrupting continuous feedings to check GRV unless required by policy or unless the client is at high risk for aspiration or exhibits signs and symptoms of not tolerating the feedings [e.g., pain, nausea, abdominal distention, feeling of fullness] [McClave et al. 2016].)

Follow-up Care During and After Enteral Feedings

27. **SAF** During and after feedings, leave the client's HOB elevated according to facility policy. *This is a safety measure that reduces the risk of reflux and aspiration of enteral feedings.*

28. **EVAL** Monitor the client for tolerance of feedings. If the client has severe cramping, nausea or vomiting, or any other problems, stop feedings immediately and notify the authorized healthcare provider. *Prevents aspiration or other complications.*

29. **EVAL** If the client has a nasally inserted tube, monitor placement and ensure that the tape remains intact at the nose. *Helps ensure the tube does not migrate during feedings.*

30. **EVAL** If the client has a gastrostomy, jejunostomy, or PEG, monitor the adapter and the area around the stoma to ensure that there is no leakage or other problem with feedings.

31. **ACC** If the client has a low-profile gastrostomy feeding button, disconnect the adapter or extension set (after it is flushed), and replace the button safety plug per the manufacturer instructions.

32. **If the enteral feedings will be discontinued:**
    a. **SAF** Turn off the feeding pump.
    b. **ACC** Pinch, clamp, or fold over the end of the enteral tube and disconnect from the feeding set or adapter without allowing air to enter the tube.
    c. **ACC** After placement is verified, flush the feeding tube with 30 mL of sterile water (or whatever is ordered) per facility policy into the main lumen of the tube. *Prevents clogging of tube.*

d. **ACC** Place an integral plug or cap on the main lumen of the enteral tube.

33. **If the nasally inserted feeding tube will be removed:**

    a. **ACC** Ensure that the client's HOB is elevated, clear the feeding tube of gastric contents or residual formula, and follow the procedure as outlined in Skill 5.8. **WARNING:** Ensure that the tube is clamped or folded before removing it. *This prevents dripping of residual formula or aspiration into the lungs.*

    b. **SAF** Ensure the tip or weight on the end of the feeding tube is intact and not broken off. (Note: If the tip is broken off, notify the authorized healthcare provider immediately.)

34. **CCC** Provide comfort care to the client by cleaning any spillage.

35. **INF** Provide oral care to the client. If the client has a high risk for aspiration, consider using chlorhexidine mouthwash if ordered. *Diligent oral care prevents bacterial contamination in the oropharynx that could lead to aspiration pneumonia (McClave et al., 2016).*

36. **INF** Dispose of equipment according to facility policy.

FINISHING THE SKILL

37. **INF** Remove gloves and perform hand hygiene.

38. **SAF** Ensure safety and comfort. Ensure that the bed is in the lowest position and verify that the client can identify and reach the nurse call system. *These safety measures reduce the risk of falls.*

39. **EVAL** Evaluate the outcomes. Is the client tolerating the feedings? Does the client have signs of nutritional improvement, such as weight gain and improved lab values?

40. **COM** Document assessment findings, care given, and outcomes in the legal healthcare record:
    - verification of placement of tube or enteral device used for feeding
    - method used to administer feeding (syringe method, bag/tubing set)
    - brand or generic name of formula and amount of time to administer
    - amount and type of fluid used for flushing
    - any unusual or adverse reactions or complication, such as diarrhea.

■ SKILL 5.12 Using a Kangaroo Feeding Pump

This skill has been adapted from the Joey Kangaroo pump operating manual. Follow your facility policy and the manufacturer's instructions for the specific pump you will be using.

EQUIPMENT

Enteral feeding pump and pole
EN administration set
EN formula for open or closed system (room temperature)
Sterile water (if needed)
Labels for feeding bags, containers, and tubing

BEGINNING THE SKILL

1. **ACC** Review order for:
   a. type of tube feeding to be administered (open or closed)
   b. rate of infusion (intermittent or continuous)
   c. any instructions or order for specific feeding pump.
2. **INF** Perform hand hygiene.
3. **CCC** Introduce yourself to the client and family and explain the procedure.
4. **SAF** Identify the client using two identifiers.
5. **CCC** Provide privacy if needed.

PROCEDURE

6. **ACC** Prepare and check the feeding pump.
   a. Attach a power cord to the back of the pump and plug into A/C wall outlet.
   b. Press power button ON and inspect the screen on the pump. (Note: There should be an audible tone,

hopping kangaroos, or some type of indication that the pump is working.)
   c. Ensure that there are functional batteries in the pump.
7. **SAF** If using an IV pole to hold the pump, use a clamp that will hold the pump securely.
8. **ACC** Prepare the administration set and insert into the pump. (Note: Ensure that the feeding administration set is compatible with the feeding pump.)
   a. Perform hand hygiene again and apply clean gloves.
   b. Hang the feeding administration set or feed/flush set on the IV pole. Pour formula into the feeding bag or use a closed system container. (Note: Ensure that the top or starting volume of formula within the feeding bag is approximately 25 to 45 cm [10–18 inches] above the top of the pump per manufacturer instructions. *The proper height facilitates accurate feeding.*)
   c. Open the door of the pump and load the feeding administration set.
   d. Insert the tubing into the pump per manufacturer instructions and stretch the silicone tubing around the rotor of the pump. Ensure that the valve on the tubing is fully inserted and secure. **WARNING:** Do not overstretch the silicone tubing.
   e. Close the door of the pump and inspect the screen to determine if the set is properly loaded. If the tubing is not loaded properly, the door of the feeding pump will not close. (Note: The display screen on the pump will usually say "set loaded.")

9. **ACC** Prime feeding administration set using on-screen prompts. **WARNING:** Do not attach the feeding to the client until after the administration set is fully primed.

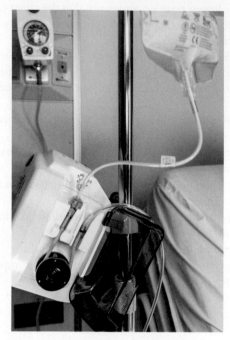

STEP 9 Prime the tubing with formula.

10. **ACC** If automatic priming is used, push the button for automatic priming. (Note: For feed/flush systems, the flush line will usually prime prior to the feeding line.)
11. **ACC** If manual priming is used, press and hold the prime buttons. If a feed/flush system is used, prime the flush line first before priming the feeding line.
12. **SAF** Ensure that feeding line is primed past the valve and to the end of the connector. *This technique ensures that minimal air will inadvertently enter into the client.*
13. **ACC** Select intermittent or continuous mode on the pump and follow the on-screen prompts.
14. **ACC** Connect and administer the tube feeding as described in Skill 5.11. (Note: Ensure that the tubing administration set and feeding bag/container are properly labeled.)
15. **ACC** Program the pump per the manufacturer instructions and ordered parameters, including the rate and volume to be delivered.

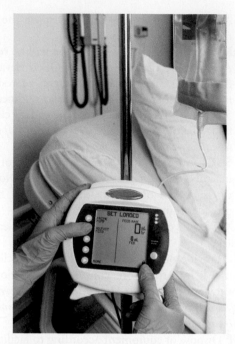

STEP 15 Adjust pump settings.

16. **ACC** If using a feed/flush system, set the volume and frequency of flushes and the flush intervals to be delivered per policy and order (e.g., every 4 hours).
17. **ACC** Select RUN on the pump and ensure that the tube feeding is infusing properly.
18. **EVAL** Continue to monitor the client and volume of feeding that has been infused. *Ongoing monitoring is essential to ensure the pump is working properly.*

FINISHING THE SKILL

19. **INF** Perform hand hygiene.
20. **SAF** Ensure safety and comfort. Ensure that the bed is in the lowest position and verify that the client can identify and reach the nurse call system. *These safety measures reduce the risk of falls.*
21. **EVAL** Evaluate the outcomes. Did the pump deliver the tube feeding accurately?
22. **COM** Document assessment findings, care given, and outcomes in the legal healthcare record:
    - type of feeding pump used (feeding only or feed/flush system)
    - pump mode (intermittent or continuous)
    - program parameters (e.g., rate, volume of fluid to be delivered).
    - volume of feeding delivered as expected and ordered.

■ CASE STUDY

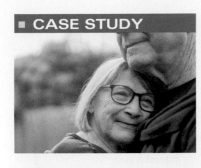

Mrs. Sharp is a 74-year-old retired teacher with a history of esophageal cancer who is being admitted for weight loss and mucositis pain. She is alert and oriented and has been living at home with her husband of 40 years. On admission, she has a height of 162.56 cm (5 ft, 4 inches) and a weight of 46.36 kg (102 lb). She reports a 9.1 kg (20-pound) weight loss over the last several months. In addition, she is immunocompromised, with a white blood cell (WBC) count of 2.5. Her vital signs are within expected parameters. During her screening, Mrs. Sharp states that she hasn't had much of an appetite and that "everything tastes like cardboard." She also tells the nurse that "it hurts to swallow." Her pain rating is 7 on a scale of 1 (least pain) to 10 (most pain).

After completing the admission assessment, the nurse implements measures to provide comfort and control Mrs. Sharp's pain. The nurse also refers Mrs. Sharp for a dietary consult. The authorized healthcare provider orders a texture modified-consistency, minced and moist diet. Over the next several days, the nurses on the medical-surgical unit carefully record Mrs. Sharp's food and fluid intake while continuing to provide care and control her pain. They also allow flexible visiting hours and encourage her husband to remain at the bedside during her meals at Mrs. Sharp's request. Mrs. Sharp's pain is now more controlled (rating of 2), and her appetite improves slightly. However, her intake is still not adequate, and she continues to lose weight. The authorized healthcare provider then decides to place a PEG tube for enteral feedings. Before the tube is placed, the nurse ensures that Mrs. Sharp consents to the PEG tube as well as to EN. After the PEG tube is placed, the nurses notice a small amount of serous drainage around the PEG tube exit site. Before the nurses initiate feedings, they verify the placement of Mrs. Sharp's PEG tube and prepare for her enteral nutrition. When Mrs. Sharp is discharged to home, the nurses provide teaching to Mrs. Sharp and her husband. They both express some anxiety about the PEG tube.

Case Study Questions

1. Considering Mrs. Sharp's nutritional screening and signs and symptoms on admission, what are the priorities regarding her care? What immediate interventions does the nurse do in this case to care for Mrs. Sharp? What additional measures could the nurse do?

2. The authorized healthcare provider places Mrs. Sharp on a texture modified-consistency, minced and moist diet. Describe this type of diet and how it may help Mrs. Sharp.

3. In order to prevent further weight loss, the nurse does several things in this case to improve Mrs. Sharp's appetite and encourage eating. Describe these measures and any additional interventions the nurse could do to improve Mrs. Sharp's intake of food.

4. How would the nurse accurately monitor Mrs. Sharp's oral intake? Describe additional ways the nurse can assess Mrs. Sharp's tolerance and intake of food.

5. Because Mrs. Sharp's weight continues to decline, the authorized healthcare provider places a PEG tube for enteral feedings. Describe what a PEG tube is and where it is inserted. Why would a PEG tube be a better choice for Mrs. Sharp than a nasally inserted tube? Will it be possible for Mrs. Sharp to eat orally and receive oral care while she has a PEG tube?

6. After the PEG tube is inserted, the nurses observe a small amount of drainage around the insertion site. What are possible complications Mrs. Sharp might be at risk for? How can the nurse prevent these complications and provide optimal care for Mrs. Sharp?

7. Before initiating feedings, the nurses verify the placement of Mrs. Sharp's PEG tube. How often must the nurses check the placement of her tube, and what methods should they use? What is the gold standard for verifying the placement of enteral feeding tubes?

8. Before Mrs. Sharp is discharged to home, the nurses will be involved in teaching Mrs. Sharp and her husband how to prepare and self-administer her enteral feedings. Considering Mrs. Sharp's history, what teaching is critical to prevent complications?

9. **Application of QSEN Competencies:** One of the Quality and Safety Education for Nurses (QSEN) skills for Patient-Centered Care is to "Remove barriers to presence of families and other designated surrogates based on patient preferences" (Cronenwett et al., 2007). How did the nurse in this case honor Mrs. Sharp's preferences, and how did it help her? What other QSEN patient-centered skill did the nurse demonstrate before Mrs. Sharp's PEG tube was placed?

■CONCEPT MAP

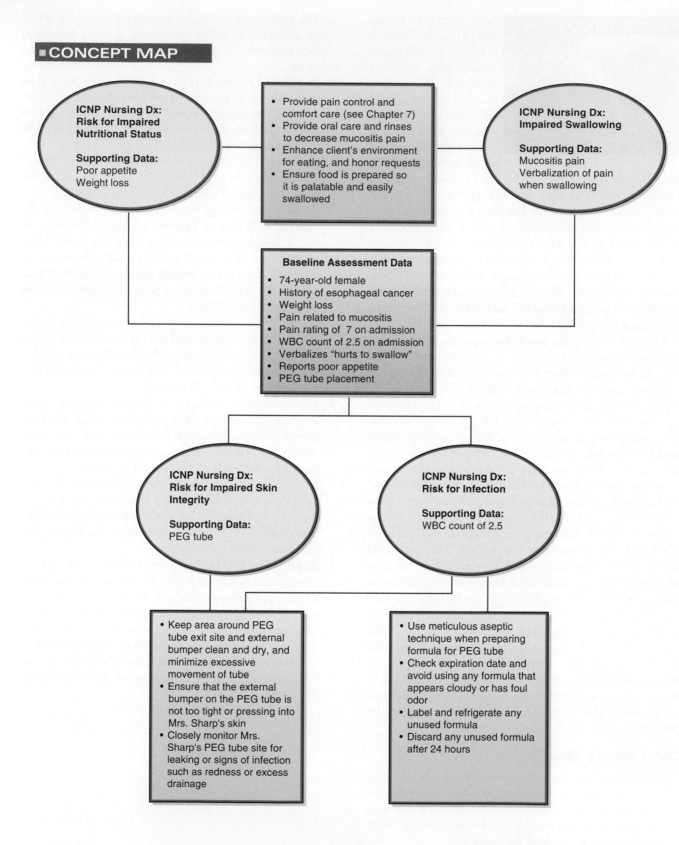

ICNP Nursing Dx: Risk for Impaired Nutritional Status

Supporting Data:
Poor appetite
Weight loss

- Provide pain control and comfort care (see Chapter 7)
- Provide oral care and rinses to decrease mucositis pain
- Enhance client's environment for eating, and honor requests
- Ensure food is prepared so it is palatable and easily swallowed

ICNP Nursing Dx: Impaired Swallowing

Supporting Data:
Mucositis pain
Verbalization of pain when swallowing

Baseline Assessment Data

- 74-year-old female
- History of esophageal cancer
- Weight loss
- Pain related to mucositis
- Pain rating of 7 on admission
- WBC count of 2.5 on admission
- Verbalizes "hurts to swallow"
- Reports poor appetite
- PEG tube placement

ICNP Nursing Dx: Risk for Impaired Skin Integrity

Supporting Data:
PEG tube

ICNP Nursing Dx: Risk for Infection

Supporting Data:
WBC count of 2.5

- Keep area around PEG tube exit site and external bumper clean and dry, and minimize excessive movement of tube
- Ensure that the external bumper on the PEG tube is not too tight or pressing into Mrs. Sharp's skin
- Closely monitor Mrs. Sharp's PEG tube site for leaking or signs of infection such as redness or excess drainage

- Use meticulous aseptic technique when preparing formula for PEG tube
- Check expiration date and avoid using any formula that appears cloudy or has foul odor
- Label and refrigerate any unused formula
- Discard any unused formula after 24 hours

References

Academy of Nutrition and Dietetics. (2019). *Nutrition care manual.* Retrieved from https://www.nutritioncaremanual.org/adult-nutrition-care.

American Association of Critical Care Nurses (AACN). (2016a). *Initial and ongoing verification of feeding tube placement in adults.* Retrieved from https://www.aacn.org/~/media/aacn-website/clincial-resources/practice-alerts/feedingtubepa.pdf.

American Association of Critical Care Nurses (AACN). (2016b). *AACN practice alert: Prevention of aspiration in adults.* Retrieved from https://www.aacn.org/clinical-resources/practice-alerts/prevention-of-aspiration.

Boullata, J. I., Carrera, A. L., Harvey, L., Hudson, L., McGinnis, C., & Wessell, J. J. (2017). ASPEN safe practices for enteral nutrition therapy. *Journal of Parenteral and Enteral Nutrition, 41*(1), 15–103.

Brown, L. D., Hendrickson, K., Evans, R., Davis, J., Anderson, M. S., & Hay, W. W. (2016). Enteral nutrition. In S. L. Gardner, B. S. Carter, M. E. Hines, & J. E. Hernandez (Eds.), *Merenstein & Gardner's handbook of neonatal intensive care* (8th ed.). St. Louis, MO: Mosby.

Brown, T. L. (2017). Pediatric variations in nursing interventions. In M. J. Hockenberry, D. Wilson, & C. C. Rodgers (Eds.), *Wong's essentials of pediatric nursing* (10th ed.) (pp. 575–635). St. Louis, MO: Elsevier.

Chang, C. C., & Roberts, B. L. (2011). Strategies for feeding patients with dementia. *American Journal of Nursing (AJN), 111*(4), 36–44.

Covidien. (n. d.) *Nursing care. Enteral access.* Retrieved from http://medicalsupplies.medtronic.com/products/enteral-feeding.

C. R. Bard. (2017). *Gastric management.* Retrieved from https://www.crbard.com/en-US/Product-Search?pg=1&category=gastric+management.

Cronenwett, L., Sherwood, G., Barnsteiner, J., Disch, J., Johnson, J., Mitchell, P., ... Warren, J. (2007). Quality and safety education for nurses. *Nursing Outlook, 55*(3), 122–131. Retrieved from http://qsen.org/competencies/pre-licensure-ksas/.

De Alaiz, A. (2018). *Carbohydrate counting.* Retrieved from http://www.clinidiabet.com/en/infodiabetes/pumps/41.htm.

Dudek, S. G. (2018). *Nutrition essentials for nursing practice* (8th ed.). Philadelphia, PA: Lippincott, Williams, & Wilkins.

Ecklund, M. M. (2017). Percutaneous endoscopic gastrostomy (PEG), gastrostomy, and jejunostomy tube care. In D. L. Wiegand (Ed.), *AACN procedure manual for high acuity, progressive, and critical care* (7th ed.) (pp. 1216–1220). St. Louis, MO: Saunders Elsevier.

International Classification for Nursing Practice. (n.d.). *eHealth & ICNP.* Retrieved from https://www.icn.ch/what-we-do/projects/ehealth-icnp.

Irving, S. Y., Rempel, G., Lyman, B., Sevilla, W. M. A., Northington, L., Guenter, P., & American Society for Parenteral and Enteral Nutrition. (2018). Pediatric nasogastric tube placement and verification: Best practice recommendations from the NOVEL Project. *Nutrition in Clinical Practice, 33*(6), 921–927.

Lyman, B., Yaworski, J. A., Duesing, L., & Moore, C. (2016). *Verifying NG feeding tube placement in pediatric patients.* Retrieved from https://www.americannursetoday.com/verifying-ng-feeding-tube-placement-pediatric-patients/.

Mann, E. (2016). Nasoenteric tube feeding. Monitoring and care. Retrieved from *The Joanna Briggs Institute EBP Database,* JBI@OVID.

Mazur, E. E., & Litch, N. A. (2019). *Lutz's Nutrition & diet therapy* (7th ed.). Philadelphia: F.A: Davis Company.

McClave, S. A., Taylor, B. E., Martindale, R. G., Warren, M. M., Johnson, D. R., Braunschweig, C., American Society for Parenteral and Enteral Nutrition. (2016). Guidelines for the provision and assessment of nutrition support therapy in the adult critically ill patient: Society of Critical Care Medicine (SCCM) and American Society of Parenteral and Enteral Nutrition (A.S.P.E.N). *Journal of Parenteral and Enteral Nutrition, 40*(2), 159–211.

McGinnis, C. (2017). Nasogastric and orogastric tube insertion, care and removal. In D. L. Wiegand (Ed.), *AACN procedure manual for high acuity, progressive, and critical care* (7th ed.) (pp. 1011–1019). St. Louis, MO: Elsevier.

Metheny, N. A. (2018). *Preventing aspiration in older adults with dysphagia.* Retrieved from https://consultgeri.org/try-this/general-assessment/issue-20.pdf.

Metheny, N. A., Krieger, M. M., Healy, F., & Meert, K. L. (2019). A review of guidelines to distinguish between gastric and pulmonary placement of nasogastric tubes. *Heart and Lung, 48*(2019), 226–235.

Morley, J. E. (2018). *Overview of undernutrition.* Retrieved from http://www.merckmanuals.com/professional/nutritional_disorders/undernutrition/overview_of_undernutrition.html.

Nasogastric tube misplaced: Large verdict for patient's death. (2008). *Legal Eagle Eye Newsletter for the Nursing Profession.* Retrieved from http://www.nursinglaw.com/.

Nestlé. (2017). *Nutrition support information.* Retrieved from http://www.nestlenutritionstore.com/Pages/WhatIsDysphagia.aspx.

Paik, N. J. (2017). *Dysphagia.* Retrieved from https://emedicine.medscape.com/article/2212409-overview.

Santos, S. C., Woith, W., Freitas, M. I., & Zeferino, E. B. (2016). Methods to determine the internal length of nasogastric feeding tubes: An integrative review. *International Journal of Nursing Studies, 61,* 95–103.

Shlamovitz, G. Z., & Kulkarni, R. (2018). *Nasogastric tube.* Retrieved from https://emedicine.medscape.com/article/80925-technique.

Taylor, S. J., Allan, K., McWilliam, H., & Deirdre, T. (2014). Nasogastric tube depth: The "NEX" guideline is incorrect. *British Journal of Nursing, 23,* 641–644.

U.S. Department of Agriculture. (2016). *Food composition.* Retrieved from https://www.nal.usda.gov/fnic/food-composition.

U.S. Department of Agriculture. (2017). *MyPlate resources.* Retrieved from http://www.choosemyplate.gov/information-healthcare-professionals.html.

World Health Organization. (2017). *Nutrition health topics.* Retrieved from http://www.who.int/nutrition/topics/en/.

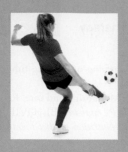

CHAPTER 6

Supporting Mobility and Immobilization

"Walking is man's best medicine." | **Hippocrates, 370 BCE**

LEARNING OBJECTIVES

By the end of this chapter, the reader will be able to:

1. Assist the client with active or passive range of motion.
2. Assist the client with ambulation using a transfer belt.
3. Describe client abilities required for different assistive devices: cane, walker, and crutches.
4. Identify the criteria for the correct size cane, walker, and crutches.
5. Teach the client to use a cane for ambulation and getting in and out of a chair.
6. Teach the client to use a walker for ambulation and getting in and out of a chair.
7. Teach the client to use crutches for ambulation and getting in and out of a chair.

248

8 Perform a neurovascular assessment.
9 Discuss different methods of extremity immobilization.
10 Discuss different methods of cervical spine immobilization.
11 Apply a variety of bandages, including a spiral bandage, a reverse spiral bandage, and a figure-8 bandage.
12 Assess a client in a cast.
13 Identify client education related to cast care at home.
14 Assess the client with traction.
15 Describe critical elements of managing care for a client in skin traction and in skeletal traction.

16 Perform pin-site care.
17 Apply a cervical collar.
18 Prioritize care for a client who has halo traction.
19 Discuss issues related to caring for a client with a limb loss, including phantom limb pain.
20 Assist the client with exercise and positioning following an amputation.
21 Demonstrate how to apply a compression bandage or commercial shrinker to the affected extremity following an amputation.

TERMINOLOGY

Abduction Movement of a limb away from the body's midline.

Adduction Movement of a limb toward the body's midline.

Arthroplasty Repair or replacement of a joint.

Atrophy Decrease in size of organ or tissue.

Circumduction Moving an extremity in such a manner that it makes the shape of a cone; the apex of the cone is the proximal joint, and the distal end of the extremity moves in full circles.

Compartment syndrome Cluster of signs and symptoms that occur when circulation and function of tissue are compromised by swelling within a muscle group or compartment surrounded by fascial membranes, putting further pressure on the arterioles, eventually resulting in ischemia and necrosis.

Contracture Permanent shortening or tightening of a muscle.

Dorsiflexion Flexion toward the posterior of that body part; opposite of palmar flexion or plantar flexion.

Eversion Turning outward; eversion of the ankle is moving the ankle so that the sole of the foot turns inward.

Extension Straightening a limb, increasing the angle of the joint.

Fascia A fibrous membrane covering, supporting, and dividing muscles.

Fasciotomy Surgical opening of the fascia.

Flexion Decreasing the angle of a joint; bending a limb at the joint.

Fracture A break in a bone.

Hemiparesis Paralysis affecting only one side of the body.

Hemiparetic A person with partial paralysis.

Hemiplegia Paralysis affecting only one side of the body.

Hyperextension Extending a joint past 180 degrees.

Hypertrophy Enlargement of muscles.

Inversion To turn inward; moving the ankle so that the sole of the foot turns inward.

Opposition Touching the thumb to each finger.

Peripheral vascular disease Disease of the arteries and veins of the extremities resulting in poor circulation.

Petaling Applying cut pieces of silk tape or moleskin with rounded edges in an overlapping pattern on the edge of a cast.

Pronation Moving the body or a part of the body to face downward, such as moving the forearm so that the palms of the hands face downward.

Rotation Circular movement around a central axis.

Spasticity Increase in muscle tension.

Sprain Trauma to a joint resulting in pain, disability, and the possibility of torn ligaments.

Strain Joint injury resulting from stretching the muscles and tendons surrounding the joint.

Supination Moving the body or a part of the body to face upward, such as moving the forearm so that the palms of the hands face upward.

ACRONYMS

AKA Above-the-knee amputation
BKA Below-the-knee amputation
ORIF Open reduction and internal fixation
PLP Phantom limb pain

SECTION 1 Supporting Mobility

Mobility is the ability to move freely and easily. In the healthcare setting, supporting mobility means ensuring the client engages in sufficient movement to maintain muscle mass and strength, prevent bone absorption, and maintain joint flexibility. Supporting mobility also often means supporting the ability to walk, one of the defining movements of human beings.

Walking keeps bones and muscles strong, helps to control body weight and reduce body fat, and improves blood lipids and blood pressure. The Centers for Disease Control and Prevention identifies walking as the most commonly reported physical activity performed by adults in the United States. Americans report that they are walking for leisure or transportation more frequently than in years past, with a little over 65% of women and 62% of men reporting they walked more than 10 minutes within the last 7 days (Ussery et al., 2017). Being physically active is one of the most important ways that we can improve our health. Physical activity improves sleep and decreases depression. According to the Physical Activity Guidelines Advisory Committee (2018), regular moderate to vigorous physical activity can reduce the risk for many types of cancers, including breast, colon, endometrium, esophagus, kidney, lung, and stomach cancer. For those individuals with an existing chronic condition, regular physical activity can reduce the risk of progression of the condition and reduce the risk of developing a new condition. This includes hypertension, type 2 diabetes, and osteoarthritis, which are a few of the more common chronic conditions in our country today.

Mobility enhances the physiologic functions not only of the musculoskeletal system but also of many other body systems. Physical activity improves respiratory function by increasing oxygen intake and gas exchange and mobilizing secretions. Physical activity benefits the cardiovascular system by increasing the heart rate, heart muscle contractility, cardiac output, and circulation. Activity benefits the gastrointestinal system by increasing intestinal motility, helping to prevent constipation. The endocrine system benefits because exercise stabilizes blood sugar and improves insulin uptake. Being upright and active improves blood flow to the urinary system and prevents stasis of urine in the bladder. Moderate exercise even seems to improve immune system function. In short, mobility is an important aspect of optimal health and health maintenance. Teaching clients how to use assistive devices that support their ability to walk therefore enhances many other aspects of their health (Fig. 6.1).

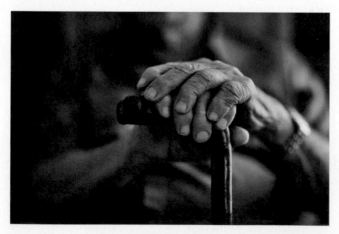

FIG. 6.1 The use of assistive devices that support individuals' ability to walk enhances many other aspects of their health.

Following illness and surgery, a rapid return to mobility and ambulation are often a priority nursing goal. Many years of research demonstrate that early ambulation is an effective method for reducing the complications of severe illness or surgery and improving long-term outcomes. Restoring a client's mobility follows a progression of repositioning before ambulating. Repositioning begins with sitting the client up in bed and progresses to dangling and sitting in a chair before beginning ambulation. The positioning of the client before ambulation is described in the "Moving Clients Safely" section of Chapter 1. Postsurgical units and intensive care units will have early activity and mobility protocols. Early activity and ambulation have been demonstrated to be safe and beneficial even in clients who are receiving mechanical ventilation (Negro et al., 2018). Early ambulation of critically ill clients requires collaboration, time, and effort on the part of a multidisciplinary team, including physicians, respiratory therapy, physical therapy, and nursing, in order to ambulate the client.

COLLABORATIVE CARE FOR CLIENTS WITH ASSISTIVE DEVICES

Restoration of walking is one of the most important goals of rehabilitation. Assistive devices support independent walking. They relieve some of the client's weight and provide stability so that clients can walk without falling. Falling is a significant source of injury in older adults. Rehabilitation with an assistive device is a multidiscipline endeavor that includes medicine, physical therapy, occupational therapy, and nursing.

The Role of the Nurse

The type of assistive device selected for ambulation depends on the strength and abilities of the client. Although nurses do not select the type of device, nurses' documentation of nursing assessments of the client's strengths and abilities can assist the healthcare provider in determining the timing to initiate ambulation and the type of assistive device prescribed. For example, in order to ambulate, clients must be able to bear their weight, have hip stability, and be cooperative. Therefore, documented nursing assessments about clients' successes in standing (weight bearing and hip stability) and degree of cooperation will assist the authorized healthcare provider in determining the type of assistive device required.

After an appropriate device has been selected for a client, nurses teach the client how to use it. Thereafter, nurses monitor and document the client's gait while he or she is using the assistive device. Gait reflects the client's core strength, posture, coordination, balance, and neuromuscular status. Nurses may teach clients ways to adjust their natural gait when they are learning to use an assistive device. Nurses also evaluate the speed and endurance of the client when ambulating with or without an assistive device. Finally, nurses evaluate the client's understanding of the safe use of an assistive device.

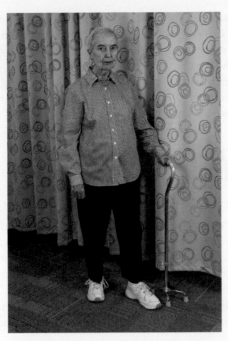

FIG. 6.2 Cane with a quad foot and an offset handle.

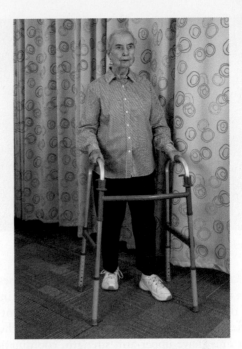

FIG. 6.3 Walkers provide more stability than canes.

Canes

A cane is an appropriate assistive device for a client who can bear weight and ambulate but requires assistance to maintain balance. Canes are also appropriate to assist a client with weakness in one leg but adequate balance, arm, and hand strength to use a cane successfully.

There are several types of canes. A standard cane has a rounded handle and a single tip or "foot." A tripod cane, or crab cane, has three feet. A quad cane provides the most support and has four feet. The use of rubber caps on cane feet provides traction and helps prevent slipping. Canes are the correct length if they extend from the client's greater trochanter to the floor. When the client holds the cane, the client's elbow should flex 20 to 30 degrees (Fig. 6.2).

Walkers

Walkers provide more stability than canes. They have four legs, which are usually adjustable, and handgrips, and they are made of lightweight metal. Legs may have rubber caps, wheels, or slides, which are sometimes made from tennis balls. Walkers are appropriate for people with bilateral weakness and less balance but who are still able to stand and walk. Walkers relieve more body weight than canes. Walkers come in a variety of frame sizes. The walker should be large enough that the client can step into the frame of the walker. The walker should extend from the floor to the client's greater trochanter. When the client holds the walker, the client's elbow should flex 20 to 30 degrees. As adults age, the use of walkers becomes more prevalent (Fig. 6.3).

Crutches

The two types of crutches are forearm crutches (also called Lofstrand crutches) and axillary crutches. Forearm crutches

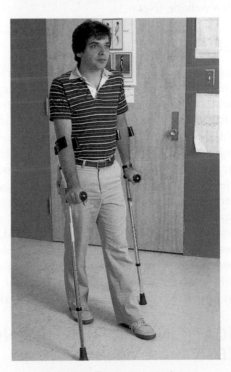

FIG. 6.4 Forearm crutches.

are more common for long-term use. They are metal and are shorter than axillary crutches, coming only to the forearm, with metal bands encircling the forearm. They distribute weight along the forearm and do not put stress on the wrists and shoulders (Fig. 6.4). Axillary crutches may be made of aluminum or wood. They reach from the floor to just under the axilla, but they should not touch the axilla. They are frequently used when a lower-extremity injury, such as a broken ankle, prevents full weight bearing on the injured extremity.

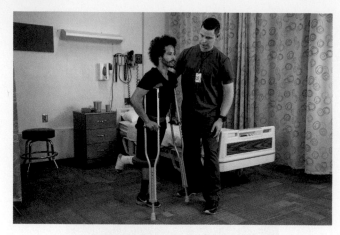

FIG. 6.5 Axillary crutches.

Axillary crutches should extend from 5 cm (2 inches) below the axilla to the floor when placed about 15 cm (6 inches) in front of the client in line with the axilla. The client's elbow should flex 15 to 30 degrees. In order to use crutches safely, a person must have upper-arm strength, coordination, and good balance. Using crutches is strenuous, requiring more energy than walking (Fig. 6.5).

RANGE OF MOTION

Some clients are not able to ambulate. For those clients, the immediate goal may be to maintain muscle integrity and joint flexibility. Nurses assist these clients with range-of-motion (ROM) exercises, which systematically move joints in their full range of motion through all appropriate planes. For example, the cervical joints of the neck are flexed, extended, and rotated. If the client is able to perform ROM independently, the nurse instructs and encourages the client to perform a series of active ROM movements from head to toe. If the client is unable to participate, the nurse or physical therapist may provide passive ROM, moving the client's joints him- or herself. The goals of performing ROM exercises are to promote circulation, prevent thrombophlebitis, maintain muscle strength, prevent contractures, and promote body alignment and joint flexibility.

APPLICATION OF THE NURSING PROCESS

Examples of Related International Classification for Nursing Practice (ICNP) Nursing Diagnoses, Expected Client Outcomes, and Nursing Interventions:

Nursing Diagnosis: Impaired walking

Supporting Data: Client requires an assistive device for safe ambulation.

Expected Client Outcomes: The client will increase walking distances as appropriate:
- Demonstrate the correct use of assistive devices to increase mobility.
- Use safety measures to minimize potential for injury.
- Demonstrate measures to safely increase mobility.

- Evaluate pain rating and quality of pain management.

Nursing Intervention Examples: Use safety measures, such as a transfer belt. Evaluate the client's gait, walking pace, and endurance.

Reference: International Classification for Nursing Practice. (n.d.). *eHealth & ICNP.* Retrieved from https://www.icn.ch/what-we-do/projects/ehealth-icnp.

CRITICAL CONCEPTS
Mobility

Accuracy (ACC)

Supporting mobility is subject to the following variables:
- assessment of the client, including alignment, capabilities and limitations for movement, cooperation and orientation, strength, mobility, level of discomfort, and activity intolerance
- identification of anatomical landmarks
- identification of accurate musculoskeletal movement
- understanding of the procedure by the client and family.

Client-Centered Care (CCC)

When supporting mobility, respect for the client is demonstrated through
- promoting autonomy
- providing privacy
- ensuring comfort
- arranging for an interpreter, if needed.

Infection Control (INF)

When supporting mobility, healthcare-associated infection is prevented by reducing the number and transfer of microorganisms, primarily through hand hygiene.

Safety (SAF)

When supporting mobility, safety measures prevent harm and provide a safe care environment, including:
- using a transfer belt and encouraging the client to wear nonslip shoes
- securing all medical lines and checking patency.

Communication (COM)
- Communication exchanges information (oral, written, nonverbal, or electronic) between two or more people.
- Documentation records information in a permanent legal record.
- Collaboration with the client and healthcare professionals improves mobility outcomes.

Health Maintenance (HLTH)

Nursing is dedicated to the promotion of health and abilities related to mobility, including ambulation and full ROM.

Evaluation (EVAL)

When supporting mobility, evaluation of outcomes enables the nurse to determine the efficacy of the care provided.

■ SKILL 6.1 Assisting With Ambulation Using a Transfer Belt

EQUIPMENT

Sit to stand lift, if indicated
Appropriate-size sling
Transfer belt
Nonslip shoes or slippers
Age-appropriate, facility-approved pain assessment tool
Clean gloves, if there is a risk of exposure to body fluids

BEGINNING THE SKILL

1. **INF** Perform hand hygiene.
2. **INF** Apply gloves if there is a risk of exposure to body fluids.
3. **CCC** Introduce yourself to the client and family and explain the procedure.
4. **SAF** Identify the client using two identifiers.
5. **CCC** Provide privacy. Close the door; pull the curtain until the client is dressed and standing.

PROCEDURE

6. **SAF** Review order. *Verifying the plan of care and possible limitations prevents injury to the client.*
7. **ACC** Assess the following:
   a. client's level of orientation and ability to follow instructions and cooperate
   b. client's ability to bear weight and upper-extremity strength in order to determine the need for assistive lifting equipment to assist the client to stand
   c. **CCC** client's pain-intensity rating, the character of the pain, and the exact location of the pain.
   The client must be able to bear weight, have hip stability, and be cooperative in order to successfully ambulate. See Chapter 1 and follow the Algorithm for Transfer to or From a Seated Position to determine the need for assistive lifting equipment to assist the client to stand. Assistive equipment is necessary anytime a nurse is lifting more than approximately 16 kg (35 lb). Implementing safe handling and movement standards prevents injury to the nurse and client.
8. **SAF** Assess for the presence of intravenous (IV) lines, catheters, and other equipment that might be an impediment to movement.
9. **SAF** Lock the wheels of the bed.
10. **SAF** Lower the bed to the lowest position.
11. **SAF** Move client into a sitting position and ensure the client can place both feet firmly on the floor.
12. **SAF** Observe the client's color. Make eye contact and ask how the client feels. Remain standing in front of the client. *Clients may experience orthostatic hypotension. Symptoms may include changes in color, an unfocused gaze, complaints of dizziness, and fainting.*
13. **SAF** Assist the client to put on nonslip shoes or slippers and a robe. Ensure the client can place both feet firmly on the floor.
14. **SAF** Secure a transfer belt around the client's waist. *The use of a transfer belt allows a safer hold while guiding a client from one position to another and assisting with ambulation.*

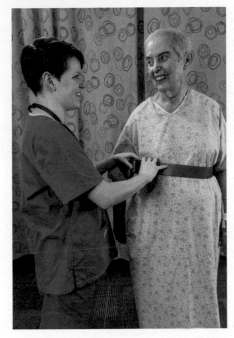

STEP 14 Secure a transfer belt around the client's waist.

15. **SAF** Grasp the transfer belt with one hand and assist the client to a standing position.
16. **SAF** Again observe the client's color for signs of pallor. Assess the client's balance. Ask how the client feels. *Clients may experience orthostatic hypotension and become light-headed or may be too unsteady to ambulate. Symptoms may include changes in color, an unfocused gaze, and complaints of dizziness.*
17. **SAF** Position yourself to the side and slightly behind the client, and then grasp the transfer belt.

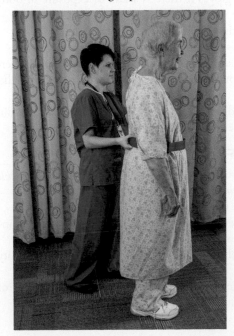

STEP 17 Maintain a hold on the transfer belt.

18. **EVAL** While continuing to grasp the transfer belt, encourage the client to walk. Match your pace to the client's steps. Monitor the client's balance and strength.
19. **ACC** Ambulate the identified distance and return to the client's bed or chair.
20. **SAF** Assist the client to a seated position and remove the transfer belt.
21. **EVAL** Evaluate the client's activity tolerance.

FINISHING THE SKILL

22. **CCC** Provide comfort. Assist the client with positioning, replace the pillows, and rearrange the bedding.

23. **SAF** Secure and check for patency of any medical equipment attached to the client, such as IV lines and Foley catheters.
24. **SAF** Ensure client safety. Ensure that the bed is in the lowest position and verify that the client can identify and reach the nurse call system. *These safety measures reduce the risk of falls.*
25. **INF** Remove gloves, if used. Perform hand hygiene.
26. **EVAL** Evaluate outcomes, including pain rating after walking, client gait, and how far and how fast the client walked.
28. **COM** Document assessment findings, care given, and outcomes in the legal healthcare record.

▪ SKILL 6.2 Teaching the Client to Use a Cane

EQUIPMENT

Cane
Transfer belt, if indicated
Nonslip shoes or slippers
Age-appropriate, facility-approved pain assessment tool
Clean gloves, if there is a risk of exposure to body fluids

BEGINNING THE SKILL

1. **INF** Perform hand hygiene.
2. **INF** Apply gloves if there is a risk of exposure to body fluids.
3. **CCC** Introduce yourself to the client and family.
4. **SAF** Identify the client using two identifiers.
5. **COM** Explain the procedure. Ensure the client understands the purpose of using a cane to assist with walking.
6. **CCC** Provide privacy. Close the door; pull the curtain until the client is dressed and standing.

PROCEDURE

7. **SAF** Review order. *Verifying the plan of care and possible limitations prevents injury to the client.*
8. **ACC** Assess the following:
   a. client's level of orientation and ability to follow instructions
   b. client's ability to bear weight and upper-extremity strength
   c. **CCC** client's pain-intensity rating, the character of the pain, and the exact location of the pain.

Clients must be able to bear weight, have hip stability, and be cooperative in order to successfully use a cane. Clients must have sufficient handgrip and arm strength for the cane to provide stability. A client's pain may prevent successful ambulation and interfere with learning the use of the cane.

9. **SAF** Assess for the presence of IV lines, catheters, and other equipment that might be an impediment to movement.
10. **SAF** If the client is in a bed, lock the wheels of the bed and lower the bed to the lowest position.
11. **SAF** Move the client into a sitting position and ensure the client can place both feet firmly on the floor.
12. **SAF** Assess for orthostatic hypotension. Observe the client's color and make eye contact. Ask how the client feels. Remain standing in front of the client. *Clients may experience orthostatic hypotension, and older adults are at increased risk. Symptoms may include changes in color, an unfocused gaze, complaints of dizziness, and fainting.*
13. **SAF** Assist the client to put on nonslip shoes or slippers and a robe.
14. **SAF** Secure a transfer belt around the client's waist, if indicated. *The use of a transfer belt allows a safer hold while guiding a client from one position to another and assisting with ambulation.*
15. **EVAL** Instruct the client to stand. If the client requires assistance to stand, a cane is probably not an adequate assistive device.

16. **ACC** Assess the fit of the cane. The cane should extend from the floor to the client's greater trochanter. When the client holds the cane, the client's elbow should flex 20 to 30 degrees.

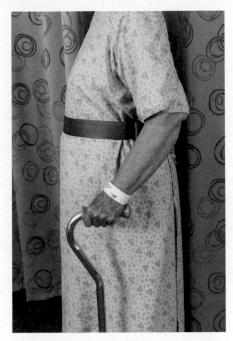

STEP 16 The elbow should flex 20 to 30 degrees.

17. **ACC** Instruct the client to hold the cane on the stronger side. *Holding on the stronger side improves support and prevents leaning into the cane.*

Walking

18. **ACC** Instruct the client to advance the cane a comfortable distance, between 15 and 30 cm (6–12 inches) depending on the height and strength of the client, directly in front of the hand holding the cane.
19. **ACC** Instruct the client to advance the foot on the weaker side even with the cane. *This provides a base of support combining the cane and foot of the weaker side.*
20. **ACC** Instruct the client to step forward with the foot on the stronger side even with or in front of the cane. Encourage the client to adjust the length of the step according to the client's balance and strength.
21. **EVAL** Accompany the client to practice the sequence (cane, weak side, strong side). If the client is walking well, the client may advance the cane and the foot of the weaker side together and then bring the foot of the strong side forward. Encourage the client to practice until a smooth gait is established.

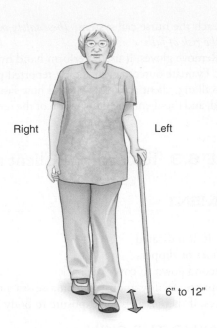

STEP 21 Step sequence is cane, weak side, and then strong side.

Getting in and out of a Chair

22. **ACC** Teach the client how to rise from a chair. Beginning with the client seated, instruct the client to hold the cane on the stronger side and hold the arm of the chair with the weaker side.
23. **ACC** Instruct the client to place the foot of the stronger side ahead of the foot of the weaker side.
24. **ACC** Instruct the client to push up out of the chair, distributing body weight between the feet and the cane.
25. **ACC** Teach the client how to sit down in a chair. Position the client standing directly in front of the chair. Grasp the transfer belt, if worn. Instruct the client to set aside the cane (hang the cane over the back or arm of the chair).
26. **ACC** Instruct the client to turn so that his or her back is to the chair, and then grasp the chair arms with both hands and lower into the chair. Release the transfer belt.
27. **EVAL** Observe the client get into and out of a chair using the cane.
28. **SAF** Assist the client to return to bed or chair and remove the transfer belt, if used.
29. **EVAL** Evaluate the client's activity tolerance, and reassess the client's pain level.

FINISHING THE SKILL

30. **CCC** Provide comfort. Assist the client with positioning, replace the pillows, and rearrange the bedding.
31. **SAF** Secure and check for the patency of any medical equipment attached to the client, such as IV lines and Foley catheters.
32. **SAF** Ensure client safety. Ensure that the bed is in the lowest position and verify that the client can identify

and reach the nurse call system. *These safety measures reduce the risk of falls.*

33. **INF** Remove gloves, if used. Perform hand hygiene.
34. **EVAL** Evaluate outcomes, including reported pain rating after walking, client gait, how far and how fast the client walked, and the client's demonstration of the use of a cane.

35. **COM** Document assessment findings, including client strength, balance, and reported pain level; care given, including cane fitting and instruction in the use of the cane; and outcomes in the legal healthcare record.

▪ SKILL 6.3 Teaching the Client to Use a Walker

EQUIPMENT

Walker
Transfer belt, if indicated
Nonslip shoes or slippers
Robe or second gown to cover the back
Age-appropriate, facility-approved pain assessment tool
Clean gloves, if there is a risk of exposure to body fluids

BEGINNING THE SKILL

1. **INF** Perform hand hygiene.
2. **INF** Apply gloves if there is a risk of exposure to body fluids.
3. **CCC** Introduce yourself to the client and family and explain the procedure. Ensure the client understands the purpose of using a walker to assist with walking.
4. **SAF** Identify the client using two identifiers.
5. **CCC** Provide privacy. Close the door; pull the curtain until the client is dressed and standing.

PROCEDURE

6. **SAF** Review order. Check if the indication for the walker is noted. *Verifying the plan of care prevents injury to the client.*
7. **ACC** Assess the following:
   a. client's level of orientation and ability to follow instructions
   b. client's ability to bear weight and upper-extremity strength
   c. **CCC** client's pain-intensity rating, the character of the pain, and the exact location of the pain.

Clients must be able to bear weight, walk, and cooperate in order to successfully use a walker. Clients must have sufficient handgrip and arm strength to lift or push the walker forward. A client's pain may prevent successful ambulation and interfere with learning the use of the walker.

8. **SAF** Assess for the presence of IV lines, catheters, and other equipment that might be an impediment to movement.
9. **SAF** If the client is in a bed, lock the wheels of the bed and lower the bed to the lowest position.
10. **SAF** Move the client into a sitting position and ensure the client can place both feet firmly on the floor.
11. **SAF** Assess for orthostatic hypotension. Observe the client's color and make eye contact. Ask how the client feels. Remain standing in front of the client. *Clients may experience orthostatic hypotension, and older adults are at*

increased risk. Symptoms may include changes in color, an unfocused gaze, complaints of dizziness, and fainting.

12. **SAF** Assist the client to put on nonslip shoes or slippers and a robe. If the client does not have a robe, put a second gown on backward to help cover the client's backside.
13. **SAF** Instruct the client to stand. If the client requires some assistance, secure a transfer belt around the client's waist. *The use of a transfer belt allows a safer hold while guiding a client from one position to another and assisting with ambulation.*
14. **ACC** Assess the fit of the walker. The walker should be large enough that the client can step into the frame of the walker. The walker should extend from the floor to the client's greater trochanter. When the client holds the walker, the client's elbow should flex 20 to 30 degrees.

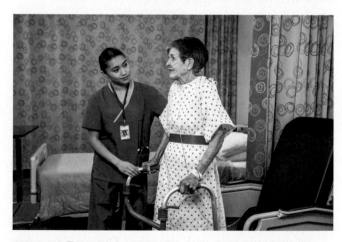

STEP 14 The elbow should flex approximately 20 degrees.

Walking

15. **SAF** Stand to one side and a little behind the client. Hold on to the transfer belt if the client is unsteady.
16. **ACC** Instruct the client to hold on to the handgrips and advance the walker a comfortable distance, between 15 and 30 cm (6–12 inches), by lifting or pushing depending on the type of walker.
17. **ACC** Instruct the client to step into the walker while all four feet are firmly on the floor. *This provides a broad base of support.*
18. **ACC** If the client has one side that is stronger, instruct the client to step forward with the foot on the weaker side first and then the stronger side.

19. **EVAL** Accompany the client to practice the sequence (walker forward, weak side, strong side), and evaluate the client's use of the walker.

Getting in and out of a Chair

20. **ACC** Teach the client how to get out of a chair. Grasp the transfer belt if the client is unsteady while practicing getting in and out of a chair. Instruct the client to do the following:
    a. Position the walker in front of the chair.
    b. Slide forward in the chair and place the foot of the stronger side ahead of the foot of the weaker side.
    c. Place both hands on the arms of the chair and push up out of the chair. **WARNING:** Do not pull up using the walker. *Using the walker to pull up does not provide sufficient stability and may cause the client to fall.*

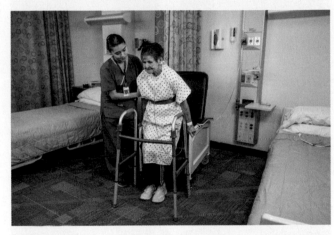

STEP 20C Encourage the client to place both hands on the arms of the chair to stand up.

    d. Distribute weight evenly between the feet and hold on securely to the walker handgrips.

    e. Advance the walker and step into it.
21. **ACC** Teach the client how to sit down in a chair. Instruct the client to do the following:
    a. Back up to the chair until the client feels the back of the legs touching the chair.
    b. Release the walker handgrips.
    c. Hold the chair arms with both hands and lower into the chair.
22. **EVAL** Observe the client get into and out of a chair using the walker.
23. **SAF** Assist the client to return to the bed or a chair and remove the transfer belt, if used.
24. **EVAL** Evaluate the client's activity tolerance, and reassess the client's pain level.

FINISHING THE SKILL

25. **CCC** Provide comfort. Assist the client with positioning, replace the pillows, and rearrange the bedding.
26. **SAF** Secure and check for the patency of any medical equipment attached to the client, such as IV lines and Foley catheters.
27. **SAF** Ensure client safety. Ensure that the bed is in the lowest position and verify that the client can identify and reach the nurse call system. *These safety measures reduce the risk of falls.*
28. **INF** Remove gloves, if used. Perform hand hygiene.
29. **EVAL** Evaluate outcomes, including reported pain rating after walking, client gait, how far and how fast the client walked, and the client's demonstration of the use of a walker.
30. **COM** Document assessment findings, including client strength, balance, and reported pain level; care given, including walker fitting and instruction in the use of the walker; and outcomes in the legal healthcare record.

■ SKILL 6.4 Teaching the Client to Use Crutches

EQUIPMENT

Crutches
Nonslip shoes or slippers
Robe or second gown to cover the back
Age-appropriate, facility-approved pain assessment tool
Clean gloves, if there is a risk of exposure to body fluids

BEGINNING THE SKILL

1. **INF** Perform hand hygiene.
2. **INF** Apply gloves if there is a risk of exposure to body fluids.

3. **CCC** Introduce yourself to the client and explain the procedure. Ensure the client understands the purpose of walking with crutches.
4. **SAF** Identify the client using two identifiers.
5. **CCC** Provide privacy. Close the door; pull the curtain until the client is dressed and standing.

PROCEDURE

6. **SAF** Review order. Check if the indication for the crutches is noted. *Verifying the plan of care prevents injury to the client. The amount of weight bearing that is allowed determines the appropriate gaits for the client to use.*

7. **ACC** Assess the following:
   a. client's level of orientation and ability to follow instructions
   b. client's ability to bear weight, coordination, balance, and upper-extremity strength
   c. **CCC** client's pain-intensity rating, the character of the pain, and the exact location of the pain.

   Clients must have sufficient arm strength, coordination, and balance to successfully use crutches. Different gaits are indicated for clients bearing weight on both legs as compared to just one. A client's pain may prevent successful ambulation and interfere with learning the use of the crutches.

8. **SAF** Assess for the presence of IV lines, catheters, and other equipment that might be an impediment to movement.

9. **SAF** If the client is in a bed, lock the wheels of the bed and lower the bed to the lowest position.

10. **SAF** Move the client into a sitting position and ensure the client can place both feet firmly on the floor.

11. **SAF** Assess for orthostatic hypotension. Observe the client's color and make eye contact. Ask how the client feels. Remain standing in front of the client. *Clients may experience orthostatic hypotension. Symptoms may include changes in color, an unfocused gaze, complaints of dizziness, and fainting.*

12. **SAF** Assist the client to put on nonslip shoes or slippers and a robe. If the client does not have a robe, put a second gown on backward to help cover the client's backside.

13. **SAF** Instruct the client to stand. Secure a transfer belt around the client's waist until you have evaluated the client's upper-arm strength, coordination, and balance. *The use of a transfer belt allows a safer hold while guiding a client from one position to another and assisting with ambulation. In order to use crutches safely, a person must have upper-arm strength, coordination, and good balance.*

14. **ACC** Assess the fit of the crutches. The crutches should extend from 5 cm (2 inches) below the axilla to the floor, placed about 15 cm (6 inches) in front of the client in line with the axilla.

15. **ACC** When the client holds the crutches, the client's elbow should flex 15 to 30 degrees. Adjust the handgrips for the crutches to enable the client to achieve this degree of flexion.

16. **SAF** Stand to one side and a little behind the client. Hold on to the transfer belt if the client is unsteady.

17. **ACC Teaching four-point gait (weight-bearing on both feet):**

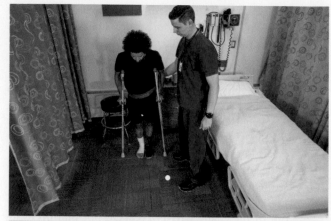
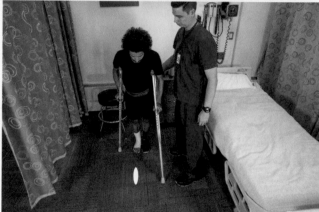
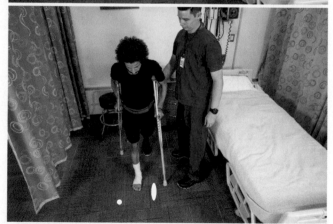
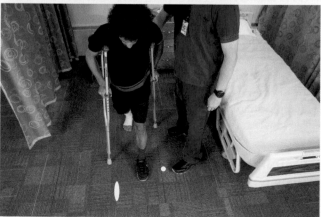

STEP 17 Four-point gait.

a. Instruct the client to place the crutch tips just in front of the feet.

b. Instruct the client to advance the left crutch a comfortable distance, between 15 and 30 cm (6–12 inches) depending on the height and strength of the client, and then to advance the right foot even with the tip of the crutch.

c. Instruct the client to advance the right crutch the same distance, and then advance the left foot even with the tip of the crutch.

d. Accompany the client as he or she practices the sequence (crutch tip, foot, crutch tip, foot), evaluating the client's gait. Encourage the client to practice until a smooth gait is established.

18. **ACC Teaching three-point gait (non–weight bearing on one foot):**

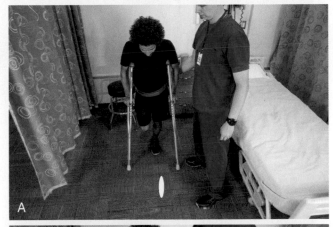

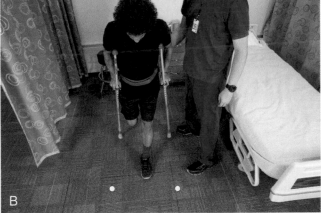

STEP 18 Three-point gait (non–weight bearing).

a. Instruct the client not to put weight on the non–weight-bearing foot.

b. Instruct the client to place the crutch tips 10 to 15 cm (4–6 inches) in front of the feet.

c. Instruct the client to support his or her weight on the crutches and advance the weight-bearing foot a comfortable distance, between 15 and 30 cm (6–12 inches), depending on the height and strength of the client.

d. Instruct the client to transfer his or her weight to the strong foot and then advance the crutch tips 10 to 15 cm (4–6 inches) in front of the feet. Instruct the client to support his or her weight on the crutches and advance the strong (weight-bearing) foot forward.

e. Accompany the client as he or she practices the sequence (crutch tips, strong foot, crutch tips, strong foot), evaluating the client's gait. Encourage the client to practice until a smooth gait is established.

19. **ACC Teaching three-point plus gait (partial weight bearing):**
a. Instruct the client to avoid putting full weight on the partial–weight-bearing foot.

b. Instruct the client to place the crutch tips 10 to 15 cm (4–6 inches) in front of the feet.

c. Instruct the client to support his or her weight on the crutches and the partial–weight-bearing foot while advancing the weight-bearing foot a comfortable distance, between 15 and 30 cm (6–12 inches), depending on the height and strength of the client.

d. Instruct the client to transfer his or her weight to the strong foot and then advance the crutch tips 10 to 15 cm (4–6 inches) in front of the feet. Instruct the client to support his or her weight on the crutches and advance the partial–weight-bearing foot, then advance the weight-bearing foot forward.

e. Accompany the client as he or she practices the sequence (crutch tips with weak foot, strong foot, crutch tips with weak foot, strong foot), evaluating the client's gait. Encourage the client to practice until a smooth gait is established.

20. **ACC Teaching swing-to gait or swing through**
a. Instruct the client to place the crutch tips just in front of the feet.

b. Instruct the client to advance both crutches a comfortable distance, between 15 and 30 cm (6–12 inches), depending on the height and strength of the client. The client is bearing his or her weight independently.

c. **Swing to:** Instruct the client to transfer his or her weight onto the crutches and advance both feet even with the tips of the crutches.

d. **Swing through:** Instruct the client to transfer his or her weight onto the crutches and advance both feet to a point between 15 and 30 cm (6–12 inches) in front of the tips of the crutches. The safe distance will vary according to the height and strength of the client.

e. Accompany the client as he or she practices the sequence (crutch tips, both feet to crutch tips), evaluating the client's gait. Encourage the client to practice until a smooth gait is established.

21. **ACC Using crutches to ascend and descend stairs:**
    a. **Ascending:** Instruct the client to transfer his or her weight onto the crutches and arm rail if available.
    b. Place the unaffected foot on the step and step up, bringing the affected foot to the step. Bring the crutches to the level of the unaffected foot.

    c. **Descending:** Instruct the client to transfer his or her weight onto the unaffected foot/leg.
    d. Instruct the client to position both crutches on the lower stair and step down with the affected foot/leg while supporting his or her weight on the crutches.
    e. Place the unaffected foot/leg alongside the crutches. Transfer the weight to the unaffected foot/leg.
    f. Position both crutches on the next lower step. Repeat as needed.

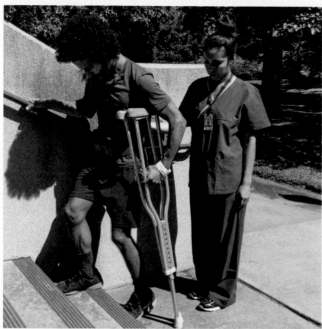

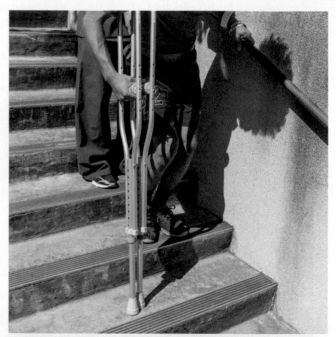

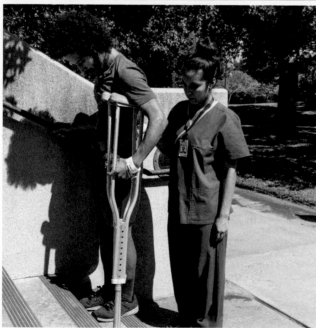

STEPS 21A AND 21B Using crutches to ascend stairs.

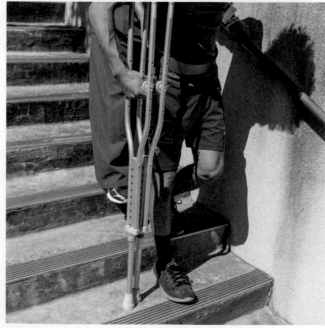

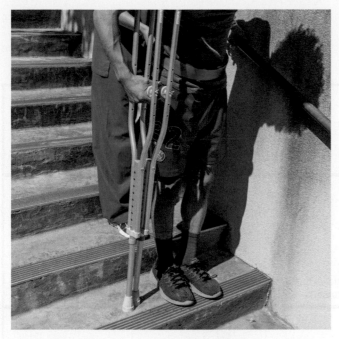

STEP 21F Using crutches to descend stairs.

g. Accompany the client as he or she practices the sequence, evaluating the client's gait. Encourage the client to practice until a smooth gait is established.

22. **SAF** Assist the client to return to bed or chair and remove the transfer belt, if used.
23. **EVAL** Evaluate the client's activity tolerance, and reassess the client's pain level.

FINISHING THE SKILL

24. **CCC** Provide comfort. Assist the client with positioning, replace the pillows, and rearrange the bedding.
25. **SAF** Secure and check for the patency of any medical equipment attached to the client, such as IV lines and Foley catheters.
26. **SAF** Ensure client safety. Ensure that the bed is in the lowest position and verify that the client can reach the nurse call system. *These safety measures reduce the risk of falls.*
27. **INF** Remove gloves, if used. Perform hand hygiene.
28. **EVAL** Evaluate outcomes, including reported pain rating after walking with crutches, client gait, how far and how fast the client walked, and the client's demonstration of the use of crutches.
29. **COM** Document assessment findings, including client strength, balance, and reported pain level; care given, including crutches fitting and instruction in the use of crutches; and outcomes.

▪ SKILL 6.5 Performing Active and Passive Range-of-Motion (ROM) Exercises

EQUIPMENT

Clean gloves, if there is a risk of exposure to body fluids

BEGINNING THE SKILL

1. **INF** Perform hand hygiene.
2. **INF** Apply gloves if there is a risk of exposure to body fluids.
3. **CCC** Introduce yourself to the client and family and explain the procedure.
4. **SAF** Identify the client using two identifiers.
5. **CCC** Provide privacy. Close the door, pull the curtain, and cover the client with a gown or blanket.

PROCEDURE

6. **SAF** Set up an ergonomically safe space. Raise the bed to a comfortable working height. Raise one side rail. *Setting up an ergonomically safe space prevents injury to the nurse and client.*
7. **SAF** Review order. *Verifying the plan of care and possible limitations prevents injury to the client.*
8. **ACC** Assess the following:
   a. client's level of orientation and ability to follow instructions
   b. client and family's understanding of ROM exercises

   c. **CCC** client's pain-intensity rating, the character of the pain, and the exact location of the pain.
   Your assessment is to determine the client's ability to perform and/or participate in ROM exercises.
9. **CCC** Premedicate client, if indicated and ordered.. *Pain limits mobility and can be triggered by movement.*
10. **SAF** Assess for the presence of IV lines and other equipment that might be an impediment to movement, such as a Foley catheter, ventilator tubing, or electrocardiogram (ECG) wires.
11. **ACC** Instruct or assist the client to perform the ROM movements:
    a. flexion by tucking the chin down to the chest
    b. extension by lifting the chin toward the ceiling
    c. rotation by turning the chin toward first one shoulder then the other
    d. and lateral flexion by tilting the head first to one shoulder and then the other shoulder.
12. **ACC** Support the client's arm, first one and then the other, and instruct or assist the client to perform shoulder rotation:
    a. external rotation by raising the arm, bending the elbow to a 90-degree angle, and moving the forearm and hand up to the shoulder

b. internal rotation by maintaining the 90-degree angle and moving the forearm and hand down toward the client's hip.

13. **ACC** Support the client's arm, first one and then the other, and instruct or assist the client to perform arm motions:
   a. flexion by lifting the arm toward the ceiling then above the client's head

Head	Flexion/extension · Rotation · Lateral flexion
Shoulder	Flexion/extension · Internal/external rotation · Adduction · Abduction
Elbow	Flexion/extension · Pronation/supination
Wrist	Rotation · Abduction/adduction · Flexion/extension
Hand	Flexion/extension · Abduction/adduction · Opposition · Rotation
Hip and knee	Flexion/extension · Abduction/adduction · Internal rotation · External rotation
Ankle, foot, and toe	Flexion/extension · Abduction/adduction · Rotation

Range of motion for body joints.

b. extension by returning the arm to the client's side

c. abduction by moving the arm laterally out to the side then above the client's head

d. adduction by returning the arm to the client's side and moving the arm across the body.

14. **ACC** Support the client's elbow, first one and then the other, and instruct or assist the client to perform elbow motions:

a. flexion and extension of the elbow by bending and straightening the elbow

b. supination and pronation of the elbow by supporting the elbow, maintaining the 90-degree angle, and turning the palm up and then the palm down.

15. **ACC** Support the client's forearm and wrist, first one and then the other, and instruct the client to perform wrist motions:

a. flexion and extension by bending the palm down toward the forearm, straightening the wrist, and then bending the dorsal aspect of the hand back toward the forearm

b. abduction and adduction by turning the fingers and moving the wrist away from the body and then toward the body

c. rotation by turning the hand in a circle.

16. **ACC** Support the client's hand, first one and then the other, and instruct or assist the client to perform hand motions:

a. extension and flexion by extending all of the fingers and then flexing them into a fist

b. abduction and adduction by spreading the fingers wide and bringing them together

c. opposition by touching the thumb to each finger

d. rotation by turning the thumb in a circle.

17. **ACC** Support the client's lower leg, first one and then the other, and instruct or assist the client to perform hip and knee motions:

a. flexion by raising the leg, bending the knee, and moving the knee toward the chest

b. extension by straightening the knee and hip and bringing the leg back to the bed

c. abduction by moving the leg laterally out to the side and away from the body

d. adduction by returning the leg to midline and moving the leg across the other leg

e. internal rotation by turning the leg so that the knee and toes point to the other leg

f. external rotation by turning the leg so that the knee and toes point away from the body.

18. **ACC** Support the client's lower leg, or if the client is able to perform independently, allow the client's leg to rest on the bed, first one and then the other, and instruct or assist the client to perform ankle and foot motions:

a. flexion and extension by alternating pointing the toes downward and dorsiflexing by pulling the toes upward toward the shin

b. abduction and adduction by turning the toes and moving the foot away from the body and then toward the body

c. rotation by turning the ankle in a circle.

FINISHING THE SKILL

19. **CCC** Provide comfort. Assist the client with positioning, replace the pillows, and rearrange the bedding.

20. **SAF** Secure and check for the patency of any medical equipment attached to the client, such as IV lines and Foley catheters.

21. **SAF** Ensure client safety. Ensure that the bed is in the lowest position and verify that the client can identify and reach the nurse call system. *These safety measures reduce the risk of falls.*

22. **INF** Remove gloves, if used. Perform hand hygiene.

23. **EVAL** Evaluate outcomes, including the client's pain rating after ROM; the client's ability to assist; and the client's ability to flex, extend, abduct, adduct, and rotate body joints.

24 **COM** Document assessment findings, care given, and outcomes in the legal healthcare record.

SECTION 2 Supporting Immobilization

The previous section discusses the methods and rationale for nurses to support mobility; however, nurses also support immobilization. When there has been an injury to the bone or the soft tissue around the bone, immobilizing the affected area keeps it appropriately aligned and allows it to heal without further injury.

SUPPORTING IMMOBILIZATION OF A LIMB OR JOINT

Immobilization is used in the treatment of injuries to ligaments, tendons, muscles, and bones in limbs and joints. As discussed in the following sections, slings, bandages, casts, fixation, and traction may be used.

TABLE 6.1 Five Ps of Neurovascular Assessment

Five Ps	Assessment	Symptoms of
Pain	Assess level of pain using an appropriate pain scale. Assess pain location, radiation, frequency, and quality.	Pain may be a symptom of pressure on a nerve, pressure on skin and tissue, or the formation of a thrombus.
Paralysis	Assess the client's ability to move the distal portion of the extremity. Ask the client to wiggle toes or fingers.	Paralysis may be a symptom of pressure on nerves.
Paresthesia	Ask the client if he or she has any altered sensations, such as tingling or "pins and needles."	Altered sensation is a symptom of pressure on a nerve.
Pulses	Palpate pulses distal to the immobilization device. Compare the pulse on the affected limb to the pulse on the other limb. Check capillary refill. Use a Doppler if you are unable to palpate a pulse.	Absent pulses and decreased capillary refill are symptoms of compromised circulation.
Pallor	Assess the color of the affected extremity distal to the immobilization device and compare the color to the other hand or foot.	Changes in color are a symptom of compromised circulation.

Reference: Peters, 2017.

A critical aspect of nursing care supporting the immobilization of a limb or joint is the neurovascular assessment. Orthopedic immobilizers can potentially place pressure on nerves or the vascular supply of the affected extremity. The neurovascular assessment has traditionally included the "five Ps": pain, paralysis, paresthesia, pulses, and pallor (Peters, 2017). Knowing that there are five signs to assess helps to prevent overlooking one sign. Review Table 6.1 for more details regarding the neurovascular assessment. Communicate any changes in the neurovascular assessment immediately to the authorized healthcare provider because interventions may need to occur. As described in Box 6.1, the failure to relay changes in the neurovascular assessment can have tragic outcomes.

In addition, the nurse uses an age-appropriate, culturally sensitive pain assessment tool that is facility approved to assess the client's pain related to the injury. See Chapter 7 for further descriptions of pain assessment tools. The nurse also performs a skin assessment to determine the status of the skin related to the injury and continues to monitor the skin to determine if the immobilization of the limb or joint or the pressure from the immobilizing device is resulting in skin injury.

Slings

A sling is a simple device commonly used to immobilize an upper extremity and provide support to relieve the weight of the arm. Slings are typically used for wrist, forearm, elbow, arm, and shoulder injuries. Immobilization in a sling allows

BOX 6.1 Lessons From the Courtroom: Failure to Report Assessment Findings Results in Amputation of Pediatric Client's Leg

A jury in the Superior Court of Dougherty County, Georgia, awarded over $24 million to a 14-year-old male who lost his leg following care for a fractured distal femur. The fracture was repaired with a closed reduction with an external fixator.

The night following the surgery, the midnight assessment performed by the nurse noted the client complained that his leg was numb and that he could not move his toes. The next morning, the 0800 assessment noted the toes were cool to touch, there was no palpable pulse, and the client complained of increasing pain. The changes in the neurovascular assessment were never reported to the orthopedic surgeon. By the afternoon, an arteriogram showed no blood flow below the knee. Because there was not a vascular surgeon available to try to reestablish perfusion, the leg was amputated that afternoon.

The attorney for the family brought in an outside nursing expert and established that the nurses providing care to the young man did not adequately assess the neurovascular status of the extremity, did not understand the significance of the warning signs they documented, and did not notify the orthopedic surgeon in time to save the boy's leg.

Reference: Post-op care: Failure to monitor leads to amputation of pediatric patient's leg, 2008.

the bone to maintain alignment as remodeling occurs and soft tissue and muscle heal. Sling use can also prevent dependent edema by positioning the hand slightly above the elbow and maintaining elbow flexion of 90 degrees (Obeid, 2017). Slings may be used to keep a client from using the arm following pacemaker or cardioverter implantation. Slings have also been shown to improve walking for clients with hemiparesis. In this situation, immobilizing an extremity helps the client's mobility. Supporting the affected arm results in a decrease in the work of walking and a smoother gait. See Box 6.2 for information on the research.

Nursing care for a client with a sling includes assessment for dependent edema and skin breakdown beneath the sling, in the axilla, and along the neck where the sling strap is positioned (Obeid, 2017). Nurses also assess the fit of the sling: There are many different brands and types; however, sling size is determined by the distance from the client's wrist to the elbow. The fit is correct if the elbow is firmly in the cuff of the sling and the forearm, wrist, and hand are supported. Nursing assessments may also include observation of the client's gait with the sling. One area of investigation regarding the use of slings is the effect of an arm sling on walking in clients with hemiplegia. One study found that gait efficiency and speed were increased when a sling was used on the affected arm for clients with hemiplegia following stroke (Han et al., 2011; Obeid, 2017).

BOX 6.2 Lessons From the Evidence: Improving Mobility With Immobilization

The Effect of Arm Slings on Walking in Clients With Hemiplegia

This study examined the impact of wearing an arm sling on the affected side during walking training in clients with hemiplegia following a stroke.

Characteristics of a typical hemiplegic gait include slow speed, a short stance, poorly coordinated movements deviating from the person's center of gravity, and decreased weight bearing of the weak leg. Thirty-one clients with hemiparesis caused by stroke and 31 able-bodied individuals matched for age, sex, height, and weight participated in the study. All participants wore a single-strap arm sling during the gait trials. To analyze gait, reflective markers were placed on anatomic landmarks, and five cameras recorded the location of the markers. Additionally, three-dimensional gait data were collected with the Vicon system.

The study by Han et al. (2011) investigated the effect of an arm sling on energy consumption while walking. Data were collected on walk speed, oxygen rate, heart rate, and oxygen cost on 37 hemiparetic clients by walking with and without an arm sling. Half walked with the arm sling first, rested 20 minutes, and then walked without the arm sling. The other half of the group walked without the arm sling first, rested, and then walked with the arm sling. The results of the study showed significantly increased gait speed, and the oxygen consumption rate (mL/kg min) and oxygen cost (mL/kg m) were decreased when walking with the arm sling. In fact, the oxygen cost in clients with hemiplegia when walking without the arm sling was 1½ times greater than in those walking with the arm sling. This decreased energy use when walking with an arm sling has implications for the performance of activities of daily living and independence.

Bandages

Bandages may be applied for a variety of reasons: to support a wound, to immobilize a wound, to apply pressure, or to secure a dressing. Like a sling, a bandage may immobilize tissues to support healing and provide comfort. Bandages can also be used to compress tissues in order to prevent swelling, promote venous return, or to apply pressure to a wound. However, the use of a compression bandage in older adults with peripheral vascular disease may be contraindicated (Giles, 2018). Bandages may be applied in the following manner:

- spiral bandage around a cylindrical extremity
- reverse spiral around an extremity with increasing diameter
- figure-8 bandage over a joint.

When bandaging ankles, the figure-8 method is preferred over the spiral because less pressure is applied to the Achilles tendon (Giles, 2018).

There are many different sizes and types of bandages, including elasticized bandages and gauze bandages. Elasticized bandages, such as an Ace bandage, come in rolls, and a variety of different widths are available, from 1 inch to 6 inches. Elasticized bandages can be used to protect the skin, stabilize a splint, or secure hot or cold therapy. They can be wrapped to apply pressure to reduce swelling, such as wrapping a sprained ankle, or to prevent dependent edema, for example, when a client has venous insufficiency. However, applying a compression dressing for a venous ulcer is discussed in Chapter 16, Wound Care. If bandages are not wrapped correctly, they can have a tourniquet effect, resulting in places where high pressure is exerted and, as a result, cause tissue damage and necrosis. Therefore, a bandage should be removed if the client experiences any changes in warmth, color, or sensation or increased pain. The older adult is more susceptible to tissue damage and should be assessed frequently (Giles, 2018).

At times, there should be a layer of padding applied before the bandage is wrapped; this is especially true for older adults. For example, when an ankle is bandaged, the Achilles tendon should be padded because it is an area of high-pressure concern (Giles, 2018). Elasticized bandages are secured with Velcro, tape, or safety pins. The use of metal clips is discouraged because they can injure the skin. In the past, elasticized bandages commonly contained latex; however, most elasticized bandages today are latex-free. For clients who are allergic to latex, ensure that the bandage is latex-free before application.

Gauze bandages can also protect the skin and secure wound dressings. Gauze bandages are very absorbent and can be impregnated with a medication or other substance; for example, impregnating with petroleum jelly creates a bandage through which air cannot pass. Like elasticized bandages, gauze bandages come in rolls of various widths. They have different amounts of stretch, compression, and durability depending on the amount and combination of cotton, polyester, and elastic in the bandage.

Nurses assess the site each time bandages are changed. The nursing assessment includes a pain assessment, an assessment of skin condition, and neurovascular checks to ensure sufficient blood flow to the affected site. Signs of compromised blood flow include color change, edema, coolness to the touch, decreased pulses, and client report of a tingling sensation.

Casts

Casts are rigid structures applied to immobilize bones and soft tissue in a specific position to promote optimal healing. They are applied with a variety of types of fractures. In a closed fracture, a bone is broken but the skin is intact; thus, there is less of a risk for infection. An open fracture refers to a break in the bone that protrudes through the skin. When swelling is anticipated, a splint may be used until the swelling subsides, and then a cast may be applied.

The purposes of casts are to maintain anatomical alignment and protect the bone and soft tissue as they heal. Casts may include the joint closest to the fracture to increase stability. Although casts are most commonly used with fractured bones, they may also be used to reposition soft tissue,

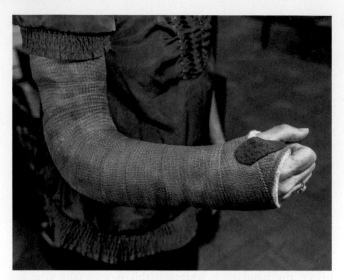

FIG. 6.6 Casts maintain anatomical alignment and protect the bone and soft tissue.

BOX 6.3 Lifespan Considerations: Pediatric and Geriatric Considerations in Cast Care

Pediatric Considerations

Pediatric clients are at increased risk for developing complications from casts. Pediatric clients who are nonverbal, have developmental delays, and/or have muscle spasticity are at particularly high risk. Within a rigid cast, ischemia occurs very quickly if there is swelling of the soft tissues. Because of this potential in children, nurses immediately investigate the skin and neurovascular status when children demonstrate overt signs of pain, such as crying, and subtler signs of pain, such as agitation and sleeplessness.

Children are at risk for putting items into their casts. Older children may be trying to scratch an itch, and younger children may insert a small toy or other object, much as they will put objects in the ears, nose, or mouth. An object inside a cast may result in ischemia, skin breakdown, infection, and very serious consequences. Children and parents need to be told to never put an object inside a cast.

Geriatric Considerations

Older adults have less elasticity in their skin and are at greater risk for skin tears. Nurses emphasize, both within the healthcare setting and when the client is home, the importance of assessing and caring for skin. Observing and reporting any redness or skin breakdown around the edge of the cast or within the casted area is important to prevent infection or further skin breakdown.

---

such as casting for clubfoot (Fig. 6.6). Sometimes casts are made with a "window," which is an open area that serves to relieve pressure or allow visualization of a wound.

Casts may be formed with several different types of materials, with each type having advantages and disadvantages. A traditional Plaster of Paris cast is heavy, takes at least 24 hours to completely harden and dry, and must be kept dry. Before a plaster cast is completely dry, care must be taken to prevent any accidental pressure on the cast that might in turn put pressure on the tissue and skin underneath the cast. When a plaster cast is applied, the heat released from the exothermic process can result in skin burns. On the positive side, plaster casts are inexpensive and provide strong, rigid support for broken bones. In contrast, fiberglass casts are lighter than plaster, harden very quickly, tolerate getting wet, and are less likely to injure the skin; however, they are more expensive. Today, fiberglass casts are much more commonly used as a result of their durability, ease of removal, and, greater client satisfaction (Chu, 2017; Wollan, 2017).

Nursing care associated with casts includes vigilant assessment to ensure any complications related to the cast are reported immediately and addressed. Regular skin assessment is performed to detect skin breakdown or pressure injury resulting from the rigid structure of the cast. If undetected, these can quickly lead to an infection. Pediatric and geriatric clients have specific age-related cast care considerations, as described in Box 6.3.

Assessment for swelling is critical because if an extremity swells significantly, the cast can impair circulation or compress nerves. When an extremity is casted following a surgical repair, assess for bleeding by observing for any blood absorbed by the cast.

A severe potential complication of a fracture or soft tissue injury is compartment syndrome. Compartment syndrome is swelling within the muscle compartment restricted by fascia. When swelling occurs in an enclosed space, venous return is decreased. This further exacerbates the edema, which in turn exerts even greater pressure, including on the arterioles. Eventually, the result is ischemia and necrosis. Pain is an early warning sign of compartment syndrome, whereas pallor and diminished pulses in the affected limb are late signs. If the healthcare team suspects compartment syndrome, the cast is removed immediately. If compartment syndrome is occurring, a fasciotomy is performed as soon as possible to relieve pressure within the soft tissue. A delayed response can result in ischemia and necrosis, possibly requiring amputation of the limb (Gyi, 2018).

Fixation

Severe fractures, especially those that involve fragmentation of bone, may require a surgical repair known as an open reduction and internal fixation (ORIF). The procedure begins with reduction, or realignment of the structures, followed by fixation, or stabilization and joining of the bone ends or pieces with screws, pins, rods, or plates.

Sometimes, external fixation is used instead of ORIF. An external fixation device is a rigid metal frame that maintains alignment of the bone while it heals. It is attached to the healthy bone on either side of the break with pins, bolts, or wires inserted through small incisions in the skin and soft tissue (Wollan, 2017). An external fixation device can be used temporarily until the client is determined to be able to tolerate ORIF, which is a longer surgery, or when there has been significant soft tissue damage. A skill related to the nursing

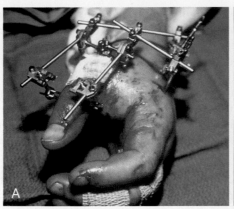
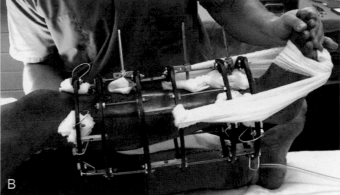

FIG. 6.7 External fixation device.

care of a client with an external fixation device is pin-site care, which is described in more detail later in the chapter (Fig. 6.7).

Traction

Traction, the application of a pulling force, is another method used to immobilize fractured bones. Although current orthopedic management more frequently uses internal and external fixation, traction may still be used as a temporary measure before surgery or as a conservative, noninvasive treatment for femur or hip fractures. Traction may also be used in children, either for femur fracture or congenital hip dislocation. Traction is also sometimes used to reduce pain and muscle spasm for individuals with back pain unrelated to fracture.

Two methods for applying traction are skeletal and skin traction. Skeletal traction involves the placement of skeletal pins by an orthopedic surgeon. The skeletal pins are then attached to a frame and are used to provide the pulling force. Although this technique firmly immobilizes the bone, it is invasive and puts the client at risk for infection. However, skeletal traction is less invasive and less expensive than external fixation (Fig. 6.8).

In contrast, skin traction is noninvasive and does not increase the risk of infection. The weights are attached to the skin either by an adhesive method, such as tape, or a non-adhesive method, such as straps or a boot. Skin traction can only be used if the individual's skin is intact and healthy. Skin traction cannot support as much weight as skeletal traction. Skin breakdown is a disadvantage of skin traction (Fig. 6.9).

Nursing care for a client in traction involves maintaining the pulling force of the weights; maintaining the alignment of the extremity; and if skeletal traction is involved, providing pin-site care. As with other methods of immobilization, assessment of skin and neurovascular function is a critical nursing function.

SUPPORTING CERVICAL IMMOBILIZATION

In addition to extremities requiring immobilization, the cervical spine may also need immobilization, commonly

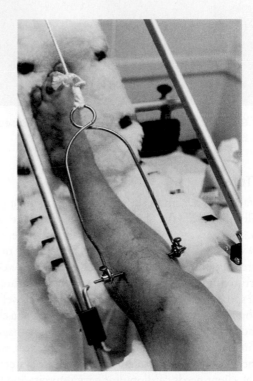

FIG. 6.8 Skeletal traction involves the placement of skeletal pins attached to a pulling force.

as a result of an injury sustained during a motor vehicle collision; a fall; or while skiing, diving, or playing team sports.

Cervical Collar

A cervical collar stabilizes and maintains the alignment of the cervical spine. There are two types:
- Two-piece rigid collars prevent neck flexion, extension, and rotation, thereby maintaining anatomical alignment, promoting healing, and preventing injury to the spinal cord.
- One-piece soft collars provide gentle neck support (Fig. 6.10).

Nursing care includes pain management, skin assessment under the collar, and client education about the cervical collar.

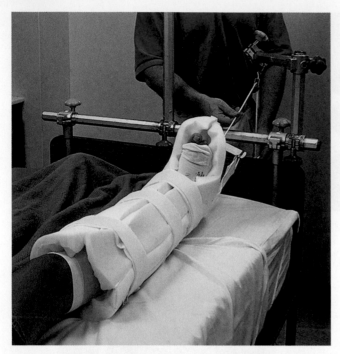

FIG. 6.9 Skin traction is noninvasive and involves securing a wrap, straps, or a boot to a pulling force.

Halo Traction

Halo traction is a form of skeletal traction in which pins are surgically placed in the skull. The halo apparatus is made up of a vest, bars attached to the vest, a halo device, and the pins in the skull. Halo traction may be used to maintain the correct alignment for healing when the cervical vertebrae are fractured. It provides even greater immobilization of the cervical spine than the two-piece cervical collar, as well as stabilization and support of the head. Nursing care of a client in halo traction includes providing pin care, pain management, and skin and neurovascular assessment. The vest worn in halo traction should have an emergency release system in the event the client needs cardiopulmonary resuscitation (CPR).

PIN CARE

Pin care is an important aspect of nursing care for clients with external fixation devices, skeletal traction, and halo traction. The approach to pin-site care has been debated and researched for many years; however, the methods and types of studies are so heterogeneous that there are still no clear recommendations for evidence-based practice (Lethaby, Temple, & Santy-Tomlinson, 2013; Mann, 2016). Typically with pin care, a sterile cotton-tipped applicator is dipped into a solution and then used to clean around the insertion site of a pin. The type of solution varies and may include sterile normal saline, hydrogen peroxide, half-strength hydrogen peroxide, and chlorhexidine. The National Association of Orthopaedic Nurses currently recommends cleaning with chlorhexidine 2 mg/mL. Iodine has been shown to interfere with normal healing and is not used for pin care (Lagerquist

et al., 2012). A dressing is sometimes applied to the pin sites and sometimes not. On external fixator devices, leaving the initial dressing on from surgery for 1 week before removing it and initiating any pin care was shown to improve outcomes (Mann, 2016).

Another area of research has been the frequency of pin care. Pin-site care once a week may be appropriate on uninfected sites (Mann, 2016). Pin sites that are red and tender are likely to have daily cleaning ordered (Lagerquist et al., 2012).

APPLICATION OF THE NURSING PROCESS

Examples of Related ICNP Nursing Diagnoses, Expected Client Outcomes, and Nursing Interventions:

Nursing Diagnosis: Risk for ineffective tissue perfusion

Supporting Data: Injury and/or immobilizing devices can result in edema, constriction, and ineffective tissue perfusion.

Expected Client Outcomes: The client will have adequate tissue perfusion with palpable pulses, brisk capillary refill, pink underlying color, and warm and dry skin.

Nursing Intervention Examples: Perform neurovascular checks and maintain the correct elevation of the extremity.

Reference: International Classification for Nursing Practice. (n.d.). *eHealth & ICNP*. Retrieved from https://www.icn.ch/what-we-do/projects/ehealth-icnp.

CRITICAL CONCEPTS
Immobilization

Accuracy (ACC)

The accuracy of limb and cervical spine immobilization is subject to the following variables:

- assessment of the client's pain, including pain intensity, character of the pain, and exact location of the pain
- peripheral blood flow and neurovascular assessment
- skin integrity assessment
- identification of anatomical landmarks
- measurement to determine appropriate sling, bandage, and cervical collar size
- position of the affected limb
- pressure and force applied to immobilize
- understanding of procedure by client and family.

Client-Centered Care (CCC)

When immobilizing a limb or cervical spine, respect for the client is demonstrated through:

- promoting autonomy
- providing privacy
- ensuring comfort
- answering questions that the client or family may have
- honoring cultural preferences
- arranging for an interpreter, if needed
- advocating for the client and family.

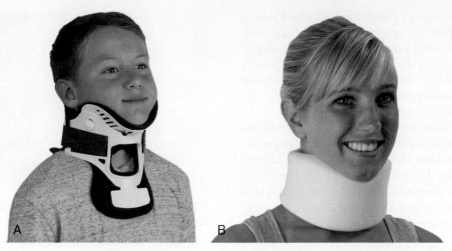

FIG. 6.10 A, Two-piece rigid collars provide more immobilization. **B,** One-piece soft collars provide gentle neck support.

Infection Control (INF)

When immobilizing a limb or cervical spine, healthcare-associated infection and client infection are prevented by reducing the number and transfer of microorganisms.

Safety (SAF)

When immobilizing a limb or cervical spine, safety measures prevent harm and provide a safe care environment, including:
• verifying client identity, allergies, and plan of care.

Communication (COM)

• Communication exchanges information (oral, written, nonverbal, or electronic) between two or more people.

• Documentation records information in a permanent legal record.

Health Maintenance (HLTH)

Nursing is dedicated to the promotion of health and abilities related to healing through immobilization, including self-management of health and protecting skin integrity.

Evaluation (EVAL)

When immobilizing a limb or cervical spine, evaluation of outcomes enables the nurse to determine the efficacy of the care provided.

■ SKILL 6.6 Applying a Sling

EQUIPMENT

Arm sling, commercial or triangle
Age-appropriate, facility-approved pain assessment tool
Appropriate skin assessment form, if indicated
Neurovascular assessment flow sheet, if indicated
Written educational material on wearing a sling, if available
Clean gloves, if there is a risk of exposure to body fluids

BEGINNING THE SKILL

1. **INF** Perform hand hygiene.
2. **INF** Apply gloves if there is a risk of exposure to body fluids.
3. **CCC** Introduce yourself to the client and family and explain the procedure.
4. **SAF** Identify the client using two identifiers.

5. **SAF** Determine if the client has any pertinent allergies.

PROCEDURE

6. **SAF** Review order. *Verifying the plan of care and possible limitations prevents injury to the client.*
7. **ACC** Position the client comfortably and measure the distance from the elbow to the wrist. *Your measurement will verify you have the appropriate-size sling.*
8. **ACC** Assess the following:
   a. client's pain-intensity rating, the character of the pain, and the exact location of the pain
   b. neurovascular status of the affected arm
   c. skin integrity of the affected arm
   d. client and family's knowledge or anxiety related to sling application.

These assessments establish a baseline against which you can compare data from subsequent assessments of pain, neurovascular status, skin integrity, and client knowledge.

9. **ACC** Instruct or assist the client to remove any jewelry or wristwatch on the affected arm. *Jewelry and watches may impair circulation and/or place pressure on the skin, especially if swelling is present.*

10. **ACC** Instruct or assist the client to position the affected arm across the chest with the elbow flexed 90 degrees.

11. **ACC** Instruct or assist the client to insert the affected arm into the sling. Position the hand with the thumb up, and maintain the elbow flexed 80 to 90 degrees with the hand slightly elevated above the elbow. *Positioning the hand slightly above the elbow helps to prevent swelling of the hand.*

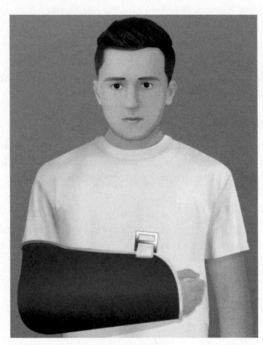

STEP 11 Position the hand with thumb up and the elbow flexed 80 to 90 degrees.

12. **ACC** Adjust the sling shoulder strap to maintain the elbow flexion of 80 to 90 degrees.

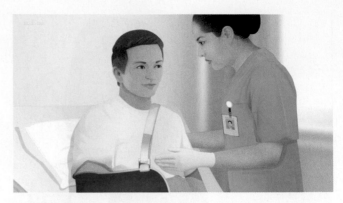

STEP 12 Adjust the sling shoulder strap to maintain the elbow flexion.

13. Adjust and secure the second strap around the unaffected shoulder.

14. **COM** Answer questions the client and family may have about wearing a sling. Provide verbal and written information if available. *Client education is improved when clients receive verbal and written information.*

FINISHING THE SKILL

15. **SAF** Ensure client safety and comfort. If in a healthcare facility, ensure that the bed is in the lowest position and verify that the client can identify and reach the nurse call system. *These safety measures reduce the risk of falls.*

16. **EVAL** Evaluate outcomes. Evaluate the angle of the elbow and the pressure on the skin. Evaluate neurovascular status by checking pulses and capillary refill. Evaluate pain status after sling application.

17. **INF** Remove gloves, if used. Perform hand hygiene.

18. **COM** Document the following in the legal healthcare record:
    - client's level of pain
    - neurovascular and skin assessment findings
    - date and time sling applied
    - size of sling applied
    - education provided to the client and family.

18. **HLTH** Provide follow-up care by discussing how long the sling is to be worn, physical therapy (if prescribed), and follow-up appointments. *Nursing supports individuals to achieve self-management of health.*

■ **SKILL 6.7** Applying Bandages

EQUIPMENT

Elastic bandage or gauze bandage; type, width, and length as prescribed
Safety pins or self-closures or tape
Gauze pads
Washcloth or disposable wipes
Cleanser or soap
Age-appropriate, facility-approved pain assessment tool
Appropriate skin assessment form

Neurovascular assessment flow sheet, if indicated
Clean gloves, if there is a risk of exposure to body fluids

BEGINNING THE SKILL

1. **INF** Perform hand hygiene.
2. **INF** Apply gloves if there is a risk of exposure to body fluids.
3. **CCC** Introduce yourself to the client and family and explain the procedure.

4. **SAF** Identify the client using two identifiers.
5. **SAF** Determine if the client has any pertinent allergies, such as latex. *Elastic bandages may contain latex.*
6. **CCC** Provide privacy. Close the door; pull the curtain if the client will be exposed while applying the bandage.
7. **ACC** Position the client comfortably with the extremity to be bandaged exposed.

PROCEDURE

8. **SAF** Review order. *Verifying the plan of care and possible limitations prevents injury to the client.*
9. **ACC** Remove any existing bandages and clean the area to be bandaged, if indicated.
10. **ACC** Assess the following:
    a. client's pain-intensity rating, the character of the pain, and the exact location of the pain
    b. neurovascular status of the affected extremity
    c. skin integrity of the affected extremity.
    These assessments establish a baseline against which you can compare data from subsequent assessments of pain, neurovascular status, and skin integrity.
11. **ACC** Instruct or assist the client to remove jewelry, including a watch, on the affected extremity. *Jewelry and watches may impair circulation and/or place pressure on the skin, especially if swelling is present.*
12. **CCC** Place absorbent gauze or cotton between the toes or fingers to absorb moisture, if indicated.
13. **ACC** Hold the bandage roll in your dominant hand close to the client. Keep the bandage rolled up, unwrapping only a short length of bandage at a time. Never unroll the entire length of bandage. *Unwrapping a short length of bandage helps to maintain a constant amount of tension and therefore an even application of pressure. Uneven pressure may impair circulation.*
14. **ACC** Identify the area to begin bandaging distal to the affected joint or area being wrapped.
15. **ACC** To apply a spiral bandage around a cylindrical extremity:
    a. Using even tension, wrap the bandage around the extremity over itself two times to anchor the end of the bandage.
    b. Wrap around the extremity from distal to proximal, overlapping the previous wrap by one-third to one-half of the bandage width.

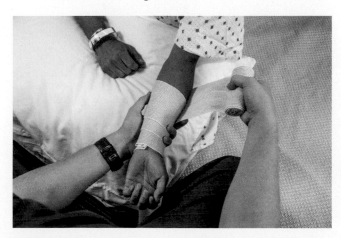

STEP 15B Wrap from distal to proximal.

c. Secure the bandage by wrapping it over itself two times and anchoring the end of the bandage with tape, safety pins, or Velcro closures. Metal clips are not recommended.
16. **ACC** To apply a reverse spiral around an extremity with increasing diameter:
    a. Using even tension, wrap the bandage around the extremity over itself two times to anchor the end of the bandage.
    b. Wrap around the extremity from distal to proximal, reversing direction halfway through the turn and overlapping the previous wrap by one-third to one-half of the bandage width. *A reverse spiral maintains a secure bandage when the extremity is not of a consistent diameter.*

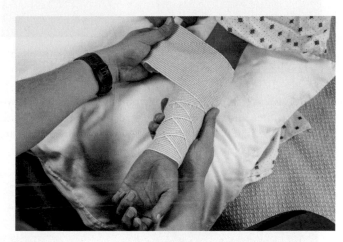

STEP 16B Reverse direction halfway through the turn.

c. Secure the bandage by wrapping it over itself two times and anchoring the end of the bandage with tape, safety pins, or Velcro closures. Metal clips are not recommended.
17. **ACC** To apply a figure-8 bandage over a joint:
    a. Using even tension, wrap the bandage around the extremity over itself two times to anchor the end of the bandage.

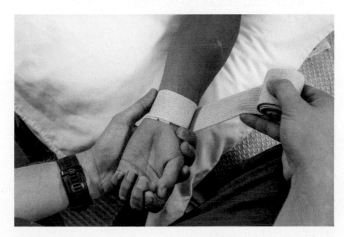

STEP 17B Anchor the end of the bandage.

b. Wrap by alternating ascending and descending turns, making a figure 8 overlapping the previous wrap by one-half to two-thirds of the bandage width.

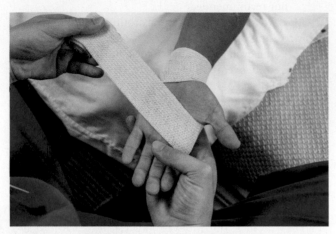

STEP 17B Make a figure 8 overlapping the previous wrap by one-half to two-thirds.

c. Secure the bandage by wrapping it over itself two times and anchoring the end of the bandage with tape, safety pins, or Velcro closures. Metal clips are not recommended.

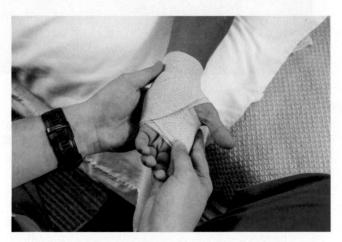

STEP 17C Secure the bandage.

d. If wrapping the foot, do not wrap the toes. Provide padding over the Achilles tendon.

18. **COM** Answer questions and address concerns that the client and family may have about the bandage. Determine if written information is available regarding the type of bandage the client has received. *Client education is improved when clients receive verbal and written information.*

FINISHING THE SKILL

19. **SAF** Ensure client safety and comfort. If in a healthcare facility, ensure that the bed is in the lowest position and verify that the client can identify and reach the nurse call system. *These safety measures reduce the risk of falls.*
20. **EVAL** Elevate the extremity for 30 minutes after bandaging to facilitate venous return.
21. **EVAL** Evaluate outcomes. Evaluate neurovascular status by checking pulses and capillary refill.
22. **INF** Remove gloves, if used. Perform hand hygiene.
23. **COM** Document the following in the legal healthcare record:
    - client's level of pain
    - neurovascular and skin assessment findings
    - date and time bandage was applied
    - type, size, and location of bandage applied
    - client's response to the bandaging.
24. **HLTH** Provide follow-up care by discussing how long the bandage is to be worn, physical therapy (if prescribed), and follow-up appointments. *Nursing supports individuals to achieve self-management of health.*

■ SKILL 6.8 Providing Cast Care

EQUIPMENT

Clean gloves, if there is a risk of exposure to body fluids
Age-appropriate, facility-approved pain assessment tool
Appropriate skin assessment form
Neurovascular assessment flow sheet, if indicated
Cast tape or moleskin
Hairdryer, if indicated
Written educational material on cast care, if available

BEGINNING THE SKILL

1. **INF** Perform hand hygiene.
2. **INF** Apply gloves if there is a risk of exposure to body fluids.
3. **CCC** Introduce yourself to the client and family and explain the procedure.
4. **SAF** Identify the client using two identifiers.
5. **SAF** Determine if the client has any pertinent allergies.

6. **SAF** Determine the type of cast the client has and whether or not it is waterproof.
7. **CCC** Provide privacy. Close the door; pull the curtain if the client will be exposed while providing cast care.
8. **ACC** Position the client comfortably with the casted extremity exposed.

PROCEDURE

9. **SAF** Review order. *Verifying the plan of care and possible limitations prevents injury to the client.*
10. **ACC** Perform a systematic neurovascular assessment, including the five Ps:

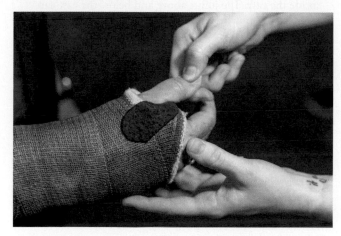

STEP 10 Perform a systematic neurovascular assessment

   a. Pain. Assess client's pain-intensity rating, the character of the pain, and the exact location of the pain. Pain maybe a sign of pressure on skin or tissue or of compartment syndrome. Compartment syndrome is an emergency. Notify the healthcare provider immediately. *If compartment syndrome is suspected, the cast will be removed immediately.*
   b. Paralysis. Ask the client to move the digits distal to the cast. *Altered movement may indicate pressure on the nerves.*
   c. Paresthesia. Ask the client if he or she has any tingling or feeling of pins and needles. *Altered sensation may indicate pressure on the nerves.*
   d. Pulses. Assess pulses distal to the cast and compare the quality of the pulse to the same pulse on other extremity. If the pulse is difficult to feel, check capillary refill and obtain a Doppler to assess the pulse. *Pulses should be symmetrical. Capillary refill should be less than 3 seconds. Diminished pulses and/or slowed capillary refill may indicate compromised circulation and/or compartment syndrome.*

   e. Pallor. Assess the color of the extremity distal to the cast and compare the color to the other extremity to determine the symmetry of coloration. *Color should be a healthy pink and the same in both extremities. Pallor may indicate compromised blood flow; bluish or purple coloration may indicate venous stasis.*
11. **ACC** Perform a skin assessment of the affected extremity. Inspect the skin for any evidence of skin irritation or breakdown, and feel the skin to assess warmth or coolness.
12. **CCC** If the edges of the cast are rubbing the skin, tape or moleskin can be applied to the cast. Cut pieces of silk tape or moleskin with rounded edges and apply them in an overlapping pattern. This technique is called petaling because the pieces of tape or moleskin lie in a pattern like the petals of a flower.
13. **COM** Assess the client and family for knowledge deficits and anxiety related to cast care at home. Answer client and family questions and concerns. Discuss strategies for cast care at home, including pain, swelling, itching, neural signs, vascular signs, rest, and exercise (see Box 6.4 for specific information). Provide verbal and written information on cast care. *Client education is improved when clients receive verbal and written information. Your assessment is also to determine knowledge deficits in order to develop a teaching plan and/or anxiety level in order to determine the type of emotional support that would be most helpful.*

FINISHING THE SKILL

14. **SAF** Ensure client safety and comfort. Verify that the client and family can identify the nurse call system if you leave the room. *These safety measures reduce the risk of falls.*
15. **EVAL** Evaluate outcomes, including client/family education.
16. **INF** Remove gloves, if used. Perform hand hygiene.
17. **COM** Document the following in the legal healthcare record:
    • client's level of pain
    • neurovascular and skin assessment findings
    • date and time cast care was provided
    • client's response to cast care
    • client/family education provided.
18. **HLTH** Provide follow-up care by discussing how long the cast is to be worn, physical therapy (if prescribed), and follow-up appointments. *Nursing supports individuals to achieve self-management of health.*

BOX 6.4 Home Care Considerations for Cast Care

Most of the time, cast care takes place in the home. Nurses are often the person explaining and emphasizing care and potential complications. Potential complications of casts run the gamut from potentially life-threatening events such as increased risk for deep vein thrombosis (DVT), thromboembolic events, compartment syndrome, and infection to less severe but very aggravating events such as skin ulcerations, itching, rashes, and contact dermatitis.

Topics of information to be shared with families who will be caring for a cast at home include pain, swelling, cast care, itching, neural signs, vascular signs, and exercise/rest.

- Pain is a warning sign. Increased pain in the affected extremity is a reason to seek care from a healthcare provider.
- Swelling can be reduced by elevating the extremity, using cold therapy, and moving unaffected fingers or toes distal to the cast.
- Cast care includes emphasizing that plaster casts must be kept dry. If the client is going to shower, the cast can be covered with a plastic bag and secured with a large rubber band.
- Itching can be managed with antihistamines or by blowing cool air under the cast with a fan or hair dryer set on a cool setting. Objects should never be put into the cast to try to scratch. Lotions and powers should not be applied under the cast.

- Neural signs that clients should know include changes in the ability to move the fingers or toes distal to the cast, changes in sensation sensitivity distal to the cast, and a tingling feeling or "pins and needles" in the affected extremity.
- Vascular signs that the client should know include changes in color, the extremity feeling cool to the touch, and slow refill when a finger or toe is blanched.
- Exercise and rest: The client should know that in order to prevent muscle atrophy, daily exercises should be performed by contracting and relaxing the muscles inside the cast. The joints above and below the cast can be exercised, but the joints within the cast cannot be exercised until the cast is removed. The client should be informed as to whether or not weight bearing on the affected extremity is allowed. If the client is allowed to walk on the cast, a cast boot is often given to keep from wearing the bottom of the cast and to provide more traction.
- Resting: If swelling is noted, the affected extremity may need to be elevated when resting. This is more common in the first 48 hours after the injury. Elevating the extremity on a pillow can reduce swelling and pain. Applying ice for 15 minutes when resting is also an effective method of reducing swelling.

■ SKILL 6.9 Managing Traction

EQUIPMENT

Appropriate traction hardware: traction cord, pulleys, prescribed weights
Frame attached to the bed
For skin traction: adhesive traction tape or elastic bandage
Washcloth or disposable wipes
Cleanser or soap
Moisturizer or skin barrier
Age-appropriate, facility-approved pain assessment tool
Appropriate skin assessment form
Neurovascular assessment flow sheet, if indicated
Written educational material on traction, if available
Clean gloves, if there is a risk of exposure to body fluids

BEGINNING THE SKILL

1. **INF** Perform hand hygiene.
2. **INF** Apply gloves if there is a risk of exposure to body fluids.

3. **CCC** Introduce yourself to the client and explain your role in the management of traction.
4. **SAF** Identify the client using two identifiers.
5. **SAF** Determine if the client has any pertinent allergies.
6. **CCC** Provide privacy. Close the door; pull the curtain.

PROCEDURE

7. **SAF** Review order and note the type of traction and amount of weight. Review notes regarding client abilities and limitations. *Verifying the plan of care and possible limitations prevents injury to the client.*
8. **ACC** Assess the following:
   a. client's pain-intensity rating, the character of the pain, and the exact location of the pain (Administer pain medication if indicated.)
   b. neurovascular status of the affected extremity
   c. skin integrity of the affected extremity, especially over bony prominences

d. fracture site, if a fracture is present

e. client's knowledge and anxiety related to traction.

Your assessment is to monitor any changes in pain, neurovascular status, and skin integrity. Your assessment is also to determine knowledge deficits in order to develop a teaching plan and/or anxiety level in order to determine the type of emotional support that would be most helpful.

9. **ACC** Examine the traction setup.

a. Ensure weights are hanging freely and are the prescribed amount. Weights must not be resting on the floor or bed.

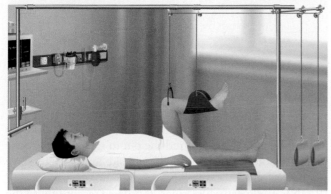

STEP 9A Ensure that the weights are hanging freely.

b. Ensure ropes move freely through the pulleys.

c. Ensure the client is positioned in the center of the bed, providing the countertraction to the weights.

The traction setup determines the force of pull on the affected extremity.

10. **ACC** For skin traction:

a. Remove the boot or straps and footplate every 4 to 8 hours per orders to perform a neurovascular and skin assessment.

b. Clean the extremity before reapplying straps or boots, if indicated.

c. Reapply boot or straps and footplate. If using a traction boot, ensure the fit is snug but not too tight. *The use of skin traction requires vigilant assessment and care of skin integrity.*

11. **ACC** For skeletal traction:

a. Examine all pins and connections within the traction setup.

b. Assess all pin sites.

c. **INF** Provide pin care as ordered.

The use of skeletal traction requires vigilant assessment of pin sites and pin care to provide accurate force and to prevent infection.

12. **CCC** Provide verbal and written educational material on traction. Answer questions and address concerns that the client and family may have about traction. *Client education is improved when clients receive verbal and written information.*

FINISHING THE SKILL

13. **CCC** Ensure client comfort. (Note: Raised side rails may assist the client with self-positioning. A trapeze also allows clients to assist with positioning, as described in Chapter 2 in Types of Beds.)

14. **SAF** Ensure client safety. Verify that the client can identify and reach the nurse call system. *These safety measures reduce the risk of falls.* (Note: The bed is locked but not in the lowest position because the weights must hang freely and not touch the floor.)

14. **EVAL** Evaluate outcomes, such as changes in pain level if medication was administered. Evaluate neurovascular status by checking pulses and capillary refill.

15. **INF** Remove gloves, if used. Perform hand hygiene.

16. **COM** Document the following in the legal healthcare record:

- client's initial level of pain
- neurovascular and skin assessment findings
- status of traction (e.g., amount of weight hanging freely)
- client's response to traction
- traction education provided
- outcomes, client's pain, and neurovascular status after traction management.

■ **SKILL 6.10** Providing Pin-Site Care

EQUIPMENT

Prescribed cleaning agent
Sterile cup
Sterile cotton-tipped applicators
Prescribed dressing, if ordered
Clean gloves, if there is a risk of exposure to body fluids

BEGINNING THE SKILL

1. **INF** Perform hand hygiene.
2. **INF** Apply gloves if there is a risk of exposure to body fluids.
3. **CCC** Introduce yourself to the client and explain the procedure.
4. **SAF** Identify the client using two identifiers.
5. **SAF** Determine if the client has any pertinent allergies.
6. **CCC** Provide privacy. Close the door; pull the curtain if the client will be exposed while providing pin care.
7. **ACC** Position the client comfortably with the extremity exposed.

PROCEDURE

8. **SAF** Review order. *Verifying the plan of care and possible limitations prevents injury to the client.*
9. **ACC** Assess the client's pain-intensity rating, the character of the pain, and the exact location of the pain. Administer pain medication if indicated. *The initial assessment allows you to establish a baseline from which you can monitor any changes in pain.*
10. **ACC** Assess the client's knowledge and anxiety related to pin care. *Identifying knowledge deficits will enable you to develop a teaching plan, and identifying the client's anxiety level will help you to determine the type of emotional support that would be most helpful.*
11. **ACC** Assess pin sites for the following:
    a. discoloration, pain, and swelling
    b. redness and heat
    c. type and color of discharge (Note: Pins inserted through fat may leak yellowish discharge.)
    d. pin movement
    e. skin growth on the pin or crusting around the pin.
    Your assessment is to monitor pin position and any signs of infection.
12. **ACC** Provide pin care per order. *There is no conclusive evidence supporting one cleansing solution or frequency of cleaning for pin care. Nurses are responsible for following the provider's orders and hospital policy.*
13. **INF** If the sterile cleansing agent is not in a single-use dose, pour a small amount of the prescribed cleansing agent into a sterile cup or sterile specimen container.
14. **INF** Wet the sterile cotton-tipped applicator in the prescribed cleansing agent. (The National Association of Orthopedic Nurses currently recommends the use of chlorhexidine 2 mg/mL solution for this purpose.)
15. **INF** Clean one time around the pin site in a circular motion, and then discard the cotton-tipped applicator.

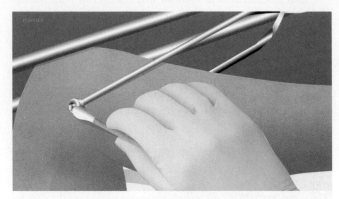
STEP 15 Clean one time around the pin site.

16. **ACC** If skin growth is visible on the pin, use a sterile cotton-tipped application to remove the skin.
17. **INF** If crusts have formed around the pin, continue to moisten and clean around the pin to remove the crusts.
18. **INF** Continue cleaning each pin site until all sites have been cleaned.
19. **INF** Apply gauze dressings, if ordered, according to the authorized healthcare provider's orders and hospital policy.
20. **CCC** Share information about pin care with the client. Answer questions the client may have about pin care. Listen to the client's perceptions of healing versus the presence of infection. *Clients are often the first to notice changes in symptoms (Timms & Pugh, 2012).*

FINISHING THE SKILL

21. **CCC** Ensure client comfort. (Note: Raised side rails may assist the client with self-positioning. A trapeze also allows clients to assist with positioning, as described in Chapter 2 in Types of Beds.)
22. **SAF** Ensure client safety. Verify that the client can identify and reach the nurse call system. Perform a safety check on the bed. *These safety measures reduce the risk of falls.* (Note: If the client has skeletal traction, the bed is locked but not in the lowest position because the weights must hang freely and not touch the floor. If the client has an external immobilizer, the bed is placed in the lowest position.)
23. **INF** Remove gloves, if used. Perform hand hygiene.
24. **EVAL** Evaluate outcomes, such as changes in pain level if medication was administered.
25. **COM** Document the following in the legal healthcare record:
    - client's initial level of pain
    - pin-site assessment findings
    - date, time, and type of pin care provided
    - client's response to pin care
    - client's knowledge and anxiety related to pin care
    - pin-care education provided
    - client's pain status after pin care.

■ SKILL 6.11 Applying a Cervical Collar

EQUIPMENT

Cervical collar, appropriate size per measurements
Clean gloves, if there is a risk of exposure to body fluids

BEGINNING THE SKILL

1. **INF** Perform hand hygiene.
2. **INF** Apply gloves if there is a risk of exposure to body fluids.
3. **CCC** Introduce yourself to the client and family and explain the procedure.
4. **SAF** Identify the client using two identifiers.
5. **SAF** Determine if the client has any pertinent allergies.
6. **CCC** Provide privacy. Close the door; pull the curtain if the client will be exposed while cleaning and applying the cervical collar.
7. **ACC** Position the client comfortably seated upright and facing forward.

PROCEDURE

8. **CCC** Clean the client's neck and face, if indicated. *The client may have experienced trauma, such as a motor vehicle collision. Look for blood and fragments of glass or debris.*
9. **ACC** Measure the client's neck circumference and the distance from the client's sternum to the bottom of the chin. *These measurements are necessary to select the correct-size cervical collar.*
10. **SAF** Review order and manufacturer's size chart for the selection of the correct-size collar. *Verifying the plan of care and possible limitations prevents injury to the client.*
11. **ACC** Assess the following:
    a. client's pain-intensity rating, the character of the pain, and the exact location of the pain
    b. neurologic status
    c. skin integrity of the face and neck.
    Your assessment is to determine a baseline as you continue to evaluate pain, neurologic status, and skin integrity.
12. **SAF** If indicated, another caregiver may be needed to safely apply the collar. Ask the second caregiver to hold the client's head.
13. **ACC** Place the back half of the collar along the back of the neck. Ensure the center of the collar is in alignment with the client's spine.

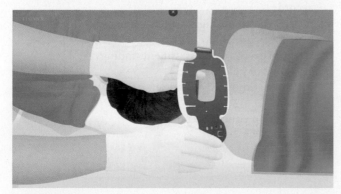

STEP 13 Ensure that the center of the collar is in alignment with the client's spine.

14. **ACC** Place the front half of the collar on the neck, ensuring that the center of the collar is centered under the client's chin and that the client's chin fits snugly in the designated indentation.
15. **ACC** Secure the Velcro fasteners on each side. Allow one finger's breadth between the collar and the neck.

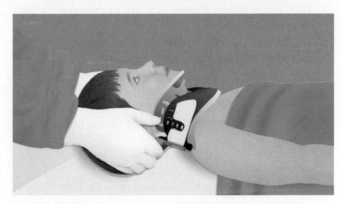

STEP 15 Secure the Velcro fasteners on each side.

16. **COM** Assess the client and family for knowledge deficits and anxiety related to the cervical collar. Answer client and family questions and concerns. Provide verbal and written information on wearing a cervical collar. *Client education is improved when clients receive verbal and written information. Your assessment is also to determine knowledge deficits in order to develop a teaching plan and/or anxiety level in order to determine the type of emotional support that would be most helpful.*

FINISHING THE SKILL

17. **SAF** Ensure client safety and comfort. If in a healthcare facility, ensure that the bed is in the lowest position and verify that the client can identify and reach the nurse call system. *These safety measures reduce the risk of falls.*
18. **INF** Remove gloves, if used. Perform hand hygiene.
19. **EVAL** Evaluate outcomes. Evaluate pain and neurologic status regularly.
20. **COM** Document the following in the legal healthcare record:
    - client's initial level of pain
    - neurovascular and skin assessment findings
    - date and time cervical collar was applied
    - type and size of collar applied
    - client's response to the collar application
    - client's pain and neurologic status after cervical collar application.
21. **HLTH** Provide follow-up care by discussing how long the cervical collar is to be worn, the importance of inspecting the skin under the collar, and follow-up appointments. *Cervical collars are often worn 24 hours a day. Pressure ulcers may appear on the occipital area of the skull, chin, ears, or suprascapular area as a result of pressure from the cervical collar. Nursing supports individuals to achieve self-management of health.*

■ SKILL 6.12 Managing Halo Traction

EQUIPMENT

Written educational material on halo traction, if available
Clean gloves, if there is a risk of exposure to body fluids

BEGINNING THE SKILL

1. **INF** Perform hand hygiene.
2. **INF** Apply gloves if there is a risk of exposure to body fluids.
3. **CCC** Introduce yourself to the client and explain your role in the management of halo traction.
4. **SAF** Identify the client using two identifiers.
5. **SAF** Determine if the client has any pertinent allergies.
6. **CCC** Provide privacy. Close the door; pull the curtain.

PROCEDURE

7. **SAF** Review order and notes regarding the halo traction. *Verifying the plan of care and possible limitations prevents injury to the client.*
8. **SAF** Examine the halo traction to ensure all connections within the halo traction are secure and no pins or bars have loosened.

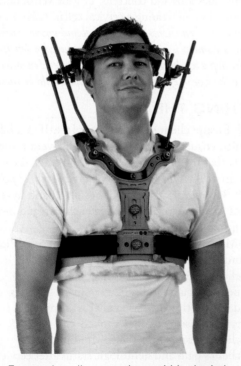

STEP 8 Ensure that all connections within the halo traction are secure.

9. **ACC** Assess the following:
   a. client's cervical spine alignment
   b. client's pain-intensity rating, the character of the pain, and the exact location of the pain. (Administer pain medication if indicated.)
   c. client's skin at each pin site for signs of infection, such as redness, swelling, drainage, or tenderness; changes in the pin site, such as skin growth on the pin or crusting around the pin
   d. skin integrity around and under the vest; shoulders, chest, and back for skin irritation
   e. client's knowledge and anxiety related to halo traction.
   The initial assessment allows you to establish a baseline from which you can monitor any changes in cervical spine alignment, pain, and pin-site status. Identifying knowledge deficits will enable you to develop a teaching plan, and identifying the client's anxiety level will help you to determine the type of emotional support that would be most helpful.
10. **INF** Perform pin-site care (see Skill 6.10). Apply dressings, per agency policy.
11. **HLTH** Apply skin moisturizer or barrier to areas under the vest to enhance skin integrity as indicated. Apply padding if indicated.
12. **CCC** Provide verbal and written educational material on halo traction. Caution the client that seeing items on the ground or stairs is not possible in halo traction; therefore, all walkways must be kept clear. *Client education is improved when clients receive verbal and written information.*

FINISHING THE SKILL

13. **CCC** Ensure client comfort. Assist the client with self-positioning.
14. **SAF** Ensure client safety. Ensure that the bed is in the lowest position and verify that the client can identify and reach the nurse call system. *These safety measures reduce the risk of falls.*
15. **INF** Remove gloves, if used. Perform hand hygiene.
16. **EVAL** Evaluate client outcomes.
17. **COM** Document the following in the legal healthcare record:
    - cervical spine alignment assessment findings
    - client's initial level of pain
    - pin-site and skin assessment findings
    - status of halo traction
    - client's knowledge and anxiety related to halo traction
    - traction education provided.

BOX 6.5 Lessons from the Evidence: Efficacy of Client Instruction Concerning Casts

According to the literature review by Hossieny, Carey Smith, Yates, and Carroll (2012), at least 2 decades of research demonstrate that clients have very poor recall of medical information and instruction. Studies have shown that clients will state that they understand what they have been told even when they are unable to recall the specific points. The research of Hossieny et al. examined the effectiveness of verbal and written client instruction concerning the following aspects of cast self-care: pain, swelling, itching, neural signs, vascular signs/symptoms, cast care, exercise/rest. Study participants had a face-to-face interview to collect information on their awareness of signs and symptoms of possible complications and whether they had received written or verbal instruction. A follow-up phone call was made after the cast was removed. Although the hospital policy was to provide a written information sheet to all clients with casts, in fact, not all clients received written instruction.

In the face-to-face interview, 5% of people stated they received no instruction at all, 33% of people stated they received only verbal instruction, 27% of people stated they had received verbal and written instructions but had not read the written instructions, and 35% of people stated they had received verbal and written instructions and that they had read the information.

The findings in the follow-up phone call were consistent with other studies' findings. The recall of information regarding cast care and cast complications was less than 60%. Those people who received and read the instruction sheet had the highest rate; those who had received verbal instruction only had the lowest recall. Casts remain on the affected extremity for 4 to 6 weeks, and complications can occur at any time; however, pressure ulcers, deep vein thrombosis, and nerve damage are associated with longer casting time.

This study took place in Western Australia, but the findings are consistent with the findings of other studies from a variety of countries. The conclusion was that recall of medical information regarding casts applied after a fracture was less than 60%. People who received and read the instruction sheet had the highest level of recall. The importance of understanding cast complications was reinforced by the fact that among the study participants, four individuals had complications resulting from the cast. Proposed strategies to improve the understanding of medical information included ensuring that everyone receives the written instruction sheet, ensuring that people receive written instruction at a time during the casting process when they would have time to read it, and ensuring the development of simple and easy-to-read instruction sheets.

Reference: Hossieny et al., 2012.

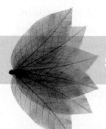

SECTION 3 Caring for a Client With an Amputation

In the United States, approximately 1.6 million people have experienced limb loss. Major amputations include below-the-elbow, above-the-elbow, below-the-knee, and above-the-knee amputations. Minor amputations include the loss of toes or fingers and hand or mid-foot amputations (Varma, Stineman, & Dillingham, 2014). Most of the literature focuses on lower-extremity limb loss. Although leg and foot amputations have decreased in the past decade due to improvements in diabetes management, the majority of lower-extremity amputations are a result of chronic diseases, primarily peripheral vascular disease as a consequence of diabetes, and occur in older populations. Traumatic injuries resulting in amputation can happen to anyone but occur more frequently in young men (Virani, Green, & Turin, 2014). In addition, more than 1700 American service members lost limbs in the last decade (Wollan, 2017), and approximately 6000 amputations occurred in the Vietnam War (Varma et al., 2014). African Americans experience limb loss at least two times more frequently than Caucasian Americans. Vascular disease and diabetes occur more frequently in minorities, and limb-sparing procedures are done less frequently on minorities (Lefebvre & Lavery, 2011).

The care of clients who have experienced limb loss is complex. For those who experienced a traumatic amputation, they may also experience posttraumatic stress disorder as a result of the traumatic experience (Wollan, 2017). The majority of those recovering from a limb loss have comorbidities associated with chronic vascular disease. The client will need to continue to manage his or her chronic disease in addition to the new challenges of an amputation. Thirty-five percent of people have major depression following an amputation, which can negatively impact their motivation during rehabilitation (Slade, 2018). Nursing care following limb loss involves caring for the residual limb as it heals. In addition to the residual limb, other issues related to caring for a client with a limb loss include the following:
- addressing and managing phantom limb pain
- addressing the emotional, social, and psychological impact of limb loss
- balance training and gait training
- muscle strengthening, including aerobic capacity
- regaining mobility
- adaptive equipment options
- operation of a prosthetic and incorporating one into daily living (Sharma, 2016)

POSTOPERATIVE CARE

Exercising and Positioning the Residual Limb

The postoperative care of the residual limb includes wound care (covered in Chapter 16), positioning of the residual limb in order to prevent edema, and exercising the residual limb to prevent contractures and to enhance extensor muscle strength. Edema and pain are likely to occur if the residual limb is in a dependent position. Flexor muscles are stronger than extensor muscles; if the limb is in a flexed position and the extensor muscles are not exercised, contractures may develop. Hip-flexion contracture is the most common contracture. It may result from prolonged sitting or keeping the leg elevated, thus flexing the hip. In order to use a prosthesis, clients need muscle retraining and mobility training (Wollan, 2017).

Applying a Compression Bandage or Commercial Shrinker to a Residual Limb

Another aspect of postoperative care is to mold the shape of the residual limb in order to achieve a shape that is optimal for prosthetic use. The goal is to use pressure to achieve a conical shape. Only pressure bandages are used initially while the amputation site is healing; later, when the site has healed, a commercial shrinker is applied. Bandages are wrapped diagonally, starting at the distal end of the limb, and medially, moving from the outer side of the leg to the inner side of the leg. Wrapping medially helps to prevent the residual limb from turning outward. To prevent the bandage from sliding off, the bandage is wrapped up the leg and then around the client's waist. The pressure bandage should provide even pressure and not impair circulation. A commercial shrinker is similar to an elasticized sock for a residual limb. The shrinker prevents swelling, promotes healing, and shapes the residual limb. Initially, the nurse applies the commercial shrinker; however, as soon as the client is able, the client may apply the commercial shrinker.

Addressing Pain

Pain assessments following limb loss have identified three types of pain. First, clients experience pain at the wound site and residual limb as it heals and they adapt to a prosthesis. Second, they experience aches and strains in other parts of their body as they compensate for the limb loss. Third, a unique source of pain for people with limb loss is known as phantom limb pain (PLP). Medical terminology sometimes uses *phantom* to refer to something that does not exist, such as a phantom pregnancy, but PLP is very real. Of people with a limb loss, 65% to 75% experience some type of pain, including phantom limb pain (Slade, 2018). PLP is neuropathic pain with varied and subjective descriptors. Some people describe it as burning or stabbing; others describe it as throbbing or crushing. Reports of PLP intensity usually decrease over time. The location of the pain varies: about half of clients say the pain is in the entire missing limb, and about half report it is in the most distal part of the missing limb, such as the toes (Virani et al.,

2014). Most people with an amputation do experience PLP, but the pain experience has great variability in intensity, frequency, and quality between individuals (Fuchs, Flor, & Bekrater-Bodmann, 2018).

Addressing and resolving pain following a limb loss is critical for a healthy recovery. Following the loss of a limb, an individual's pain experience has a negative impact on recovery. Pain frequently interferes with the use of a prosthesis, which is important for an individual with an amputation to return to activities of daily living, work participation, and leisure activities. Nurses can help by assessing for pain; believing the client's reports of pain; and determining if the pain is resulting from the residual limb, PLP, or secondary pain musculoskeletal pain resulting from changes in posture and strain in other areas. Managing PLP is very challenging because analgesics are not always effective. Pharmacological and nonpharmacological treatments may be explored to reduce the client's pain. Other pain treatments shown to be effective in pain reduction include transcutaneous electrical nerve stimulation (TENS) (see Skill 7.6) and mirror therapy (Sharma, 2016). Other treatments that have been explored include acupuncture, sympathetic nerve blocks, and hypnotherapy (Virani et al., 2014).

COMMUNICATION: CLIENT EDUCATION AND COLLABORATION

Limb loss necessitates multiple life changes and adaptations. Effectively communicated client education, including education for physical activity and pain management, must be integrated into each stage of the client's amputation care: preoperative care education for all nontraumatic amputations, hospital education, rehabilitation education, and home education (Slade, 2018).

Multidisciplinary therapeutic education programs assist clients in returning to an active home life and improve self-management. Training programs for lower-limb rehabilitation recommend including flexibility, gait and balance training, muscle strength, and cardiovascular training (Sharma, 2016). This may seem daunting to an older individual with chronic disease. Encouragement and emotional support is needed to regain strength and mobility and learn new skills.

Information is needed about prosthetics. There are many different types of prosthetics. Traditionally, socket-suspended prostheses are worn by individuals with a lower-limb loss, but a new type of prosthetic is now available with a direct skeletal attachment via an osseointegrated fixation implanted directly in the residual bone. This new type is called a bone-anchored prosthesis (Pather, Vertriest, Sondergeld, Ramis, & Frossard, 2018). Education programs help clients integrate a prosthesis into daily life.

Nurses can provide support and resources for clients as they transition from inpatient care to the community. Nurses can help to develop enhanced collaboration and lead multidisciplinary programs to help clients manage pain and cope with the physical, emotional, social, and psychological consequences of limb loss. The introduction of collaborating multidisciplinary programs has shown a reduction in time to independent walking (Sharma, 2016).

APPLICATION OF THE NURSING PROCESS

Examples of Related ICNP Nursing Diagnoses, Expected Client Outcomes, and Nursing Interventions:

Nursing Diagnosis: Impaired physical mobility

Supporting Data: Client has a lower limb amputation

Expected Client Outcomes: Client will set and meet mutually established goals for exercise and positioning in order to increase strength and endurance of limbs and prevent contractures.

Nursing Intervention Example: Assist and encourage the client to perform the prescribed stretching, extension, adduction, abduction, and strengthening exercises for the prescribed number of repetitions and prescribed time of muscle contraction.

Reference: International Classification for Nursing Practice. (n.d.). *eHealth & ICNP.* Retrieved from https://www.icn.ch/what-we-do/projects/ehealth-icnp.

CRITICAL CONCEPTS
Client With an Amputation

Accuracy (ACC)

Providing care for a client with an amputation is subject to the following variables:

- assessment of client, including capabilities and limitations for movement, cooperation, strength, mobility, level of discomfort, and activity intolerance
- identification of anatomical landmarks
- position of the affected limb
- pressure applied to the affected limb
- identification of accurate musculoskeletal movement
- number of repetitions and prescribed time of muscle contraction
- understanding of procedures and purpose of exercise, positioning, and wrapping by client and family.

Client-Centered Care (CCC)

When providing care for a client with an amputation, respect for the client is demonstrated through:

- promoting autonomy
- providing privacy
- ensuring comfort
- providing encouragement and emotional support
- honoring cultural preferences
- arranging for an interpreter, if needed
- advocating for the client and family.

Infection Control (INF)

When providing care for a client with an amputation, healthcare-associated and client infection are prevented by reducing the number and transfer of microorganisms.

Safety (SAF)

When providing care for a client with an amputation, safety measures prevent harm and provide a safe care environment, including:

- identifying client identity, allergies, and plan of care
- securing all medical lines and checking patency.

Communication (COM)

- Communication exchanges information (oral, written, nonverbal, or electronic) between two or more people.
- Documentation records information in a permanent legal record.
- Collaboration with the client and members of a multidisciplinary team improves client outcomes.

Health Maintenance (HLTH)

When providing care for a client with an amputation, nursing is dedicated to the promotion of health and abilities, including regaining strength and mobility, supporting health-seeking behaviors, and seeking community resources.

Evaluation (EVAL)

When providing care for a client with an amputation, evaluation of outcomes enables the nurse to determine the efficacy of the care provided.

■ SKILL 6.13 Exercising and Positioning the Residual Limb

EQUIPMENT

Clean gloves, if there is a risk of exposure to body fluids
Age-appropriate, facility-approved pain assessment tool
Small pillow
Written educational material on exercises following amputation, if available

BEGINNING THE SKILL

1. **INF** Perform hand hygiene.

2. **INF** Apply gloves if there is a risk of exposure to body fluids.
3. **CCC** Introduce yourself to the client and family and explain the procedure and purpose of exercising and positioning.
4. **SAF** Identify the client using two identifiers.
5. **CCC** Provide privacy. Close the door and pull the curtain.

PROCEDURE

6. **SAF** Review order or unit protocols for exercise and positioning. Review physical therapy notes regarding client progress and plan. *Verifying the plan of care and possible limitations prevents injury to the client.*

7. **ACC** Assess the following:
   a. the incision site of amputation, presence of edema, color, and skin integrity of the residual limb
   b. positioning of the residual limb
   c. client's ability and willingness to follow instructions
   d. client and family's understanding of extension and adduction exercises and the importance of positioning
   e. client's pain-intensity rating, the character of the pain, and the exact location of the pain.

   The initial assessment allows you to establish a baseline from which you can monitor any signs or symptoms of infection, changes in pain, skin breakdown, dependent edema, flexion deformities, or contractures. Your assessment is also to determine the motivation of the client and the extent to which the client will be able to cooperate and/or participate during the extension and adduction exercises. If the client is unwilling to participate in exercises, he or she may be experiencing altered body image, grief for the lost limb, or depression.

EXERCISING

8. **CCC** Premedicate client, if indicated and ordered. *Pain limits mobility and can be triggered by movement.*

9. **SAF** Assess for the presence of IV lines and other equipment that might be an impediment to movement, such as a Foley catheter, and secure them out of the way.

10. **ACC** Assist the client to perform the prescribed stretching, extension, adduction, abduction, and strengthening exercises for the prescribed number of repetitions and prescribed time of muscle contraction.
    a. Stretching exercises may include the following: In the supine position, bring both legs to the chest, and then lower the affected leg to the bed surface, thus stretching the hip flexor muscles.

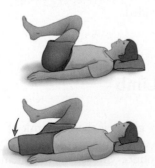

STEP 10A Hip flexor muscle stretches.

b. Extension exercises may include the following: In the prone position, contract the gluteal muscles to lift to the affected leg off the bed surface, holding for 10 seconds.

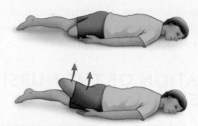

STEP 10B Extension exercises.

c. Adduction exercises may include the following: In the supine or sitting position, squeeze a small pillow between the thighs for 10 seconds, and then release the contraction for 10 seconds; repeat as prescribed.

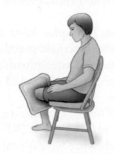

STEP 10C Adduction exercises

d. Abduction exercises may include the following: In the side-lying position, lift the affected leg and hold for 10 seconds.

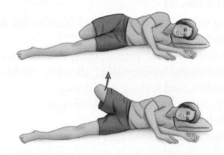

STEP 10D Abduction exercises

e. Strengthening exercises may include the following: In a seated position at the end of a surface, straighten the affected leg and hold that position for 5 to 10 seconds, and then release.

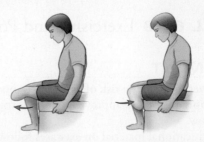

STEP 10E Strengthening exercises

11. **ACC** Encourage the client to practice for the prescribed number of repetitions and prescribed time of muscle contraction.

12. **EVAL** Evaluate the client's activity tolerance, and reassess the client's pain level. *Many clients have an amputation as a result of chronic vascular disease and may have significant activity intolerance. Exercise may trigger pain.*

13. **SAF** Inspect any medical equipment attached to the client, such as IV lines and Foley catheters, to ensure it remains secure and patent. *Maintaining the patency of existing lines provides a safe care environment.*

14. **CCC** Assist the client with positioning.

POSITIONING

15. **ACC** For the first 24 hours, elevate the foot of the bed to prevent edema in the residual limb. Do not place the residual limb on a pillow. After 24 hours, do not elevate the foot of the bed.

16. **ACC** Encourage the client to rest in the prone position for about an hour several times a day. *The prone position promotes hip extension and prevents hip-flexion contractures.*

17. **ACC** Encourage clients with a below-the-knee amputation (BKA) to rest with the knee extended. *Extension of the knee prevents hamstring contractures.*

18. **ACC** Encourage the client to make frequent position changes. *Position changes and movement prevent skin breakdown and promote the maintenance of healthy muscle tone.*

19. **ACC** Encourage the client to time how long the limb is in a flexed position and then provide an equal amount of time with the limb in an extended position. *Flexor muscles are stronger than extensor muscles. Providing equal time in an extended position helps to maintain full ROM and prevent contraction.*

20. **COM** Provide verbal and written educational material on exercising and positioning following an amputation. *Client education is improved when clients receive verbal and written information.*

FINISHING THE SKILL

21. **CCC** Ensure client comfort. Provide encouragement and emotional support. *Active encouragement supports client motivation in exercise and positioning following limb loss.*

22. **SAF** Ensure client safety. Ensure that the bed is in the lowest position and verify that the client can identify and reach the nurse call system. *These safety measures reduce the risk of falls.*

23. **INF** Remove gloves, if used. Perform hand hygiene.

24. **EVAL** Evaluate outcomes, including reported pain level after exercising and with specific positions, the client's ability to perform the prescribed number of repetitions and prescribed time of muscle contraction, and activity tolerance.

25. **COM** Document the following in the legal healthcare record:
    - client's initial pain rating
    - physical and emotional assessment findings
    - date and time of care given
    - pain medication administered
    - exercises performed and client position
    - client tolerance of exercise and positioning
    - client's pain and status after exercising and positioning
    - education provided to the client and family.

26. **HLTH** Provide follow-up care and observe to ensure that the client continues to exercise and optimally position the affected limb.

27. **HLTH** Refer the client and family to local support groups and community services for individuals with amputations. *Supportive services within the community are a vital part of restoring the client's health.*

■ SKILL 6.14 Applying a Compression Bandage and Commercial Shrinker to a Residual Limb

EQUIPMENT

Elastic bandage, type, width, and length as prescribed or Commercial shrinker

Wash basin, soap, and warm water or warm prepackaged bath cloths

Tape or safety pins

Age-appropriate, facility approved pain assessment tool

Clean gloves, if there is a risk of exposure to body fluids

Written educational material on applying bandages or commercial shrinker following amputation, if available

BEGINNING THE SKILL

1. **INF** Perform hand hygiene.
2. **INF** Apply gloves if there is a risk of exposure to body fluids.
3. **CCC** Introduce yourself to the client and family and explain the procedure.
4. **SAF** Identify the client using two identifiers.
5. **SAF** Determine if the client has any pertinent allergies, such as latex. *Elastic bandages may contain latex.*

6. **CCC** Provide privacy. Close the door; pull the curtain if the client will be exposed while you apply the bandage or shrinker.

7. **ACC** Position the client comfortably with the extremity to be bandaged exposed.

PROCEDURE

8. **SAF** Review order. *Verifying the plan of care and possible limitations prevents injury to the client.*

9. **CCC** Remove the existing bandages. Clean and dry the area to be bandaged, if indicated. Do not apply powders or lotions.

10. **ACC** Assess the following:
    a. the incision site of the amputation
    b. the shape and appearance of the residual limb, including the presence of edema, color, and skin integrity
    c. **CCC** client's pain-intensity rating, the character of the pain, and the exact location of the pain
    d. client and family's understanding of limb molding.

The initial assessment allows you to establish a baseline from which you can monitor changes in the incision site; the shape and appearance of the residual limb; and the level, character, and location of the pain. Your assessment of the client's understanding of limb molding evaluates the client's readiness to learn and the education the client has received.

PRESSURE BANDAGE

11. **ACC** Hold the bandage roll in your dominant hand close to the client. Keep the bandage rolled up, unwrapping only a short length of bandage at a time. *Unwrapping a short length of bandage helps to maintain a constant amount of tension and therefore an even application of pressure. Uneven pressure may impair circulation.*

12. **ACC** With your nondominant hand, wrap from the lateral side of the thigh over the medial distal end of the residual limb.

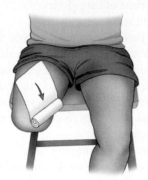

STEP 12 Ensure that the first wrap includes the distal end of the limb.

13. **ACC** Using your dominant hand and maintaining even tension about two-thirds of the capacity of the elastic stretch. Use alternating ascending and descending turns to apply a figure-8 bandage. Wrap medially and diagonally from the distal end to the proximal end of the limb. Overlap the previous wrap by one-half to two-thirds of the bandage width. Do not allow the bandage to wrap around the limb in a circular fashion.

14. **ACC** Wrap up the leg to the groin, and then wrap from the outside of the thigh, across the lower abdomen to the waist, and around the waist.

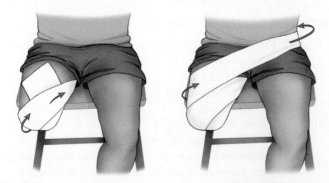

STEP 14 Wrap up the leg to the groin and then around the waist.

15. **SAF** If there is enough length remaining in the bandage, wrap from lateral to medial and anterior to posterior around the distal end of the of the wrapped limb. Secure the bandage by anchoring the end of the bandage with tape, safety pins, or Velcro closures. Metal clips are not recommended.

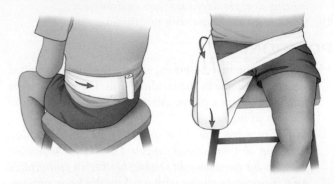

STEP 15 Secure the end of the bandage.

COMMERCIAL SHRINKER

16. **ACC** Using both hands, roll the open end of the shrinker toward the closed end.

17. **ACC** Position the shrinker over the distal end of the residual limb.

18. **ACC** Roll the shrinker smoothly along the leg. *Folds or wrinkles in the shrinker may promote skin breakdown.*

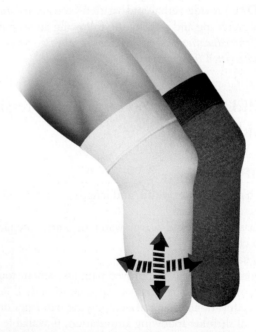

STEP 18 Roll the shrinker smoothly along the leg.

19. **COM** Provide verbal and written educational material on applying a compression bandage and/or commercial shrinker following an amputation. *Client education is improved when clients receive verbal and written information. The client will apply the commercial shrinker himself or herself, when the client is able to do so.*

FINISHING THE SKILL

20. **CCC** Ensure client comfort. Provide encouragement and emotional support. *Active encouragement supports client motivation in learning self-care skills following limb loss.*

21. **SAF** Ensure client safety. Ensure that the bed is in the lowest position and verify that the client can identify and reach the nurse call system. *These safety measures reduce the risk of falls.*

22. **INF** Remove gloves, if used. Perform hand hygiene.

23. **EVAL** Evaluate outcomes, including client pain level and the shape and appearance of the residual limb.

24. **COM** Document the following in the legal healthcare record:
    - client's initial pain rating
    - limb assessment findings
    - date and time pressure bandage or shrinker was applied
    - client's response to the bandaging or application of the commercial shrinker
    - pain medication, if administered
    - client tolerance of pressure bandage or shrinker application
    - client's pain and status after pressure bandage application
    - education provided to the client and family.

■ CASE STUDY

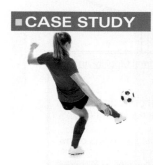

Samantha Tosatto is a 17-year-old high school athlete living just outside of a large metropolitan midwestern city. She has played soccer since she was 4 years old. She is team captain and plays forward on both her high school soccer team and a traveling club team. During a weekend soccer game, she and another player are both going for the soccer ball, and Samantha receives a hard kick to her right ankle. She feels intense, sharp pain and is unable to bear weight on her right leg. Her parents are able to support her, and she is able to use just her uninjured leg to get to the car. Her parents drive her to a nearby hospital with a reputation for excellent orthopedic care.

In the emergency department, x-ray confirms that the distal end of the fibula is broken, a lateral malleolus fracture, but the bone is not displaced. Samantha's ankle is swollen to approximately twice the size of her left ankle and bruised. Samantha also complains of significant pain. She rates her pain a 7 out of 10. Samantha is given oral pain medication. Her ankle is elevated, and ice packs are placed on each side of her ankle. Previously, several members of Samantha's athletic family had been treated by an orthopedic surgeon, Dr. Bronson, and her parents requested that he be notified of Samantha's injury. Samantha and her parents want to discuss options with Dr. Bronson for managing her broken fibula that would get her back on the soccer field the fastest. This is an important season for Samantha to be seen by college scouts and, hopefully, be offered an athletic scholarship.

When Dr. Bronson arrives, he explains that Samantha does not need surgery because the bone is not displaced and the ankle is stable. There is also injury to the ankle ligaments. His recommendation is to manage the break with a short leg cast. However, Samantha will not be returning to the soccer field very quickly. She will not be weight bearing on the right leg for at least 2 weeks and possibly for as long as 6 weeks. He recommends applying a fiberglass cast as soon as the swelling subsides, and he tells Samantha she will be able to pick the color. In the meantime, he will put a splint on Samantha's ankle, and she can go home. He asks the nurse to teach Samantha how to use crutches without bearing any weight on her right foot.

Five days later, Samantha's ankle is much less edematous, and Dr. Bronson applies a fiberglass cast. He tells Samantha that she will need to not bear weight at all on her right foot for the next 2 weeks. After 2 weeks, another x-ray will be taken to determine bone placement. The nurse instructs her on home cast care before sending her home. The nurse also asks Samantha what she is most concerned about regarding her broken ankle. Samantha said that she already noticed "things were different" with her teammates, who are also her closest friends. As a team member and leader, she is accustomed to being in the middle of things, on and off the soccer field. Now she feels sidelined and discouraged about her whole junior year of high school.

Case Study Questions

1. While waiting for Dr. Bronson to come to the emergency department, what is the priority regarding Samantha's nursing care?

2. Pain and edema are early warning signs of compartment syndrome. Samantha complains of significant pain, and her ankle is very edematous. What other assessments could the nurse perform to establish the presence or absence of compartment syndrome?

3. What information should the nurse share with Samantha while monitoring Samantha's neurovascular status? What instructions should the nurse provide after the cast is applied?

4. How will the nurse establish the correct-size crutches for Samantha?

5. What type of crutch gait is most appropriate for Samantha to use?

6. What safety precautions would the nurse select when first teaching Samantha to walk with her crutches?

7. What strategies for effective client education would the nurse consider when teaching Samantha about caring for her cast at home?

8. **Application of QSEN Competencies:** One of the Quality and Safety Education for Nurses (QSEN) skills for Safety is to use appropriate strategies to reduce reliance on memory (Cronenwett et al., 2007). In addition

to a written instruction sheet for Samantha, what strategies would assist the nurse who is providing care for Samantha in the ER and providing client and family education in preparation for her discharge home?

9. Situational changes in mobility can impact a person's self-concept. What could the nurse say or suggest that might be helpful for Samantha?

■ CONCEPT MAP

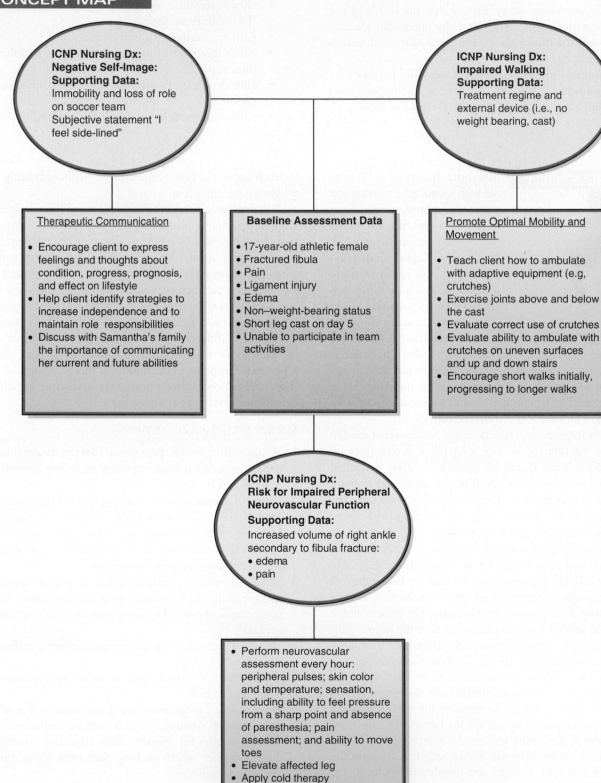

ICNP Nursing Dx:
Negative Self-Image:
Supporting Data:
Immobility and loss of role on soccer team
Subjective statement "I feel side-lined"

ICNP Nursing Dx:
Impaired Walking
Supporting Data:
Treatment regime and external device (i.e., no weight bearing, cast)

Therapeutic Communication

- Encourage client to express feelings and thoughts about condition, progress, prognosis, and effect on lifestyle
- Help client identify strategies to increase independence and to maintain role responsibilities
- Discuss with Samantha's family the importance of communicating her current and future abilities

Baseline Assessment Data

- 17-year-old athletic female
- Fractured fibula
- Pain
- Ligament injury
- Edema
- Non–weight-bearing status
- Short leg cast on day 5
- Unable to participate in team activities

Promote Optimal Mobility and Movement

- Teach client how to ambulate with adaptive equipment (e.g, crutches)
- Exercise joints above and below the cast
- Evaluate correct use of crutches
- Evaluate ability to ambulate with crutches on uneven surfaces and up and down stairs
- Encourage short walks initially, progressing to longer walks

ICNP Nursing Dx:
Risk for Impaired Peripheral
Neurovascular Function
Supporting Data:
Increased volume of right ankle secondary to fibula fracture:
- edema
- pain

- Perform neurovascular assessment every hour: peripheral pulses; skin color and temperature; sensation, including ability to feel pressure from a sharp point and absence of paresthesia; pain assessment; and ability to move toes
- Elevate affected leg
- Apply cold therapy
- Encourage wiggling toes several times an hour

References

Chu, W. H. (2017). *Plaster of Paris: Clinician information.* [Evidence summary]. The Joanna Briggs Institute EBD Database, JBI@Ovid. JBI527.

Cronenwett, L., Sherwood, G., Barnsteiner J., Disch, J., Johnson, J., Mitchell, P., ... Warren, J. (2007). Quality and safety education for nurses. *Nursing Outlook, 55*(3),122–131. Retrieved from http://qsen.org/competencies/pre-licensure-ksas/.

Fuchs, X., Flor, H., & Bekrater-Bodmann, R. (2018). Psychological factors associated with phantom-limb pain: A review of recent findings. *Pain Research and Management, 2018,* 1–12. Retrieved from doi.org/10.1155/2018/5080123.

Giles, K. (2018). *Bandaging: Basic principles for the older person.* [Evidence summary]. The Joanna Briggs Institute EBD Database, JBI@Ovid. JBI1494.

Gyi, A. A. (2018). *Forearm compartment syndrome: Management.* [Evidence summary]. The Joanna Briggs Institute EBD Database, JBI@Ovid. JBI19809.

Han, S. H., Kim, T., Jang, S. H., Kim, M. J., Park, S. B., & Yoon, S. I. (2011). The effect of an arm sling on energy consumption while walking in hemiplegic patients: A randomized comparison. *Clinical Rehabilitation, 25*(1), 36–42.

Hossieny, P., Carey Smith, R., Yates, P., & Carroll, G. (2012). Efficacy of patient information concerning casts applied post-fracture. *ANZ Journal of Surgery, 82*(3), 151–155.

International Classification for Nursing Practice. (n.d.). *eHealth & ICNP.* Retrieved from https://www.icn.ch/what-we-do/projects/ehealth-icnp.

Lagerquist, D., Dabrowski, M., Dock, C., Fox, A., Daymond, M., Sandau, K. E., et al. (2012). Care of external fixator pin sites *American Journal of Critical Care, 21*(4), 288–292.

Lethaby, A., Temple, J., & Santy-Tomlinson, J. (2013). Pin site care for preventing infections associated with external bone fixators and pins. [Review]. *The Cochrane Library, 12.* Retrieved from https://www.cochranelibrary.com.

Lefebvre, K. M., & Lavery, L. A. (2011). Disparities in amputations in minorities. *Clinical Orthopaedics and Related Research, 469,* 1941–1950.

Mann, E. (2016). *External skeletal pin: Site care.* [Evidence summary]. The Joanna Briggs Institute EBD Database, JBI@Ovid. JBI171.

Negro, A., Cabrini, L., Lembo, R., Monti, G., Dossi, M., Perduca, A., ... Zangrillo, A. (2018). Early progressive mobilization in the intensive care unit without dedicated personnel. *Canadian Journal of Critical Care Nursing, 29*(3), 26–31.

Obeid, S. (2017). *Slings: Clinician information.* [Evidence summary]. The Joanna Briggs Institute EBD Database, JBI@Ovid. JBI1555.

Pather, S., Vertriest, S., Sondergeld, P., Ramis, M. A., & Frossard, L. (2018). Load characteristics following transfemoral amputation in individuals fitted with bone-anchored prostheses a scoping review protocol. [Systematic review protocol]. *JBI Database of Systematic Reviews and Implementation Reports, 16*(6), 1286–1310.

Peters, M. D. J. (2017). *Neurovascular assessment: Clinician information.* [Evidence summary]. The Joanna Briggs Institute EBD Database, JBI@Ovid. JBI188.

Physical Activity Guidelines Advisory Committee. (2018). *Physical activity guidelines advisory committee scientific report.* Washington, DC: U.S. Department of Health and Human Services.

Post-op care: Failure to monitor leads to amputation of pediatric patient's leg. (2008, June). *Legal Eagle Eye Newsletter for the Nursing Profession.* Retrieved from http://www.nursinglaw.com

Sharma, L. (2016). *Lower limb amputation: Rehabilitation.* [Evidence summary]. The Joanna Briggs Institute EBD Database, JBI@Ovid. JBI3428.

Slade, S. (2018). *Amputation: Patient education.* [Evidence summary]. The Joanna Briggs Institute EBD Database, JBI@Ovid. JBI10926.

Timms, A., & Pugh, H. (2012). Pin site care: Guidance and key recommendations. *Nursing Standard, 27*(1), 50–55.

Ussery, E. N., Carlson, S. A., Whitfield, G. P., Watson, K. B., Berrigan, D., & Fulton, J. E. (2017, June 30). Walking for transportation or leisure among U.S. women and men—National Health Interview Survey, 2005–2015. *Morbidity and Mortality Weekly Report, 66*(25), 657–662.

Varma, P., Stineman, M. G., & Dillingham, T. R. (2014). Epidemiology of limb loss. *Physical Medicine and Rehabilitation Clinics of North America, 25*(1), 1–8.

Virani, A., Green, T., & Turin, T. C. (2014). Phantom limb pain: A nursing perspective. *Nursing Standard, 29*(1), 44–50.

Wollan, M K. (2017). Musculoskeletal trauma and orthopedic surgery. In S. L. Lewis, L. Bucher, M. M. Heitkemper, M. M. Harding, J. Kwong & D. Roberts (Eds.), *Medical-surgical nursing: Assessment and management of clinical problems* (10th ed.) (pp. 1462–1495). St. Louis, MO: Elsevier.

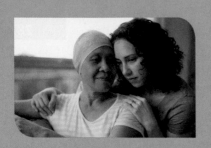

CHAPTER 7

Comfort Care

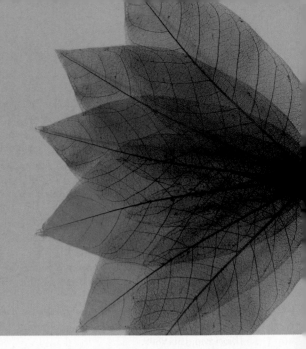

"First and foremost, human beings—worldwide—want to be comforted and kept safe by nursing care."

Author Unknown

LEARNING OBJECTIVES

By the end of this chapter, the reader will be able to:

1 Identify major concepts related to providing comfort.
2 Differentiate between acute and chronic pain.
3 Discuss assessment of pain and discomfort.
4 Enhance the client's environment.
5 Assist client with controlled-breathing exercises.
6 Assist client with guided imagery exercises.
7 Provide a back massage.
8 Use a TENS unit.
9 Use a heat or cold pack (instant or nondisposable)
10 Use a cold therapy ice bag.
11 Use a portable sitz bath.
12 Use localized circulating (aqua) heat or cold therapy
13 Assess a client for appropriateness of PCA therapy.
14 Teach the client and family about PCA therapy.
15 Initiate and monitor PCA therapy.
16 Prioritize care for a client with an epidural catheter.

TERMINOLOGY

Analgesic Medication (opioid or nonopioid) used for relief of pain.

Breakthrough pain Temporary increase in pain that "breaks through" during persistent pain that has been otherwise controlled (Pasero & McCaffery, 2011).

Distillation Process by which fluids are purified.

Heal To restore a person's body, mind, and spirit back to health (Dossey, 2016).

Invasive Entering a body cavity or vein.

Intermittent pain Pain that is not continuous.

Multimodal Refers to the use of more than one analgesic or modality for pain control.

Non pharmacologic Measures that do not involve the administration of drugs.

Opioid Characteristic of drugs that relieve pain by binding to opioid receptors.

Opioid naïve Description of clients who are not receiving opioid analgesics on a regular (daily) basis and have not developed a tolerance for opioids (NCCN, 2019).

Pain An unpleasant sensory and emotional experience associated with actual or potential tissue damage (International Association for the Study of Pain, 2012).

ACRONYMS

ADL Activities of daily living
CNPI Checklist of Nonverbal Pain Indicators
EFIC European Federation of IASP chapters
EtCO$_2$ End-tidal carbon dioxide
IASP International Association for the Study of Pain
TENS Transcutaneous electrical nerve stimulation
NACAM National Association of Complementary and Alternative Medicine
PCA Patient-controlled analgesia
PCEA Patient-controlled epidural analgesia
UPAT Universal Pain Assessment Tool

It is the beginning of your shift, and you walk into your client's room. As you look around, one of the first things you notice is the darkness of the room (even though it is daytime), and the shades are tightly shut. Your client, Mrs. Lopez seems restless; she is tossing side to side and pulling her covers up and down. When you ask how she is doing, she replies, "I'm fine." But when you take a closer look, you notice that Mrs. Lopez' face appears tense and drawn.

Discomfort can have a profound effect on a person's sense of well-being. Every client has a unique story. Some clients, such as Mrs. Lopez may not always be able to openly express their discomfort. The nurse, as an advocate for the client, has an important role in identifying subtle clues, as well as obvious signs of discomfort, and intervening accordingly. Florence Nightingale wrote extensively about the role of the nurse in providing comfort and creating an environment of healing (Nightingale, 1860). In every setting, comfort must be a high priority, regardless of a client's condition.

This chapter discusses basic skills and procedures that may be used by nurses to promote comfort and relieve pain including (but not limited to) nonpharmacologic methods such as relaxation techniques, massage, transcutaneous electrical nerve stimulation (TENS), and hot/cold therapy. This chapter also discusses caring for clients who are receiving patient-controlled analgesia (PCA) and those who have epidural catheters. However, the chapter is not intended to be an advanced pain management manual. The client's needs, abilities, and level of interest determine which skills and procedures are most effective (Fink, Gates, & Montgomery, 2015).

THE IMPACT OF PAIN

One of the most distressing symptoms a client can experience is unrelieved pain. According to the European Federation of IASP Chapters (EFIC, 2016), pain continues to be a significant problem worldwide. Unrelieved pain can interfere with a client's quality of life as well as a client's ability to function. Pain can also interfere with a client's relationships and cause severe anxiety, fear, and depression, possibly leading to suicide (EFIC, 2016). To promote the client's comfort and reduce pain, an understanding of the major classifications and categories of pain is essential.

TABLE 7.1 Nociceptive and Neuropathic Pain

Nociceptive Pain		Neuropathic Pain[a]
Definition	Normal processing of stimulus that damages normal tissue or has the potential to do so if prolonged	Abnormal processing of sensory input by the peripheral or central nervous system
Treatment	Usually responsive to nonopioid and/or opioid drugs	Treatment usually includes adjuvant analgesics.
Types	**Superficial Somatic Pain** Pain arising from skin, mucous membranes, and subcutaneous tissue Tends to be well localized *Examples:* sunburn, skin contusions **Deep Somatic Pain** Pain arising from muscles, fasciae, bones, and tendons Localized or diffuse and radiating *Examples:* arthritis, tendonitis, myofascial pain **Visceral Pain** Pain arising from visceral organs, such as the GI tract and bladder Well or poorly localized often referred to cutaneous sites *Examples:* appendicitis, pancreatitis, cancer affecting internal organs, irritable bowel and bladder syndromes	**Central Pain** Caused by primary lesion or dysfunction in the CNS *Examples:* poststroke pain, pain associated with multiple sclerosis **Peripheral Neuropathies** Pain felt along the distribution of one or many peripheral nerves caused by damage to the nerve *Examples:* diabetic neuropathy, alcohol-nutritional neuropathy, trigeminal neuralgia, postherpetic neuralgia **Deafferentation Pain** Pain resulting from a loss of or altered afferent input *Examples:* phantom limb pain, postmastectomy pain, spinal cord injury pain **Sympathetically Maintained Pain** Pain that persists secondary to sympathetic nervous system activity *Examples:* phantom limb pain, complex regional pain syndrome

[a]Note: Some types of neuropathic pain (e.g., postherpetic neuralgia) are caused by more than one neuropathologic mechanism.
CNS, Central nervous system; *GI,* gastrointestinal.
Adapted from National Institute of Neurological Disorders and Stroke. (2017). *Complex regional pain syndrome fact sheet.* Retrieved from http://www.ninds.nih.gov/disorders/reflex_sympathetic_dystrophy/detail_reflex_sympathetic_dystrophy.htm.

NOCICEPTIVE AND NEUROPATHIC PAIN

Pain may be described in a variety of ways based on the pathophysiology of the source of the pain. The International Association for the Study of Pain (IASP) describes nociceptive pain as related to damage to nonneural tissue and activation of nociceptors (IASP, 2012). This category of pain may affect visceral organs and may be thought of as having a focal or discrete cause (e.g., postoperative pain; pain related to trauma, an infection, or an abscess).

Neuropathic pain is a process that affects the somatosensory nervous system. Examples of neuropathic pain include neurological disease, diabetic neuropathy, sensory neuropathy from chemotherapy, and trigeminal neuralgia. The pain is often described as shooting, prickly, burning, tingling, or like an electric shock (Polomano & Fillman, 2017). A comparison of nociceptive and neuropathic pain is provided in Table 7.1.

ACUTE AND CHRONIC PAIN

The two main temporal categories of pain are acute and chronic pain, as described in Table 7.2. Acute pain usually occurs for a short amount of time after a specific incident or event, such as an acute or unexpected injury, or after a surgical

TABLE 7.2 Major Temporal Categories of Pain

Pain	Major Characteristics
Acute pain	Sudden onset Often well defined Shorter duration (days, weeks, <3 months) Usually caused by acute illness or injury
Chronic pain	Persistent, continuous, or recurrent Often vague and poorly relieved Longer duration (usually >6 months) Etiology may be unknown or poorly understood

References: Coyle et al., 2015; Fink et al., 2015; Polomano & Fillman., 2017.

procedure. Acute pain may also be a warning sign of possible injury if the cause of pain is not identified and resolved. When clients have chronic pain, they may not have some of the expected physical signs of pain, such as increased blood pressure (BP) or increased heart rate, because the autonomic nervous system may have adapted over time. In addition, clients with chronic pain may be more difficult to assess and may be at a higher risk of being undertreated (Fink et al., 2015).

Regardless of whether the client's pain is acute or chronic, it is important to remember that the absence of physiologic or behavioral indicators of pain does not necessarily mean that the client is not having pain. Further assessment is usually warranted (McCaffery et al., 2011).

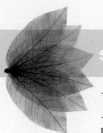

Inadequate assessment of pain continues to be a primary barrier to effective pain management (National Comprehensive Cancer Network [NCCN], 2019). However, the nurse at the bedside can help prevent this barrier by performing thorough and timely pain assessments for clients who are at risk for having pain. As discussed shortly, it is also important to use a consistent pain tool that is facility approved and appropriate for the individual client. This will enhance communication and collaboration between the nurse, the client, and other healthcare providers. To further facilitate communication, the client's pain assessment must be clearly documented as part of the electronic healthcare record.

SUBJECTIVE AND OBJECTIVE ASSESSMENT OF PAIN

Assessing a client's pain requires attention to subjective symptoms (e.g., self-report) as well as objective signs of pain (see Chapter 4). For example, the client's self-report of pain, such as "I feel uncomfortable when I turn on my side," is part of subjective assessment, and it is usually the most reliable indicator of pain. It is also important to believe the client's pain (Horgas, Grall, & Yoon, 2016). Only the client can truly understand his or her pain. As noted, the client's self-report is the gold standard as the best way to assess the client's pain (American Association of Critical Care Nurses [AACN], 2018).

Objective signs of pain include behavioral indicators and/or physiologic reactions. Behavioral indicators may include restlessness, facial grimacing, muscle tension, or other nonverbal expressions. For clients who cannot communicate verbally, it may be helpful to ask family or friends how the client communicates that he or she is in pain. In addition, be alert for changes in the client's usual behavior patterns, and intervene accordingly (AACN, 2018; Horgas et al., 2016). Physiologic reactions or autonomic responses, such as changes in vital signs may also be present. However, current evidence notes that vital sign changes are not a reliable indicator of pain (AACN, 2018). There are variables other than pain that may affect vital signs. Moreover, some clients in pain may not have vital sign changes at all. Nevertheless, when a client is unable to report pain (e.g., newborns, nonverbal critically ill clients), physiologic clues may alert the nurse that further assessment using behavioral indicators is needed.

EXAMPLES OF PAIN TOOLS USED FOR ASSESSMENT OF PAIN

To assess and measure pain accurately, pain tools are used. *Pain tool* is a generic term that may include scales, images, or questionnaires. Because various pain tools are available,

the nurse must choose the most appropriate tool. The tool must also be facility approved and consistently used. Clients who are alert and oriented may use a visual analog scale (VAS) or numerical rating scale (NRS). However, nonverbal clients or clients who have a cognitive impairment may require behavioral scales, such as the Checklist of Nonverbal Pain Indicators (CNPI), which quantifies pain behaviors. The components of the CNPI are as follows: (a) vocal complaints (e.g., moans, groans, cries, gasps, or sighs), (b) facial grimaces (e.g., furrowed brow or clenched teeth), (c) bracing (e.g., clutching or holding onto bedrails), (d) restlessness (e.g., constant shifting, rocking, or hand motions), (e) rubbing or massaging affected area, and (f) verbal expressions (e.g., "ouch" or " that hurts"). When selecting a behavioral tool, consider the setting as well as the client's clinical status. For example, critically ill, nonverbal clients in the intensive care unit (ICU) may require tools specifically designed for clients in critical care areas (see Chapter 18).

For clients who have language difficulties or difficulty understanding numerical rating scales, the Wong-Baker Faces Pain Rating Scale (FACES) or the Faces Pain Scale—Revised (FPS-R) may be appropriate. The FACES scale shows different expressions with corresponding numbers and descriptions such as 0 ("no hurt") to 10 ("biggest hurt"). When the FACES scale is used, the client is instructed to pick the face that best reflects how the pain feels. Although the FACES scale was developed to assess pain in children, evidence has shown that it is also preferred by some adults. In addition, the FACES scale has demonstrated cultural sensitivity for children and adults from different ethnicities and cultures (Hockenberry, 2017; McCaffery et al., 2011).

It is important to note that quantitative pain scales don't always tell the whole story. In other words, a pain-intensity rating alone without further evaluation is *not* an adequate assessment of the client's pain (McCaffery et al., 2011). In addition, linear quantitative scales may not be appropriate for some clients who conceptualize pain in a different way or clients who have a high pain tolerance and are not able to quantify their pain. Whatever scale is used, the client's ability to function and perform activities of daily living must be assessed. It is also helpful to ask the client open-ended statements or questions, such as "Tell me about your pain" or "How do you feel today?" or "How is the pain affecting your ability to do your normal activities?"

One scale that may be appropriate for clients who prefer several options is the Universal Pain Assessment Tool (UPAT). This tool includes (a) a numerical rating scale (0-10), (b) a verbal descriptor scale, (c) the FACES scale with descriptive terms, and (d) an activity tolerance scale. If a client cannot use the numerical scale, he or she can choose one of the other scales to communicate the pain. The UPAT is also available in many different languages and may be used in various settings (Yoost & Crawford, 2016) (Fig. 7.1).

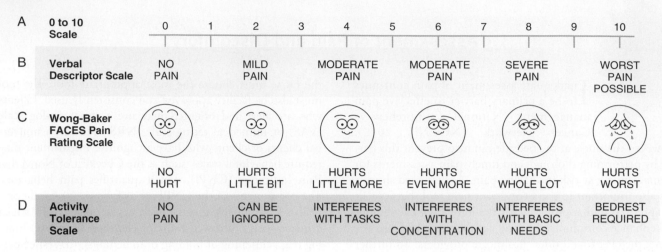

FIG. 7.1 Universal Pain Assessment Tool (UPAT). Instruct the client to use the scale (or scales) that best describes his or her pain.

ASSESSMENT OF PAIN FOR DIVERSE POPULATIONS

When assessing pain among diverse populations, use a tool that is culturally sensitive, consistently applied and appropriate for the individual client. Verify that the client can understand the tool and that it makes sense to the client. If there is a language barrier, obtain assistance from a trained interpreter and use a pain tool with written translations if available. In addition, the client's culture may influence the client's interpretation of pain scales. For example, some clients may prefer to describe pain intensity by using metaphors and images from nature as opposed to linear scales with numbers. For additional cultural considerations, see Box 7.1.

LIFESPAN CONSIDERATIONS: OLDER ADULTS AND PEDIATRIC CLIENTS

During a pain assessment, it is important to allow the client an adequate amount of time to respond to your questions and not to rush. Many clients, particularly older adults, may process information slower in stressful or uncertain situations (Horgas et al., 2016). In addition, older adult clients may have difficulty understanding the pain tool due to alterations in vision and hearing. If possible, provide a pain tool with large print and numbering, and ensure that the client has any needed visual aids and hearing aids during the pain assessment. It is also important to sit at eye level with the client and face the client directly as you ask questions. This is particularly helpful if the client has a hearing impairment.

Among pediatric clients, pain may be difficult to understand or quantify, depending on the age and developmental level of the child. Children who are 4 years of age or older may use self-report scales such as the FACES scale (see Fig. 7.1). For children between the ages of 0 and 4, behavioral and observational scales are usually used (Hockenberry,

BOX 7.1 Cultural Considerations: Acknowledging the Cultural Impact of Pain

Clients' beliefs related to pain management and their responses to pain are influenced by their culture. Key considerations when providing culturally sensitive comfort care include the following:

- Identify your feelings and attitudes about pain and pain management. Provide comfort measures based on clients' needs rather than your personal beliefs.
- Avoid making judgments about what clients feel about pain or particular treatments for pain. Remember, every client is different.
- Offer a variety of nonpharmacologic interventions (such as music or relaxation techniques) and select one that the client chooses.
- Assess what type of comfort measures have worked for the client in the past.
- Ask family members and significant others how they would like to help, and involve them as much as possible.
- If a client has asked to work with his or her traditional spiritual healer, such as a *shaman* or *curandero*, involve the healer in the client's care as much as possible.
- Assess the client's pain at frequent intervals using a culturally sensitive tool.

References: Andrews, 2016; Coyle et al., 2015.

2017). However, a disadvantage of behavioral scales is that it may be difficult to differentiate pain behaviors from other causes of stress, such as hunger or anxiety (Hockenberry, 2017). One behavioral pain scale that may be used (among others) is the FLACC Pain Assessment tool, which considers the child's facial expression, leg movement, activity, cry, and consolability. A tool often used for neonates is the CRIES scale. The acronym CRIES correlates with the following metrics: **c**rying, **r**equiring increased oxygen, **i**ncreased vital signs; **e**xpression; and increased **s**leeplessness.

SUMMARY OF BEST PRACTICE RECOMMENDATIONS FOR ASSESSMENT OF PAIN

With respect to best-practice recommendations, a multifaceted approach must be used that includes evaluation of the client's response to pharmacologic and nonpharmacologic interventions (NCCN, 2019). This is particularly important if the client has an opioid addiction. Due to the increased number of overdose-and opioid-related deaths in recent years, the opioid crisis has been declared a public health emergency (Centers for Disease Control and Prevention [CDC], 2017). Thus, it is important to carefully assess and identify clients who may be at risk for opioid abuse and opioid use complications. Because opioids may cause respiratory depression, assess the client's respiratory status at frequent intervals, including the rate and depth of respirations (The Joint Commission, 2017). This assessment *must* be done prior to giving any additional doses of opioids. In addition, the client's sedation level must be assessed. (For more information on evaluating the client's sedation, see Section 5 of this chapter).

Current best-practice guidelines note that the goal of comprehensive pain assessment is to determine the cause of the client's pain and to reassess the client's pain at frequent intervals to determine if the interventions the client is receiving are safe and effective (NCCN, 2019). The client's personal goals regarding pain control and function are a critical part of the assessment (The Joint Commission, 2017). What is an acceptable amount of pain from the client's point of view, and how does pain affect the client's life? For example, how does the client's pain affect his or her ability to perform activities of daily living (ADLs)? Does the pain interfere with the client's sleep or appetite? The client can collaborate with the nurse and the healthcare team to determine what functional/daily living goals are important to the client.

SUMMARY OF APPLICATION OF CRITICAL CONCEPTS FOR ASSESSMENT OF PAIN

The registered nurse is responsible for the assessment, monitoring, and evaluation of the client's pain. When performing a pain assessment, accuracy, client-centered care, communication, and safety are some of the most important critical concepts to consider. In particular, effective communication and documentation are essential. For clients at risk for pain, perform a baseline assessment and reassess the client at regular intervals and during activities that may cause discomfort. In addition, evaluate the client's pain after the administration of analgesics and reassess the client at the bedside during hand-off communication (AACN, 2018). This will enhance accuracy as well as safety and client-centered care.

APPLICATION OF THE NURSING PROCESS

Examples of Related International Classification for Nursing Practice (ICNP) Nursing Diagnoses, Expected Client Outcomes, and Nursing Assessment:

Nursing Diagnosis: Discomfort

Supporting Data: Client has increased restlessness and increased pain-intensity score.

Expected Client Outcomes: Client will have decreased discomfort, as seen by:
- decreased restlessness
- self-report of decreased pain and decreased pain-intensity rating
- absence of nonverbal indicators of pain, such as facial grimacing
- ability to achieve personal goals regarding function and performance of ADLs.

Nursing Assessment Example: Use a consistent, culturally sensitive, and age-appropriate tool for pain assessments.

Reference: International Classification for Nursing Practice. (n.d.). *eHealth & ICNP*. Retrieved from https://www.icn.ch/what-we-do/projects/ehealth-icnp.

CRITICAL CONCEPTS
Assessment of Pain and Discomfort

Accuracy (ACC)

Assessment of pain and discomfort is sensitive to the following variables:

Client-Related Factors
- Level of consciousness and orientation
- Sedation level and effect of analgesics
- Culture and language
- Ability to understand the pain tool
- Age and developmental level
- Vision, hearing, or any pertinent disabilities

Nurse-Related Factors
- Personal biases or assumptions about pain
- Selection of an appropriate pain assessment tool that is based on the clinical status, client's cognitive ability, development level, age, language, and culture
- Use of a consistent tool and consistent technique for pain assessments for the client
- Ability to verify findings and perform further pain assessments, as needed

Client-Centered Care (CCC)

Respect for the client when performing a pain assessment is demonstrated through:
- promoting autonomy and ensuring comfort; allowing client to identify personal goals
- providing privacy during the pain assessment

- honoring cultural preferences and using a pain tool that is culturally sensitive
- advocating for the client and family and explaining the pain tool
- arranging for an interpreter and providing an appropriate written translation of the pain tool if available.

Infection Control (INF)

Healthcare-associated infection when performing a pain assessment is prevented by:
- reducing the transfer and number of microorganisms, primarily through hand hygiene.

Safety (SAF)

Safety measures when performing a pain assessment prevent harm and provide a safe care environment, including:
- frequent assessment of sedation and respiratory rate for clients receiving analgesics.

Communication (COM)

- Communication exchanges information (oral, written, nonverbal, or electronic) between two or more people.
- Documentation records information in a permanent legal record.
- Collaboration between the nurse, client, and other members of the healthcare team facilitate an accurate pain assessment and clarify the client's goals.

Evaluation (EVAL)

Evaluation of the outcomes allows the nurse to determine the effectiveness of the pain tool. Follow-up evaluations help determine if the client's goals are met regarding reduction of pain and ability to function (e.g., walk to bathroom, turn in bed, cough and deep breathe)

▪ SKILL 7.1 Performing a Pain Assessment

EQUIPMENT

Appropriate pain assessment tool
Reading glasses for the client if necessary to see pain tool

BEGINNING THE SKILL

1. **ACC** Review client's medical/surgical history and review previous tool used to perform client's pain assessments. *Using a consistent and appropriate tool will ensure accuracy.*
2. **INF** Perform hand hygiene.
3. **CCC** Provide privacy. Introduce yourself to the client and family and explain the procedure.
4. **SAF** Identify the client using two identifiers.

PROCEDURE

5. **ACC** Assess factors that may influence the client's report of pain:
   - orientation to person, time, place, and situation
   - age, condition, and ability to understand the pain tool
   - vision and hearing
   - language and culture
   - cognitive and developmental level.
6. **ACC** Provide glasses, hearing aids, and written instructions in large print. *Some clients, particularly older clients, may have difficulty hearing instructions or reading small print.*
7. **ACC** Observe the client's objective behaviors (e.g., restlessness, grimacing). *Although these signs are not absolute indicators of pain, they may provide clues that the nonverbal client needs further pain assessment.*

8. **CCC** Ask the client if pain is being experienced at the present time or if pain has been experienced within the last 24 hours. *The client's self-report is the gold standard for pain assessment.* (Note: If the client is not able to communicate verbally, a behavioral tool such as the CNPI may need to be used.)
9. **CCC** Believe the client's pain. *This demonstrates respect for the client as an individual.*
10. **ACC** Assess alternative pain terminology that may be used by the client. *Many clients may use terms other than "pain" when they are uncomfortable.*
11. **ACC** Select a pain assessment tool that is based on the client's clinical status, cognitive ability, developmental level, language, and culture. Use the same tool each time for each individual client. *Using the same tool each time an individual client's pain is assessed enhances consistency between pain assessments among members of the healthcare team.*
12. **ACC** Ask the client about the intensity of the pain by using an appropriate pain rating scale (e.g., "What do you rate your pain?"). (Note: Measuring the client's pain-intensity rating alone is not an adequate assessment. Other factors, such as the client's ability to function [e.g., turning in bed, walking to the bathroom, performing exercises] must also be considered.)
13. **ACC** Ask the client about the location of the pain (e.g., "Where is your pain?"). Ask the client to identify on a diagram or drawing where the pain is located or to place one finger on the part of the body that hurts the most. *Locating the pain facilitates an assessment of the underlying cause of the pain. A diagram allows the client to communicate the location of the pain.*

14. **ACC** Ask the client about the duration and the frequency of the pain (e.g., "How long have you had the pain, and how often are you having the pain?"). *Assessing how long and how often the client has been experiencing the pain facilitates an accurate assessment of whether the pain is chronic or acute.*

15. **ACC** Ask the client about the quality of the pain (e.g., "Is your pain sharp or dull, tingling, or achy?"). *Assessing the quality of the pain facilitates an assessment of the character of the pain.*

16. **ACC** Ask the client if there are activities or "triggers" that seem to make the pain worse. *Assessing the aggravating or mitigating factors can help determine the etiology of the client's pain. Understanding the client's point of view is crucial in order to accurately assess the client's pain.*

17. **COM** Assess the client's personal goals regarding his or her pain and function. If the client is having pain, assess how it is affecting the client's ability to function or perform ADLs.

18. **CCC** Assess the client for pain relief and effects of treatment. If the client's pain is not relieved, follow up with further assessment and interventions if indicated.

19. **SAF** If the client is taking analgesics or pain medication (such as opioids), assess the client at frequent intervals for respiratory depression or other adverse effects of pain medication. *Certain medication, particularly opioids, may cause adverse side effects.*

FINISHING THE SKILL

20. **INF** Perform hand hygiene.
21. **SAF** Ensure safety and comfort. Ensure that the bed is in the lowest position and verify that the client can identify and reach the nurse call system. *These safety measures reduce the risk of falls.*
22. **EVAL** Evaluate the outcomes. Did the client understand the pain tool? Is the healthcare team using a consistent pain tool for the client that is age appropriate and culturally sensitive?
23. **COM** Document assessment findings, care given, and outcomes in the legal healthcare record:
    - results and detailed description of the client's pain assessment
    - time, location, and tool used for pain assessment
    - vital signs, including respirations and sedation level
    - client's functional abilities and ability to perform ADLs.
24. **EVAL** Provide follow-up evaluations and determine whether or not the client feels that his or her pain and functional goals were achieved. *Follow-up evaluations about pain and function from the client's point of view facilitate communication and client-centered care.*

SECTION 2 Using Relaxation Measures to Promote Comfort

To reduce pain and promote comfort, nonpharmacologic (nondrug) measures such as relaxation techniques may be helpful for many people. These measures are cost-effective and have minimal side effects. They may be especially helpful for clients who have intermittent or breakthrough pain or for clients who cannot tolerate analgesic medication. However, helping a client relax can be a challenge in our hectic society. Nursing measures such as using touch and therapeutic communication, making eye contact, and offering support can make a difference (Fig. 7.2). Repositioning clients and using distraction (e.g., music, humor, prayer, reading) may also be effective. In addition, measures such as controlled-breathing and imagery exercises, massage, and other techniques may help promote comfort and relaxation. One of the most compelling advantages of these techniques is that they encourage the client and family to participate and be actively involved in the client's care (National Cancer Institute [NCI], 2019; NCCN, 2019). The techniques discussed in this section include enhancement of the client's environment, controlled breathing, guided imagery, and performing a basic massage.

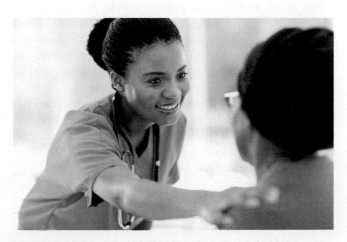

FIG. 7.2 Use touch and therapeutic communication to promote comfort.

ENHANCING THE CLIENT'S ENVIRONMENT

One nonpharmacologic approach to pain management is the assessment and appropriate modification of the client's environment. Dossey (2016) notes that a person's ability to heal is influenced by both the internal and external environment. For the client in a hospital, the external environment includes the images, smells, and sounds within the room. Florence Nightingale discussed the effect that these factors can have on a client's health. In particular, she expressed concern about the need for natural light and good ventilation, as well as the negative effect of noise (Nightingale, 1860). Aspects of the environment that promote comfort depend on the individual client. Assess your client's preferences regarding lighting, temperature, and seating for loved ones, as well as visual features such as where cards, flowers, and pictures of loved ones are placed.

CONTROLLED BREATHING

The technique of controlled breathing promotes slower, deeper respirations that facilitate relaxation. Controlled breathing may also reduce the client's stress and anxiety during painful procedures. As with guided imagery, assess the client ahead of time and explore what type of controlled breathing may be helpful from the client's point of view. Before the controlled breathing exercise, ask the client if listening to music or audiotapes or using aromatherapy or something else during the exercise might help. Assess the client continuously to ensure the client does not hyperventilate or experience any other type of physical or emotional distress.

GUIDED IMAGERY

The guided imagery technique promotes relaxation by using the power of the client's imagination to create a daydream in which the client rests in a safe, tranquil place (NCI, 2019). All of the client's senses may be involved: touch, sound, sight, taste, and smell (Fitzgerald & Langevin, 2018). Use a calm voice, and keep the exercise simple, age appropriate, and personally meaningful. For example, rather than closing their eyes, some clients may prefer to focus on a photo of a loved one or an image that is special to them. It may also help to personalize the session by referring to the client by his or her name (Schaub & Burt, 2016).

Guided imagery can be done with deep breathing or while listening to music. Assess the client for contraindications, such as a history of hallucinations or psychosis, and consult with other professionals as necessary (Coyle, Layman-Goldstein, & Hunter-Johnson, 2015).

MASSAGE THERAPY

Massage therapy, which has been used for thousands of years, promotes relaxation by using the power of touch. It is defined by the American Massage Therapy Association (AMTA) as the promotion of health and well-being by the manipulation of the

BOX 7.2 Lessons From the Evidence: The Effect of Back Massage

In a review of the evidence, Harris and Richards (2010) found that multiple studies support the use of slow-stroke back massage and slow-stroke hand massage in older clients to promote relaxation. The authors limited their review to studies that met qualifications for rigorous research. According to the authors, the recurring theme and general consensus among these studies is that back massage (that ranged from 3 to 10 minutes) significantly improved psychologic indicators of relaxation (e.g., anxiety levels) among participants between the ages of 65 and 100. The authors also reported an improvement or trend toward improvement of physiologic indicators (e.g., vital signs) after back massage, with heart rate being the strongest indicator of relaxation. More recent studies related to massage show similar results.

In a recent study conducted by Miladinia, Baraz, Shariati, and Melehi (2017), slow-stroke back massage significantly reduced a symptom cluster of pain, fatigue, and sleep disorders over time among a group of 60 adult participants with acute leukemia. In the study (which took place in oncology and hematology clinics), participants were randomly assigned to a control group or intervention group. The intervention group received 10-minute massage sessions by trained nurses three times a week over a 4-week period. The results reinforced findings from previous studies that back massage may be beneficial for clients in different settings. However, the researchers also reported that the symptom cluster scores increased or worsened a week after the intervention, which suggests the effect might be short term (Miladinia et al., 2017). One limitation the authors cited is that music was used during the massage sessions, which may or may not be a confounding variable. More studies are needed in a variety of settings with participants from different cultures and age groups.

soft tissues and the movement of the body (AMTA, 2017). As discussed in Box 7.2, slow-stroke back massage may improve both psychologic and physiologic indicators of relaxation. In addition to reducing anxiety, improving mood, and promoting sleep, massage may also enhance the client's circulation, reduce tension, and relax muscles and nerves (Kravits, 2015; NCI, 2019). Massage can be especially comforting for clients who need human contact and touch (Coyle et al., 2015).

Although back massage is often done during or after a client's bath or to promote sleep, the timing, location, and frequency of massage are up to the client. Use gentle pressure and carefully assess for the contraindications and precautions listed in Box 7.3. A variety of strokes can be used (Table 7.3). Finally, do not assume that the client wants to be touched. Ask the client's permission, and involve the family as much as possible (Jackson & Latini, 2016).

SUMMARY

When using relaxation measures, nonpharmacologic techniques (including the initial and ongoing assessments) are usually initiated by the registered nurse. However, assistive

BOX 7.3 Major Precautions and Contraindications for Massage

- Avoid areas with open wounds, bruises, lesions, rashes, or skin breakdown.
- Avoid areas with deep vein thrombosis (DVT) or possible blood clots in a vein.
- Avoid deep tissue massage, especially for frail clients or clients with end-stage cancer; use gentle, light massage only (Kravits, 2015).
- Avoid areas over bones where there may be metastatic sites due to the risk for bone fractures (Kravits, 2015).
- Avoid areas of soft tissue where the skin is sensitive after radiation therapy.
- Use precautions with clients who have low platelet counts (Kravits, 2015).
- Use precautions with clients who have a history of thrombophlebitis.

References: Jackson & Latini, 2016; Kravits 2015; NCI, 2019.

TABLE 7.3 Examples of Different Stroke Techniques in Massage

Stroke Technique	Description
Effleurage	Long rhythmic, circular stroking motions
Petrissage	• Kneading motion over an area on the client's body that involves lifting and squeezing underlying muscles and tissues • Limited to tissues having significant muscle mass
Tapotement	Tapping an area, such as up and down the spinous muscles
Vibration	Rapid, continuous stroke; used with entire hand or fingers

References: Harris, 2018; NCI, 2019.

personnel can assist with monitoring and obtaining vitals signs as allowed by the state nurse practice act and facility policy. One of the most important critical concepts is client-centered care, particularly as it relates to autonomy. The client must feel empowered to choose the relaxation techniques that are most effective, and the client's family must be allowed to participate as desired by the client. This strategy also requires excellent communication.

APPLICATION OF THE NURSING PROCESS

Examples of Related ICNP Nursing Diagnoses, Expected Client Outcomes, and Nursing Interventions:
Nursing Diagnosis: Anxiety
Supporting Data: Increased agitation and expression of anxiety; altered vital signs
Expected Client Outcomes: Client will have decreased anxiety, as seen by:
- decreased objective signs of anxiety (e.g., agitation,

pacing, fidgeting with bedsheets)
- verbalization of decreased anxiety
- BP, pulse, and respirations within expected parameters.
Nursing Intervention Example: Use relaxation measures such as massage as desired by client.

Nursing Diagnosis: Impaired sleep
Supporting Data: Client is tossing and turning at night and complains of inability to fall asleep.
Expected Client Outcomes: Client will have improved sleep, as seen by:
- self-report of improved ability to fall asleep and stay asleep at night
- decreased restlessness, tossing and turning, and agitation at night.
Nursing Intervention Examples: Enhance client's environment (e.g., decrease ambient noise, reduce bright lights) and provide back massage and other measures as desired by the client.
Reference: International Classification for Nursing Practice. (n.d.). *eHealth & ICNP*. Retrieved from https://www.icn.ch/what-we-do/projects/ehealth-icnp.

CRITICAL CONCEPTS
Using Relaxation Measures to Promote Comfort

Accuracy (ACC)

Using relaxation measures is sensitive to the following variables:
- assessment of client, including pain assessment using an appropriate pain tool
- client's level of consciousness and orientation and ability to follow instructions
- client's medical/surgical history, age, clinical status, and developmental level
- technique and tools used for massage and other relaxation measures
- client's readiness to learn and level of interest in relaxation measures
- family involvement in and support for relaxation measures.

Client-Centered Care (CCC)

Respect for the client when using relaxation measures is demonstrated through:
- promoting autonomy by allowing client to choose preferred techniques
- providing privacy during massage and other relaxation measures
- ensuring a comfortable environment during relaxation measures
- honoring cultural preferences and arranging for an interpreter if necessary
- advocating for the client and family and explaining procedures.

Infection Control (INF)

Healthcare-associated infection when using relaxation measures is prevented by:
- reducing the transfer and number of microorganisms, primarily through hand hygiene.

Safety (SAF)

Safety measures prevent harm and provide a safe care environment when using relaxation measures.
- Assessment of contraindications for relaxation measures prevents injury to the client.

Communication (COM)

- Communication exchanges information (oral, written, nonverbal, or electronic) between two or more people.
- Documentation records information in a permanent legal record.
- Collaboration between the client, nurse, and other healthcare providers enhance the effectiveness of the relaxation measures for the client.

Evaluation (EVAL)

Evaluation of the outcomes related to relaxation measures allows the nurse to determine the efficacy of the care provided.

■ SKILL 7.2 Enhancing a Client's Environment

BEGINNING THE SKILL

1. **ACC** Review the client's medical and surgical history. *Understanding the client's history could provide clues regarding needs the client may have that could enhance the client's environment.*
2. **INF** Perform hand hygiene.
3. **CCC** Introduce yourself to the client and family.
4. **SAF** Identify the client using two identifiers.
5. **CCC** Provide privacy when needed and per the client's request.
6. **ACC** Assess the client's orientation to person, time, place, and situation. *A baseline assessment of the client's level of consciousness and orientation must be done in order to determine the appropriate interventions for enhancing the client's environment and promoting relaxation.*

PROCEDURE

7. **CCC** Assess the client for cultural and spiritual preferences, and allow objects that have special meaning for the client to remain in the room. *Facilitates cultural sensitivity and client-centered care.*
8. **CCC** Explore the client's preferences regarding:
   a. sights (e.g., nature scenes, pictures of loved ones, colors)
   b. sounds (e.g., nature sounds, favorite music)
   c. smells (e.g., fragrances, air fresheners).
9. **CCC** Provide thermal comfort and adequate ventilation:
   a. Adjust the temperature in the room for client comfort if possible.
   b. Allow client control over the temperature in the room if possible.
   c. Offer extra blankets and pillows to the client if needed.
   d. Offer a soft blowing fan if allowed by your facility.
10. **CCC** Provide lighting that the client prefers for reading and activities. Provide natural light when possible.

Avoid bright lights. *Bright lights may cause glare and stress (Dossey, 2016).*

11. **CCC** Move the client's chairs and bed near a window and natural light if desired.
12. **CCC** Provide landscape images with soothing colors or nature scenes. Offer to arrange pictures of loved ones or cards on the wall if desired by the client. *This may relax the client.*
13. **CCC** Remove unnecessary clutter and debris from the room as soon as possible.
14. **CCC** Arrange furniture with plenty of seating and areas for family/friends.
15. **CCC** Reduce noise and avoid loud talking, chatter, and laughter outside of the client's room. Decrease noise inside the client's room (e.g., a loud television) if possible. *Excessive noise may increase the client's stress and interfere with healing (Dossey, 2016; Nightingale, 1860).*
16. **CCC** Avoid smells of cleaning sprays or other strong chemicals if possible.
17. **CCC** Allow flexible visiting hours, and allow the client to decide who can visit. *Allowing the client to decide who can visit and allowing visitors provides support and facilitates client autonomy.*
18. **CCC** Ensure the client has access to personal items. *Enhances the client's feelings of security.*

FINISHING THE SKILL

19. **INF** Perform hand hygiene.
20. **SAF** Ensure safety and comfort. Ensure that the bed is in the lowest position and verify that the client can identify and reach the nurse call system. *These safety measures reduce the risk of falls.*
21. **EVAL** Evaluate the outcomes. Does the client appear less agitated or restless? Does the client report less pain or anxiety? Is the client sleeping better at night?
22. **COM** Document assessment findings, care given, and outcomes in the legal healthcare record.

■ SKILL 7.3 Assisting a Client With Controlled-Breathing Exercises

BEGINNING THE SKILL

1. **ACC** Review the client's medical and surgical history. *Understanding the client's history can help determine the client's needs and the appropriateness of controlled-breathing exercises.*
2. **ACC** Review the client's oxygen use: type, amount, and how often used. *Oxygen therapy could be affected by controlled breathing and should be considered before beginning exercises.*
3. **INF** Perform hand hygiene.
4. **CCC** Introduce yourself to client and family and explain the procedure.
5. **SAF** Identify the client using two identifiers.
6. **CCC** Provide privacy. (Note: If requested by the client, place a "Do Not Disturb Sign" on the door.) *Preventing interruptions will enhance relaxation (Dossey, 2016).*
7. **ACC** Assess the client's level of orientation and ability to follow instructions. *This will help determine if the client is able to perform the controlled-breathing and relaxation exercises.*
8. **CCC** Obtain consent before beginning breathing exercises. *Promotes client autonomy.*

PROCEDURE

9. **COM** Ask the client what types of breathing and relaxation exercises have worked in the past and if there are certain breathing or relaxation exercises the client prefers. *Collaboration with the client regarding personal choices enhances the effectiveness of the exercises.*
10. **CCC** Assess the client for preferences regarding:
    a. time of day to do deep-breathing exercises
    b. lighting and temperature in room during exercise
    c. choice of music, images, aromatherapy, or anything else during exercise
    d. any cultural, social, or spiritual considerations.
11. **CCC** If the client has a recent surgical incision, provide a pillow to support the incision. *Deep breathing may precipitate coughing that could increase incisional pain.*
12. **CCC** Assess the client's pain management needs and intervene appropriately. (Note: If the client has analgesics ordered, administer medication 30 minutes prior to activity if needed.)
13. **CCC** Ensure that the client is in a comfortable position. Reposition as needed and provide support under the client's joints with pillows. *Positioning may enhance relaxation (NCI, 2019).*
14. **ACC** Instruct the client to breathe in (inhale) slowly through the nose and out (exhale) through the mouth. *This technique enhances the client's relaxation.*
15. **ACC** Instruct the client to continue slow, deep breaths and to slowly relax different parts of the body from head to toe or toe to head depending on preference.
16. **CCC** Instruct the client to imagine tension leaving the body while breathing out and to envision pain leaving the body with each breath. *Promotes relaxation while breathing.*
17. **CCC** Instruct the client to count slowly (i.e., 1, 2, 3 ...) if it helps the client's rhythm.
18. **SAF** If the client feels out of breath or begins to breathe too fast, instruct the client to slow down the rate of breathing. *Some clients, especially those in pain, may hyperventilate (NCI, 2019).*
19. **SAF** Reassess the client during and after the breathing exercise for response. Instruct the client to let you know if he or she experiences distress or discomfort.
20. **EVAL** Encourage the client to write in diary or journal how the controlled breathing made him or her feel if the client chooses to do so. *Journaling encourages the client to self-reflect on goals.*
21. **CCC** Provide follow-up information with the appropriate written translations for the client and family as needed.

FINISHING THE SKILL

22. **INF** Perform hand hygiene.
23. **SAF** Ensure safety and comfort. Ensure that the bed is in the lowest position and verify that the client can identify and reach the nurse call system. *These safety measures reduce the risk of falls.*
24. **EVAL** Evaluate the outcomes. Did the client tolerate the controlled-breathing exercises? Does the client report improved relaxation or less anxiety, stress, or discomfort?
25. **COM** Document assessment findings, care given, and outcomes in the legal healthcare record.

■ SKILL 7.4 Assisting a Client With Guided Imagery Exercises

BEGINNING THE SKILL

1. **ACC** Review the client's medical and surgical history. *Understanding the client's history can help determine the client's needs and the appropriateness of guided imagery exercises.*
2. **SAF** Note any possible contraindications for guided imagery, such as schizophrenia, hallucinations, or other severe psychiatric disorders (Coyle et al., 2015).
3. **INF** Perform hand hygiene.
4. **CCC** Introduce yourself to the client and family and explain the procedure.
5. **SAF** Identify the client using two identifiers.
6. **CCC** Provide privacy. (Note: If requested by the client and allowed by facility policy, place a "Do Not Disturb" sign on the door.) *Preventing interruptions will enhance relaxation (Dossey, 2016).*
7. **ACC** Assess the client's level of orientation and ability to follow instructions. This will help determine if the client

is able to perform the guided imagery and relaxation exercises.

8. **CCC** Obtain consent before beginning guided imagery. *Promotes client autonomy.*

PROCEDURE

9. **COM** Ask the client what types of guided imagery exercises have worked in the past and if there are certain preferred guided imagery or relaxation exercises. *Collaboration with the client regarding personal choices enhances the effectiveness of guided imagery.*

10. **CCC** Assess the client for preferences regarding:
    a. time of day to do guided imagery exercises
    b. lighting and temperature in room during guided imagery
    c. choice of music, images, aromatherapy, or anything else
    d. any cultural, social, or spiritual considerations.

11. **CCC** Ensure that the client is in a comfortable position. Reposition the client as needed, and provide support under the client's joints with pillows. *Positioning may enhance relaxation (NCI, 2019).*

12. **ACC** Instruct the client to close his or her eyes or concentrate on an object important to him or her. *Centering may help the client focus (Fitzgerald & Langevin, 2018; Schaub & Burt, 2016).*

13. **ACC** Instruct the client to create an image in his or her mind and think of a place that makes him or her feel happy. Instruct the client to explore this place further, to imagine pain leaving the body, and to remember how the image made him or her feel. *Creates self-feedback for the client (NCI, 2019).*

14. **ACC** Instruct the client to note what he or she sees, hears, tastes, smells, and feels. *Using all five of the senses will enhance the client's experience (Fitzgerald & Langevin, 2018).*

15. **ACC** Observe the client's body language and nonverbal clues. If the client shows signs of tension, ask, "What are you experiencing?" *Explores the client's feelings (Schaub & Burt, 2016).*

16. **ACC** If the client chooses to do controlled breathing during guided imagery, follow the assessment and procedure for breathing exercises as outlined in Skill 7.2.

17. **EVAL** Continue to monitor the client during the guided imagery exercise for response. Instruct the client to let you know if he or she experiences distress or discomfort.

18. **EVAL** Encourage the client to write in diary or journal how the massage made him or her feel if the client chooses to do so. *Journaling encourages the client to self-reflect about pain-control goals.*

19. **CCC** Provide follow-up information with the appropriate written translations for the client and family as needed.

FINISHING THE SKILL

20. **INF** Perform hand hygiene.

21. **SAF** Ensure safety and comfort. Ensure that the bed is in the lowest position and verify that the client can identify and reach the nurse call system. *These safety measures reduce the risk of falls.*

22. **EVAL** Evaluate the outcomes. Did the client tolerate the guided imagery exercises? Does the client report less anxiety, stress, or discomfort? Is the client reporting improved sleep?

23. **COM** Document assessment findings, care given, and outcomes in the legal healthcare record.

■ SKILL 7.5 Providing a Back Massage

EQUIPMENT

Towels or linens
Alcohol-free lotions or emollients (if client prefers)
Music CDs, videos, or other relaxation devices of client's choice

BEGINNING THE SKILL

1. **ACC** Review the client's medical and surgical history. *Understanding the client's history can help determine the client's needs and the appropriateness of back massage.*

2. **SAF** Note any contraindications for back massage, such as musculoskeletal or back injuries, open wounds or lesions, low platelet count, or deep vein thrombosis (DVT) (see Box 7.3).

3. **INF** Perform hand hygiene.

4. **CCC** Introduce yourself to the client and family.

5. **SAF** Identify the client using two identifiers.

6. **CCC** Provide privacy and explain the procedure.

7. **ACC** Assess the client's level of consciousness and ability to follow instructions. *This will help determine if the client is able to understand the procedure and consent to the massage.*

8. **CCC** Obtain consent or ask the client's permission before massage. (Note: In some cultures, the client's spouse

or family may have to give consent before the client can be touched.)

PROCEDURE

9. **COM** Ask the client what area or muscles he or she prefers to have massaged (e.g., shoulders, back). *Collaboration with the client ahead of time will increase the effectiveness of the massage.*

10. **ACC** Assess the client for any mobility limitations and the ability to turn on his or her side for massage. *This will help determine if the client can tolerate certain positions or being moved during massage.*

11. **CCC** Assess the client for preferences regarding:
    a. time of day and timing to do massage
    b. lighting and temperature in room during massage
    c. choice of music or aromatherapy or any cultural, social, or spiritual needs
    d. use of lotion or other emollient during massage (Note: It is important to note any allergies to specific emollients or lotions before using any product on the client.)

12. **CCC** Assess the client's pain management needs and intervene appropriately. (Note: If the client has analge-

sics ordered, administer medication 30 minutes prior to massage if needed.)

13. **SAF** Ask the client if there is any area or part of the back that is tender or painful, and assess the client's skin for any redness, wounds, bruises, or tender areas. Avoid touching these areas. *Massaging over tender areas could cause pain and harm.*

14. **CCC** Ask the client to empty the bladder. *This will reduce the chance of interruption during the massage and make the client feel more comfortable (Jackson & Latini, 2016).*

15. **CCC** Ensure that the room is quiet and lights are per the client's preferences.

16. **SAF** Set up an ergonomically safe space. Raise the bed to a comfortable working height. Raise one side rail. *Prevents injury to the nurse and client.*

17. **CCC** Before beginning massage, warm your own hands. *Warming your hands before beginning the massage promotes comfort and prevents the client from being startled.*

18. **CCC** If using lotion, warm it in your hands prior to touching the client.

19. **CCC** Expose only the area of the back that you will be massaging, and begin the massage on the right or left side. *Limiting exposure protects privacy and prevents chilling.*

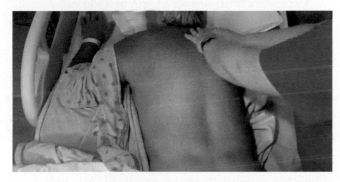

STEP 19 Begin massage.

20. **ACC** Using light pressure, massage with long, circular motions (effleurage). Use the palmar (front) part of the hand for larger surfaces and the thumbs and fingers for smaller surfaces. *Effleurage is an effective method for optimal pain relief (NCI, 2019; Harris, 2018).*

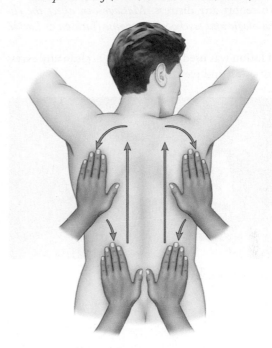

STEP 20 Use effleurage.

21. **ACC** During the massage, keep at least one hand on the client at all times (e.g., the right hand will begin a stroke as the left hand completes a stroke). *If both hands are removed during the massage, the client may think that the massage is over (Coyle et al., 2015).*

22. **ACC** Continue the massage using additional strokes, such as petrissage if tolerated.

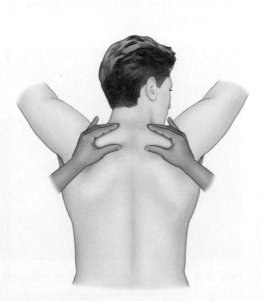

STEP 22 Use petrissage.

23. **CCC** When turning the client during the massage, keep the body covered with a sheet or blanket. *This increases comfort and prevents the client from chilling during the massage.*
24. **SAF** Reassess the client during the massage. Instruct the client to report any distress. *Massage can affect the client's physiologic and psychologic response (Jackson & Latini, 2016).*
25. **CCC** If lotion was used for the massage, clean any excess off client's skin and pat dry.

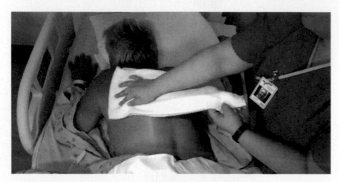

STEP 25 Remove excess lotion.

26. **CCC** Position the client in a comfortable position and use pillows to support joints.
27. **SAF** Lower the client's bed back to the lowest position. *Prevent falls and injury to the client.*
28. **EVAL** Encourage the client to write in a diary or journal how the massage made him or her feel if the client chooses to do so. *Journaling encourages the client to self-reflect about pain-control goals.*

FINISHING THE SKILL

29. **INF** Perform hand hygiene.
30. **SAF** Ensure safety and comfort. Ensure that the bed is in the lowest position and verify that the client can identify and reach the nurse call system. *These safety measures reduce the risk of falls.*
31. **EVAL** Evaluate the outcomes of the effectiveness of the massage. Did the client tolerate the procedure? Does the client report less anxiety and stress and improved sleep at night?
32. **COM** Document assessment findings, care given, and outcomes in the legal healthcare record:
    - type of lotion or oil used for massage
    - appearance and condition of skin
    - presence of any lesions or skin breakdown.

SECTION 3 Using a TENS Unit to Promote Comfort

A TENS procedure is a nonpharmacologic intervention that controls pain by delivering pulsations of electrical current that stimulate nerve pathways. The TENS unit contains a battery, one or more electrical signal generators, and a set of electrodes (Fig. 7.3). It is attached to the client by cables that are connected to electrodes that have been placed on the client's skin around the area of pain or discomfort. The electrical output or impulses of the TENS (both the intensity and the duration) can be adjusted as needed or as prescribed by the authorized healthcare provider.

Advantages of TENS include the fact that it is noninvasive, it may be helpful in managing both acute and chronic pain, and it can be used continuously or intermittently. The TENS unit may also be used as an adjunct for pharmacologic pain management, and it does not usually interfere with the client's ADLs (Coyle et al. 2015; TENSproducts, n.d.).

Although TENS therapy may be effective for many clients, it does require an order. In addition, the nurse must be aware of possible contraindications and special precautions. TENS may be contraindicated for clients who have internal defibrillators, electrocardiogram (ECG) monitoring, or demand-type pacemakers. In addition, TENS should not be used for clients who have an altered level of consciousness

and are unable to communicate. Clients who have a history of epilepsy, transient ischemic attacks (TIAs), strokes, or myocardial disease should not have electrodes applied to the head, neck, or chest. Moreover, the TENS electrodes should NOT be placed:
- over tumors or near cancerous lesions
- on the eye

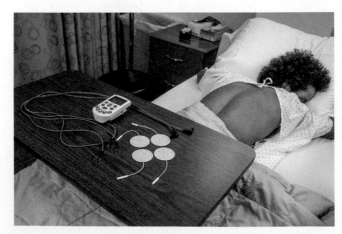

FIG. 7.3 Transcutaneous electrical nerve stimulation (TENS) unit, cables, and electrodes.

- over or around the carotid sinus, as this placement could stimulate the vagus nerve and precipitate dysrhythmias (see Chapter 19)
- on the anterior side of the neck or mouth, as this placement could cause airway problems (Coyle et al., 2015; TENSproducts, n.d.)

Because the TENS unit is an electrical device, there are additional precautions that must be considered. For example, the unit should not be submerged in water or allowed to get wet. In addition, the unit must be turned off and removed if the client is bathing or showering.

For the TENS unit to be effective, the electrode placement and adjustment of the output must be accurate, and the unit should be used as directed by the manufacturer. Therefore, accuracy is one of the most important critical concepts to consider. Good communication and health maintenance are also important. When teaching about TENS therapy, remind the client and family that it may take several fine-tunings within the prescribed settings to determine what provides the best pain relief (Coyle et al., 2015). If the client will be continuing TENS therapy in the home, ensure that he or she is changing the electrodes at regular intervals and prepping and caring for the skin at the electrode sites as recommended by the manufacturer.

APPLICATION OF THE NURSING PROCESS

Examples of Related ICNP Nursing Diagnoses, Expected Client Outcomes, and Nursing Interventions:

Nursing Diagnosis: Pain

Supporting Data: Increased agitation and verbalization of pain

Expected Client Outcomes: Client will exhibit decreased pain, as seen by:
- decreased pain rating on pain-intensity scale
- ability to achieve functional and pain-control goals
- ability to perform ADLs.

Nursing Intervention Example: Use TENS as prescribed and follow manufacturer guidelines.

Reference: International Classification for Nursing Practice. (n.d.). *eHealth & ICNP.* Retrieved from https://www.icn.ch/what-we-do/projects/ehealth-icnp.

CRITICAL CONCEPTS
Using a TENS Unit to Promote Comfort

Accuracy (ACC)

Accuracy when using a TENS unit is affected by the following variables:
- client's level of consciousness and orientation and ability to follow instructions
- client's medical/surgical history, age, clinical status, and developmental level

- assessment of client, including pain assessment using an appropriate pain tool
- selection and preparation of sites on client for electrode placement
- placement of the electrodes on client
- adjustment of TENS intensity settings.

Client-Centered Care (CCC)

Respect for the client when using a TENS unit is demonstrated through:
- promoting autonomy by encouraging client to set his or her own functional and pain-control goals when using the TENS unit
- providing privacy during the TENS procedure if needed
- ensuring comfort when placing the TENS electrodes and using the unit
- honoring cultural preferences and arranging for an interpreter if necessary
- advocating for the client and family and explaining the procedure.

Infection Control (INF)

Healthcare-associated infection when caring for clients when using a TENS unit is prevented by
- reducing the transfer and number of microorganisms, primarily through hand hygiene.

Health Maintenance (HLTH)

Nursing is dedicated to the promotion of health when using a TENS unit by:
- protecting client's skin when electrodes are placed
- caring for client's skin after electrodes are removed.

Safety (SAF)

Safety measures when using a TENS unit will prevent harm and provide a safe care environment.
- Assessment of contraindications or allergies to adhesive when using a TENS unit prevents injury to the client.
- Ensuring that the TENS unit is functioning properly prevents injury to the client.

Communication (COM)

- Communication exchanges information (oral, written, nonverbal, or electronic) between two or more people.
- Documentation records information in a permanent legal record.
- Collaboration with the client regarding personal goals related to pain and function will facilitate the effectiveness and proper use of the TENS unit.

Evaluation (EVAL)

Evaluation of the outcomes allows the nurse to determine the efficacy of the care provided.

■ SKILL 7.6 Applying and Discontinuing a TENS Unit

EQUIPMENT

TENS unit, lead wires, and cables
Electrodes (reusable or disposable)
Electrode gel (if electrodes are nonadhesive)
Alcohol wipes or prep pads (per manufacturer)
Battery (AA rechargeable or 9 V); battery recharger
Hypoallergenic tape or adhesive patch
Towels and washcloths
Adhesive remover
Skin care product or cleaner, if needed and ordered

BEGINNING THE SKILL

1. **SAF** Review the order for TENS, including number and placement of electrodes and duration of therapy. (Note: The duration of the therapy will vary depending on the client's pain.)
2. **ACC** Review the client's medical and surgical history. *Understanding the client's history can help determine the client's needs and the appropriateness of the TENS unit.*
3. **SAF** Note any contraindications for using a TENS unit, such as the presence of internal defibrillators or pacemakers or ECG monitoring.
4. **INF** Perform hand hygiene.
5. **CCC** Introduce yourself to the client and family.
6. **SAF** Identify the client using two identifiers.
7. **CCC** Provide privacy and explain the procedure.
8. **ACC** Assess the client's level of consciousness and ability to follow instructions. *This will help determine if the client is able to understand the procedure and consent to the TENS unit.*
9. **SAF** Assess the client's history of allergies to adhesive backing or gel.
10. **CCC** Obtain consent for the procedure. *Protects client autonomy.*

PROCEDURE

11. **ACC** Assess the following:
    a. client and family's understanding of the TENS procedure
    b. client's pain-intensity rating, character of pain, and exact location of pain.
12. **COM** Ask the client about his or her personal pain and functional goals with the TENS unit. *It is important to collaborate with the client to help him or her achieve personal goals.*
13. **SAF** Examine the TENS unit, electrodes, and leads for broken cords or other defects.
14. **SAF** If the battery is not already installed, insert a battery into the TENS unit. Ensure that the battery cover is on the battery terminals so that they are not in direct contact with the client's skin. *Unprotected battery terminals may cause burns and trauma to the skin.*

15. **ACC** Prepare the TENS unit setup. Attach lead cables to electrodes and insert the cables with the attached electrodes securely into the TENS unit.

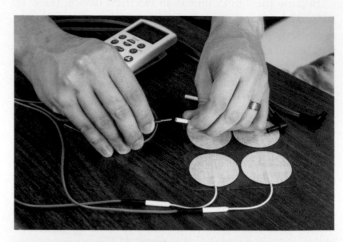

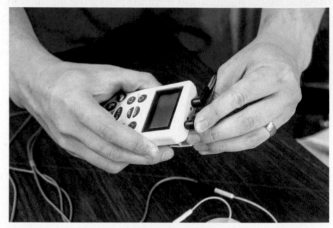

STEP 15 Prepare the TENS setup

16. **HLTH** Identify where electrodes will be placed, and assess the client's skin for any lesions, rashes, or signs of irritation. Avoid these areas if possible. *Electrode placement on areas of irritation can cause additional irritation and disruption of the client's skin.*
17. **ACC** Clean and prep skin where electrodes will be placed per manufacturer instructions. Pat dry. *Enhances contact and increases effectiveness of TENS.*
18. **ACC** Prepare the electrodes as recommended by the manufacturer. If the electrodes do not have an adhesive backing, apply electrode gel to the bottom of each electrode.
19. **CCC WARNING**: Ensure that the TENS unit is turned off. *Prevents startling of the client.*
20. Place electrodes on skin at least 5 cm (2 inches) apart around area of pain as prescribed. *Spacing electrodes will create an even distribution of the stimulation.*

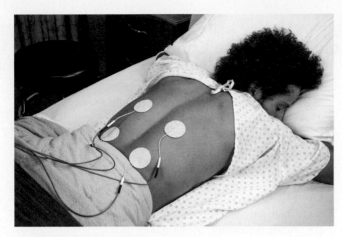

STEP 20 Place electrodes.

21. **CCC** Before turning the TENS unit on, warn the client that he or she will feel a tingling sensation, although it should not feel painful. Ensure that the unit is initiated at the lowest possible setting. *An initial high setting on the TENS would startle the client.*
22. **ACC** Turn the unit on. Instruct the client to tell you when he or she feels a tingling sensation.
23. **ACC** Adjust the channel control (beginning at lowest level) per manufacturer instructions. Slowly increase the intensity according to order and client comfort.

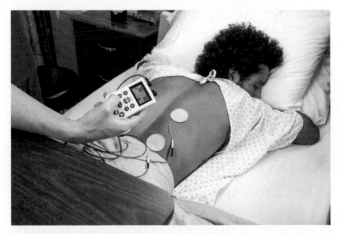

STEP 23 Adjust settings.

24. **COM** Instruct the client to maintain the intensity of the TENS at the highest level he or she can tolerate in order to achieve his or her personal goals regarding pain relief.
25. **CCC** If the client is ambulatory, provide carrying pouch or bag per facility policy.
26. **COM** Instruct the client to report severe pain, twitching, or any distress. Tell the client that the tingling sensation should NOT feel painful (TENSproducts, n.d.).
27. **CCC** If the client complains of discomfort, slowly decrease the stimulation level.
28. **SAF** Monitor the client for excessive stimulation. If the client complains of intense burning or shock-like sensation, decrease the stimulation and notify the authorized healthcare provider.

29. **ACC** If the client complains of inadequate pain relief or inability to feel tingling, check to see if the battery is still charged and check the electrodes, lead wires, cables, and TENS unit.
30. **ACC** If electrodes come off accidentally, are removed, or have to be replaced, turn TENS off. When restarting the TENS, start at the lowest setting and then increase the intensity again.
31. **HLTH** If TENS is used continuously, remove the electrodes periodically, clean skin, and replace gel per policy. *Intermittently removing electrodes will prevent skin breakdown.*
32. **CCC** During TENS therapy, monitor the integrity of client's skin and comfort level. Instruct the client to notify you of any discomfort. *Prevents injury and promotes comfort.*

DISCONTINUING THE TENS UNIT

33. **ACC** Ensure that the TENS therapy duration (usually about 20 minutes) was completed as ordered. (Note: The duration will vary depending on the setting and needs of the client.)
34. **EVAL** Evaluate the client for his or her response to the TENS therapy. Encourage the client to write down in a pain journal how the TENS unit made him or her feel.
35. **CCC** Warn the client that you will be turning off the TENS unit.
36. **ACC** Turn off the channels on the TENS unit.
37. **HLTH** Carefully remove the electrodes, using adhesive remover if needed.
38. **HLTH** Reinspect the skin where electrodes were placed for redness, irritation, or breakdown. (Note: If skin breakdown is noted, notify the authorized healthcare provider.)
39. **HLTH** Clean the client's skin and provide skin care per facility policy. Pat the skin dry.
40. If the electrodes are reusable, place on the plastic liner provided by the manufacturer.
41. If the battery is rechargeable, recharge per facility policy.
42. **INF** Clean the TENS unit and other equipment per facility policy.

FINISHING THE SKILL

43. **INF** Perform hand hygiene.
44. **SAF** Ensure safety and comfort. Ensure that the bed is in the lowest position and verify that the client can identify and reach the nurse call system. *These safety measures reduce the risk of falls.*
45. **EVAL** Evaluate the outcomes. Did the client tolerate the TENS? Did the client achieve his or her personal goals regarding pain relief? Is the client's skin intact without signs of irritation?
46. **COM** Document assessment findings, care given, and outcomes in the legal healthcare record:
    - placement and number of electrodes used
    - duration of TENS therapy treatment
    - type of skin prep used for electrodes
    - level of intensity required to control the client's pain.

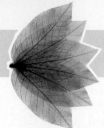

Heat and cold therapy are physical methods used to provide comfort. Although both heat and cold can reduce muscle spasm and pain, they usually have opposite effects that complement each other. Immediately after an injury, cold therapy is typically used because it causes vasoconstriction and decreases inflammation and swelling at the site. Heat therapy is often used for chronic pain or pain that does not involve acute inflammation. Heat may be particularly helpful for muscle, joint, or arthritic pain. Because heat increases swelling and bleeding, it should typically not be used for the first 24 to 48 hours after an acute injury (Polomano & Fillman, 2017).

SAFETY CONSIDERATIONS AND PRECAUTIONS FOR HEAT AND COLD THERAPY

In the healthcare setting, the use of heat or cold therapy requires an order by the authorized healthcare provider. When using heat or cold, consider client safety: both heat and cold can cause impaired skin integrity, tissue damage, and an altered sensitivity to pain. For example, cold therapy may cause freeze burns or frostbite if left in place too long. Heat therapy requires extreme caution, especially among young children and older adults, both of whom tend to have fragile, delicate skin that may burn easily. These populations may have difficulty communicating and alerting the nurse if they feel pain or discomfort. The nurse can reduce the risk of thermal injury by using shorter application times and carefully observing these clients at more frequent intervals. Heat or cold should also be avoided or used cautiously for people who are confused or have an altered level of consciousness (Stryker, 2017). See Box 7.4 for a list of additional contraindications and precautions for heat and cold therapy.

Other client safety measures to consider when providing heat therapy include the following:
- Vary the location of the heating device on the client's skin.
- Ensure that the temperature of the heating device does not exceed the temperature recommended by the manufacturer or facility policy (Stryker, 2017).
- Avoid microwaving any heat device that will be placed on the client.
- Avoid using heat over areas where menthol ointments (used frequently by older adults) or other oils have been applied. Oil intensifies heat (Polomano & Fillman, 2017).
- Avoid getting moisture between the heat device and the client's skin because moisture intensifies the effect of heat and increases the chance of injury (Stryker, 2017).
- Remove the heat device immediately if redness, pain, swelling, blistering, or pale skin (blanching) occurs. Educate the client and family to alert you for these changes.

BOX 7.4 Major Contraindications and Precautions for Heat and Cold Therapy

---

CONTRAINDICATIONS AND/OR PRECAUTIONS FOR HEAT THERAPY
- Acute injury (first 24 hours)
- Impaired circulation
- Bleeding or hematoma
- Open wounds
- Acute dermatitis
- Damaged or infected tissue
- High body temperature (Stryker, 2017)

CONTRAINDICATIONS AND/OR PRECAUTIONS FOR COLD THERAPY
- Cold hypersensitivity
- Cryoglobulinemia (hyperviscosity of the blood)
- Peripheral vascular disease
- Cardiac disease
- Sickle cell anemia
- Raynaud's disease (Stryker, 2017)
- Tissue damage from radiation therapy (NCI, 2019)

References: NCI, 2019; Polomano & Fillman, 2017; Stryker, 2017.

- Carefully assess and document skin condition before and after therapy as well as the type of heat device, method, temperature setting, and client response (Polomano & Fillman, 2017).

DIFFERENT TYPES OF HEAT AND COLD THERAPY

Instant Single-Use Cold or Heat Packs

Instant single-use cold or heat packs are handy when no ice or heating element is available. Instant packs contain chemicals that are released within the pack when compressed and shaken or folded. When activated, the chemical in the cold pack creates an endothermic reaction within the pouch, causing a cool temperature. The chemical in the heat pack creates an exothermic reaction within the pouch that causes a warm temperature. The disadvantage of instant packs is that they do not stay cold or warm for long, and they can be difficult to activate. Before using an instant cold or heat pack, check the outside liner and ensure that none of the chemicals, which could cause burns, have leaked. For examples of instant cold and hot packs, see Fig. 7.4.

Nondisposable Cold Gel Packs

Nondisposable cold gel packs are reusable packs that are kept in the freezer until ready for use. They contain a gelatinous substance that prevents the packs from freezing

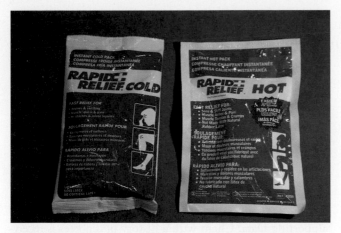

FIG. 7.4 Examples of disposable instant cold and hot packs.

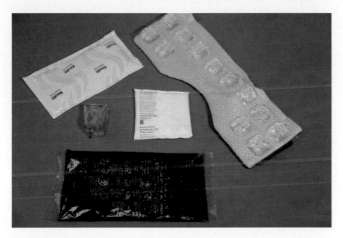

FIG. 7.5 Examples of cold gel packs in various sizes.

solid. An advantage of gel packs is that they are flexible and conform to the area of the body where the pack is placed. Gel packs come in a variety of shapes and sizes for the individual needs of the client (Fig. 7.5). If the gel pack does not have a built-in liner, it may need to be wrapped in a light cloth before application to prevent tissue damage. Gel packs can also be placed in holders that can be secured around the face or jaw (Fig. 7.6).

Ice Bags

Ice bags are another reusable option. They are made by placing cold water, crushed ice, or cubed ice inside a commercial ice bag, a zipper-top plastic bag (preferably leakproof), stocking, disposable glove, or anything that can hold ice. If using a commercial ice bag, place fluid in it first, turn it upside down, and check for leaks in the bag before filling with ice. An advantage of ice bags is that they tend to stay colder longer than instant cold packs, and like the gel pack, they can conform to the body's contours. A disadvantage of ice bags is that they can accumulate condensation or leak as soon as the ice starts to melt. It may be helpful to provide extra towels or a pad with a liner to help keep the client dry.

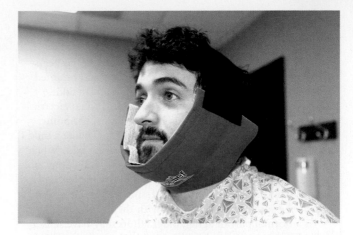

FIG. 7.6 Example of a cold gel pack for jaw and face.

Dry Heat Therapy (Heating Pads and Infrared Heat Lamps)

Heat therapy can involve the use of dry heat or moist heat. An example of dry heat is the electric heating pads or heating blankets that clients may use in the home setting. For safety, the newer electric heating pads have several levels of heat controls and an automatic shut-off timer to avoid burns. When doing discharge planning or home teaching, instruct the client and family about precautions for these devices in order to prevent burn injuries (Box 7.5).

Another example of dry heat is an infrared heat lamp. Heat lamps require an order by the authorized healthcare provider. These devices work by warming the client's tissues through conversion by converting radiant energy into heat. They are not as commonly used as in the past because of the increased drying effects and potential damage to the client's skin. Because of the intense heat generated, use a heat lamp with an automatic timer, and limit the therapy to no more than 15 to 20 minutes. If a heat lamp is used, ensure that it is at least 45 to 60 cm (18–24 inches) away from the client, and ensure the client's eyes and genitalia are protected. As with other types of heat, there are precautions/contraindications to consider. For example, heat lamps should not be used with clients who are unconscious or incapacitated. In addition, they should be used with caution with clients who have poor circulation or who may burn easily.

Moist Heat Therapy

A type of moist heat or immersion therapy that may be used is a sitz bath, which immerses only the client's perineal area in warm water. It is often used to decrease inflammation and promote healing in the client's perineal area after childbirth or in the rectal area after surgery. Although there is no evidence that sitz baths are more effective than other treatments for pain relief and wound healing, there is some evidence of improved client satisfaction after using sitz baths and water-spray methods (Fong, 2018).

If the client is able to stand without difficulty, a shower spray nozzle could be used to create the warm-water spray for the client's affected area. If this method is used, stay with the client, and ensure that he or she does not become dizzy or lightheaded while standing.

BOX 7.5 Home Care and Geriatric Considerations: Using Heat Safely at Home

Ms. Long, an 84-year-old client who lives alone, has been discharged to home after surgery. She is alert and oriented and has a history of osteoporosis and hip pain. In addition to oral analgesics, she uses warm packs and an electric heating pad for pain. During a follow-up visit, the home care nurse notices that Ms. Long has what looks like a mild sunburn on her side in the shape of her heating pad. When the nurse asks if the area hurts, Ms. Long replies, "Why, no! In fact, I have to leave the pad on for a long time because it stops working!" After further assessment, Ms. Long also admits she sometimes falls asleep with the heating pad on.

As a normal part of aging, older adults may have sensory alterations that cause a decreased sensitivity to heat. This may explain why Ms. Long stated that the heating pad seemed to "stop working." When she increased the setting on the pad to get the same effect, she also increased her risk of getting a burn.

As part of home teaching, the nurse instructs Ms. Long about limiting the time that the heating pad is on her skin to 15 minutes, then leaving it off for 15 minutes, as well as alternating the location of the pad. In addition, the nurse advises Ms. Long to avoid lying directly on the pad and to make sure that the pad does not have any damage or tears. The nurse also advises Ms. Long to avoid using other heat devices, such as a warm pack or hot water bottle, with the electric pad and to use the lowest heat level possible. She also suggests using an electric pad with a built-in timer and automatic shut-off. As part of follow-up care, the nurse refers Ms. Long to the appropriate healthcare provider and instructs her to avoid placing a heating pad or anything else on her skin in the location of the burn injury.

Circulating Cold or Heat Therapy

Circulating cold or heat therapy, also known as aquatherapy, is used for some clients to provide comfort by locally applying cold or heat to a certain part of the body. It is most often used for localized pain or discomfort. The pump for this system contains distilled water that is warmed or cooled by the pump, depending on the client's needs, and then circulates through a pad that is placed on the client. An advantage of this type of therapy is that the pads can be wrapped and molded closely around the client's specific area of pain. To prevent skin damage, keep the area between the client and aqua pad dry. Excessive moisture and prolonged pressure from the client can cause injury. In addition, assess the client and ensure that therapy is appropriate. The length of treatment may vary. Follow the manufacturer's instructions and facility policy closely.

SUMMARY

In summary, heat and cold therapy may be an effective non-pharmacologic method for reducing pain and discomfort. When using heat and cold therapy, three of the most important critical concepts are accuracy, safety, and health maintenance. These critical concepts are also interrelated. To reduce the risk of injuries and impaired skin integrity, heat and cold therapy must be used accurately and according to the manufacturer instructions. The client's history and the presence of contraindications must also be considered. In addition, the client must be taught how to accurately use heat and cold therapy if he or she will be using these products at home.

APPLICATION OF THE NURSING PROCESS

Examples of Related ICNP Nursing Diagnoses, Expected Client Outcomes, and Nursing Interventions:

Nursing Diagnosis: Risk for impaired skin integrity

Supporting Data: Client with a history of diabetes is receiving hot/cold therapy.

Expected Client Outcomes: Client will have no evidence of impaired skin integrity, as seen by:
- intact skin
- absence of redness and blisters on skin
- absence of burn patterns or markings on skin.

Nursing Intervention Examples: Monitor the client's skin frequently during heat or cold therapy. Maintain a dry barrier between the client's skin and the devices used for heat or cold therapy.

Reference: International Classification for Nursing Practice. (n.d.). *eHealth & ICNP*. Retrieved from https://www.icn.ch/what-we-do/projects/ehealth-icnp.

CRITICAL CONCEPTS
Using Heat or Cold to Promote Comfort

Accuracy (ACC)

Accuracy when using heat or cold is affected by the following variables:
- assessment of client including pain assessment using an appropriate pain tool
- client's medical/surgical history, including age, clinical status, indications for heat and cold therapy, and presence of impaired circulation or any contraindications (see Box 7.4)
- preparation and technique used to apply heat or cold therapy
- selection of site on client for placement of heat or cold therapy
- duration and length of treatment for heat or cold therapy
- positioning of client for heat or cold therapy.

Client-Centered Care (CCC)

Respect for the client when using heat or cold is demonstrated through:
- promoting autonomy by allowing client to participate in the choice of heat or cold therapy
- providing privacy when applying heat or cold therapy devices
- ensuring comfort by following guidelines for heat or cold therapy applications

- honoring cultural preferences and explaining the procedure
- advocating for the client and family.

Infection Control (INF)

Healthcare-associated infection when using heat or cold is prevented by:
- preventing and reducing the transfer of microorganisms
- reducing the number of microorganisms.

Safety (SAF)

When using heat or cold therapy, safety measures prevent harm and provide a safe care environment.
- Assessment of contraindications and following manufacturer guidelines when using heat and cold reduce the risk of injuries.

Communication (COM)

- Communication exchanges information (oral, written, nonverbal, or electronic) between two or more people.

- Documentation records information in a permanent legal record.
- Collaboration with the client regarding personal goals and personal preferences related to comfort facilitate the effectiveness of the heat or cold therapy.

Health Maintenance (HLTH)

Nursing is dedicated to the promotion of health and self-care abilities when using heat or cold by:
- caring for client's skin during heat or cold therapy
- preventing skin injury from burns during heat or cold therapy.

Evaluation (EVAL)

Evaluation of the outcomes when using heat or cold therapy allows the nurse to determine the efficacy of the care provided.

▪ SKILL 7.7 Using a Heat or Cold Pack (Instant or Reusable)

EQUIPMENT

Clean gloves, if there is risk of exposure to body fluids
Hypoallergenic tape
Washcloth, towel, or soft cloth liner
Instant cold or heat pack (compressible or fold-to-activate style)
Reusable cold gel pack

BEGINNING THE SKILL

1. **SAF** Review the order for heat or cold pack (instant or reusable).
2. **ACC** Review the client's medical and surgical history. *Understanding the client's history can help determine the client's needs and the appropriateness of the heat or cold pack.*
3. **SAF** Identify indications and contraindications for using heat or cold therapy (see Box 7.4).
4. **INF** Perform hand hygiene.
5. **CCC** Introduce yourself to the client and family
6. **SAF** Identify the client using two identifiers.
7. **SAF** Provide privacy and explain the procedure.
8. **ACC** Assess the client's level of consciousness and ability to follow instructions. *This will help determine if the client is able to understand and consent to the heat or cold pack.*
9. **CCC** Obtain consent for the procedure. *Promotes autonomy.*

PROCEDURE

10. **ACC** Assess the following:
    a. client and family's understanding of procedure for heat or cold pack
    b. client's sensitivity to pain, exact location of pain, and sensation or feeling in area where treatment will be targeted with heat or cold pack.
11. **COM** Ask the client about his or her personal pain and functional goals with heat or cold therapy. *Collaborating with the client facilitates the effectiveness of the heat or cold intervention.*
12. **HLTH** Examine the skin where heat or cold pack will be placed for any lesions, rashes, or signs of irritation. Avoid these areas if possible. *Placement of a cold or heat pack on areas of irritation can cause additional disruption of the client's skin.*
13. **SAF** Apply gloves if there is a risk of exposure to chemicals or body fluids.

If Using an Instant (Fold-and-Activate) Heat or Cold Pack

14. **ACC** Remove instant heat or cold pack from manufacturer packaging.
15. **SAF** Examine the pack before use. **WARNING:** If there are any punctures, tears, or leaking of chemicals, *do not use;* dispose of the pack immediately. If any chemical leaks directly on the client's skin, flush skin immediately with cool water (Medline, n.d.).

16. **ACC** Prepare instant cold or heat pack:
    a. If using the fold-to-activate style, fold the bag from top to bottom to "pop" the inner fluid bag.
    b. If using the compressible style, locate inner pouch and squeeze firmly to rupture inner pouch.
17. **ACC** Shake pack briefly to mix the contents and ensure activation of the chemical.
18. **HLTH** Wrap pack in a lightweight, soft cloth liner.
19. **ACC** Assist the client to an appropriate position for placement of the pack.
20. **ACC** Apply pack to treatment area on the client for 15 to 20 minutes per order. (Note: Application of cold or heat pack should be limited to a maximum of 20 minutes or per manufacturer recommendations to prevent burns or damage to skin.)
21. **HLTH** Monitor the client's skin frequently for redness, irritation, or other skin changes.
22. **HLTH** If there is no sign of irritation, gently secure pack in place with hypoallergenic tape or instruct the client to hold the pack in place using firm, but gentle pressure per client comfort.
23. **CCC** Instruct the client to notify you immediately of any pain or discomfort.
24. **ACC** If using an instant cold pack, do not place in refrigerator or freezer. *Attempting to refreeze an instant cold pack could cause damage to the skin and frostbite (Medline, n.d.).*
25. **SAF** If using an instant heat pack, do not place in microwave. *This could cause severe burns.*
26. **ACC** After the designated treatment time, remove and dispose of the instant pack.
27. **EVAL** Ask the client if the instant cold or heat pack helped with the client's pain or discomfort.
28. **HLTH** Reassess skin for any sign of redness or irritation.

If Using a Reusable Cold Gel Pack

29. **ACC** Prepare gel pack by placing in the freezer for a minimum of 2 hours or per guidelines.
30. **SAF** Inspect pack before use. If there are defects, tears, or ruptures, dispose of the pack.
31. **HLTH** If cold gel pack does not have a cloth liner or soft-touch fabric, wrap the pack in a soft cloth or towel. *Prevents freeze burns or frostbite of the client's skin.*
32. **ACC** Assist the client to an appropriate position for placement of the cold gel pack.
33. **INF** If there is a risk of exposure to body fluids, apply gloves.
34. **ACC** Apply cold gel pack to client's treatment area for 15 to 20 minutes per order. *Application of cold gel packs should be limited to a maximum of 20 minutes or per manufacturer recommendations in order to prevent freeze burns or frostbite.*

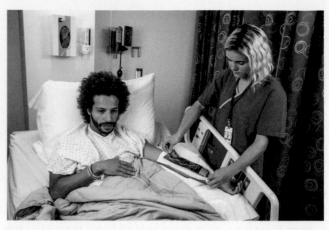

STEP 34 Apply gel pack.

35. **HLTH** Monitor the client's skin frequently for redness, irritation, or other skin changes. (Note: If there is no sign of irritation, secure cold gel pack in place with a compress holder [if available] or instruct the client to hold the pack in place using firm, but gentle pressure).
36. **CCC** Instruct the client to notify you immediately of any pain or discomfort.
37. **ACC** After the designated treatment time, remove the cold gel pack.
38. **INF** Clean the nondisposable cold gel pack with warm water and allow it to air dry.
39. **ACC** Keep the nondisposable cold gel pack in the freezer. *Gel packs must be in the freezer for a minimum of 2 hours before using again per manufacturer instructions.*
40. **EVAL** Ask the client if the heat or cold pack (instant or reusable) helped with the client's pain or discomfort.
41. **HLTH** Reinspect the client's skin to evaluate if there is any sign of redness or irritation.

FINISHING THE SKILL

42. **INF** Remove gloves if used and perform hand hygiene.
43. **SAF** Ensure safety and comfort. Ensure that the bed is in the lowest position and verify that the client can identify and reach the nurse call system. *These safety measures reduce the risk of falls.*
44. **EVAL** Evaluate the outcomes and effectiveness of the heat or cold pack. Did the heat or cold pack reduce the client's pain? Is the client's skin intact, without redness or irritation?
45. **COM** Document assessment findings, care given, and outcomes in the legal healthcare record:
    • duration of treatment time with a heat or cold pack
    • condition of the client's skin before and after removal of the heat or cold pack.

■ SKILL 7.8 Using an Ice Bag

EQUIPMENT

Clean gloves, if there is risk of exposure to body fluids
Crushed or cubed ice
Washcloth, towel, or cloth cover
Absorbent disposable protective pads
Commercial ice bag, zipper-top plastic bag, glove, or stocking

BEGINNING THE SKILL

1. **SAF** Review the order for the ice bag.
2. **ACC** Review the client's medical and surgical history. *Understanding the client's history can help determine the client's needs and the appropriateness of the ice bag.*
3. **SAF** Identify indications and contraindications for using cold therapy (see Box 7.4).
4. **INF** Perform hand hygiene.
5. **CCC** Introduce yourself to the client and family
6. **SAF** Identify the client using two identifiers.
7. **CCC** Provide privacy if needed and explain the procedure.
8. **ACC** Assess the client's level of consciousness and ability to follow instructions.
9. **SAF** Obtain consent for procedure. *Promotes autonomy.*

PROCEDURE

10. **ACC** Assess the following:
    a. client and family's understanding of procedure for ice bag
    b. client's sensitivity to pain, exact location of pain, and sensation or feeling in area where treatment will be targeted with ice bag.
11. **HLTH** Examine the skin where the ice bag will be placed and assess for any lesions, rashes, or signs of irritation. Avoid these areas if possible. *Placement of the bag on areas of irritation can cause additional disruption of the client's skin.*
12. **ACC** Prepare ice bag:
    a. If using a reusable commercial ice bag, fill the bag two-thirds full with cold water, crushed ice, or ice cubes. Do not force ice cubes through the opening. *Forcing ice through the opening could damage the bag.*

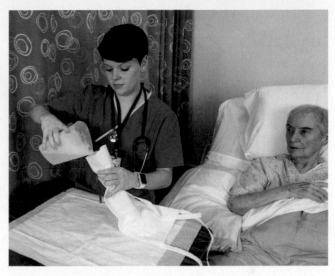

STEP 12A Prepare the ice bag.

    b. Close the bag securely and turn upside down to test for leaking.
    c. If using a zipper-top freezer bag or stocking, fill the bag one-half to two-thirds full of crushed ice or ice cubes. Seal the top of the freezer bag or secure and tie the opening of the stocking.
13. **SAF** Inspect the ice bag. If there are tears, ruptures, or defects, do not use the bag.
14. **HLTH** If the ice bag does not have a cloth liner or soft-touch fabric, wrap in soft cloth or towel. *Prevents freeze burns and/or frostbite.*
15. **ACC** Assist the client to an appropriate position for placement of the ice bag.
16. **INF** If there is a risk of exposure to body fluids, apply gloves.
17. **ACC** Apply ice bag to the client's treatment area for 15 to 20 minutes per order. *Application of an ice bag should be limited to a maximum of 25 minutes or per manufacturer recommendations in order to prevent freeze burns or frostbite.*

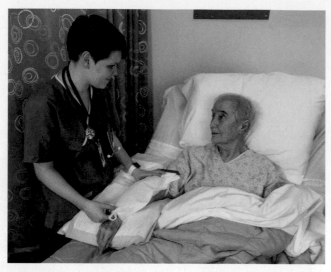

STEP 17 Apply the ice bag.

18. **HLTH** Monitor the client's skin frequently for redness, irritation, or other skin changes.
19. **ACC** If there is no sign of irritation, hold or loosely tie ice bag in place and secure with pillows on each side, or instruct the client to hold in place using firm, but gentle pressure.
20. **CCC** Instruct the client to notify you immediately of any pain or discomfort.

21. **CCC** Monitor ice bag for condensation or leaking. If this occurs, provide a disposable absorbent pad or towel and replace the ice bag if necessary.
22. **ACC** If ice melts or is no longer cold, replace ice as necessary.
23. **ACC** After the designated treatment time, remove the ice bag.
24. **INF** Clean ice bag per manufacturer instructions and allow to air dry.
25. **EVAL** Ask the client if the ice bag helped with his or her pain or discomfort.
26. **HLTH** Reassess the client's skin for any sign of redness or irritation.

FINISHING THE SKILL

27. **INF** Remove gloves if used and perform hand hygiene.
28. **SAF** Ensure safety and comfort. Ensure that the bed is in the lowest position and verify that the client can identify and reach the nurse call system. *These safety measures reduce the risk of falls.*
29. **EVAL** Evaluate the outcomes and effectiveness of ice bag therapy. Did the client tolerate the procedure? Does the client have reduced swelling and report less pain after ice bag therapy?
30. **COM** Document assessment findings, care given, and outcomes in the legal healthcare record:
    • duration of treatment time with an ice bag
    • condition of the client's skin before and after removal of the ice bag.

▪ SKILL 7.9 Using a Portable Sitz Bath

EQUIPMENT

Clean gloves
Washcloth and towels
Intravenous (IV) pole for water bag
Disposable absorbent protective pads
Portable over-the-toilet sitz bath basin
Sitz bath tubing and water bag
Water bath thermometer

BEGINNING THE SKILL

1. **SAF** Review the order for the sitz bath.
2. **ACC** Review the client's medical and surgical history. *Understanding the client's history can help determine the client's needs and the appropriateness of the sitz bath.*
3. **SAF** Identify indications and contraindications/precautions for the sitz bath, including frequent urinary tract infections, cardiovascular disease, diabetes, or diseases and conditions that might place the client at increased risk for fainting or dizziness (see Box 7.4).
4. **INF** Perform hand hygiene.
5. **CCC** Introduce yourself to the client and family.

6. **SAF** Identify the client using two identifiers.
7. **CCC** Provide privacy and explain the sitz bath procedure.
8. **ACC** Assess the client's level of consciousness and ability to follow instructions.
9. **SAF** Obtain consent for the procedure. *Promotes autonomy.*

PROCEDURE

10. **ACC** Assess the following:
    a. client and family's understanding of procedure for a sitz bath
    b. client's sensitivity to pain, exact location of pain, and sensation or feeling in area where treatment will be targeted with sitz bath
    c. client's mobility and ability to sit, stand, and ambulate and whether or not the client has orthostatic hypotension (see Chapter 3) when sitting up or standing.
11. **INF** Apply gloves.

12. **HLTH** Inspect the client's skin in the area that will be immersed in the sitz bath (i.e., perineal or rectal area). Note any redness or irritation in these areas.

13. **ACC** Encourage the client to empty the bladder. *Emptying the bladder will enhance comfort and prevent the client's sitz bath treatment from being interrupted.*

14. **ACC** Prepare over-the-toilet basin for sitz bath:
    a. Raise client's toilet seat and toilet bowl cover.
    b. Insert the end of the tubing (that is attached to water bag) through the entry hole in the basin and snap and secure the tubing into the channel at the bottom of the basin.
    c. Place the sitz bath basin on the toilet bowl by placing the part of the basin labeled as "Front" facing toward the front of the toilet bowl.
    d. Ensure that the three drainage holes at the back side of the basin are facing toward the back so that overflow water can easily drain into the toilet bowl.

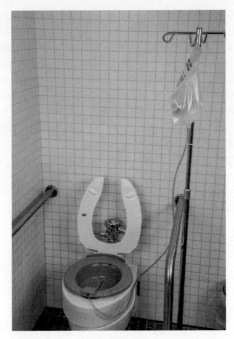

STEP 17 Adjust the height of the water bag.

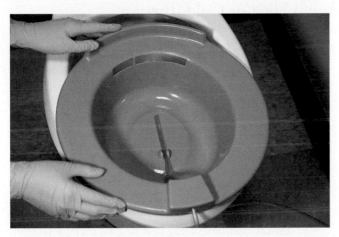

STEP 14D Prepare the sitz bath.

15. **INF** Remove gloves and perform hand hygiene.

16. **ACC** Prepare sitz bath water bag and tubing:
    a. Place sitz bag water bag with attached tubing and components on the IV pole and inspect for defects. If there are any defects, do not use.
    b. Move the flow control clamp closer to the bag and close the clamp. To open the clamp, slide it from the narrow to the wide side. To close the clamp, slide from the wide to the narrow side.
    c. Open the top of the water bag and fill it with warm water at a temperature of no more than 40°C to 43°C (105°F –110°F) or per facility policy.

17. **ACC** Adjust the height of the water bag and tubing on the IV pole high enough above the basin so that water can flow from the bag into the basin. If water is flowing too fast, lower the bag. If it is flowing too slow, raise the bag. *Height determines flow rate by gravity.*

18. **SAF** Slowly open the clamp on water bag tubing and fill the basin with water 1/2 to 2/3 full. Ensure that the water is at the proper temperature per manufacturer recommendation and facility policy. Measure the temperature with a bath thermometer if necessary.

19. **ACC** Assist the client to an appropriate position seated on the sitz bath basin.

20. **CCC** Ask the client if the water in the sitz bath basin is a comfortable temperature (not too hot or cold), and ensure that the client's treatment area is completely submerged in water.

21. **CCC** Cover the client with a blanket for warmth or offer the client extra towels for comfort.

22. **CCC** Ensure that the clamp on the tubing for the water bag is in a convenient location for the client.

23. **COM** Teach the client how to adjust the clamp on the sitz bath, and have the client demonstrate how to do this. *This will validate the client's understanding of the procedure.*

24. **ACC** Instruct the client to unclamp the tubing attached to the water bag and allow warm water to flow into the sitz bath basin if the water in the basin becomes too cool. Remind the client that as warm water flows in, overflow water will drain out the back through the drainage holes.

25. **SAF WARNING:** Ensure that the client is tolerating the sitz bath without feeling dizzy or lightheaded, and ensure that the client has access to the emergency call light in the bathroom.

26. **SAF** During the sitz bath (usually about 20 minutes), continue to monitor the client at frequent intervals. *The client could become dizzy during the treatment and require assistance.*

27. **INF** Perform hand hygiene and apply gloves again. Then assist the client off the sitz bath.
28. **SAF** Instruct the client to stand up slowly, and reassess the client for dizziness or discomfort. *Clients who have been in a sitting or lying position for a long time are at risk for orthostatic hypotension upon standing up. Rising up slowly prevents this.*
29. **CCC** Assist the client to gently pat the treatment area dry and return to bed if desired.
30. **HLTH** Reinspect the client's skin to evaluate if there is any sign of redness or irritation.
31. **INF** Empty the water bag and rinse the client's reusable basin; allow the basin to air dry.

FINISHING THE SKILL

32. **INF** Remove gloves and perform hand hygiene.

33. **SAF** Ensure safety and comfort. Ensure that the bed is in the lowest position and verify that the client can identify and reach the nurse call system. *These safety measures reduce the risk of falls.*
34. **EVAL** Evaluate the outcomes and the effectiveness of the sitz bath. Did the client tolerate the sitz bath? Does the client report decreased pain and discomfort after the sitz bath?
35. **COM** Document assessment findings, care given, and outcomes in the legal healthcare record:
    - appearance and condition of client's skin in treatment area
    - presence of any redness or irritation in treatment area
    - duration of treatment time for the sitz bath and client's tolerance of the treatment

■ SKILL 7.10 Using Localized Circulating (Aqua) Heat or Cold Therapy

EQUIPMENT

Clean gloves, if risk of exposure to body fluids
Washcloth and towels
Disposable absorbent protective pads
Cover, pillowcase, or other barrier
Distilled water
Automatic timer (if pump doesn't have one)
Circulating hot/cold localized therapy pump
Disposable or reusable pads for therapy pump

BEGINNING THE SKILL

1. **SAF** Review the order for localized circulating heat or cold therapy, including the setpoint. *The setpoint is the desired water temperature in the reservoir (Stryker, 2017).*
2. **ACC** Review the client's medical and surgical history.
3. **SAF** Identify indications and contraindications/precautions. (Note: Clients who have diabetes or circulation disorders are at increased risk of ischemic injury.) (See Box 7.4.)
4. **INF** Perform hand hygiene.
5. **CCC** Introduce yourself to the client and family
6. **SAF** Identify the client using two identifiers.
7. **CCC** Provide privacy if needed and explain the procedure.

PROCEDURE

8. **SAF** Obtain consent for procedure. *Promotes autonomy.*
9. **ACC** Assess the following.
    a. client and family's understanding of circulating heat or cold therapy
    b. client's level of pain/discomfort, exact location of pain, and sensation or feeling in area where treatment will be applied with localized circulating heat or cold therapy.

10. **HLTH** Examine the skin where the localized circulating hot or cold therapy pump will be placed and assess for any irritation or breakdown. Avoid these areas if possible. *Placement of hot or cold therapy on areas of irritation can cause additional disruption or damage to the skin.*
11. **SAF** Check circulating heat or cold therapy equipment for the following:
    a. Ensure that plug outlets and wire connections are intact, without breaks or frays.
    b. Ensure that pads and connectors are clean and intact, without tears.
    c. Ensure that circulating heat or cold therapy pump is not leaking.
12. **ACC** Prepare circulating heat or cold therapy per guidelines:
    a. **WARNING:** To reduce the risk of electrical shock, ensure that the pump is *not* plugged into an electrical outlet until after the reservoir is filled with water (Stryker, 2017).
    b. Before filling the pump, attach the pad to the connector hose of the pump.
    c. Ensure there are no kinks in the hose or pad and open the hose clamps.
    d. Open the fill cap on the top of the pump and fill the reservoir.
    e. If the client is receiving circulating heat therapy, fill the pump reservoir with room-temperature (not hot) distilled water to the water line marked "Heating."
    f. If the client is receiving circulating cold therapy, fill the pump with distilled cold water to the line marked "Cooling," or fill with ice to the full capacity of the reservoir.
13. **SAF** Plug the pump into an appropriate outlet (after unit has been prepared) and ensure that the cords are

not in an area that can be tripped over or bumped by the client.

14. **ACC** Press the on/standby button of the pump.
15. **ACC** Set the temperature setpoint on the pump as ordered (cooling, low heat, or high heat). (Note: Some pumps have a lock for the setpoint [desired temperature] and light indicator that indicates that water has reached the desired temperature [Stryker, 2017].)
16. **SAF** Allow water to flow through the circulating therapy pads to ensure that it is warming or cooling properly and that there are no leaks.
17. **ACC** Check the water level in the pump. If it drops below operating level, add water. *The pump will not work properly if there is insufficient water (Stryker, 2017).*
18. **SAF** If pads do not have a built-in barrier, place a light cover on the pad.
19. **INF** Apply gloves if there is a risk of exposure to body fluids.
20. **ACC** Assist the client to a position that will provide optimal access to the treatment area, and ensure that the area that will be treated is clean and dry.
21. **ACC** Place pad on treatment area. If pads need to be secured, use flexible gauze or hypoallergenic tape. Avoid pins or anything sharp that could puncture the pads.
22. **SAF** If the pump does not have an automatic timer, set the manual timer per order and facility policy. *A timer can prevent injury from prolonged exposure to heat or cold.*
23. **ACC** Position the pump at or above the level of the pad and the client.

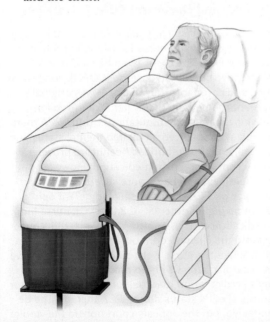

STEP 23 Position pump.

If the pump is placed below the level of the pad, water could flow back into the pump when off and create a leak, particularly if there is an excess of water (Stryker, 2017).

24. **CCC** Ask the client if the circulating heat or cold therapy is helping to ease the pain.
25. **SAF** Instruct the client to report any discomfort or any other problem with therapy.
26. **SAF** Instruct the client not to lie on the pad (particularly if the client is receiving heat). *Direct pressure of skin on the heating pad could trap heat and cause burns (Stryker, 2017).*
27. **SAF** Instruct the client and family not to change the pump settings or the placement of the pads.
28. **HLTH** Continue to monitor the client's skin in the treatment area at frequent intervals (at least every 15–20 minutes). Ensure that there are no areas of redness, irritation, or burns.
29. **SAF** Continue to monitor the pump for leaks during therapy, and monitor the water level in the reservoir. *If the water level becomes too low, mechanisms could overheat and be damaged.*
30. **ACC** If the ice melts during cooling, place the pump on standby, unplug from power outlet, drain reservoir, and refill with ice per manufacturer guidelines.
31. **ACC** If the pump will not heat or cool the pad, check the reservoir to make sure there is water or ice, and ensure that flow to the pad is not blocked or kinked. *This troubleshoots the system.*
32. **ACC** At the end of the circulating heat or cold therapy, discontinue the pump and do the following:
    a. Press the off or standby button and unplug the pump.
    b. Close all of hose clamps and disconnect the pads from the pump.
    c. Disconnect the pad from the pump with the connectors raised above the level of the pad and pump. *Prevents water from spilling out of the connectors.*
    d. **INF** Clean and store equipment per facility policy.
33. **HLTH** Reinspect the client's skin to evaluate if there is any sign of redness or irritation.

FINISHING THE SKILL

34. **INF** Remove gloves if used and perform hand hygiene.
35. **SAF** Ensure safety and comfort. Ensure that the bed is in the lowest position and verify that the client can identify and reach the nurse call system. *These safety measures reduce the risk of falls.*
36. **EVAL** Evaluate the outcomes and effectiveness of the aquatherapy. Did the client tolerate the procedure? Does the client report decreased pain and discomfort after aquatherapy?
37. **COM** Document assessment findings, care given, and outcomes in the legal healthcare record:
    • appearance and condition of the client's skin in treatment area
    • presence of redness or irritation of the client's skin before and after treatment
    • duration of treatment time for circulating heat or cold therapy

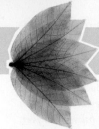

SECTION 5 Using Patient-Controlled Analgesia to Promote Comfort

When managing a client's pain, it is optimal to use the least invasive methods possible. However, some clients require intravenous (IV) administration of pharmacologic analgesics, including via patient-controlled analgesia (PCA). As the name suggests, PCA allows clients to administer their own analgesia and experience pain relief in a timely manner.

PCA therapy can be used in a variety of different settings, including acute care, home health, or hospice. In the acute care setting, PCA therapy is often administered into the client's vein through an IV catheter, but it may also be given by other routes, including an epidural catheter. The use of an epidural catheter is discussed in the next section. For the purpose of this section, IV PCA is discussed. Because IV PCA requires entry into the client's vein, sterile technique must be followed (see Chapters 10 and 12).

An intravenous PCA system consists of an electronic portable infusion PCA pump that is lockable and has an automated timing system. As shown in Fig. 7.7, there is also an area inside the locked pump for an analgesic vial/syringe or cartridge. The PCA pump is used with special disposable tubing that can be attached to the syringe and the client's main infusion line. To give the client control, there is an attached PCA dosing button that the client can press and release when he or she wishes to obtain or "demand" analgesia.

The order for PCA usually includes an initial bolus dose or loading dose, the PCA dose (which is the dose received when the client presses the dosing control button), and the mode (which is either continuous or intermittent). A continuous dose may also be known as the basal rate. If a client is opioid naïve, a continuous mode may not be recommended because of the cumulative effect of opioids and the risk for respiratory depression. There may also be an order for the upper limits of analgesic medication and the lockout interval. During the lockout, the client cannot receive any more medication even if the PCA dosing button is pushed. This prevents the client from getting an analgesic overdose and becoming overly sedated.

SAFETY CONSIDERATIONS WHEN USING PCA THERAPY

The analgesics used for PCA therapy usually include high-alert medications, such as opioids, that can cause respiratory depression and other serious side effects. Thus, there are critical safety issues to consider with PCA therapy. Life-threatening errors have occurred that are related to violations of the medication safety checks and rights of medication administration (see Chapter 11), as well as communication and pump programming errors. Errors have also occurred

BOX 7.6 Lesson From the Courtroom: Failure to Properly Monitor and Document PCA

In a Texas lawsuit *(McAllen Hospitals v. Muniz et al.)*, a jury ruled against a hospital and nurse for failing to monitor a client receiving PCA. The client (who had a history of chronic obstructive pulmonary disease [COPD], congestive heart failure, and coronary artery disease) was originally placed on IV morphine (an opioid) per PCA pump for postoperative pain after leg amputation. During PCA therapy, the nursing staff observed an altered mental status and blood pressure, and the authorized healthcare provider switched the client to oral pain medication. However, after 3 days, the client began to have more severe pain and was placed back on PCA therapy using a different opioid (Dilaudid) with a higher potency. At 8:00 PM, a nurse initiated the medication by PCA pump. At 9:00 PM, the same nurse went into the client's room only to draw blood for a glucose test. When the nurse went back in at 10:54 PM, the client was in cardiac arrest with no pulse and respirations.

The jury's verdict found that the nurse failed to monitor and record the client's status during PCA therapy. The defendant appealed, but the appeals court upheld the verdict and stated that the nurse should have considered that the client's medical history and previous sensitivity to opioids placed him at increased risk for sedation and respiratory depression. When the PCA medication was restarted, the nurse had a responsibility to monitor and document the client's condition, including his vital signs, oxygen saturation, and respirations.

Reference: *Patient-controlled analgesia: Jury relates patient's death to nursing negligence,* 2008.

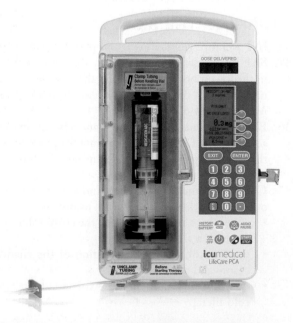

FIG. 7.7 Example of a locked PCA pump/infuser.

due to inadequate assessment and monitoring (Grissinger, 2016). See Box 7.6.

During PCA therapy, the nurse must closely monitor the client's pain, respiratory status, and sedation using a reliable sedation scale. When monitoring the client's respiratory status, it is important to not only count the rate but also to assess the depth, character, and quality of the client's respirations. Because sedation usually precedes respiratory depression, the client's level of sedation is the most critical parameter for predicting respiratory depression in clients receiving IV opioids (Grissinger, 2016). One scale that is often used is the Pasero Opioid-Induced Sedation Scale (POSS) that scores sedation based on the arousability of the client. The score components include **S** (sleeping, easy to arouse); **1** (awake and alert); **2** (slightly drowsy, easily aroused), **3** (frequently drowsy, arousable, but drifts off to sleep during conversation, and **4** (somnolent, minimal or no response to physical stimulation). A score of 3 or 4 is considered unacceptable and requires immediate action, such as holding the opioid dose, administering oxygen, providing airway support, and notifying the authorized healthcare provider (McCaffery et al., 2011). Another scale that may be used is the Richmond Agitation and Sedation Scale (RASS). Different facilities will use specific tools and protocols. Regardless of which tool is used, it is important to use the scale consistently and to intervene in a timely manner.

An additional tool that may be used is capnography monitoring to measure end-tidal carbon dioxide ($EtCO_2$), which facilitates early detection of respiratory depression. If the client has respiratory depression, carbon dioxide levels will rise, leading to further deterioration in the client's level of consciousness. Capnography monitoring may be particularly helpful for clients who are opioid naïve or clients who have sleep apnea or other risk factors. For more information about capnography monitoring, see Chapter 18. Oxygen saturation may also be monitored. However, oxygen saturation levels may not show abnormalities until the client is already in severe distress (Grissinger, 2016). For clients at risk for respiratory depression related to opioids, an opioid antagonist such as naloxone (Narcan) may be on standby (see Chapter 11).

PCA by Unauthorized Proxy

Another issue that can cause complications is PCA by unauthorized proxy (ISMP, 2016). In this situation, someone (who is not authorized to do so) is pushing the PCA dosing control button instead of the client. Sometimes family members with good intentions may do this because the client is unable to push the button on his or her own or they are afraid their loved one will be in pain (Box 7.7). The Joint Commission and the American Society for Pain Management Nursing (ASPMN) do *not* support the use of PCA by unauthorized proxies. However, the ASPMN supports the practice of authorized agent-controlled analgesia (AACA) under strict guidelines. As the ASPMN guidelines note, AACA can only be done by a person, such as a nurse

BOX 7.7 Lessons From Experience: PCA by Unauthorized Proxy

> Kimmy is a 16-year-old client who is receiving pain medication via a PCA pump for acute pain following abdominal surgery. Her PCA orders indicate that she may receive a demand (bolus) dose of 1 mg of morphine with a lockout of 20 minutes. On admission, she is alert and oriented, and her vital signs and sedation level are within expected parameters. Later during the shift, Kimmy becomes increasingly drowsy. Although her respirations and vital signs are still at baseline, Kimmy quickly falls back to sleep after briefly being awakened for her assessment. Her sedation level has also increased. The nurse asks Kimmy's mother (who is at her bedside) if Kimmy has been waking up and complaining of pain. Her mother states, "No, I have been pushing that button on the machine regularly so that she won't wake up and have pain."
>
> In this scenario, the client is being given doses of analgesics (via the PCA demand button) by an unauthorized proxy (the client's mother). Because oversedation often precedes respiratory depression, Kimmy is at risk for respiratory compromise. One of the safeguards of PCA is that the client can only push the control button when awake (which will prevent oversedation). Although Kimmy's mother meant well, she circumvented that safeguard when she pushed the button herself. The nurse explained to Kimmy's mother that only Kimmy was allowed to push her PCA control button. The nurse also contacted the prescribing healthcare provider and continued to watch Kimmy's vital signs, respiratory effort, sedation, and oxygen saturation closely. Most institutions do *not* allow PCA by an unauthorized proxy. When caring for clients who have attentive family members (e.g., parents), it is a good idea to involve them in client teaching about PCA (see Skill 7.14) as much as possible and then reinforce this information at regular intervals.

or caregiver, who is (a) consistently available, (b) competent, (c) properly trained to activate the dosing button, and (d) authorized by the prescriber in accordance with facility policy. In addition, the use of an AACA must be limited to clients who are unable to self-administer their pain medication to control their pain (Cooney et al., 2013).

In order for PCA to be safe, it must be appropriate for the client. Clients who are confused or too young to understand how PCA works may not be good candidates for PCA. Many facilities have protocols for selection criteria to ensure the client can safely receive PCA. As a result of potential risks with PCA, key risk reduction strategies have been developed (Box 7.8).

To further facilitate safety, PCA pumps that contain barcode technology and other features are available (Fig. 7.8). Some PCA pumps are now integrated into electronic health records and client monitoring. However, the PCA pump doesn't replace the nurse's clinical judgment at the bedside. One of the most important things the nurse can do is double-check and ask questions. Nurses reduce risk by being aware of the hazards and looking for warning signs.

BOX 7.8 Summary of Risk Reduction Strategies for PCA Therapy

- Standardize whenever possible. Use standardized orders/policies, automated dispensing systems, and prefilled cartridges/syringes per facility guidelines.
- Identify and clearly label where the client's IV line and PCA line are infusing.
- Use independent checks at the bedside with a second nurse. Many facilities require that a second nurse double-check and verify the client's ID, PCA pump settings (initially and with any changes), PCA analgesic label, and dosage.
- Before the infusion starts, ensure that the information on PCA analgesic label is identical with the information displayed on the PCA pump screen.
- Do not allow the free flow of medication to the client. Ensure that the anti-siphon device on the PCA tubing (that prevents free flow) is intact and working properly.
- Keep a close watch on the client. Monitor sedation, respiratory rate/effort and depth, vital signs, oxygen saturation, $EtCO_2$, and other parameters required by the facility.
- Monitor the client's IV site and ensure that it is patent and working properly.
- Keep track of how much PCA medication is actually going into the client.

References: Grissinger, 2016; ISMP, 2016.

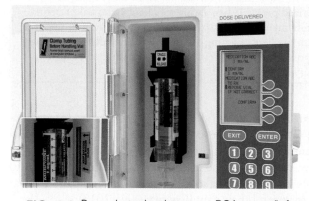

FIG. 7.8 Barcode technology on a PCA pump/infuser.

- Is there a change in your client's orientation level from baseline?
- Is your client becoming increasingly more sedated or difficult to wake up?
- Are your client's respirations slowing down or becoming more shallow?
- Has a large volume of PCA medication in the cartridge, syringe, or bag infused in a short amount of time or at a faster rate than expected?
- Is the high-pressure alarm or other alarm on the pump going off, which could indicate an infiltrated IV line, blocked or kinked tubing, or a closed clamp?

BOX 7.9 Expect the Unexpected: Problems With PCA Therapy

Mr. Willis is a 74-year-old man admitted to your med-surg unit following lung resection. On admission, the hospitalist placed Mr. Willis on PCA therapy. Before PCA was initiated, his assessment indicated he was awake, alert, and oriented, with a pain rating of 5. When the nurse did client teaching, Mr. Willis was able to demonstrate an understanding of how to use the PCA dosing button, and he was physically able to push the dosing button. Several hours into the night shift (approximately 2 AM), Mr. Willis's wife comes out to the nurses' station and states, "I don't know what is wrong with my husband. He is hurting, and it seems to be getting worse." When the nurse checks Mr. Willis, she notes that his pain rating is now 7. However, the analgesic history on the PCA pump indicates that Mr. Willis has not made any recent demands or pushes on the PCA control button. When the nurse asks Mr. Willis to show her again how to use the PCA dosing button, he holds it up in the air and states "I am ready to go to the store now!" On further assessment, Mr. Willis is not oriented to place, time, or situation.

   Although Mr. Willis was initially a good candidate for PCA, he has now become confused. In addition, he is not able to self-administer his own pain medication. When the nurse realizes this, she makes arrangements to give Mr. Willis his pain medication herself as an authorized proxy. Clients who are confused are at increased risk for PCA complications and undertreatment for pain. The stressful hospital environment and other factors may cause clients to become confused (especially at night). During PCA therapy, continue to watch the client closely, and be alert for any changes in the client's clinical condition.

- Does the client seem to be having trouble remembering how to use the PCA control button, or is your client becoming increasingly more confused?
- Is the client complaining of increased pain or discomfort?

   Many facilities have policies regarding monitoring for PCA therapy. Some facilities also have electronic flow sheets that document critical parameters, including sedation ratings, vital signs, respiratory effort/quality, and side effects. Before, during, and after the PCA therapy, monitor the client's level of pain using a consistent, reliable, and culturally appropriate pain tool (see Section 1 of this chapter). If your client is not getting adequate pain relief, troubleshoot and intervene appropriately. Likewise, it is important to continuously assess and reassess your client to ensure the client remains alert and oriented and can properly use PCA (Box 7.9).

SUMMARY

In summary, the registered nurse is responsible for the assessment and care of clients who are receiving PCA therapy. This is not a procedure that can be delegated to assistive personnel. Because of the risks associated with the use of opioids and other analgesics, safety and accuracy are two of the most important critical concepts to consider when using PCA. In addition, excellent communication, client-centered care, and collaboration with the client and family are essential to improve knowledge about PCA and to maintain optimal pain control for the client.

APPLICATION OF THE NURSING PROCESS

Examples of Related ICNP Nursing Diagnoses, Expected Client Outcomes, and Nursing Interventions:

Nursing Diagnosis: Inadequate pain control

Supporting Data: Client reports increased pain and inability to perform normal activities.

Expected Client Outcomes: Client will have adequate pain control:
- decreased pain rating on pain-intensity scale
- ability to achieve functional and pain-control goals
- ability to perform ADLs.

Nursing Intervention Examples: Ensure that PCA pump is working properly and client's IV access is patent. Use a consistent, culturally sensitive tool for pain assessments.

Nursing Diagnosis: Lack of knowledge of PCA

Supporting Data: Client expresses lack of understanding regarding PCA dosing control button.

Expected Client Outcomes: Client will have increased understanding of PCA, as seen by:
- ability to verbalize purpose of PCA pump and demonstrate how to use PCA dosing button
- acknowledgment by client that PCA dosing button should only be used when he or she has pain
- acknowledgment by client that only the client can push the PCA dosing button, not others.

Reference: International Classification for Nursing Practice. (n.d.). *eHealth & ICNP*. Retrieved from https://www.icn.ch/what-we-do/projects/ehealth-icnp.

CRITICAL CONCEPTS
Using Patient-Controlled Analgesia to Promote Comfort

Accuracy (ACC)

Accuracy when using PCA therapy is affected by the following variables:
- assessment of client, including age, medical/surgical history, clinical status, level of consciousness/orientation, and pain assessment

- appropriateness of PCA therapy for client
- patency and integrity of IV site for PCA therapy
- preparation, setup, and programming for PCA therapy
- adherence to medication safety checks and the rights of medication administration: right drug, right dose, right time, right client, right route, and right documentation (see Chapter 11).
- understanding of procedure by client, family, and/or authorized proxy.

Client-Centered Care (CCC)

Respect for the client during PCA therapy is demonstrated through:
- promoting autonomy by allowing client to self-administer PCA medication
- providing privacy and ensuring comfort
- honoring cultural preferences and arranging for an interpreter if necessary
- advocating for the client and family and explaining the procedure.

Infection Control (INF)

Healthcare-associated infection during PCA therapy is prevented by:
- preventing and reducing the transfer of microorganisms
- reducing the number of microorganisms.

Safety (SAF)

Safety measures and adherence to safety guidelines during PCA therapy prevent harm and provide a safe care environment.
- Performing medication safety checks, assessing for allergies and contraindications, and closely monitoring the client reduces the risk of complications.

Communication (COM)

- Communication exchanges information (oral, written, nonverbal, and electronic) between two or more people.
- Documentation records information in a permanent legal record.
- Collaboration and instruction with the client and family and follow-up teaching during PCA therapy will facilitate safe and effective pain management and care.

Evaluation (EVAL)

Evaluation of the outcomes of PCA allows the nurse to determine the efficacy and safety of the care provided.

▪ SKILL 7.11 Assessing a Client for Appropriateness of PCA Therapy

(Note: Many facilities have approved protocols or criteria for assessment and qualification of clients for PCA therapy. Consult your facility PCA policies and guidelines.)

EQUIPMENT

Sedation assessment scale (used by facility)
Pain-intensity scale (age/culturally appropriate)
Screening tool (used by facility)
BP cuff and stethoscope
Antimicrobial wipes

BEGINNING THE SKILL

1. **SAF** Review the order for PCA therapy.
2. **SAF** Review the following criteria:
   a. client's medical history and indications for PCA therapy. *Clients who have a history of cognitive disorders or other medical disorders may not be good candidates for PCA.*
   b. client's history of previous analgesic or opioid use. *Clients who are opioid naïve will be more sensitive and at a higher risk for respiratory depression than clients who have a long history of analgesic use.*
3. **INF** Perform hand hygiene.
4. **CCC** Introduce yourself to the client and family.
5. **SAF** Identify the client using two identifiers.
6. **CCC** Provide privacy.
7. **COM** Explain to the client and family that you will be evaluating the client for PCA therapy. Assess the client's personal goals regarding pain and function. *Facilitates collaboration.*

PROCEDURE

8. **ACC** Assess baseline vital signs. *Baseline vital signs are important for future comparisons.*
9. **ACC** Assess the following:
   a. client's understanding and willingness to use PCA therapy
   b. client's level of pain/discomfort and exact location of pain (see Section 1).
10. **ACC** Evaluate the client's cognitive and neurologic function:
    a. Is the client oriented to person, time, place, and situation?
    b. Does the client follow commands and instructions appropriately?
    c. Does the client have any periods of confusion or disorientation?
    d. Does the client have an understanding of the relationship between pushing the dosing button on the PCA machine and relief of his or her pain?
11. **ACC** Assess the client's respiratory function:
    a. Does the client have any difficulty breathing or shortness of breath?
    b. Are respirations shallow, labored, or noisy?
    c. Does the client have periods of sleep apnea or loud snoring?
    d. Does the client require oxygen or monitoring of the oxygen saturation level?
    e. What is the client's respiratory rate? *Many facilities do not allow clients with a respiratory rate of less than 10 to 12 breaths/minute to be on PCA therapy. Check facility policy.*
12. **ACC** Assess the client's mobility:
    a. Is the client able to squeeze your hands on command without pain or difficulty?
    b. Can the client demonstrate the ability to press and release the PCA dosing button?
13. **SAF** Assess the client's sedation level:
    a. Does the client sleep excessively during the daytime?
    b. Does the client fall back easily into sedation after being aroused? *A client may be starting to become oversedated if he or she is easily falling back into sedation (Grissinger, 2016).*
    c. What is the client's score on the standardized sedation assessment scale used by the facility?
14. **SAF** If the client does not meet selection criteria or appears to be a high risk for PCA, notify the authorized healthcare provider. *Clients who are high risk or don't meet criteria may need additional safety measures, such as oxygen saturation or capnography monitoring, to measure ventilation and early detection of respiratory depression. The client may also need to have an authorized proxy (AACA) for administering the analgesic according to the facility policy.*

FINISHING THE SKILL

15. **INF** Perform hand hygiene.
16. **SAF** Ensure safety and comfort. Ensure that the bed is in the lowest position and verify that the client can identify and reach the nurse call system. *These safety measures reduce the risk of falls.*
17. **EVAL** Evaluate the outcomes. Is the client a good candidate for PCA? What is the client's sedation level? What are the client's oxygen saturation and $EtCO_2$?
18. **COM** Document assessment findings, care given, client and family education provided, and outcomes in the legal healthcare record.

■ SKILL 7.12 Initiating and Managing PCA Therapy

EQUIPMENT

PCA pump and PCA pump key
PCA electronic record and/or flowsheet
Pain-intensity rating scale and sedation scale
PCA tubing administration set
Injector for PCA analgesic vial
PCA analgesic vial/syringe
Clean gloves
BP cuff and stethoscope
Antiseptic wipes
Oxygen and naloxone (Narcan) (standby if needed)
IV line, normal saline bag, Y connector, and IV pole
Oxygen saturation monitor and capnography monitor (if ordered)

BEGINNING THE SKILL

1. **SAF** Review order for PCA, including the mode (PCA, continuous, or combination), type of analgesia, PCA dose, lockout interval, dose limit, or initial bolus dose.
2. **ACC** Review and verify the client's selection criteria and client assessment (see Skill 7.11).
3. **INF** Perform hand hygiene.
4. **CCC** Introduce yourself to the client and family.
5. **SAF** Identify the client using two identifiers.
6. **CCC** Provide privacy and explain the procedure.
7. **SAF** Assess for allergies, including allergies to PCA analgesics and other medications.
8. **CCC** Ensure that client consent has been obtained. *Promotes autonomy.*

PROCEDURE

9. **ACC** Assess current pain level, baseline vital signs, and sedation level. (Note: The client must be awake and alert and able to follow instructions to receive PCA. See Skill 7.11.)
10. **ACC** Inspect the infusion site where PCA therapy will be infused, and ensure that the catheter is patent and without signs of infiltration or phlebitis (see Chapter 12).

Preparing PCA Therapy

11. **ACC Prepare PCA pump:**
    a. Plug the PCA pump into the electrical outlet and ensure that the battery is fully charged.
    b. Ensure that the key for the PCA pump is working properly. *The key is used to unlock the door to the pump and allows the analgesic syringe to be secured and locked.*
    c. Using the key, adjust the PCA pump on the pole if needed, and open the door.
    d. Turn the pump on and allow it to go through all self-checks if necessary.
    e. Ensure that all alarms and safety features on the pump are working properly.

f. If the PCA pump has a barcode reader on the side of the pump, clean with a dry soft cloth. *A clean barcode scanner facilitates accurate reading.*

12. **SAF** Prepare PCA medication vial/syringe or cartridge:
    a. Check label on vial or cartridge and ensure that it matches client ID and order and perform independent safety checks with a second healthcare provider. (Note: Follow the safety checks by ensuring medication administration rights discussed in Chapter 11.)

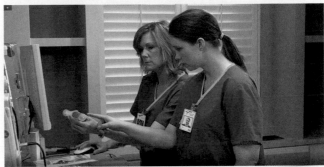

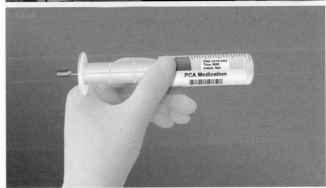

STEP 12A Check analgesia and perform safety checks.

b. Inspect vial and tubing and ensure they are free from cracks or defects.
c. Using sterile technique, remove or "pop off" caps from PCA vial/syringe and attach to PCA injector. *This will supply your PCA medication.*

13. **ACC Prepare PCA tubing:**
    a. Attach long length of PCA tubing to PCA vial/syringe.
    b. Prime PCA tubing and label tubing according to policy (see Chapter 12).
    c. If the client has existing IV with fluid, check compatibility with PCA medication.
    d. If the client does not have an existing IV with fluid, start an IV (see Chapter 12), prime regular tubing with fluid that is compatible with the analgesic, and insert primed tubing into a separate IV pump. If allowed by facility policy, attach the end of the regular tubing to the short piece of PCA tubing with a Y connector. *This line with compatible fluid will serve as the "keep open line" for the client's IV when PCA medication is not infusing.*

14. **ACC** Load PCA vial/syringe with tubing into the pump according to manufacturer instructions. You may hear a "click" sound to indicate insertion is secure.

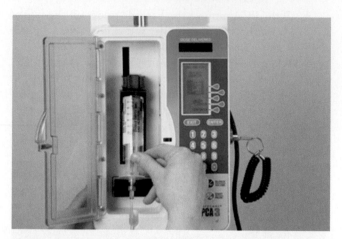

STEP 14 Load the PCA vial/syringe.

15. **ACC** After insertion of the vial into the pump, reinspect the vial for any crack or breaks in the glass. *Sometimes the pressure from insertion can damage the vial.*
16. **ACC** Ensure that graduated markings on vial/syringe are facing front in clear view and that the barcode (if there is one) is facing toward the scanner. *The barcode has to be lined up properly to be read by the scanner. Facing the graduated markings on the vial/syringe toward window allows the nurse to see how much medication has infused into the client* (see Fig. 7.7).
17. **ACC** Ensure that the tubing is lined up in the track of the pump before the door is closed. *Prevents PCA infusion tubing from being blocked or kinked.*
18. **SAF** Close and lock pump door. (Note: The key will have to be secured in a safe place.)
19. **ACC** Set PCA settings (mode, dose, volume, lockout, limit) according to order. **WARNING:** Before starting the infusion, verify the client's ID, PCA pump settings, PCA analgesic label, and dosage with a second nurse. *When PCA is initiated or changed, these parameters must be double-checked.*

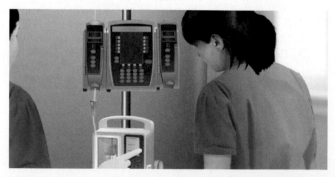

STEP 19 Set PCA settings and verify with a second nurse.

20. **ACC** Open the clamp on the tubing. If there is air in the bottom portion of the tubing, purge the air out with fluid *before* the tubing is attached to the client. *Prevents air from going into the client.*

Connecting PCA Tubing to the Client

21. **INF** Perform hand hygiene again.
22. **INF** Apply gloves.
23. **INF** Clean lowest connection port or cap on the client's IV with an antiseptic wipe.
24. **SAF** Connect primed PCA tubing to the client using sterile technique. **WARNING:** Before connecting the PCA tubing to the client's IV, trace the IV line from the client's insertion site to the connection or fluid source. *Tracing a line from client's insertion site to the connection is a safety strategy to prevent misconnection errors.*
25. **SAF** Begin infusion and observe the client's IV site at frequent intervals for leaking, pain, or other problems. *These signs could indicate that the IV is infiltrated or loose at the hub.*
26. **SAF** If giving an initial bolus dose, give dose slowly and observe the client closely.
27. **ACC** Continue to monitor the client's pain, sedation level, ability to be aroused, orientation, vital signs, and respiratory function at frequent intervals. (Note: This is particularly important if the client is opioid naïve.)
28. **ACC** During infusion, continue to inspect the vial/syringe for any leaks. *Sometimes cracks and leaks will not be obvious until the vial/syringe is under pressure from the pump.*
29. **ACC** Continue to monitor the client's IV site and keep track of the total amount of analgesic received. *This verifies that the client is receiving the medication as intended.*
30. **SAF** Place a label on the PCA tubing close to the source and close to the client that states "PCA." *Proper labeling prevents misconnection errors.*

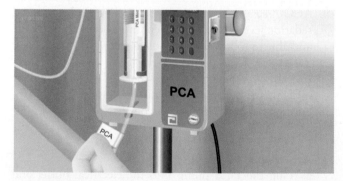

STEP 30 Place labels.

31. **COM** Place a bold label on the PCA cord that states the following: **WARNING: DOSING BUTTON IS TO ONLY BE PRESSED BY THE CLIENT.** *Placing a label on the cord provides a caution for family and friends that only the client must push the PCA button (ISMP, 2016).*
32. **COM** Teach the client (or authorized proxy) about PCA (see Skill 7.13), including how to use the dosing button. Reiterate that only the client may push the dosing button.

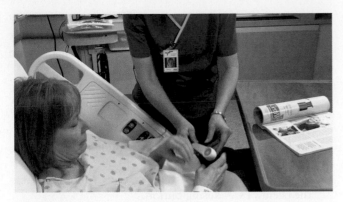

STEP 32 Provide client teaching.

33. **CCC** Ensure that the client has access to the PCA dosing button and call light. Avoid placing the PCA dosing button in a location that would cause confusion with the call button.

34. **CCC** Instruct the client to contact you if pain is not relieved.

FINISHING THE SKILL

35. **INF** Remove gloves and perform hand hygiene.

36. **SAF** Ensure safety and comfort. Ensure that the bed is in the lowest position and verify that the client can identify and reach the nurse call system. *These safety measures reduce the risk of falls.*

37. **EVAL** Evaluate the outcomes. Is the client tolerating PCA therapy, without signs of oversedation or respiratory depression? Does the client have reduced pain and discomfort?

38. **COM** Document assessment findings, care given, client and family education provided, and outcomes in the legal healthcare record:
    - appearance and patency of client's IV catheter site
    - pain-intensity ratings and other pain assessment parameters, such as whether or not client is able to meet his or her functional and pain control goals with PCA therapy
    - sedation level, ability to be aroused, orientation level, vital signs, respiratory function, and character/quality of respirations during PCA therapy
    - pulse oximetry reading and $EtCO_2$ if done

Follow-up Care and Monitoring During PCA Therapy

39. **SAF** Review PCA orders and perform hand hygiene.

40. **EVAL** Monitor the client's pain level, vital signs, sedation level, and respiratory effort and document per facility policy. *PCA infusions require continuous monitoring.* (Note: Oxygen saturation and $EtCO_2$ may also be monitored during PCA therapy for some clients.)

41. **EVAL** Monitor the IV site where PCA therapy is infusing and ensure that catheter is patent, without signs of infiltration or phlebitis. Apply gloves if needed (see Chapter 12).

42. **If a replacement vial is required during PCA therapy:**
    a. **SAF** Inspect new replacement vial for any cracks or leaks.
    b. **SAF** Close slide clamp of PCA tubing, and then use the key to open the pump door. **WARNING:** Do not allow analgesic to "free flow" into the client's IV line.
    c. **SAF** Remove old vial and disconnect from plunger per manufacturer instructions. **WARNING:** If an alarm goes off when the vial is removed, temporarily reset, but do not deactivate, the alarm. *Alarms are safety features that must remain activated.*
    d. **ACC** Using sterile technique, place the new vial on the plunger and load the vial/syringe into the pump per manufacturer instructions (see steps 11 to 17).
    f. **SAF** Verify the client's ID, PCA settings, analgesic label, and dosage with a second nurse. *Replacing narcotic vials require independent checks by a second nurse.* (Note: Follow the safety checks by ensuring medication administration rights, as discussed in Chapter 11.)
    g. **SAF** Close and lock the PCA pump door.
    h. **ACC** Unclamp the slide clamp on the PCA tubing and restart the PCA pump.

43. **Disposing of a removed PCA vial:**
    a. **SAF** If the removed vial is empty, dispose of it in the sharps container box per policy.
    b. **SAF** If the removed vial has analgesic remaining (waste), discard the vial and sign out with a second nurse as a witness, or send the medication to the pharmacy according to policy.
       (Note: Some facilities use automated dispensing systems for medications.)

44. **INF** Remove gloves if worn and perform hand hygiene. Follow finishing steps 35 to 38. (Note: Document information related to discarded waste electronically if required by policy.)

■ SKILL 7.13 Teaching the Client and Family About PCA Therapy

(Note: Some facilities require that PCA teaching must be done prior to initiating PCA therapy. Check facility policy.)

EQUIPMENT

Pain-intensity scale and sedation-level scale

Written materials about PCA therapy (as needed)

BEGINNING THE SKILL

1. **SAF** Review and verify the order for the current PCA therapy.

2. **ACC** Review and verify the client's selection criteria and assessment (see Skill 7.11). *The client's assessment, including level of consciousness, orientation, and sedation level, will determine the client's ability to participate in the learning process about PCA.*
3. **INF** Perform hand hygiene.
4. **CCC** Introduce yourself to the client and family.
5. **SAF** Identify the client using two identifiers.
6. **CCC** Provide privacy.

PROCEDURE

7. **CCC** Assess the client's pain using a consistent, culturally sensitive tool that is facility approved. *Verifies effectiveness of PCA therapy and identifies need for further intervention or teaching.*
8. **COM** Assess the client and family's readiness to learn about the client's PCA therapy, and explore any particular areas of concern they have about PCA therapy. *Adult learners are most receptive to learning about issues that are important to them personally.*
9. **COM** Teach the client or authorized proxy how to control pain by pressing and releasing the PCA dosing button. Have the client demonstrate pressing and releasing the dosing button.
10. **COM** Instruct the client to listen for a beep sound when pressing the PCA dosing button, and explain to the client that the beep sound indicates that the client is receiving a dose of medication.

11. **COM** Explain to the client that there will be a period of time during which he or she will not be able to get any more medication according to the doctor's order so that the client doesn't get overly sleepy.
12. **COM** Instruct the client to press the PCA dosing button only when experiencing pain and not to just "watch the clock" and press the button when the lockout interval is over.
13. **CCC** Instruct the client to notify you if he or she is not receiving pain relief.
14. **SAF** Reiterate to family/friends that they must *not* press the client's PCA dosing button.
15. **COM** Provide written information and materials about PCA as needed.

FINISHING THE SKILL

16. **INF** Perform hand hygiene.
17. **SAF** Ensure safety and comfort. Ensure that the bed is in the lowest position and verify that the client can identify and reach the nurse call system. *These safety measures reduce the risk of falls.*
18. **EVAL** Evaluate the outcomes. Do the client and family express an understanding of PCA therapy? Is the client able to demonstrate how to use the PCA dosing button properly?
19. **COM** Document assessment findings, care given, client and family education provided, and outcomes in the legal healthcare record.

■ SKILL 7.14 Discontinuing PCA Therapy

EQUIPMENT

PCA record and key
PCA electronic record
Clean gloves

BEGINNING THE SKILL

1. **SAF** Review order to discontinue PCA therapy.
2. **INF** Perform hand hygiene.
3. **CCC** Introduce yourself to the client and family.
4. **SAF** Identify the client using two identifiers.
5. **CCC** Provide privacy and explain the procedure.
6. **COM** Assess the client to determine if his or her personal goals regarding pain control and function have been met. *Assessing the client's personal goals facilitates collaboration and communication.*
7. **CCC** Assess the client's ability to tolerate oral analgesics if needed. *Before discontinuing IV analgesics, it is important to verify if the client can tolerate oral analgesics.*

PROCEDURE

8. **SAF** Review the analgesic history on the PCA pump for the following:

a. number of times PCA dose delivered
b. volume of analgesic used by client each shift
c. total number of vial/syringe changes each shift
d. number of denials or demands during lockout interval.

9. **SAF** Record analgesic history on the PCA electronic medication administration record per policy. (Note: Some of the current PCA pumps record and transmit PCA information to electronic medical records.)
10. **SAF** Discard and sign out waste (analgesic remaining in syringe) with a second nurse as a witness, or send the medication to the pharmacy according to the facility policy.
11. **SAF** Document waste information electronically if required by the facility.
12. **SAF** Turn off the PCA pump and close the slide clamp.
13. **INF** Apply gloves and disconnect the PCA tubing from the client's IV.
14. If the client's IV line is to remain intact, secure a normal saline line at the keep-open rate per order. *Maintaining IV fluid at a keep open rate will prevent the client's IV from clotting.*

15. **INF** Dispose of equipment and clean the PCA pump per facility policy.

FINISHING THE SKILL

16. **INF** Remove gloves and perform hand hygiene.
17. **SAF** Ensure client safety and comfort. Ensure that the bed is in the lowest position and verify that the client can identify and reach the nurse call system. *These safety measures reduce the risk of falls.*
18. **EVAL** Evaluate the outcomes. What is the client's attitude about discontinuing PCA? Is the client able to achieve pain control with oral analgesics after PCA therapy is discontinued?
19. **COM** Document assessment findings, care given, and outcomes in the legal healthcare record:
    - condition of IV catheter tip (note any breakage)
    - appearance of IV insertion site where catheter was removed
    - pain-intensity rating and other pain assessment parameters after PCA is discontinued.
20. **EVAL** Continue to monitor the client for pain control with oral analgesics and monitor the client's ability to function and perform ADLs.

SECTION 6 Using Epidural Analgesia to Promote Comfort

Another method for delivering analgesia is through an epidural catheter. This device is placed directly through the client's back into the epidural space (usually at the L3-L4 interspace or L4-L5 interspace) located in the spinal canal superficial to the dura mater (Fig. 7.9). For clients who may need a long-term epidural catheter, and to provide stability and reduce the risk of complications, the catheter may be tunneled underneath the skin to a side entry location.

Analgesia administered in the epidural space controls pain by blocking transmission of pain signals. It is commonly used in the obstetrics unit to provide pain relief or anesthesia to block sensations during labor. Epidural analgesia may also be used after surgery or for pain that does not respond to alternative methods. It can be given by bolus (one-time dose), continuous administration, or by patient-controlled epidural analgesia (PCEA).

In most facilities, the anesthesiologist, nurse anesthetist, or other specially trained healthcare provider will insert the epidural catheter and give the client the initial analgesic bolus. This individual may also initiate continuous epidural therapy. The nurse at the bedside is responsible for continuously monitoring the client, including vital signs, pain level, sedation level, and respiratory status/function. The client's upper and lower extremities should also be assessed and reassessed at appropriate intervals for motor function, sensation level, and level of paresthesia.

SAFETY CONSIDERATIONS FOR EPIDURAL CATHETERS

As with PCA therapy, caring for clients who have an epidural catheter requires the consideration of safety issues. Fatal errors have occurred when medication was inadvertently administered through the epidural catheter instead of the client's peripheral IV line or, conversely, when medication or anesthesia was administered through the client's IV line when it was supposed to be given through the epidural catheter. Place brightly colored labels on the epidural catheter that clearly say **"EPIDURAL LINE ONLY"** and/or **"NOT FOR INTRAVENOUS USE"** so that the client's IV line does not get accidentally mixed up or switched with an epidural catheter line. Many facilities have specialized epidural tubing without injection ports or Y connectors that have color coding such as a yellow line within the length of the tubing. However, if the epidural tubing does have ports or Y connectors, they must be taped off in order to prevent administration of medications into the epidural catheter that were intended for the IV line. Look closely at the labels on the epidural infusion bags. In some cases, the epidural infusion bag may look almost identical to normal saline bags. For an illustration of these potential hazards, see Box 7.10.

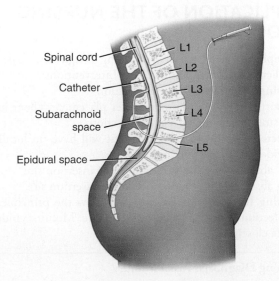

FIG. 7.9 Placement of epidural catheter.

Spinal cord — L1

— L2

Catheter — L3

Subarachnoid space — L4

— L5

Epidural space —

BOX 7.10 Expect the Unexpected: Caring for a Client With an Epidural Catheter

Mandy, a nursing student, is caring for Ms. Bell, a 54-year-old client who is being admitted to the med-surg unit after surgery. On admission, Ms. Bell is awake and alert. She has a peripheral IV line and an epidural catheter that was placed by the anesthesiologist in post-anesthesia recovery (PAR).

While assisting with the admission, Mandy notices that the tubing for the client's peripheral IV has a bright yellow line within it and does not look like regular IV tubing. When Mandy traces the tubing back to the attached bag of fluid, she is immediately alarmed. The epidural medication (a potent drug intended for the epidural space) is accidentally going into the client's peripheral IV line instead of into the epidural catheter. Likewise, the regular IV tubing with normal saline (intended for the client's peripheral IV) is infusing into the epidural catheter! Realizing this mix-up, Mandy immediately reported it to the client's nurse and checked the client's vital signs. The client's nurse stopped the epidural medication from infusing into the client's IV line, contacted the anesthesiologist, and corrected the error. The nurse also placed bold, bright labels on the epidural medication and epidural tubing. To further reduce risks and prevent errors, the nurse placed the infusion pump for the epidural catheter on one side of the bed and the pump for the client's IV line on the other side of the bed (Williams, 2017).

Accidental administration of epidural medication into a client's IV line can cause seizures, oversedation, and respiratory and/or cardiac arrest. In this case, the error occurred just before the client came up from the PAR. The nursing student's astute observation and the quick actions of the client's nurse and student prevented the client's death.

BOX 7.11 Lessons From The Courtroom: Heparin Started Too Soon After Epidural Catheter Was Removed

In a lawsuit filed in Oakland County, Michigan (*Confidential v. Confidential*), a 54-year-old client had received an epidural anesthetic through an epidural catheter for a procedure to remove a blood clot from his leg. After the client was moved to the post-anesthesia care unit (PACU), the anesthesiologist removed the epidural catheter. Just 12 minutes later, the PACU nurse started the client on a continuous infusion of IV heparin (that may have been ordered by a different authorized healthcare provider) through an IV line. The heparin (which affects the clotting mechanisms of the blood) was continued for 24 hours until the client was found to have become quadriplegic. It was determined that the paralysis was caused by bleeding into the epidural space as a result of heparin being started too soon after the epidural catheter was removed. The client, who is now permanently paralyzed, was awarded a 1.9-million-dollar settlement.

During settlement negotiations, it was reported by the circuit court that there was no dispute it was an error to start heparin less than an hour after the epidural catheter was discontinued. The court also stated there had been a serious breakdown in communication that contributed to the error.

Reference: *Heparin: Nurse started infusion too soon after epidural,* 2009.

SUMMARY

When using an epidural catheter and epidural analgesia, the registered nurse is responsible for the assessment, monitoring, care, and evaluation of pain for these clients. As with PCA therapy (see Section 5 of this chapter), safety and accuracy are two of the most important critical concepts to consider. In addition to injury, the client with an epidural catheter may be at risk for a catheter-related infection. Thus, risk reduction strategies such as using sterile technique and monitoring the epidural insertion site are imperative.

APPLICATION OF THE NURSING PROCESS

Examples of Related ICNP Nursing Diagnoses, Expected Client Outcomes, and Nursing Interventions:

Nursing Diagnosis: Risk for infection

Supporting Data: Epidural catheter placement; client has a history of a catheter-related infection.

Expected Client Outcomes: Client will have no localized evidence of infection, as seen by:

- absence of redness or drainage at insertion site
- absence of induration or pain at insertion site.

Nursing Intervention Examples: Follow the principles of infection control and sterile technique. Monitor epidural site closely.

Nursing Diagnosis: Risk for injury

Supporting Data: Client is receiving opioid analgesics through an epidural catheter.

POTENTIAL COMPLICATIONS OF EPIDURAL CATHETERS

Because of the location of the epidural catheter and the increased vascularity in that area, some of the medication or anesthesia can be absorbed systemically (depending on the dosage and type of medication). For example, clients receiving analgesics such as opioids must be monitored for opioid side effects, such as nausea, pruritus (itching), urinary retention, respiratory depression, or oversedation. Clients may also experience hypotension (low blood pressure) as well as other vital sign changes. Avoid rapid position changes (e.g., moving from supine to upright), and position the client in bed according to order or protocol.

Although not common, epidural catheters can cause complications such as bleeding and hematoma formation. Many facilities have protocols for clients who are on anticoagulants such as enoxaparin (Lovenox) or heparin. As discussed in Box 7.11, adverse consequences have occurred when heparin was started too quickly after the epidural catheter was removed. Because epidural catheters are invasive, use sterile technique (see Chapter 10), and monitor your client closely for any signs of infection.

Expected Client Outcomes: Client will have no evidence of injury from the epidural catheter or analgesia, as seen by:
- vital signs, sedation level, and respiratory status within established parameters
- no sign of bleeding, leaking, or hematoma at epidural insertion site
- intact epidural catheter tip on catheter after removal.

Nursing Intervention Examples: Monitor client's vital signs, sedation level, and respiratory status. Assess epidural catheter insertion site and movement of upper and lower extremities.

Reference:International Classification for Nursing Practice. (n.d.). *eHealth & ICNP*. Retrieved from https://www.icn.ch/what-we-do/projects/ehealth-icnp.

CRITICAL CONCEPTS
Using Epidural Analgesia to Promote Comfort

Accuracy (ACC)

Accuracy when using epidural analgesia is affected by the following variables:
- assessment of client, including clinical status, age, medical history, level of consciousness/orientation, and pain assessment using consistent tool
- appropriateness of epidural analgesia for client
- technique used when caring for a client with an epidural catheter
- patency and integrity of catheter used for epidural analgesia
- understanding of procedure by client, family, and/or authorized proxy.

Client-Centered Care (CCC)

Respect for the client when using epidural analgesia is demonstrated through:

- promoting autonomy and providing privacy when using an epidural catheter
- ensuring comfort when using an epidural catheter
- honoring cultural preferences and arranging for an interpreter if necessary
- advocating for the client and family and explaining procedures.

Infection Control (INF)

Healthcare-associated infection when using epidural analgesia is prevented by:
- preventing and reducing the transfer of microorganisms
- reducing the number of microorganisms.

Safety (SAF)

Safety measures when using epidural analgesia prevent harm and provide a safe care environment, including:
- adherence to medication safety guidelines and assessment of allergies and contraindications
- proper labeling and prevention of misconnection errors.

Communication (COM)

- Communication when using epidural analgesia exchanges information (oral, written, nonverbal, or electronic) between two or more people.
- Documentation records information in a permanent legal record.
- Communication with the client, family, and healthcare team prevents misconnection errors and other complications and increases effectiveness of client's epidural analgesia.

Evaluation (EVAL)

Evaluation of the outcomes when using epidural analgesia allows the nurse to determine the efficacy and safety of the care provided.

■ SKILL 7.15 Caring for a Client With an Epidural Catheter

EQUIPMENT

Epidural electronic record or flowsheet (if used by facility)
Pain-intensity rating scale and sedation scale
Epidural infusion tubing (without ports)
Epidural analgesic vial, syringe, or bag
Epidural pump and equipment
Clean gloves
Nonalcohol and nontoxic antiseptic wipes (preservative-free)
Labels for epidural line
Hypoallergenic tape
BP cuff and stethoscope
Oxygen and naloxone (Narcan) (standby if needed)
Oxygen saturation and capnography monitors (if ordered)

BEGINNING THE SKILL

1. **SAF** Review the orders for epidural therapy.

2. **ACC** Review the client's medical/surgical history. Consider the client's age, condition, and indications for epidural analgesia. *These factors can influence epidural therapy.*

3. **SAF** Identify contraindications and precautions for an epidural catheter or epidural analgesia, which may include the following: clients who are on anticoagulants or have bleeding disorders, systemic infections, meningitis, spinal disorders, hypovolemia, or cardiac disorders.

4. **ACC** Review the client's history of previous analgesic or opioid use. *Clients who are opioid naïve will be more sensitive and prone to respiratory depression than clients who have a long history of analgesic use (Grissinger, 2016).*

5. **INF** Perform hand hygiene.

6. **CCC** Introduce yourself to client and family.

7. **SAF** Identify the client using two identifiers.
8. **CCC** Provide privacy and explain the procedure.
9. **ACC** Assess the client's level of consciousness and orientation to person, time, place, and situation. If the client will be receiving PCA therapy through the epidural catheter, the client must be awake and alert and able to understand instructions.
10. **SAF** Assess the client for allergies, including epidural anesthesia and other medications.
11. **CCC** Ensure that informed consent has been obtained. *Promotes autonomy.*

PROCEDURE

12. **ACC** Assess the client for the following:
    a. level of pain/discomfort and exact location of pain using a consistent tool
    b. baseline vital signs, respiratory status (including rate, depth, quality, and function), and baseline oxygen saturation and $EtCO_2$ if ordered.
    c. mobility, warmth, color, sensation, and movement of all four extremities
    d. client and family's understanding of the procedure for epidural analgesia.
13. **ACC** If the client will be receiving PCA through the epidural catheter (PCEA), see Skills 7.11 to 7.14 for PCA therapy.
14. **INF** Apply clean gloves.
15. **INF** Assess catheter exit site and ensure that catheter is intact and taped securely, without signs of leaking or infection, such as redness, swelling, induration, or pain.

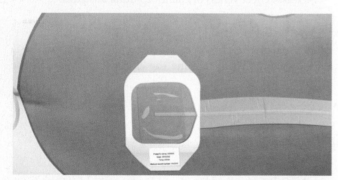

STEP 15 Inspect exit site.

16. **SAF** If required by facility policy, place a sign in large print over the client's bed that alerts other healthcare providers that the client is receiving epidural analgesia.
17. **SAF** Ensure that emergency equipment, naloxone (Narcan), oxygen, and oxygen saturation and capnography monitors are nearby according to your facility policy.
18. **SAF** Trace the epidural line from the client's epidural insertion site to the connection or epidural medication source. If the tubing for the epidural line or catheter has injection ports, tape them off. *These measures reduce the risk of misconnection errors and inadvertent administration of medications into the catheter that was not intended for the epidural route.*

19. **SAF** Place a label on the epidural catheter tubing per facility policy that states **NOT FOR INTRAVENOUS USE** and/or **EPIDURAL LINE ONLY.** Ensure that the labels are close to the client's insertion site and close to the source of the epidural pump and medication. *Proper labeling reduces the risk of misconnection errors.*

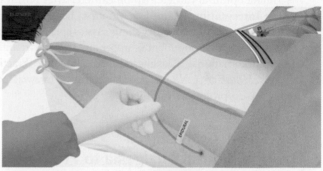

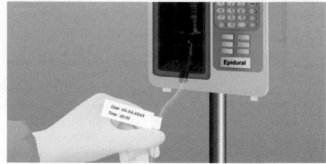

STEP 19 Place labels.

20. **ACC** If the client will be receiving analgesia or anesthesia through the epidural catheter:
    a. Assist the anesthesiologist or other authorized healthcare provider as needed.
    b. **WARNING:** Ensure that only nonalcohol, nontoxic, and preservative-free antimicrobial wipes are used for injections. Alcohol and preservatives may be toxic to neural tissues.
    c. Ensure that micron filters are used for injections per the facility policy.
    d. Ensure that all fluids for injection and infusions are free from preservatives. *Preservatives may cause neuronal injury (Williams, 2017).*
21. **SAF** During and after epidural infusions, observe the client closely for vital sign changes (particularly low blood pressure), shallow or difficult respirations, oversedation, or other possible side effects (e.g., nausea/vomiting, itching, or urinary retention).
22. **ACC** Ensure that catheter remains intact with a transparent dressing per your facility policy. *A transparent dressing facilitates monitoring of the epidural catheter exit site.*
23. **SAF** Tape the epidural tubing securely to the client so that there is not direct tension on the catheter site. *Prevents dislodgement or accidental removal of the epidural catheter.*

24. **SAF** Assess the client's motor strength and sensation in the extremities, and continue to monitor the client's vital signs, respiratory function, and sedation. Document these parameters on the electronic record per facility policy. *Epidural analgesia can affect clients for hours, and assessments must be repeated at appropriate intervals (Williams, 2017).*

25. **SAF** If the client is on anticoagulants (e.g., enoxaparin [Lovenox], heparin), observe the exit site closely for bleeding or hematoma. Avoid removing the catheter for at least 12 hours after the anticoagulant is discontinued. *Reduces the risk of bleeding into the epidural space.*

26. **SAF** If the client becomes hypotensive (low blood pressure), contact the authorized healthcare provider and place the client in a supine position if tolerated (Williams, 2017).

27. **CCC** Ask the client about his or her pain. If epidural therapy is not helping the client's pain, troubleshoot for kinked or clamped tubing or other technical problems. If technical problems are ruled out, notify the anesthesiologist or other designated healthcare provider.

28. **COM** Client/family teaching: Provide verbal and written instructions about the epidural catheter as indicated. Instruct the client to report any problems or discomfort.

FINISHING THE SKILL

29. **INF** Remove gloves and perform hand hygiene.
30. **SAF** Ensure client safety and comfort. Ensure that the bed is in the lowest position and the call light is within reach. *Analgesics can alter a client's spatial awareness and increase the risk for falls.*
31. **EVAL** Evaluate the outcomes. Is the client tolerating the procedure? Does the client have decreased pain? Are the client's vital signs and other variables within established parameters?
32. **COM** Document assessment findings, care given, and outcomes in the legal healthcare record:
    - appearance of client's epidural catheter site
    - pain-intensity ratings and other pain assessment parameters, such as whether or not client's pain-control goals and functional goals have been met
    - sedation-level score, ability to be aroused, orientation level, vital signs, respiratory function, and character/quality of respirations
    - motor function, warmth, color, and sensation in lower extremities.
33. **EVAL** Continue to monitor the client for side effects, allergic reactions, or adverse reactions to the epidural medication. *Adverse effects of analgesics can occur at any time.*

■ SKILL 7.16 Assisting With Removal of an Epidural Catheter

EQUIPMENT

Gauze
Clean gloves
Transparent dressing

BEGINNING THE SKILL

1. **ACC** Review the order to remove the epidural catheter.
2. **SAF** Review policy regarding who may remove an epidural catheter. *Some facilities allow only an authorized healthcare provider or specially trained nurse to remove epidural catheters.*
3. **SAF** Review the client's history for bleeding disorders or recent anticoagulants. *Anticoagulants can increase the risk of bleeding or hematoma. Some facilities require clients to be off anticoagulants for at least 12 hours prior to the removal of the catheter.*
4. **INF** Perform hand hygiene.
5. **CCC** Introduce yourself to the client and family.
6. **SAF** Identify the client using two identifiers.
7. **CCC** Provide privacy and explain the procedure.

PROCEDURE

8. **INF** Apply clean gloves.
9. **CCC** Assist the client to a comfortable position on the side with the spine flexed. *Positioning the client with the back flexed provides access and opens up the intervertebral spaces.*
10. **INF** Carefully remove dressing and assess exit site per protocol using aseptic technique.
11. **SAF** Remove or assist with the removal of the catheter (depending on facility policy) while keeping the tip sterile. **WARNING:** If there is resistance, do not remove the catheter.
12. **CCC** Inspect the end of catheter to ensure the tip is intact and without breakage. The blue tip should be intact. (Note: If the catheter tip is missing, notify the authorized healthcare provider.)

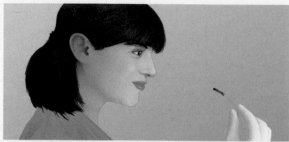

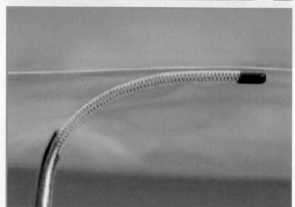

STEP 12 Check catheter tip.

13. **INF** If signs of infection/inflammation are present, save the catheter tip in a sterile container and notify the appropriate healthcare provider.

14. **SAF** Apply pressure as long as needed with gauze and apply transparent dressing on epidural catheter site per protocol. *Clients who have previously been on anticoagulants may require longer pressure application in order to prevent hematoma formation.*

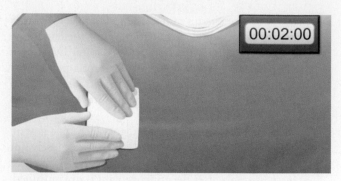

STEP 14 Apply pressure.

15. **CCC** Assist the client to a comfortable position.
16. **INF** Dispose of and/or clean equipment per facility policy.
17. **SAF** Observe catheter site for leaking, drainage, bleeding, or signs of infection.

FINISHING THE SKILL

18. **INF** Remove gloves and perform hand hygiene.
19. **SAF** Ensure client safety and comfort. Ensure that the bed is in the lowest position and verify that the client can identify and reach the nurse call system. *These safety measures reduce the risk of falls.*
20. **EVAL** Evaluate the outcomes. Did the client tolerate the procedure?
21. **COM** Document assessment findings, care given, and outcomes in the legal healthcare record:
    • time that client's epidural catheter was removed
    • condition of epidural catheter tip (note any breakage)
    • appearance of site where catheter was removed.
22. **SAF** Provide follow-up monitoring for at least 24 hours after removal of the epidural catheter. Assess the client for back pain, changes in sensory and motor function (e.g., client's ability to move extremities), or sudden loss in bowel and bladder function. *Complications such as hematoma formation can cause paralysis if undetected (Williams, 2017).*

■ CASE STUDY

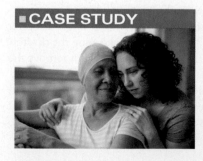

Mrs. Lopez is a 58-year-old female with a history of multiple myeloma, lytic bone lesions, and diabetes. She has been on oral analgesics for chronic back pain for more than 6 months. She has recently been admitted to the medical unit for renal insufficiency. Prior to admission, Mrs. Lopez fell at home. Although Mrs. Lopez has no evidence of fractures, she is having increased left arm and back pain, with a pain rating of 7 on a scale of 1 to 10. She also states that her pain is making her feel really "tired" and preventing her from doing usual activities, such as dressing herself and sitting up on the side of the bed. In addition, she is becoming increasingly restless and agitated.

Because it has been more than 24 hours since her fall, the authorized healthcare provider orders localized circulating heat for her arm. In addition, a TENS unit is ordered for her back pain. Mrs. Lopez's daughter, who is at her bedside, has tears in her eyes and states, "I can't stand to see my mom hurting like this!" Recognizing her distress, the nurse offers support and explains the comfort measures they will be using for her mother. The nurse also explores what Mrs. Lopez's goals are for her pain control and daily activities by using open-ended questions and other strategies.

Although the nonpharmacologic measures (TENS and heat therapy) seem to help Mrs. Lopez relax, she still rates her pain as a 6 on a scale of 1 to 10. The authorized healthcare provider orders PCA therapy to help maintain a steady blood level of pain medication. After PCA therapy is initiated, the nurse discovers that Mrs. Lopez is pushing her PCA dosing button frequently but still complaining of increased pain. The nurse checks Mrs. Lopez's IV to make sure it is still intact, and she ensures that the PCA tubing is not clamped or kinked inside the PCA pump.

After troubleshooting and verifying the PCA pump is working properly, the nurse notifies the authorized healthcare provider about adjusting Mrs. Lopez's pain medication. In addition, the nurse enhances Mrs. Lopez's environment by reducing the noise and bright lights in her room and offers additional comfort measures such as relaxation exercises. The nurse also maintains close observation of Mrs. Lopez while continuing to provide support and care to her daughter.

Case Study Questions

1. Considering Mrs. Lopez's medical history and signs and symptoms on admission, what is the highest priority regarding her care?

2. Why is it important to incorporate nonpharmacologic methods as adjuncts to Mrs. Lopez's pharmacologic pain regimen?

3. The authorized healthcare provider has ordered localized circulating heat therapy (also known as aqua therapy) for Mrs. Lopez's arm pain. Before implementing this therapy, what interventions are important for the nurse to do? How could the nurse further individualize localized heat therapy for Ms. Lopez in order to maximize effectiveness and ensure safety?

4. The authorized healthcare provider later orders a TENS unit to be placed on Mrs. Lopez for her increased back pain. What should the nurse do to ensure effectiveness when applying the TENS?

5. Describe the teaching the nurse would do regarding the TENS unit. How can the nurse ensure that Mrs. Lopez has an understanding of how to use the TENS unit?

6. Because Mrs. Lopez continues to have significant pain, the authorized healthcare provider decides to order PCA. What interventions must be done prior to initiating PCA therapy? How can the nurse ensure safety and effectiveness with PCA therapy?

7. After Mrs. Lopez's PCA is initiated, she continues to have significant pain despite making increased demands (frequently pushing the PCA control button) for her pain. What troubleshooting measures and timely interventions does the nurse do in this case?

8. What interventions can the nurse do to provide comfort for Mrs. Lopez and her daughter or any other family members the client may have?

9. What additional interventions could the nurse do to help Mrs. Lopez with comfort and relaxation? What follow-up measures must the nurse do to promote comfort?

10. **Application of QSEN Competencies:** One of the Quality and Safety Education for Nurses (QSEN) skills for Patient-Centered Care is to "Elicit expectations of patient and family for relief of pain, discomfort, or suffering" (Cronenwett et al., 2007). How did the nurse in this case demonstrate these competencies?

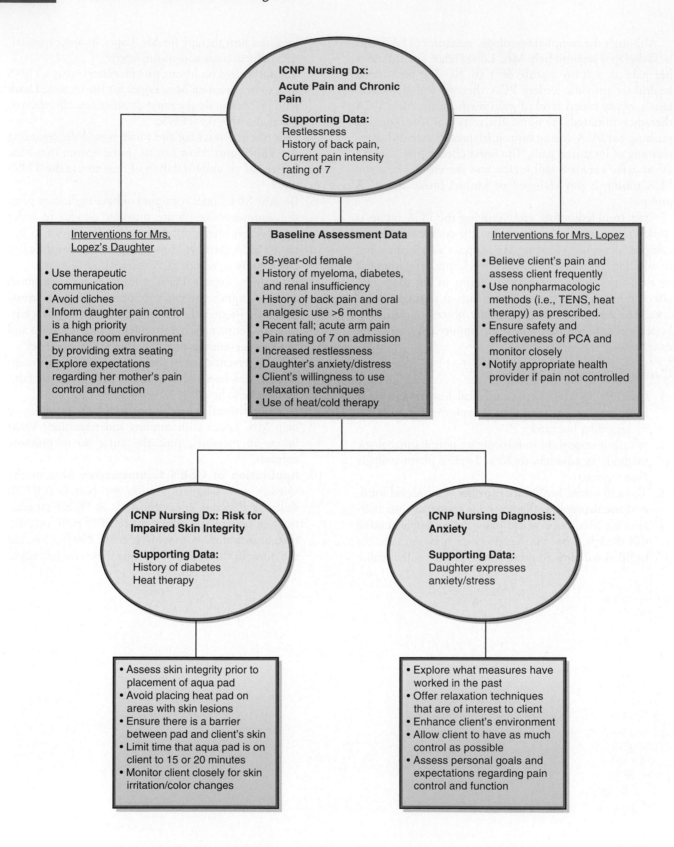

ICNP Nursing Dx:

Acute Pain and Chronic Pain

Supporting Data:
Restlessness
History of back pain,
Current pain intensity
rating of 7

Interventions for Mrs. Lopez's Daughter

- Use therapeutic communication
- Avoid cliches
- Inform daughter pain control is a high priority
- Enhance room environment by providing extra seating
- Explore expectations regarding her mother's pain control and function

---

Baseline Assessment Data

- 58-year-old female
- History of myeloma, diabetes, and renal insufficiency
- History of back pain and oral analgesic use >6 months
- Recent fall; acute arm pain
- Pain rating of 7 on admission
- Increased restlessness
- Daughter's anxiety/distress
- Client's willingness to use relaxation techniques
- Use of heat/cold therapy

Interventions for Mrs. Lopez

- Believe client's pain and assess client frequently
- Use nonpharmacologic methods (i.e., TENS, heat therapy) as prescribed.
- Ensure safety and effectiveness of PCA and monitor closely
- Notify appropriate health provider if pain not controlled

ICNP Nursing Dx: Risk for Impaired Skin Integrity

Supporting Data:
History of diabetes
Heat therapy

ICNP Nursing Diagnosis: Anxiety

Supporting Data:
Daughter expresses anxiety/stress

- Assess skin integrity prior to placement of aqua pad
- Avoid placing heat pad on areas with skin lesions
- Ensure there is a barrier between pad and client's skin
- Limit time that aqua pad is on client to 15 or 20 minutes
- Monitor client closely for skin irritation/color changes

- Explore what measures have worked in the past
- Offer relaxation techniques that are of interest to client
- Enhance client's environment
- Allow client to have as much control as possible
- Assess personal goals and expectations regarding pain control and function

References

American Association of Critical Care Nurses (AACN). (2018). *AACN practice alert: Assessing pain in critically ill adults.* Retrieved from https://www.aacn.org/clinical-resources/practice-alerts/assessing-pain-in-critically-ill-adults.

American Massage Therapy Association (AMTA). (2017). *Glossary of terminology.* Retrieved from https://www.amtamassage.org/infocenter/research_glossary-of-research-terminology.html.

Andrews, M. M. (2016). The influence of culture and health belief systems on health care practices. In M. M. Andrews, & J. S. Boyle (Eds.), *Transcultural concepts in nursing care* (7th ed.) (pp. 102–119). Philadelphia: Lippincott, Williams & Wilkins.

Centers for Disease Control and Prevention (CDC). (2017). *Opioid overdose: Understanding the epidemic.* Retrieved from https://www.cdc.gov/drugoverdose/epidemic/index.html.

Cooney, M. F., Karnack, M., Dunwoody, C., Eksterowicz, N., Merkel, S., & Oakes, L. (2013). American Society for Pain Management Nursing position statement with clinical practice guidelines: Authorized agent controlled analgesia. *Pain Management Nursing, 14*(3). Retrieved from http://www.aspmn.org/Documents/AuthorizedAgentControlledAnalgesia_PMN_August2013.pdf.

Coyle, N., Layman-Goldstein, M., & Hunter-Johnson, J. L. (2015). Pain assessment and pharmacological/non-pharmacological interventions. In M. Matzo, & D. Witt-Sherman (Eds.), *Palliative care nursing: Quality care to the end of life* (4th ed.) (pp. 431–486). New York: Springer.

Cronenwett, L., Sherwood, G., Barnsteiner, J., Disch, J., Johnson, J., Mitchell, P., ... Warren, J. (2007). Quality and safety education for nurses. *Nursing Outlook, 55*(3), 122–131. Retrieved from http://qsen.org/competencies/pre-licensure-ksas/.

Dossey, B. M. (2016). Nursing: holistic, integral, and integrative. In B. M. Dossey, L. Keegan, C. C. Barrere, M. A. Blaszko Helming, D. A. Shields, & K. M. Avino (Eds.), *Holistic nursing: A handbook for practice* (7th ed.) (pp. 3–49). Sudbury, MA: Jones and Bartlett.

European Federation of IASP Chapters (EFIC). (2016). *People with pain.* Retrieved from http://www.europeanpainfederation.eu/people-with-pain/.

Fink, R. M., Gates, R. A., & Montgomery, R. K. (2015). Pain assessment. In B. R. Ferrell, N. Coyle, & J. A. Paice (Eds.), *Textbook of palliative nursing* (4th ed.) (pp. 113–134). New York: Oxford University Press.

Fitzgerald, M., & Langevin, M. (2018). Imagery. In R. Lindquist, M. F. Tracy, & M. Snyder (Eds.), *Complementary & alternative therapies in nursing* (8th ed.) (pp. 81–108). New York, NY: Springer.

Fong, E. (2018). Anorectal disorders: Sitz bath. [Evidence Summary.] Retrieved from The Joanna, Briggs Institute EBD Database. JBI@OVID. JB13703.

Grissinger, M. (2016). Fatal PCA adverse events continue to happen: Better patient monitoring is essential to prevent harm. *Pharmacy and Therapeutics, 41*(12), 736–737, 800. Retrieved from https://www.ncbi.nlm.nih.gov/pmc/articles/PMC5132411/.

Harris, M. (2018). Massage. In R. Lindquist, M. F. Tracy, & M. Snyder (Eds.), *Complementary & alternative therapies in nursing* (8th ed.) (pp. 249–264). New York: Springer.

Harris, M., & Richards, K. C. (2010). The physiological and psychological effects of slow-stroke back massage and hand massage on relaxation in older people. *Journal of Clinical Nursing, 19*(7-8), 917–926.

Heparin: Nurse started infusion too soon after epidural. (2009, September). *Legal Eagle Eye Newsletter for the Nursing Profession, 18*(4). Retrieved from http://www.nursinglaw.com/.

Hockenberry, M. J. (2017). Pain assessment and management in children. In M. J. Hockenberry, D. Wilson, & C. C. Rodgers (Eds.), *Wong's essentials of pediatric nursing* (10th ed.) (pp. 114–129). St. Louis, MO: Elsevier.

Horgas, A. L., Grall, M. S., & Yoon, S. L. (2016). Pain Management. In M. Boltz, E. Capezuti, T. Fulmer, & D. Zwicker (Eds.), *Evidence-based geriatric nursing protocols for best practice* (5th ed.) (pp. 263–282). New York: Springer Publishing Company.

Institute For Safe Medication Practices (ISMP). (2016). Worth Repeating. *Recent PCA by proxy event suggests reassessment of practices that may have fallen by the wayside.* Retrieved from https://www.ismp.org/resources/worth-repeating-recent-pca-proxy-event-suggests-reassessment-practices-may-have-fallen?id=1149.

International Association for the Study Of Pain (IASP). (2012). *Pain terms.* Retrieved from http://www.iasp-pain.org/Education/Content.aspx?ItemNumber=1698.

International Classification for Nursing Practice. (n.d.). *eHealth & ICNP.* Retrieved from htps://www.icn.ch/what-we-do/projects/ehealth-icnp.

Jackson, C., & Latini, C. (2016). Touch and hand mediated therapies. In B. M. Dossey, L. Keegan, C. C. Barrere, M. A. Blaszko Helming, D. A. Shields, & K. M. Avino (Eds.), *Holistic nursing: A handbook for practice* (7th ed.) (pp. 299–318). Sudbury, MA: Jones and Bartlett.

The Joint Commission (August, 2017). Pain assessment and management standards for hospitals. *R3 Report Requirement, Rationale, Reference.* (Issue 11). Retrieved from https://www.jointcommission.org/r3_issue_11/.

Kravits, K. (2015). Complementary and alternative therapies in palliative care. In B. R. Ferrell, N. Coyle, & J. A. Paice (Eds.), *Textbook of palliative nursing* (4th ed.) (pp. 449–462). New York: Oxford University Press.

McCaffery, M., Herr, K., & Pasero, C. (2011). Assessment. In M. McCaffery, & C. Pasero (Eds.), *Pain assessment and pharmacologic management* (pp. 2–48). St. Louis, MO: MosbyElsevier.

Medline Industries (n.d.). Product insert and brochure. Hot and cold therapy. Retrieved from https://www.medline.com/category/Hot-Cold-Therapy/cat350058.

Miladinia, M., Baraz, S., Shariati, A., & Malehi, A. S. (2017). Effects of slow-stroke back massage on symptom cluster in adult patients with acute leukemia. Supportive care in cancer nursing. *Cancer Nursing, 40*(1), 31–38.

National Cancer Institute (NCI). (2019). *Cancer pain control: Support for people with cancer.* Retrieved from http://www.cancer.gov/cancertopics/coping/paincontrol.

National Comprehensive Cancer Network (NCCN). (2019). *Guidelines for supportive care. Adult Cancer Pain.* Retrieved from https://www.nccn.org/professionals/physician_gls/default.aspx#supportive.

Nightingale, F. (1860). *Notes on nursing: What it is and what it is not. [first American edition].* New York: NY: D. Appleton & Company. Retrieved from http://digital.library.upenn.edu/women/nightingale/nursing/nursing.html.

Patient-controlled analgesia: Jury relates patient's death to nursing negligence. (2008, January). *Legal Eagle Eye Newsletter for the Nursing Profession, 16*(1). Retrieved from http://www.nursinglaw.com/.

Pasero, C., & McCaffery, M. (2011). *Pain assessment and pharmacologic management.* St. Louis, MO: MosbyElsevier.

Polomano, R. C., & Fillman, M. (2017). Pain. In S. L. Lewis, L. Bucher, M. M. Heitkemper, M. M. Harding, J. Kwong, & D. Roberts

(Eds.), *Medical-surgical nursing: Assessment and management of clinical problems* (10th ed.) (pp. 102–127). St. Louis, MO: Saunders Elsevier.

Schaub, B. G., & Burt, M. M. (2016). Imagery. In B. M. Dossey, L. Keegan, C. C. Barrere, M. A. Blaszko Helming, D. A. Shields, & K. M. Avino (Eds.), *Holistic nursing: A handbook for practice* (7th ed.) (pp. 269–294). Sudbury, MA: Jones and Bartlett.

Stryker Inc. (2017). Product Brochure and Operators Manual. *TP700 & TP700C Series Localized Temperature Therapy.* Retrieved from https://techweb.stryker.com/Temp_Management/Tpump/index.html and https://techweb.stryker.com/Temp_Management/Tpump/Operations/101515E.1.pdf.

TENSproducts. (n.d.). *Products and info: Electrotherapy explained.* Retrieved from http://www.tensproducts.com/Electrotherapy-Basics/Electrotherapy-Explained/.

Williams, K. (2017). Epidural catheters: Assisting with insertion and pain management. In D. L. Wiegand (Ed.), *AACN procedure manual for high acuity, progressive, and critical care* (7th ed.) (pp. 929–994). St. Louis, MO: Saunders Elsevier.

Yoost, B. L., & Crawford, L. R. (2016). *Fundamentals of nursing: Active learning for collaborative practice.* St. Louis, MO: Saunders Elsevier.

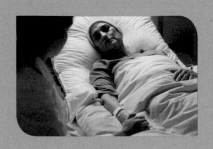

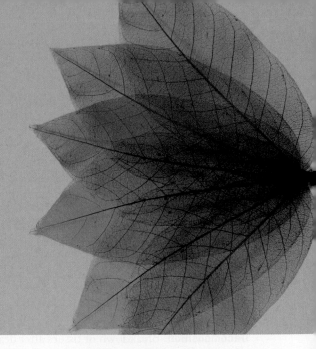

CHAPTER 8

End-of-Life Care

"You matter because you are you, and you matter until the last moment of your life. We will do all we can, not only to help you die peacefully, but to also live until you die." | **Dame Cicely Saunders, Founder of St. Christopher's Hospice (Established in 1967)**

LEARNING OBJECTIVES

By the end of this chapter, the reader will be able to:

1   Identify key concepts related to end-of-life care and palliative care.
2   Identify guidelines and initiatives related to end-of-life care and palliative care.
3   Discuss the role of the nurse in end-of-life care and palliative care.
4   Discuss the grieving process and concepts related to grief.
5   Demonstrate the critical elements of caring for the client and family who are grieving.
6   Perform a spiritual assessment of the client and family.
7   Discuss the importance of advance care planning (ACP).

8   Provide assistance with advance directives and do-not-resuscitate (DNR) orders.
9   Provide physical care for the client who is nearing the end of life.
10 Discuss care for the client and family at the time of the client's death.
11 Perform postmortem care for the deceased client (autopsy and nonautopsy).
12 Analyze a case study and concept map related to death and dying.

TERMINOLOGY

Advance care planning Refers to the entire process of discussion of end-of-life care that involves ongoing communication between the client, family, and healthcare team.

Advance directive A legal document that is one of the tools for advance care planning. Allows clients to stipulate their wishes regarding treatment in the event they are unable to communicate these wishes themselves. It does not replace advance care planning or ongoing communication.

Autopsy Examination of a client's body after death that usually requires consent from family or significant other and is performed by a medical specialist in order to determine the cause of death.

Bereavement Period following loss, characterized by manifestations of grief.

Decomposition Breakdown of tissues after death that occurs in stages and causes odor.

Do-not-resuscitate (DNR) order Legal order written by the authorized healthcare provider that instructs healthcare team not to initiate cardiopulmonary resuscitation (CPR).

Family Includes individuals who are legally bound by marriage or linked by "biology or affection." "Family is whomever the client says it is" (American Nurses Association, 2016).

Healthcare proxy (also known as durable power of attorney) Individual designated by a client to make legal decisions regarding medical care for the client in the event the client is unable to make decisions or communicate on his or her own behalf.

Hospice Concept of care that focuses on quality of life, pain and symptom management, and optimal comfort at the end of life. Hospice care can be provided in a facility or in the home.

Informed consent Clients' legal right to determine their care and treatment after the appropriate healthcare provider explains the risks and answers questions to the satisfaction of the client.

Medical examiner Public official, usually a licensed physician with specialized medical forensics training, who investigates a death that may not be due to natural causes.

Mourning Process and outward expression of grief that is influenced by a client's culture, rituals, and societal norms.

ACRONYMS

AACN American Association of Colleges of Nursing
ANA American Nurses Association
ACP Advance care planning
AD Advance directives
DNAR Do not attempt resuscitation
DPOA Durable power of attorney
DNR Do not resuscitate
ELNEC End-of-Life Nursing Education Consortium
IOM Institute of Medicine
NAM National Academy of Medicine
NCI National Cancer Institute
NCP National Consensus Project
NCHPC National Coalition for Hospice and Palliative Care
POLST Physician orders for life-sustaining treatment
PSDA Patient Self-Determination Act
WHO World Health Organization

Death is a universal phenomenon that personally touches all of us. At some point in our lives, most of us will experience the loss of a loved one. It is estimated that each year, over 56 million people die worldwide, and this number is expected to rise as the population continues to age (World Health Organization [WHO], 2018). As the need for end-of-life care increases, the nurse is the professional who is most likely to be with the client during all phases of the dying process. Therefore, the quality of nursing care is one of the most important factors that will determine whether or not the client has a "good death" that is peaceful as well as comfortable.

Providing excellent, culturally sensitive end-of-life care is not only important for older adults, but for all clients of all ages in every setting across the healthcare spectrum. As the American Nurses Association (ANA) notes, nurses have an obligation to provide comprehensive and compassionate care, and they must collaborate with other members of the healthcare team to ensure optimal symptom management and support for the client and family (ANA, 2016).

DEFINITION OF END OF LIFE

End of life is difficult to define. According to a classic position statement by the National Institutes of Health (NIH), there is no exact definition. In other words, you cannot define *end of life* within a rigid or set time frame. It is different for each person. However, evidence supports that it may be characterized by the presence of irreversible disease with symptoms or impairments that persist and may limit function, requiring ongoing care and ultimately leading to death. This process could last days, weeks, months, or even years. The duration and intensity of this transition from illness to death will vary, depending on the individual client (NIH, 2004).

END-OF-LIFE CARE AND PALLIATIVE CARE

To provide optimal care, the client's palliative care needs must be addressed. Although the terms *end-of-life care* and *palliative care* are often used interchangeably, they are different. End-of-life care falls under the larger umbrella of palliative care. *Palliative* comes from the word *palliate*, which means "to make a person comfortable and relieve symptoms." The WHO defines palliative care as "an approach that improves the quality of life of patients and their families facing the problem associated with life-threatening illness, through the prevention and relief of suffering by means of early identification and impeccable assessment and treatment of pain and other symptoms, physical, psychosocial, and spiritual" (WHO, n.d.). Although palliative care is crucial at the end of life, it is *not* used exclusively for clients who are facing imminent death.

As palliative care has evolved, evidence-based guidelines have been developed. For example, the National Consensus Project (NCP) has identified domains of palliative care that reflect evidence-based practice and expert consensus. These domains include structural processes of care; physical, psychological, cultural, spiritual, social, and ethical/legal aspects of care; and caring for the client who is nearing the end of life. A more detailed description of the domains can be found on the National Coalition for Hospice and Palliative Care (NCHPC) website at http://www.nationalcoalitionhpc.org/ncp/. As noted by the guidelines, palliative care should be based on the client and family goals, and it must be available to seriously ill clients across the lifespan, regardless of the setting or the client's prognosis (National Consensus Project for Quality Palliative Care, 2018).

NURSING INITIATIVES AND END-OF-LIFE CARE

Nursing care of the client who is dying can occur in a variety of areas. It may take place in a palliative care unit, a critical care unit, the emergency room, a medical-surgical unit, a neonatal unit, a nursing home, an ambulatory clinic, a community setting, or a private home with hospice support (Fig. 8.1). Teamwork and collaboration are essential. As part of the healthcare team, nurses work closely with other professionals to meet the needs of the client and family.

One nursing initiative that strives to improve end-of-life care in every healthcare setting is the End-of-Life Nursing Education Consortium (ELNEC) project, administered through the City of Hope (COH) and the American Association of Colleges of Nursing (AACN, 2019). The ELNEC curriculum mirrors core areas essential for end-of-life care as outlined in the AACN's *2016 Competencies and Recommendations for Educating Undergraduate Nursing Students* (CARES), which was previously the 1998 publication *Peaceful Death: Recommended Competencies and Curricular Guidelines for End of Life Nursing Care*. The major themes of these competencies include, but may not be limited to, the following:

- recognizing the client and family as the unit of care
- the role of the nurse as the client and family advocate
- recognition of the client's culture and spirituality
- attention to vulnerable populations
- interdisciplinary cooperation
- financial and legal aspects of end-of-life care
- supporting the family in cases of sudden or unexpected death.

In summary, the ELNEC initiatives and NCP guidelines emphasize that palliative care may be the main focus of care, or it may be provided while the client is receiving other therapies, regardless of the stage of the client's disease. Likewise, the Institute of Medicine (IOM), now renamed the National Academy of Medicine, asserts that palliative care must occur "upstream" and begin early after the client's diagnosis. The IOM report *Dying in America: Improving Quality and Honoring Individual Preferences Near the End of Life* notes that palliative care must be individualized and flexible (IOM, 2015). As with other guidelines, the primary goal is to promote *person-centered care* with a focus on the client/family unit. The core concepts articulated by these initiatives (Fig. 8.2) serve as the framework for the skills in this chapter.

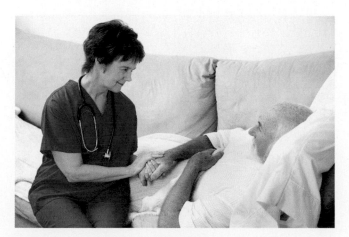

FIG. 8.1 Hospice care is often delivered in a home environment.

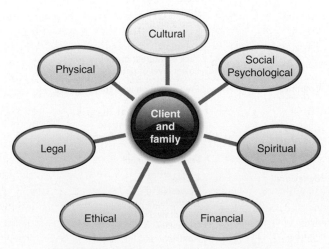

FIG. 8.2 Core concepts in palliative care.

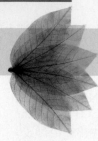

SECTION 1   Bereavement and Spiritual Care

CARING FOR A CLIENT AND FAMILY WHO ARE GRIEVING

Imagine how it must feel to lose a friend, a family member, a cohort, or even a cherished pet. The feelings associated with grieving can be significant, as well as highly personal, for those who experience it. The nurse can help the client and family during this difficult time. In order to understand grieving, it is important to review the concepts associated with this process:

- **Loss:** The impact of loss occurs when we lose something of value to us. It may be the loss of a loved one, a job, a marriage, or something else. When a parent loses a child, the feelings may be compounded by the loss of a dream of what that child could be. Loss can also trigger grief and mourning (COH & AACN, 2018a). Possible reactions to loss are listed in Table 8.1.
- **Grief:** Grief is a *normal* reaction to loss. It is also a feeling of sadness or emotional pain that often begins before the client's death. Grief may be experienced by the client, family, personal caregivers, or the nurse. The intensity and the expression of the grief reaction will vary, depending on the person and his or her support systems (COH & AACN, 2018a).
- **Mourning:** Mourning is the process of adjusting to the loss and the outward expression of grief, including burials and funerals. Mourning practices and behavior are influenced by a person's culture, rituals, norms, and values (Corless, 2015) (Fig. 8.3). The period of mourning may consist of several different phases that may include a desire to bring back the deceased person, intense sadness, disorganization, and reorganization and healing (National Cancer Institute [NCI], U.S. National Institutes of Health, 2019a).
- **Bereavement:** The NCI defines bereavement as the time following the loss. This will vary with each individual. The duration depends on many factors, including age, gender, culture, and socioeconomic status, among others. Bereavement is also influenced by how much time the bereaved person had to prepare for the loss as well as the circumstances of the loss. For example, if the death is caused by a tragic and sudden accident, the bereavement period may be more prolonged and complicated (Corless, 2015; NCI, U.S. National Institutes of Health, 2019a).

THEORIES OF GRIEVING

Kübler-Ross's Stages of Grief

One of the most well-known stage theories of grief is the stages of grief model developed by Elisabeth Kübler-Ross (1969). A criticism of this model and other stage models is that they may not always be valid for certain clients. Some people do not pass through the stages at the same rate, in the same sequence, or with the same intensity. Some people may go back and forth, whereas others may skip over some of the stages entirely. Kübler-Ross's stages are as follows:

TABLE 8.1 Possible Reactions to Loss

Affected Domain	Signs and Symptoms
Physical	Tightness in the chest and throat Oversensitivity to noise Breathlessness Muscular weakness Lack of energy Fatigue Sleep disturbances Changes in appetite
Emotional	Numbness Loneliness Sadness Sorrow Guilt Shock Anxiety Depression Anger Agitation Lack of interest or motivation Lower level of patience or tolerance
Cognitive	Preoccupation with the deceased Forgetfulness Preoccupation with the loss Inability to concentrate Inability to retain information Disorganization Feeling confused
Behavioral	Crying Insomnia Restlesness Withdrawal Irritability Apathy Impaired work performance

From Yoost & Crawford, 2016.

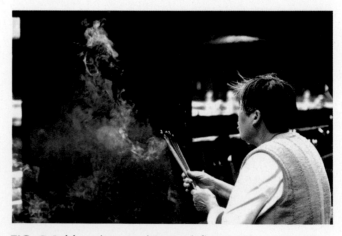

FIG. 8.3 Mourning practices are influenced by a person's culture. A woman at a Buddhist temple mourns the death of her loved one with special rituals.

- Denial—"This can't be happening."
- Anger—"Why did God let this happen?"
- Bargaining—"I promise I'll be better!"
- Depression—"I just want to be alone."
- Acceptance—"I need to get my things in order."

Kübler-Ross's theory has made a significant contribution to our knowledge about grief. However, many researchers now believe the evidence supports individual pathways and accomplishment of tasks of grieving as opposed to stage theories of grief (COH & AACN, 2018a).

Tasks of Grieving

The underlying premise of accomplishing the tasks of grieving is that people deal with grief in their own way and at their own pace. This is often determined by our culture and our personal experiences as to how we cope with stress. Although individual clients will vary in the way they grieve, most of the grief theories describe a process with the following tasks or events:

1. The person becomes aware of the death or impending death, which is followed by emotional shock. The reality of the situation must be acknowledged.
2. The person will experience the loss emotionally and intellectually.
3. The person will begin to reorganize his or her life and form new bonds and relationships.
4. The person will reintegrate into society. A critical component of this task is finding hope and meaning in the future. The survivors can participate in life and accept the death while still remembering and honoring their loved one's memory (Corless, 2015; COH & AACN, 2018a).

Grieving is hard work. When clients and families are working through grief, there will be good days and bad days, and they may go back and forth between the tasks. This is perfectly normal. However, if individuals are unable to work through grief, they may lash out or have difficulty coping. By carefully assessing the verbal and nonverbal reactions of clients and families, the nurse can have a better understanding of how they are moving through the process.

TYPES OF GRIEF

Uncomplicated Grief

Uncomplicated grief encompasses a wide variety of reactions. These may include temporarily feeling stunned or physically ill or having feelings of sadness, anxiety, or frustration. The person may also have problems focusing on a task and may find it difficult to concentrate (NCI, U.S. National Institutes of Health, 2019a). Uncomplicated grief responses can occur if the loss is expected and there is time to adjust (as in a terminal illness) or when the loss is unexpected, as in the case of a trauma or unforeseen accident. However, when the loss is unexpected, the survivors may be at more risk for complicated grieving. Uncomplicated grieving may last for more than a year, and it is not unusual for family and friends to continue rituals for years, such as visiting a loved one's gravesite (Fig. 8.4). Whatever the circumstances, duration, or difficulty of the recovery process in uncomplicated grief, eventually the loss is accepted (Corless, 2015).

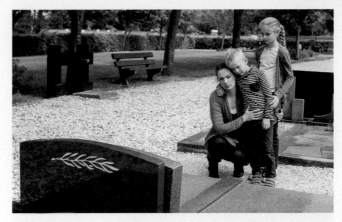

FIG. 8.4 Visiting the graveside of a loved one is a normal part of grieving.

Anticipatory Grief

Anticipatory grief occurs before the death when the client and family become aware of the impending loss. This type of grief may begin when the client and family are confronted with bad news or information that is distressing (Corless, 2015). Anticipatory grief may include sadness and extreme concern for the dying person. It may also help the significant others complete "unfinished business" and give them more time to get used to life without their loved one. However, anticipatory grief may not occur at all, and the grief that is experienced before a death may have no effect on the grief responses experienced after death (NCI, U.S. National Institutes of Health, 2019a).

Complicated or Dysfunctional Grief

Complicated grief occurs when grief responses do not seem to resolve or improve over time (NCI, U.S. National Institutes of Health, 2019a). This type of grief may interfere with a person's ability to function, and symptoms may include severe anxiety, depression, and suicidal thoughts. Factors that are especially likely to lead to complicated grief are sudden death, the death of a child, or death out of time (i.e., a teenager killed in a car accident). When there is a disaster that results in numerous unexpected and violent deaths, such as those that occur during a natural disaster, terrorist attack, or mass shooting, the community at large is at risk for complicated grief (Fig. 8.5). This type of grief may overwhelm the ability to cope and result in a feeling that the world is chaotic and hopeless. Complicated grief may not resolve easily, and some people may need to seek professional help. The major types of complicated grief are listed in Box 8.1.

Disenfranchised Grief

Disenfranchised grief is grief that cannot be expressed openly because of some complication surrounding the loss, such as HIV infection, the commission of a crime, or other information that cannot be shared with others. Nurses may experience this type of grief if they find it difficult to talk about it with their peers or feel that they are supposed to accept grief as just part of their job. Grieving in secret can make the grieving process more difficult and may cause unresolved grief (Corless, 2015). Nurses

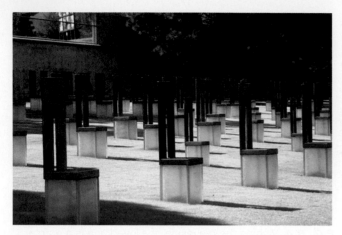

FIG. 8.5 Grief can affect an entire community. Memorial site of the Oklahoma City bombing. The chairs represent each of the victims who were killed in the bombing.

BOX 8.1 Major Types of Complicated or Dysfunctional Grief

- **Chronic grief**: Grief reactions that do not resolve or improve over a long period of time. Example: Julia, a 63-year-old woman, lost her husband over 2 years ago. She has been diagnosed with depression, and she rarely socializes with friends or family.
- **Exaggerated grief**: Grief accompanied by destructive or inappropriate behavior. Example: Michael, a 15-year-old student, lost his dad in a car accident 6 months ago. He has been getting into fights frequently at school, and he is in and out of detention.
- **Delayed grief**: There is an absence or suppression of grief reactions, or grief may be postponed. Example: Kate's mom died of cancer last year. Kate is having feelings of sadness, but she doesn't want to attend support groups or discuss her mom's death.
- **Masked grief**: A refusal to acknowledge grief or that it is interfering with daily life. Example: Dan and Beth lost their newborn infant from a rare genetic condition. They insist they are doing fine, and they quickly went back to work. However, Dan has started having frequent headaches, and Beth is having difficulty sleeping at night.

References: COH & AACN, 2018a; NCI, U.S. National Institutes of Health, 2019a.

must be sensitive to individuals who are at risk of disenfranchised grief. For example, restrictive visiting hours or limiting visitors to only blood relatives or legally sanctioned spouses may make the grief worse and cause unnecessary distress for the client and significant others. Good communication ahead of time with the client regarding personal preferences about visitors is the key to preventing this cause of disenfranchised grief.

CHILDREN AND GRIEF

When children are grieving, they may not want others to know they are sad, and they may have trouble putting feelings about

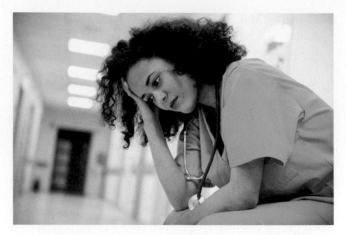

FIG. 8.6 A nurse grieves after the loss of a client.

loss and grief into words. They may express anxiety through play or games in order to work out feelings. Because children may be egocentric (particularly among the younger age groups), they may also believe they have supernatural powers and caused the death of their loved one. The child's expressions of grief may include the following:
- "I think maybe I made this happen."
- "Is it going to happen to me, too?"
- "Who will take care of me now?" (NCI, 2019a)

Expressions of grief in children depend on their age and developmental level. Children may grieve longer than adults, but their understanding of death may vary. For example, children who are aged 2 to 6 years may think that death is like sleeping and not final. Children over the age of 6 may understand that death is final, but they are not sure it could ever happen to them. By the time children are 9 years old, they usually understand that death is final (NCI, U.S. National Institutes of Health, 2019a).

When helping children with grief, use clear, age-appropriate language that is easy to understand. Allow expressions of grief through art, pictures, and play. Be honest and open about the death of their loved one without using euphemistic language. For example, instead of saying, "Aunt Jane is sleeping now," be truthful and say, "Aunt Jane has died" (NCI, U.S. National Institutes of Health, 2019a).

NURSES AND GRIEF

Caring for clients who are dying and helping them experience a peaceful death is a privilege that can be highly rewarding. However, the nurse may also experience a tremendous amount of personal grief (Fig. 8.6). Nurses are problem solvers, and they may perceive the death of a client as a personal failure. Other emotions experienced by the nurse may include frustration, distress, anger, and a feeling of hopelessness and powerlessness.

If the nurse works in an area where clients die often, there may not be enough time to resolve grief before having to move on to the next client (COH & AACN, 2018a). Likewise, nursing students may experience grief if they are caring for a client in a clinical situation who dies. Nurses and students need to examine and discuss their own feelings, reach out to each other, and take care of themselves.

BOX 8.2 Therapeutic Communication During the Grieving Process

- *Convey empathy.* If you express your sorrow in a sincere way, it sends the message, "I care about you.".
- *Use humor.* Laughing in an appropriate way and remembering humorous qualities about the deceased loved one can "break the ice" and help everyone relax.
- *Use touch.* When used appropriately, holding a hand or giving someone a hug to convey your concern for the individual's loss can say more than a thousand words.
- *Be patient.* It takes time to work through the grieving process (Bowden & Greenberg, 2014).
- *Use active listening.* Maintain eye contact at the person's level, with attentive posture, and *listen* carefully to what the individual is saying.
- *Use open-ended questions, and give the person time to respond.* Examples of open-ended questions are "How are you feeling?" or "What is it like…?"
- *Use silence and presence.* Sometimes just being there for someone is helpful.
- *Allow the client and family to share their stories.* This facilitates empathy and allows the nurse to "bear witness" and understand their fears and experiences (COH & AACN, 2018a).
- *Avoid clichés.* Boilerplate responses such as "I know how you feel" or "At least you have other children" are *not* helpful and may cut off communication.
- *Avoid judgments.* There is no "right" or "wrong" way to grieve; the experience and expression of grief are unique to the individual and to the situation (COH & AACN, 2018a).

References: Bowden & Greenberg, 2014; COH & AACN, 2018a; Yoost & Crawford, 2016.

Continuing education, counseling, and spiritual care may also help.

The work of grieving can be a difficult process. As described in Box 8.2, nurses can provide therapeutic communication and support in a variety of ways that will help clients and families cope. To further facilitate the grieving process, nurses can encourage families to share stories, interact, and spend time with their loved one, even if they become less responsive (Box 8.3). Clients and families remember the details. Careful assessment and thoughtful nursing care can make a significant difference for your client and his or her family.

PROVIDING SPIRITUAL CARE FOR A CLIENT AND FAMILY

Providing spiritual care for clients and families involves more than just calling the chaplain or asking about religious preferences (Baird, 2015). Spiritual care is an inseparable part of care for the client and family during the entire dying process. It must be initiated early and reevaluated on an ongoing basis (Johnston-Taylor, 2015). The nurse can facilitate spiritual care by establishing trust and maintaining excellent communication. Allowing the family members to stay at the client's bedside and continue rituals that are important to them is also helpful (Fig. 8.7).

BOX 8.3 Lessons From Experience: Facilitating the Grieving Process

Mrs. Smith, a 64-year-old retired schoolteacher, is dying of a terminal lung disorder in the palliative care unit. Before Mrs. Smith's illness, one of her primary roles in the family had been to help raise and care for her 9-year-old granddaughter Melissa (whose mother had died in an accident). Mrs. Smith took great pride in helping her granddaughter learn how to read. When Mrs. Smith was admitted, she told the nurse that helping Melissa read was "the highlight of her day." Since Mrs. Smith's admission, the staff has offered flexible visiting hours and allowed Melissa to visit her grandma anytime her father was able to bring her. On weekends, Melissa would often sit for hours reading and talking to her grandma. Mrs. Smith became progressively less alert and less responsive, and eventually, she was not able to talk or interact with Melissa.

One day, Melissa sadly looked up at the nurse and said, "What's the point? She probably doesn't know I'm here." Mrs. Smith's nurse sat down with Melissa at eye level and explained that her grandma might be able to hear even though she could not say anything back. The nurse encouraged Melissa to continue talking and reading to her grandma. The nurse also told Melissa how lucky her grandma was to have her as a granddaughter. In addition, the nurse made sure there was comfortable seating and encouraged Melissa to snuggle close to her grandma.

When a dying client becomes less responsive, the family, especially children, are often reluctant or fearful about interacting with the client. The family may also have feelings of intense sadness and loss about how things used to be with their loved one. In this situation, the nurse's thoughtful care, including the use of therapeutic communication, offering helpful suggestions, and enhancing the environment (e.g., offering comfortable seating), facilitated Melissa's grieving.

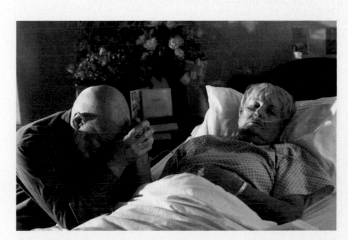

FIG. 8.7 A person's spiritual practices can help the individual cope with grieving.

Definition of Spirituality

Spirituality is a difficult term to define. It has different meanings for different people, and it is defined by the individual. Although *spirituality* and *religion* are often used interchangeably, they are not the same. *Religion* refers to a set of organized beliefs, values, and rules. *Spirituality* is a broader term that refers to how individuals find inner peace, comfort, and a sense of purpose. Although there may be some overlap, spirituality may or may not involve religion. When providing individualized spiritual care, it is important to understand the difference between these concepts (Baird, 2015). Clients who are approaching death begin to look at their lives and come to terms with spirituality. Likewise, nurses who care for the dying often become more aware of their own feelings about spirituality. Everyone is unique when it comes to spiritual needs, and this is influenced by culture. Spiritual awareness helps clients and families find hope, strength, and meaning in the dying process (Johnston-Taylor 2015; Witt-Sherman & Free, 2015).

Guidelines Related to Spiritual Care

Various guidelines stipulate that the spiritual needs of clients must be addressed. For example, The Joint Commission requires that a spiritual assessment be conducted on all clients who enter an approved healthcare facility. At a minimum, this must include the client's denomination, beliefs, and spiritual practices and the process used to complete the spiritual assessment. Although The Joint Commission does not require a specific tool, it offers suggestions that could be included in the spiritual assessment (Box 8.4).

The Hospice and Palliative Nurses Association (HPNA) position statement notes that assessing spirituality and spiritual distress in clients and families is an essential component of spiritual care. However, nurses must also recognize the rights of people to decline spiritual care (HPNA, 2015; Ganz, 2019). Before contacting the chaplain, first explore the preferences of the client and family. Cultural considerations are discussed further in Box 8.5.

It is important to bear in mind that different clients will derive comfort from different types of literature, from scriptures and prayers to essays and poems. Specific requests can be referred to the healthcare facility's chaplain with the permission of the client. Chaplains are members of the healthcare team and may be able to offer prayers, scripture readings, counseling, or a referral to the client's spiritual leader at the client's request. The chaplain may also provide religious services or other rituals in the client's room or in the facility's chapel.

Spiritual care, like spirituality, may or may not involve religion. It can be provided simply by sitting with your clients, talking to them at their level, and listening to their stories (Fig. 8.8). It may also include reading, playing music, or singing songs (Baird, 2015). Some clients may enjoy spending time in a garden or viewing peaceful nature scenes outside the window. A client who is dying often wants to stay connected to family. For example, a mother may find comfort in hearing a recording of her child's recital or looking at a photo album. Listen carefully to your client. As Baird relates, spiritual care is about connecting to the person in a way that says, "I see you. I hear your concerns. You matter. You are important. You are not alone. I care" (Baird, 2015).

BOX 8.4 Major Elements of a Spiritual Assessment Recommended by The Joint Commission

COPING
- How has the illness affected the client and the family?
- What helps the client keep going from day to day?
- How does the client find strength and hope?

PERSONAL BELIEFS
- What does suffering mean to the client?
- What does dying mean to the client?
- What are the client's goals related to spirituality?
- How does the client describe a personal philosophy of life?

SPIRITUAL OR RELIGIOUS PRACTICES
- How does the client express spirituality?
- Does the client use prayer?
- Who is the client's clergy, ministers, chaplain, pastor, or rabbi?
- Does the client desire or prefer a certain type of spiritual or religious support?

Reference: The Joint Commission, 2017.

BOX 8.5 **Cultural Considerations: Spirituality at the End of Life**

Spirituality and culture are closely linked (Hanson & Andrews, 2016). Because we live in an increasingly diverse multicultural society, the nurse's thoughtfulness regarding a client's culture and spirituality facilitates the grieving process and determines whether or not the client has a peaceful death. As part of culturally sensitive care, assess the client and family for spiritual ceremonies and rituals that are important and help them to cope. The most accurate way to assess the spiritual needs of clients and families from different cultures is to ask them directly. One of the first questions to ask may be, "Do you have a spiritual leader you would like for us to contact or to be present?" The client's spiritual advisor may be a priest, rabbi, minister, shaman, curandero, or other spiritual leader or healer. However, it is important to avoid stereotyping or making assumptions about expected behavior based on the client's ethnicity or religion.

Every client and family are unique. Death may have a different meaning for a person from a Judeo-Christian background compared with someone from a Buddhist or Islamic background. Among Native Americans, beliefs may be based on their tribal identity rather than Native American ancestry (Witt-Sherman & Free, 2015). By asking, "Do you have any special requests or preferences?" the nurse conveys interest and concern for the person as an individual.

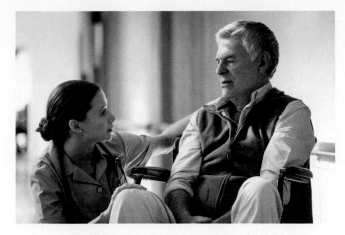

FIG. 8.8 A nurse offers spiritual support.

SUMMARY

When providing bereavement and spiritual care, client-centered care and communication are two of the most important critical concepts to consider. These critical concepts are also interrelated. Using therapeutic communication and collaborating with the client, family, and other healthcare providers will enhance client-centered care and facilitate the grieving process. This will also decrease the client and family's risk for dysfunctional or complicated grief. In addition, self-care and self-examination of your own feelings about grief will help facilitate the grieving process.

APPLICATION OF THE NURSING PROCESS

Examples of Related International Classification for Nursing Practice (ICNP) Nursing Diagnoses, Expected Client Outcomes, and Nursing Interventions:

Nursing Diagnosis: Risk for dysfunctional grief

Supporting Data: Unexpected illness or sudden death of a loved one.

Expected Client Outcomes: The client/family will have no evidence of dysfunctional grief as seen by:
- willingness to discuss feelings with nurse and other healthcare providers
- ability to function and perform previous activities of daily life.

Nursing Intervention Example: Use therapeutic communication, such as active listening.

Nursing Diagnosis: Readiness for effective spiritual status

Expected Client Outcomes: The client/family will exhibit spiritual health and well-being, as seen by:
- participation in support groups and interaction with others as desired
- requests for assistance from spiritual leader or counselors as needed.

Nursing Intervention Examples: Allow flexible visiting hours for family, friends, and significant others, and allow clients to keep objects or literature with special meaning to them in their rooms.

Reference: International Classification for Nursing Practice. (n.d.). *eHealth&ICNP.* Retrieved from https://www.icn.ch/what-we-do/projects/ehealth-icnp.

CRITICAL CONCEPTS
Bereavement and Spiritual Care

Client-Centered Care (CCC)

When providing bereavement and spiritual care, respect for the client is demonstrated by:
- providing individualized, person-centered care for the client and family
- self-examination of personal beliefs about bereavement and spiritual care
- assessment of the client and family and their bereavement and spiritual needs
- promoting autonomy and allowing client and family to grieve in their own way
- providing opportunities for client and family that will meet spiritual needs
- providing privacy and ensuring comfort
- honoring cultural and spiritual preferences, and advocating for the client and family.

Infection Control (INF)

Healthcare-associated infection is prevented by reducing the number and transfer of microorganisms, primarily through hand hygiene.

Safety (SAF)

Safety measures prevent harm by maintaining a safe care environment.

Communication (COM)

- When providing bereavement and spiritual care, listening and collaboration with the client and family facilitate grieving and comfort.
- Communication exchanges information (oral, written, nonverbal, or electronic) between two or more people during the dying process.
- Documentation records information in a permanent legal record.

Evaluation (EVAL)

Evaluation of the outcomes allows the nurse to determine the efficacy of the care provided.

■ SKILL 8.1 Caring for a Client and Family Who Are Grieving

Before caring for a client and family who are grieving, it is important to examine your own feelings about grief and spirituality, as well as your feelings about death and dying.

BEGINNING THE SKILL

1. **INF** Perform hand hygiene.
2. **COM** Introduce yourself to the client and family.
3. **SAF** Identify the client using two identifiers.

PROCEDURE

Before the Client's Death

4. **CCC** Assess the client's orientation to person, time, place, and situation. *A baseline assessment of the client's level of consciousness and orientation must be done in order to determine appropriate interventions for providing assistance with the grieving process.*
5. **CCC** Assess the client's comfort and pain management needs and intervene appropriately. *Pain and discomfort may interfere with the grieving process. (See Chapter 7.)*
6. **COM** Use therapeutic communication with client and family, such as silence, active listening, and open-ended questions (e.g., "What is important to you at this time?"). *Therapeutic communication facilitates the grieving process by helping the nurse establish trust.*
7. **CCC** Assess the client and family's desire and need for bereavement care and their cultural and spiritual preferences. *Provides a baseline assessment and determines if referrals, interpreters, or other resources are needed.* (Note: For more information on spiritual assessment and care, see Skill 8.2 and Box 8.4.)
8. **COM** Ask the client and family to give you a list of friends and other family members, including children, whom they want to be with them at the time of his or her death. *Allowing the client to decide who is in the room during this time facilities dignity and autonomy.*
9. **CCC** Allow flexible visiting hours for family, friends, and religious advisors as desired by the client and allowed by facility policy. *Flexible visiting hours facilitate the grieving process by supporting client autonomy and allowing family, friends, and others to be with the client.*
10. **CCC** Encourage the client's family to spend time talking with, reading to, cuddling, and holding their loved one as long as they wish, regardless of the client's level of consciousness. Tell the family that their loved one may still hear them even if the individual does not respond. *Families may be reluctant to talk to a loved one who is unconscious or critically ill.* (Note: This point is illustrated in Box 8.3.)
11. **CCC** Provide extra seating, sleeping couches, and other items for the family as appropriate and allowed by policy. *Helping family members remain with the client and making them comfortable facilitates the grieving process (COH & AACN, 2018a).*

At the Time of the Client's Death

12. **CCC** Allow the client's family members to be with the client at the time of death (if they choose to do so). If the client's death was unexpected or traumatic, prepare the family by explaining the situation and the physical appearance of their loved one before they see the individual. *A tragic, unexpected death can be particularly distressing for loved ones. This might be compounded by the appearance of the body if the death was violent. Preparing the family before they see the body may be helpful.*
13. **CCC** Stay with the family members or arrange for someone to be with them if they wish. If the family members want to be alone with their loved one, honor their wishes. *This facilitates autonomy.*
14. **CCC** Allow the family to stay with the deceased client as long as they desire. If the client is a child, an infant, or a stillbirth, allow the parents to hold the child if they desire.
15. **CCC** Encourage family members to share special memories, photo albums, and journals about their loved one who has died. *Facilitates memories and grief resolution (COH & AACN, 2018a).*
16. **COM** Avoid clichés and artificial consolations, such as "Look at the bright side." *Communication that is not therapeutic will interfere with the grieving process.*
17. **CCC** Allow family members the opportunity to provide the "last bath" and other kinds of personal care for the deceased client if they wish. *Providing the final bath to their loved one may provide comfort for family members and facilitate the grieving process (Matzo & Hill, 2015).* (Note: In some cultures, there may be certain rituals that are performed during the client's final bath.)
18. **CCC** Encourage the family to keep items that hold memories of the deceased client, such as locks of hair, identification bands, photographs, handprints, footprints, and so forth.
19. **CCC** Provide positive feedback to the client's family about their role as supportive caregivers (e.g., "You did a good job taking care of your dad and making him comfortable"). (Note: See Box 8.2 for additional suggestions and examples of therapeutic communication during the grieving process.)
20. **CCC** Encourage the client's bereaved family to verbalize feelings and discuss their loss.

FINISHING THE SKILL

21. **INF** Perform hand hygiene.
22. **SAF** Ensure safety and comfort of the family after the client's death.
23. **EVAL** Evaluate the outcomes. Are the family members able to verbalize their feelings? Are they interacting with each other and other people? Are they participating in support groups?

24. **COM** Document your assessment findings, care given, and outcomes in the legal healthcare record.

Follow-up Care With the Family After the Client's Death

25. **CCC** Assist the bereaved family with funeral arrangements or other services as allowed by facility policy.

26. **COM** Continue to encourage the family to verbalize their feelings, and provide information and materials about grief as appropriate. Refer the family for bereavement counseling or support groups if indicated or requested. *Facilitates the grieving process.*
27. **CCC** If allowed by facility policy, follow up with the bereaved family via phone calls or cards after the client's death and at special holidays and events.

■ SKILL 8.2 Providing Spiritual Care for a Client and Family

BEGINNING THE SKILL

1. **INF** Perform hand hygiene.
2. **CCC** Introduce yourself to the client and family.
3. **SAF** Identify the client using two identifiers.

PROCEDURE

4. **CCC** Assess the client and family's desire and need for spiritual care and their cultural and spiritual preferences. *Provides a baseline spiritual assessment of the client and family.* (Note: Some clients and families may not want spiritual care, and this must be respected [Ganz, 2019].)
5. **CCC** Perform a spiritual assessment using a facility-approved tool (see Box 8.4). Make referrals to clergy as indicated and desired by the client and family.
6. **COM** Use therapeutic communication, such as silence, active listening, and open-ended questions (e.g., "What is important to you at this time?"). *This will facilitate spiritual care by helping the nurse establish trust (Johnston-Taylor, 2015).*
7. **CCC** Explore what is comforting for the client and family. For example, do they like nature? Do they enjoy meditation? *Facilitates assessment of what is meaningful to the client.*
8. **COM** Ask the client and family if they have a religious or spiritual advisor they wish to contact. Respect the client's desire to not speak to a chaplain if that is the client's preference.
9. **CCC** Allow flexible visiting hours for family, friends, and religious advisors as desired by the client and allowed by policy. *Flexible visiting hours facilitate spiritual care by supporting client autonomy and allowing family, friends, clergy, and others to be with the client.*
10. **COM** Assess nonverbal clues about the client's practices, such as the presence of religious symbols, books, cards, or other objects among the client's personal possessions.

Assessment of the client's environment and nonverbal behavior provides information about spiritual preferences.

11. **COM** Ask clients if they have rituals, traditions, or ceremonies that are important to them.
12. **CCC** Allow the client to continue with normal rituals as much as possible, such as birthdays, celebration of special holidays, religious activities, and so forth, as tolerated and appropriate. *Allowing the client to maintain as many rituals and practices as possible can help preserve personal identity and meet spiritual needs (Baird, 2015; COH & AACN, 2018a).*
13. **CCC** Allow client to keep religious objects and other items that are important to them close by. *Personal items provide comfort and a feeling of safety.*
14. **CCC** If desired by the client, assist the client to chapel for religious services or ceremonies.
15. **CCC** Offer prayer, scripture reading, singing, or other spiritual activities if desired by the client. Explore with clients what scriptures are most important to them personally.
16. **CCC** Offer CDs, religious tapes, meditation recordings, or other music or spiritual guides as desired by the client. If the client has a book he or she likes, offer to read it aloud. *Nurses are invaluable in offering suggestions that are comforting (Baird, 2015).*

FINISHING THE SKILL

17. **INF** Perform hand hygiene.
18. **SAF** Ensure safety and comfort of the client and family.
19. **EVAL** Evaluate the outcomes. Are the client and family interacting with one another in a meaningful way? Are they participating in support groups or other activities?
20. **COM** Document the assessment findings, care given, and outcomes in legal healthcare record.

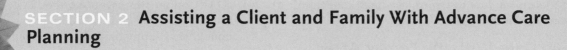

The topic of death and dying is often avoided in our society. Many people feel uncomfortable with this issue. However, clients and families frequently trust nurses to help them understand and navigate through the options. To facilitate this process, advance care planning (ACP) is becoming increasingly important. ACP allows clients to discuss their healthcare goals and values and preferences that are important to them. These discussions should not be a one-time activity, nor should they wait until the client is dying (IOM, 2015). The key is early, ongoing communication between the client, family, and healthcare providers.

TOOLS USED FOR ADVANCE CARE PLANNING

Several tools that may be used as part of ACP include advance directives and do-not-resuscitate (DNR) orders, among others. It is important to note that these tools do *not* replace ongoing discussions.

Advance directives are legal documents that allow clients to make their wishes known ahead of time. The major types of advance directives are the living will and the medical power of attorney. A living will is a legal document that stipulates what treatments the client may or may not want to receive. A medical power of attorney is often called a durable power of attorney (DPOA). With the DPOA, clients appoint an individual or healthcare proxy to make decisions for them in the event they are incapacitated and cannot speak for themselves. A healthcare proxy (also known as healthcare surrogate) can interpret the client's wishes and make decisions. The advantage of having a healthcare proxy is that this individual has some flexibility with treatment decisions as the client's condition and circumstances change. The language that authorizes this type of advance directive may vary for each state (NCI, U.S. National Institutes of Health, 2015; Perrin, 2015).

DNR or do-not-attempt-resuscitation (DNAR) orders are medical orders that document the client's desire not to have cardiopulmonary resuscitation (CPR). Advance directives are not automatically DNR orders. A specific DNR order must be written by the authorized healthcare provider. Some states have passed legislation that requires DNR orders to be portable or travel with the client from one setting to another. Various states may also require an additional DNR consent form for clients who have DNR orders.

Because advance directives and DNR orders have dramatic consequences, accurate communication is essential so that a client's wishes regarding resuscitation are not misunderstood. Miscommunication or lack of communication can result in harm. Therefore, clarification of a client's DNR status as soon as possible is a top priority. As discussed in Box 8.6, there is no time to look for paperwork in an emergency.

Advance directives and DNR orders are closely related to the principle of autonomy. They are both voluntary, and they can both be retracted at any time (NCI, U.S. National Institutes of Health, 2015). According to the ANA *Code of Ethics,* nurses have a clear responsibility to preserve the client's right to autonomy and self-determination. Nurses must be aware that culture, ethnicity, and religion can affect a client's decision making, and the principle of autonomy may not be applicable. For example, in some cultures, it is often the family who determines whether or not the client is resuscitated. Some ethnic groups prefer to shield their loved ones from the burden of decision making. However, this does not necessarily mean that clients who are from non-Western cultures don't want to be involved in their own treatment and care decisions (Post & Boltz, 2016).

In 1991, the Patient Self-Determination Act (PSDA) was enacted, requiring healthcare facilities that are certified by Medicare and Medicaid to notify adults who enter their facility of their right to refuse or receive medical care and their right to have an advance directive (Perrin, 2015). Likewise, The Joint Commission requires facilities to determine whether a client has an advance directive and provide assistance to those who do not. A copy of the client's advance

BOX 8.6 Lessons From the Courtroom: DNR—Nurse Faulted for Delay in Care of Client While Looking for DNR Paperwork

In a Texas lawsuit *(IHS Acquisition v. Crowson),* a client was in a skilled facility following hip surgery. While her son was in the room, the client began to gasp for breath. The son called for the nurse, who, upon arrival, discovered that the client had no palpable pulse. According to testimony, the nurse waited 8 minutes to begin resuscitation while checking to see if there were do-not-resuscitate (DNR) orders. The client later died in a hospital. The court of appeals ruled against the nurse and skilled facility and in favor of the family. When a client is in cardiac or respiratory arrest and the DNR status is unknown, the legal standard of care requires providers to begin cardiopulmonary resuscitation (CPR) and call a code or 911 immediately (Do not resuscitate: Nurse faulted for delay while looking for patient's code paperwork, 2010).

This case is a good example of why it is so critically important to have complete handoff communication between shifts. To prevent this error (or other errors) from occurring, the nurses who are caring for the client on different shifts could review the client's paperwork together during the shift-change report and determine the client's DNR status. If there is any uncertainty, the authorized healthcare provider should be contacted for clarification. Maintaining ongoing communication with the family is essential. Regular family conferences may also be helpful, particularly for clients who are at increased risk for sudden illness or cardiac arrest.

directive (if there is one) must remain in the client's chart in every setting.

Assisting a client with advance directives means more than simply telling the client to fill in the blanks. It is important to assess the client and family's understanding of the document, be available for questions, and make appropriate referrals if necessary. If a client needs someone to sign as a witness for an advance directive, check your facility policy, or call the nurse supervisor. Some states stipulate certain rules about who may be a witness for an advance directive, and the signatures may have to be notarized to be legally binding. The guiding principle of advance directives is that all people, regardless of their gender, socioeconomic status, or prognosis, have a right to determine what care they will or will not receive (Post & Boltz, 2016).

Physician Orders for Life-Sustaining Treatment

A recent initiative, physician orders for life-sustaining treatment (POLST) is becoming more common. These are considered to be "controlled" orders for certain life-sustaining treatments that must be written by the authorized healthcare provider. One important distinction is that a POLST is immediately active, whereas advance directives (which are initiated by the client) are only active once the client is incapacitated. Another important distinction is that a POLST is only appropriate for clients who have a terminal, life-limiting illness. One of the advantages of POLST is portability. For example, it remains valid when the client is at home or if the client is cared for in different healthcare facilities (IOM, 2015).

It is important to remember that advance directives, DNR orders, and medical directives are not plans of care. There may also be conflicts, disagreements, and arguments between family members. Some of these conflicts are related to a lack of knowledge or fear and can be resolved with more information and family conferences. Therefore, the critical concepts of communication and client-centered care are imperative. Nurses must be alert for possible breakdowns in communication and make referrals as needed. The questions clients often ask are "Will I still get care?" and "Can I change my mind?" As advocates, nurses can reassure clients they will continue to receive care, and they can always change their minds.

APPLICATION OF THE NURSING PROCESS

Examples of Related ICNP Nursing Diagnoses, Expected Client Outcomes, and Nursing Interventions:

Nursing Diagnosis: Lack of Knowledge

Supporting Data: The client and family have verbalized that they have a lack of understanding regarding ACP and end-of-life care options.

Expected Client Outcomes: The client and family will seek knowledge and demonstrate an increased understanding of ACP and end-of-life care options:

- willingness to discuss and ask questions related to advance directives

- requests for follow-up materials and/or referrals regarding advance directives.

Nursing Intervention Examples: Provide information and literature related to advance directives. Make referrals and collaborate with other healthcare professionals as needed.

Reference: International Classification for Nursing Practice. (n.d.). *eHealth & ICNP*. Retrieved from https://www.icn.ch/what-we-do/projects/ehealth-icnp.

CRITICAL CONCEPTS
Assisting With Advance Care Planning

Client-Centered Care (CCC)

When assisting a client and family with ACP, respect for the client is demonstrated through:

- providing individualized person-centered care for the client and family
- promoting autonomy and ensuring there is informed consent for procedures
- allowing self-determination regarding treatment options and advance care planning
- providing education and follow-up related to advance care planning
- providing privacy and ensuring comfort
- honoring cultural and spiritual preferences, arranging for an interpreter, and providing the appropriate written translations if needed
- advocating for the client and family.

Infection Control (INF)

Healthcare-associated infection is prevented by reducing the number and transfer of microorganisms, primarily through hand hygiene.

Safety (SAF)

Safety considerations with advance care planning prevent harm and maintain a safe care environment.

Communication (COM)

- When assisting a client and family with ACP, collaboration with other healthcare professionals enhances decision making.
- Communication exchanges information (oral, written, nonverbal, or electronic) between two or more people.
- Documentation records information in a permanent legal record.
- Communication and documentation regarding advance directives improves care for the client.

Evaluation (EVAL)

Evaluation of the outcomes with ACP allows the nurse to determine the efficacy of the care provided.

▪ SKILL 8.3 Assisting With Advance Directives and Do-Not-Resuscitate (DNR) Orders

BEGINNING THE SKILL

1. **INF** Perform hand hygiene.
2. **SAF** Introduce yourself to the client and family.
3. **CCC** Identify the client using two identifiers.

PROCEDURE

4. **CCC** Assess the client's orientation to person, time, place, and situation. *A baseline assessment of the client's level of consciousness and orientation must be done in order to determine appropriate interventions for assisting with advance directives and DNR orders.*
5. **CCC** Assess the client's comfort and pain management needs and intervene appropriately. *Pain and discomfort are a distraction and may interfere with the client's decision making.*
6. **CCC** Assess the client and family's desire and need for advance directives and their cultural and spiritual preferences. Make referrals to clergy or other professionals as indicated.
7. **CCC** Verify that an explanation has been provided to the client upon admission of the client's right to have an advance directive and the client's right to refuse or accept medical treatment. *This is required by the PSDA and The Joint Commission for clients in certified healthcare facilities (Post & Boltz, 2016).*
8. **COM** Ask whether the client has an existing advance directive or a designated durable power of attorney or healthcare proxy. Determine if the client has a wallet-size card, bracelet, or necklace that contains advance directive information. *This will ensure that the client's advance directives and treatment decisions are honored in case the client is unable to speak on his or her own behalf.*
9. **COM** If the client has an existing advance directive and healthcare proxy/agent:
   a. Ensure that a copy of the documents, the durable power of attorney, healthcare proxy, and other instructions are in the client's chart. (Note: Some jurisdictions require that an informed consent form be signed in addition to the advance direction. Check facility policy.)
   b. Ensure that the attending physician or authorized healthcare provider and healthcare proxy/agent have a copy of the advance directive.
   c. Return the original advance directive to the client.

10. **COM** If the client does *not* have an advance directive or designated healthcare proxy/agent:
    a. Offer assistance or make referrals as indicated by facility policy and state law.
    b. Contact the nursing supervisor per facility policy to determine who may act as a witness for the client's advance directive and whether or not the signatures must be notarized.
11. **COM** If the client has a written DNR order from the authorized healthcare provider:
    a. Determine that the DNR order is signed and witnessed as indicated by facility policy.
    b. Determine that the informed consent form and rationale for the DNR order is signed and on the client's chart as indicated by facility policy.
    c. Review the DNR order periodically and before invasive procedures.
    d. Notify the authorized healthcare provider if the DNR order is expired.
12. **CCC** If the client asks to change the advance directives or DNR orders, honor the client's requests and notify authorized healthcare provider as soon as possible. *Clients have a right to change their minds regarding previous decisions about advance directives or DNR orders.*
13. **COM** Consult with the appropriate committee or other professionals if indicated or if a conflict arises regarding advance directives or DNR orders. *Nurses must be aware of their facility policy and other available resources for resolving conflict (Post & Boltz, 2016).*
14. **CCC** Provide follow-up educational information to the client and family as indicated or requested. *This facilitates culturally sensitive care and promotes understanding of advance directives and DNR orders among clients of different cultural backgrounds.*

FINISHING THE SKILL

15. **INF** Perform hand hygiene.
16. **SAF** Ensure safety and comfort of the client and family.
17. **EVAL** Evaluate the outcomes. Is a current advance directive on the client's chart? Do the client and family express an understanding of and knowledge about the advance directive?
18. **COM** Document the assessment findings, care given, and outcomes in the legal healthcare record.

SECTION 3 Caring for a Client Near the End of Life

When the client approaches imminent death, the priority is comfort care. Nurses must be able to recognize the signs and symptoms of impending death and know how to offer support to the client and family (ANA, 2016). Although dying is a natural part of life, it may be difficult for families to witness the physical changes. Family members want to know that their loved one is not suffering and will not be abandoned (COH & ACCN, 2018b).

The dying process is unique for each person. Some people experience all of the typical signs and symptoms. However, some of these changes may not occur at all or in any particular sequence. Although every death is different, it can be helpful for families to know what to expect. If clients and families are prepared, the changes that do occur may seem less frightening (Matzo & Hill, 2015). As discussed in Box 8.7, this preparation may be especially helpful for family members who are caring for loved ones at home.

As death approaches, clients will experience a natural slowing of their physical and mental functioning (Matzo & Hill, 2015). This often leads to increased sleepiness, lethargy, and eventually death. Some of the most common symptoms that occur are noisy and difficult breathing, increasing restlessness/agitation, and increased incontinence. Signs that death may be only days away may include severe fatigue and weakness, pale physical appearance, lack of interest in food, and increased difficulty swallowing (Berry & Griffie, 2015).

Changes in the cardiovascular system are also common. Tachycardia, which slowly changes to bradycardia, can occur. Dyspnea (difficulty breathing) or other changes in the breathing pattern can occur as the chest wall muscles become weaker and oxygen exchange becomes impaired (Berry & Griffie, 2015; Matzo & Hill, 2015). In addition, the client's breathing may become more shallow (see Chapter 3).

Changes in the client's brain and central nervous system function may cause agonal respirations or gasping. As a result of the body shutting down, there may be a decreased blood flow to the kidneys and brain, resulting in decreased urine output and increased confusion, respectively. During the dying process, some clients may not have any pain at all. If a client does have pain, the level of pain may change or worsen as death approaches. Thus, the management of distressing symptoms is a top priority (Berry & Griffie, 2015; Matzo & Hill, 2015).

Although clients who are dying may have changes in hearing and vision, remind families that their loved ones may still hear them even though they cannot respond. Encourage the family to hold, cuddle, and talk to their loved one (Fig. 8.9). Attention to emotional responses is also important. Fear is a common emotion for the client and the family. In particular, they may have a fear of pain and fear of the unknown. The discomfort associated with the dying process can also cause other reactions such as severe depression or anxiety (Berry & Griffie, 2015; COH & AACN, 2018b). Client-centered care, particularly ensuring comfort to the client and family, is critically important during this difficult time. Excellent communication is also important.

BOX 8.7 Home Care Considerations: Supporting Family Caregivers Who Are Caring for Their Loved Ones at Home

Glenn Smith, who has been diagnosed with a terminal illness, was discharged from the hospital. Twenty-four hours after Mr. Smith was discharged, his wife calls the hospital unit, distressed and crying. She states, "I'm not sure what is going on with Glenn. He is breathing hard, and his arms and hands are so cold. Is this normal? I can't handle this!" When a client who is dying is discharged to the home, it is often stressful for caregivers. Many family members feel inadequate and unsure of what to expect. To reduce anxiety, it is important for the nurse to educate the client and family prior to discharge about these possible changes.

One of the most frightening changes for family caregivers to witness is dyspnea and increased respiratory congestion from secretions. This can create noisy and labored breathing. The client at the end of life will also experience changes in cardiac output. As the body attempts to compensate for a decreased circulating blood volume, blood will divert to vital organs and away from extremities. This change may be what caused Mr. Smith's arms and hands to feel cold.

To provide support for caregivers in the home, many facilities offer educational materials that alert caregivers about the possible changes their loved one may experience as they approach death. For some clients and families, hospice care may be preferred. Hospice care usually requires a referral and can be provided in an inpatient facility or occur in the home setting.

In addition to alterations in skin temperature and breathing patterns, some other possible changes caregivers should be aware of include the following:

- increasing fear and anxiety
- drowsiness and lethargy
- withdrawal from family and friends
- changes in sleep patterns or excessive sleeping
- increasing weakness and fatigue
- changes in appetite or decreased appetite
- refusal to eat or decreased oral intake
- dysphagia (difficulty swallowing)
- decreased urination and bowel changes
- increased confusion or delirium
- near-death awareness or dreams about loved ones who have died.

Reference: NCI, U.S. National Institutes of Health, 2019b.

APPLICATION OF THE NURSING PROCESS

Examples of Related ICNP Nursing Diagnoses, Expected Client Outcomes, and Nursing Interventions:

Nursing Diagnosis: Discomfort

Supporting Data: Discomfort associated with the dying process, such as dyspnea (difficulty breathing), pain, restlessness, confusion, and other distressing symptoms

Expected Client Outcomes: The client will exhibit decreased discomfort, as demonstrated by:
- decreased restlessness
- decreased dyspnea
- decreased pain-intensity rating.

Nursing Intervention Examples: Provide nonpharmacologic and pharmacologic comfort measures and pain control. Provide a therapeutic environment (see Chapter 7).

Nursing Diagnosis: Anxiety

Supporting Data: Increased physical signs of anxiety, such as agitation, shaking, and tremors

Expected Outcomes: The client and family will exhibit decreased anxiety as demonstrated by:
- decreased agitation
- verbalization of decreased anxiety.

Nursing Intervention Example: Provide information about expected physical changes that may occur with the dying process and allow the client and family to ask questions.

Reference: International Classification for Nursing Practice. (n.d.). *eHealth & ICNP*. Retrieved from https://www.icn.ch/what-we-do/projects/ehealth-icnp.

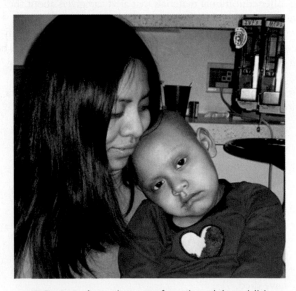

FIG. 8.9 A mother comforts her dying child.

CRITICAL CONCEPTS
Caring for a Client Near the End of Life

Client-Centered Care (CCC)

Respect when caring for a client near the end of life is demonstrated through:
- providing individualized, person-centered care for a client and family
- promoting autonomy and ensuring there is informed consent for procedures
- providing privacy and protecting a client's dignity near the end of life
- monitoring client's clinical status and comfort needs, and ensuring comfort by using nonpharmacologic and pharmacologic comfort measures
- honoring cultural preferences and arranging an interpreter if necessary
- being an advocate for the client and family.

Infection Control (INF)

When caring for the client near the end of life, healthcare-associated infection is prevented by:
- containment of microorganisms
- preventing and reducing the transfer of microorganisms
- reducing the number of microorganisms.

Safety (SAF)

Safety measures when caring for the client near the end of life prevent harm by maintaining a safe care environment.

Communication (COM)

- When caring for the client near the end of life, collaboration with other members of the healthcare team improves care.
- Communication exchanges information (oral, written, nonverbal, or electronic) between two or more people.
- Documentation records information in a permanent legal record.
- Communication about expected signs and symptoms near the end of life enhances care.

Evaluation (EVAL)

Evaluation of the outcomes allows the nurse to determine the efficacy of the care provided.

▪ SKILL 8.4 Providing Physical Care for a Client Who Is Dying

EQUIPMENT

Clean gloves and PPE, if there is a risk of exposure to body fluids
Disposable absorbent protective pads
Moist cloths and towels if needed
Paper tape
Soft circular bandages
Oral care supplies

BEGINNING THE SKILL

1. **INF** Perform hand hygiene.
2. **CCC** Introduce yourself to the client and family.
3. **SAF** Identify the client using two identifiers.

PROCEDURE

4. **INF** Apply gloves and PPE if indicated and if there is a risk of exposure to body fluids.

5. **CCC** Assess the client's orientation to person, time, place, and situation. *A baseline assessment of the client's level of consciousness and orientation must be done in order to determine appropriate interventions and care for the client who is near the end of life.*

6. **CCC** Assess the client's comfort and pain management needs and intervene appropriately. *When death is imminent, pain and other signs and symptoms may intensify. Inadequate management of pain and symptoms creates distress for the client and family (Berry & Griffie, 2015).*

7. **COM** Inform the client and family about the possible physical changes that can occur when death is imminent. *Conveying information about possible physical changes their loved one may experience in the last days may decrease their anxiety and sense of panic.* (See Box 8.7.)

8. **SAF** Assess the client for increased delirium, hallucinations, or seizures. If this occurs, provide close observation; arrange for someone to sit with the client if possible (Berry & Griffie, 2015). *Changes in mental status or increased seizure activity can increase the client's risk for falls and injury.*

9. **CCC** Assess the client for dyspnea and respirations caused by increased secretions. If the client has signs and symptoms of dyspnea or difficulty breathing:
   a. Reposition and elevate the client's head of the bed or turn the client to the side. *Elevating the head of the bed or repositioning client can improve drainage and help lung expansion.*
   b. Use a fan to provide a gentle breeze. *Using a fan improves ventilation and decreases the client's sense of suffocating* (Berry & Griffie, 2015; Matzo & Hill, 2015).
   c. Avoid suctioning or suction only when necessary (see Chapter 9). *Suctioning is harsh on mucosa and may stimulate more secretions (Berry & Griffie, 2015; NCI, U.S. National Institutes of Health, 2019b).*
   d. Avoid overloading the client with fluids. *Increased fluids can increase secretions and place stress on the client's weakened cardiovascular system* (Berry & Griffie, 2015).

10. **SAF** Assess the client for increased difficulty swallowing. If the client has difficulty, elevate the head of the bed and allow the client more time to swallow. Avoid giving the client foods that are difficult to swallow. *Swallowing too fast or while lying flat increases the risk of choking.*

11. **CCC** Assess the client for changes in bowel and bladder function. If the client is at risk for incontinence, provide absorbent protective pads. *Bowel changes, such as constipation, can occur due to decreased intake of food and water. Absorbent protective pads will provide comfort and prevent skin breakdown.*

12. **CCC** Assess the client for decreased fluid/food intake and dry mouth. If the client has dry mouth, provide meticulous mouth care by keeping the lips moist, and consider a room humidifier. Use soft-bristle toothbrushes or oral swabs, rinse the mouth frequently, offer sips of fluids, or allow ice chips to melt in the mouth. Provide normal saline mouth sprays. *Moisture and mouth care prevent further drying of the client's mouth and oral mucosa. As imminent death approaches, the client is at an increased risk for dry mouth because of decreased intake, mouth breathing, and changes in the level of consciousness (Berry & Griffie, 2015; Matzo & Hill, 2015).*

13. **CCC** Provide soothing eye care, such as moist cloths or artificial tears. *As the client approaches imminent death, the blink reflex may be altered, or the eyes may remain partially open, particularly if the client has a decreased level of consciousness (Berry & Griffie, 2015).*

14. **CCC** Provide support under the client's joints when turning or bathing. If turning the client on his or her side, place a pillow between the knees to promote alignment. *Promotes comfort and protects the spine.*

15. **CCC** Provide therapeutic massage, touch, music, or other relaxation techniques. Provide relaxation tools (e.g., client's favorite CDs, warm blanket, poetry). *Alternative therapies and relaxation techniques may ease distressing symptoms* (see Chapter 7).

16. **CCC** Provide a soothing, nonstimulating room environment with temperature control and low-level lighting. *A therapeutic environment will help reduce anxiety and discomfort.*

17. **CCC** Encourage family members to interact with and talk *to* the client, not over the client. Remind families that their loved ones may be able to hear even if they don't respond. Encourage families to touch or hold their loved ones if they wish and tell them they are loved.

18. **COM** Communicate to the family that everything possible is being done for their loved one and that the client's comfort needs are being addressed. *Provides reassurance and decreases anxiety.*

FINISHING THE SKILL

19. **INF** Remove gloves and PPE (if used), and perform hand hygiene.

20. **SAF** Ensure safety and comfort for the client and family. Ensure that the bed is in the lowest position and verify that the client and family can identify and reach the nurse call system. *These safety measures reduce the risk of falls.*

21 **EVAL** Evaluate the outcomes. Have the client's distressing symptoms (e.g., pain, dyspnea, nausea) decreased in intensity? Does the client appear to be less agitated and restless?

22. **COM** Document the assessment findings, care given, and outcomes in the legal healthcare record.

23. **CCC** Provide follow-up care and refer the family for spiritual or bereavement care, social services, or chaplain services as needed. (see Section 1, Bereavement and Spiritual Care.)

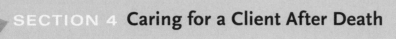

SECTION 4   Caring for a Client After Death

When a client dies, the nurse's job continues. The death of a client may be traumatic for the family and create severe anxiety as well as other strong emotions such as grief and fear, particularly if the client's death was sudden or unexpected. The nurse can offer support to the family by showing respect and providing culturally sensitive care and communication (Berry & Griffie, 2015; Fig. 8.10).

Communication with the family about the client's death should be done in a quiet, private setting with comfortable seating if possible. If the family has limited English proficiency, arrange for an interpreter to be present. It may also be helpful to prepare the family ahead of time regarding the appearance of their deceased loved one. To facilitate the grieving process and create lasting memories, the nurse can provide an opportunity for the family, including siblings, to hold, and even photograph, their deceased loved one if they wish. This may be especially helpful in the case of a deceased child or stillborn infant with whom the family has bonded (Fig. 8.11).

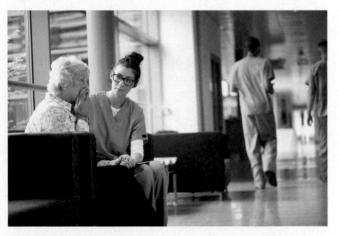

FIG. 8.10 Nurse offering support to a family member in distress.

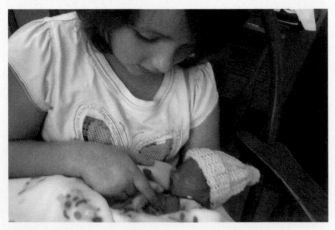

FIG. 8.11 Big sister holding her stillborn baby brother. (Courtesy of Shannon Davis.)

To further facilitate the grieving process, convey to the family that their loved one has value. Care after death should be family centered, not nurse directed (Berry & Griffie, 2015). The nurse's care at this time can affect the family forever. Communicate closely with the family members to determine their beliefs and preferences about death and the care of their loved one's body (Box 8.8). For example, the family may prefer that only people of the same gender and religion perform postmortem care or bathe and prepare the body for viewing. In addition, some families may believe their loved one's body must face east immediately after death or that the loved one's head must be elevated above the body (Witt-Sherman & Free, 2015). Respect these requests if possible.

In most states, the physician or authorized healthcare provider must pronounce the client's death and sign the death certificate. The signs of death are relaxed jaws, absent carotid and apical pulses and heart rate, absent lung sounds and breathing, fixed and dilated pupils, no reaction to sound or touch, and loss of control of bowel and bladder. In addition, blood will begin to pool by gravity and accumulate in the dependent areas of the body (Berry & Griffie, 2015).

The three main physiologic changes that occur are rigor mortis, algor mortis, and livor mortis (Table 8.2). Rigor mortis (also referred to as postmortem rigidity) can occur within 2 to 4 hours of death (Berry & Griffie, 2015). If the family's viewing of the body will be delayed, it is helpful to keep the room cool and notify the funeral home. If the client has died at home or in a hospice, the funeral home may pick up the client after the family gives consent. In the hospital, the nurse may prepare the body for transfer to the morgue.

When performing postmortem care, treat the deceased client with the same care and respect you would give a client who is alive. Routinely wearing gloves without a good reason

BOX 8.8 Cultural Considerations: Identifying Cultural Preferences Regarding Postmortem Care

- Identify preferences and beliefs related to autopsy and organ donation.
- Identify rituals and customs that are important to the client's family.
- Identify objects of spiritual importance that need to remain with the client's body.
- Identify specific practices related to positioning or caring for the client's body.
- Identify specific practices related to bathing the client's body, such as the use of incense or herbs. Determine if there are cultural restrictions as to who may bathe the body.
- Identify if there are gender preferences as to who may handle the body.
- Identify preferences related to ceremonies such as baptism and identify whether or not these ceremonies need to be conducted before or after the client's death.

TABLE 8.2 Physiologic Changes That Occur After Death

Change	Timeline and Characteristics	Possible Nursing Measures
Livor Mortis, also known as postmortem lividity	• Begins shortly after death • Purple-red discoloration of the skin caused by breakdown of red blood cells and hemoglobin; may appear to be mottled • Blood will begin to pool in dependent areas of the body or parts of the body where the skin has been punctured by tubes.	• Avoid heavy blankets or anything that would place excess pressure on the deceased client's skin. • Use light clothing and sheets. • Elevate the head of the deceased client's bed 20–30 degrees.
Algor mortis	• The internal body temperature may decrease by approximately 1°C per hour until it is at room temperature. • The skin becomes more fragile and loses natural flexibility as the body cools. • The deceased client may appear to be sweating as the body continues to cool.	• Handle the body with gentle care to avoid tearing the skin. • Use paper tape and circular loose bandages if needed. • Inform the family that skin may feel cool and moist to the touch.
Rigor mortis	• May begin within 2–4 hours after death and last 24–48 hours, depending on ambient room temperature • Joints and muscles become rigid with muscle fiber contraction. • The body becomes stiff, beginning with the eyelids, neck, and jaw and eventually extending to the client's internal organs.	• Place the deceased client in a natural and relaxed position. • Close the deceased client's eyes, mouth, and jaw. • Reposition the body to the side if needed and carefully fold the hands.

References: Berry & Griffie, 2015; Matzo & Hill, 2015.

may depersonalize your care and give the family a sense that their deceased loved one is not valued. However, if there is a risk of exposure to body fluids, mucous membranes, or non-intact skin (e.g., replacing dentures, removing or adjusting tubes, placing absorbent pads under the client), the nurse will need to wear gloves according to standard precautions. If the client is in isolation, other precautions may have to be used during postmortem care, such as the use of personal protective equipment (PPE). Check your facility's policy and the guidelines of the Centers for Disease Control and Prevention (CDC) regarding additional precautions.

In addition to caring for the client and supporting the family, the nurse must ensure that facility policy and regulations are followed. Under U.S. federal law 99-5-9 of the Medicare regulations, hospitals must give family members an opportunity to authorize the donation of their loved one's organs or tissues as outlined by the Anatomical Gift Act. This should be done at the time of death or immediately after the client's death (Berry & Griffie, 2015). Depending on your facility policy and the laws in your state, only a person who is officially trained and authorized is allowed to approach the family for permission regarding organ donation.

Before preparing the client's body for viewing, the nurse must first verify with the authorized healthcare provider whether the body will be undergoing an autopsy or be sent to the medical examiner, as this will determine the procedure for postmortem care. Check the facility policy regarding postmortem care for deceased clients who are receiving autopsies. Regardless of whether or not the deceased client will be a medical examiner case or is receiving an autopsy, continue to provide thoughtful care for the deceased client and to the client's family. These measures will help the family as they continue to work through the grieving process.

APPLICATION OF THE NURSING PROCESS

Examples of Related ICNP Nursing Diagnoses, Expected Client Outcomes, and Nursing Interventions:

Nursing Diagnosis: Family grief

Supporting Data: Family expresses distress and withdrawal after the death of their loved one.

Expected Client Outcomes: The family will demonstrate effective coping mechanisms that will facilitate grief resolution as demonstrated by:

• willingness to verbalize and express feelings regarding loss of deceased loved one

• willingness to participate in support groups and bereavement care.

Nursing Intervention Examples: Ask family members if they would like to help give the "last bath" to their loved one, and ask the family members about any other preferences or special requests they may have. Allow the family to stay with their loved one as long as they wish.

Reference: International Classification for Nursing Practice. (n.d.). *eHealth & ICNP.* Retrieved from https://www.icn.ch/what-we-do/projects/ehealth-icnp.

CRITICAL CONCEPTS
Caring for a Client After Death

Client-Centered Care (CCC)

Respect for the client after death and during postmortem care is demonstrated through:

• protecting the integrity and dignity of the deceased client's body

• proper and respectful handling of the client's personal belongings

• providing bereavement and spiritual care for the family

• promoting autonomy for the client's family

• providing privacy and ensuring comfort for the client's family

• honoring cultural preferences and requests

• advocating for the family of the deceased client.

Infection Control (INF)

Healthcare-associated infection during postmortem care is prevented by:

- containment of microorganisms
- preventing and reducing the transfer of microorganisms
- reducing the number of microorganisms.

Safety (SAF)

Safety measures when providing postmortem care prevent harm by maintaining a safe care environment.

Communication (COM)

- When providing postmortem care, timely communication with and from other members of the healthcare team improves care and support of the client's family.
- Communication exchanges information (oral, written, nonverbal, or electronic) between two or more people.
- Documentation records information in a permanent legal record.

Evaluation (EVAL)

Evaluation of the outcomes allows the nurse to determine the efficacy of the care provided.

■ SKILL 8.5 Providing Postmortem Care

EQUIPMENT

Clean gloves and PPE, if there is a risk of exposure to body fluids
Bathing supplies (see Chapter 2)
Washcloths and towels
Shroud or morgue bag, if indicated by facility policy
ID tags, if indicated by facility policy
Secure bag for client's valuables
Disposable absorbent protective pads
Paper tape and soft circular bandages
Oral care supplies
Soft eye patches, if needed

BEGINNING THE SKILL

1. **SAF** Perform hand hygiene.
2. **CCC** Introduce yourself and explain the procedure to the family.
3. **SAF** Identify the deceased client by using at least two identifiers as required.

PROCEDURE

4. **SAF** Establish that death has occurred and that the client has no signs of life. Determine that the client is pronounced dead by the authorized healthcare provider. *Safety measures regarding the pronouncement of death by the authorized healthcare provider and identification of the deceased before and during postmortem care prevents harm and misidentification of the client.*
5. **CCC** Provide support to the deceased client's family and address their bereavement and spiritual needs. (see Skills 8.1 and 8.2.) (Note: Ask the family members if they have a spiritual leader or someone whom they prefer to be contacted.) *Promotes autonomy and shows respect.*
6. **COM** If family members are not present, verify that they have been notified by the authorized healthcare provider. Notify the facility chaplain if indicated and required by policy.
7. **COM** Ensure that the appropriate person (e.g., a certified organ donation requester) has been notified of the

death per facility policy. (Note: This procedure may vary depending on the facility.)

8. **COM** Determine from the authorized healthcare provider (prior to postmortem care) whether the deceased client's body will be autopsied or sent to the medical examiner.
9. **SAF** If the body will be autopsied or sent to the medical examiner:
   a. Leave all of the tubes in the client's body intact according to facility policy.
   b. Ensure that the original chart and consent forms remain with the client.
   c. Ensure that client identifications and all documentation remain with the client. *This prevents misidentification of the body in the morgue or medical examiner's office.*
10. **CCC** Ask the client's family members if they have preferences for the following:
    a. care of their loved one's body or special clothing they wish the client to wear
    b. how the bath is done or if they would like to help with the deceased client's final bath
    c. whether or not jewelry, such as a wedding ring, is to be left on deceased client
    d. how the room where the client will be viewed is set up (e.g., special flowers, music)
    e. if the deceased client needs to be placed in a certain position or face a certain direction
    f. if there are other family members or friends who will want to view the deceased client's body before transfer to morgue or funeral home
    g. if they have any other special requests for the care of their loved one's body.
11. **INF** Perform hand hygiene again and gather equipment.
12. **INF** Apply gloves and PPE if there is risk of exposure to body fluids and before removing any tubes. (Note: Check facility policy and CDC guidelines to determine if PPE is needed).

13. **CCC** Clean up any clutter in the room and ensure that environment is presentable to the family. *Cleaning up the room environment reduces the psychological stress of the death for the family.*

14. **CCC** Elevate the head of the deceased client's bed 20 to 30 degrees. *This prevents pooling of blood and discoloration of the face (Berry & Griffie, 2015; Matzo & Hill, 2015).*

15. **CCC** Place disposable absorbent pads under the deceased client as needed. *This prevents soiling and odor when the urinary and rectal sphincters relax (Berry & Griffie, 2015).*

16. **CCC** Remove heavy blankets or clothing and place a light sheet over the deceased client. *This prevents further discoloration and pressure on client's fragile skin (Berry & Griffie, 2015).*

17. **CCC** If the deceased client will not be sent to the medical examiner or receive an autopsy, remove, tie, or saline-lock the client's tubes and remove equipment as outlined by facility policy. If the client is in a home setting, double bag and dispose of tubes according to policy.

18. **CCC** Place dentures in the mouth and close the mouth and jaw. *Having the dentures in place will preserve the natural appearance of the client's face, and they must be put in before rigor mortis sets in.*

19. **CCC** Provide oral care and keep the mouth and lips moist. *This prevents mouth odor, irritation, and flaking caused by dryness of the mouth and improves the appearance of the mouth.*

20. **CCC** Close the deceased client's eyes and provide eye care. If you have difficulty closing the eyes, gently use soft gauze soaked in saline. *This preserves the client's natural appearance.*

21. **CCC** Use circular bandages and paper tape for draining wounds. Clean adhesive from the client's skin. *The deceased client's skin is fragile and tears easily. Circular bandages and paper tape will be easier on the skin than adhesive tape. Previous intravenous sites and puncture wounds from catheters may leak fluid after the client's tubes are removed (Matzo & Hill, 2015).*

22. **CCC** Bathe the deceased client with plain water and pat dry. Support the joints, straighten the extremities, and turn the client gently while bathing. Use aromatic tea or herbs if the family desires.

23. **CCC** Provide clean linens and pillows to gently position the client as the family desires.

24. **CCC** Encourage the family to comb the deceased loved one's hair and to keep a lock of hair as a keepsake if they wish. If the deceased client is a child, encourage the family to cuddle the child in a blanket. *This allows the family to participate in the loved one's care and facilitates the grieving process.*

25. **CCC** Ask the client's family if they would like for you to refer to the deceased client by name. *This shows the family that you respect and value their deceased loved one.*

26. **CCC** Allow family members to stay with their deceased loved one as long as they desire. *This may help the family's grieving and facilitate grief resolution.*

27. **CCC** Place jewelry or other valuables in a secure bag. If the family prefers that the client's wedding ring remain on the finger, tape it gently in place (Matzo & Hill, 2015). (Note: Some facilities require placing valuables in a safe until they can be signed out by the family.)

28. **CCC** Avoid using regular trash bags for the deceased client's personal belongings. *Placing the client's belongings in regular trash bags may be perceived by the family as disrespectful.*

29. **SAF** If the deceased client is in a home setting, offer to dispose of the client's medications according to the agency policy. Document a complete list (especially narcotics) of the client's medications, and ensure that another authorized person is a witness for the disposal. *Safety measures regarding proper disposal of medications after a client's death prevent harm to others.*

30. **CCC** Prepare the body for transfer to the morgue or contact the funeral home (that the client has selected) after the family and others have the opportunity to view the body. (Note: Ensure that the family has given permission for the transfer.) *Demonstrates respect for family autonomy.*

31. **CCC** Avoid tying the deceased client's extremities tightly across the body. *Using ropes or tight strings on a deceased client's extremities can cut into the skin, causing wounds.*

32. **SAF** Ensure that the deceased client has identification forms and tags as determined by facility policy, and ensure that identification is securely fastened. *This prevents misidentification.*

33. **CCC** If the deceased client is going to the morgue, place the body gently on a gurney. Cover the body with sheets or place in a shroud. (Note: This may vary depending on the facility.)

34. **CCC** Attend the client's transfer to the morgue by using a private elevator as indicated by policy. *This protects the client and family's privacy and prevents the distress of other people in the facility.*

35. **INF** Remove linens and clean gurney after use as indicated by facility policy.

FINISHING THE SKILL

36. **INF** Remove gloves and PPE (if worn for removing tubes or due to risk of exposure to body fluids).

37. **INF** Perform hand hygiene.

38. **EVAL** Evaluate the outcomes. Did the client's skin remain intact during postmortem care?

39. **COM** Document the assessment findings, care given, and outcomes in the legal record.

40. **CCC** Provide follow-up care for the family, if allowed by facility policy, which may include:
    a. assisting the family with phone calls or contacting other family members and friends
    b. assisting the family with further arrangements for memorial services or a funeral home
    c. assessing the family for grief reactions and referring for further services if indicated
    d. sending cards and making follow-up calls if indicated and allowed by policy.

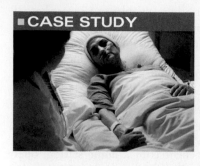

■ CASE STUDY

Beth Cavuto is a 47-year-old woman admitted to the medical-surgical unit from the intensive care unit (ICU) with a diagnosis of terminal metastatic lung cancer. She has an advance directive and a DNR order on her chart. She is also a single mother of two children, ages 8 and 10. The transfer report from the ICU indicates that Ms. Cavuto's mother and children visit frequently.

On admission, the nurse performs a comprehensive assessment. Ms. Cavuto has mild dyspnea, and her respiratory rate is approximately 25 to 28 per minute. In addition, Ms. Cavuto is complaining of having some trouble "catching my breath." She is becoming increasingly restless and has an anxious look on her face. As part of the spiritual assessment, the nurse asks Ms. Cavuto if she has a spiritual leader she would like to have contacted. The nurse also notes that Ms. Cavuto has a small Bible, a colorful scarf, and numerous cards on her bedside table. During the assessment, Ms. Cavuto asks, "What are your visiting hours? My kids need me!"

Several days after Ms. Cavuto is admitted, she becomes increasingly unresponsive. The nurse continues to provide comfort care to Ms. Cavuto, and she addresses her by name. She also allows flexible visiting hours. In addition, extra seating is provided in the room. While Ms. Cavuto's mother is in the room, she asks the nurse, "Do you think Beth can hear me?"

After 4 days on the medical-surgical unit, Ms. Cavuto dies while her family is at her bedside. Ms. Cavuto's young son runs out of the room, and her daughter clutches her mother's scarf and wraps it tightly around her shoulders. The nurse comforts Ms. Cavuto's family and offers to stay and contact their spiritual leader. After first determining from the authorized healthcare provider that Ms. Cavuto will not need an autopsy, the nurse begins to prepare Ms. Cavuto's body for viewing by other family and friends. Before beginning her postmortem care, the nurse asks Ms. Cavuto's mother if she has any special requests or preferences regarding her care.

Case Study Questions

1. Considering Ms. Cavuto's diagnosis of terminal cancer, her signs and symptoms on admission, and her DNR status, what is the nurse's immediate priority regarding her care?
2. Identify spiritual, bereavement, or possible referral needs Ms. Cavuto and her family may have.
3. During the initial assessment, Ms. Cavuto asks the nurse about visiting hours and states, "My children need me!" How can the nurse respond in a therapeutic way?
4. As Ms. Cavuto faces imminent death, she becomes increasingly unresponsive. How can the nurse respond to Ms. Cavuto's mother when she asks, "Do you think Beth can hear me when I talk to her?" What additional advice and care could the nurse offer to the family?
5. Immediately after Ms. Cavuto's death, the children have an emotional response. Considering their age, how is their reaction helping them cope with the death of their mother? How can the nurse respond in a therapeutic way at this time?
6. Before and after Ms. Cavuto's death, the nurse does several things that show respect and cultural/spiritual sensitivity for Ms. Cavuto and her family. Describe these interventions, and describe additional ways the nurse could help Ms. Cavuto and her family.
7. Describe how the nurse can prepare Ms. Cavuto's body after death for viewing in order to optimize her physical appearance.
8. Evidence has shown that providing bereavement support after a client's death may be helpful (Box 8.9). In this scenario, discuss how the nurse can facilitate the grieving process for Ms. Cavuto's family after her death and during postmortem care. What are some possible follow-up interventions the nurse might do to facilitate the family grieving process?
9. **Application of QSEN Competencies:** Two of the Quality and Safety Education for Nurses (QSEN) skills for Patient-Centered Care are to "Assess levels of physical and emotional comfort" and to "Provide patient-centered care with sensitivity and respect for the diversity of human experience" (Cronenwett et al., 2007). How does the nurse demonstrate these competencies with respect to Ms. Cavuto and her family?

BOX 8.9 Lessons From the Evidence: Bereavement Support for the Family

Although more research is needed, there is evidence that family members may benefit from bereavement care after the death of their loved ones in the intensive care unit (ICU). This care may include, but not be limited to, bereavement support from ICU staff, follow-up family meetings and bereavement services, and staff debriefing. It should also be noted that bereavement support must begin before the client has died (Ganz, 2019).

A recent pilot investigation (which examined prolonged grief, posttraumatic stress, depression, anxiety, and ICU satisfaction), found that a group of family members (N = 30) who received bereavement support interventions after the death of their loved ones in an ICU setting had significantly reduced prolonged grief compared with a group of family members who had not received the bereavement support interventions (N = 10). Although not statistically significant, the findings also revealed that the family members who had received the bereavement support interventions had lower posttraumatic stress disorder (PTSD) scores than the group that did not receive support interventions (McAdam & Puntillo, 2018). The bereavement support interventions consisted of receiving a brochure that contained information related to grieving and other information such as funeral and financial arrangements. The bereavement support group also received condolence cards signed by ICU staff, resource packets with practical information and referral information regarding support groups. In addition, the bereavement support group received follow-up calls from the ICU staff within 4 to 5 weeks. Both groups completed and returned surveys 13 months after the deaths of their loved ones. The investigators acknowledged that this study had some limitations due to the small sample sizes. In addition, the study took place in one large academic center on the West Coast (McAdam & Puntillo, 2018).

In summary, follow-up bereavement care may be beneficial for many families. However, more studies are needed in different clinical settings with larger sample sizes and diverse populations.

■ CONCEPT MAP

ICNP Nursing Dx: Risk for Dysfunctional Grief

Supporting Data:
Single mother
Concern about children
Anxiety

Facilitate Grieving Process for Client and Family Before Death

- Allow flexible visiting hours
- Use therapeutic communication
- Encourage family to talk to and read with the client
- Provide comfortable seating and sleeping couches
- Answer questions

Facilitate Grieving for Family Near the Time of Death and After Death

- Allow family to stay as long as desired with client
- Refer to client by name if okay with family
- Show respect during care
- Encourage family to keep mementos, such as a lock of hair

Baseline Assessment Data

- 47-year-old female with terminal metastatic cancer
- Written DNR order
- Two minor children
- Presence of spiritual and religious objects
- Increased restlessness
- Increased dyspnea
- Respirations 25-28/minute
- Stated concern about children/visiting hours
- Anxious expression

ICNP Nursing Dx: Discomfort

Supporting Data:
Respirations 25-28/minute
Complains of difficulty "catching my breath"
Increased restlessness
Anxious expression

Provide Spiritual Care

- Allow flexible visiting hours
- Contact chaplain or spiritual leader of client's choice if desired by client
- Allow client to keep personal, spiritual, and religious objects in room
- Offer prayer or scripture reading if desired by client

ICNP Nursing Dx: Readiness for Effective Spiritual Status

Supporting Data:
Spiritual objects in room

Promote Comfort

- Elevate head of bed
- Reposition or turn client to improve lung expansion
- Provide fan and direct cool air towards face
- Use relaxation techniques
- Enhance environment
- Confirm that oxygen is working properly

References

American Association of Colleges of Nursing. (2019). *End of life nursing education consortium (ELNEC) factsheet*. Retrieved from https://www.aacnnursing.org/Portals/42/ELNEC/PDF/ELNEC-Fact-Sheet.pdf.

American Nurses Association. (2016). *Nurses' roles and responsibilities in providing care and support at the end of life*. Retrieved from https://www.nursingworld.org/~4af078/globalassets/docs/ana/ethics/endoflife-positionstatement.pdf.

Baird, P. (2015). Spiritual care intervention. In B. R. Ferrell, N. Coyle, & J. A. Paice (Eds.), *Oxford textbook of palliative nursing* (4th ed.) (pp. 546–553). New York, NY: Oxford University Press.

Berry, P., & Griffie, J. (2015). Planning for the actual death. In B. R. Ferrell, N. Coyle, & J. A. Paice (Eds.), *Oxford textbook of palliative nursing* (4th ed.) (pp. 515–530). New York, NY: Oxford University Press.

Bowden, V. R., & Greenberg, C. S. (2014). *Children and their families: A continuum of care* (3rd ed.). Philadelphia, PA: Lippincott, Williams & Wilkins.

City of Hope (COH) & American Association of Colleges of Nursing (AACN). (2018a). ELNEC: End-of-Life Nursing Education Consortium–Core, Module 7: Loss, Grief, & Bereavement. Duarte, CA: Authors.

City of Hope (COH) & American Association of Colleges of Nursing (AACN). (2018b). ELNEC: End-of-Life Nursing Education Consortium–Core, Module 8: Final Hours of Life. Duarte, CA: Authors.

Corless, I. B. (2015). Bereavement. In B. R. Ferrell, N. Coyle, & J. A. Paice (Eds.), *Oxford textbook of palliative nursing* (4th ed.) (pp. 487–499). New York, NY: Oxford University Press.

Cronenwett, L., Sherwood, G., Barnsteiner J., Disch, J., Johnson, J., Mitchell, P., … Warren, J. (2007). Quality and safety education for nurses. *Nursing Outlook, 55*(3), 122–131. Retrieved from http://qsen.org/competencies/pre-licensure-ksas/.

Do not resuscitate: Nurse faulted for delay while looking for patient's code paperwork. (2010, April). *Legal Eagle Eye Newsletter for the Nursing Profession, 18*(4). Retrieved from http://www.nursinglaw.com/.

Ganz, F. D. (2019). Improving family intensive care unit experiences at the end of life: barriers and facilitators. *Critical Care Nurse, 39*(3), 52–58.

Hanson, P. A., & Andrews, M. M. (2016). Religion, culture, and nursing. In M. M. Andrews, & J. S. Boyle (Eds.), *Transcultural concepts in nursing care* (7th ed.) (pp. 394–446). Philadelphia, PA: Lippincott, Williams & Wilkins.

Hospice and Palliative Nurses Association. (2015). *HPNA position statement: Spiritual care*. Retrieved from https://advancingexpertcare.org/position-statements.

Institute of Medicine. (2015). *Dying in America: Improving quality and honoring individual preferences near the end of life*. Washington, DC: National Academies Press.

International Classification for Nursing Practice. (n.d.). *eHealth & ICNP*. Retrieved from https://www.icn.ch/what-we-do/projects/ehealth-icnp.

The Joint Commission. (2017). *Standards, FAQ details. Medical record—spiritual assessment*. Retrieved from https://www.jointcommission.org/standards/standard-faqs/hospital-and-hospital-clinics/provision-of-care-treatment-and-services-pc/ka0440000004rbh/.

Johnston-Taylor, E. (2015). Spiritual assessment. In B. R. Ferrell, N. Coyle, & J. A. Paice (Eds.), *Oxford textbook of palliative nursing* (4th ed.) (pp. 531–545). New York, NY: Oxford University Press.

Kübler-Ross, E. (1969). *On death and dying*. New York, NY: Macmillan.

Matzo, M., & Hill, J. A. (2015). Peri-death nursing care. In M. Matzo, & D. Witt-Sherman (Eds.), *Palliative care nursing: Quality care to the end of life* (pp. 649–674). New York, NY: Springer.

McAdam, J. L., & Puntillo, K. (2018). Pilot study assessing the impact of bereavement support on families of deceased intensive care unit patients. *American Journal of Critical Care, 27*(5), 372–380.

National Cancer Institute, U.S. National Institutes of Health. (2015). *Advance directives*. Retrieved from https://www.cancer.gov/about-cancer/managing-care/advance-directives.

National Cancer Institute, U.S. National Institutes of Health. (2019a). *Grief, bereavement, and coping with loss. PDQ® health professional version*. Retrieved from https://www.cancer.gov/about-cancer/advanced-cancer/caregivers/planning/bereavement-hp-pdq.

National Cancer Institute, U.S. National Institutes of Health. (2019b). *Last days of life. PDQ® health professional version*. Retrieved from https://www.cancer.gov/about-cancer/advanced-cancer/caregivers/planning/last-days-hp-pdq.

National Consensus Project for Quality Palliative Care. (2018). *Clinical practice guidelines for quality palliative care* (4th ed.). Richmond, VA: National Coalition for Hospice and Palliative Care, 2018. Retrieved from https://www.nationalcoalitionhpc.org/ncp/.

National Institutes of Health. (2004). *National Institutes of Health state of the science conference statement on improving end of life care*. Retrieved from http://consensus.nih.gov/2004/2004EndOfLifeCareSOS024html.htm.

Perrin, K. O. (2015). Legal aspects of end-of-life decision making. In M. Matzo, & D. Witt-Sherman (Eds.), *Palliative care nursing: Quality care to the end of life* (pp. 61–90). New York, NY: Springer.

Post, L. F., & Boltz, M. (2016). Advance directives. In M. Boltz, E. Capezuti, T. Fulmer, & D. Zwicker (Eds.), *Evidence-based geriatric nursing protocols for best practice* (5th ed.) (pp. 691–701). New York, NY: Springer.

Witt-Sherman, D., & Free, D. (2015). Culture and spirituality as domains of quality palliative care. In M. Matzo, & D. Witt-Sherman (Eds.), *Palliative care nursing: Quality care to the end of life* (pp. 91–128). New York, NY: Springer.

World Health Organization. (n.d.). *WHO definition of palliative care*. Retrieved from http://www.who.int/cancer/palliative/definition/en/.

World Health Organization. (2018). *The top 10 causes of death. Fact sheet*. Retrieved from http://www.who.int/mediacentre/factsheets/fs310/en/.

Yoost, B. L., & Crawford, L. R. (2016). *Fundamentals of nursing. Active learning for collaborative practice*. St. Louis, MO: Elsevier.

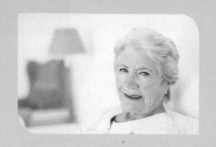

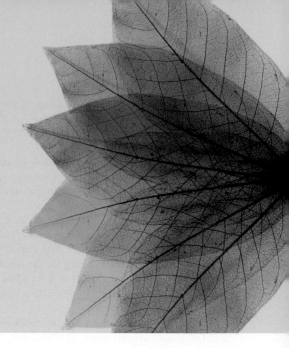

CHAPTER 9

Airway and Breathing

"How do you tell if something's alive? You check for breathing." | **Markus Zusak, Author of *The Book Thief***

LEARNING OBJECTIVES

By the end of this chapter, the reader will be able to:

1 Discuss principles of respiration, ventilation, and oxygenation.

2 Describe a nursing assessment of a client's respiratory status.

3 Instruct the client in appropriate methods for deep-breathing and coughing exercises.

4 Instruct the client in the use of an incentive spirometer.

5 Perform manual chest physiotherapy, percussion, and vibration with postural drainage.
6 Demonstrate safe use of a pressurized oxygen cylinder.
7 Identify key features when using an oxygen regulator and flowmeter.
8 Demonstrate administration of oxygen by nasal cannula.
9 Compare the advantages and disadvantages between oxygen administration by the following masks: simple face mask, OxyMask™, Venturi mask, nonrebreather, face tent, and tracheostomy collar.
10 Describe principles of administering oxygen using continuous positive airway pressure (CPAP).

11 Insert an oropharyngeal or nasopharyngeal airway.
12 Suction a nasopharyngeal airway.
13 Suction an artificial airway: endotracheal tube or tracheostomy.
14 Identify indications for and complications of airway suctioning.
15 Collect a sputum specimen using a sputum trap.
16 Identify and describe appropriate responses to tracheostomy emergencies.
17 Provide routine care for a client with a tracheostomy, including cleaning the stoma site and changing tracheostomy ties.

TERMINOLOGY

Alveoli (alveolus) A thin-walled, saclike terminal dilation of the respiratory bronchioles, alveolar ducts, and alveolar sacs across which gas exchange occurs between alveolar air and pulmonary capillaries.

Apnea Temporary cessation of breathing and, therefore, of the body's intake of oxygen and release of carbon dioxide.

Atelectasis Loss of air in all or part of the lung as a result of collapsed alveoli, with resulting loss of lung volume.

Carina (tracheae) Ridge at the lower end of the trachea that separates the left and right bronchi.

Consolidation Solidification into a mass; most often applied to the swelling and hardening of lung tissue as a result of inflammation and exudate in the alveoli, as commonly seen in pneumonia.

Cyanosis Characterized by blue, gray, dark purple, or slate coloration of the skin and/or mucous membranes secondary to unoxygenated hemoglobin.

Dyspnea Shortness of breath, a subjective difficulty or distress in breathing.

Expectorate To spit out saliva or cough up mucus or phlegm from the air passageways leading to the lungs.

Flange A border that projects above the main structure, such as a rim. Artificial airways may have a flange to help keep the airway in place.

Manometer An instrument for measuring the pressure of gases and vapors (e.g., a pressure gauge).

Splinting Stabilizing the abdominal area during coughing to minimize pain.

Stoma An artificially created opening between two passages or body cavities or between a cavity or passage and the body's surface.

Tidal volume The volume of air displaced between inhalation and exhalation (i.e., a normal breath volume); the average volume for an adult male is 500 mL and for an adult female is 400 mL.

Tidaling Periodically rising and falling, increasing and decreasing.

Tracheostomy A surgical procedure performed to create an opening into the trachea.

Tracheal necrosis Death of cells or tissues in the trachea.

Tracheal stenosis Narrowing of the trachea.

Vital capacity The greatest volume of air that can be exhaled from the lungs after a maximum inspiration.

ACRONYMS

BiPAP Bilevel positive airway pressure
BVM Bag-valve mask; also called a manual resuscitator
COPD Chronic obstructive pulmonary disease
FiO$_2$ The fractional concentration of oxygen
LTOT Long-term oxygen therapy
MDI Metered-dose inhalers
NPA Nasopharyngeal airway
OPA Oropharyngeal airway
OSA Obstructive sleep apnea
SO$_2$ Oxygen saturation

This chapter discusses basic skills related to supporting and maintaining the client's respiratory system: breathing, oxygenation, and establishing and maintaining an open airway. This chapter describes tracheostomy care, including postoperative and routine care, suctioning, and collecting a sputum sample. Advanced skills related to respiratory care, such as mechanical ventilation and obtaining arterial blood gases, are discussed in Chapter 18.

The process of breathing, or ventilation, allows gaseous exchange through the movement of air into and out of the lungs. Inhaled oxygen from the atmosphere passively diffuses from the alveoli of the lungs into the pulmonary capillaries and then binds to hemoglobin in the red blood cells or dissolves into the plasma. Once the oxygen is bound to the hemoglobin, it is transported to the body's tissues via the blood in a process known as perfusion. The vital function of breathing and perfusion is to provide oxygen to the body's organs and tissue.

Oxygen is removed from the blood by the tissues through the process of cellular respiration. The by-products of cellular respiration are carbon dioxide and water, along with energy. These by-products are transported back to the lungs,

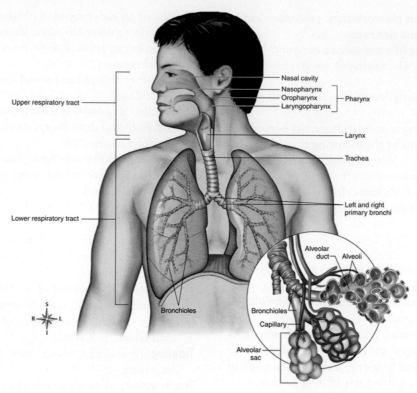

FIG. 9.1 Anatomy of the lungs and associated structures. The respiratory tract includes the nasal cavity, pharynx, larynx, trachea, bronchi, and lungs. The inset shows the alveolar sacs, where the grape-like alveoli interface with the pulmonary vasculature for the gaseous exchange of oxygen and carbon dioxide.

where carbon dioxide diffuses across the alveoli and is removed during exhalation. In order for this to occur, the anatomical and functional structures of the lung and airways must be intact (Fig. 9.1). The structures at risk are the alveoli, which may collapse, resulting in a loss of air volume, or fill with secretions. Nurses assist the client in keeping the grape-like alveoli fully inflated and free of secretions. Fig. 9.2 shows illustrations of alveoli.

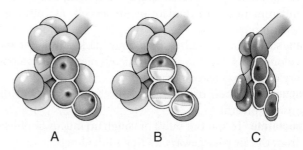

FIG. 9.2 A, Normal bronchiole and alveoli. **B,** Fluid filling alveoli. **C,** Collapse of alveoli.

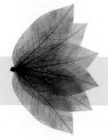

SECTION 1   Maintaining the Health of the Respiratory System

In order to facilitate optimal ventilation and oxygenation and to prevent respiratory disorders, it is important to maintain the integrity of the respiratory system and the effectiveness of the client's breathing pattern. In this text, one of the critical concepts is health maintenance. The American Nurses Association (ANA) scope of practice includes the statement that nursing is the optimization of health and abilities (ANA, 2017). In this section of the chapter, the health maintenance critical concept applies to

optimizing the health of the respiratory system. Teaching client ways to provide self-care, such as deep breathing and splinting when coughing, arms the client with the strategies to improve or maintain the physical health of the body. This section covers instructing the client in deep-breathing and coughing exercises, instructing the client to use incentive spirometry, and performing pulmonary chest physiotherapy, all of which are useful tools in maintaining the respiratory system by promoting oxygenation, expanding the alveoli, and mobilizing secretions. Client education is typically not delegated; therefore, instructions would be given by a registered nurse. Performing chest physiotherapy may be delegated, but the assessment and evaluation of the client's respiratory status must be performed by the registered nurse.

Clients most at risk include those coming to the hospital for surgery. Postoperative pulmonary complications account for 25% of deaths following surgery. Pulmonary complications occur with variations in likelihood based on the type of surgery and history of the client (Beddoe & Engelke, 2018). Clients may be weak after surgery, and incision sites are often painful. This may prevent clients from wanting to engage in deep-breathing and coughing exercises. In fact, when people are in pain, their inspiratory capacity may be only one-half to three-quarters of the preoperative measurement (Beddoe & Engelke, 2018). Shallow breathing is ineffective for inflating the alveoli and mobilizing secretions.

DEEP BREATHING AND COUGHING

Deep-breathing and coughing exercises help keep the client's lungs inflated and prevent pulmonary complications. Teaching the client to splint the incision with a pillow and providing pain medications prior to the exercises can help the client actively participate. Pursed-lip breathing can also assist the client who is having difficulty breathing because it maintains the pressure in the airways and thereby prevents the collapse of the airways. While doing the exercises, the client may naturally cough or should be encouraged to cough because this will help mobilize secretions. As secretions are mobilized, it is important to provide the client tissues, an emesis basin, and/or a Yankauer suction catheter to remove the secretions from the oral cavity. This will help promote comfort and contain microorganisms present in the secretions. If the client has an infection that can be transmitted by droplets, then the client will be placed on Transmission-Based Precautions, and the nurse's PPE will include wearing a mask.

INCENTIVE SPIROMETRY

Deep breathing with a visual and objective measurement of the inspiratory volume is accomplished with an incentive spirometer. The incentive spirometer is a device that contains one or more chambers, a mouthpiece, and a scale of inspiratory volumes where goals can be marked. There are two types of inspiratory

spirometers. One is based on airflow and has a freely moving plastic ball. As the client inhales, the ball rises. The goal for the client is to both reach a specific level and hold the ball. The second type is an air-volume model equipped with a small bellow that raises up as the client inhales to reach a specific desired level. The incentive spirometer is often used after surgery or after a respiratory illness such as pneumonia in order to improve the functioning of the client's lungs. The client is encouraged to set goals and inhale at a predetermined flow or target volume. The American Association of Respiratory Care has established the following clinical guidelines for the use of incentive spirometry:

- Use every hour when awake for 10 breaths.
- Hold an inhalation for 3 to 5 seconds.
- Provide adequate pain management to promote deep breathing.
- Incentive spirometry should not be used alone but, rather, in conjunction with deep breathing, coughing, and early ambulation.

Incentive spirometry is contraindicated for those who lack the fine motor skills, those who are confused or uncooperative, and those who are unable to generate adequate inspiration to move the ball or bellows. Although incentive spirometry is widely used, there is no sound evidence supporting improved outcomes with the use of incentive spirometry over deep breathing and coughing alone (Beddoe & Engelke, 2018).

CHEST PHYSIOTHERAPY

A third strategy to optimize the health of the respiratory system is chest physiotherapy. *Chest physiotherapy* (CPT) is a collective term that includes the use of percussion, vibration, forced expiration or huffing, and a series of positions that allow gravity to assist in the clearance of airway secretions. The first of these, manual percussion, is administered by the caregiver rhythmically clapping each lung lobe in a systematic pattern. The clapping is done with a cupped hand to create a gentle vibration of the chest wall. The client is then positioned to maximize secretion drainage from each lobe during the percussion. Fig. 9.3 shows how positioning the client can facilitate the movement and expulsion of secretions. CPT was once prescribed to individuals with many different pulmonary diagnoses. Today, rigorous evidence-based research has shown that although it is an

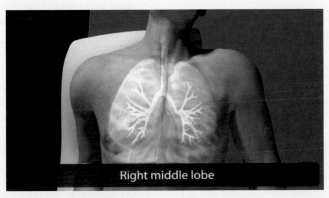

Right middle lobe

FIG. 9.3 Postural drainage positions the client to facilitate the movement and expulsion of secretions during chest physiotherapy.

effective intervention to assist individuals in transporting and expelling sputum, it also has limitations. It has long been and continues to be an effective intervention for those with cystic fibrosis (Warnock & Gates, 2015). It is recommended for those with bronchiectasis and may help those with chronic obstructive pulmonary disease (COPD) (Obeid, 2018a). Even when manual CPT is indicated, it has significant limitations, including how time consuming it is to complete in all of the postural drainage positions and that the efficacy is tied to the skill and strength of the caregiver. It is not recommended as a routine intervention for either adults or children with pneumonia, and it is not recommended for infants with bronchiolitis or those on mechanical ventilation (Giles, 2018a, 2018b; Paull, 2017; Slade, 2018). The use of metered-dose inhalers (MDIs) and nebulizer procedures, which are also strategies to improve lung function, are covered in the medication administration chapter (see Chapter 11).

RESPIRATORY SYSTEM-SPECIFIC ASSESSMENT

After completing any of the three interventions described previously, your evaluation of the client's respiratory system is critical to determine the impact of the intervention on the client's respiratory health. Objective parameters such as respiratory rate, inspiratory volume, and oxygen saturation are compared with your pre-intervention assessment data. Observation of the client's respiratory effort and use of accessory muscles to assist with breathing is noted. Auscultation of bilateral breath sounds in all lobes is another means of evaluation as you compare air movement and the presence of adventitious breath sounds before and after the intervention. Subjective assessments are also important because clients are often the best source of determining changes in the status of their respiratory systems. Lastly, you evaluate how the client tolerated the skills related to maintaining the integrity and effectiveness of the respiratory system. A chapter section on assessing respirations is located in Chapter 3.

APPLICATION OF THE NURSING PROCESS

Examples of Related International Classification for Nursing Practice (ICNP) Nursing Diagnoses, Expected Client Outcomes, and Nursing Interventions:

Nursing Diagnosis: Impaired breathing

Supporting Data: Client has shallow breathing, dyspnea, and decreased vital capacity.

Expected Client Outcomes: Client will resume effective breathing.

- Client's respiration rate will return to baseline.
- Client will demonstrate increased depth and ease of breathing without shortness of breath.
- Client will demonstrate effective deep breathing and coughing and/or effective use of incentive spirometer and achieve recommended goal.

Nursing Intervention Example: Instruct the client in deep-breathing and coughing exercises and in the use of incentive spirometry.

Reference: International Classification for Nursing Practice. (n.d.). *eHealth & ICNP.* Retrieved from https://www.icn.ch/what-we-do/projects/ehealth-icnp.

CRITICAL CONCEPTS
Maintaining the Health of the Respiratory System

Accuracy (ACC)

Accuracy in maintaining the health of a client's respiratory system is affected by the following variables:

Client-Related Factors
- Client's age, medical history, and medical status
- Client's level of consciousness and orientation
- Client's ability to follow instructions
- Client's fine motor skills
- Client's pain/discomfort level
- Hydration and ability to mobilize secretions

Nurse-Related Factors
- Positioning of the client
- Assessment of the client's respiratory status, oxygenation status, and breath sounds
- Assessment and treatment of the client's level of pain/discomfort
- Assessment of the client's level of cooperation, understanding, and fine motor skills
- Proper placement of cupped hands for percussion and vibration
- Instructing the client in the proper technique (e.g., deep breathing and using incentive spirometry)

Equipment-Related Factors
- Identifying volume to be achieved for incentive spirometry

Client-Centered Care (CCC)

Respect for the client when maintaining the health of a client's respiratory system is demonstrated through:
- explaining the procedure, providing instruction, and promoting autonomy
- providing culturally sensitive explanations and arranging for an interpreter, if needed
- answering questions that the client or family may have
- providing privacy and ensuring comfort.

Infection Control (INF)

Healthcare-associated infection when maintaining the health of a client's respiratory system is prevented by:
- containment of microorganisms in pulmonary secretions
- preventing and reducing the transfer of microorganisms
- reducing the number of microorganisms.

Safety (SAF)

When maintaining the health of a client's respiratory system, safety measures prevent harm and provide a safe care environment, including:
- providing working suction for airway clearance.

Communication (COM)

- Communication exchanges information (oral, written, nonverbal, or electronic) between two or more people.
- Documentation records information in a permanent legal record.
- Collaboration with the client, the client's family, and other healthcare professionals improves care when maintaining the health of the respiratory system.

Health Maintenance (HLTH)

Nursing is dedicated to the promotion of health and abilities related to maintaining the health of a client's respiratory system.

Evaluation (EVAL)

Evaluation of outcomes enables the nurse to determine the efficacy of the care provided, including:

- monitoring client for secretion mobilization and deep breathing
- monitoring the client's respiratory and oxygenation status

■ SKILL 9.1 Instructing a Client in Deep-Breathing and Coughing Exercises

EQUIPMENT

Stethoscope
Tissues
Emesis basin
Personal protective equipment, if transmission precautions are ordered
Clean gloves
Pillow for splinting, if indicated
Yankauer suction catheter with wall suction set-up for oral secretions, if needed
Pulse oximeter and sensor

BEGINNING THE SKILL

1. **INF** Perform hand hygiene and apply personal protective equipment (PPE) if indicated.
2. **INF** Apply gloves, if the client has a productive cough and you handle soiled tissues.
3. **CCC** Introduce yourself to the client and family and explain the procedure.
4. **SAF** Identify the client using two identifiers.
5. **CCC** Provide privacy. Close the door and pull the curtain.

PROCEDURE

6. **ACC** Assist the client to a comfortable sitting position. The bed may be in the semi-Fowler (head of bed 30 degrees) or Fowler position (head of bed ≥45 degrees). *Allows optimal lung expansion and improved ventilation, which increases blood oxygenation.*
7. **ACC** Assess the client for the following:
   - respiratory rate, effort, and use of accessory muscles
   - bilateral breath sounds
   - any pain or discomfort (using a facility-approved pain tool)
   - oxygen saturation.
8. **CCC** If the client is having pain, provide pain medication at least 30 minutes before the procedure.
9. **ACC** Instruct the client to place the palms of his or her hands along lower borders of the anterior rib cage, with the tips of middle fingers lightly touching each other.

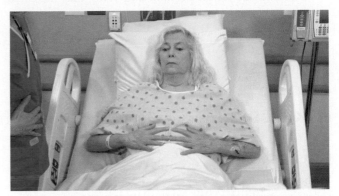

STEP 9 Place palms along lower borders of anterior rib cage, with tips of middle fingers lightly touching.

10. **ACC** Instruct the client to take slow, deep breaths, inhaling through the nose and pushing the abdomen with his or her hands. *Prevents hyperventilation, and breathing through the nose warms, humidifies, and filters air.*
11. **ACC** Instruct the client to hold his or her breath for 3 seconds and slowly exhale through the mouth using pursed-lip breathing. *Maintains the pressure in the airway to prevent large airways from collapsing.*
12. **HLTH** Encourage the client to cough after exercise. *To expectorate secretions.*
13. **CCC** Provide pillow splinting to support the incision, if indicated. Instruct the client to hold the pillow over the incision while coughing. *Provides comfort and support.*

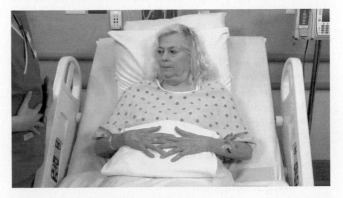

STEP 13 Provide pillow splinting.

14. **INF** Provide emesis basin and tissues for the client to expectorate secretions. Place trash container within reach to discard tissues as needed. Instruct the client in the importance covering his or her mouth and disposing of tissues.

15. **ACC** Encourage the client to practice this exercise 10 times each hour while awake.

16. **ACC** Assess the client's ability to mobilize secretions.

17. **SAF** Use a Yankauer suction catheter to assist the client with secretion removal, if needed. See Skill 2.8, Providing Oropharyngeal Suctioning With a Round-Tip Suction Tip (Yankauer).

FINISHING THE SKILL

18. **SAF** Ensure client safety and comfort. Ensure that the bed is in the lowest position and verify that the client

can identify and reach the nurse call system. *These safety measures reduce the risk of falls.*

19. **INF** Remove soiled gloves, remove PPE if worn, and perform hand hygiene.

20. **EVAL** Evaluate the outcomes.

21. **COM** Document assessment findings, care given, and outcomes in the legal healthcare record:
    * respiratory rate, depth, and effort
    * breath sounds
    * pulse oximetry values
    * instruction provided
    * how the client tolerated the procedure
    * sputum color, volume, and consistency if the client has a productive cough.

22. **EVAL** Monitor the client for ability to clear secretions from the airway and how the client is tolerating the activity.

■ SKILL 9.2 Instructing a Client to Use Incentive Spirometry

EQUIPMENT

Stethoscope
Incentive spirometer with appropriate mouthpiece
Tissues
Emesis basin
Pillow, if needed for splinting
PPE, if transmission precautions are ordered
Clean gloves
Yankauer suction catheter with wall suction set-up for oral secretions, if needed
Pulse oximeter and sensor

BEGINNING THE SKILL

1. **INF** Perform hand hygiene. Apply gloves, if client has a productive cough and you handle soiled tissues.

2. **CCC** Introduce yourself to the client and family and explain the procedure.

3. **SAF** Identify the client using two identifiers.

4. **CCC** Provide privacy. Close the door and pull the curtain.

PROCEDURE

5. **ACC** Position the client as upright as possible. *Allows optimal lung expansion and improved ventilation, which increases blood oxygenation.*

6. **ACC** Assess the client for the following:
   * respiratory rate, effort, and use of accessory muscles
   * bilateral breath sounds
   * any pain or discomfort (using a facility-approved pain tool)
   * oxygen saturation.

7. **CCC** Provide the client with a pillow for splinting, if indicated. *Splinting reduces pain and provides support by decreasing muscle movement at the incision site.*

8. **CCC** Instruct the client that the purpose of incentive spirometry is to prevent atelectasis (the loss of lung volume) and consolidation (fluid in the lungs).

9. **ACC** Show the client how to seal the mouthpiece.

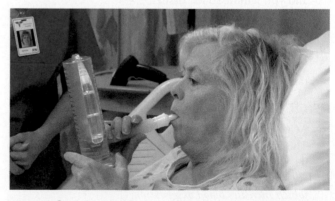

STEP 9 Seal the mouthpiece of the incentive spirometer.

10. **ACC** Encourage the client to exhale completely through the mouth before placing the lips around the mouthpiece.

11. **ACC** Identify the client's target volume on the incentive spirometer.

12. **ACC** Instruct the client to hold the incentive spirometer upright and to slowly, deeply, and continuously inhale.

13. **ACC** Inform the client that it is more beneficial to sustain maximum inhalation for 5 seconds than to quickly inhale and exhale. *The indicator should slowly rise to the*

level of the target set for the client. This facilitates slow, deep breathing.

14. **ACC** Instruct the client to hold his or her breath for 3 to 5 seconds or until reaching the maximum inhalation. *This allows for extended, maximum expansion of the lungs.*

15. **ACC** Advise the client to remove the mouthpiece and exhale completely.

16. **SAF** Allow the client to rest a for few seconds before resuming incentive spirometry, if necessary. *This prevents hyperventilation and fatigue.*

17. **ACC** Instruct the client to repeat the technique for the prescribed number of times, usually 10.

18. **HLTH** Instruct the client to cough at the end of the activity. *This helps the client expel mucus from the deeper airways.*

19. **INF** Provide an emesis basin and tissues for the client to expectorate secretions. Place trash container within reach to discard tissues as needed. Instruct the client in the importance covering his or her mouth and disposing of tissues.

20. **SAF** Use a Yankauer suction catheter to assist the client with secretion removal, if needed. (See Skill 2.8.)

21. **ACC** Encourage the client to use the incentive spirometer every hour while awake or as ordered.

22. **SAF** Instruct the client to notify the nurse if he or she experiences chest pain or an increase in sputum produc-

tion. *Chest pain may indicate a collapsed lung. Excessive sputum production may indicate infection.*

FINISHING THE SKILL

23. **SAF** Ensure client safety and comfort. Ensure that the bed is in the lowest position and verify that the client can identify and reach the nurse call system. *These safety measures reduce the risk of falls.*

24. **INF** Remove gloves, if worn. Perform hand hygiene.

25. **EVAL** Evaluate the outcomes.

26. **COM** Document assessment findings, care given, and outcomes in the legal healthcare record:
    * respiratory rate, depth, and effort
    * breath sounds
    * pulse oximetry values
    * instruction provided
    * how the client tolerated the procedure
    * sputum color, volume, and consistency, if the client has a productive cough.

27. **EVAL** Follow up to confirm that the client is using the spirometer correctly and to evaluate the effectiveness of the activity.

28. **EVAL** Determine if the client is able to increase the inspired volume with regular use.

■ SKILL 9.3 Performing Chest Physiotherapy (CPT)

EQUIPMENT

PPE, if transmission precautions are ordered

Clean gloves, if there is a risk of exposure to body fluids

Yankauer suction catheter with wall suction set-up for oral secretions, if needed

Tissues

Emesis basin

Towel

Stethoscope

Pulse oximeter and sensor

BEGINNING THE SKILL

1. **INF** Perform hand hygiene and apply PPE if transmission precautions are ordered.

2. **INF** Apply clean gloves if there is a risk of exposure to body fluids.

3. **CCC** Introduce yourself to the client and family and explain the procedure.

4. **SAF** Identify the client using two identifiers.

5. **CCC** Provide privacy. Close the door and pull the curtain.

PROCEDURE

6. **CCC** Assess the client for the following:
   * respiratory rate, effort, and use of accessory muscles
   * bilateral breath sounds
   * any pain or discomfort (using a facility-approved pain tool)
   * oxygen saturation.

7. **CCC** Administer prescribed pain medication if indicated.

8. **CCC** If the client is having pain, provide pain medication at least 30 minutes prior to initiating CPT.

9. **SAF** Determine time of most recent food intake. **WARNING:** If the client is receiving continuous tube feeding, discontinue at least 30 minutes prior to CPT

and wait 1.5 to 2 hours after meals for those receiving oral feedings. *Time without feeding before CPT prevents aspiration and emesis (Caple & Schub, 2017).*

10. **SAF** Apply pulse oximeter probe. Monitor vital signs and oxygen saturation throughout the procedure. If the client's oxygen saturation decreases or respiratory rate increases, this suggests the client is not tolerating the procedure and CPT should stop.

Percussion

11. **CCC** Cover the area to be percussed with a towel or gown to reduce discomfort.
12. **CCC** Encourage the client to breathe slowly and deeply to promote relaxation.
13. **ACC** Cup the hand with the fingers and thumbs held together and flexed slightly.
14. **ACC** Flex and extend the wrists rapidly, clapping the hands against the chest, alternating the hands in a rhythmic manner.

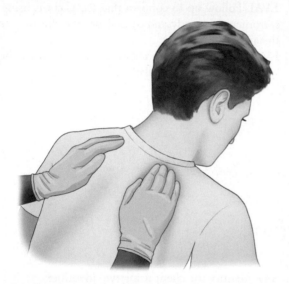

STEP 14 Flex and extend the wrists rapidly.

15. **ACC** Percuss each affected lung segment. **WARNING:** Avoid the spine, liver, kidneys, and spleen. *These areas are not lung segments, and percussing organs may cause damage.*

Vibration

16. **ACC** Place your hands, one over the other, palms down, on the chest area to be drained.

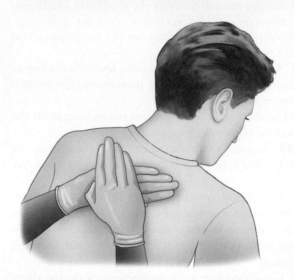

STEP 16 Place hands, one over the other, on the area of the chest to be vibrated.

17. **ACC** Keep fingers extended and together.
18. **ACC** Ask the client to inhale deeply and exhale slowly through the nose or pursed lips.
19. **ACC** During exhalation, tense your hand and arm muscles, and vibrate the heel of the hand, moving your hands downward over the ribs.
20. **ACC** Stop the vibration when the client inhales. *This allows maximum expansion of the lungs.*
21. **ACC** Repeat the procedure five times over the affected lung segment.
22. **CCC** Encourage the client to cough and expectorate into tissue or emesis basin.

Postural Drainage

The following positions are used for postural drainage.

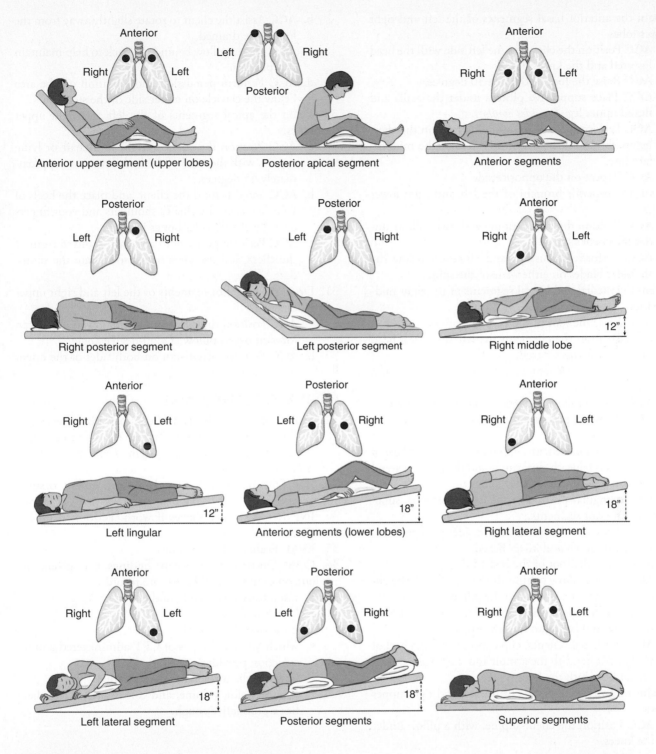

STEPS 23 TO 31 Positions for postural drainage

23. Drain the posterior basal segments of the left and right lower lobes.
    a. **ACC** Position the client prone, with the client's head lowered.
    b. **CCC** Place pillows under the chest and abdomen.
    c. **ACC** Raise the foot of the bed 30 degrees.
    d. **ACC** Perform percussion and vibration over the lower posterior ribs on either side of the spine
24. Drain the lateral basal segments of the lower lobes.

    a. **ACC** Position the client prone, with the head lowered and the upper leg flexed over a supportive pillow.
    b. **ACC** Assist the client in rotating a quarter of a turn upward.
    c. **ACC** Raise the foot of the bed 30 degrees.
    d. **ACC** Administer percussion and vibration on the lateral chest wall over the uppermost part of the lower ribs.

25. Drain the anterior basal segments of the left and right lower lobes.
    a. **ACC** Position the client on the left side with the head lowered and the knees flexed.
    b. **ACC** Raise the foot of the bed 30 degrees.
    c. **CCC** Place supportive pillows under the axilla and flexed upper leg. *Provides comfort.*
    d. **ACC** Perform percussion and vibration on the chest below the shoulder blades posterior to the midaxillary line.
    e. **ACC** Repeat on the opposite side.
26. Drain the superior bronchi of the left and right lower lobes.
    a. **ACC** Position the client supine with two pillows under the client's hips.
    b. **ACC** Perform percussion and vibration below the shoulder blades on either side of the spine.
27. Drain the medial and lateral segments of the right middle lobe.
    a. **ACC** Raise the foot of the bed 15 degrees.
    b. **ACC** Position the client on the left side, with head lowered and knees flexed.
    c. **ACC** Assist the client in rotating one-quarter of a turn backward.
    d. **ACC** Place a pillow beneath the client for support.
    e. **ACC** Perform percussion and vibration under the right nipple.
    f. **CCC** For female clients, cup hand so that the heel of the hand is beneath the armpit and the fingers extend forward beneath the breast.
28. Drain the lingular portion of the left upper lobe, superior and inferior segments.
    a. **ACC** Assist the client into a right side-lying position, with head down and knees flexed.
    b. **ACC** Raise the foot of the bed 15 degrees.
    c. **ACC** Place a pillow behind the back, and roll the client a quarter of a turn onto the pillow.
    d. **ACC** Perform percussion and palpate the area below the axilla and lateral to the left nipple.
    e. **ACC** For female clients, cup hand so that the heel of the hand is beneath the armpit and the fingers extend forward beneath the breast.
29. Drain the anterior segments of the left and right upper lobes.
    a. **ACC** Position the client supine, with a pillow under the knees.

    b. **ACC** Assist the client to rotate slightly away from the lobe to be drained.
    c. **ACC** Place a pillow behind the back to help maintain this position.
    d. **ACC** Perform percussion and vibration on the area below the clavicle on either side of the sternum.
30. Drain the apical segments of the left and right upper lobes.
    a. **ACC** Position the client upright in a chair or lying supine, with the head of the bed elevated to approximately 45 degrees.
    b. **ACC** Stand behind the client, and place the heels of your hands on the client's shoulders and your fingers over the client's collarbones in front.
    c. **ACC** Perform percussion, and then stand in front of the client and use your hands to vibrate the shoulders.
31. Drain the posterior segments of the left and right upper lobes.
    a. **ACC** Position the client in a sitting position, to lean forward over a pillow at a 30-degree angle.
    b. **ACC** Perform percussion on both sides of the upper spine.

FINISHING THE SKILL

32. **SAF** Ensure client safety and comfort. Place the bed in the lowest position and verify that the client can identify and reach the nurse call system. *These safety measures reduce the risk of falls.*
33. **INF** Discard soiled tissues. Rinse out emesis basin if necessary.
34. **INF** Remove soiled gloves if worn. Perform hand hygiene.
35. **EVAL** Evaluate the outcomes.
36. **COM** Document assessment findings, care given, and outcomes in the legal healthcare record:
    • respiratory rate, depth, and effort
    • breath sounds
    • pulse oximetry values
    • which lobes and types of CPT administered and instruction provided
    • how the client tolerated the procedure
    • sputum color, volume, and consistency, if the client has a productive cough.

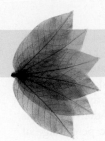

SECTION 2 **Administering Oxygen**

Oxygen is one of the essential elements for life. It is necessary for cellular metabolism. Without it, the body's tissues and organs cannot function or maintain homeostasis.

IMPAIRED GAS EXCHANGE

Acute conditions and chronic diseases can result in impaired gas exchange of oxygen and carbon dioxide, resulting in hypoxemia, a decreased level of oxygen in arterial blood, and/or carbon dioxide retention. Acute disorders that can cause hypoxia include pneumonia, burns, trauma, surgery, fever, and infections. Chronic pulmonary conditions such as COPD, pulmonary fibrosis, cystic fibrosis, asthma, and obstructive sleep apnea may interfere with both oxygenation and the elimination of carbon dioxide. Oxygen has historically been administered as a part of therapy for traumatic brain injuries, emergency surgery, resuscitation during cardiac arrest, and during episodes of hemorrhagic shock (Chu et al., 2018). In addition, impaired gas exchange can be the result of inadequate ventilation, which can occur during medical sedation, during anesthesia, or by drug overdose.

Inadequate oxygen triggers compensatory mechanisms. When our bodies identify the need for more oxygen, the first compensatory action is to breathe faster. (Imagine yourself running up a flight of stairs.) If an increase in respiratory rate does not provide the needed gas exchange, there will be an increase in the work of breathing. Our bodies will work hard and enlist the assistance of accessory muscles and strategies to pull air into the lungs and push air out.

When a client is at risk for impaired gas exchange, the nurse vigilantly assesses the respiratory system. Assess the client's respiratory status at regular intervals. Inspect the client's general appearance, posture, and breathing effort. The brain is a very sensitive organ. Note any changes in the client's behavior or mental status, such as confusion or changes in orientation. Assess and note the respiration rate, depth, and effort, noting any accessory muscle use. Auscultate breath sounds bilaterally and in all lung fields. Obtain a pulse oximeter and monitor oxygen saturation. An oxygen saturation of less than 90% in an individual without lung disease indicates hypoxia. Perfusion is dependent on adequate circulation, so the assessment of pulse, blood pressure, circulating blood volume, and anemia is also essential. Inspect the client's nailbeds for capillary refill, and inspect the client's skin and mucous membranes for discoloration. However, be aware that cyanosis is a very late sign of hypoxia. If the authorized healthcare provider is concerned about the degree of hypoxia, an arterial blood gas might be ordered. Arterial oxygenation is measured by the partial pressure of oxygen in the blood.

If compensatory mechanisms are insufficient, the person will become hypoxic. Untreated hypoxia can impair the physiologic function of all organ systems, trigger cardiac arrhythmias and/or heart failure, and cause the client's death.

Fortunately, the intervention of providing supplemental oxygen often relieves hypoxemia. Oxygen administration is measured in either the rate of flow (liters/minute) or the fractional concentration of oxygen measured as a percentage. The percentage of oxygen in room air is 21%. Providing supplemental oxygen can increase the fractional concentration of oxygen, which is referred to as the FiO_2.

Oxygen is considered a medication and must be administered within the parameters of the authorized healthcare provider's orders. However, emergent situations allow the administration of oxygen to sustain life. Oxygen can be lifesaving, but it is important to recognize that it can cause toxicity if high concentrations are administered for extended periods (Khanh-Dao Le, 2018). Sustained high concentrations of oxygen cause vasoconstriction and inflammation, resulting in stress to the pulmonary, cardiovascular, and neurological systems. A recent review of 16,000 records found clear evidence that the liberal use of oxygen is harmful. In fact, the liberal use of oxygen has a dose-dependent increased risk of short-term and long-term mortality (Chu et al., 2018). Thus, supplemental oxygen therapy should be administered at the lowest concentrations possible in order to achieve an oxygen saturation that is appropriate for the client's needs.

At-Risk Populations: COPD and Premature Infants

Some clients need lower oxygen levels than others. Two populations warrant additional discussion: clients with COPD and premature infants. Clients with COPD should not be given liberal supplemental oxygen. COPD encompasses a number of disease processes that are manifested in chronic, progressive, and irreversible limitations of airflow. Clients with COPD may have a high level of impaired gas exchange, with particular difficulty expelling carbon dioxide. For some clients, short-term oxygen therapy during activity or periods of shortness of breath may suffice. For other clients with advanced COPD, long-term oxygen therapy (LTOT) is generally used. Although some supplemental oxygen is beneficial and may prevent hypoxia, caution must be exercised. In healthy individuals, the respiratory drive is the result of hypercapnia (CO_2). However, in some individuals with COPD, the respiratory drive is based on hypoxia. If they are given too much oxygen, they lose the drive to breathe and will experience respiratory arrest. The guidelines for maintaining oxygen saturations for clients with COPD are often at lower levels, such as 89% to 92% (Fong, 2018). The second population is premature infants. Liberal supplemental oxygen is associated with retinopathy of prematurity (ROP), which can result in impaired vision or blindness. Although recent evidence indicates there may be a genetic risk in the development of ROP, there continues to be a correlation between higher oxygen saturations and higher incidence of ROP (Giles, 2018b).

USING A HIGH-PRESSURE OXYGEN CYLINDER

Pressurized oxygen cylinders (Fig. 9.4) are used when supplemental oxygen is needed for client transport or for clients who require home oxygen. The cylinder contains 100% pressurized oxygen gas. A regulator and flowmeter, along with tubing and a designated oxygen-delivery device, are connected to the cylinder to deliver the prescribed amount of oxygen. For additional safety guidelines when using a high-pressure oxygen cylinder, see Box 9.1.

Attaching the regulator to the oxygen cylinder and accurate use of the flowmeter are standard nursing activities. Leaks from the oxygen cylinder can generally be detected by listening for a hissing sound or checking to see whether or not the gauge reflects a loss of the oxygen when it is in the off position. Whenever possible, it is important to ensure ahead of time that the oxygen equipment is working properly and troubleshoot any problems delivering oxygen to the client.

ADMINISTERING SUPPLEMENTAL OXYGEN

The goal for oxygen therapy is to maintain adequate oxygenation of tissues and organ systems. If there is an increased demand for oxygen as a result of pain, fever, or agitation, then managing the source may lower oxygen demands and reduce oxygen consumption in some situations. When those interventions are not effective, supplemental oxygen is necessary.

In acute care settings, oxygen is available in wall outlets. A flowmeter is plugged into the wall outlet that regulates the flow of oxygen. A nut and nipple adapter, called a "Christmas tree," is screwed onto the flowmeter to connect to the client's oxygen tubing (Fig. 9.5). By regulating the rate on the flowmeter and using selected oxygen-delivery masks, supplemental oxygen can be administered from just slightly above room air to virtually 100% oxygen. These oxygen-delivery masks combine air and oxygen to deliver a specific percentage of oxygen to the client. The major types of supplemental oxygen-delivery devices are discussed in this section.

Oxygen Humidification

Humidification is sometimes added to oxygen therapy to moisturize the mucous membranes of the nose and mouth and to prevent the thickening of respiratory secretions. Only sterile deionized water is used for humidification. The

BOX 9.1 Safety Elements for Using High-Pressure Oxygen Cylinders

- Check the surroundings to verify that it is safe for oxygen usage.
- Post safety signage such as "Oxygen in Use" and "No Smoking."
- Secure the high-pressure oxygen cylinder in a designated oxygen stand.
- Assess the functioning of the cylinder valve by opening the regulator. Ensure the flowmeter is turned off if one is attached.
- Identify the amount of oxygen in the cylinder and determine that it is sufficient for the client during transport. (There should be >500 psi for client transport.) Determine if there is an oxygen source at the client's destination.
- Handle cylinders with care. Do not carry them, drag them, or roll them because damage may occur to the cylinder valve. A damaged valve may rapidly release oxygen and turn the high-pressure cylinder into a dangerous projectile.

Reference: Schub & Caple, 2018.

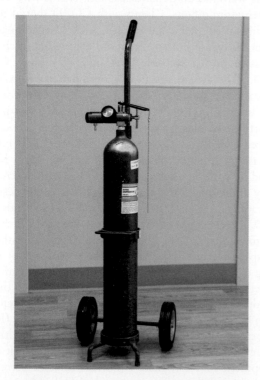

FIG. 9.4 Pressurized oxygen cylinder.

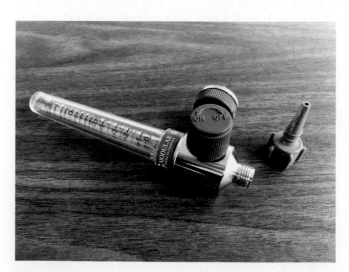

FIG. 9.5 Oxygen flowmeter and nut and nipple adapter (Christmas tree adapter).

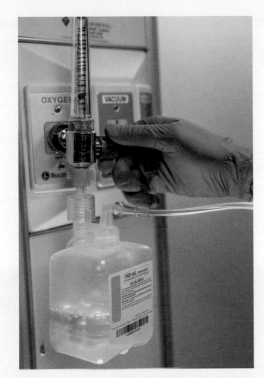

FIG. 9.6 A sterile water reservoir adds humidification to oxygen.

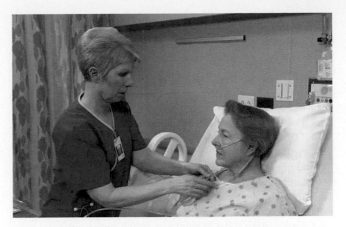

FIG. 9.7 Nasal cannula placed on a client.

TABLE 9.1 Nasal Cannula Flow Rate and Corresponding FiO₂

Flow rate	FiO$_2$
1 L/min	24%
2 L/min	28%
3 L/min	32%
4 L/min	36%
5 L/min	40%
6 L/min	44%

Reference: Schub & Heering, 2017.

reservoir connects to the oxygen flowmeter and has a connection for the oxygen tubing (Fig. 9.6). Humidity added to oxygen-delivery devices must be ordered by the authorized healthcare provider. One risk of using humidity reservoirs is that the tubing and/or the reservoirs may also become reservoirs for microorganisms, including bacteria or mold. Humidification is usually not indicated unless the oxygen flow is high enough to be very drying to the mucous membranes and to prevent condensation in the tubing (Smith, 2017).

Safety Measures

When oxygen is in use, safety measures include posting an "Oxygen in Use" sign and teaching clients and family members about avoiding smoking and open flames when using supplemental oxygen. Oxygen is not flammable, but it accelerates and supports combustion.

Nasal Cannula

Nasal cannulas consist of tubing that has two hollow prongs that fit into the client's nares. The tubing is connected to an oxygen source, and oxygen flows through the tubing into the nose (Fig. 9.7). The tubing for the nasal cannula is placed behind the ears, and this can cause skin irritation. Commercially prepared foam devices that connect to the oxygen tubing to protect the ears are available, but the use of a 2 × 2 gauze pad is also an effective intervention to prevent skin breakdown. The nasal cannula can be used for acute care situations or long-term administration of oxygen at home. The oxygen therapy delivered using a nasal cannula is from 0.5 to 6 L at concentrations less than or equal to 44% (Schub & Heering, 2017). Table 9.1 shows the percentage of oxygen delivered at each liter of flow.

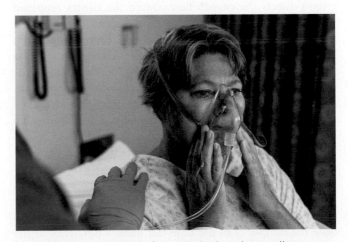

FIG. 9.8 A simple face mask placed on a client.

Simple Face Mask

A simple face mask, as seen in Fig. 9.8, is placed primarily over the client's nose and mouth. This type of oxygen mask is seen in acute care settings, outpatient clinics, or in emergency situations during care and transport to the hospital. The oxygen flowmeter is set at 5 to 10 liters per minute to deliver oxygen therapy at 40% to 60%. There are also vent holes located on each side of the simple face mask that allow the client to inhale room air (21% oxygen) that mixes with the supplemental oxygen. Notice that the lowest flow is much higher for a simple mask than for a nasal cannula.

BOX 9.2 Lessons From the Evidence: OxyMask™ Compared With Nonrebreather Mask

A study was conducted with manikin heads and carbon dioxide flow and oxygen delivery to compare oxygen administration and carbon dioxide clearance between the OxyMask™ and the nonrebreather mask. The masks were each tested at three different simulated respiratory rates (15, 20, and 24 breaths/min) and at two very different oxygen flow rates (2 and 15 L/min). The results show that at the higher rate of flow, both masks provide accurate oxygen and flush out the carbon dioxide. Note that this is within the recommended flow per minute for the nonrebreather mask. However, at 2 L/min, the fraction of inspired carbon dioxide level was much higher with the nonrebreather (4.9%) compared with the OxyMask™ (2.9%). (The carbon dioxide level in room air is less than 0.04%.) This study reinforced the need to be watchful for signs of imbalanced gas exchange in closed masks, especially at lower rates of flow.

Reference: Lamb & Piper, 2016.

TABLE 9.2 OxyMask™ Adult, Plus, and Kid Flow Rate and Approximate Corresponding FiO$_2$

Flow rate	FiO$_2$
1 L/min	24–27%
2 L/min	27–32%
3 L/min	30–60%
4 L/min	33–65%
5 L/min	36–69%
7 L/min	48–80%
10 L/min	53–85%
12 L/min	57–89%
>15 L/min	60–90%

Reference: Southmedic, n.d.

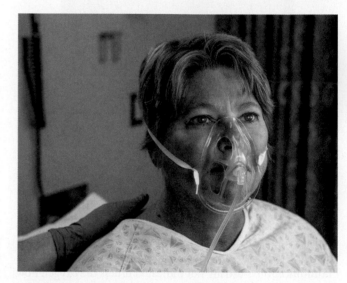

FIG. 9.9 OxyMask™ on a client.

There must be enough oxygen flow to chase out the expired carbon dioxide (Schub & Balderrama, 2017).

OxyMask™

There is a new type of open mask on the market that can deliver between 24% and 90% oxygen, and the rate of flow for the oxygen can range from 1 to 15 L/min. A pin and diffuser system directs the oxygen flow toward the client's nose and mouth. It comes in four sizes: adult, plus size, children aged 3 to 10 years, and infants and young children aged 6 months to 3 years. A significant advantage of OxyMask™, beyond the flexible oxygen delivery, is that carbon dioxide cannot accumulate, which is a safety concern with closed masks and inadequate flow. Box 9.2 presents a comparison of the OxyMask™ with a nonrebreather. In addition, clients can drink through a straw, do not have claustrophobic complaints, and can be easily understood when talking and wearing the mask. The open design allows humidity from the room to enter so that humidification may not be needed. The wide oxygen concentration range at each liter of flow is due to the individual characteristics of the client's breathing: respiratory rate, depth, and how close the diffuser is to the nose can make a difference in the percentage received. Table 9.2 shows the approximate percentage of oxygen delivered at each liter of flow for the Adult, Plus, and Kid masks. The OxyMask™ Tyke has a different rate of flow to oxygen percentage.

Venturi Face Mask

A Venturi face mask differs from a simple mask in that it fits over the client's nose, mouth, and chin. The mask has a large tube at the bottom that is connected to a Venturi valve. The valve may be adjustable or may be color-coded based on the percentage of oxygen delivery (Fig. 9.9). The settings on the valve are adjusted to determine the percentage of oxygen delivered, and the valve identifies the required liter/minute rate of flow needed to achieve that percentage. The Venturi mask can deliver between 24% and 50% oxygen, and the rate of flow for the oxygen meter can be set at 4 to 12 liters per minute depending on the required oxygen. Clients with CO$_2$ retention may benefit from this type of therapy because CO$_2$ escapes from the holes on the side of the mask (Schub & Balderrama, 2017).

Nonrebreather Mask

A nonrebreather mask looks like a simple mask but has a reservoir bag attached at the bottom, as well as one-way valves on the vent holes located on each side of the mask (Fig. 9.10). The bag is inflated using 6 to 15 liters per minute of oxygen flow for a full nonrebreather, and the mask delivers between 60% and 100 % oxygen therapy.

The one-way valves are removed from the vented holes of a nonrebreather mask for partial nonrebreather mask therapy. A partial nonrebreather requires the oxygen flowmeter to be set at 6 to 10 liters per minute for 40% to 70% oxygen therapy. Like the simple mask, the flow of oxygen must be set high enough to prevent the accumulation of carbon dioxide. The removal of one of the one-way valves increases the mixing of room air and increases the release of carbon dioxide. This type of oxygen therapy mask should be used only for short-term management of hypoxia because oxygen therapy in excess of 60% for extended periods can result in oxygen toxicity (Schub & Balderrama, 2017) (Fig. 9.11).

Face Tent

The face-tent mask provides oxygen therapy to the nose and mouth without the discomfort of a mask on the nose (Fig. 9.12). Clients who have facial trauma or burns or have had oral surgery may benefit from this method of oxygen delivery. Clients who feel claustrophobic with masks may also be more comfortable using face tents. The face tent allows clients to see and speak without the obstruction of a mask. The flow rate for face tents is 8 to 15 liters per minute at concentrations of 21% to 40%.

Tracheostomy Collar

Tracheostomy collars, also known as tracheal masks or T-pieces (Fig. 9.13), deliver continuous oxygen therapy to a client with a tracheostomy. The collar attaches to an oxygen source and may use a Venturi valve to adjust the oxygen percentage. Venturi valves allow the nurse to regulate oxygen delivery between 24% and 50%. Because a tracheostomy does not allow for the typical warming and humidification of air inspired through the nose and mouth, oxygen delivered via tracheostomy collar or T-piece is often humidified (Schub & Walsh, 2017).

Continuous Positive Airway Pressure

Continuous positive airway pressure (CPAP) delivers pressurized air that prevents airway collapse during inspiration and expiration (Fig. 9.14). CPAP is the first-line treatment for obstructive sleep apnea (OSA) (Slade, 2017). CPAP may also assist clients with respiratory insufficiency to continue breathing without the need for intubation. CPAP can be administered with room air or with supplemental oxygen. CPAP can be delivered using a full-face mask, a nasal mask, or specially designed nasal prongs/pillows (Fig. 9.15). For

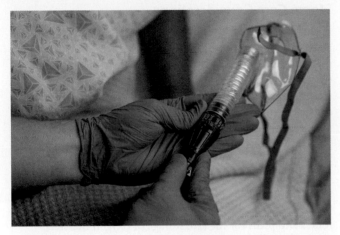

FIG. 9.10 Venturi mask with an adjustable valve.

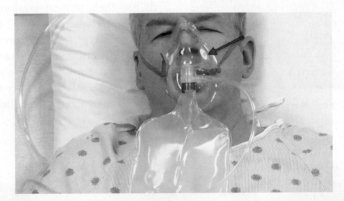

FIG. 9.11 Nonrebreather (reservoir) mask on a client. (Note: When the one-way valves (identified by the *red arrow*) are removed, this mask is a partial nonrebreather.)

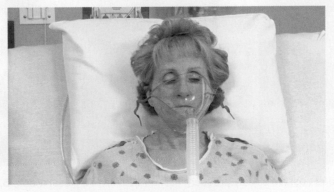

FIG. 9.12 A face tent on a client.

effective therapy, the seal must be secure between the mask and the client's skin. The position of the mask around the client's eyes and the straps around the head may give the client a sense of claustrophobia, which may prevent the client from using CPAP. Mask modifications or large-cannula

CPAP devices may enhance client compliance with therapy. Skin irritations, rashes, or breakdown from the CPAP mask are also potential adverse effects (Caple & Schub, 2017).

There is also an invasive CPAP mode, or setting, that is used for a client who is intubated, sometimes when weaning from a mechanical ventilator. The prescribing healthcare provider determines the client's suitability for CPAP therapy and prescribes the airway pressure and FiO_2 to be delivered. For more information on CPAP and mechanical ventilation, see the discussion of advanced respiratory management in Chapter 18.

Home Care Considerations

Home oxygen use has several safety considerations and requires additional client education and a thorough home assessment prior to discharge. Education covers the explosive dangers of oxygen and includes purchasing and maintaining functional smoke detectors, as well as small fire extinguishers. Parents/caregivers must be warned against the danger of oxygen in contact with fire, such as candles, stove burners, and cigarettes. The importance of posting signs in the home is covered; "Oxygen in Use" and "No Smoking" signs alert individuals to refrain from smoking. Additionally, if a fire is present, signs alert emergency personnel to proceed with caution to remove the oxygen source. Instruct families in developing evacuation routes and plans for the safe storage of oxygen canisters. Education also covers the oxygen administration equipment and planning involved in caring for and traveling with a person on oxygen. Older children should be instructed on how to use their oxygen equipment. Parents of children and infants on oxygen must be educated regarding the transportation of oxygen during travel. During air travel, the airline must be informed in advance. Parents must know with whom to communicate or where to go in case of emergencies and must be able to identify empty cylinders, displaced cannulas, and blocked valves (Jayasekara, 2018).

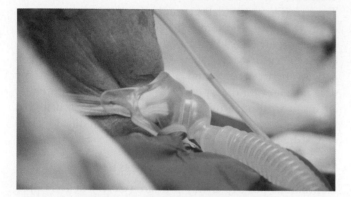

FIG. 9.13 Tracheostomy collar on a client.

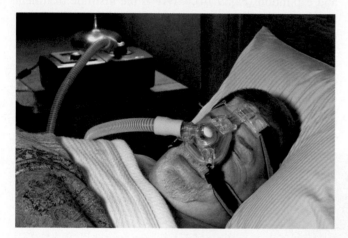

FIG. 9.14 A man sleeping with a nasal mask and headgear to prevent sleep apnea.

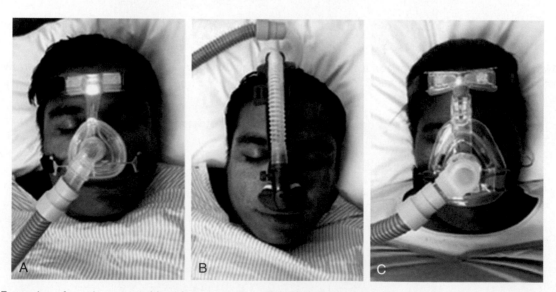

FIG. 9.15 Examples of continuous positive airway pressure (CPAP) delivery. **A,** Nasal mask; **B,** nasal prongs/pillows; and **C,** full-face mask.

SUMMARY

Administering oxygen to safely provide a therapeutic level of oxygenation requires the consistent use of safety measures and knowledge of several accuracy-related variables identified in the accompanying Critical Concepts. The nurse must accurately assess the client's oxygenation status and use the correct techniques and equipment to administer supplemental oxygen. The nurse evaluates the client's response to oxygen therapy to determine if the client has achieved the expected outcomes. Collaboration and teamwork among healthcare providers and the client are required to deliver the safe administration of oxygen. Delegation of tasks related to the administration of oxygen is based on the stability and predictability of the client as well as the training and competence of the delegatee. For example, if a client has been on 2 L of oxygen via nasal cannula with no change in oxygenation status for many months, that is a stable situation and different from a situation where the client's condition is not stable. Regardless, the licensed nurse remains accountable for the client, whereas the person to whom the skill or task is delegated is responsible for completing the task or procedure.

APPLICATION OF THE NURSING PROCESS

Examples of Related ICNP Nursing Diagnoses, Expected Client Outcomes, and Nursing Interventions:

Nursing Diagnosis: Impaired gas exchange

Supporting Data: Respiratory rate greater than five breaths per minute from baseline and oxygen saturation less than 95%

Expected Client Outcome: The client will have improved gas exchange.
- Client will maintain respiratory rate within five breaths per minute of established parameters for the client.
- Client's oxygen saturation will return to 95% or greater.
- Client will have breath sounds demonstrating air movement.
- Client will express feelings of comfort in breathing.

Nursing Intervention Example: Administer oxygen via the method prescribed by the authorized healthcare provider at the correct flow rate/ percentage of oxygen.

Reference: International Classification for Nursing Practice. (n.d.). *eHealth & ICNP*. Retrieved from https://www.icn.ch/what-we-do/projects/ehealth-icnp.

CRITICAL CONCEPTS
Administering Oxygen

Accuracy (ACC)

Accuracy in administering oxygen is affected by the following variables:

Client-Related Factors
- Client's age, medical history, and medical status
- Client's level of consciousness and orientation
- Client's understanding of and capacity to tolerate the oxygen-delivery device
- Client's activity level

Nurse-Related Factors
- Assessment of the client's respiratory status, oxygenation status, and breath sounds
- Appropriate preparation, setup, and adjustment of the oxygen-delivery system
- Assessment of the client's level of cooperation and understanding of oxygen therapy

Equipment-Related Factors
- Proper functioning of oxygen delivery on wall unit and portable oxygen tank

Client-Centered Care (CCC)

Respect for the client when administering oxygen is demonstrated by:
- explaining the procedure
- providing culturally sensitive explanations and arranging for an interpreter, if needed
- answering questions that the client or family may have
- providing privacy and ensuring comfort
- advocating for the client and family.

Infection Control (INF)

Healthcare-associated infection when administering oxygen is prevented by reducing the transfer and number of microorganisms, primarily through hand hygiene.

Safety (SAF)

When administering oxygen, safety measures prevent harm and maintain a safe care environment, including:
- the use of signage and safety equipment at the bedside
- teaching the client and family about safety measures when using oxygen.

Communication (COM)

- Communication exchanges information (oral, written, nonverbal, or electronic) between two or more people.
- Documentation records information in a permanent healthcare record.
- Collaboration with other healthcare providers is essential to achieve safe administration of oxygen.

Health Maintenance (HLTH)

Nursing is dedicated to the promotion of health and abilities when using oxygen therapy including:
- protecting client's skin when oxygen delivery devices are in use
- providing humidity to protect nasal mucosa and alveoli.

Evaluation (EVAL)

Evaluation of outcomes when administering oxygen enables the nurse to determine the efficacy of the care provided and includes:
- monitoring the respiratory and oxygenation status of the client.

■ SKILL 9.4 Using a High-Pressure Oxygen Cylinder

EQUIPMENT

Clean gloves, if there is a risk of exposure to body fluids.
Pulse oximeter
Oxygen-delivery device per authorized healthcare provider's orders
Oxygen cylinder
Oxygen regulator and flowmeter
Christmas tree nut and nipple adapter
Portable oxygen carrier

BEGINNING THE SKILL

Preparation

Prior to entering the client's room with the portable high-pressure oxygen cylinder:

1. **SAF** Turn the flowmeter to the "off" position.
2. **SAF** Assess valve functioning by attaching the regulator/flowmeter to the cylinder.
3. **SAF** Tighten the regulator/cylinder connection by turning the screw clockwise to the right. (Note: Do not overtighten. *This may cause excessive pressure or make it difficult for the next person to loosen.*)
4. **SAF** Quickly open and close the post valve using the regulator attachment screw by turning the screw counterclockwise, then clockwise. *Allows oxygen to be released from the canister, verifies the valve is functioning, and clears debris from the valve.*
5. **SAF** Open the post valve until the regulator pressure gauge stops rising. *This will indicate the amount of oxygen contained in the cylinder.*

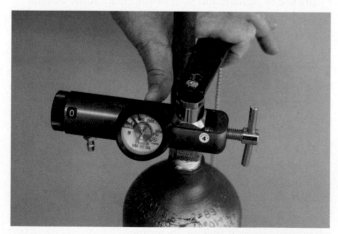

STEP 5 Open the post valve until the pressure gauge stops rising.

6. **SAF** Read the gauge. Determine if the amount of oxygen in the cylinder is adequate to support the client during transport. *Gauge should read greater than 500 psi.*

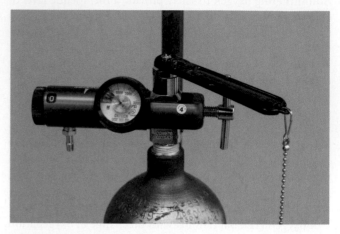

STEP 6 Read the pressure gauge.

7. **SAF** Assess the device for leaks, listening for a hissing sound or looking at the gauge.
8. **SAF** Tighten connections as needed.
9. **SAF** Transport to the client's room in a carrier per hospital protocol.
10. **INF** Perform hand hygiene. Apply clean gloves, if there is a risk of exposure to body fluids.
11. **CCC** Introduce yourself to client and family and explain the procedure.
12. **SAF** Identify the client using two identifiers.
13. **CCC** Provide privacy. Close the door and pull the curtain.

PROCEDURE

14. **ACC** Assess and document the client's vital signs and baseline oxygen saturation.
15. **SAF** Secure the oxygen cylinder within the portable oxygen stand.
16. **ACC** Connect the Christmas tree nut and nipple adapter to the regulator.
17. **ACC** Adjust the oxygen flow rate by turning the knob of the regulator until the needle or ball gauge reaches the prescribed flow rate.
18. **ACC** Connect the oxygen delivery device to the oxygen cylinder.
19. **SAF** Monitor client's oxygenation, respiration rate, and pulse.

FINISHING THE SKILL

20. **SAF** Ensure client safety and comfort. Ensure that the bed is in the lowest position and verify that the client can identify and reach the nurse call system. *These safety measures reduce the risk of falls.*
21. **INF** Remove gloves if worn and perform hand hygiene.
22. **EVAL** Evaluate the outcomes.

23. **COM** Document assessment findings, care given, and outcomes in the legal healthcare record:
   - vital signs
   - respiratory rate, depth, and effort
   - breath sounds
   - pulse oximetry values
   - color of mucous membranes.

■ SKILL 9.5 Using an Oxygen Flowmeter

EQUIPMENT

Stethoscope
Clean gloves, if there is a risk of exposure to body fluids
Pulse oximeter
Oxygen-delivery device appropriate for client's size
Extension tubing as needed
Oxygen source
Oxygen flowmeter
Sterile water reservoir, if humidity is ordered

BEGINNING THE SKILL

1. **INF** Perform hand hygiene.
2. **CCC** Introduce yourself to client and family and explain the procedure.
3. **SAF** Identify the client using two identifiers.
4. **INF** Apply clean gloves, if there is a risk of exposure to body fluids.
5. **CCC** Provide privacy. Close the door and pull the curtain.

PROCEDURE

6. **CCC** Position client in a semi-Fowler (head of bed 30 degrees) or high-Fowler position (head of bed elevated ≥45 degrees), unless contraindicated. *This reduces the work of breathing.*
7. **SAF** Verify the client's room is safe for oxygen administration. **WARNING:** Replace electrical equipment with nonelectric items if possible; avoid petroleum-based products. *The risk of fires is increased with the potential for sparks. Petroleum-based products are flammable.*
8. **SAF** Remind the client and family of the risks of open flames, such as lighters or candles.
9. **SAF** Post signs indicating "Oxygen in Use."
10. **SAF** Verify that the flowmeter is securely connected to the oxygen source. (Note: There may be a hissing noise present if the connection is not secure.)
11. **ACC** Connect the Christmas tree nut and nipple adapter, or sterile water reservoir, if ordered. *Humidification prevents drying of the mucous membranes.*
12. **SAF** Securely connect the oxygen delivery device to the oxygen flowmeter or reservoir.
13. **ACC** Begin oxygen therapy by opening the oxygen source to the flowmeter.
14. **ACC** Determine if oxygen is flowing by placing your wrist or forearm at the outlet to feel the oxygen flow.
15. **ACC** Set the oxygen flow rate to the prescribed rate by adjusting the needle or height of the ball.

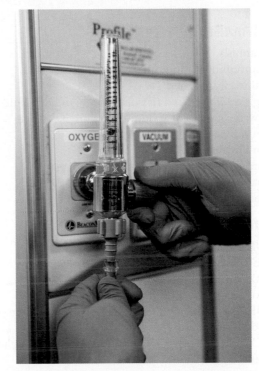

STEP 15 Set the oxygen flow rate by adjusting the height of the ball.

16. **ACC** Maintain the tubing loosely and verify that it is not pinched.
17. **CCC** Place the oxygen-delivery device on the client and adjust for comfort.
18. **EVAL** Assess the client's response to oxygen therapy by assessing vital signs, comfort level, physical appearance, and behavior for signs of improved oxygenation. *Clients will demonstrate decreased irritability and anxiety, improved skin color, and decreased heart and respiratory rate when oxygenation improves.*
19. **EVAL** Check oxygen saturation with pulse oximetry and client's capillary refill.

FINISHING THE SKILL

20. **SAF** Ensure client safety and comfort. Ensure that the bed is in the lowest position and verify that the client can identify and reach the nurse call system. *These safety measures reduce the risk of falls.*
21. **INF** Remove soiled gloves if worn. Perform hand hygiene.
22. **EVAL** Evaluate the outcomes.

23. **COM** Document assessment findings, care given, and outcomes in the legal healthcare record:
    * vital signs
    * respiratory rate, depth, and effort
    * breath sounds
    * pulse oximetry values and capillary refill time
    * color of mucous membranes
24. **COM** Notify the authorized healthcare provider if significant changes in the respiratory assessment are noted.

■ SKILL 9.6 Placing a Client on Oxygen by Nasal Cannula

EQUIPMENT

Nasal cannula
Extension tubing, if indicated
Humidifier, if indicated
Clean gloves if there is a risk of exposure to body fluid
Sterile water reservoir for humidification, if ordered
Oxygen source
Oxygen flowmeter
Christmas tree device, nut, and nipple adapter
Pulse oximeter
Appropriate oxygen safety signs

BEGINNING THE SKILL

1. **INF** Perform hand hygiene.
2. **CCC** Introduce yourself to client and family and explain the procedure.
3. **SAF** Identify the client using two identifiers.
4. **INF** Apply clean gloves, if there is a risk of exposure to body fluids.
5. **CCC** Provide privacy. Close the door and pull the curtain.

PROCEDURE

6. **ACC** Assess the client for the following:
    * respiratory rate, effort, and use of accessory muscles
    * oxygen saturation
    * bilateral breath sounds
    * contraindications, indications, and precautions
    * any pain or discomfort (using a facility-approved pain tool)
    * condition of nares; presence of any lesions or obstructions.
7. **ACC** Review the authorized healthcare provider's order to determine if humidification is ordered.
8. **ACC** Connect the end of the nasal cannula tubing to one of the following:
    * the Christmas tree adapter on the flowmeter, *or*
    * the sterile water reservoir attached to the flowmeter, if humidification is ordered
9. **ACC** Adjust oxygen flowmeter to prescribed flow rate. Verify flow out of the prongs.
10. **CCC** Place the two prongs of the cannula in the client's nares. (Note: If the prongs are curved, they should be positioned with the prong opening pointed down.)

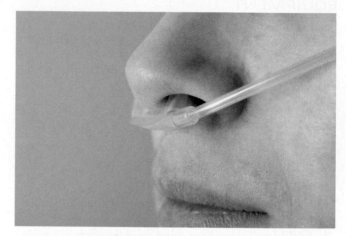

STEP 10 Place the two prongs of the cannula in the client's nares.

11. **CCC** Place the oxygen tubing over the client's ears.

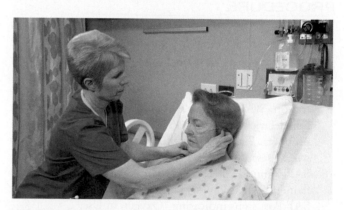

STEP 11 Place the oxygen tubing over the client's ears.

12. **CCC** Adjust the tubing to fit snugly but not tightly.
13. **HLTH** Provide padding behind ears, if indicated. *Protects against skin breakdown.*
14. **EVAL** Monitor the client's response to oxygen therapy by observing for increased oxygen saturation and capillary refill time.
15. **SAF** Post "Oxygen in Use" and "No Smoking" signs in the room and on the client's door.

FINISHING THE SKILL

16. **SAF** Ensure client safety and comfort. Ensure that the bed is in the lowest position and verify that the client

can identify and reach the nurse call system. *These safety measures reduce the risk of falls.*

17. **INF** Remove gloves if worn. Perform hand hygiene.
18. **EVAL** Evaluate the outcomes.
19. **COM** Document assessment findings, care given, and outcomes in the legal healthcare record:

- vital signs
- respiratory rate, depth, and effort
- breath sounds
- pulse oximetry values and capillary refill time
- color of mucous membranes.

■ SKILL 9.7 Placing a Client on Oxygen by Face Mask

EQUIPMENT

Clean gloves, if there is a risk of exposure to body fluid
Oxygen-delivery mask, as ordered
Extension tubing if indicated
Sterile water reservoir for humidification, if ordered
Oxygen source
Oxygen flowmeter
Christmas tree device
Pulse oximeter
Appropriate oxygen safety signs

BEGINNING THE SKILL

1. **INF** Perform hand hygiene.
2. **CCC** Introduce yourself to client and family and explain the procedure.
3. **SAF** Identify the client using two identifiers.
4. **INF** Apply clean gloves, if there is a risk of exposure to body fluid.
5. **CCC** Provide privacy. Close the door and pull the curtain.
6. **ACC** Follow authorized healthcare provider's orders for type of mask, oxygen flow rate, and FiO$_2$ to be delivered.

PROCEDURE

7. Administer oxygen using a simple face mask.
   a. **ACC** Attach the sterile water reservoir to the oxygen flowmeter, if humidification is ordered.
   b. **ACC** Connect the mask to the oxygen tubing.
   c. **ACC** Connect the tubing to the oxygen flowmeter or sterile water reservoir (if used).
   d. **ACC** Adjust the oxygen flow rate as prescribed (5–10 L/min).
   e. **ACC** Crimp the metal nosepiece to secure the mask to the nose. Ensure that the mask fits well and has a proper seal around the client's face. *This facilitates oxygen delivery to the client.*

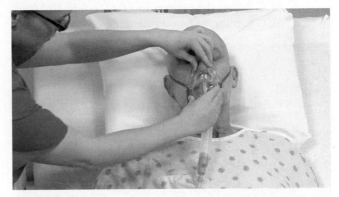

STEP 7E Crimp the metal nosepiece to fit the mask to the client's nose.

8. Administer oxygen using a Venturi face mask.
   a. **ACC** Attach the sterile water reservoir to the oxygen flowmeter, if humidification is ordered.
   b. **ACC** Select the appropriate size/color Venturi valve to administer the appropriate oxygen concentration.
   c. **ACC** Connect the Venturi valve to the mask.
   d. **ACC** Adjust the Venturi valve to the prescribed flow rate.

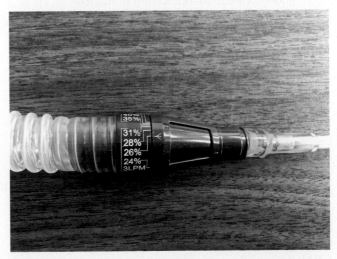

STEP 8D Adjust the Venturi valve to the prescribed flow rate.

   e. **ACC** Connect the tubing to the Venturi valve.
   f. **ACC** Connect the tubing to the oxygen flowmeter or sterile water reservoir, if used.

g. **CCC** Crimp the metal nosepiece to secure the mask to the nose.
h. **ACC** Adjust the oxygen flow rate as prescribed.
i. **CCC** Adjust straps over the client's ears.
j. **ACC** Verify that all air entry and exit holes are open and that there are no kinks.

9. Administer oxygen using a nonrebreather mask.
   a. **ACC** Connect the mask to the oxygen tubing.
   b. **ACC** Connect the tubing to the oxygen flowmeter.
   c. **CCC** Crimp the metal nosepiece to secure the mask to the nose.
   d. **ACC** Adjust the oxygen flow rate to 6 to 10 L/min.
   e. **ACC** Ensure the bag is fully inflated, as shown.

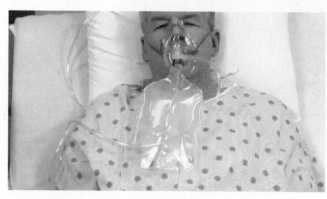

STEP 9E Ensure the bag for the nonrebreather is fully inflated.

   f. **CCC** Adjust the straps over the client's ears.
   g. **ACC** Verify that all air entry and exit holes are open and that there are no kinks.

10. Administer oxygen using a face-tent mask.
    a. **ACC** Attach the sterile water reservoir to the oxygen flow meter, if humidification is ordered.
    b. **ACC** Connect the face tent to the oxygen tubing.
    c. **ACC** Connect the tubing to the oxygen flowmeter.
    d. **ACC** Adjust the oxygen flow rate as prescribed.
    e. **ACC** Place the face tent in front of the client's face, ensuring fit under the chin.
    f. **ACC** Adjust the straps over the client's ears, as shown.

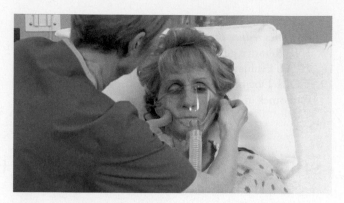

STEP 10F Adjust the straps over the client's ears.

11. Administer oxygen using a tracheostomy collar mask.
    a. **ACC** Attach the sterile water reservoir to the oxygen flow meter, if humidification is ordered.
    b. **ACC** Attach tube adapter to a humidification drainage bag.
    c. **ACC** Connect the Venturi valve to the oxygen tubing.
    d. **ACC** Adjust oxygen flow rate as prescribed.
    e. **ACC** Adjust Venturi flow rate as prescribed.
    f. **ACC** Apply collar loosely around tracheostomy.

FINISHING THE SKILL

12. **SAF** Ensure client safety and comfort. Ensure that the bed is in the lowest position and verify that the client can identify and reach the nurse call system. *These safety measures reduce the risk of falls.*
13. **INF** Remove gloves if worn. Perform hand hygiene.
14. **EVAL** Evaluate the outcomes.
15. **COM** Document assessment findings, care given, and outcomes in the legal healthcare record:
    • vital signs
    • respiratory rate, depth, and effort
    • breath sounds
    • pulse oximetry values and capillary refill time
    • color of mucous membranes.
16. **COM** Notify the authorized healthcare provider if significant changes in the respiratory assessment are noted.

■ SKILL 9.8 Placing a Client on Continuous Positive Airway Pressure (CPAP)

EQUIPMENT

Clean gloves, if there is a risk of exposure to body fluid
CPAP device
Oxygen source and appropriate tubing
Nasal prongs, nose mask, or full-face mask, as ordered
Pulse oximeter

BEGINNING THE SKILL

1. **INF** Perform hand hygiene.

2. **CCC** Introduce yourself to client and family and explain the procedure.
3. **SAF** Identify the client using two identifiers.
4. **INF** Apply clean gloves, if there is a risk of exposure to body fluids or mucous membranes.
5. **CCC** Provide privacy. Close the door and pull the curtain.

PROCEDURE

6. **ACC** Assess the client for the following:
   - respiratory rate, effort, and use of accessory muscles
   - oxygen saturation
   - bilateral breath sounds
   - contraindications, indications, and precautions
   - any pain or discomfort (using a facility-approved pain tool).
7. **HLTH** Note the condition of the client's skin over the nose and mouth. *The risk for skin breakdown exists with CPAP masks.*
8. **ACC** Connect the large-bore tubing to the pressure generator, and connect the oxygen source and flowmeter to the flow generator.
9. **ACC** Place the mask on the client so that it fits snugly over the client's nose and/or mouth to create a tight seal.
10. **ACC** Set the initial CPAP setting per order (e.g., 4–8 cm H_2O).
11. **ACC** Adjust the oxygen flowmeter to deliver the prescribed amount of oxygen.

FINISHING THE SKILL

12. **SAF** Ensure client safety and comfort. Ensure that the bed is in the lowest position and verify that the client can identify and reach the nurse call system. *These safety measures reduce the risk of falls.*
13. **INF** Remove gloves if worn and perform hand hygiene.
14. **EVAL** Evaluate the outcomes.
15. **EVAL** Monitor the client's response to CPAP:
    - Observe for signs of anxiety and claustrophobia.
    - Monitor vital signs and pulse oximetry.

- Monitor the skin around the client's nose and mouth for signs of impaired skin integrity.

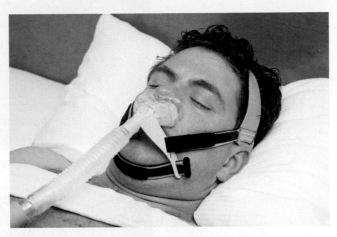

STEP 16 Monitor the client's response to CPAP.

16. **COM** Document assessment findings, care given, and outcomes in the legal healthcare record:
    - vital signs
    - respiratory rate, depth, and effort
    - breath sounds
    - pulse oximetry values and capillary refill time
    - color of mucous membranes
    - type of oxygen mask used and how the client tolerated the procedure
    - condition of the client's skin underneath the mask.
17. **COM** Notify the authorized healthcare provider if significant changes in the respiratory assessment are noted.

SECTION 3 Establishing and Maintaining an Open Airway

Clients who are experiencing respiratory distress may require interventions to establish or maintain an open airway. This can be achieved using oropharyngeal and nasopharyngeal airways. Both the oropharyngeal and nasopharyngeal airways prevent the tongue from occluding the airway, allowing air to pass to the trachea. These airways should only be used as a temporary means of maintaining an airway because they put pressure on soft tissue. A more permanent airway is a tracheostomy, which provides direct access from the neck to the trachea. These three types of airways, as well as suctioning the nasopharynx and obtaining a sputum specimen with a suction catheter, are discussed in this section.

OROPHARYNGEAL AIRWAY

An oropharyngeal airway (OPA) is a curved, firm, hollow tube with a rectangular hole in the center. When inserted, the OPA allows air to flow from the mouth and glottis and prevents the tongue from obstructing the upper airway (Fig. 9.16). OPAs have a flange, or circular disk, that rests at the client's lips to prevent further insertion of the OPA. When the airway is in position, the airway should extend from the front of the teeth to the end of the jawline (AACN, 2017). An OPA that is too large can cause damage or obstruct the airway.

OPAs are typically used only with unresponsive clients who cannot protect their own airway. OPAs are used as a bite block. They may be inserted along with endotracheal tubes or oral gastric tubes to prevent the client from biting the tube. OPAs are not used in a conscious client because they can stimulate the gag reflex and cause vomiting with subsequent aspiration. OPAs are also contraindicated with recent oral surgeries, dentures, and when the client has loose teeth. This is to prevent loose teeth from becoming dislodged and falling into the airway. OPAs are seldom inserted in children. Children's airways are very narrow, and the OPA may block the airway (Walsh & Woten, 2018).

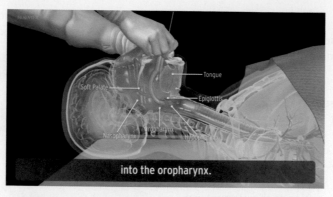

FIG. 9.16 Oropharyngeal airway (OPA) in position.

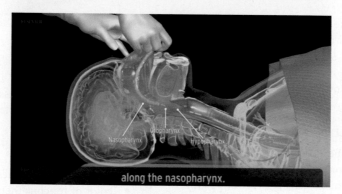

FIG. 9.17 Nasopharyngeal airway (NPA) in position.

NASOPHARYNGEAL AIRWAY

A nasopharyngeal airway (NPA), also known as a nasal trumpet, is a soft rubber or plastic tube with a flared end. NPAs are inserted into one of the client's nares and advanced into the posterior pharynx (Fig. 9.17). An NPA offers several advantages. It is the least invasive means of protecting an airway and is more comfortable than an OPA. If there is a large amount of secretions, the NPA provides a pathway to suction the pharynx because a catheter can be passed down inside the NPA. The NPA can be used when a client's jaw is clenched, surgically wired shut, or if the client is semiconscious and would not tolerate the insertion of an OPA. However, just as with an OPA, an NPA is a temporary intervention until the obstruction is removed or a more permanent airway is inserted.

NPAs are available in many sizes. Determine the appropriate size by holding the airway beside the client's jaw. Place the flared end of the NPA at the tip of the client's nose, and place the distal tip at the client's earlobe. Lubricate the tube generously to reduce discomfort and minimize trauma to the client's nasopharyngeal mucosa (Jaffe & Balderrama, 2017).

NASOPHARYNGEAL SUCTIONING

Nasopharyngeal suctioning is passing a catheter into a nostril, advancing it to the nasopharynx, and applying suction as the catheter is withdrawn. This procedure is usually performed in conjunction with oropharyngeal suctioning, the much more frequently performed and safer suctioning skill, which is described in Chapter 2. Nasopharyngeal suctioning is only performed if the client cannot clear secretions without assistance. Pharyngeal suctioning is performed to prevent the aspiration of secretions, vomit, or blood. Nasopharyngeal suctioning can trigger gagging and vomiting. The catheter should not enter the trachea because tracheal stimulation can trigger a vasovagal response resulting in arrhythmias, bradycardia, and hypotension. Furthermore, nasopharyngeal suctioning may result in swelling of the nasal mucosa and more difficulty maintaining airway patency. This procedure is performed with a sterile suction catheter to prevent the introduction of microorganisms (Sharma, 2018a).

TRACHEOSTOMY

A tracheostomy is a surgically created opening, or stoma, in the trachea through the anterior portion of the neck inferior to the vocal cords (Fig. 9.18). The purpose of creating a surgical airway is usually related to easier access to the tracheobronchial tree. Most frequently, a tracheostomy is created to facilitate ventilation for those on mechanical ventilation. However, a tracheostomy is also performed to prevent upper airway obstruction. It can be used to manage secretions, provide an airway, or prevent aspiration in clients with neurological trauma or disease. Clients who have head and neck cancer may also require a tracheostomy when tumors, swelling, or strictures jeopardize the airway. Tracheostomies may be performed urgently at the bedside but are more typically performed as planned surgical procedures. Once the incision is created, a tracheostomy appliance is

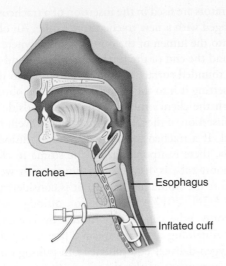

FIG. 9.18 Tracheostomy—an artificial airway from the anterior portion of the neck into the trachea.

Trachea

Esophagus

Inflated cuff

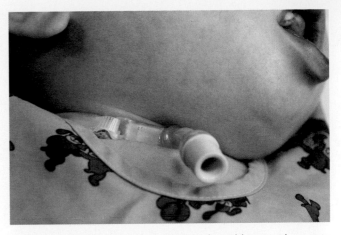

FIG. 9.19 A simple tracheostomy tube without an inner cannula.

inserted. A planned surgical procedure allows for a controlled environment, and temporary stay sutures could be used to assist with reinsertion of the tracheostomy tube should it come out in the postoperative period.

Oxygen and Breathing With a Tracheostomy

Clients with a tracheostomy may have a variety of degrees of oxygen and respiratory support. The greatest amount of support is for those requiring mechanical ventilation. In fact, the most common reason a tracheostomy is performed is for long-term mechanical ventilation. For clients who require mechanical ventilation greater than 7 days, the Council on Critical Care of the American College of Chest Physicians recommends a tracheostomy (Lindman, Peralta, Elluru, & Khan, 2017). Ventilation via a tracheostomy rather than an endotracheal tube provides several advantages for long-term care, including decreased airway resistance, improved comfort, less risk of damage to the vocal cords, and facilitating speech and feedings. Others who require oxygen but not mechanical ventilation may be placed on a tracheostomy oxygen collar or t-piece, discussed earlier in this chapter. Some clients (particularly those who have a long-term tracheostomy) may not require any supplemental oxygen at all.

Types of Tracheostomy Tubes

There are a number of different variations in tracheostomy tubes. As shown in Fig. 9.19, the most simplistic version of a tracheostomy is a hollow curved tube with a flange to prevent it from slipping into the trachea. Tracheostomy tubes may be made from the following materials: polyvinyl chloride, silicone, stainless steel, and silver. Tracheostomy tubes come in different sizes, and the size is generally indicated on the neck plate. In addition to the size number, the neck plate or a new tracheostomy box will show the cannula outer diameter (OD), inner diameter (ID), and length. This information is important to know when determining the appropriate suction catheter size and the depth to which to pass

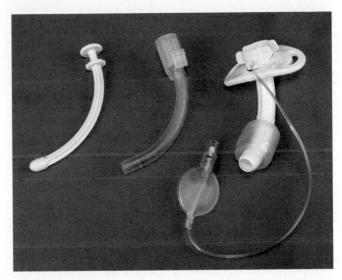

FIG. 9.20 From left to right: An obturator, a disposable inner cannula, and a cuffed tracheostomy tube with an inflation valve.

the suction catheter. Ideally, the tracheostomy tube is approximately three-quarters the diameter of the trachea and sits 2 to 3 cm above the carina. A typical size for a woman is a size 6 Shiley and for a man is an 8 Shiley. Although sizes differ, the outer adapter is one universal size, a 15-mm hub that fits onto ventilator tubing or a resuscitation bag for emergency situations.

One variation is whether or not the tube is a single cannula or whether it has an inner and outer cannula. Most adult tracheostomy tubes contain an inner and outer cannula. The outer cannula is inserted directly into the trachea during surgery and is a continuation of the neck plate located outside the client's tracheal stoma. The inner cannula can be removed and cleaned, or it may be disposable and can be replaced.

A second variation in tracheostomy tubes is cuffed versus uncuffed. The cuffed tracheostomy has an inflatable balloon, or cuff, near the base surrounding the outer cannula (Fig. 9.20). The cuff creates a seal and exerts gentle pressure against the tracheal wall. Thus, when a positive-pressure breath is

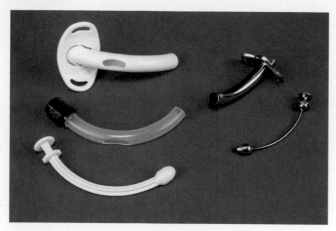

FIG. 9.21 *Left,* An uncuffed fenestrated tracheostomy tube with an inner cannula and obturator. *Right,* A stainless-steel tracheostomy tube with obturator.

delivered, the air does not leak back out. In addition, the cuff prevents secretions from entering the trachea and lungs. The cuff is inflated by attaching an air-filled syringe to the distal end of the inflation line, where a small external balloon also inflates. The cuff pressure is measured using a manometer every shift. Cuff pressure is usually between 20 and 25 cm H_2O. Routine cuff deflation is no longer recommended (American Association of Critical-Care Nurses [AACN], 2017). Indications for using a cuffed tracheostomy tube include the following:

- positive pressure ventilation
- risk of aspiration
- newly established tracheostomy (Lindman et al., 2017).

However, in infants and children less than 12 years of age, only uncuffed tracheostomy tubes are used because their airways are small, and inflating a cuff poses greater risks of trauma to the trachea.

Another variation in tracheostomy tubes is whether they are fenestrated or not. A fenestrated tube has an opening that allows air to pass by the vocal cords, making speech and coughing easier. Fig. 9.21 shows an example of a fenestrated tracheostomy tube. Fenestrated tracheostomy tubes are contraindicated for clients on mechanical ventilation.

Tracheostomy Safety Measures

Maintaining a secure and patent airway is a priority. At the bedside of a client with a tracheostomy, there should be the necessary emergency equipment to respond to the problems of replacing the tracheostomy tube should it become dislodged. In addition, there must be the routine safety equipment that provides the means to suction and ventilate the client. A new tracheostomy tube of the appropriate size and type, and one size smaller, should always be kept at the client's bedside in case the tracheostomy tube has to be replaced immediately. This is particularly important because mechanical ventilation tubing and the mechanical ventilation bag will only attach to the inner cannulas. Keeping a smaller-size appliance allows for ease of insertion in case the stoma starts to close. If the client has a cuffed tube, you will also need a 10-mL syringe to inflate the cuff.

Obturators are used in the insertion of a tracheostomy and are packaged with a new tracheostomy tube. An obturator is placed into the lumen of the outer cannula, where it extends just beyond the end of the tracheostomy tube and provides a smooth, rounded surface to minimize trauma to the trachea when inserting it into the client's trachea. The obturator that came with the client's tube is kept at the bedside for emergency reinsertion of the tracheostomy in the event it becomes dislodged. If a tracheostomy tube becomes dislodged from the stoma, there is a potential for the stoma to close. If the tracheostomy tube is dislodged within the first week of surgery (before the stoma has healed), it is considered an emergency (AACN, 2017). The risk for dislodgement of the tracheostomy tube can be minimized by keeping the ties secure, maintaining cuff pressure, and preventing the ventilator or oxygen-delivery equipment from pulling on the tube. Frequent assessment of the client's tracheostomy tube minimizes the risk of dislodgement as well, as discussed in Box 9.3.

Routine safety equipment to maintain a patent airway includes having working suction set up, suction catheters the correct size for the tracheostomy, a Yankauer catheter for oropharyngeal suctioning, a replacement inner cannula, and sterile water or normal saline to rinse the catheter and suction tubing. Having a manual resuscitation bag and an oxygen source allows emergency breaths and oxygen to be administered. Specific details on suctioning follow.

Postoperative Care for the Client With a Tracheostomy

Immediate postoperative care for the client with a tracheostomy includes assessing for and preventing the three most common postoperative emergencies: hemorrhage, tube obstruction, and tube dislodgement. Bleeding at the stoma site is a risk during the immediate postoperative period. Some bleeding is expected at the new surgical site, but blood-soaked drain sponges or blood-filled secretions returned when suctioning indicate a problem, and the surgeon should be notified immediately. In addition, maintaining a patent airway is critical. Postoperative nursing care includes keeping the inner cannula free from secretions, either by suctioning or by removing and replacing a disposable inner cannula or cleaning an inner cannula that is not disposable. Humidification is usually provided with or without supplemental oxygen to help keep secretions thin.

Maintaining a neutral midline position is also vital to prevent accidental dislodgement or trauma to the trachea and stoma. Palpate for crepitus around the insertion site. Crepitus is the crackling sound made when air is trapped in subcutaneous tissue. The presence of crepitus could indicate the tube is dislodged. Assess for the loss of breath sounds, increased work of breathing, or cyanosis, which may indicate tube obstruction.

Postoperative care in the days to follow includes assessing the stoma for signs of infection, including redness, inflammation, odor, and drainage (Lewis, Bucher, Heitkemper, & Harding, 2017). Additional information regarding

BOX 9.3 Expect the Unexpected: Forceful Coughing Ejects Tracheostomy Tube

Carol Keith is a 58-year-old female who has a temporary size 7 tracheostomy tube that was placed after facial trauma due to a motor vehicle accident and the inability to secure an oral airway. She is currently two weeks postop. The tracheostomy site requires dressing changes every 8 hours to manage copious secretions; moreover, Mrs. Keith had been on warfarin prior to the collision, and now small amounts of blood are oozing at the tracheostomy site. She is alert and oriented but has a persistent, strong cough secondary to bronchitis that has not resolved while hospitalized. She is currently receiving 30% flow-by oxygen via tracheostomy collar. The trauma floor is extremely busy, and the nurse is providing tracheostomy care alone while changing the tracheal ties on the tracheostomy neck plate. During the procedure, Mrs. Keith coughs forcefully, and the tracheostomy tube is ejected from her trachea and onto the floor.

In response to this emergency, the nurse immediately calls for emergency assistance and remains calm while reassuring Mrs. Keith and telling her what is about to occur. The nurse has a new tracheostomy tube with an obturator at the bedside. She removes the inner cannula from the new tracheostomy tube, replacing the inner cannula with the obturator. A respiratory therapist and another nurse respond to the emergency. The nurse visualizes the trachea and inserts the new tracheostomy tube at a right angle and gently twists the device to align with the trachea, then removes the obturator. The respiratory therapist confirms bilateral breath sounds while the second nurse assists with securing the tracheal ties. The authorized healthcare provider was notified of this occurrence, and the nurse acknowledged that she was attempting to change the ties without assistance.

This situation could have been catastrophic, but quick recognition and responsive action allowed the nurse and other staff to manage the situation. However, this situation could have been prevented. Always keep extra tracheostomy tubes—one of the same size and one that is one size smaller—with an obturator at the bedside. Specially trained nurses, respiratory therapists, and other advanced healthcare providers can reinsert the tracheostomy should it become dislodged. This will maintain the client's surgically created airway.

tracheostomy emergencies and complications is presented in Box 9.4.

Routine Tracheostomy Care: Cleaning the Stoma and Changing Ties

Routine care for the client with a tracheostomy includes assessing and cleaning the stoma site, cleaning or replacing inner cannulas, and changing the tracheostomy ties, as needed. Tracheostomy ties secure the tracheostomy neck plate to the client and wrap around the client's neck. Velcro ties are most commonly used (Fig. 9.22). However, cotton twill ties may also be used. Changing tracheostomy ties is a skill that generally requires two individuals to perform the

change safely. One nurse or assistant holds the tracheostomy appliance in place while the second nurse secures the twill or Velcro tracheostomy ties. The ties must *not* be removed before the new ones are securely in place. One finger (or two small fingers) should fit snugly under the tie when determining if the tracheostomy appliance is secured.

When replacing the disposable inner cannula, it is important to have readily available the correct size and style that will fit into the client's outer cannula. If cleaning and replacing a nondisposable inner cannula, use caution regarding the type of solution. Use only sterile normal saline, and avoid hydrogen peroxide. Some types of inner cannulas, such as those made of silicone or metal, may be damaged by hydrogen peroxide. Follow the manufacturer guidelines and facility policy (AACN, 2017).

SUCTIONING AN ARTIFICIAL AIRWAY

Maintaining the patency of an artificial airway is critical. Suctioning removes substances that may obstruct an artificial airway. Pulmonary secretions easily accumulate within the artificial airway because it takes a very forceful cough to expel secretions completely out of the tracheostomy tube. In addition, assisting the client with an artificial airway to mobilize secretions is an important aspect of nursing care. Providing humidity, ensuring adequate hydration, and encouraging physical mobility can help mobilize secretions. Mobilizing and suctioning secretions prevent the accumulation of fluids in the lower lobes of the lungs that could result in pneumonia. However, clients are only suctioned when the need for suctioning is clinically indicated.

The goal of suctioning is primarily to clear only the artificial airway while not damaging the tracheal mucosa. There are two techniques of airway suctioning: (1) minimally invasive, which suctions the predetermined depth of the airway, and (2) deep suctioning, which suctions within the bronchotracheal tree. The minimally invasive method has long been endorsed for children and infants by the American Thoracic Society (ATS) (2000). The American Association for Respiratory Care (AARC, 2010) recommends using the minimally invasive method for adults as well. The American Association of Critical Care Nurses (AACN, 2017) states that due to inconsistencies in the definitions, there is no conclusive evidence to support the practice of minimally invasive suctioning versus deep suctioning.

When using the minimally invasive method, you must determine the appropriate depth to which to insert the suction catheter. If the depth was not given to you in the nursing handoff, then you must determine the length of the artificial airway. For a tracheostomy tube, the suction catheter is to extend not more than 0.5 cm for pediatrics and 1.0 cm for adults beyond the end of the tracheostomy tube. There are several sources within the client's room where you can confirm the exact distance that the suction catheter should enter the tracheostomy tube. The spare tracheostomy tube that is at the bedside for emergencies will have the length, ID, and OD of the tube. Note that this length does not include the height of the inner cannula

BOX 9.4 Tracheostomy Emergencies and Complications

TRACHEOSTOMY EMERGENCIES

Hemorrhage
- At stoma
  - Small amount is expected and is normally self-limiting.
  - Management: continue to assess
  - Large amounts or continuous bleeding
  - Management: contact surgeon
- Into trachea
  - Tracheoinnominate fistula (rare)—artery erodes through trachea with subsequent exsanguination (rare)
  - Management
  - Contact surgeon
  - Provide oxygenation.

Tube Dislodgement
- Displaced completely (decannulation)
  - Management for new stoma (less than 1 week old)—stoma will close rapidly
  - Provide bag mask ventilation
  - Prepare for endotracheal intubation
- Management for mature stoma
  - Dependent on age of stoma (stoma will close 50% within 12 hours, 90% within 24 hours)
  - Keep two tracheostomy appliances at bedside (one of same size and one that is one size smaller)
  - Remove inner cannula and replace with obturator
  - Insert at a 90-degree angle to decrease likelihood of entering false passage
  - Twist gently to align vertically with trachea; remove obturator
  - Displaced partially (dislodgement)—tip lies with false passage anterior to trachea
  - Management for dislodgement
  - Quick recognition and action
  - Supplies needed for advanced healthcare provider
  - Suctioning equipment, oxygen
  - New tracheostomy tube with obturator
  - Equipment for inserting endotracheal tube

Tube Obstruction
- Management
  - Remove, inspect, and clean or replace inner cannula
  - If client is in continued distress, call for help
  - Attempt to insert suction catheter (resistance indicates potential for obstruction)
  - Mature stoma—entire tube is replaced by qualified personnel
  - Immature stoma

- Deflate cuff and provide mask ventilation
- Advanced healthcare provider will orally intubate

COMPLICATIONS OF TRACHEOSTOMIES
- Infection
  - At stoma site
  - Treat with topical anti-infectives and wound care dressings
  - Ventilator-associated pneumonia—systemic antibiotics
- Small amounts of bleeding
  - From tracheostomy suctioning
  - Continue to suction to prevent accumulation of thick secretions
  - Change to red rubber suction catheters to reduce irritation
  - Avoid use in those with latex allergies
  - At stoma
  - Provide careful tracheostomy care
  - Request special dressings to help with coagulation
- Tracheomalacia—breakdown of rigid structures of trachea
  - Occurs with overinflation of cuff or weight of ventilator circuit
  - Prevention
  - Maintain tracheostomy tube in neutral position
  - Limit traction against the tube and avoid overinflation of the cuff
  - Short-term treatment
  - Placement of longer tracheostomy tube to bypass affected area
- Skin breakdown
  - Management
  - Maintain tracheostomy tube in neutral position
  - Keep site as dry as possible with drain sponges or skin barriers
- Tracheoesophageal fistula
  - Causes
  - Overinflation of cuff
  - Direct trauma during the tracheotomy procedure
  - Signs and symptoms
  - Copious secretions, dyspnea
  - Signs and symptoms of aspiration
  - Cuff leak
  - Gastric distention
  - Treatment
  - Placement of double stent in both esophagus and trachea
  - Surgical repair

Adapted from Morris, Whitmer, & McIntosh, 2013.

external adapter. Therefore, the length plus 2 cm for the adapter plus 1 cm to extend past will be the total length the suction catheter is passed. Use a suction catheter with centimeter markings visible on its surface.

In addition to determining the distance to pass the suction catheter, the size of the suction catheter is determined based on the diameter of the tracheostomy tube. For adults, the OD of the suction catheter should not be greater than 50% of the

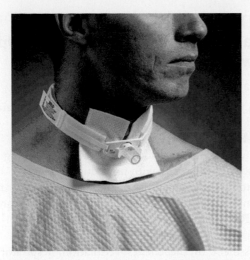

FIG. 9.22 Velcro ties secure to the tracheostomy faceplate.

ID of the tracheostomy tube (AACN, 2017). For children with a tracheostomy, the current recommendation is to use a catheter that inserts easily but is close in size and to suction for only 5 seconds (Boroughs & Dougherty, 2015). Catheters should have side holes close to the distal end and not simply one hole at the distal end. The side holes do a better job of removing secretions from the wall of the inner cannula.

There is an aspect of suctioning where the authorities are currently all in agreement, and that is that normal saline should not be instilled into the artificial airway before suctioning. Decades ago, this was thought to help loosen secretions. Years of research and client testimony of anxiety and fear are finally stopping this practice. See Box 9.5 for more information on why instillation of normal saline into an airway is harmful.

Suctioning: Inline and Open

In the acute care setting, the suction regulator is mounted on the wall, although portable models may be available. Suction regulators are calibrated to deliver specific amounts of suction in millimeters of mercury (mm Hg). The wall regulator is connected to the suction canister, which may be disposable or reusable, to which a longer suction tubing is attached for use with the suction catheter.

It is critical to check the wall regulator and suction equipment ahead of time to ensure that it is working and ready in case of an emergency. Pressure settings used for suctioning will vary, depending on the client's age and the route of suctioning:

- Newborns: 60 to 80 mm Hg
- Infants: 80 to 100 mm Hg
- Children: 80 to 100 mm Hg
- Adolescents: 80 to 120 mm Hg
- Adults: 80 to 150 mm Hg (use the least amount of suction that removes secretions [Boroughs & Dougherty, 2015]).

Pressures greater than 150 mm Hg have been shown to cause tracheal mucosal damage (AACN, 2017; Sharma, 2018b).

Prior to suctioning, clients receiving ventilation and oxygenation require hyperoxygenation. This is best provided with a mechanical ventilator, increasing the baseline FiO_2 to

---

BOX 9.5 Lessons From the Evidence: Putting a Stop to Instilling Normal Saline Into the Airways of Our Clients

Many decades ago, it was thought that instilling normal saline into an artificial airway would help to thin the pulmonary secretions. However, the simple life experience of coughing up sputum and spitting it into the toilet shows those secretions do not quickly dissolve! The evidence has been mounting for decades that instilling normal saline into an artificial airway:
- does not thin secretions
- decreases oxygen saturation
- causes hemodynamic changes: increased heart rate, increased mean arterial BP, increased intracranial pressure
- increases the risk of infection
- causes pain, anxiety, and dyspnea.

Despite this evidence, removing the instillation of normal saline from clinical practice has been slow.

The evidence-informed methods to mobilize and thin secretions include the following:
- Maintain the client's hydration status
- Maintain airway humidification
- Provide prescribed treatments and medications
- Use cough assistive devices, such as a vibration vest.

References: AARC, 2010; Boroughs & Dougherty, n.d., 2015; Halm & Krisko-Hagel, 2008.

100% or to the level ordered, rather than using a manual resuscitation bag (AACN, 2017). Hyperoxygenating before suctioning helps to prevent the hypoxia associated with suctioning. However, most of the research has been conducted on clients with tracheostomies on ventilators. For clients who do not require ventilator support, the need for hyperoxygenation should be determined by individual client assessment and agency policy (AACN, 2017).

Suctioning can be performed by the open method, in which a single-use catheter is passed into the artificial airway by the nurse using sterile technique. Suction is applied by occluding the opening as the catheter is rotated and pulled out of the tracheostomy tube. Rotation helps to clean off the inner walls of the tracheostomy tube and maintains the patency of the tube. The catheter is then discarded.

Inline suctioning is performed with a catheter in a plastic sleeve that remains attached to the tracheostomy opening. This method of suctioning is most often used when the client is receiving mechanical ventilator support. The advantage is that the client is not removed from the positive pressure or oxygen of the ventilator for suctioning and therefore is not exposed to a decrease in airway pressure and is less likely to have atelectasis. Another advantage is that the closed system protects the catheter from microorganisms.

Complications and Contraindications

Suctioning clients can cause serious complications, including hypoxia, cardiac dysrhythmias, laryngospasm or bronchospasm, damage to the tracheal mucosa, increased intracranial pressure, and pneumothorax. Suctioning is not a benign procedure; however, it may be essential to maintain an open airway. Thus, it is important to assess the client carefully for indications of the need for suctioning; review the authorized healthcare provider's orders for hyperoxygenating; and monitor the client's oxygen saturation, respiratory status, and hemodynamic status during suctioning.

COLLECTING SPUTUM SAMPLES

Sputum samples are collected either by having a client cough and expectorate (or spit) into a sterile container or by using a sterile sputum trap attached to a suction catheter. Samples are generally collected early in the morning. Sputum samples are collected to grow and isolate microorganisms and to guide the treatment of infections. The laboratory will identify the pathogen responsible for the infection and will complete culture and sensitivity testing to determine the most effective antibiotic. As the nurse, if you notice changes in the color of pulmonary secretions, especially when accompanied by other clinical changes, notify the authorized healthcare provider because he or she may wish to order a sputum sample.

SUMMARY

An oropharyngeal or nasopharyngeal airway may be used to establish or maintain a patent airway. Both of these are temporary strategies that require accurate assessment of the client and measurement of the size of the airway for safe and effective insertion. A tracheostomy is a surgically created opening with direct access to the tracheobronchial tree. Key critical concepts for caring for the client with a tracheostomy tube include client-centered care, safety measures, and accurate knowledge of the type of equipment and means of reducing risk. Establishing and maintaining a patent airway may require suctioning to prevent airway obstruction. Airway maintenance is a healthcare priority and requires clear communication and collaboration among members of the healthcare team.

APPLICATION OF THE NURSING PROCESS

Examples of Related ICNP Nursing Diagnoses, Expected Client Outcomes, and Nursing Interventions:

Nursing Diagnosis: Impaired airway clearance

Supporting Data: Presence of a tracheostomy, ineffective cough, and/or difficulty removing airway secretions

Expected Client Outcome: The client will have a clear airway, as seen by clear air exchange and the lack of secretion buildup on the inner cannula.

Nursing Intervention Example: Assess airway patency and suction inner cannula when indicated.

Reference: International Classification for Nursing Practice. (n.d.). *eHealth & ICNP*. Retrieved from https://www.icn.ch/what-we-do/projects/ehealth-icnp.

CRITICAL CONCEPTS
Establishing and Maintaining an Open Airway

Accuracy (ACC)

Accuracy in establishing and maintaining an open airway is affected by the following variables:

Client-Related Factors
- Client's level of consciousness and understanding of and capacity to cooperate with procedures
- Anatomical abnormalities or trauma to mouth or trachea
- Client's ability to communicate with the healthcare team

Nurse-Related Factors
- Positioning the client
- Assessment of the client's ventilation, respiratory, and pulmonary secretion status
- Proper setup and settings of suction equipment
- Identifying the appropriate size of the artificial airway
- Correct placement, maintenance, and securement of artificial airway or tracheostomy tube
- Proper technique used for suctioning

Equipment-Related Factors
- Proper functioning of suction equipment

Client-Centered Care (CCC)

Respect for the client when establishing and maintaining an open airway is demonstrated by:
- explaining the procedure
- providing culturally sensitive explanations and arranging for an interpreter, if needed
- answering questions of the client and family
- providing privacy and ensuring comfort
- advocating for the client and family.

Infection Control (INF)

Healthcare-associated infection when establishing and maintaining an open airway is prevented by:
- containment of microorganisms
- preventing and reducing the transfer of microorganisms
- reducing the number of microorganisms.

Safety (SAF)

When establishing and maintaining an open airway, implementing safety measures prevent harm and maintain a safe care environment, including:
- ensuring safety equipment and emergency equipment are at the bedside.

Communication (COM)

- Communication exchanges information (oral, written, nonverbal, or electronic) between two or more people.
- Documentation records information in a permanent healthcare record.

Evaluation (EVAL)

Evaluation of outcomes when establishing and maintaining an open airway enables the nurse to determine efficacy of care provided and includes:
- monitoring the patency of the airway.

▪ SKILL 9.9 Inserting an Oropharyngeal Airway

EQUIPMENT

Clean gloves
Oropharyngeal airway
Suction source, tubing, and catheter
Yankauer suction catheter with wall suction set-up for oral
    secretions (if needed)
Tongue depressor
Pulse oximeter

BEGINNING THE SKILL

1. **INF** Perform hand hygiene.
2. **INF** Apply clean gloves.
3. **CCC** Introduce yourself to the client and family and explain the procedure.
4. **SAF** Identify the client using two identifiers.
5. **CCC** Provide privacy. Close the door and pull the curtain.

PROCEDURE

6. **CCC** Determine the client's level of consciousness. **WARNING**: A client who is conscious and has a gag reflex should not receive an oropharyngeal airway. In addition, oropharyngeal airways should not be placed for a client who is actively seizing.
7. **ACC** Assess the client to confirm need for OPA:
   - absent cough or gag reflex
   - excessive oral secretions, drooling
   - labored or absent respirations, or tachypnea.
8. **ACC** Place the client in a supine position.
9. **ACC** Determine appropriate size for oral airway.
   - Flange is at the corner of the mouth.
   - Tip of curved section reaches the earlobe.

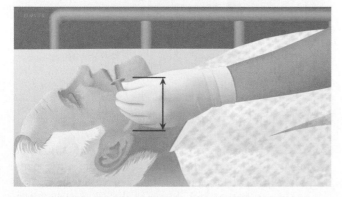

STEP 9 Measure from the corner of the mouth to the earlobe.

10. **ACC** If not contraindicated, hyperextend the client's neck, or gently tilt client's head back, and open the client's mouth. **WARNING**: Clients with suspected cervical spine injury should not have their necks hyperextended.
11. **SAF** Assess the client's mouth and remove the following objects if possible:
    - oral appliances
    - dentures
    - foreign objects.
12. **ACC** Initially insert the airway into the mouth with the tip of the curved end pointing upward until the tip reaches the soft palate.

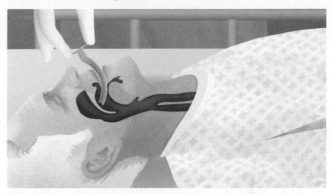

STEP 12 Initially insert the airway with the tip of the curved end pointing upward until it reaches the soft palate, and then rotate.

   a. **ACC** Rotate the airway 180 degrees into the correct position over the back of the tongue.
13. **INF** Remove gloves. Perform hand hygiene.
14. **EVAL** Assess the client's respiratory status with the OPA in position:
    - respiratory rate, depth, and effort
    - breath sounds
    - pulse oximetry readings
    - color of mucous membranes. *Your assessment of the client's respiratory status evaluates the effectiveness of the OPA in establishing a patent airway.*
15. **CCC** Suction mouth and throat secretions with Yankauer suction tip as needed.

FINISHING THE SKILL

16. **SAF** Ensure client safety and comfort. Reposition client as needed. Place the bed in the lowest position. If family members are present verify that they can identify and reach the nurse call system. (Note: An OPA is only recommended in instances when the client has a low level of consciousness and therefore may not be able to call for assistance.) *These safety measures reduce the risk of falls.*
17. **INF** Perform hand hygiene.
18. **EVAL** Evaluate and monitor the client outcomes.
19. **COM** Document assessment findings, care given, and outcomes in the legal healthcare record:
    - vital signs
    - respiratory rate, depth, and effort
    - breath sounds
    - pulse oximetry values and capillary refill time
    - color of mucous membranes
    - type of oral airway used and how the client tolerated the procedure.

■ SKILL 9.10 Inserting a Nasopharyngeal Airway

EQUIPMENT

Clean gloves

Stethoscope and pulse oximeter

Nasopharyngeal airway, appropriately sized (Note: It may be necessary to bring more than one airway to the client's bedside for accurate sizing.)

Topical anesthetic (if ordered)

Yankauer suction catheter with wall suction set-up for oral secretions, if needed

Tongue depressor

Water-soluble lubricant

Washcloth

BEGINNING THE SKILL

1. **INF** Perform hand hygiene.
2. **INF** Apply clean gloves.
4. **CCC** Introduce yourself to the client and family and explain the procedure.
3. **SAF** Identify the client using two identifiers.
5. **CCC** Provide privacy. Close the door and pull the curtain.

PROCEDURE

6. **ACC** Position client in the semi-Fowler (head of bed 30 degrees) or high-Fowler position (head of bed elevated ≥45 degrees), unless contraindicated.
7. **SAF** Set up an ergonomically safe space. Raise the bed to a comfortable working height. Raise one side rail. *Setting up an ergonomically safe space prevents injury to the nurse and client.*
8. **SAF** Assess the client's nares for obstructions or deviations. Ask if there is a history of nose fracture or deviated septum.
9. **SAF** Assess the client's mouth and remove the following objects if possible:
   - oral appliances and braces
   - dentures
   - foreign objects.

   This prevents foreign objects from being forced into the airway.
10. **CCC** Prepare the client for the procedure:
    a. If the client is able to assist, have the client blow his or her nose. If the client is unable to assist, suction the nares. Note the amount, color, and viscosity of secretions.
    b. Assess one naris at a time for patency. Ask the client to place his or her finger on the side of each naris while breathing through the other.
    c. Provide tissues and emesis basin for client.
    d. If ordered, spray topical anesthesia as needed for comfort and wait for the medication to take effect.

11. **ACC** Prepare the equipment.
    a. Determine that the nasopharyngeal airway is the appropriate size by measuring it from the tip of the client's nostril to the earlobe.

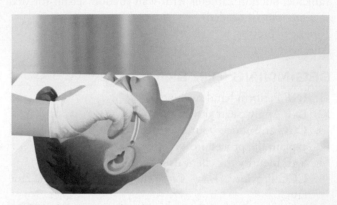

STEP 11A Confirm NPA is appropriate size by measuring it from the tip of the nostril to the earlobe.

    b. Lubricate the nasopharyngeal airway generously with water-soluble lubricant.
12. **ACC** Insert the nasopharyngeal airway with the angled side facing the nasal septum into the selected naris. Gently advance the tube back toward the nasopharynx. Do *not* angle up into the nose. *Reduces the risk of injuring the turbinates.*

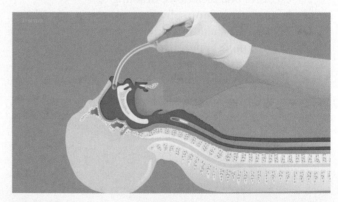

STEP 12 Insert NPA into the selected nostril.

13. **ACC** Advance the nasopharyngeal airway by rotating the NPA until the flange reaches the outer naris. **WARNING:** If resistance is felt, verify that the client is not in any distress and change to the other naris.
14. **CCC** Provide comfort care to the client by cleaning off secretions.
15. **CCC** Suction the oropharynx with a Yankauer suction tip to remove secretions, as necessary.
16. **EVAL** Evaluate placement by looking in the client's mouth. Look for the distal end of the NPA below the client's uvula.

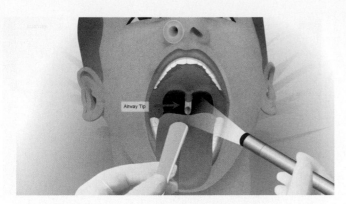

STEP 16 Look for the distal end of the NPA below the client's uvula.

17. **EVAL** Evaluate the patency of the client's airway by assessing the client's respiratory status:
    - respiratory rate, depth, and effort
    - breath sounds
    - pulse oximetry readings
    - color of mucous membranes.

18. **CCC** Suction mouth and throat secretions with a Yankauer suction tip as needed.

FINISHING THE SKILL

19. **INF** Remove gloves and perform hand hygiene.
20. **SAF** Ensure client safety and comfort. Place the bed in the lowest position and verify that the client can identify and reach the nurse call system. *These safety measures reduce the risk of falls.*
21. **EVAL** Evaluate the outcomes.
22. **COM** Document assessment findings, care given, and outcomes in the legal healthcare record:
    - respiratory rate, depth, and effort
    - breath sounds
    - pulse oximetry values
    - color of mucous membranes
    - size of nasal airway inserted
    - how the client tolerated the procedure.

■ SKILL 9.11 Performing Nasopharyngeal Suctioning

EQUIPMENT

PPE, face shield, or mask and goggles
Clean gloves
Topical analgesic, if ordered
Sterile gloves (may be included in the suction catheter package)
Sterile suction catheter(s) of the appropriate size (as determined by the client's size and physiology; e.g., use #10–16 French catheter for an adult, #8 or #10 French catheter for a child)
Sterile normal saline and sterile container (container may be included in suction catheter kit)
Wall suction with suction regulator
Connection tubing (4–6 feet)
Sterile water-soluble lubricant (to facilitate passage of the catheter)
Pillow or folded blanket
Towel
Oxygen saturation monitor

BEGINNING THE SKILL

1. **SAF** Review the order and review the client's medical/surgical history for contraindications to nasopharyngeal suctioning (e.g., nasal or sinus surgery, nasal septum defects, basilar skull fracture, or risk for bleeding [e.g., coagulation laboratory test results]).
2. **INF** Perform hand hygiene and apply clean gloves. Obtain a face shield or mask and goggles and place on a clean surface. *Standard Precautions identify the need for a mask and eye protection (a face shield provides both) during procedures that may generate sprays of respiratory secretions, especially suctioning (Centers for Disease Control and Prevention [CDC], 2016).*
3. **CCC** Introduce yourself to the client and family and explain the procedure. Ensure the client consents to the suctioning procedure.
4. **SAF** Identify the client using two identifiers. Assess for pertinent allergies.
5. **CCC** Provide privacy. Close the door and pull the curtain.

PROCEDURE

6. **SAF** Assess the client's degree of cooperation. Assess the client's degree of discomfort, using an age-appropriate, facility-approved pain tool. *Your assessment is to determine the extent to which the client can cooperate during the procedure and tolerate suctioning.*
7. **ACC** Assess the client's respiratory status for indications that suctioning is needed:
    - client's report of difficulty breathing or need for suctioning
    - change in vital signs, such as a change in respiratory rate, depth, and effort
    - breath sounds
    - pulse oximetry values.
Changes in respiratory rate are an early indicator of increased oxygen demand. Changes in oxygen saturation will occur before color changes to mucous membranes or nailbeds.

8. **ACC** Position the client sitting up (90 degrees) or in the high-Fowler positions (≥45 degrees), unless contraindicated. *Sitting up is much more effective than reclining. (Consider how you position yourself to cough.)*

9. **ACC** Assess the client's ability to cough or expectorate. Use a Yankauer catheter to suction the oropharynx. *If the client is able to cough and expectorate sputum, suctioning is not necessary.*

10. **SAF** Set up an ergonomically safe space. Raise the bed to a comfortable working height. Raise one side rail. Place an over-the-bed table at a right angle to the bed by your dominant hand. Set up a workspace according to your hand dominance; that is, if you are right-handed, stand on the client's right side. *Setting up an ergonomically safe space prevents injury to the nurse and client.*

11. **CCC** Prepare the client:
    a. Place a disposable absorbent pad or towel across the client's chest to catch secretions.
    b. Provide a pillow or folded blanket for splinting if the client has an abdominal or chest surgical incision or wound. *Prevents discomfort during coughing.*

12. **SAF** Prepare the suction equipment:
    a. Turn on wall suction regulator and adjust suction to 80 to 120 mm Hg or as prescribed. *Higher suction pressure reduces airway pressure, increasing the risk of atelectasis.* (Note: Variations regarding the amount of suction are dependent on the client's age, secretion amount, and viscosity or facility protocol. Use the least amount of suction necessary to remove secretions.)
    b. Ensure tubing is securely connected to vacuum canister and distal end of tubing is within easy reach.
    c. Occlude the end of the connection tubing with the thumb and observe the gauge to verify maximum suction pressure.

13. **INF** Remove soiled gloves. Perform hand hygiene.

14. **SAF** Apply face shield or mask/goggles.

PROCEDURE

15. **INF** Prepare a sterile field:
    a. Open the sterile suction catheter package and use the inner wrapper to create sterile field.
    b. Extract the sterile container, open it, and set it on the over-the-bed table.
    c. Pour a small amount (~100 mL) of sterile water or saline into the sterile basin.
    d. Squeeze a small amount of water-soluble lubricant onto the sterile packaging, using the nondominant hand.
    e. Apply sterile gloves.

16. **INF** Pick up the suction catheter package and remove the catheter, maintaining sterility of the catheter.

17. **ACC** Determine the appropriate depth to which the suction catheter will be inserted by measuring from the tip of the nose to the tragus of the ear.

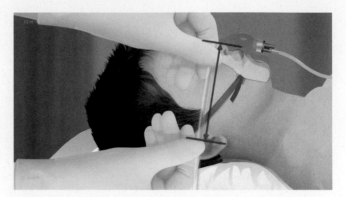

STEP 17 Determine the appropriate depth to which the suction catheter will be inserted.

18. **INF** Coil the suction catheter around the dominant hand, with the suction port between the thumb and forefinger.

19. **INF** Grasp the connecting tubing with the nondominant hand. *Your nondominant hand is no longer sterile, but your dominant hand will remain sterile.*

20. **INF** Attach the suction port to the connecting tubing using the sterile hand, keeping the suction catheter and the fingertips of your dominant hand sterile. Ensure that the suction catheter and connecting tubing are snugly attached. *Stabilizes the catheter and prevents the catheter from becoming disconnected during suctioning.*

21. **INF** Hold the connecting tubing with the nonsterile hand to control the suction port during the procedure.

22. **SAF** Test equipment by suctioning a small amount of solution from the sterile container by occluding the suction vent with the thumb to create suction. *Confirms functioning of equipment.*

23. **ACC** Coat the end of the catheter lightly with the lubricant. Visualize the client's nostrils to determine the most easily accessible passage and insert the suction catheter tip gently into the client's nostril.

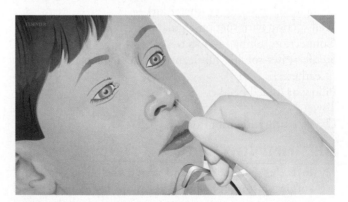

STEP 23 Insert the suction catheter tip gently into the client's nostril.

24. **CCC** Rotate the tip gently to help it advance through the selected nostril.

25. **ACC** Advance the catheter tip slowly into the client's pharynx while instructing him or her to inhale without swallowing. **WARNING:** Do not apply suction while introducing the catheter because it may damage the mucosa.

26. **SAF** Withdraw the catheter slowly, rotating it gently while suctioning. Apply continuous suction and limit suctioning to a few seconds.
27. **INF** Suction a small amount of sterile saline into the catheter to clear the catheter lumen, if necessary. *Clearing the catheter and tubing contains secretions and microorganisms in the suction canister.*
28. **EVAL** Evaluate client's oxygenation status. Determine whether secretions have been adequately removed from the nasopharynx:
    a. Occlude each of the client's nostrils individually while instructing the client to breathe through the opposite nostril.
29. **SAF** Provide supplemental oxygen if necessary and if permitted by the authorized healthcare provider's orders.
30. **ACC** Repeat the procedure only as needed.
31. **INF** Disconnect the suction catheter from the connection tubing and twist the suction catheter around the fingers of one gloved hand.

32. **INF** Remove glove, pulling over suction catheter to encase the catheter in the glove. Remove other soiled glove. *This contains the soiled catheter and microorganisms from the nasopharynx inside the glove.*
33. **INF** Perform hand hygiene.

FINISHING THE SKILL

34. **SAF** Ensure client safety and comfort. Place the bed in the lowest position. Verify that the client can identify and reach the nurse call system. *These safety measures reduce the risk of falls.*
35. **EVAL** Evaluate the outcomes.
36. **COM** Document assessment findings, care given, and outcomes in the legal healthcare record:
    * vital signs, including respiratory rate, depth, and effort
    * ability to breathe through nostrils
    * amount, color, and consistency of secretions
    * pulse oximetry values.

■ SKILL 9.12 Suctioning an Artificial Airway: Tracheostomy or Endotracheal Tube

EQUIPMENT

PPE, face shield, or mask and goggles
Clean gloves
Sterile suction catheter kit (sterile gloves, sterile suction catheter, and sterile container)
Sterile suction catheter(s) of the appropriate size (as determined by the ID of client's tracheostomy tube or endotracheal tube [ETT])
Sterile normal saline
Wall suction and suction regulator
Suction canister and connection tubing
Oxygen saturation monitor
Toothbrush or oral rinse, as needed

BEGINNING THE SKILL

1. **SAF** Review the order. Determine if specific hyperoxygenation parameters are given. Determine if minimally invasive suctioning or deep suctioning will be performed. (Note: For minimally invasive suctioning, you must determine how far to advance the suction catheter. This measurement is the length of the tracheostomy tube and adapter or length of the ETT plus approximately 1 cm.)
2. **INF** Perform hand hygiene and apply clean gloves. Obtain a face shield or mask and goggles and place on a clean surface. *Standard Precautions indicate the need for a mask and eye protection (a face shield provides both) during procedures that may generate sprays of respiratory secretions, especially suctioning (CDC, 2016).*
3. **CCC** Introduce yourself to the client and family and explain the procedure. Ensure the client consents to the suctioning procedure.

4. **SAF** Identify the client using two identifiers.
5. **CCC** Provide privacy. Close the door and pull the curtain.

PROCEDURE

6. **SAF** Assess the client's degree of cooperation. Assess the client's degree of discomfort, using a facility-approved pain tool. *Your assessment is to determine the extent to which the client can cooperate during the procedure and tolerate suctioning.*
7. **SAF** Assess the client's means of communication. If the client has no means of verbalizing needs, establish a signal to alert you if he or she experiences any distress or significant discomfort during procedure. *A preestablished means of communication prevents harm to the client.*
8. **ACC** Assess the client's respiratory status for indications that suctioning is needed:
    * client's report of difficulty breathing or need for suctioning
    * change in vital signs, such as a change in respiratory rate, depth, and effort
    * breath sounds; audible secretions over trachea
    * pulse oximetry values.
    Changes in respiratory rate are an early indicator of increased oxygen demand. Oxygen saturation changes will occur before color changes to mucous membranes or nailbeds.
9. **ACC** Position client sitting up (90 degrees) or in the high-Fowler positions (≥45 degrees), unless contraindicated. *Sitting up is much more effective than reclining. (Consider how you position yourself to cough.)*
10. **SAF** Set up an ergonomically safe space. Raise the bed to a comfortable working height. Raise one side rail.

Place an over-the-bed table at a right angle to the bed by your dominant hand. Set up a workspace according to your hand dominance; that is, if you are right-handed, stand on the client's right side. *Setting up an ergonomically safe space prevents injury to the nurse and client.*

11. **SAF** Prepare the suction equipment:
    a. Turn on wall suction regulator and adjust suction to 80 to 120 mm Hg or as prescribed. *Higher suction pressure reduces airway pressure, increasing the risk of atelectasis.* (Note: Variations regarding the amount of suction are dependent on client age, secretion amount and viscosity, or facility protocol. Use the least amount of suction necessary to remove secretions.)
    b. Ensure tubing is securely connected to vacuum canister and distal end of tubing is within easy reach.
    c. Occlude the end of the connection tubing with the thumb and observe the gauge to verify maximum suction pressure.

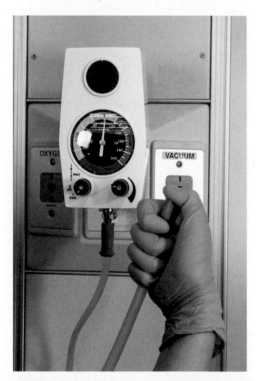

STEP 11C Verify maximum suction pressure by occluding the end of the tubing.

Suctioning an Artificial Airway (Open Method)

12. **CCC** Prepare the client:
    a. Place a disposable absorbent pad or towel across the client's chest to catch secretions.
    b. Provide a pillow or folded blanket for splinting if the client has an abdominal or chest surgical incision or wound. *Prevents discomfort during coughing.*
13. **INF** Remove soiled gloves. Perform hand hygiene.

14. **SAF** Apply face shield or mask/goggles.
15. **INF** Prepare a sterile field:
    a. Open the sterile suction catheter package and use the inner wrapper to create a sterile field.
    b. Extract the sterile container, open it, and set it on the over-the-bed table.
    c. Pour a small amount (~100 mL) of sterile water or saline into the sterile basin.
    d. Apply sterile gloves.
16. **INF** Pick up the suction catheter package, and remove the catheter, maintaining sterility of the catheter. Coil the suction catheter around the dominant hand, with the suction port between the thumb and forefinger.
17. **INF** Grasp the connecting tubing with the nondominant hand. Your nondominant hand is no longer sterile, but your dominant hand will remain sterile.
18. **INF** Attach the suction port to the connecting tubing using the sterile hand, keeping the suction catheter and the fingertips of your dominant hand sterile. Ensure that the suction catheter and connecting tubing are snugly attached. *Stabilizes the catheter and prevents the catheter from becoming disconnected during suctioning.*
19. **INF** Hold the connecting tubing with the nonsterile hand to control the suction port during the procedure.
20. **SAF** Test equipment by suctioning a small amount of solution from the sterile container by occluding the suction vent with the thumb to create suction. *Confirms functioning of equipment.*

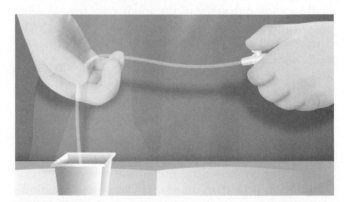

STEP 20 Test equipment by suctioning a small amount of solution from the sterile container.

21. **ACC** Hyperoxygenate the client according to the authorized healthcare provider's guidelines.
    a. If the client is receiving humidified oxygen via a trach collar, encourage the client to take deep breaths, if able, and to cough during tracheostomy suctioning. *This allows the client to oxygenate and expectorate sputum.*
    b. If the client is receiving mechanical ventilation, use the ventilator to provide airway pressure and increase oxygen per authorized healthcare provider's guidelines (Note: If increasing oxygen incrementally, be

careful to return oxygen to presuctioning level after suctioning.)

22. **ACC** Observe the client's pulse oximeter and obtain a respiratory rate in order to have a baseline assessment prior to suctioning.

23. **CCC WARNING:** Do *not* instill sterile normal saline into the client's airway. This has been determined *not* to be effective (AACN, 2017).

24. **ACC** Insert the suction catheter quickly but gently into the tracheostomy tube. With the open method, your dominant hand and the catheter must remain sterile.

    a. **Minimally invasive suctioning**: Insert catheter to the predetermined distance: the length of the tracheostomy tube and adapter or ETT plus 0.5 to 1 cm. (0.5 for children and 1 for adults). *This length clears the artificial airway but does not touch the tracheal mucosa. This method is recommended for children and infants.*

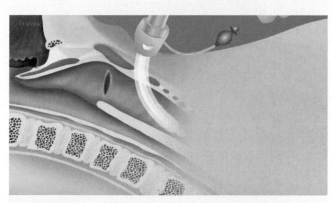

STEP 24A Minimally invasive suctioning. The catheter clears the artificial airway but does not touch the tracheal mucosa.

    b. **Deep suctioning:** Insert catheter until resistance is met (this is the carina), and then withdraw the catheter 1 cm (0.5 inch). **WARNING**: Do not apply suction until after withdrawing the catheter 1 cm (0.5 inch). *Suction is not applied until after withdrawing 1 cm to avoid contact with the mucosal wall during suctioning.*

25. **ACC** Place the thumb of your nondominant hand over the suction catheter vent to create suction. Rotate the catheter between the fingers and thumb of your dominant hand while withdrawing the suction catheter. Your nondominant hand can help withdraw the catheter. Limit suctioning to a 10-second period for adults and a 5-second period for children (AACN, 2017) *Rotating the catheter allows the holes on the suction catheter to more effectively clean the inner surface of the cannula.*

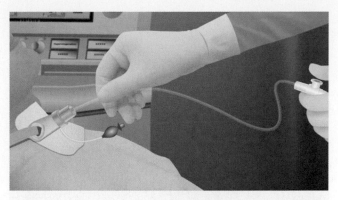

STEP 25 With the open method, keep your dominant hand and the catheter sterile.

26. **CCC** Observe the client's pulse oximeter for desaturation and observe the client for any signs of distress during suctioning. If the client shows signs of hypoxia or distress, quickly withdraw the catheter and reattach oxygen.

27. **SAF** Apply oxygen to the client to as soon as the suction catheter is removed.

28. **INF** Rinse the catheter and tubing by placing the catheter into the container of sterile solution and suctioning up enough solution to clear the catheter and tubing.

29. **EVAL** Assess how well the client tolerated suctioning. How quickly is the client's oxygen saturation returning to baseline? Assess breath sounds to determine if the secretions are cleared or if further suctioning is required.

30. **SAF** Repeat procedure no more than two additional times, and only as needed.

    a. Wait at least 30 seconds to 1 minute between suction passes.

    b. If the client is receiving pulse oximetry monitoring, wait until readings return to the client's presuctioning baseline. *This reduces the client's risk of hypoxia.*

    c. Disconnect the suction catheter from the connection tubing and discard.

Suctioning an Artificial Airway (Closed Method)

31. **CCC** Prepare the client: Provide a pillow or folded blanket for splinting if the client has an abdominal or chest surgical incision or wound. *Prevents discomfort during coughing.*

32. **INF** Remove soiled gloves. Perform hand hygiene.

33. **INF** Apply clean gloves. Apply face shield or mask/goggles, if indicated.

34. **ACC** Connect the suction tubing to the closed system suction port.

35. **ACC** Rotate the thumb valve to unlock suction according to the manufacturer's guidelines.

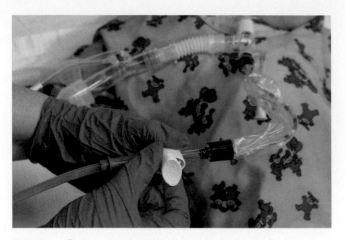

STEP 35 Rotate the thumb valve to unlock suction.

36. **ACC** Hyperoxygenate the client according to the authorized healthcare provider's guidelines.
    a. If the client is receiving mechanical ventilation, use the ventilator to provide airway pressure and increase oxygen per the authorized healthcare provider's guidelines (Note: If increasing oxygen incrementally, be careful to return oxygen to presuctioning level after suctioning.)
    b. If the client is receiving humidified oxygen via a trach collar, encourage the client to take deep breaths, if able, and to cough during tracheostomy suctioning. *This allows the client to oxygenate and expectorate sputum.*
37. **ACC** Observe the client's pulse oximeter and obtain a respiratory rate in order to have a baseline assessment prior to suctioning.
38. **ACC** Insert the suction catheter quickly but gently into the tracheostomy or ETT. With the closed method, the catheter is within a sleeve that protects the sterility of the catheter. Your other hand stabilizes the artificial airway.

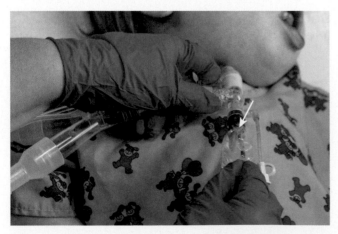

STEP 38 Insert the catheter to a predetermined mark.

    a. **Minimally invasive suctioning**: Insert catheter to the predetermined distance: the length of the trache-

ostomy tube and adapter or ETT plus 0.5 to 1.0 cm. (0.5 for children and 1.0 for adults). *This length clears the artificial airway but does not touch tracheal mucosa. This method is recommended for children and infants.*
    b. **Deep suctioning:** Insert catheter until resistance is met (this is the carina), and then withdraw the catheter 1 cm (0.5 inch). **WARNING**: Do not apply suction until after withdrawing the catheter 1 cm (0.5 inch). *Suction is not applied until after withdrawing 1 cm to avoid contact with the mucosal wall during suctioning.*
39. **ACC** Place your dominant thumb over the thumb valve to create suction and withdraw the suction catheter. Stabilize the connection of the adapter to the tracheostomy or ET tube with your other hand. Limit suctioning to a 10-second period for adults and a 5-second period for children (AACN, 2017).

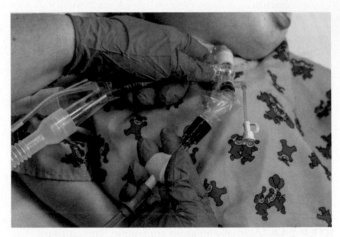

STEP 39 Apply suction and withdraw the catheter.

40. **CCC** Observe the client's pulse oximeter for desaturation and observe the client for any signs of distress during suctioning. If the client shows signs of hypoxia or distress, quickly withdraw the catheter.
41. **EVAL** Evaluate how well the client tolerated suctioning. How quickly is the client's oxygen saturation returning to baseline? Evaluate breath sounds to determine if the secretions are cleared or if further suctioning is required.
42. **SAF** Repeat the procedure no more than two additional times, and only as needed.
    a. Wait at least 30 seconds to 1 minute between suction passes.
    b. If the client is receiving pulse oximetry monitoring, wait until readings return to the client's presuctioning baseline. *This reduces the client's risk of hypoxia.*
43. **INF** Rinse the catheter and tubing by attaching a saline bullet to the side port of the inline suction catheter. Align the suction port of the catheter with the side port.
44. **INF** Instill sterile saline into the side port while applying continuous suction until the catheter is clear; be careful *not* to allow saline to enter the tracheostomy tube/ETT. Note color, consistency, and volume of secretions.

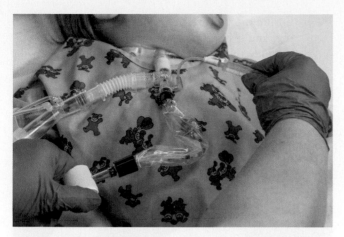

STEP 44 Instill sterile saline into the side port while applying continuous suction.

45. **ACC** Rotate the thumb valve back to locked position. *This prevents accidental suctioning.*
46. **ACC** Disconnect the suction tubing from the closed system suction port if providing oral care.

Providing Oral Care With an Artificial Airway (Suctioning Open or Closed)

47. **INF** Attach the suction catheter to a Yankauer.
48. **HLTH** Suction the client's mouth using a Yankauer and provide oral care as needed.

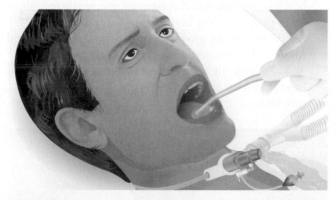

STEP 48 Suction the client's mouth using a Yankauer and provide oral care as needed.

49. **INF** Remove gloves and PPE. Perform hand hygiene.

FINISHING THE SKILL

50. **SAF** Ensure the client's oxygen administration is returned to the appropriate FiO_2 after suctioning.
51. **SAF** Ensure client safety and comfort. Place the bed in the lowest position and verify that the client can identify and reach the nurse call system. *These safety measures reduce the risk of falls.*
52. **INF** Perform hand hygiene.
53. **EVAL** Evaluate the following outcomes after suctioning:
    - client's report of difficulty breathing
    - respiratory rate, depth, and effort
    - breath sounds over trachea and lobes
    - pulse oximetry values.
54. **COM** Document assessment findings, care given, and outcomes in the legal healthcare record:
    - vital signs, including respiratory rate, depth, and effort before and after suctioning
    - breath sounds before and after suctioning
    - pulse oximetry values before and after suctioning
    - sputum color, consistency, and volume
    - size of suction catheter used
    - how the client tolerated the procedure.

■ SKILL 9.13 Obtaining a Sputum Sample From a Client With an Artificial Airway

EQUIPMENT

PPE, face shield, or mask and goggles
Clean gloves
Laboratory identification labels with appropriate client identifiers
Laboratory requisition, including appropriate client identification, date, time, name of test, and source of culture
Sterile specimen sputum trap
Wall suction and suction regulator

Suction canister and connection tubing (4–6 feet)
Biohazard bag

BEGINNING THE SKILL

1. **SAF** Review the order. Determine if specific hyperoxygenation parameters are given for suctioning. Determine if minimally invasive suctioning or deep suctioning will be performed. (Note: For minimally invasive suctioning, you must determine how far to advance the

suction catheter. This measurement is the length of the tracheostomy tube and adapter or length of the ETT plus approximately 1 cm.)

2. **INF** Perform hand hygiene.

3. **INF** Apply clean gloves. Obtain a face shield or mask and goggles and place on a clean surface. *Standard Precautions indicate the need for a mask and eye protection (a face shield provides both) during procedures that may generate sprays of respiratory secretions, especially suctioning (CDC, 2016).*

4. **CCC** Introduce yourself to the client and family and explain the procedure. Ensure that the client gives verbal consent for the suctioning procedure and specimen collection.

5. **SAF** Identify the client using two identifiers.

6. **CCC** Provide privacy. Close the door and pull the curtain.

PROCEDURE

7. **SAF** Assess the client's degree of cooperation and degree of discomfort, using a facility-approved pain tool. *Your assessment is to determine the extent to which the client can cooperate during the procedure and tolerate suctioning.*

8. **ACC** Assess the client's respiratory status prior to obtaining a sputum specimen:
   - client's report of difficulty breathing
   - respiratory rate, depth, and effort
   - breath sounds
   - pulse oximetry values.

Changes in respiratory rate are an early indicator of increased oxygen demand. Oxygen saturation changes will occur before color changes to mucous membranes or nailbeds.

9. **ACC** Position client sitting up (90 degrees) or in the high-Fowler's position (≥45 degrees), unless contraindicated. *Sitting up is much more effective than reclining. (Consider how you position yourself to cough.)*

10. **SAF** Set up an ergonomically safe space. Raise the bed to a comfortable working height. Raise one side rail. *Setting up an ergonomically safe space prevents injury to the nurse and client.*

11. **CCC** Prepare the client:
    a. Place a disposable absorbent pad or towel across the client's chest to catch secretions.
    b. Provide a pillow or folded blanket for splinting if the client has an abdominal or chest surgical incision or wound. *Prevents discomfort during coughing.*

12. **SAF** Prepare the suction equipment:
    a. Turn on wall suction regulator and adjust suction to 80 to 120 mm Hg or as prescribed. *Higher suction pressure reduces airway pressure, increasing the risk of atelectasis.* (Note: Variations regarding the amount of suction are dependent on client age or facility protocol. Use the least amount of suction necessary to remove secretions.)

b. Ensure tubing is securely connected to vacuum canister and distal end of tubing is within easy reach.
    c. Occlude the end of the connection tubing with the thumb and observe the gauge to verify maximum suction pressure.

13. **INF** Remove soiled gloves. Perform hand hygiene. Apply face shield or mask and goggles.

14. **ACC** Connect suction tube to adapter on sputum trap while maintaining sterility of sputum trap.

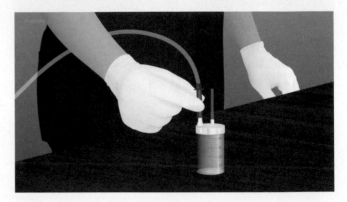

STEP 14 Connect the suction tube to the adapter on the sputum trap.

15. **INF** Prepare a sterile field:
    a. Open the sterile suction catheter package using sterile technique to create sterile field.
    b. Open the suction catheter and use sterile technique to place it on the sterile field.

16. **SAF** Apply sterile gloves; consider the dominant hand sterile and the nondominant hand nonsterile.

17. **ACC** Pick up the catheter and coil it in your dominant hand. Connect suction port of suction catheter to sputum trap.

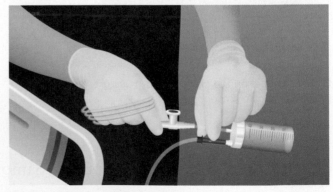

STEP 17 Connect the suction port of the suction catheter to the sputum trap.

18. **SAF** Insert tip of suction catheter through tracheostomy tube or ETT without applying suction and without touching the surface of the tube to the identified depth.

19. **ACC** Apply suction for 5 to 10 seconds to collect sufficient sputum. (Note: Check with the laboratory for the amount of sputum needed for the laboratory test ordered.)
20. **ACC** Release suction and withdraw the catheter. (Note: Do not apply suction as you withdraw the catheter. This would allow the specimen to be contaminated with flora from the upper airway.)
21. **ACC** Do not flush the catheter and tubing with sterile water. Detach catheter from specimen trap and dispose of catheter in appropriate container.
22. **ACC** Secure tubing on specimen sputum trap over the adapter to seal the container.
23. **ACC** Label specimen container in the presence of the client and place in a biohazard bag for immediate transport to the laboratory. *National safety guidelines recommend labeling specimens in the presence of the client.*

FINISHING THE SKILL

24. **INF** Remove gloves and perform hand hygiene.
25. **SAF** Ensure client safety and comfort. Place the bed in the lowest position and verify that the client can identify and reach the nurse call system. *These safety measures reduce the risk of falls.*
26. **EVAL** Evaluate the outcomes.
27. **COM** Document assessment findings, care given, and outcomes in the legal healthcare record.
    * respiratory rate, depth, and effort
    * breath sounds
    * pulse oximetry values
    * how the client tolerated the procedure
    * amount, color, and consistency of sputum collected
    * time specimen was transported to lab.

■ SKILL 9.14 Cleaning a Tracheostomy and Replacing Tracheostomy Ties

EQUIPMENT

Clean gloves, sterile gloves, and other PPE
Vital sign monitoring equipment, including stethoscope and pulse oximeter
Sterile normal saline (NS) for stoma site care and for cleaning nondisposable inner cannula
Prepackaged tracheostomy kit, or sterile containers if not using a kit
Small percolator brush, inner cannula brush, or sterile pipe cleaners, if not included in kit
Sterile cotton-tipped swabs
Sterile 4 × 4 gauze pads
Drain sponges
Sterile disposable inner cannula of appropriate size
Two replacement tracheostomy tubes of same type as the one inserted (one of the same size and one that is one size smaller) and obturators in a readily available location
Emergency equipment: suction, resuscitation bag-valve mask (BVM), and obturator positioned nearby
Tracheostomy ties
* Adjustable Velcro-secured collar
* Ribbon-like cotton (twill tie) of appropriate length
Scissors

BEGINNING THE SKILL

1. **INF** Perform hand hygiene and apply mask and goggles or a face shield. *Standard Precautions identify the need for a mask and eye protection (a face shield provides both) during procedures that may generate sprays of respiratory secretions, especially suctioning (CDC, 2016).*
2. **INF** Apply clean gloves and face shield.
3. **CCC** Introduce yourself to the client and family and explain the procedure.
4. **SAF** Identify the client using two identifiers.
5. **CCC** Provide privacy. Close the door and pull the curtain.

PROCEDURE

If replacing a disposable inner cannula, perform the following steps. If cleaning a nondisposable inner cannula, skip to step 16.
6. **ACC** Check the size of the inner cannula to determine it is the appropriate size.
7. **INF** Open the package containing the disposable inner cannula. Do not remove the cannula from the package. (Note: Double-check that the size and type of the inner cannula are the same as the one in the packaging. Do not discard old cannula until the new one is confirmed.).
8. **ACC** Remove tracheostomy oxygen collar or detach ventilator circuitry from tracheostomy tube. *Allows access to the inner cannula for removal from tracheostomy appliance.*
9. **SAF** Secure neck plate of tracheostomy with nondominant hand.

10. **ACC** Remove inner cannula from outer cannula of tracheostomy tube.
   a. **For clasp lock connector:** Pinch the clasps and withdraw the cannula. Stabilize the tracheostomy faceplate with your nondominant hand. *Reduces the risk of excess pressure being applied to tracheostomy site and prevents dislodgement.*

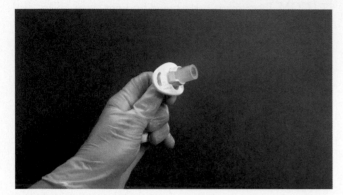

STEP 10A For a clasp lock connector, pinch the clasps and withdraw the cannula.

   b. **For adaptor lock:** Rotate the adaptor counterclockwise with your dominant hand. Stabilize the tracheostomy faceplate with your nondominant hand. *Reduces the risk of excess pressure being applied to tracheostomy site and prevents dislodgement.*

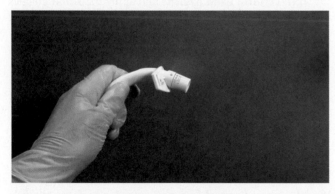

STEP 10B For an adaptor lock, rotate adaptor counterclockwise with your dominant hand.

11. **INF** Discard into an appropriate container or transfer the soiled inner cannula into your nondominant hand and place it in the new cannula package after removing the new cannula.
12. **INF** Remove the new, sterile inner cannula from the package, grasping *only* the adaptor or connector. *The inner cannula will be contaminated if touched with nonsterile gloves.*
13. **SAF** Stabilize the tracheostomy neck plate with your nondominant hand. *Reduces the risk of excess pressure being applied to tracheostomy site and prevents dislodgement.*
14. **ACC** Insert the new, sterile inner cannula into the outer cannula. Rotate or click lock into place.

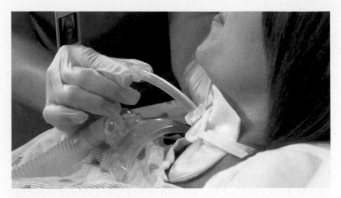

STEP 14. Insert a new, sterile inner cannula into the outer cannula.

15. **SAF** Reapply tracheostomy collar or ventilator circuitry.
If cleaning a nondisposable inner cannula, perform the following steps:
16. **INF** Open tracheostomy care kit or two individual sterile containers onto a sterile field.
17. **INF** Open the recommended sterile solution (usually sterile normal saline solution) and pour into a compartment of the tracheostomy care kit. Keep the container open to rinse scrubbed cannula. **WARNING:** Check the manufacturer guidelines before using hydrogen peroxide because it may damage some types of tracheostomy tubes. Follow facility protocol.

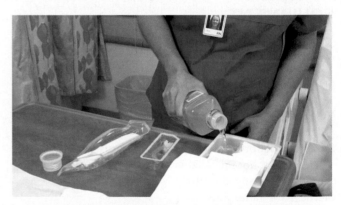

STEP 17 Pour sterile solution (normal saline) into a compartment of the sterile tracheostomy care kit.

18. **ACC** Remove tracheostomy oxygen collar or detach ventilator circuitry from tracheostomy tube. *Allows access to inner cannula for removal from tracheostomy appliance.*
19. **SAF** Position oxygen source close to outer cannula until procedure is completed. Maintain oxygen supply. (Note: Work quickly to avoid prolonged time off the ventilator or humidification source. Monitor the client's condition and oxygen saturation. If the client cannot tolerate disconnection from the oxygen source, insert the new inner cannula and reattach the oxygen source immediately, and then clean the soiled cannula and store in sterile container for later use.)
20. **INF** Remove existing inner cannula, touching only the outer adapter, and immerse in solution of sterile saline.
21. **INF** Remove clean gloves. Perform hand hygiene and apply sterile gloves.

22. **INF** Insert percolator brush and scrub clean the inner cannula.

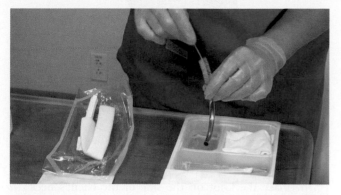

STEP 22 Insert a percolator brush and scrub the inner cannula clean.

23. **INF** Rinse inner cannula by pouring sterile saline with your nondominant hand. Maintain the sterility of your dominant hand. Shake off excess saline solution.

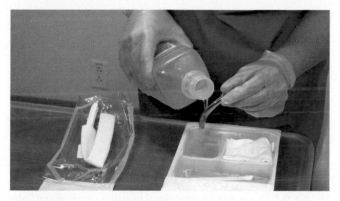

STEP 23 Rinse with sterile saline.

24. **SAF** Reinsert inner cannula into outer cannula and lock into place. Reassess the client's oxygenation status before moving on to cleaning the stoma site. Reapply the tracheostomy collar and allow recovery time if needed.

Cleaning the Stoma Site

25. **INF** Remove the soiled drainage sponge. (Note: If the dressing is soiled, remove gloves, perform hand hygiene, and reapply clean gloves.)
26. **ACC** Assess the stoma site and skin under the neck plate for inflammation, edema, or signs of discolored secretions. *This skin is at risk for moisture-associated dermatitis. Your assessment of the stoma site determines approximately how many cotton-tipped applicators will be needed to clean the area.*
27. **INF** Pour sterile normal saline into a container or an unused compartment in your kit. Add several cotton-tipped applicators. Reapply cap to sterile normal saline solution.
28. **HLTH** Clean around tracheostomy stoma and under the neck plate with the cotton-tipped applicators dipped in

sterile saline. Clean from the stoma outward. Discard in an appropriate container. *Cleaning removes any secretions.*

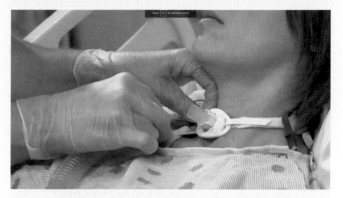

STEP 28 Clean around the tracheostomy stoma with cotton-tipped applicators.

29. **HLTH** Dry skin thoroughly with gauze sponges. Discard gauze sponges.

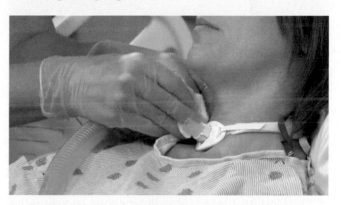

STEP 29 Dry skin thoroughly with gauze sponges.

30. **SAF** Slide the new drain sponge into place under the neck plate. **WARNING**: Do not cut a gauze sponge to use around a tracheostomy because the cotton fibers can enter the trachea (Obeid, 2018b).

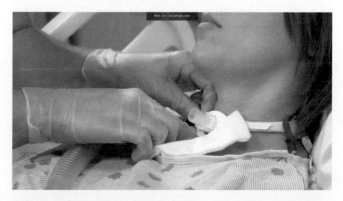

STEP 30 Slide the new drain sponge into place under the neck plate.

Replacing Tracheostomy Ties

This procedure has the inherent risk of causing movement of the tracheostomy tube, which can trigger forceful coughing.

The procedure is safely accomplished with two caregivers, one to stabilize and minimize movement of the tracheostomy tube and the other to replace the tracheostomy ties. **WARNING:** If you are changing ties alone, do not remove the old ties until the new ties are securely in place.

31. **ACC If you are replacing tracheostomy ties using a Velcro tracheostomy tube holder:**
    a. Place the new strap under the client's neck.
    b. Place the narrow end of the Velcro tie under and through the opening on one side of neck plate. Attach the narrow end to the strap. Ensure it is secure.
    c. Insert the narrow end of the strap on the other side of the neck plate and adjust the tension. (Note: The tension should allow just two fingerwidths.)

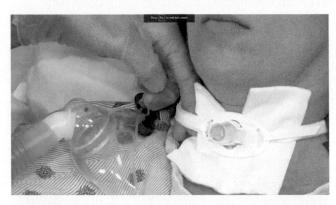

STEP 31 Adjust the tension to allow just two fingerwidths.

32. **ACC If you are replacing tracheostomy ties using twill ties:**
    a. Measure a length of twill tape long enough to encircle the client's neck twice.
    b. Cut ends diagonally.
    c. Insert one end through the neck place eyelet and pull the ends even.
    d. Bring to other side underneath the client.
    e. Instruct assistant to apply clean gloves and securely hold the tracheostomy tube in place. (Note: Do not apply pressure to the tracheostomy tube because this will cause the client to cough.)
    f. Thread one end through the neck plate's second eyelet.
    g. Secure with a double square knot on the side of the client's neck. *To reduce the potential of losing the tracheostomy tie and to prevent irritation on the client's neck.*

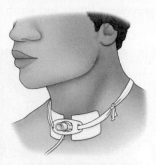

STEP 32G Secure with a double square knot on the side of the client's neck.

    h. Place the knot on the side of the client's neck. *To prevent irritation at neck or tracheostomy insertion site.*
    i. Carefully cut the old ties from the neck plate. **WARNING:** Do not remove the old ties until the new ties are securely in place.
33. **SAF** Reattach tracheostomy oxygen collar or ventilator or ventilator circuitry if it has been removed.

FINISHING THE SKILL

34. **INF** Remove gloves. Remove face shield/eye protection and any other PPE worn.
35. **INF** Perform hand hygiene.
36. **SAF** Ensure client safety and comfort. Place the bed in the lowest position and verify that the client can identify and reach the nurse call system. *These safety measures reduce the risk of falls.*
37. **EVAL** Evaluate the outcomes. Ask the client how the new tracheostomy ties feel. What is the client's respiratory status after tracheostomy care?
38. **COM** Document assessment findings, care given, and outcomes in the legal healthcare record:
    • amount, color, and viscosity of secretions noted on inner cannula or around the stoma
    • condition of the skin around the stoma, under the neck plate, and under the tracheostomy ties
    • respiratory status, including respiratory rate, depth, and effort
    • pulse oximetry values and capillary refill time
    • type and size of inner cannula (disposable or nondisposable)
    • type of ties used (Velcro or twill)
    • how the client tolerated the procedure
39. **EVAL** Monitor the client's production of secretions and how secure the tracheostomy ties are keeping the tracheostomy tube. *The inner cannula must remain patent, and the tracheostomy ties are to prevent movement of the tracheostomy tube.*

■ CASE STUDY

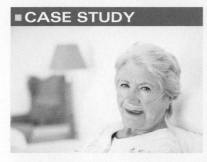

Elizabeth (Betty) Hines has a been admitted with a diagnosis of pneumonia with exacerbation of COPD. She is allergic to latex. Betty is a retired industrial secretary with a 40-year history of smoking two to three packs of cigarettes a day. She is currently on 2 L of oxygen via nasal cannula. Her orders are to maintain her oxygen saturation between 89% and 94%. If oxygen stays below 89% for >15 minutes, increase oxygen to 3 L/min. She has incentive spirometry ordered 10 times an hour. She has a history of COPD for over 10 years. To treat her pneumonia, she is on Cefazolin 500 mg q 6 hours intravenous piggyback (IVPB).

When you enter the room, you find that Betty has her legs out of the bed and her purse clutched in her hand. "I am so glad to see you!" she says. "You can help me get out of here and go for a smoke!" Her breathing is audible and labored. You do not see her nasal cannula. Her complexion is pale, with a gray cast.

"I am here to help you, Mrs. Hines, but first let me help you catch your breath! Where is your nasal cannula?"

"Oh, that thing! I have such a time keeping it on my face when I sleep," Betty says.

You trace the oxygen tubing from the flowmeter down the tubing and find the end of the nasal cannula under Betty's pillow. You slip your pulse oximeter on Mrs. Hines's finger, noting that without oxygen, her oxygen saturation is about 85%. You put her nasal cannula in position and check the oxygen flow. Her oxygen saturation increases to 91%. You help position her back in bed, explaining that your hospital has a no smoking policy. You can see and hear that as Mrs. Hines's oxygenation status improves, her breathing is less audible and is slowing down. She is also becoming more cooperative.

"What position is most comfortable for you to catch your breath, Mrs. Hines?" you ask.

"I like that little table right in front so I can lean forward on it if I need to," Mrs. Hines says.

Next, you ask about the incentive spirometer: "Have you been taking deep breaths using this device?"

"It's like taking a drag on a cigarette, except it gets me coughing so hard sometimes that I can't catch my breath," Mrs. Hines says.

"Tell me more about your cough, Mrs. Hines. Are you bringing any sputum up when you cough?"

"Yes. It just started breaking up last night," she says.

At that moment, her breakfast tray arrives, and she seems delighted to get some hot coffee, so you leave her to drink her coffee and eat her breakfast.

Case Study Questions

1. What was your top priority when you entered Betty Hines's room? Why?
2. Is there a correlation between Betty's erratic behavior in trying to leave for a cigarette and her hypoxia?
3. Betty has a diagnosis of pneumonia, an acute problem, and COPD, a chronic disease. What measures can the nurse or nursing student take collaboratively with the client to improve her respiratory status?
4. What are some ideas for keeping Betty's nasal cannula in place while she sleeps?
5. Is Betty Hines a fall risk? If so, what safety measures would you implement to help prevent her from falling?
6. Betty has said that she now has a productive cough. What are strategies to contain the sputum and microorganisms from her cough?
7. **Application of QSEN Competencies:** There are several attitude competencies in the Quality and Safety Education for Nurses (QSEN) Patient-Centered Care (which we call client-centered care) area that may apply to providing care for Betty; for example: "Recognize personally held attitudes about working with patients from different ethnic, cultural, and social backgrounds. Willingly support patient-centered care for individuals and groups whose values differ from own" (Cronenwett et al., 2007). Do you have personally held attitudes about cigarette smokers? How do you feel about the fact that Betty's habit of smoking two to three packs of cigarettes a day has impacted her health? How will you show respect for Betty's preferences, values, and needs? Look over the other attitude competencies and discuss other potential conflicts.

■ CONCEPT MAP

Baseline Assessment Data

- Client is not wearing her nasal cannula
- Client's breathing is audible and labored
- Color is pale, with a grey cast
- Oxygen saturation without supplemental oxygen is 85%
- Client is trying to leave her room to go smoke
- Diagnosis of pneumonia
- History of COPD
- 40-year history of smoking 2-3 packs of cigarettes/day
- Age >65 years

ICNP Nursing Dx: Impaired Gas Exchange

Supporting Data:
History of COPD
Oxygen saturation without oxygen is 85% and breathing is labored

ICNP Nursing Dx: Acute Confusion

Supporting Data:
When her nasal cannula is off, Betty tries to leave the facility
When her oxygen is on, she is cooperative and states she understands she cannot smoke in the room and must have assistance getting out of bed

ICNP Nursing Dx: Risk for Fall

Supporting Data:
Age, acute illness, and recent change in cognition
Client tried to leave her room to go smoke

Administer Oxygen and Optimize Gas Exchange

- Administer 2 L oxygen via nasal cannula
- Maintain oxygen saturation between 89% and 94%
- Use the incentive spirometer 10 times/hour
- Assist the client into a comfortable position that facilitates gas exchange

Reduce Risk for Hypoxic Episodes

- Provide client-centered communication with frequent orientation to place and time
- Provide Mrs. Hines several choices to secure the nasal cannula to her face, especially while sleeping, such as transparent dressing, a small piece of Duoderm, or paper tape
- Communicate client status to all members of the healthcare team
- Encourage healthcare team members to check on Mrs. Hines frequently, especially at night to verify the nasal cannula is in place
- Promote continuity of caregivers

Reduce Risk for Falls

- Keep bed in lowest position and locked
- Provide hourly rounding and ask about assistance with elimination
- Ensure Mrs. Hines can identify and demonstrate the nurse call system
- Complete a fall risk assessment for older adults

References

American Association of Critical-Care Nurses. (2017). In D. L. Weigand (Ed.), *AACN Procedure manual for high acuity, progressive, and critical care* (7th ed.). St. Louis, MO: Elsevier.

American Association for Respiratory Care (2010). AARC clinical practice guidelines. Endotracheal suctioning of mechanically ventilated patients with artificial airways 2010. *Respiratory Care, 55*(6), 758–764.

American Nurses Association (2017). *Scope of practice.* Retrieved from https://www.nursingworld.org/practice-policy/scope-of-practice/.

American Thoracic Society (2000). Care of the child with a chronic tracheostomy. Official statement of the American Thoracic Society. *American Journal of Respiratory and Critical Care Medicine, 161*(1), 297–308.

Beddoe, A. E., & Engelke, Z. (2018). *Patient education: Incentive spirometry at the bedside. Nursing practice & skill.* Ipswich, MA: EBSCO Publishing. Retrieved from Cinahl Information Systems.

Boroughs, D., & Dougherty, J. (n.d.). *Evidence-based pediatric secretion management.* Retrieved from https://www.nurse.com/ce/evidence-based-pediatric-secretion-management.

Boroughs, D., & Dougherty, J. (2015). Pediatric tracheostomy care: What home care nurses need to know. *American Nurse Today, 10*(3), 8–10.

Caple, C., & Schub, E. (2017). Chest physical therapy: Performing- an overview. *Nursing practice & skill.* Ipswich, MA: EBSCO Publishing. Retrieved from Cinahl Information Systems.

Centers for Disease Control and Prevention. (2016). *Protecting healthcare personnel.* Retrieved from https://www.cdc.gov/hai/prevent/ppe.html.

Chu, D. K., Kim, L. H., Young, P. J., et al. (2018). Mortality and morbidity in acutely ill adults treated with liberal versus conservative oxygen therapy (IOTA): A systematic review and meta-analysis. *Lancet, 391*, 1693–1705.

Cronenwett, L., Sherwood, G., Barnsteiner, J., Disch, J., Johnson, J., Mitchell, P., ...Warren, J. (2007). Quality and safety education for nurses. *Nursing Outlook, 55*(3), 122–131.

Giles, K. (2018a). *Bronchiolitis (acute): Chest physiotherapy for infants.* [Evidence summary]. Retrieved from The Joanna Briggs Institute EBP Database, JBI@Ovid. JBI940.

Giles, K. (2018b). *Infant (preterm low birth weight): Supplemental oxygen.* [Evidence summary]. Retrieved from The Joanna Briggs Institute EBP Database, JBI@Ovid. JBI1968.

Halm, M. A., & Krisko-Hagel, K. (2008). Instilling normal saline with suctioning: Beneficial technique or potentially harmful sacred cow? *American Journal of Critical Care, 17*(5), 469–472.

International Classification for Nursing Practice. (n.d.). *eHealth & ICNP.* Retrieved from https://www.icn.ch/what-we-do/projects/ehealth-icnp.

Jaffe, S. E., & Balderrama, D. (2017). *Nasopharyngeal airway: Inserting in adults. Nursing practice and skill.* Ipswich, MA: EBSCO Publishing. Retrieved from Cinahl Information Systems.

Jayasekara, R. (2018). *Home oxygen therapy (pediatrics).* [Evidence summary]. Retrieved from The Joanna Briggs Institute EBP Database, JBI@Ovid. JBI1722.

Khanh-Dao Le, L. (2018). *Oxygen therapy: Hospital setting.* [Evidence summary]. Retrieved from The Joanna Briggs Institute EBP Database, JBI@Ovid. JBI164.

Lamb, K., & Piper, D. (2016). Southmedic Oxymask™ GM compared with the Hudson RCI Non-Rebreather Mask MT safety and performance comparison. *Canadian Journal of Respiratory Therapy, 52*(1), 13–15.

Lewis, S., Butcher, L., Heitkemper, M., & Harding, M. M. (2017). In J. Kwong, & D. Roberts (Eds.), *Medical-surgical nursing: Assessment and management of clinical problems* (10th ed.). St. Louis, MO: Elsevier.

Lindman, J. P., Peralta, R., Elluru, R. G., & Khan, M. K. (2017). *Tracheostomy. Medscape drugs & diseases.* Retrieved from https://emedicine.medscape.com/article/865068-overview#a2.

Morris, L. L., Whitmer, A., & McIntosh, E. (2013). Tracheostomy care and complications in the intensive care unit. *Critical Care Nurse, 33*(5), 18–30.

Obeid, S. (2018a). *Chest physiotherapy: Chronic obstructive pulmonary disease and bronchiectasis.* [Evidence summary]. Retrieved from The Joanna Briggs Institute EBP Database, JBI@Ovid. JBI262.

Obeid, S. (2018b). *Tracheostomy (older adults): Dressing.* [Evidence summary]. Retrieved from The Joanna Briggs Institute EBP Database, JBI@Ovid. JBI1774.

Paull, T. (2017). *Chest physiotherapy: Clinician information.* [Evidence summary]. Retrieved from The Joanna Briggs Institute EBP Database, JBI@Ovid. JBI196.

Schub, E., & Balderrama, D. (2017). Providing oxygen therapy by face mask: Adult patient. *Nursing practice & skill.* Ipswich, MA: EBSCO Publishing. Retrieved from Cinahl Information Systems.

Schub, T., & Caple, C. (2018). Oxygen cylinder, high pressure: Using. *Nursing practice & skill.* Ipswich, MA: EBSCO Publishing. Retrieved from Cinahl Information Systems.

Schub, E., & Heering, H. (2017). Providing oxygen therapy by nasal cannula. *Nursing practice & skill.* Ipswich, MA: EBSCO Publishing. Retrieved from Cinahl Information Systems.

Schub, T., & Walsh, K. (2017). Administration of oxygen therapy by T-piece. *Nursing practice & skill.* Ipswich, MA: EBSCO Publishing. Retrieved from Cinahl Information Systems.

Sharma, L. (2018a). *Pharyngeal suction: Clinician information.* [Evidence summary]. Retrieved from The Joanna Briggs Institute EBP Database, JBI@Ovid. JBI237.

Sharma, L. (2018b). *Tracheostomy and endotracheal tube suctioning.* [Evidence summary]. Retrieved from The Joanna Briggs Institute EBP Database, JBI@Ovid. JBI1357.

Slade, S. (2017). *Continuous positive airway pressure (CPAP) for obstructive sleep apnea in adults: Clinician information.* [Evidence summary]. Retrieved from Joanna Briggs Institute EBP Database, JBI@Ovid. JBI129.

Slade, S. (2018). *Chest physiotherapy: Pneumonia.* [Evidence summary]. Retrieved from The Joanna Briggs Institute EBP Database, JBI@Ovid. JBI1009.

Smith, N. (2017). Humidification therapy: Using a diffusion head humidifier. *Nursing practice & skill.* Ipswich, MA: EBSCO Publishing. Retrieved from Cinahl Information Systems.

Southmedic. (n.d.). *OxyMask.* Retrieved from http://thebetteroxygenmask.com/oxymask/.

Walsh, K., & Woten, M. (2018). Oropharyngeal airway: Insertion in adults. *Nursing practice and skill.* Ipswich, MA: EBSCO Publishing. Retrieved from Cinahl Information Systems.

Warnock, L., & Gates, A. (2015). Chest physiotherapy compared to no chest physiotherapy for cystic fibrosis. *Cochrane Database of Systematic Reviews, 2015* (12), 1-44.

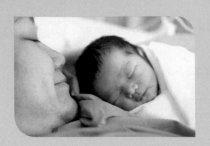

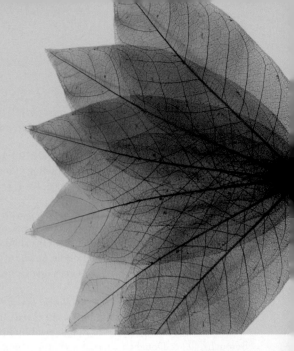

CHAPTER 10

Sterile Technique

"Louis Pasteur's theory of germs is ridiculous fiction." | **Pierre Pachet, Professor of Physiology, 1872**

SECTION 1 Preparing a Sterile Field

- **SKILL 10.1** Opening a Sterile Pack
- **SKILL 10.2** Applying and Removing Sterile Gloves
- **SKILL 10.3** Opening a Sterile Barrier and Setting Up a Sterile Field
- **SKILL 10.4** Adding Sterile Items to a Sterile Field and Draping a Sterile Field
- **SKILL 10.5** Pouring a Sterile Liquid

SECTION 2 Preparing to Enter a Sterile Perioperative Setting

- **SKILL 10.6** Performing a Surgical Handrub
- **SKILL 10.7** Performing a Surgical Hand Scrub
- **SKILL 10.8** Performing Surgical Gowning
- **SKILL 10.9** Performing Closed Surgical Gloving

LEARNING OBJECTIVES

By the end of this chapter, the reader will be able to:

1. Discuss the difference between sterile technique and clean technique.
2. Identify and apply principles of sterile technique.
3. Open a sterile pack.
4. Perform sterile gloving.
5. Open a sterile barrier and set up a sterile field.
6. Add sterile items to a sterile field.
7. Cover a sterile field with drapes.
8. Pour a sterile liquid.
9. Perform a surgical handrub and hand scrub.
10. Perform surgical gowning.
11. Perform surgical gloving.

TERMINOLOGY

Draping Technique involving covering a patient and surrounding the patient area with a sterile barrier to minimize the potential transmission of microorganisms from nonsterile to sterile areas.

Persistent activity Ability of an antimicrobial product to prevent or inhibit the growth or survival of microorganisms after the initial application of the product; also known as residual activity.

Sterile Free from all living microorganisms, including bacteria, viruses, and fungi and their spores.

Sterile barrier Drape used to separate a sterile area from a nonsterile area.

Sterile field Specified area, such as within a tray or on a sterile barrier, which is considered free of microorganisms.

Sterile technique Technique to maintain a sterile surface of an object.

Subungual Under the nail.

Surgical hand antisepsis Antiseptic hand scrub or antiseptic handrub performed preoperatively by surgical personnel to eliminate transient hand flora and reduce resident hand flora.

Surgical handrub Surgical hand preparation with a waterless, alcohol-based handrub.

Surgical hand scrub Surgical hand preparation with antimicrobial soap and water.

Wick (wicking) To draw liquid by capillary action.

ACRONYMS

AORN Association of PeriOperative Registered Nurses
SSI Surgical-site infection

The term *sterile* refers to the complete absence of microorganisms and spores and thus is different from the term *clean,* which refers to a decrease in microorganisms but not their complete elimination. *Sterile technique,* also called *surgical asepsis,* is a set of procedures designed to keep sterile items sterile and to minimize contamination. The ultimate goal of sterile technique is to prevent healthcare-associated infection (HAI).

Approximately 1 out of every 25 persons hospitalized will develop an HAI (Centers for Disease Control and Prevention [CDC], 2018c). Prevention is critical because HAIs can sometimes be fatal. They also result in longer hospital stays and increased costs, and third-party payers may not cover the extra patient costs related to an HAI (Paull, 2017).

The development of sterile technique has mirrored the development of surgical advances, which changed and progressed as our understanding of microorganisms expanded. Several notable scientists are credited with our understanding of microorganisms and infection. The French chemist and biologist Louis Pasteur (1822–1895) established the link between microorganisms and disease and was responsible for the widespread acceptance of the germ theory of disease. As you can see by the quote from Pierre Pachet at the beginning of this chapter, many of Pasteur's contemporaries were not immediately persuaded that microorganisms could cause disease. However, Pasteur's ideas were eventually accepted because his application of germ theory resulted in visibly successful techniques, such as preventing milk from spoiling through pasteurization, preventing wine from souring, and the development of a rabies vaccine.

Lord Joseph Lister (1827–1912), an English doctor, applied the germ theory to medical procedures. He developed a carbolic acid mixture to kill microorganisms and sprayed it on surgical instruments and directly into wounds. He instituted hygienic practices within the surgical area and was rewarded with dramatically lower infection rates. His success was noted by Queen Victoria, and he became her personal surgeon.

Not all advocates of infection control met with success. The sad story of the Austrian physician Ignaz Semmelweis (1818–1865) is often repeated by infection control nurses. Before the achievements of Pasteur and Lister, Semmelweis came to the conclusion that hand washing could prevent the transfer of infectious material. He began the practice of hand washing with a lime chloride solution between autopsies and seeing his patients. Despite a dramatic decrease in infection rates, he found no support for his ideas. Mocked by his colleagues and demoted at his hospital, Semmelweis became severely depressed. He was committed to a mental institution where, ironically, he died from septicemia from a cut on his finger.

Preparing a Sterile Field

When surgery or any other procedure requires the penetration of body tissue or contact with mucous membranes, sterile technique is used to prevent the introduction of microorganisms into the body. It begins with the sterilization of objects and surfaces, typically by exposure to high heat, steam, or gases such as formaldehyde or ethylene oxide that kill microorganisms. When a surface cannot be sterilized, it is cleaned with a substance that kills microorganisms. For example, human skin is not sterilized but cleaned with antiseptic agents, such as chlorhexidine gluconate, or isopropyl alcohol (70%–90%), to reduce the number of microorganisms. Large items that cannot be sterilized, such as tables, chairs, walls, and imaging equipment, are cleaned with disinfectants to reduce the number of microorganisms. Skin and nonsterile equipment and furniture are then draped to prevent transferring microorganisms to sterile surfaces. See Chapter 1 for more information on disinfectants.

Preventing the contamination of sterile items is the driving goal behind the principles of sterile technique, which are identified in Box 10.1. To prevent surgical-site infections, strict adherence to these principles is essential for all members of the surgical team (Paull, 2017). For example, sterile gloved hands remain above the waist and within view at all times so that all members of the team are confident of their sterility. Protocols for sterile procedures indicate the role of a scrubbed and gloved individual as well as the role of an unscrubbed assistant. Nurses fill both of these roles and need to be adept at the techniques and procedures within both roles. Nurses also verify the sterility of instruments and equipment. For example, nurses check sterile packages for any potential breaks in sterility, such as moisture or tears in the wrapping, and check the sterilization expiration date marked on the packages. Inspection of equipment and adherence to sterile technique by nurses can prevent many breaks in sterile technique. Box 10.2 lists common breaks in sterile technique.

Sterile technique is also practiced in areas beyond the perioperative setting. As just noted, any procedure that requires the penetration of body tissue, such as starting an intravenous line, or insertion into a sterile area, such as inserting a urinary catheter, requires sterile technique in order to prevent the introduction of microorganisms. Practice and protocols may differ, however, according to the environment because the perioperative setting, hospital, long-term care facility, and home each have different factors influencing the risk for infection. Variables in the home environment are discussed in Box 10.3.

Today, there is a concerted national effort to research HAIs and develop trial sterility protocols to reduce their number. As a result, nursing practice continues to evolve. For example, research evidence indicates that nurses should prepare sterile fields as close in time to when they will be used and in the location where they will be used (Association of PeriOperative Registered Nurses [AORN],

---

BOX 10.1 Principles of Sterile Technique

- Sterile drapes are used to create a sterile field.
- Sterile only touches sterile.
- All items introduced onto a sterile field are opened, dispensed, and transferred by methods that maintain sterility and integrity.
- A sterile field is monitored at all times.
- Contaminated items must be removed immediately from the sterile field.
- When a sterile barrier becomes wet, it is no longer sterile.
- Nonsterile items should not cross over a sterile field.
- Below the waist or below the tabletop is not considered sterile.
- If a drape extends over the sides of a table, the drape is sterile only at the table level.
- Always face a sterile field.
- Avoid talking, coughing, or sneezing over a sterile field.
- Do not reach over a sterile field.
- When you create a sterile field, there is a 2.5-cm (1-inch) border around the field that is not sterile.

BOX10.2 Common Breaks in Sterile Technique When Setting Up a Sterile Field

- Not checking sterility indicators
- Not noticing tears in sterile packaging
- Not recognizing soaked-through spots
- Contaminating the sterile field, instruments, or supplies
- Improperly delivering solutions
- Improperly moving tables
- Leaving sterile supplies open too long

Adapted from Hopper & Moss, 2010; Spruce, 2017.

BOX 10.3 Home Care Considerations: Preventing Infection in the Home

Although much of the discussion of sterile technique is related to surgery, it also applies to invasive procedures occurring in other settings. Home care has become increasingly complex, and today, many people with invasive devices are cared for at home. The study of home care–associated infections is still in its infancy. The home should have fewer risks for the transfer of microorganisms. For some procedures, such as intermittent catheterization, the recommendation is to perform the skill using clean technique rather than sterile technique in the non–acute care setting (CDC, 2016). When items need to be disinfected in the home, there are three methods that can be safely used: bleach, hydrogen peroxide, or 70% isopropyl alcohol (see Chapter 1, Box 1.5) (CDC, 2018b). Preventing infection in the home is based on the fundamental infection control principles, including reducing the number of microorganisms and preventing their transfer.

BOX 10.4 Lessons From the Evidence: How Quickly Do Open Trays Become Contaminated?

A study sponsored by AORN examined the rate at which uncovered sterile trays become contaminated within a 4-hour period and the effect of operating room (OR) traffic on the contamination rate. Forty-five trays were divided into three groups, and all trays were opened using sterile technique. One group of trays was covered immediately. One group was left uncovered in a room with no traffic, and the last group was left uncovered in a room with traffic. All trays were cultured upon opening and then every 30 minutes for a 4-hour period. The results of the study showed that the covered trays were not contaminated during the testing period. The results also showed a direct relationship between the contamination of an uncovered OR tray and the duration of open exposure, with 30% of the trays contaminated at 4 hours. There was no difference in the contamination rate between the uncovered trays in the room with traffic and those in the room without traffic. The evidence supports not opening trays until immediately before they are needed and, if sterile trays must be opened earlier, covering them with a sterile towel to minimize the exposure to environmental contaminants.

References: AORN, 2018; Dalstrom et al., 2008.

2018). If there is an unexpected delay after a sterile field is set up or during periods of increased activity, the sterile field is covered with sterile drapes (AORN, 2018). Box 10.4 describes how a research study informed evidence-based practice.

Nurses select the type of barrier on which to set up a sterile field. The barrier may be paper or may have a plastic film on one side making it impervious to moisture. The moisture-proof side will be slick and shiny. Nurses place the moisture-proof side down in order to prevent microorganisms from wicking through from the surface underneath. Typically, the blue side of a barrier goes down on the surface, and the white side is facing up.

Because a sterile field is a three-dimensional space, sterile technique does not allow unsterile objects or bare hands to cross over the sterile field. The sequence of opening supplies, the method of adding items to the sterile field, and the method of pouring liquid all affect the maintenance of a sterile field. For example, nurses open sterile packs before applying sterile gloves because the outer wrapper of the sterile pack is not sterile. The outside of a sterile liquid container is very seldom sterile. Therefore, nurses must plan when to open and pour the liquid within the sequence of setting up the sterile field and before putting on sterile gloves.

Sometimes wearing a surgical mask is indicated when setting up a sterile field. Examples include during preparation for surgery, for central venous catheter insertion, for peripherally inserted central catheter insertion, and for spinal canal procedures (AORN, 2018). The mask must be put on before sterile gloves are applied. Once set up, a sterile field must be monitored to ensure sterility. Conversations are kept to a minimum to prevent droplet transmission of microorganisms.

APPLICATION OF THE NURSING PROCESS

Examples of Related International Classification for Nursing Practice (ICNP) Nursing Diagnoses, Expected Client Outcomes, and Nursing Interventions:

Nursing Diagnosis: Risk for infection
Supporting Data: One in 25 hospital residents has an HAI.
Expected Client Outcome: The client will not demonstrate any signs of an HAI while in the healthcare setting.
Nursing Intervention Example: Strict adherence to principles of sterile technique when preparing a sterile field
Reference: International Classification for Nursing Practice. (n.d.). *eHealth & ICNP.* Retrieved from https://www.icn.ch/what-we-do/projects/ehealth-icnp.

CRITICAL CONCEPTS
Preparing a Sterile Field

Accuracy (ACC)

The accuracy of sterile technique is subject to the following variables:
Nurse-Related Factors
• Adherence to AORN and CDC guidelines
• Recognition of accidental contamination
Equipment-Related Factors
• Proper sterilization of liquids and equipment

Client-Centered Care (CCC)

When preparing a sterile field, respect for the client is demonstrated primarily through:
• acknowledgment of the individual
• ensuring comfort.

Infection Control (INF)

Healthcare-associated infection is prevented by:
• containment of microorganisms
• preventing and reducing the transfer of microorganisms
• reducing the number of microorganisms.

Safety (SAF)

When preparing a sterile field, safety measures prevent harm to the client and maintain a safe care environment.

Communication (COM)

• Communication exchanges information (oral, written, nonverbal, or electronic) between two or more people.
• Collaborating with the client and healthcare team facilitates preparing and maintaining a sterile field.

Evaluation (EVAL)

When preparing a sterile field, evaluation of outcomes enables the nurse to determine the efficacy of the sterile technique provided.

■ SKILL 10.1 Opening a Sterile Pack

EQUIPMENT

Sterile pack
Sterile mask, if required

BEGINNING THE SKILL

1. **INF** Perform hand hygiene.
2. **CCC** Introduce yourself to the client and family.
3. **SAF** Identify the client using two identifiers.
4. **COM** Explain the procedure and instruct the client not to touch or cross over the sterile barrier and not to touch any items on the sterile field. *A sterile pack may be opened very close to the client, and the client must be instructed not to touch the sterile pack and sterile wrapping.*
5. **ACC** Apply a sterile mask if indicated by the type of procedure or facility policy. *Wearing a sterile mask prevents contamination of the field with microorganisms from the nurse by airborne or droplet transmission. Wearing a sterile mask is required by CDC and AORN policy for specific procedures.*
6. **INF** Set a clean work surface at waist height. If needed, wipe the surface clean, dry thoroughly, and perform hand hygiene again. *Cleaning the work surface reduces the number of microorganisms. Drying prevents moisture from contaminating the pack. Setting the work surface at waist height adheres to the sterile principles.*

PROCEDURE

7. **ACC** Examine the sterile pack for proper sterile processing, package integrity, and expiration date. *Careful inspection prevents the use of a contaminated pack.*
8. If the pack has an outer wrapper, peel open the outer wrapper and discard in a trash receptacle. Place the pack on the center of the work surface.
9. **INF** Position the pack with the top flap of the wrapper set to open away from you. Do not touch any of the inside folds of the wrapper. *The sequence used to open a pack allows for each side to be unwrapped while never crossing over the sterile field.*
10. **INF** Reach around (not over) the pack and pinch the first flap on the outside of the pack wrapper between the thumb and index finger. Pull the flap away from you until open and lay it flat on the far surface. *Reaching over the pack would be a break in sterile technique.*

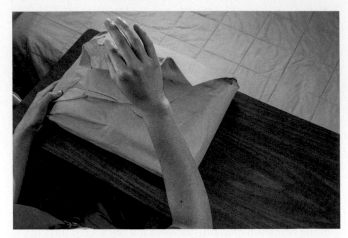

STEP 10 Pull the first flap away from you.

11. Use your left hand to pull the left flap to the left and lay it on the work surface. *Do not allow an unsterile surface, such as your sleeve, to touch the inside of the sterile pack.*

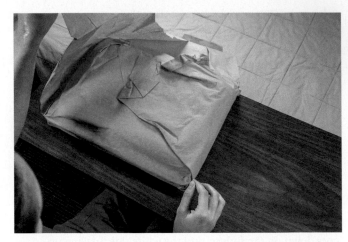

STEP 11 Use your left hand to pull the left flap to the left.

12. Use your right hand to pull the right flap to the right and lay it on the work surface.
13. **INF** Grasp the final flap and pull toward you. Lay it on the work surface. (Note: If the folded flap attempts to refold in toward the sterile field, you can rub the outside of the flap over the table edge in order to straighten out the folds.)

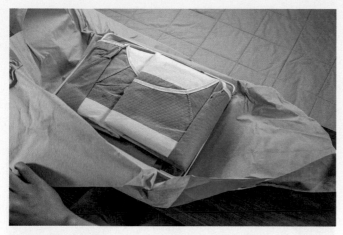

STEP 13 Grasp the final flap and pull toward you.

14. **INF** The sterile pack is now open. Wear sterile gloves if you need to touch items within the sterile pack.
15. **INF** Cover the sterile field if there is a delay in use. *The evidence supports covering open sterile trays with a sterile drape until they are needed to minimize the exposure to environmental contaminants.*

FINISHING THE SKILL

16. **INF** Remove and discard sterile mask in a trash receptacle, if used.
17. **EVAL** Evaluate the performance of the skill for adherence to sterile technique. *Are you confident there was no break in sterile technique?*

■ SKILL 10.2 Applying and Removing Sterile Gloves

EQUIPMENT

Sterile gloves

BEGINNING THE SKILL

1. **INF** Remove rings and jewelry.
2. **INF** Set a clean work surface at waist height. If needed, wipe the surface clean, and dry thoroughly. *Cleaning the work surface reduces microorganisms. Drying prevents moisture from contaminating the pack. Setting the work surface at waist height adheres to the sterile principles.*
3. **INF** Perform hand hygiene.

PROCEDURE

Applying Sterile Gloves

4. **INF** Place the wrapped sterile gloves on the work surface.
5. **INF** Peel open the outer wrapper of the glove package. Discard the outer wrapper. *The outside of the outer wrapper is not sterile. The inside glove package is sterile.*
6. **INF** Place the inner glove wrapper in front of you. The wrapper is marked to indicate where the cuffs are. Position the wrapper so that the cuff end is closest to you. *The cuffs must be closest to you in order to not reach over the sterile field.*
7. **INF** Unfold the top and bottom edges of the inner wrapper, touching only the outside of the wrapper. *These edges are now the top and bottom margins of your sterile field.*
8. **INF** Grasp the two edges in the center of the wrapper and lift the edges up and away to expose the gloves. *These edges are now the left and right margins of your sterile field. Do not touch the inside the margins of the wrapper or the sterile gloves with your unsterile hands.*
9. The gloves are positioned in the wrapper with the palms up and the thumbs facing the outer edges.

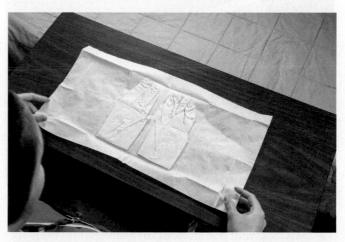

STEP 9 Gloves are positioned with the palms up and the thumbs out.

10. **ACC** If the wrapper does not easily lie flat, create a horizontal crease in the wrapper by pinching the sides of the wrapper. (Note: Wrappers sometimes refold to their previously folded position. This could contaminate the gloves if the margin of the wrapper that you touched then touches the sterile gloves.)

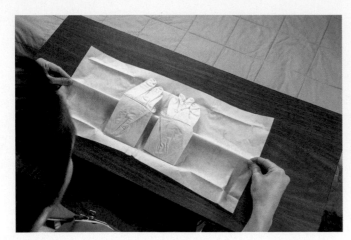

STEP 10 Create a horizontal crease in the wrapper.

11. **INF** With your nondominant hand, pinch the folded cuff (inside part of glove) of the dominant-hand glove. Lift the glove up and off the table. (Note: Do not allow the fingertips of the glove to touch any surface, and do not touch any part of the sterile outside surface of the glove with your unsterile hands.) *Gloving the dominant hand first allows it to manipulate gloving the nondominant hand, which requires a little more dexterity.*

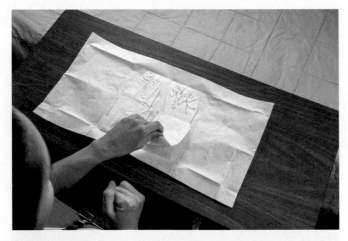

STEP 11 Pinch the folded cuff of the glove.

12. **ACC** Slip your dominant hand (palm up) into the glove.

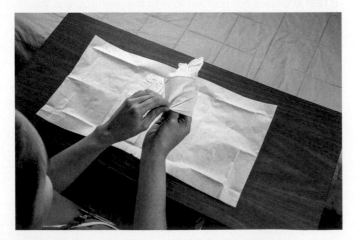

STEP 12 Slip your dominant hand into the glove.

13. **INF** Pull the glove onto your hand, touching only the folded cuff. Keep your fingers together as you slide through the palm of the glove and then spread out your fingers just before entering the glove fingers. *This will align the glove fingers with your fingers.* (Note: If the cuff does not fall into place, slip a finger under the inside of the cuff and pull it into place.) *Only the inside of the cuff can be handled with unsterile fingers.*

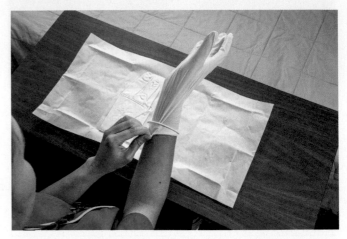

STEP 13 Pull the glove on, touching only the cuff.

14. **INF** To pick up the other glove, hold the four gloved fingers of your dominant hand together and scoop under the folded cuff of the glove lying on the wrapper. *To maintain sterile technique, the sterile gloved hand touches only the sterile outside surface of the second glove.*

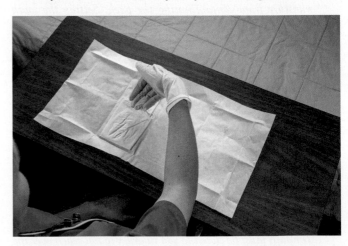

STEP 14 Scoop under the folded cuff of the glove.

15. **INF** Hold your gloved thumb out like a hitchhiker. Slip your nondominant hand, palm up, into the glove and continue to pull the glove onto your hand. Release the glove cuff over your wrist. Do not allow the sterile gloved fingers of your dominant hand to touch your wrist.

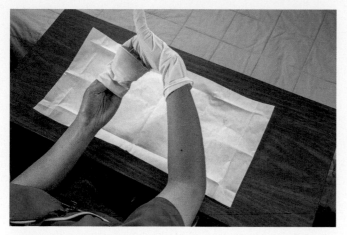

STEP 15 Hold your gloved thumb out and slip your non-dominant hand into the glove.

16. **INF** Do not touch the cuffs of the glove of your non-dominant hand. *The cuff is now against your skin, and a 2.5-cm (1-inch) margin of the cuff is considered contaminated.*

17. **INF** You may adjust your gloves as long as sterile only touches sterile. Plucking the gloves at the palm and pressing between your fingers with the fingertips of the other hand will adjust the fit of the gloves.

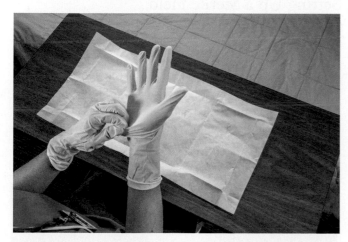

STEP 17 Adjust your gloves.

18. **INF** Hold your hands up and away from the table and your body. **WARNING:** Do not touch any unsterile object or person with your sterile gloves.

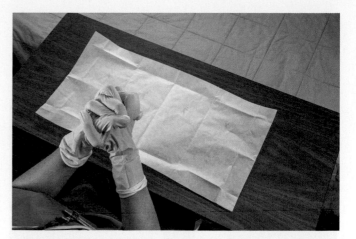

STEP 18 Hold your hands away from your body.

Removing Sterile Gloves

19. **INF** With one hand, grasp the glove on your other hand near the cuff. Do not touch your skin with the soiled glove.

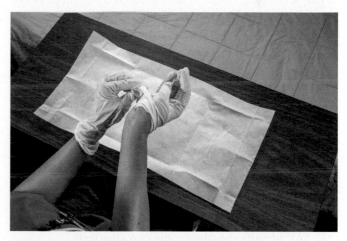

STEP 19 Grasp the glove near the cuff.

20. **INF** Pull the glove off your hand. The glove will turn inside out as you pull it off. Bunch up the soiled glove in your gloved hand.

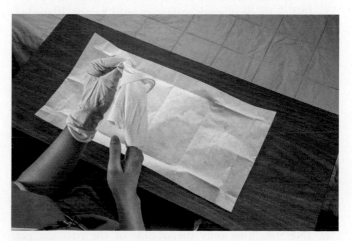

STEP 20 Pull the glove off your hand.

21. **INF** Slip a bare finger or thumb under the cuff of the gloved hand. Pull the glove off your other hand. The glove will turn inside out, and the glove from the first hand will be contained within it. *Turning the gloves inside out contains the microorganisms on the soiled gloves within the gloves.*

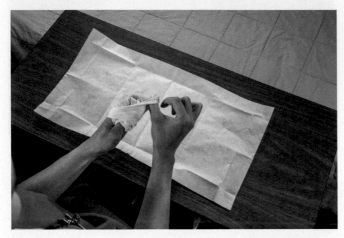

STEP 21 Slip your finger under the cuff and pull the glove off.

22. **INF** Dispose of the gloves in a trash receptacle.

FINISHING THE SKILL

23. **INF** Perform hand hygiene.
24. **EVAL** Evaluate the performance of the skill for adherence to sterile technique. *Are you confident there was no break in sterile technique?*

■ SKILL 10.3 Opening a Sterile Barrier and Setting Up a Sterile Field

EQUIPMENT

Sterile barrier
Sterile mask, if required

BEGINNING THE SKILL

1. **INF** Perform hand hygiene.
2. **CCC** Introduce yourself to the client and family.
3. **SAF** Identify the client using two identifiers.
4. **COM** Explain the procedure and instruct the client not to touch or cross over the sterile barrier and not to touch any items on the sterile field. *A sterile barrier may be opened very close to the client, and the client is instructed not to touch the sterile barrier and sterile field.*
5. **INF** Set a clean work surface at waist height. If needed, wipe the surface clean, dry thoroughly, and perform hand hygiene again. *Cleaning the work surface reduces the number of microorganisms. Drying prevents moisture from contaminating the pack. Setting the work surface at waist height adheres to the sterile principles.*
6. **ACC** Apply a sterile mask if indicated by the type of procedure or facility policy. *Wearing a sterile mask prevents contamination of the field with microorganisms from the nurse by airborne or droplet transmission. Wearing a sterile mask is required by CDC and AORN policy for specific procedures.*

PROCEDURE

7. Place the wrapped sterile barrier on the work surface.
8. **INF** Touching only the outside of the package, peel open the outside wrapper of the sterile barrier package to completely expose the sterile barrier. Do not allow the sterile barrier to touch the table surface. *The inside of the package is sterile; the outside is not. The sterile barrier is folded and placed on the opened wrapper.*
9. **ACC** Examine the folded sterile barrier and determine which corner is folded and which corner is "free."
10. **INF** Pinch the free corner between your thumb and index finger and lift the barrier up and away from the table so that the barrier does not touch the table surface as it unfolds.

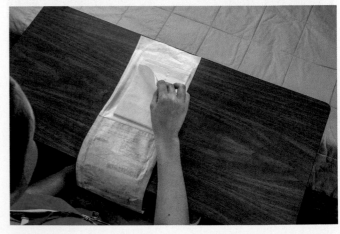

STEP 10 Pinch the free corner and lift the barrier up.

11. **ACC** Locate an adjacent corner. With your other hand, pinch that corner and fully open the sterile barrier. Keep in mind that your sterile barrier has a 2.5-cm (1-inch) border. If the barrier refuses to unfold smoothly, find the next free corner and rotate the barrier, pulling the folds open.

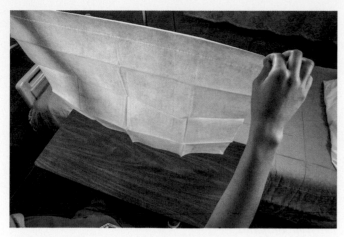

STEP 11 Pinch the adjacent corner and fully open the sterile barrier.

12. **ACC** Determine if there is an absorbent side and a moisture-proof side. Turn the barrier so that the absorbent side or white side will be up and the moisture-proof side or blue side will be down. *The moisture-proof side will be slick and shiny. Not all barriers have a moisture-proof side. The advantage of having a moisture-proof side is to prevent contamination of the sterile field if there is a spill or splash. If there is not a moisture-proof barrier, the microorganisms will wick through a wet barrier.*

13. **ACC** Place the barrier on the work surface by placing the hanging free corners away from you and placing the corners that you are holding on the work surface closest

to you. Do not allow your hands or forearms to cross over the sterile barrier. *You now have a three-dimensional sterile field.*

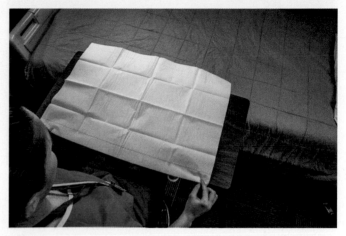

STEP 13 Place the barrier on the work surface.

FINISHING THE SKILL

14. **EVAL** Evaluate the sterile field for evidence of adherence to sterile principles. *Evidence of moisture or items within the 2.5-cm (1-inch) border would indicate a break in sterile technique.*

15. **EVAL** Evaluate the performance of the skill for adherence to sterile technique. *Are you confident there was no break in sterile technique?*

■ SKILL 10.4 Adding Sterile Items to a Sterile Field and Draping a Sterile Field

EQUIPMENT

Sterile barrier
Sterile items
Sterile mask, if required

BEGINNING THE SKILL

1. **INF** Perform hand hygiene.
2. **CCC** Introduce yourself to the client and family.
3. **SAF** Identify the client using two identifiers.
4. **COM** Explain the procedure and instruct the client not to touch or cross over the sterile barrier and not to touch any items on the sterile field. *A sterile barrier may be opened very close to the client, and the client must be instructed not to touch or cross over the sterile barrier and not to touch any items on the sterile field.*
5. **INF** Set a clean work surface at waist height. If needed, wipe the surface clean, dry thoroughly, and perform hand hygiene again. *Cleaning the work surface reduces the number of microorganisms. Drying prevents moisture from*

contaminating the pack. Setting the work surface at waist height adheres to the sterile principles.
6. **INF** Prepare the sterile barrier (see Skill 10.3).
7. **ACC** Apply a sterile mask if indicated by the type of procedure or facility policy. *Wearing a sterile mask prevents contamination of the field with microorganisms from the nurse by airborne or droplet transmission. Wearing a sterile mask is required by CDC and AORN policy for specific procedures.*

PROCEDURE
Adding Sterile Items to a Sterile Field

8. **INF** Step back from the sterile field so that as you open items, your hands are not over the sterile barrier. *The sterile barrier creates a three-dimensional sterile space.*
9. **INF** Touching only the outside of the package, peel open the outside wrapper of the sterile item to expose the sterile item. *The inside of the package is sterile; the outside is not.*

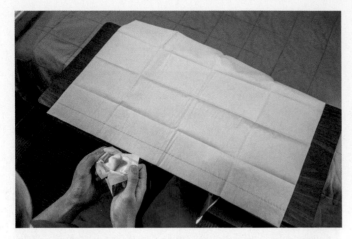

STEP 9 Peel open the outside wrapper of the sterile item.

10. **ACC** Step toward the sterile field. Invert the wrapper and drop the sterile item onto the sterile field. *Do not touch the sterile field with the nonsterile packaging or any other nonsterile object.*

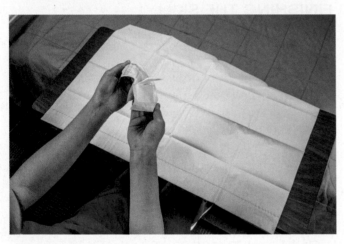

STEP 10 Invert the wrapper and drop the sterile item onto the sterile field

11. **INF** Step back from the sterile field.
12. **INF** Cover the sterile field if indicated by facility policy.

Draping a Sterile Field

13. **INF** Place a large drape with one edge cuffed back horizontally over the sterile field, covering about two-thirds of the sterile field.
14. **INF** Place the second cuffed drape from the opposite side of the sterile field and position it to cover the cuff of the first drape. *The two cuffed drapes are placed so that when they are removed, the section of the drape that was below the sterile field is never brought back to the level of the sterile field (AORN, 2018). The evidence supports immediately covering open sterile trays with a sterile towel and keeping them covered until they are needed to minimize the exposure to environmental contaminants.*

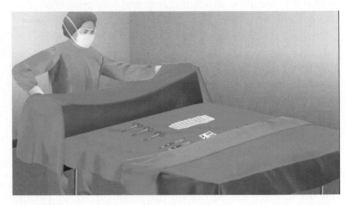

STEP 14 Place the second cuffed drape to cover the cuff of the first drape.

FINISHING THE SKILL

15. **EVAL** Evaluate the sterile field for evidence of adherence to sterile principles. *Evidence of moisture or items within the 2.5-cm (1-inch) border would indicate a break in sterile technique.*
16. **EVAL** Evaluate the performance of the skill for adherence to sterile technique. *Are you confident there was no break in sterile technique?*

■ SKILL 10.5 Pouring a Sterile Liquid

EQUIPMENT

Sterile pack
Sealed sterile liquid
Sterile receiving container
Sterile mask, if required

BEGINNING THE SKILL

1. **INF** Perform hand hygiene.
2. **CCC** Introduce yourself to the client and family.
3. **SAF** Identify the client using two identifiers.
4. **COM** Explain the procedure and instruct the client not to touch or cross over the sterile barrier and not to touch any items on the sterile field. *A sterile barrier may be opened very close to the client, and the client must be instructed not to touch or cross over the sterile barrier and not to touch any items on the sterile field.*
5. **INF** Set a clean work surface at waist height. If needed, wipe the surface clean, dry thoroughly, and perform hand hygiene again. *Cleaning the work surface reduces the number of microorganisms. Drying prevents moisture from contaminating the pack. Setting the work surface at waist height adheres to the sterile principles.*
6. **INF** Prepare the sterile barrier (see Skill 10.3).

7. **ACC** Apply a sterile mask if indicated by the type of procedure or facility policy. *Wearing a sterile mask prevents contamination of the field with microorganisms from the nurse by airborne or droplet transmission. Wearing a sterile mask is required by CDC and AORN policy for specific procedures.*

PROCEDURE

8. **ACC** Identify the sterile receiving container. Determine if the container is sterile only on the inside and the outside can be handled or if the entire container is sterile. If the liquid is to be poured into a container on a sterile field, position the container to one side of the field close to the edge. (Note: Sterile liquid is added to a variety of containers. The receiving container may be an open tray in a kit. A sterile container may need to be added to the sterile field. At times, you may need to put on sterile gloves in order to keep the container sterile—for example, if the lid needs to be unscrewed. Sometimes the container is not sterile on the outside and can be handled but is sterile on the inside. In this case, do not touch the inside of the sterile container.) *Touching the inside of the container without sterile gloves would contaminate it.*

9. **ACC** Examine the sterile fluid, checking the fluid type against the orders. Check for any signs of contamination. *Only liquid in a sealed container is considered sterile.*

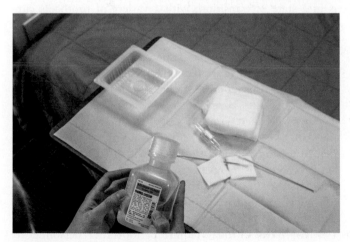

STEP 9 Examine the sterile fluid.

10. **INF** Open the container of sterile liquid. Invert the cap before placing it on the work surface. *Once liquid has been poured over the lip of a container, the lip of the container is considered contaminated. The outside of the container of sterile liquid is very seldom sterile.* (Note: It takes some planning in the sequence of setting up a sterile field with a liquid so that the liquid is poured before putting on sterile gloves.)

11. **ACC** Hold the container in the palm of your dominant hand with the label facing toward you. Double-check the contents of the container. *Keeping the label facing you allows you to see the name of the solution at all times and may prevent errors.*

12. **INF** Approach the sterile field on the same side the container is positioned. Do not reach over the sterile field in order to pour the liquid.

13. **INF** Pour the liquid. Do not allow the container to touch the receiving container, but hold the container close enough to the receiving container so that the liquid does not splash. *Splashing can contaminate the sterile field.*

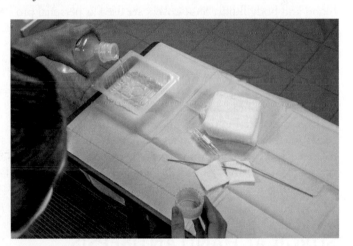

STEP 13 Pour the liquid.

FINISHING THE SKILL

14. **EVAL** Evaluate the sterile field for evidence of adherence to sterile principles. *Evidence of moisture would indicate a break in sterile technique.*

15. **EVAL** Evaluate the performance of the skill for adherence to sterile technique. *Are you confident there was no break in sterile technique?*

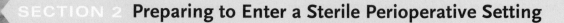

Perioperative team members entering a sterile perioperative setting must first change into surgical attire; then perform surgical hand antisepsis; and finally, put on gowns, head coverings, masks, and surgical gloves.

SURGICAL ATTIRE

When preparing to enter a sterile perioperative setting, you should change from street clothes into facility-approved, clean surgical attire that is either freshly laundered or disposable. When changing clothes, don't allow the surgical attire to touch the floor. If the attire is two pieces, tuck the top into the pants. The appropriate shoes for the perioperative setting are clean; have closed toes and backs, low heels, and non-skid soles; and are able to protect your feet from exposure to blood and body fluids. Shoe covers are used as personal protective equipment (PPE) if shoe contamination with body fluids can be reasonably anticipated. Do not wear jewelry in the perioperative setting, including finger rings, nose rings, earrings, necklaces, bracelets, and watches. Cover head and facial hair, including sideburns and the base of the neck, with a clean surgical head covering or hood.

Everyone entering the perioperative setting should wear a mask when open sterile supplies are present. A mask is worn to protect the client from infectious agents in the nurse's mouth or nose and to protect the nurse from sprays or splashes of body fluids during surgical procedures (AORN, 2018).

SURGICAL HAND ANTISEPSIS

Long recognized as the most important means of decreasing HAIs, surgical hand antisepsis is critical before entering a perioperative setting. Despite the use of sterile gloves, microorganisms from hand contamination are one of the leading sources of surgical-site infection (SSI) (Tanner, Dumville, Norman, & Fortnam, 2016). Skin contains both transient and resident microorganisms. The goal of surgical hand antisepsis is, first, to eliminate transient hand flora and reduce the number of resident hand flora and, second, to keep the total number of microorganisms very low for the duration of the surgical procedure.

Although surgical gloves greatly reduce the risk of bacterial contamination, gloves are not completely effective at preventing bacteria from contaminating a surgical procedure. Studies have demonstrated that after surgery is complete, gloves often have a wide range of tiny punctures, most of which are undetected by the surgeons wearing them. Such punctures double the risk of SSIs (Tanner et al., 2016). Additionally, a review of the scientific evidence by the World Health Organization (WHO) found several reports of infection traced to contaminated hands among members of the

surgical team despite the fact that they had been wearing surgical gloves (WHO, 2009).

Maintaining healthy skin and fingernails is also essential to surgical hand antisepsis. AORN (2018) recommends maintaining healthy, natural nails no longer than 2 mm in length. The subungual (under fingernails) area on the hands is the site with the highest microorganism count. Long fingernails give microorganisms more room to multiply and also are more likely to tear gloves. Artificial nails and extensions should not be worn in the perioperative setting. Artificial nails demonstrated higher pathogen colony counts. The CDC and many professional nursing organizations recommend that healthcare workers who provide care for high-risk populations do not wear artificial nails or extensions (AORN, 2018; CDC, 2018a). In years past, there are accounts of hospitalized patient infections and even death as a result of the transfer of microorganisms colonized in artificial nails (Gordin et al., 2007). Although wearing nail polish may be against policy, the evidence is currently inconclusive on the impact of nail polish and hand bacteria counts (Arrowsmith & Taylor, 2014).

The technique recommended for surgical hand antisepsis is in a state of transition, with a variety of protocols currently being used around the world. For the last century, the standard of practice had been a water-based surgical hand scrub with a brush and sponge. Although some institutions and healthcare practitioners still use a water-based hand scrub, brushes are no longer recommended, even for the nails. Studies have associated vigorous scrubbing with a brush with increased skin-cell shedding and irritation of the skin. This decreases the effectiveness of the skin as a barrier. At this time, there is not clear evidence that one type of hand antisepsis is more effective than any other. Neither is it clear whether the use of nail brushes and nail picks is effective in decreasing bacteria numbers (Tanner et al., 2016), as described in Box 10.5.

Many facilities today require perioperative personnel to use a waterless, alcohol-based surgical handrub. Preparations typically include long-acting compounds such as chlorhexidine gluconate or quaternary ammonium compounds that limit the regrowth of bacteria on the skin inside the glove. The criteria for antimicrobial agents are that they should have a nonirritating antimicrobial preparation with broad-spectrum, fast-acting, and persistent antimicrobial activity, lasting at least 6 hours.

Once a facility selects the alcohol-based surgical handrub, the manufacturer's recommendations must be followed. The manufacturer's recommendations will include the amount of product to use, the time needed for a surgical hand-antisepsis agent to be effective, and the most effective method of application. Currently, many of the products available recommend a 3-minute exposure. Although alcohol-based handrubs have superior antimicrobial efficacy, they are not

BOX 10.5 Lessons From the Evidence: Does Using a Nail Brush or Pick During Surgical Scrub Provide Additional Decontamination?

Scrub brushes are no longer used on the skin, but they are still used to decontaminate fingernails. Investigators wanted to determine if using a nail pick or a nail brush provided additional decontamination when compared to performing a surgical handrub without a pick or brush. Three scrub groups were selected. One group performed a surgical handrub with aqueous chlorhexidine gluconate 4%, the second group cleaned their nails with a disposable nail pick under running water before performing a surgical handrub with aqueous chlorhexidine gluconate 4%, and the third group cleaned their nails with a disposable brush before performing a surgical handrub with aqueous chlorhexidine gluconate 4%. The investigators found no statistically significant differences in bacterial counts between any two of the three intervention groups. Their conclusion was that nail brushes and nail picks used during surgical handrubs do not decrease bacterial numbers and are not necessary.

References: Tanner et al., 2009, 2016.

effective at removing spores. Therefore, a simple soap-and-water hand wash is recommended to remove any bacterial spores as a precursor to surgical hand antisepsis (see Skill 1.3). Table 10.1 presents a comparison of surgical hand-antisepsis agents.

The CDC (2018a) and WHO (2009) recommend the use of waterless antimicrobial alcohol-based surgical handrubs for the following reasons:

- They more effectively reduce the number of bacteria on the hands than other methods of surgical hand preparation.
- They reduce the bacteria count on the skin immediately and demonstrate persistent activity that prevents or inhibits the growth of microorganisms for 6 hours.
- They avoid the possibility of recontamination of the hands from contaminated water, taps, or faucets during hand rinsing. Contaminated water taps and faucets have been a recurring problem in healthcare facilities.
- They do not require large quantities of water. In many areas of the world, water is a scarce resource, and the quantity needed for a large surgical team to perform a 10- or 20-minute scrub is many gallons.

TABLE 10.1 Properties of Surgical Hand Antisepsis Agents

Antiseptic Agent	Mechanism of Action	Speed of Action	Persistent Activity	Warnings, Cautions, and Comments	Soil Removal
Soap and water	Cleansing activity due to the detergent property of soap and water as a solvent	Limited	None	Can result in an increase of bacterial counts; can result in skin dryness and irritation	Yes
Alcohol-based solutions (isopropanol, ethanol, or a combination) (concentration 60%–90%)	Denatures proteins	Excellent	None	Flammable Does not penetrate organic material Very poor activity against bacterial spores	No
Chlorhexidine (a biguanide)	Disrupts cell membrane	Slower than alcohol	Excellent	Keep out of eyes and inner ears Known sensitivity to ingredients Activity can be affected by natural soaps, different inorganic anions, nonionic surfactants, and hand lotions Very poor activity against bacterial spores	Yes
Chlorhexidine gluconate with alcohol	Disrupts cell membrane and denatures proteins	Excellent	Excellent	Keep out of eyes and inner ears Known sensitivity to ingredients Very poor activity against bacterial spores Flammable	Limited
Chloroxylenol	Inactivates bacterial enzymes and disrupts cell walls	Intermediate (not as rapidly active as chlorhexidine or iodophors)	Good	Safe up to 5% concentration	Yes
Iodine and iodophors	Disrupts cell membrane	Intermediate	Intermediate	Sensitivity to povidone iodine products prone to contamination by gram-negative bacteria Shellfish allergy is not a contraindication	No

Adapted from AORN, 2018; Tanner et al., 2016.

SURGICAL GOWNS AND GLOVES

Following surgical hand antisepsis, nurses prepare to enter the perioperative setting by putting on surgical caps, shoe covers, masks, gowns, and surgical gloves using the principles listed in Box 10.6. Surgical gowns are one-piece garments that have long sleeves with tight-fitting cuffs and a wrap closure in the back. The function of the gown, head covering, mask, and gloves is to reduce exposure to microorganisms. The final preparation is completed with assistance from perioperative team members. AORN (2018) recommends a technique called *assisted closed gloving* when a new sterile gown has been put on (Fig. 10.1). In assisted closed gloving, a member of the perioperative team who is already gowned and gloved holds a sterile glove by the cuff and stretches out the opening. The ungloved team member, keeping the gown cuff beyond his or her fingertips, inserts his or her hand into the glove such that the gown cuff only touches the inside of the glove. Once a gown cuff has moved to the wrist, the cuff is never pulled down. If assisted closed gloving is not possible, the closed surgical gloving technique described in Skill 10.9 is used.

Double gloving is currently recommended during surgery and other invasive procedures with exposure to body fluids. In fact, double gloving over a colored indicator glove helps to discover if a perforation has occurred (Spruce, 2017). Box 10.7 identifies one reason that double gloving is advised. Changing gloves is recommended at regular intervals (90–150 minutes) and if any contamination or suspected contamination occurs. If nurses need to change their gloves, another scrubbed team member holds the sterile glove by the cuff and stretches out the opening so that the nurse may insert her or his hand without contaminating the assistant.

APPLICATION OF THE NURSING PROCESS

Examples of Related ICNP Nursing Diagnoses, Expected Client Outcomes, and Nursing Interventions:

Nursing Diagnosis: Risk for infection

Supporting Data: Surgery has a risk of SSI.

Expected Client Outcome: The client will not demonstrate any signs of an HAI while in the healthcare setting.

Nursing Intervention Example: Adhere to sterile technique and AORN guidelines when preparing to enter a sterile perioperative area

Reference: International Classification for Nursing Practice. (n.d.). *eHealth & ICNP.* Retrieved from https://www.icn.ch/what-we-do/projects/ehealth-icnp.

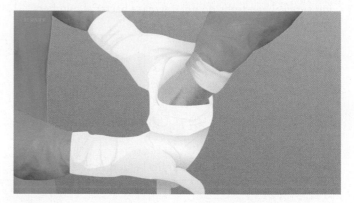

FIG. 10.1 In assisted closed gloving, a member of the perioperative team who is already gowned and gloved assists the newly gowned perioperative member to glove by holding open each glove.

BOX 10.6 Principles of Sterile Technique for Surgical Gowning and Gloving

- Surgical gowns must be sterile. Gowns should be large enough to close completely in the back, with sleeves long enough to prevent exposure of glove cuffs.
- Touch only the inside of the neck when the gown is picked up.
- Touch only the inside of gown when assisting someone to pull it up on the shoulders and tie the gown.
- Once put on, a surgical gown is considered sterile on the front from table height to the shoulders, and the sleeves are considered sterile from 5 cm (2 inches) above the elbow to the sleeve cuff.
- The neckline and cuffs are areas of increased friction with the skin and are not considered sterile.
- Ensure the surgical gloves completely cover the cuffs of the wrists of the gown.
- The back of a surgical gown is not considered sterile because it cannot be monitored.
- Once surgical gowns and gloves have been put on, the hands are kept in view above the waist and below the neckline.
- Once surgical gowns and gloves have been put on, the hands are never tucked under the armpits. This area is not considered sterile.

BOX 10.7 Lessons From Experience: Double Gloving

Christina has been recently oriented to work in the operating room (OR) in an outpatient surgical center. She has 2 years of surgical outpatient care experience but has never worked in the OR. Her preceptor, Sandy, has been an OR nurse for about 20 years. On Christina's first day to assist as a scrub nurse, Christina performs her surgical hand antisepsis and puts on her surgical gown and gloves. As she adjusts her gloves, she notices a tiny puncture. Christina asks Sandy how to handle the situation. Sandy is working as the circulating nurse (unscrubbed) this morning and removes the punctured glove without contaminating Christina's sterile gown. Then the scrub nurse assists Christina to apply two gloves on her hand that had the punctured glove and one additional glove for her other hand. Sandy suggests to Christina that she always double glove. The practice of double gloving during invasive procedures is recommended by the Centers for Disease Control and Prevention, the American College of Surgeons, and the American Academy of Orthopaedic Surgeons (Spruce, 2017).

CRITICAL CONCEPTS
Preparing to Enter a Sterile Perioperative Area

Accuracy (ACC)

When preparing to enter a sterile perioperative area, the accuracy of sterile technique is subject to the following variables:

Nurse-Related Factors
- Adherence to AORN guidelines
- Adherence to the antiseptic manufacturers' instructions for use
- Recognition of accidental contamination

Equipment-Related Factors
- Proper sterilization of liquids and equipment

Infection Control (INF)

When preparing to enter a sterile perioperative area, healthcare-associated infection is prevented by:

- containment of microorganisms
- preventing and reducing the transfer of microorganisms
- reducing the number of microorganisms.

Communication (COM)

- Communication exchanges information (oral, written, nonverbal, or electronic) between two or more people.
- Collaboration with the perioperative healthcare team facilitates maintaining sterile technique while preparing to enter the sterile perioperative area.

Evaluation (EVAL)

When preparing to enter a sterile perioperative area, evaluation of outcomes enables the nurse to determine the efficacy of the sterile technique performed.

■ SKILL 10.6 Performing a Surgical Handrub

EQUIPMENT

Nonmedicated soap
Paper towel
Surgical cap/hat
Surgical mask
Surgical shoe covers
Packaged surgical gown
Packaged surgical gloves
Alcohol-based handrub

BEGINNING THE SKILL

1. **INF** Keep fingernails trimmed short, approximately 2 mm. Do not wear artificial nails or extensions.
2. **INF** Remove watches, rings, and other jewelry.
3. **INF** Set a clean work surface at waist height. If needed, wipe the surface clean, and dry thoroughly. *Cleaning the work surface reduces the number of microorganisms. Drying prevents moisture from contaminating the pack. Setting the work surface at waist height adheres to the sterile principles.*
4. **INF** Perform hand hygiene with a nonmedicated soap, cleaning well under the nails. Dry the hands thoroughly with a disposable paper towel. (See Skill 1.3.)

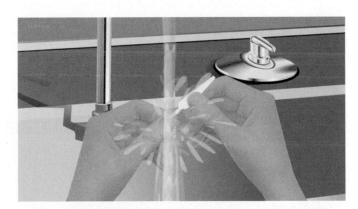

STEP 4 Clean well under the nails.

5. **INF** Put on a surgical cap/hat and mask.
6. **ACC** Place the wrapped sterile surgical gown and surgical gloves on the work surface. Check the expiration date and for signs of contamination.
7. Peel open the outside wrapper of the gown package and the glove package. Discard the outer wrapper.

PROCEDURE

8. **INF** Dispense the recommended amount of alcohol-based handrub into the palm of your nondominant hand. *Following the antiseptic manufacturer's instructions for use is critical because failure to adhere to the instructions may result in ineffectiveness of the antiseptic.*

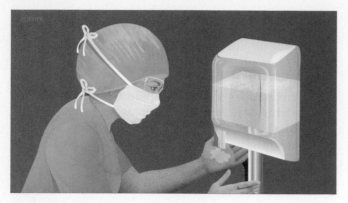

STEP 8 Dispense alcohol-based handrub into your palm.

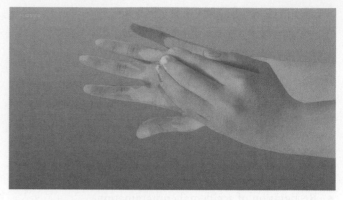

STEP 9 Systematically apply the alcohol-based handrub.

9. **ACC** Systematically apply the alcohol-based handrub on the dominant hand and forearm following the manufacturer's recommendations for method and time. *Following the antiseptic manufacturer's instructions for use is critical.*

10. **ACC** Dispense the recommended amount of alcohol-based handrub into the palm of your dominant hand and systematically apply alcohol-based handrub on your nondominant hand and forearm following the manufacturer's recommendations for method and time. *Following the antiseptic manufacturer's instructions for use is critical because failure to adhere to the instructions may result in ineffectiveness of the antiseptic.*

FINISHING THE SKILL

11. **EVAL** Evaluate the performance of the skill for adherence to sterile technique. *Are you confident there was no contamination?*

■ SKILL 10.7 Performing a Surgical Hand Scrub

EQUIPMENT

Surgical cap/hat
Surgical mask
Surgical shoe covers
Antimicrobial scrub agent
Sterile towel
Disposable nail pick
Nonabrasive antimicrobial scrub sponge
Scrub sink

BEGINNING THE SKILL

1. **INF** Keep fingernails trimmed short, approximately 2 mm. Do not wear artificial nails or extensions.
2. **INF** Remove watches, rings, and other jewelry.
3. **INF** Set a clean work surface at waist height. If needed, wipe the surface clean, and dry thoroughly. *Cleaning the work surface reduces microorganisms. Drying prevents moisture from contaminating the pack. Setting the work surface at waist height adheres to the sterile principles.*
4. **INF** Perform hand hygiene with a nonmedicated soap. Clean under each nail with a disposable nail pick. Discard the nail pick in an appropriate container. *The*

subungual area is the site with the highest microorganism count. Proper containment of contaminated objects prevents the transfer of microorganisms.
5. **INF** Dry hands thoroughly with a disposable paper towel.
6. **INF** Put on a surgical cap/hat, mask, and shoe covers.
7. **ACC** Place the wrapped sterile surgical gown and surgical gloves on work surface. Check the expiration date and for signs of contamination.
8. Peel open the outside wrapper of the gown package and the glove package. Discard the outer wrapper.

PROCEDURE

9. **INF** At the sink, adjust the water temperature to warm and the water pressure to medium using the foot lever or using a paper towel as a barrier on a hand lever. Do not touch any part of the sink or other nonsterile object once the surgical scrub has begun. *Using a foot lever prevents hand contamination, and using a paper towel as a barrier decreases the risk of contamination.*
10. **INF** Keep your hands above your elbows and away from your clothing. Rinse your hands and forearms to about 5 cm (2 inches) above your elbows.

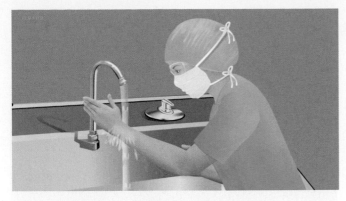

STEP 10 Keep your hands above your elbows.

11. **ACC** Dispense antimicrobial scrub agent according to the manufacturer's directions.
12. **INF** Keep your hands above your elbows and away from your clothing and apply antimicrobial agent to wet hands and forearms with a nonabrasive sponge. *Keeping your hands above your elbows allows water to flow from the cleanest area (fingers) to the least clean area (elbows). A nonabrasive sponge will not damage the skin. Surgical scrubs should not be performed with a brush that may damage the skin.*
13. **INF** Wash each thumb, finger, hand, wrist, and forearm systematically with the sponge, envisioning four sides to each digit, hand, and arm. Avoid splashing or touching your clothing. *A systematic and anatomic pattern of washing prevents inadvertently skipping over areas. A sterile gown cannot be put over damp clothing. The damp clothing would wick moisture through to the sterile gown, resulting in contamination.*

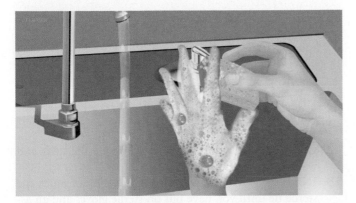

STEP 13 Wash systematically.

14. **ACC** Time the wash according to the antimicrobial manufacturer's recommendations. Avoid touching the sink or faucets. *A timed wash allows sufficient time for the antimicrobial agent to decrease microorganism counts. Touching the sink or faucets would contaminate your hands.*

15. **INF** Discard the sponge in an appropriate container. *Proper containment of contaminated objects prevents the transfer of microorganisms.*
16. **INF** Rinse the hands and forearms, keeping your hands above your elbows. *Keeping your hands above your elbows allows water to flow from the cleanest area (fingers) to the least clean area (elbows).*

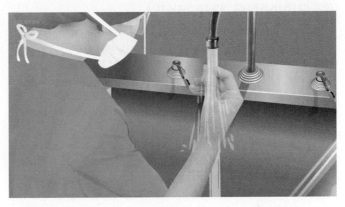

STEP 16 Rinse, keeping your hands above your elbows.

17. **INF** Dry hands and arms with a sterile towel. Dry one hand and arm at a time with each end of the towel, starting at the fingertips and moving toward the elbows in only one direction. *A sterile gown cannot be put over damp arms and hands. The moisture would wick through to the sterile gown, resulting in contamination. Drying in only one direction (from cleanest to least clean) prevents bringing microorganisms from the least clean area up to the cleanest area.*

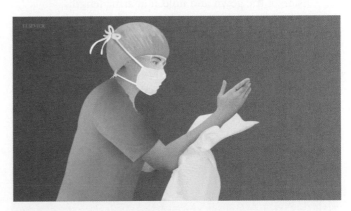

STEP 17 Dry one hand and arm at a time.

FINISHING THE SKILL

18. **EVAL** Evaluate the performance of the skill for adherence to sterile technique. *Are you confident there was no contamination?*

▪ **SKILL 10.8** Performing Surgical Gowning

EQUIPMENT

Sterile surgical gown
Surgical assistant

BEGINNING THE SKILL

1. **INF** Perform surgical handrub or hand scrub (see Skills 10.6 and 10.7) and ensure your hands are dry. *Dry hands are essential to maintain the sterility of the surgical gown.*
2. **INF** Locate the sterile surgical gown and sterile glove packages. They should be on a clean, dry surface at waist height. *Sterile principles include maintaining a sterile field at or above waist height.*
3. **INF** If the sterile surgical gown package is not open, direct an assistant to open the gown and glove packages. *Your hands are already scrubbed; therefore, you should not contaminate them by touching the outer wrapping of the package.*

PROCEDURE

4. **INF** Stand approximately 30 cm (12 inches) from the opened sterile surgical gown package. *Standing back allows enough room for the gown to unfold without touching any unsterile object.*
5. **ACC** Pick up the gown by the folded edges and lift it up directly from the package.
6. **INF** Step back from the surface. Ensure no objects are near the gown. *Sterile items can only touch other sterile items.*
7. **INF** Grasp the gown just below the neckband on the inside of the gown and hold it at arm's length.

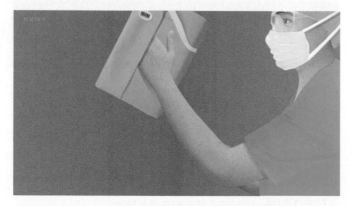

STEP 7 Grasp the gown just below the neckband.

8. **INF** Allow the gown to unfold lengthwise without touching the floor.
9. **INF** Face the inside of the gown and slide your arms into the sleeves, just to the cuffs. Keep your arms raised to prevent the gown from touching the floor.

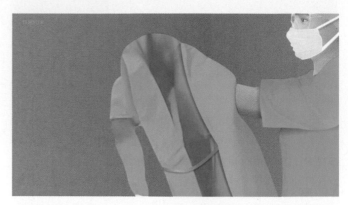

STEP 9 Slide your arms into the sleeves, just to the cuffs.

10. **INF** Do not push your hands through the cuffs of the sleeve.
11. **COM** Direct a nonsterile assistant to stand behind you and grasp the inside of the gown in order to pull the sleeves and shoulders of the gown into position. Continue to leave your hands covered by the sleeve cuffs.

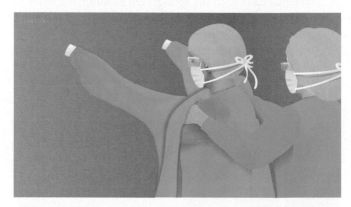

STEP 11 Direct an unsterile assistant to position and secure the gown.

12. **COM** Direct a nonsterile assistant to tie the neck and waist of the gown.
13. **INF** If the gown has a wraparound tie, do not touch the sterile tie until you have put on sterile gloves and an assistant is available. (See Skill 10.9.)
14. **COM** After you have put on sterile gloves, direct an assistant to grasp the card attached to the wraparound tie without touching any part of the sterile gown. Turn around so that the tie wraps around you. You then grasp the ends of the sterile tie and tie them in front, and the assistant pulls away the card.

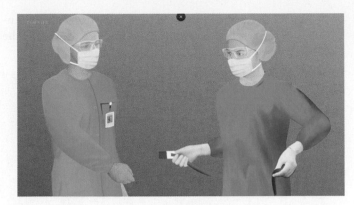

STEP 14 Direct an assistant to grasp the card.

FINISHING THE SKILL

15. **EVAL** Evaluate the performance of the skill for adherence to sterile technique. *Are you confident there was no break in sterile technique?*

■ SKILL 10.9 Performing Closed Surgical Gloving

EQUIPMENT

Package of sterile gloves, correct size

BEGINNING THE SKILL

1. **INF** Perform surgical handrub or hand scrub (see Skills 10.6 and 10.7) and ensure your hands are dry. *Dry hands are essential to maintaining the sterility of the surgical gown.*
2. **INF** Perform surgical gowning, keeping your hands covered by the surgical gown cuffs (see Skill 10.8).
3. **INF** Locate the sterile glove package. It should be on a clean, dry surface at waist height. *Sterile principles include maintaining a sterile field at or above waist height.*
4. **COM** If the sterile glove package is not open, direct an assistant to open the sterile glove package. *Your hands are already scrubbed. You should not contaminate them by touching the outer wrapping of the package.*

PROCEDURE

5. **INF** Ensure your hands and fingers are covered by the sleeve and cuff of the sterile gown.
6. **INF** Through the cuff of the sterile gown, open the inner wrapper of the sterile gloves to expose the gloves. *Sterile cuffs touch the sterile inner wrapper. Gloves are positioned in the wrapper with palms up and the thumbs to the outside.*

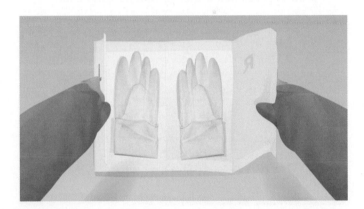

STEP 6 Through the cuffs, open the inner wrapper of the sterile gloves.

7. **INF** Using your nondominant hand (through the cuff of the sterile gown), pick up the glove of the dominant hand. The sterile cuff of the gown touches the sterile glove. Do not allow the glove to touch any unsterile surface. *Gloving the dominant hand first allows it to manipulate gloving the nondominant hand, which requires a little more dexterity.*
8. **ACC** Place the palm of the glove on the palm of your dominant hand with the fingers of the glove facing your elbow.

9. **ACC** Grasp the bottom edge of the glove with the fingers of your dominant hand through the cuff of the sterile gown.

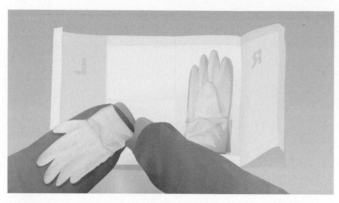

STEPS 8 AND 9 Place the palm of the glove on the palm of your hand and grasp the bottom edge of the glove.

10. **ACC** Using your nondominant hand, grasp the top part of the cuff and pull it over your dominant hand.

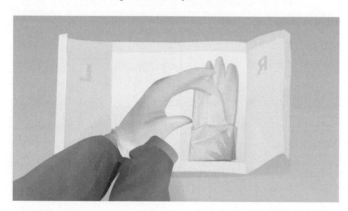

STEP 10 Grasp the top part of the cuff and pull it over your dominant hand.

11. **INF** Slip your dominant hand (palm up) into the glove and pull the glove on your hand, touching only the folded the cuff. Keep your fingers together as you slide through the palm of the glove and then spread out your fingers just before entering the glove fingers. *This will help align the glove fingers with your fingers.*
12. **INF** Pick up the other glove with the gloved hand. *The sterile gloved hand touches the sterile glove.*
13. **ACC** While maintaining the ungloved hand within the cuff of the sterile gown, place the palm of the glove on the palm of your nondominant hand with the fingers of the glove facing your elbow.

14. **ACC** Grasp the bottom edge of the glove with the fingers of your nondominant hand through the cuff of the sterile gown.

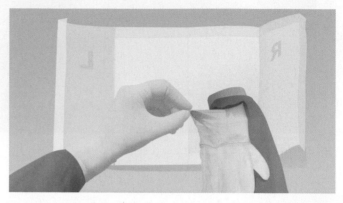

STEPS 13 AND 14 Place the palm of the glove on the palm of your dominant hand and grasp the bottom edge of the glove.

15. **ACC** Using your gloved hand, grasp the top part of the cuff and pull it over your nondominant hand.

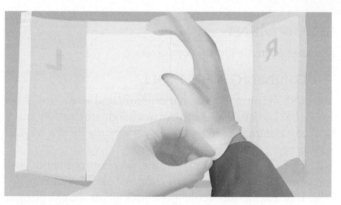

STEP 15 Grasp the top part of the cuff and pull it over your nondominant hand.

16. **ACC** Slip your nondominant hand (palm up) into the glove and pull the glove on your hand, touching only the folded cuff.
17. **INF** Adjust your gloves. Both gloves should be overlapping the lower part of the sleeves of the sterile gown. *Only allow sterile to touch sterile.*
18. **INF** Keep your sterile gloved hands in front of you, above your waist and below your shoulders. *Sterile principles specify that the hands are kept in view above the waist and below the neckline.*

FINISHING THE SKILL

19. **EVAL** Evaluate the performance of the skill for adherence to sterile technique. *Are you confident there was no break in sterile technique?*

■ CASE STUDY

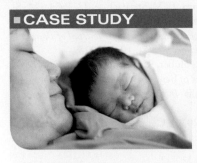

Jenny Lee is a 19-year-old who gave birth to her first baby 6 hours ago. She had an epidural for the delivery. Her baby is a big boy who weighs almost 4 kg (8 lb. 12 oz.) at birth. When Jenny's epidural wore off, she regained both sensation and movement in her lower extremities. Although she was able to get out of bed, she was not able to void. Inability to void after delivery is not an unusual phenomenon. Jenny's authorized healthcare provider ordered an intermittent catheterization. In this procedure, a straight catheter is placed in the bladder, the bladder is emptied, and then the catheter is removed. Because there is a risk of infection with any urinary catheterization, adherence to sterile technique is required.

Jenny's nurse is a recent nursing program graduate. The nurse opened the sterile pack on the bed and set up the sterile field between Jenny's legs. After putting on her sterile gloves, the nurse began to clean over the urinary meatus with an antiseptic agent. When Jenny felt the cold liquid on her perineum, she was startled and snapped her knees shut. The equipment on the sterile field scattered across the bed.

Case Study Questions

1. In this scenario, the nurse set up the sterile field on the bed between Jenny's legs. Where else could the nurse have set up the sterile field for the catheterization equipment? How could that help maintain sterile technique?
2. What instructions could the nurse have given to Jenny before setting up the sterile field? Before cleaning over the urinary meatus?
3. How would the nurse determine which items on the sterile tray could still be used to catheterize Jenny?
4. What new equipment would the nurse need to gather?
5. Does the nurse need to change sterile gloves?
6. **Application of QSEN Competencies:** Two of the Quality and Safety Education for Nurses (QSEN) competencies on attitude for Quality Improvement are "Value own and others' contributions to outcomes of care in local care settings" and "Appreciate how unwanted variation affects care" (Cronenwett et al., 2007). Discuss how variations in sterile procedures at the bedside may affect care for an individual client and affect client outcomes for an acute care facility.

■ CONCEPT MAP

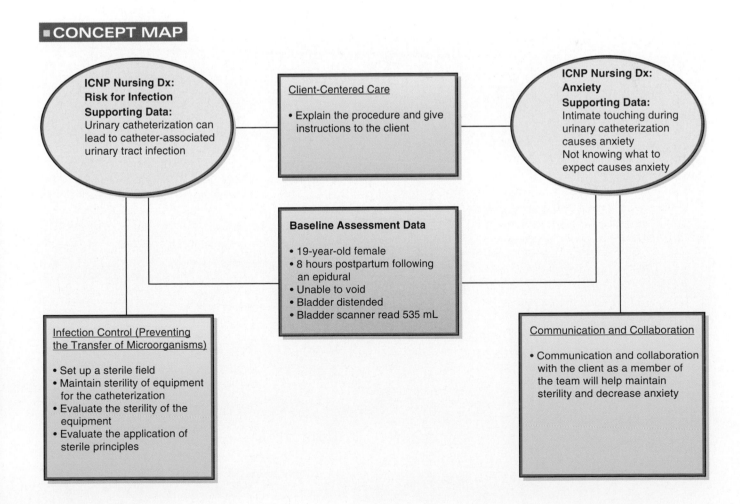

References

Arrowsmith, V. A., & Taylor, R. (2014). Removal of nail polish and finger rings to prevent surgical infection. *Cochrane Database Systemic Review, 2014*(8), CD003325. https://doi.org/10.1002/14651858.CD003325.pub3.

Association of PeriOperative Registered Nurses. (2018). *Guidelines for perioperative practice 2018*. Denver, CO: Author.

Centers for Disease Control and Prevention. (2016). *Guideline for prevention of catheter-associated urinary tract infections (2009)*. Retrieved from https://www.cdc.gov/infectioncontrol/guidelines/cauti/evidence-review.html.

Centers for Disease Control and Prevention (CDC). (2017). *National healthcare safety network*. Retrieved from https://www.cdc.gov/nhsn/about-nhsn/technology.html.

Centers for Disease Control and Prevention. (2018a). *Clean hands count for healthcare providers: Hand hygiene for surgery*. Retrieved from https://www.cdc.gov/handhygiene/providers/index.html.

Centers for Disease Control and Prevention. (2018b). *Disinfection in ambulatory care, home care, and the home*. Retrieved from https://www.cdc.gov/infectioncontrol/guidelines/disinfection/healthcare-equipment.html.

Centers for Disease Control and Prevention. (2018c). *Healthcare associated infections: HAI data and statistics*. Retrieved from https://www.cdc.gov/hai/surveillance/index.html.

Cronenwett, L., Sherwood, G., Barnsteiner J., Disch, J., Johnson, J., Mitchell, P., … Warren, J. (2007). Quality and safety education for nurses. *Nursing Outlook, 55*(3), 122–131. Retrieved from http://qsen.org/competencies/pre-licensure-ksas/.

Dalstrom, D. J., Venkatarayappa, I., Manternach, A. L., Palcic, M. S., Heyse, B. A., & Prayson, M. J. (2008). Time-dependent contamination of opened sterile operating-room trays. *Journal of Bone & Joint Surgery, American Volume, 90A*(5), 1022–1025.

Gordin, F. M., Schultz, M. E., Huber, R., Zubairi, S., Stock, F., & Karivil, J. (2007). A cluster of hemodialysis-related bacteremia linked to artificial fingernails. *Infection Control & Hospital Epidemiology, 28*(6), 743–744.

Hopper, W. R., & Moss, R. (2010). Common breaks in sterile technique: Clinical perspectives and perioperative implications. *AORN Journal, 91*(3), 350–364.

International Classification for Nursing Practice. (n.d.). *eHealth & ICNP.* Retrieved from https://www.icn.ch/what-we-do/projects/ehealth-icnp.

Paull, T. (2017). *Surgical scrubbing, gowning, and gloving.* [Evidence summary]. Retrieved from The Joanna Briggs Institute EBD Database, JBI@Ovid. JBI878.

Spruce, L. (2017). Back to basics: Sterile technique. *AORN Journal, 105*(5), 478–485.

Tanner, J., Khan, O., Walsh, S., Chernova, J., Lamont, S., & Laurent, T. (2009). Brushes and picks used on nails during the surgical scrub to reduce bacteria: A randomized trial. *Journal of Advanced Perioperative Care, 4*(1), 27–32.

Tanner, J., Dumville, J., Norman, G., & Fortnam, M. (2016). Surgical handantisepsis to reduce surgical site infection. *Cochrane Database of Systemic Reviews, 1*, CD004288. https://doi.org/10.1002/14651858.CD004288.pub3.

World Health Organization. (2009). *WHO guidelines on hand hygiene in healthcare*. Retrieved from http://whqlibdoc.who.int/publications/2009/9789241597906_eng.pdf.

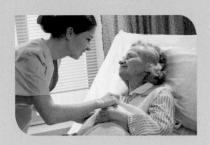

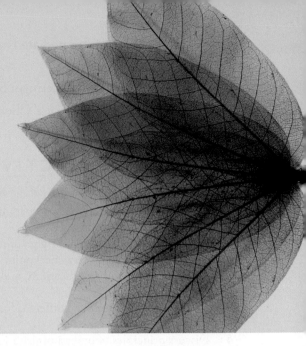

CHAPTER 11

Medication Administration

"Medicine sometimes snatches away health, sometimes gives it." | **Publius Ovidius Naso (Ovid), Roman Poet (43 BC–AD 17/18)**

431

■ **SKILL 11.19** Administering a Subcutaneous Insulin Injection

■ **SKILL 11.20** Caring for a Client With a Subcutaneous Insulin Pump (External)

LEARNING OBJECTIVES

By the end of this chapter, the reader will be able to:

1 Identify current national safety goals and best-practice initiatives related to medications.
2 Identify and discuss the "six rights of medication administration" and safety checkpoints when processing orders, preparing medications, and administering medications.
3 Compare and contrast the different formulas used for dosage calculations.
4 Discuss principles of oral administration and different types of oral medications.
5 Administer oral medications (tablets, capsules, or liquids).
6 Administer a medication through a nasogastric (NG) tube or enteral device.
7 Discuss different types of mucous membrane applications.
8 Administer a nasal spray medication.
9 Administer naloxone (Narcan) nasal spray.
10 Administer sublingual and buccal medications.
11 Administer inhaled medications.
12 Administer nebulized medications.
13 Administer rectal suppositories.

14 Administer vaginal medications (suppositories, gels, creams).
15 Discuss different types of topical medications.
16 Apply a transdermal patch.
17 Instill eye medications and eye irrigations.
18 Instill ear drops.
19 Discuss parenteral medication administration.
20 Prepare a medication from a vial and an ampule.
21 Prepare a medication that requires reconstitution.
22 Administer an intradermal injection.
23 Administer a subcutaneous injection.
24 Teach a client to self-administer an enoxaparin (Lovenox) injection.
25 Administer intramuscular injections (deltoid, vastus lateralis, and ventrogluteal).
26 Administer an intramuscular injection using the Z-track method.
27 Prepare and administer a subcutaneous insulin injection.
28 Care for a client who has an insulin pump or an insulin pen.

TERMINOLOGY

Aerosol A system or method of delivering a solid powder or suspension by an aerosol device.

Antidote Medications that help reverse the actions of other medications, usually given in emergencies where either an overdose or an error has occurred.

Buccal A medication given between the gums and the cheek of the oral cavity.

Induration Hardening of the skin, especially after reaction to an antigen or allergen injection.

Intradermal (ID) A route by which the medication is injected into the dermal layer of the skin just under the surface, commonly used for tuberculosis and allergy testing.

Intramuscular (IM) A medication route by which the medication is injected into the muscle.

Lipodystrophy Disorder of adipose tissue and accumulation of fatty deposits under the surface of the skin, caused by repeated injections. Rotation of injection sites prevents this disorder.

Localized Refers to medications that affect only a small area on the body, such as ointments.

Meniscus A crescent-shaped curve at the upper surface of a liquid caused by surface tension.

Nebulizer A machine that aerosolizes medications so that the primary effect is on the lungs.

NPO Latin phrase meaning "nil per os"; nothing by mouth.

Parenteral Refers to medications given by injection, such as intradermally, subcutaneously, intramuscularly, and intravenously.

PO Latin phrase meaning "per os"; by mouth.

PRN As needed; an indication for use and a time frame must be specified for PRN orders.

Reconstitution Process of turning a dry ingredient such as powdered medication into a liquid.

Spacer Device used with inhalers that provides a space where the aerosolized medication can reside while the client is taking in a deep breath.

STAT Immediately, without delay.

Subcutaneous A route by which a medication is injected into subcutaneous tissue.

Sublingual (SL) A route by which a medication is administered under the tongue.

Systemic effect Refers to medications that affect the entire body as opposed to having a localized effect.

Transdermal A route by which a medication is applied directly to the skin.

ACRONYMS

ADR Adverse drug reaction
ADS Automated dispensing system
EMAR Electronic medication administration record
IM Intramuscular
ISMP Institute for Safe Medication Practices
MAR Medication administration record
OTC Over the counter
SALAD Sound-alike, look-alike drugs

Medications are a central part of treatment for many clients. In addition to curing and alleviating disease, medications can relieve pain and improve a client's quality of life. Depending on the client's condition, medications can be given by a variety of routes. The major categories of medications discussed in this chapter include oral and enteral, topical, inhalation, mucous membrane, and parenteral medications. Medications administered by the intravenous (IV) route are discussed in Chapter 12. Safe administration of medications is more than just a routine mechanical task; it requires knowledge and accuracy as well as collaboration and excellent communication by the nurse and other members of the healthcare team.

MEDICATION SAFETY INITIATIVES

According to the Centers for Disease Control and Prevention (CDC), there are over 1 million emergency room visits each year in the United States related to adverse events and injury from medications (CDC, 2018). As part of the National Patient Safety Goals, The Joint Commission identifies medication safety as a top priority. As a result, guidelines continue to evolve. For example, the Institute for Safe Medication Practices (ISMP) provides a list of "confused drug names" that identifies "sound-alike/look-alike drugs (SALAD)" that can result in errors (see http://www.ismp.org/Tools/confuseddrugnames.pdf) (ISMP, 2019). The ISMP also has a table of "error-prone" abbreviations, as well as phrases that may cause confusion and must not be used (see https://www.ismp.org/recommendations/error-prone-abbreviations-list) (ISMP, 2017a).

As shown in Table 11.1, The Joint Commission (2018) has provided a condensed form of the "Do Not Use" abbreviation list that facilities must abide by to meet "minimal" standards. However, there are additional standards on the ISMP list that must be considered. For example, the abbreviation "cc" (cubic centimeters) has often been mistaken as "u" (units) or other unintended units of measure, resulting in serious dosage errors. Thus, the current recommendation is to use "mL" (milliliters) instead of "cc" (ISMP, 2017a).

Current best-practice guidelines also encourage the use of the metric system only for medications instead of nonmetric units of measure such as drams or minims. Refer to safety guidelines for updates. If any banned abbreviations or questionable units of measure have been used in the client's medication order, clarify the order before administering the medication.

RIGHTS OF MEDICATION ADMINISTRATION

As an advocate for the client at the bedside, nurses play a key role in the safe and accurate administration of medications. Before any medication can be given, there are at least five basic questions the nurse must first ask:

- Is the medication for the right client?
- Is the medication the right medication?
- Is the medication the right dose and frequency?
- Is the medication the right route?
- Is it the right time to administer the medication?

The basic "five rights" of administration are continuing to evolve. Many organizations, including the CDC, have expanded the rights to "six rights" that include "right documentation" (CDC, 2019a). The right documentation should be done *after* the medication is given in order to communicate with the healthcare team and prevent errors. Accurately document the date, time, route, and any other pertinent information, such as the client's vital signs. It is also important to consider the client's response. Did the blood pressure medication lower the client's blood pressure? Did the pain medication relieve the client's pain as expected? The rights of administration must be integrated into the entire procedure, including processing orders, safety checks, preassessments, preparation, administration, documentation, and follow-up monitoring.

SAFELY PROCESSING MEDICATION ORDERS

In most facilities, all medications, including herbal and over-the-counter (OTC) drugs, require an order by the authorized healthcare provider. At a minimum, the order must contain

TABLE 11.1 Do-Not-Use Abbreviations

Do Not Use	Potential Problem	Use Instead
U, u (unit)	Mistaken for the number 0 or 4 or for cc	Write *unit*
IU (international unit)	Mistaken for IV (intravenous) or the number 10	Write *international unit*
QD, Q.D., qd, q.d. (daily)	Mistaken for each other	Write *daily*
QOD, Q.O.D., qod, q.o.d (every other day)	Period after Q mistaken for *I*, and the O mistaken for *I*	Write *every other day*
MS, MSO$_4$, and MgSO$_4$	Confused with one another	Write *morphine sulfate*
	Can mean morphine sulfate or magnesium sulfate	Write *magnesium sulfate*
Trailing zero (X.O mg)		Write as *X mg*
Lack of leading zero (.X mg)	Decimal point is confusing	Write as *o.X mg*

Note: This is a minimal list. There may be additional abbreviations not recommended for use by the ISMP.
Reference: The Joint Commission, 2018.

the date, client's full name, name of the medication (preferably generic), dosage, time, frequency and route of administration, special instructions, and the authorized healthcare provider's signature.

An order may be written to administer the medication on a set schedule, such as twice a day or three times a day, or the order may be written to give the medication "PRN" (as needed). If an order is written as PRN, the indication of use and a minimal time frame are required on the medication order. For example, a PRN order for a client receiving pain medication might say, "Administer morphine sulfate 2 to 4 mg IV every 4 hours for breakthrough pain as needed."

Depending on the policy, the schedule of administration for each medication is entered as recurring cycles on the client's medication administration record (MAR) and/or the electronic medication administration record (EMAR). For example, if a medication is ordered to be given three times a day, the facility policy may recommend it be administered at 7 AM, 2 PM, and 9 PM. In order for medications to have an optimal therapeutic effect, medications should be given as close to the scheduled time as possible, particularly for time-critical medications such as insulin. Based on ISMP guidelines, manufacturer recommendations, and facility policy, there may be a maximum "window" allowed (e.g., 30 minutes) for administration of a timed medication.

PERFORMING PREASSESSMENTS

After the order is processed and before giving the medication, carefully assess the client. The preassessment will be based on the client's history, the medications the client is receiving, and the route by which the client is receiving the medications. Consider the client's age, level of consciousness/orientation and ability to follow instructions, motor function, ability to swallow and sit upright, and overall mental and physical condition.

One of the most critical preassessments is the client's history of allergies. To assess for allergies, review the client's chart and check the client's armband; ask the client verbally if he or she has any known allergies. The client's medication history, including herbs, vitamins, and OTC medications, is important to assess to avoid drug interactions.

If the client is receiving a medication that could affect the client's vital signs, check the vital signs before administering the medication. The authorized healthcare provider may specify parameters, such as pulse or blood pressure below a certain level, to determine if a medication needs to be held. If there is any question, or if the client has vital sign changes that significantly deviate from baseline or expected parameters, notify the authorized healthcare provider.

Another important assessment parameter is recent lab work. Lab tests such as blood chemistries include valuable information about kidney and liver function as well as blood glucose level. This is important assessment information when a client with diabetes is receiving insulin. Lab tests help to determine if the client is receiving either too much or too little of a medication. For some medications, elevated levels may be dangerous. Specific lab results may reveal that the client is becoming toxic on certain medications, such as digoxin or potassium. For example, the international normalized ratio (INR) test is a lab result for monitoring the effects of the anticoagulant medication warfarin (Coumadin). Notify the authorized healthcare provider of any INR outside of the therapeutic range and follow specific algorithms per facility policy.

SAFELY PREPARING AND DISTRIBUTING MEDICATIONS

Regardless of the route of the medication being administered, it is important to remember two key safety strategies, among others, that will prevent mistakes and medication errors:
- **Prepare only one medication at a time.**
- **Prepare medication for only one client at a time.**

Most facilities also use technology to improve medication safety, such as unit-dose systems, bar-code technology, and an automated dispensing system (ADS).
- **Unit-dose medications:** Unit doses are individually wrapped doses of medication that have been prepackaged and prelabeled by the manufacturer. Each dose is usually labeled with the name of the medication and the dose. If the facility pharmacist is involved in preparing the unit doses, the package may also include the client's name and medical record number.
- **Bar-code technology:** This technology uses a laser scanner that can be interfaced with a laptop computer, medication cart, or at the bedside. After entering a password and accessing the system, the nurse can identify the client and review the client's EMAR by scanning the bar code on the client's identification bracelet. As each unit-dose medication is verified at the cart and/or at the bedside with the client, the bar code on the medication should be scanned. This system will also note the time of administration as well as other pertinent information.
- **Automatic dispensing system:** An ADS uses medication storage devices, also known as automated dispensing cabinets (ADCs), to help dispense medications safely. As with other systems, ADS technology has safety features that can prevent medication errors. For example, some of these systems will alert the nurse about clients who have similar names to ensure that they are giving the right medication to the right client. The system can also alert the nurse to the client's allergies. Although ADS technology is not without error, it does offer safeguards. For example, most ADSs incorporate the use of bar-code technology. After the nurse performs the authorized safety checks, many systems allow for scanning of the client's armband bar code and the bar code on the medication label as each medication is verified. To prevent the risk of medication errors, avoid "overriding" the ADS. If the system does not seem to be working properly, notify the facility pharmacist per facility policy to correct the problem.

When using an ADS or ADC, the nurse will respond to standardized electronic prompts as he or she works through the system. Once it is determined which medications are needed, drawers unlock, one at a time, automatically. As medications are removed, this is recorded by the system. After the nurse has verified the medications are correct and has placed them in a medication cup (unopened), the nurse can then log-off the system before going to the client's room.

PERFORMING SAFETY CHECKS

When medications are administered, there are at least three safety checkpoints during which the rights of administration are checked (and rechecked) to ensure safety and accuracy. In this text, the three primary checkpoints are identified as occurring (1) upon accessing the medication, (2) upon preparing the medication, and (3) upon administering the medication. During the process of medication administration, stop and perform each of these safety checkpoints and avoid shortcuts in order to reduce the risk of medication errors.

First Checkpoint (Upon Accessing the Medication)

Using the rights of medication administration, the first and second checkpoints occur *before* administering the medications. The first checkpoint occurs when the nurse uses the electronic ADS to access the client's medications. In many facilities, new medication orders are checked against the MAR or EMAR to make sure they have been entered correctly. In addition, the labels on the medications obtained from the ADS need to be checked carefully against the MAR or EMAR to ensure that they are correct and there are no discrepancies. The expiration dates on the labels of the medications must also be checked. If there is any uncertainty about a medication order, contact the authorized healthcare provider *before* preparing the medication.

Second Checkpoint (Upon Preparing the Medication)

The second checkpoint occurs as the nurse is preparing the medication and before entering the client's room. As with the first check, the labels on the medications are checked against the MAR or EMAR as the medication is placed in the medication cups. Prepackaged unit doses must remain unopened in the medication cups until taken to the client's bedside. If required, the barcodes on the labels should be scanned before the unopened medications are placed in the medication cups.

If the medication is a pill or a liquid that is poured from a multidose bottle, an additional check is to verify the label of the bottle again before it is returned to storage. Once the first and second checks are completed, the medications can be taken to the client's room.

Third Checkpoint (Upon Administering the Medication)

One of the most critical aspects of medication safety is reviewing the medication with the client at the bedside. After all of the preassessments have been done (including vital signs if indicated), compare each unopened medication to the MAR or EMAR at the bedside and review it with your client. As each medication is reviewed, explain to the client what he or she is taking and why he or she is taking it. If the client expresses concern or refuses to take a medication, investigate if perhaps an error has occurred. Listen to your client. Sometimes it is the client who alerts us of a potential error. If an error has not occurred, the client may need additional information. If a client refuses to take medications that are ordered, notify the authorized healthcare provider as soon as possible.

Postadministration Checkpoint

Many facilities require a postprocedure checkpoint *after* the medication is administered to compare the MAR or EMAR to the label on the used medication packaging, container, or vial before disposal. If a medication error does occur, despite following safety checks, notify the authorized healthcare provider immediately, monitor the client closely for adverse effects, and follow facility policy regarding incident reports. As part of the rights of administration, document all medications that were administered, and document the client's response. Provide follow-up care and monitoring as indicated.

SAFETY CONSIDERATIONS FOR HIGH-ALERT MEDICATIONS

The ISMP defines high-alert medications as "drugs that bear a heightened risk of significant harm if used in error" (ISMP, 2018a). Examples of high-alert medications are digoxin, warfarin, heparin, insulin, and opioids. The ISMP provides an updated list of high-alert drugs for acute care, ambulatory care, and long-term care on its website. For a list of acute care high-alert medications, refer to the ISMP website (https://www.ismp.org/recommendations/high-alert-medications-acute-list).

Heparin and insulin, in particular, are two medications where serious drug errors have occurred, as discussed in Box 11.1. Medications that have been identified as high alert require safeguards such as standardized ordering, special labeling, automated alerts, and double-checking before administration. Most hospital facilities require that high-alert medications be verified by a second nurse during preparation. Some facilities require "independent double-checking," whereby the double check is performed separately by a second nurse without knowledge of the first person's check.

Safety Considerations for Opioids and Other Narcotics

In the United States, the number of overdose deaths and opioid-related deaths has escalated over the years. Recently, the opioid crisis has been declared a public health emergency. State and local agencies require that healthcare facilities ensure controlled substances are given as ordered. Opioids are also considered to be a high-alert medication. Any excess

BOX 11.1 Lessons From the Courtroom: Lawsuits and High-Alert Medications (Insulin and Heparin)

When medication errors occur that involve high-alert medications, such as insulin or heparin, the consequences can be devastating. As a result, litigation related to a violation of the rights of administration can occur. For example, in one lawsuit, a client was injected with insulin that was not ordered for him. Although the client's daughter reportedly informed the nurse that the client did *not* have diabetes, the nurse proceeded with the injection while failing to double check and reverify the client's identity. Although the nurse did report the error to the client's authorized healthcare provider, the client's glucose was only monitored at 8:15 PM and 10:15 PM (and not throughout the night) after the erroneous medication was given. By 6:15 AM the next morning, the client's blood glucose was only 15, and he subsequently died. Both punitive and compensatory damages may be awarded to the plaintiff in this case (Medication error: Court sees basis for liability, punitive damages, 2012). This case is a good example of why it is important to *listen* carefully to clients or family members when they try to raise a red flag and express concern about a medication that may not be appropriate for them to take.

In a high-profile lawsuit related to heparin, two infant twins were erroneously given a near-fatal dose of heparin. They received 10,000 units per mL of heparin instead of the intended heparin flush of 10 units per mL. This error occurred in a major healthcare facility and was related to look-alike vials and concentrations on the label that were easily confused. Because this type of error with heparin labels has been a recurring problem, legal action against the manufacturer was also filed. Under the guidance of the U.S. Food and Drug Administration (FDA), several manufacturers revised the labels on heparin containers to state the strength of the entire vial of medication as well as the total amount of heparin in 1 mL (U.S. FDA, 2016).

dose that is not needed should be discarded per facility policy. Many facilities use the term "wasting" for this procedure. It is required that another registered nurse (RN) witness the amount of medication that was discarded and sign off as a witness. This is usually integrated into the electronic health record.

Disposal of Medications

The CDC and U.S. Food and Drug Administration (FDA) have specific guidelines regarding the disposal of medications. For example, consumers and caregivers are encouraged to remove expired and unused medicines from the home as quickly as possible in order to decrease the risk of accidental overdose. Recent initiatives include National Prescription Drug Take-Back events and drop boxes to provide for proper disposal of medications. Current procedures for different types of medications are outlined on the FDA website (U.S. FDA, 2018). Check your facility policy. Many facilities have specific instructions regarding the proper disposal of medications.

PERFORMING DOSAGE CALCULATION

Dosage calculation is an important skill. Because the dose that is ordered is not always what is on hand in a particular setting, there are times when nurses will have to calculate the correct dosages. There are several methods that nurses can use to calculate drug dosages. It is up to the nurse to decide which method works best for him or her to facilitate accuracy.

When administering high-alert medications or working with vulnerable populations such as children, it is important to double-check all dosage calculations. Some medications, particularly for pediatric clients, may also require dosage calculation based on the client's weight and body surface area. As part of best-practice guidelines, the metric system is preferred for calculating weight in order to reduce errors. Thus, kilograms should be used instead of pounds for calculating medication dosages for both adults and children (ISMP, 2017b).

The main question to ask yourself before giving any medication is, **"Does this dosage seem reasonable for this client?"** For example, if your calculation indicates the client is to receive an unreasonable number of pills, there could have been a calculation error. Don't be afraid to ask questions. If there is any doubt, consult with other healthcare professionals.

Examples of Formulas for Dosage Calculation

The following three formulas are examples of methods commonly used for adults. For the first two formulas, ensure that all units of measure are the same. Conversions need to occur before substituting the numbers into the formulas, and any rounding of numbers in the formulas should not occur until the end of the calculation. For more information regarding pediatric formulas using weight and body surface area, consult a pediatric drug guide or textbook.

Example 1: Basic (Desired Over Have) Formula

When using the "desired over have" formula, the variables are the desired dose *(D)*; what you have on hand *(H)*; the vehicle, which is the form and amount of the drug *(V)*; and the calculated amount *(X)*. The formula is as follows:

$$\frac{D}{H} \times V = X$$

In this formula, all components must have the same unit of measurement, so conversions must be done first. Once all units of measurement are the same, they can be substituted into the formula. Example: Mr. Brown is to receive 20 mg of furosemide. However, all that is on hand is 40 mg per tablet. Solution: For this problem, 20 mg is the *D*, 40 mg is the *H*, and 1 is the *V* because the tablets are 40 mg per 1 tablet. Solve for *X* as follows:

$$\frac{20 \text{ mg}}{40 \text{ mg}} \times 1 \text{ tablet} = 0.5 \text{ tablet}$$

(Note: In this example, milligrams cancel out, and *X* will result in giving 0.5 tablet or ½ tablet.)

Example 2: Ratio-Proportion Method

Just as with the basic formula, all conversions to the same unit of measurement must occur before using the ratio-proportion formula and performing the calculations. A proportion is an equation made of two equal ratios. In this formula, desired = *D;* what is on hand = *H;* the vehicle, which is the form and amount of the drug, = *V;* and the calculated amount = *X.* In the following formula, solve for *X* by using cross-multiplication:

$$\frac{H}{V} = \frac{D}{X}$$

To repeat the previous example, the authorized healthcare provider orders 20 mg of furosemide for Mr. Brown, but all that is on hand is 40 mg per tablet. In this example, 20 mg is the *D,* 40 mg is the *H,* and 1 is the *V* because the tablets are 40 mg per 1 tablet. Solve for *X* as follows:

$$\frac{40 \text{ mg}}{1 \text{ tablet}} = \frac{20 \text{ mg}}{X}$$

To solve for *X,* cross-multiply and simplify as follows: 40 mg × *X* = 20 mg × 1 tablet.

$$X = \frac{20 \text{ mg}}{40 \text{ mg}} \text{ tablet} = \frac{1}{2} \text{ tablet}$$

Using the ratio-proportion formula, the milligrams will cancel out, and *X* will result in giving 0.5 tablet or ½ tablet.

Example 3: Dimensional Analysis Formula

When no conversion is needed, the dimensional analysis formula is set up as follows: desired = *D;* what is on hand = *H;* the vehicle, which is the form and amount available, = *V;* and the calculated amount = *X.* The dimensional analysis formula is as follows:

$$\frac{V}{H} \times \frac{D}{I} = X$$

For example, the authorized healthcare provider orders 20 mg of furosemide for the client, but all that is on hand is 40 mg per tablet. Thus, 20 mg is the *D,* 40 mg is the *H,* and 1 is the *V* because the tablets are 40 mg per 1 tablet. Solve for *X* as follows:

$$\frac{1 \text{ tablet}}{40 \text{ mg}} \times \frac{20 \text{ mg}}{1} = X$$

In this calculation, the milligrams will cancel out, and what is left is what is desired. The final answer when 20 is divided by 40 is 0.5 tablet or ½ tablet, calculated as follows:

$$\frac{1 \text{ tablet} \times 20 \text{ mg}}{40 \text{ mg}} = \frac{1 \text{ tablet} \times 20}{40} = \frac{1}{2} \text{ tablet}$$

Conversion to a Different Unit

Using this same formula, if conversion to a different unit is required, set the calculation up as follows: desired = *D;* what is on hand = *H;* the vehicle, which is the form and amount available, = *V;* the conversion factors = *C;* and the calculated amount = *X.*

$$\frac{V}{H} \times \frac{C(H)}{C(D)} \times \frac{D}{1} = X$$

If the authorized healthcare provider orders ampicillin 0.5 g, yet all that is on hand is 250 mg/mL, then how much ampicillin would be given? Set up the formula as follows:

$$\frac{1 \text{ mL}}{250 \text{ mg}} \times \frac{1000 \text{ mg}}{1 \text{ g}} \times \frac{0.5 \text{ g}}{1} = X$$

Begin the calculation by cross-canceling units (milligrams and grams cancel out), as follows:

$$\frac{1 \text{ mL}}{250 \text{ mg}} \times \frac{1000 \text{ mg}}{1 \text{ g}} \times \frac{0.5 \text{ g}}{1} = X$$

Continue the calculation by multiplying the numerator and then dividing by the denominator to solve for *X.* The final answer in this example is 2 mL of ampicillin would be given, calculated as follows:

$$X = \frac{1 \text{ mL} \times 1000 \times 0.5}{250} = 2 \text{ mL (final answer)}$$

To summarize, first it is important to recalculate the dosage whenever you are not sure of an answer. Second, consider using a different formula as your "double check," and perform a "triple check" of your calculation if needed. In addition, always look at the values you substitute into a formula to ensure they are appropriate. Third, if the result you have calculated does not seem like a reasonable dosage, recheck it. Finally, never be afraid to ask questions or ask for help. If you think an order for a dosage is incorrect, research the drug and clarify the order. As illustrated in Box 11.2, diligence and a willingness to ask questions can reduce the risk of medication errors.

BOX 11.2 Expect the Unexpected: Preventing a Potentially Fatal "Wrong-Dosage/Wrong-Route" Error

Jacob, a senior nursing student, is assigned to care for Mr. Pine, a 60-year-old gentleman who has been admitted to the cardiac unit for observation and management. An RN who has floated to the cardiac unit from another unit is assigned to care for Mr. Pine as well.

As part of his clinical assignment, Jacob is required to make a list of Mr. Pine's medications as well as the indications, contraindications, and other pertinent information about Mr. Pine's medications within the framework of the rights of medication administration.

One day, the authorized healthcare provider (who is a second-year medical resident) wrote an order to give Mr. Pine a dose of a certain medication by intravenous (IV) push that is usually given orally. As soon as Jacob saw the order for the medication, he became concerned. After researching the drug in the drug manuals on the unit and consulting with the pharmacist, Jacob discovered that the dosage was more

appropriate for an oral dose of that medication, not an IV dose. The usual dosage of the drug by IV route is 1 to 2 mg (not 20 mg as was ordered). Thus, the order did not pass the "Does this dosage seem reasonable?" test. Jacob immediately alerted Mr. Pine's nurse, who contacted the medical resident to clarify the order. The medical resident indicated he meant to write the order for "PO," not "IV." In fact, the written order was about 10 times what the parenteral (IV) dosage should be for that medication! Fortunately, the error was caught early and corrected before the medication was administered. This case is a good example of how vigilance with respect to following the rights of medication administration can reduce the risk of medication errors. Jacob's attention to detail and willingness to ask questions prevented this wrong-dosage/wrong-route error that could have had fatal consequences for Mr. Pine.

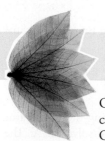

SECTION 1 Administering Oral Medications

One of the most common routes of medication administration is the oral route. Oral medications are ingested and then digested and absorbed through the gastrointestinal mucosa before being absorbed into the client's circulatory system (Caple & Schub, 2016). Thus, oral medications have one of the slowest absorption rates among all the routes; depending on the drug, they usually require 30 minutes to 1 hour to take effect (Le, 2018).

The advantage of oral medications is that they are usually the least expensive and most convenient. However, one limitation is that food and other medications in the digestive tract, as well as certain medical conditions, may affect absorption. Certain types of oral medications may cause irritation or disruption of the mucosal lining of the stomach or small intestine (e.g., aspirin or anti-inflammatory drugs). Verify if certain drugs should be given with or without food or should not be administered with other medications. It is also important to determine if oral medications are contraindicated. If the client has a decreased level of consciousness or a gastrointestinal disorder, the client may not be a good candidate for oral medications because of the risk of vomiting and aspiration. Although NPO (nothing by mouth) may be considered to be a contraindication, some authorized healthcare providers allow clients to take their medications with small sips of water rather than disrupt their schedule.

TYPES OF ORAL MEDICATIONS

The major types of oral medications are tablets, capsules, and liquids. Liquid medications include, but are not limited to, solutions, suspensions, emulsions, syrups, and elixirs (Le, 2018). One feature of tablets is that they may be cut in half if there is a specific order and if they are prescored. However, capsules or gel caps may be easier to swallow and less bitter tasting. Gel capsules are usually less irritating to the client's stomach/intestinal mucosa than tablets.

If a client has difficulty swallowing pills, a liquid version of the medication might be an appropriate alternative. If the client is receiving chewable tablets, the medication must be completely chewed first and then swallowed. A client who has poor dental health, missing teeth, or other oral issues would not be a good candidate for chewable medications. For a summary of different types of oral medications, see Table 11.2.

CRUSHING/ALTERING ORAL MEDICATIONS

In most circumstances, crushing tablets or opening capsules is *not* recommended. This is particularly true for extended/sustained release, sublingual, or enteric-coated medications because it could lead to unpredictable medication

TABLE 11.2 Common Types of Oral Medication Preparations

Category	Description
Capsule or gelcap	Shell made of gelatin, starch, or other soluble material filled with solid or liquid medicine formulation
Controlled-release tablet	Special dosage-delivery formulation to allow extended or sustained release of medicine. Should be swallowed whole. Tablet is *not* intended to be broken, chewed, crushed, or dissolved.
Elixir	Hydroalcoholic liquid containing dissolved medicinal agents
Emulsion	Two-phase system of at least two immiscible liquids; should be shaken
Enteric-coated tablet	Specially coated tablet that slows disintegration of the tablet and slows release of the medicine to allow for absorption in the small intestine rather than the stomach
Lozenge or troche	Solid medicine, in a sweetened base, intended to dissolve slowly
Orally disintegrating tablet (ODT)	Specially formulated tablet that disintegrates rapidly and allows medicine to dissolve in the oral cavity to allow for rapid absorption
Orally dissolving strip/soluble film	Thin film containing medication that dissolves quickly upon contact with a wet surface, such as the tongue or buccal mucosa
Powder	Finely ground drug frequently mixed with a diluent such as distilled or sterile water to create a suspension for oral administration
Suspension	Medication suspended in liquid; must be shaken to disperse the agent uniformly prior to administration
Syrup	Medicine dissolved in a sweet, viscous vehicle
Tablet	Solid-dosage form of medicine and diluents usually to be swallowed whole. Some may be chewed; some may be scored to allow for breaking.
Tincture	Alcoholic or hydroalcoholic solution prepared generally from vegetable material; may be potent (e.g., tincture of opium)

Reference: Le, 2018.

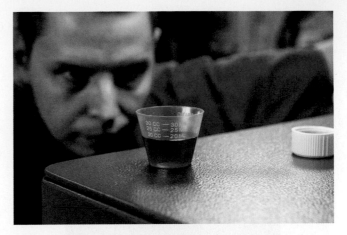

FIG. 11.1 Measure liquid at eye level.

PREPARING AND ADMINISTERING ORAL MEDICATIONS

When preparing and administering medications, use the proper technique and equipment. Prepackaged tablets must remain in their packages until ready to administer at the bedside. Once all safety verifications have been completed with the client, open the unit dose packages and place the pills in the medicine cups without touching them. When preparing liquid medications, place the liquid on a flat surface and read the bottom (U-shaped curve) of the meniscus. If using a medicine cup, measure the liquid at eye level on a flat surface to enhance accuracy (Fig. 11.1). As with pills, the liquid medication must not be touched.

BEST-PRACTICE RECOMMENDATIONS

Some liquid medications have measuring tools that must be used. Current best-practice guidelines stipulate that oral liquids not commercially available in unit doses must be given by an *oral syringe* that only displays the metric scale (ISMP, 2017b). The purpose of this guideline is to ensure accuracy. In addition, bold, bright labels that state **"ORAL USE ONLY"** may be placed on the syringe. This ensures that the oral medication is not given by the wrong route.

Clients who are being discharged or receiving home care may require additional teaching regarding the use of the oral syringe. There have been cases of serious medication errors because clients used household items such as teaspoons, tablespoons, or other devices. Ask the client to demonstrate to you how to use the oral syringe. Return demonstrations are helpful to ensure the client is accurately preparing each dose.

During administration, the client must be sitting upright if not contraindicated, and the client should be given plenty of time to take the medication. This is particularly important for an older adult client or a client who has a swallowing disorder and may need more time. Give one medication at a time, and remain with the client until each medication is

dosages. Altering medications can also increase the client's risk of complications and lead to a decreased effectiveness of the medication in the client later on. The ISMP (2018b) provides a detailed list of medications that should not be crushed (see the "Oral Dosage Forms That Should Not Be Crushed" list on the ISMP website [https://www.ismp.org/recommendations/do-not-crush]).

If a liquid form of the medication is not available and there is no alternative, a medication may only be altered if ordered by the authorized healthcare provider. In addition, use a facility-approved crusher that prevents cross-contamination of medication residue, and clean the device carefully between medications (ISMP, 2016). As recommended by The Joint Commission, the pill crusher should also be dedicated for use by only one client.

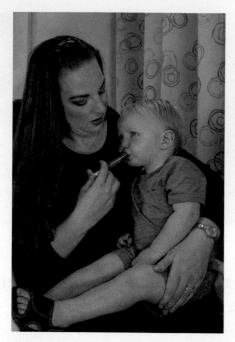

FIG. 11.2 Instruct the child's mother to use an oral syringe and hold the child securely.

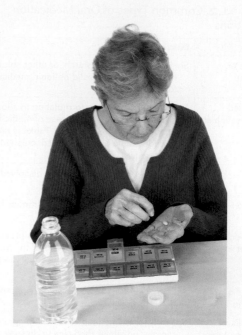

FIG. 11.4 Medication-dispensing box.

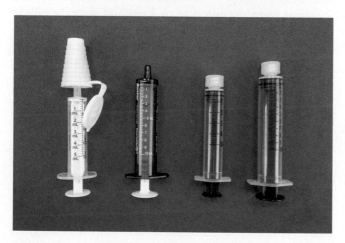

FIG. 11.3 Oral syringes.

swallowed. After the medication is administered, document appropriately and monitor the client's response.

PEDIATRIC CONSIDERATIONS

When giving oral medications to children, involve the parents as much as possible, and use techniques (such as holding) that will help the child feel more secure. As with adult clients, oral syringes must be used that display the metric scale for accuracy. After the oral syringe is secured, the medication can be slowly dripped into the child's mouth. Instruct the parent to position the infant or young child with the child's head elevated and supported while carefully administering the medication with his or her dominant hand (Fig. 11.2). If the parents will continue to give the child's medication at home, ensure that they are comfortable using an

oral syringe. Examples of oral syringes that may be used for medication are shown in Fig. 11.3.

HOME CARE AND GERIATRIC CONSIDERATIONS

In many settings, nurses will often need to provide client teaching and follow-up regarding medications in the home. For some clients, particularly older adults, maintaining a schedule for accurate self-administration of their medications can be a challenge. One device that can be helpful is a medication dispensing box that has compartments for scheduled medications, as shown in Fig. 11.4. This can be particularly useful for clients who take multiple medications at different times of the day and for clients who have difficulty remembering to take their medications. Reinforce to the client and/or the client's caretaker how to set up the compartments with the medications, and ensure they understand how to use the device.

Regardless of the setting, clients should be educated and empowered to understand their own medication regimens. This is consistent with the National Patient Safety Goals of The Joint Commission. As discussed in Box 11.3, a client's lack of understanding regarding his or her medications can lead to serious medication errors.

SUMMARY

In summary, accuracy, client-centered care, safety, infection control, communication, and evaluation are some of the most important critical concepts to consider when administering medications. The goal is safe administration of medications and improved client outcomes. To achieve this goal, effective teamwork and collaboration are essential.

BOX 11.3 Medication Confusion and "Double Dosing"

Mrs. Cumberbatch is a 69-year-old woman who has a history of hypertension and peripheral vascular disease. She has now presented to the emergency room (ER) with low blood pressure and a slow heart rate. She states that she has been feeling "lightheaded" when she sits up on the side of the bed and that she has been experiencing "near-fainting" spells at home.

During the initial assessment, the nurse caring for Mrs. Cumberbatch performs a thorough review of her medication regimen and discovers that Mrs. Cumberbatch has been taking both metoprolol (a beta blocker) and Lopressor (the brand name for metoprolol) at home from two different prescriptions. The prescriptions were written by different authorized healthcare providers at different points in time. When the nurse asked about this, Mrs. Cumberbatch replied, "Oh my, I had no idea they are the same medicine. I thought I was doing what I was supposed to do!" Because metoprolol (Lopressor) has systemic cardiovascular effects, the overdose of this medication was adversely affecting her blood pressure and hemodynamic stability.

Once the error was discovered, the dosage was adjusted by her primary authorized healthcare provider, and follow-up care was provided to ensure her condition stabilized. What is the take-away message here? This scenario underscores how important it is to educate clients and help them understand their medication regimens. The nurse in this situation caught this error because of a diligent and thorough review of the client's medications. Nurses in various settings (e.g., ambulatory care, acute care, home healthcare) can review medications with their clients and prevent errors from occurring.

In most acute care facilities, a licensed nurse usually administers medications. However, in other facilities, such as long-term care, assistive personnel who are certified may be able to administer medications under the supervision of a licensed nurse. This may vary, depending on the nurse practice act of the particular state. The registered nurse is responsible for ongoing assessment of the client. The registered nurse is also responsible for ensuring the client understands the medication regimen.

APPLICATION OF THE NURSING PROCESS

Examples of Related International Classification for Nursing Practice (ICNP) Nursing Diagnoses, Expected Client Outcomes, and Nursing Interventions:

Nursing Diagnosis: Lack of understanding of medication regime

Supporting Data: Client expresses uncertainty regarding current medications.

Expected Client Outcomes: Client will demonstrate an increased understanding of the current medication regimen, as seen by:
- ability to identify prescribed medications
- ability to identify and describe purpose of OTC medications
- ability to describe schedule and purpose of prescribed medication
- ability to demonstrate use of the sectioned pill dispenser.

Nursing Intervention Examples: Assess client's medication regimen, including prescription, herbal, and OTC medications. Teach client to use partitioned pill-dispensing box.

Reference: International Classification for Nursing Practice. (n.d.). *eHealth & ICNP.* Retrieved from https://www.icn.ch/what-we-do/projects/ehealth-icnp.

CRITICAL CONCEPTS
Administering Oral Medications

Accuracy (ACC)

Accuracy when administering oral medication is sensitive to the following variables:

Client-Related Factors
- Client's assessment, including level of consciousness and ability to take medications
- Client's ability to understand oral medication instructions
- Client's dental health and ability to swallow and/or chew oral medications
- Client's gastrointestinal, liver, and renal function

Nurse-Related and System-Related Factors
- Adherence to rights of administration, safety checks, and current safety guidelines
- Proper storage and proper labeling of oral medications
- Technique used for processing orders, preparing oral medications, administering oral medications, and providing follow-up care and monitoring
- Equipment used for administering oral medications (e.g., medication cups, special oral syringes and metric-only measuring devices, dedicated pill crushers for client)
- Correct dosage calculations and double-checking when necessary

Client-Centered Care (CCC)

Respect for the client when administering oral medications is demonstrated by:
- promoting autonomy and ensuring that verbal consent is obtained
- providing privacy and ensuring comfort
- honoring cultural preferences and arranging an interpreter if necessary
- advocating for the client and family and explaining purpose of oral medications.

Infection Control (INF)

Healthcare-associated infection when administering oral medications is prevented by:
- preventing and reducing the transfer of microorganisms
- reducing the number of microorganisms.

Safety (SAF)

Safety measures when administering oral medications prevent harm and maintain a safe care environment, including:
- checking for allergies and contraindications
- following medication safety guidelines, including the National Patient Safety Goals.

Communication (COM)

- Communication exchanges information (oral, written, nonverbal, or electronic) between two or more people.
- Documentation records information in a permanent legal record.

Evaluation (EVAL)

When administering oral medications, evaluation of the outcomes allows the nurse to determine the efficacy of the care provided, including
- monitoring the therapeutic effect of the medication
- monitoring for side effects, adverse effects, or allergic reactions.

■ SKILL 11.1 Administering Oral Medications (Tablets, Capsules, or Liquids)

EQUIPMENT

Medication cup (graduated with metric units of measure)
Cup of water and straw
Oral syringe with metric units of measure, if needed
Blood pressure (BP) cuff and stethoscope, if needed

BEGINNING THE SKILL

1. **ACC** Review the order for:
   - name of medication (generic names of medications are usually preferred)
   - dosage, time intervals, frequency, and route of administration
   - special administration instructions
   - purpose of administering medication (if PRN).
2. **ACC** Review the following:
   - **SAF** client's allergies to medications or other substances (Note: This step does not replace checking client's armband and asking the client verbally about allergies at the bedside.)
   - **SAF** indications and any contraindications for medications to be given
   - appropriateness of medication for client using the first five rights of medication administration (e.g., right client, right drug, right dose, right route, right time)
   - medical-surgical history and clinical status (particularly related to client's gastrointestinal, liver, and renal function and client's oral/dental health)
   - medication history (to check for potential drug interactions and compatibility)
   - recent lab work that would affect or be affected by the medication.
3. **INF** Perform hand hygiene.
4. **CCC** Introduce yourself to the client and family.
5. **SAF** Identify the client using at least two client identifiers. Ask the client to state his or her full name and date of birth. *Conforms with national safety standards.*

6. **CCC** Provide privacy.
7. **ACC** Assess the client's level of consciousness and orientation to person, time, place, and situation. *Provides a baseline assessment of orientation before verbal consent is obtained.*
8. **CCC** Explain the procedure and obtain verbal consent. *To provide client-centered care and prevent waste, consent should be obtained before preparing medications.*
9. **ACC** Perform client preassessments, including but not limited to the following:
   - vital signs if indicated and affected by medication (e.g., vasoactive/cardiac drugs)
   - ability to sit upright and swallow oral medications
   - presence of any abdominal distention or presence of nausea and/or vomiting.

PROCEDURE

Accessing and Preparing the Medications

10. **SAF** Perform **first safety checkpoint** when accessing the medications. (Note: If using an ADS: Log on and follow the prompts as directed.)
    a. Compare the medication orders against the MAR or EMAR (for new orders) if available, and check each of the safety administration rights (right client, drug, dose, route, and time) (Note: Many facilities require initial verification of new orders to ensure they are on the MAR or EMAR correctly.) *Provides an additional safety check.*
    b. Compare the label on the client's medication (unit-dose individual packages, multidose bottle, or liquid container) against the MAR or EMAR. Check the label for medication name, strength, expiration date, and any special precautions. (Note: Before using any medication, confirm that the medication has not expired.)

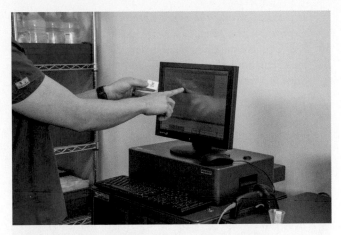

STEP 10 Perform first safety checkpoint.

11. **SAF** Perform the **second safety checkpoint** when preparing the medication. Compare the label on each unopened medication with the MAR or EMAR as it is being placed into the medication cup. Check each of the administration rights a second time. If the medication is a prepackaged unit dose, leave the packages in the medication cup (unopened) and do *not* remove from the wrappers until taken to the client's bedside. (Note: If using bar-code technology, verify the medication against the MAR or EMAR, and scan each bar code on the labels.)

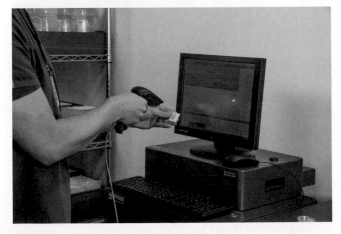

STEP 11 Perform second checkpoint and scan the bar codes.

12. **SAF WARNING:** If there is a discrepancy between the electronic medication orders or the labels and the MAR or EMAR, notify the pharmacy and the authorized healthcare provider per facility policy. *Discrepancies must be resolved before administering medications.*
13. **ACC** Perform dosage calculations if necessary, and double-check calculations.
14. **SAF** Prepare one medication at a time for one client at a time, and avoid interruptions. *These safety measures prevent distractions and medication errors.*

15. **ACC** If removing medication from a multidose bottle, pour the correct number of pills into the medication cup. (Note: Avoid directly touching medication.)
16. **ACC** If pouring a liquid medication from a bottle:
    a. Set the graduated medication cup on a flat surface.
    b. Shake the medication and place the cap, inverted, on the table.
    c. Pour the prescribed dose of medication with the label facing up against your palm.
    d. Read the level of the medication at eye level at the lowest point of the meniscus.
17. **ACC** If administering a liquid medication with a syringe, use an oral syringe per facility policy (less than 10 mL). *Using an oral syringe with metric units of measure prevents a wrong-dose or wrong-route error. An oral syringe (as opposed to parenteral) does not have a Luer-Lok tip, thus preventing a potentially fatal administration of oral medication into the client's IV line.*
18. **ACC** Recheck the label on the medication bottle (if used) against the MAR or EMAR before returning it back to storage (part of the **second safety checkpoint**).
19. **SAF WARNING:** If medications must be crushed, check order, consult facility pharmacy, and refer to ISMP "Do Not Crush" list. (Note: Refer to the ISMP website and narrative.) *Certain medications (e.g., enteric-coated, sublingual, and sustained-release forms) must not be crushed.*
20. **ACC** Avoid cutting tablets in half unless scored and authorized by the authorized healthcare provider. *Cutting a tablet in half that is not scored will result in an inaccurate dose.*
21. **SAF WARNING:** If the medication is not administered immediately, label the medication cup with the client's name, medication, time, date, and dosage (The Joint Commission, 2019).

Administering the Medications

22. **INF** Perform hand hygiene again upon entering the client's room.
23. **CCC** Maintain client privacy.
24. **SAF** Reverify the client's identity by using at least two client identifiers.
25. **SAF** Recheck the client's armband for allergies and ask the client verbally if he or she has any allergies. As you check the client's ID, compare the information against the MAR or EMAR.
26. **SAF** Perform **third safety checkpoint** by reviewing each unopened medication with the client and checking each of the labels with the client's ID band before administering. (Note: If using an ADS, scan the client's armband, and as medications are verified, scan the bar-code labels before opening packages and placing in the medicine cup.)

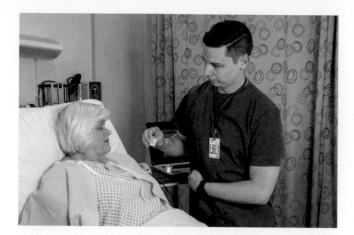

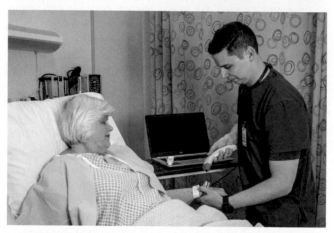

STEP 26 Perform third checkpoint at the bedside. Review each medication with the client and scan the client's armband if required.

27. **CCC** Explain the purpose of each medication with the client as needed.

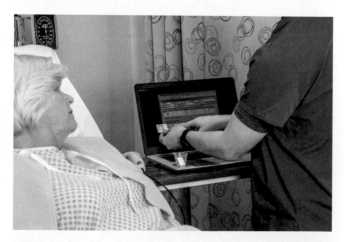

STEP 27 Provide client teaching about the medications.

28. **INF** After each medication is verified, open the medication packages (in the case of prepackaged unit doses) and drop them in the medication cup without touching them.

29. **SAF** Place the client in an upright position (if not contraindicated), provide a glass of water with a straw if needed, and instruct the client to take one medication

at a time. *Sitting the client upright and taking only one medication at a time reduces the risk of choking.*

30. **SAF** Observe the client take each medication. Remain with the client until all medications are taken. *Ensures that the client has not discarded or had difficulty with the medication.*

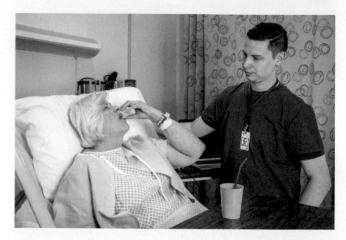

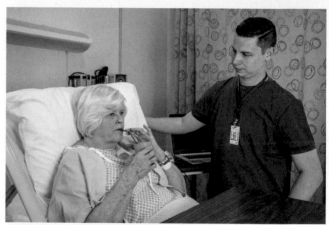

STEP 30 Observe the client take each medication. Ensure that the client can swallow the medication.

31. **SAF** If the facility has a **postadministration checkpoint,** review the empty medication package labels again (in the case of prepackaged unit doses) against the MAR or EMAR. If any errors occurred, notify the authorized healthcare provider immediately.
32. **SAF** Monitor the client for any adverse or unexpected effects of the medication.

FINISHING THE SKILL

33. **SAF** Ensure client safety and comfort. Ensure that the bed is in the lowest position, and verify that the client can identify and reach the nurse call system. *These safety measures reduce the risk of falls.*
34. **INF** Perform hand hygiene.
35. **EVAL** Monitor and evaluate the outcomes. *Was the client able to take medication without difficulty? Were the rights of administration followed (right client, drug, dose, route, time, and documentation)? Did the client respond to the medication as expected? Are there any adverse effects?*

36. **COM** Document assessment findings, medication administration, and outcomes in the legal healthcare record:
    - name of medication administered, exact time, date, and dosage
    - pertinent postassessment data, such as vital signs or pain level
    - signature and initials of the clinician who administered the medication.
37. **EVAL** Provide follow-up monitoring by continuing to evaluate the client's response to the medication and the presence of any delayed reactions. *Follow-up monitoring facilitates safety.*

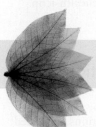

SECTION 2 Administering Enteral Medications

Although the oral route is preferred, many clients may not be able to take oral medications due to an altered level of consciousness, difficulty swallowing, or some other disorder related to the gastrointestinal system. In addition, many clients who have an enteral tube (e.g., nasogastric [NG] tube or other enteral appliance) will also need to receive enteral medications. To facilitate safe administration of enteral medications, the ISMP and the American Society for Parenteral and Enteral Nutrition (ASPEN) have provided key recommendations (Box 11.4).

When administering enteral medications, the specific characteristics of the medications being administered, as well as the route, size, and diameter of the client's tube, must also be considered (see Chapter 5). One of the most critical factors to consider is where the distal tip of the tube is located. In many cases, gastric access is preferred over jejunal access because certain drugs cannot be absorbed in the small intestine (Dudek, 2017; ISMP, 2016). In addition, giving medications through a large-bore NG sump tube may be preferred over a small-bore feeding tube because the large-bore NG tube is made of a stiffer material and is less likely to get clogged. If available, the liquid form of medication is preferred whenever possible. Some medications that are too thick may require dilution in order to avoid obstructions. Administer only one medication at a time, and flush the tube before and after *each* medication per facility policy and guidelines.

As with oral medications (see Section 1 of this chapter), medications that will be administered in an NG tube or other enteral device should not be crushed unless there is no other alternative. In particular, enteric-coated medications should *not* be crushed because doing so could alter the pharmacokinetics of the medication and cause clumping or obstruction of the tube. Enteral appliances that are smaller in diameter, such as feeding tubes or jejunostomy tubes, are particularly prone to clogging and obstruction. As noted in Section 1, the ISMP website provides a detailed list of medications that should not be crushed (ISMP, 2018b). If a medication is ordered that should not be crushed, contact the pharmacy or authorized healthcare provider.

Clients who are receiving tube feedings may require additional precautions when administering medications. If the client is receiving continuous feedings, stop the feedings, flush the tube with the ordered amount of sterile water before giving medications, flush between *each* medication that is administered, and flush after all of the medications (ISMP, 2016). Some medications may need to be administered on an empty stomach. In this situation, the feedings may need to be turned off for a certain amount of time before the medication is given. Avoid adding or mixing medications with the tube feedings (see Chapter 5, Section 6).

Prior to administration, enteral medications should be mixed in separate cups and dissolved in warm water. They may be given by gravity using the barrel of a syringe, or they may be drawn up in individual oral syringes. To maintain

---

BOX 11.4 Summary of Key Recommendations for Enteral Medication Administration

- Ensure that the drug is appropriate for enteral administration.
- Give the liquid (nonsorbitol) form of medications whenever possible.
- If medications must be given by jejunostomy, ensure they are crushed into a very fine powder. Use sterile water for jejunostomy medications.
- Do *not* crush sustained-release, sublingual, buccal, enteric-coated, hormonal, or cytotoxic drugs. Check with the pharmacist to verify if medications can be crushed.
- Prepare medications separately, crush thoroughly (or open capsule and mix contents into fluid), and allow each medication to completely dissolve or suspend.
- If medications must be reconstituted, use only sterile or purified water.
- Use only oral/enteral or ENFit syringes. Label syringe "FOR ORAL USE ONLY."
- Use caution when administering highly viscous medications. Dilute medication if possible, and instill gently to avoid rupturing the tube.
- Do *not* add medications to feedings.

References: Dudek, 2017; Institute for Safe Medication Practices, 2016.

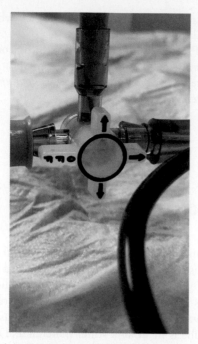

FIG. 11.5 Administering medication through a Lopez valve.

a closed system, a three-way valve or Lopez valve is often used. As shown in Fig. 11.5, a Lopez valve is used with an NG sump tube (see Chapter 5). When administering the medication, the valve can be open to allow the medication from the piston syringe to flow into the main lumen of the NG tube. After the medication is administered, the valve to the piston syringe can then be turned off to prevent air from entering the tube.

When administering medications through an enteral device, check the stoma and make sure the exit site is intact and without signs of leaking. To avoid skin irritation, use caution when giving medications such as potassium, particularly if the client has a stoma, such as a gastrostomy or a jejunostomy.

A potentially life-threatening error that can occur when giving enteral medications is inadvertent administration of medication prepared for enteral use into a client's IV line. To prevent this error, only oral medication syringes or ENFit syringes should be used that do not accept needles for IV use. Before giving any enteral medication, consult the facility pharmacy and drug administration guide, and ensure that all precautions are followed.

APPLICATION OF THE NURSING PROCESS

Examples of Related ICNP Nursing Diagnoses, Expected Client Outcomes, and Nursing Interventions:
Nursing Diagnosis: Effective response to enteral medication
Supporting Data: Client is tolerating enteral medications without complaints.
Expected Client Outcomes: Absence of signs and symptoms of adverse reactions to enteral medications:
• vital signs within expected parameters after medications

• therapeutic levels of medications achieved when applicable.
Nursing Intervention Examples: Follow standardized medication safety guidelines; flush tube between medications to prevent cross-contamination; monitor client's response to medications.
Reference: International Classification for Nursing Practice. (n.d.). *eHealth & ICNP.* Retrieved from https://www.icn.ch/what-we-do/projects/ehealth-icnp.

CRITICAL CONCEPTS
Administering Enteral Medications

Accuracy (ACC)

Accuracy when administering enteral medications is affected by the following variables, including:
• assessment of the client, including level of consciousness, medical/surgical history, clinical status, and gastrointestinal function
• adherence to rights of administration, safety checks, and standardized safety guidelines
• proper storage and proper labeling of enteral medications
• technique used for administering enteral medications
• verification of tube placement before medication administration
• frequency/timing of flushing tube with enteral administration
• equipment used for administering enteral medications (e.g., medication cups, special oral syringes and metric-only measuring devices, dedicated pill crushers for client)
• correct dosage calculations.

Client-Centered Care (CCC)

Respect for the client when administering enteral medications is demonstrated by:
• promoting autonomy and ensuring that verbal consent is obtained
• providing privacy and ensuring comfort
• honoring cultural preferences and arranging an interpreter if necessary
• advocating for the client and family and explaining purpose of enteral medications.

Infection Control (INF)

Healthcare-associated infection when administering enteral tube medications is prevented by:
• preventing and reducing the transfer of microorganisms
• reducing the number of microorganisms.

Safety (SAF)

Safety measures when administering enteral medications prevent harm and maintain a safe care environment, including:
• checking for allergies and contraindications and following safety checks and guidelines.

Communication (COM)

- Communication when administering enteral medications exchanges information (oral, written, nonverbal, and electronic) between two or more people.
- Documentation records information in a permanent legal record.
- Collaboration with the pharmacy and other members of the healthcare team regarding preparation, compatibility, and administration of medications given by the enteral route facilitates safe and effective care.

Evaluation (EVAL)

Evaluation of the outcomes when administering enteral medications allows the nurse to determine the efficacy of the care provided, including:

- monitoring the therapeutic effect of the medication.
- monitoring for side effects, adverse effects, or allergic reactions.

■ SKILL 11.2 Administering a Medication Through a Nasogastric (NG) Tube or Enteral Device

EQUIPMENT

Measuring tape, stethoscope, pH paper
Piston Toomey syringe (if indicated)
Flush solution or sterile water
ENFit or oral-tipped syringes with metric measurement markings
Disposable absorbent pads, towels, and washcloths
Client's dedicated pill crusher for single client use, if needed
Clean gloves
Medicine or water cups and labels if needed
Lopez valve for NG tube or 3-way valve if needed

BEGINNING THE SKILL

1. **ACC** Review the client's order for:
   - name of medication for enteral administration and dosage
   - route and purpose of administration and special instructions.
2. **ACC** Review the following:
   - **SAF** client's allergies to medications or other substances
   - **SAF** indications and any contraindications for medications to be given
   - client's history, lab results, and how the client is tolerating enteral feedings, if applicable
   - appropriateness of the enteral medication for the client.
3. **ACC** Review the following criteria specific to enteral medication administration:
   - Verification of initial tube placement by x-ray. **WARNING:** Before anything can be administered into an NG tube for the first time, an x-ray is usually performed to verify proper placement. *An x-ray is the gold standard for the initial placement check.*
   - **COM** Verification that the ordered medication can be administered by NG tube or other enteral device (e.g., gastrostomy, jejunostomy, or percutaneous endoscopic gastrostomy [PEG] tube). Check with the

facility pharmacist or authorized healthcare provider. *Medications that are viscous may require a larger-bore tube, such as a gastrostomy tube, and may not be able to be administered through a smaller-bore feeding tube, such as a jejunostomy, due to the risk of clogging or tube obstruction.*

   - **COM** Verification if the ordered medication can be administered with NG tube feedings (if applicable). (Note: Some medications should be given on an empty stomach. Check with the facility pharmacist or authorized healthcare provider about specific medications.)
4. **INF** Perform hand hygiene.
5. **CCC** Introduce yourself to the client and family.
6. **SAF** Identify the client using at least two client identifiers.
7. **CCC** Provide privacy.
8. **ACC** Assess the client's level of consciousness and orientation to person, time, place, and situation. *Provides a baseline assessment of orientation before verbal consent is obtained.*
9. **CCC** Explain the procedure and obtain verbal consent. *To provide client-centered care and prevent waste, consent should be obtained before preparing medications.*
10. **ACC** Perform client preassessments, including but not limited to the following:
    - vital signs if indicated and affected by medication (e.g., vasoactive drugs)
    - presence of any abdominal distention or presence of nausea and/or vomiting
    - presence of bowel sounds in all quadrants
    - appearance of the client's NG tube or enteral tube and comparison of the external tube length and external markings to those documented when placement was verified by x-ray. *A preliminary assessment of the client's NG tube or enteral tube alerts the nurse to any immediate problems or possible displacement of the tube.*

PROCEDURE

Preparing the Enteral Medication

11. **SAF** Perform the **first safety checkpoint** when accessing the enteral medication. Initiate the **second safety checkpoint** when preparing the medication. Check the rights of administration, check the expiration date, and scan the bar code on the label if required (refer to Skill 11.1). (Note: If available, consider using a liquid form of the medication whenever possible.)

12. **ACC** If the medication must be crushed, crush each medication separately into a fine powder. Clean the pill crusher between each medication. *Crushing medications into powder prevents clogging. Cleaning the pill crusher between medications prevents cross-contamination.*

13. **SAF WARNING:** Do *not* crush sustained-release, sublingual, or enteric-coated medications or gel capsules. *Crushing certain medications could cause erratic absorption or dangerous blood levels. Some medications that are crushed could obstruct tubes.*

14. **ACC** Mix each medication until dissolved or suspended in separate cups with warm water using separate straws or stirring sticks. *Mixing medications separately prevents cross-contamination of medications. Using warm water will help the medication dissolve.*

15. **ACC** If the medication is in capsule form, open the capsule and pour the powdered medication into a cup per facility policy before mixing it with warm water.

16. **SAF** Complete the **second safety checkpoint** and check the rights of administration before labeling and administering the medication. **WARNING:** If medications will be drawn up in syringes, use oral-tipped or EN-Fit syringes and label the syringes **"NOT FOR IV USE."** Label the syringe per facility policy (e.g., client's name, medication, dose, route, date, time). *Using oral syringes that will not accept an IV needle and labeling syringes properly reduce the risk of accidental administration of enteral medications into the client's IV line.*

Administering the Enteral Medication

17. **INF** Perform hand hygiene again upon entering the client's room.

18. **CCC** Maintain client privacy.

19. **SAF** Perform the **third safety checkpoint** with the client for each medication he or she is receiving and check the rights of administration again. (Note: If required, scan the client's armband and the bar code on the medication label if available.) *Facilitates client involvement.*

20. **SAF** Recheck the client's armband for allergies, and ask the client verbally if he or she has any allergies.

21. **SAF** Prepare the client for the procedure. Elevate the client's head of the bed (HOB) at least 45 degrees and place disposable absorbent pads under or around the enteral tube site. *An elevated head position prevents aspiration.*

22. **INF** Apply clean gloves.

24. **ACC** Verify placement of the NG tube or enteral tube again using a variety of methods, including checking gastric aspirate and gastric pH (refer to Chapter 5). Measure the length of the external tubing and compare it to the length on insertion of the tube. **WARNING:** If there is any doubt about the placement of the NG tube or enteral tube, do NOT administer the medication until placement can be verified. *Verifying placement before administration of the medication helps ensure the tube has not migrated or become displaced since insertion.*

25. **ACC** If the client is on NG suction, discontinue suction before administering the medication.

26. **ACC** If the client is receiving continuous feedings, stop the feeding pump, place feedings on hold, flush the enteral tube with sterile water or other fluid per facility policy, and cap the tube until enteral medications can be administered. *Flushing the enteral tube will prevent clogging and obstructions of the tube.* (Note: Some medications should be given on an empty stomach. Check with the facility pharmacist about specific medications.)

27. **ACC If administering enteral medications by gravity:**
    a. Remove the plunger from the barrel of the piston/ Toomey syringe.

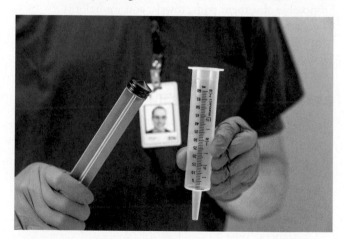

STEP 27A Remove the plunger.

(Note: The size of the syringe depends on the age of the client, the type of appliance, and the volume to be administered. For example, if the client has a gastrostomy feeding button or a jejunostomy, a smaller oral syringe may be used as opposed to larger syringes.) **WARNING:** Ensure that only oral syringes or ENFit adapters are used.

    b. Prevent air from entering the tube. Turn the Lopez valve to OFF if present. If not, clamp the tubing. *Preventing air from entering the stomach prevents abdominal distention.*
    c. Place the syringe barrel on the main port of the NG tube or the medication port of the enteral tube.
    d. Hold the syringe barrel and tube securely as a unit to prevent slipping. *Holding the syringe/tube securely prevents disconnection and loss of fluid and medication.*

e. While tubing remains clamped, pour ordered amount of flush solution or sterile water (usually 10–30 mL) into the barrel of the syringe.

f. Unclamp the tubing or open the Lopez valve (if present) and allow fluid to slowly flush the tube. *Flushing the tube prior to medication administration maintains the patency of the tube.* (Note: The amount and type of fluid for flushing the tube vary. Gastrostomy and jejunostomy tubes require less volume than NG tubes. Some facilities require sterile water for flushing a jejunostomy tube due to the risk of infection.)

g. During flushing, elevate the syringe barrel above the level of the client's stomach (no more than 45 cm [18 inches]). *The height of the syringe affects the rate of gravity flow.*

h. After flushing the tube, clamp the tubing or close the Lopez valve (if present) and pour the medication into the syringe barrel. If there is residual medication in the medication cup, add a small amount of water into the cup, stir/swirl around, and pour into the syringe barrel.

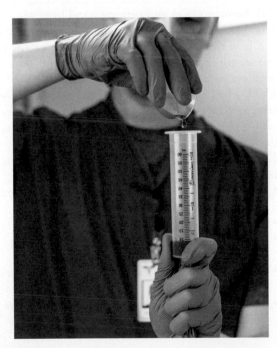

STEP 27H After checking and flushing the tube, administer medication.

i. Unclamp the tubing or open the Lopez valve (if present) and allow the medication to slowly go in by gravity. If the medication is going in too fast, lower the syringe. *Reduces risk of cramping.* (Note: Medication administration through a jejunostomy tube may take longer because of the small size of the tube. If resistance is met, more dilution may be required.)

j. Clamp the tubing before the syringe barrel is completely empty of medication. *Prevents air from entering stomach.*

k. Pour ordered flush solution or sterile water into barrel of syringe and then unclamp to allow fluid to slowly flush the tube. *Ensures all medication is administered.*

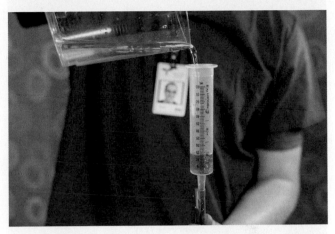

STEP 27K Flush the tube again after each medication is administered.

l. If the client is receiving more than one medication, administer *one* medication at a time and flush the tube with sterile water or another ordered fluid (usually 5–15 mL) between each medication. *Flushing between each medication will prevent cross-contamination of the medications. The amount of flush depends on the type of tube and order.* (Note: A large bore NG tube may require a higher volume of flushing than other enteral tubes.) **WARNING:** Do *not* allow air to enter the NG or enteral tube between medications or flushings. *Excess air in the client's stomach could cause distention and distress.*

m. After all medications are given, flush the NG or enteral tube according to facility policy and order. *Flushing after all of the medications will prevent clogging of the tube.*

28. **ACC If administering a medication by using syringe push method into an enteral device** (e.g., gastrostomy, PEG, jejunostomy, or low-profile gastrostomy button):

a. Ensure that an oral or ENFit syringe is used. Select the syringe size based on the volume of medication to be administered and the size of the enteral device.

b. Clamp tube and attach syringe with flush into medication port or adapter. While stabilizing the tubing/port with your nondominant hand, flush the tube (using dominant hand) with 5 to 15 mL of sterile water, as ordered.

c. After flushing, clamp the tube again, remove the flush syringe, and then attach the syringe with the medication. Open the clamp and slowly administer all of the medication by pushing the syringe plunger.

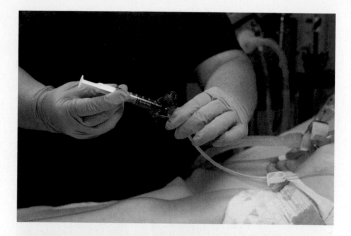

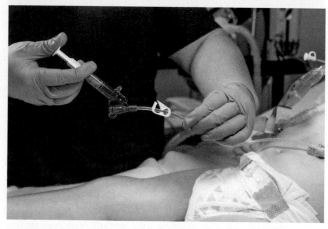

STEP 28C Attach syringe to correct port and administer medication.

    d. After the medication is administered, clamp the tube and remove the medication syringe.

    e. Attach a flush syringe and flush with 5 to 15 mL of sterile water as ordered. *Flushing the enteral tube after medication maintains patency.*

    f. After flushing, clamp the tube again and remove the flush syringe.

    g. Secure the cap on the enteral tube and ensure that the tube is clamped. (Note: Some enteral tubes, such as low-profile buttons, have attached safety caps.)

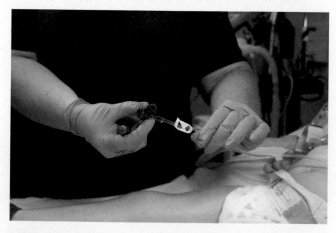

STEP 28G After flush, clamp tube and secure safety cap.

29. **SAF** After medication administration, ensure that the exit site of the enteral device or stoma is dry and intact, without signs of leaking or redness. *Ensures that integrity of tube is maintained.*

30. **SAF** Perform **postadministration safety checkpoint** if required (refer to Skill 11.1).

31. **SAF** Leave the client's HOB elevated for 1 to 2 hours according to policy after medication administration. *Prevents reflux and aspiration of medication and fluids into lungs.*

32. **ACC** If the client is on NG suction, wait at least 30 minutes before resuming suction per facility policy and the order. *Placing the client back on suction too soon will interfere with the absorption of medications.*

33. **ACC** If the client is on continuous feedings, resume feedings per facility policy. (Note: Some medications should not be mixed or taken with food and require a certain amount of wait time before feedings are resumed. Consult with the pharmacy or authorized healthcare provider.)

34. **INF** Dispose of equipment according to facility policy.

FINISHING THE SKILL

35. **INF** Remove gloves and perform hand hygiene.

36. **SAF** Ensure client safety and comfort. Ensure that the bed is in the lowest position, and verify that the client can identify and reach the nurse call system. *These safety measures reduce the risk of falls.*

37. **EVAL** Monitor and evaluate the outcomes. Did the enteral tube remain patent? Were the rights of administration followed (right client, drug, dose, route, time, and documentation)?

38. **COM** Document assessment findings, care given, and outcomes in the legal healthcare record:

    • method used to administer medications (e.g., gravity, syringe method)

    • name, dosage, and route of each medication

    • type of enteral tube used for medications (e.g., gastrostomy or jejunostomy)

    • verification of placement of tube used for medications

    • client's response to the medication (immediate and delayed).

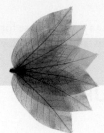

SECTION 3   Administering Mucous Membrane Applications

When a client cannot take an oral/enteral medication, or if the client needs a medication with a more rapid action, a medication via the mucous membrane tissue may be indicated. Mucous membranes are the cells that line the inside of the body. Because mucous membrane applications circumvent the gastrointestinal system and first-pass metabolism, medications delivered through this route enter the systemic circulation at a faster rate than those using the oral or enteral route. Common mucous membrane applications include sublingual or buccal medications, nasal medications, metered-dose inhalers (with and without spacers), and nebulizers. Additional mucous membrane applications that can be administered include rectal and vaginal medications.

As with other medications, the critical concepts of accuracy, safety, client-centered care, infection control, evaluation, and communication are applicable. In addition, it is important to protect the client's tissue integrity during the administration of mucous membrane medications.

SUBLINGUAL AND BUCCAL MEDICATIONS

Sublingual medications are placed under the client's tongue so that they can be absorbed directly by the small blood vessels in this area; buccal medications are placed between the client's gums and cheeks. These medications may be commonly available in the form of pills or sprays, and they may have systemic effects. Depending on the medication, some sublingual and buccal applications can take effect in several minutes. For example, nitroglycerin is commonly given to clients by the sublingual route for immediate relief of cardiac chest pain (see Chapter 19). In addition, this medication can have a systemic effect on the client's blood pressure.

For both sublingual and buccal medications, the client must allow the medication to completely dissolve and not chew or swallow the medication. Although sublingual and buccal medications usually have a rapid onset of action, many drugs cannot be given by this route because absorption may be erratic or incomplete (Le, 2018). This route may also be contraindicated for clients who have had oral surgery or those who have oral lesions.

NASAL INSTILLATIONS

The nasal mucosa is a highly vascular surface, which facilitates increased absorption into the circulatory system. Nasal medications are often used to treat nasal congestion, or they may be prescribed by the authorized healthcare provider for certain systemic conditions. One of the most common types of nasal medications is nasal sprays (either pump bottles or pressurized containers). Sprays must be transformed or atomized into small particles in the air as a mist to be absorbed (Le, 2018). In addition, atomization can improve the bioavailability of the medication due to the expansion of the surface area on the nasal mucosa for drug distribution (Corrigan, Wilson, & Hampton, 2015). This technology can potentially provide rapid and life-saving benefits. For example, naloxone (Narcan) nasal spray, an opioid antagonist, is now available and can temporarily reverse the effects of an opioid overdose. However, the pharmacologic action of the opioids may exceed the effects of the naloxone (Narcan) spray. Thus, emergency medical assistance must still be contacted immediately. Although naloxone (Narcan) may be administered by other routes (e.g., IV), the intranasal route provides easy access and rapid absorption (see Skill 11.4).

Nasal drops are another type of nasal medication that may be administered. However, this method is not as commonly used as nasal sprays due to the decreased surface area for absorption. In addition, nasal drops can result in a loss of the medication outside of the nasal passage or by run-off to the client's oropharynx (Corrigan et al., 2015). If nasal drops are used, avoid touching the dropper to the client's naris, and ensure the client's head is tilted back appropriately. It is also important to instruct the client to remain in place for several minutes and to not blow the nose.

Contraindications to nasal instillations include clients who have had nasal or sinus surgery or nasal trauma. If nasal medications are mixed, use distilled or sterile water. *Never* use tap water because tap water nasal sprays could lead to serious infections. Before administering a nasal medication, ensure that it is at room temperature to prevent discomfort. After instillation, monitor the client for side effects, such as inflammation or bleeding (Richards & Heering, 2017).

INHALERS AND NEBULIZERS

Medications that are delivered by inhalation, and thus applied directly to mucous membranes, are generally absorbed quickly and have a rapid onset of action. Various types of medications are commonly delivered in this manner, particularly bronchodilators and corticosteroids, which exert their actions quickly to dilate the airways and reduce inflammation for the management of multiple types of respiratory conditions.

Some common methods for the delivery of inhaled medications include pressurized metered-dose inhalers, dry-powder inhalers, and nebulizers. These are handheld devices that can be used by the client. A pressurized metered-dose inhaler (pMDI) has a pressurized canister that fits into a mouthpiece. When the button is pressed, the pMDI releases the medication in a propellant (liquefied compressed gas) that is aerosolized for an inhaled breath (Gardenhire, Burnett, Strickland, & Myers, 2017).

A variation of the traditional pMDI is a breath-activated inhaler that does not have a button to compress.

Depending on the needs of the client and specific orders, a traditional metered-dose inhaler can be used with or without a spacer. Spacers allow a place for the aerosolized medication to reside while the client is breathing in. This is particularly helpful for children and older adults, as well as clients who are new to inhalers, to decrease the loss of medication. The pMDI apparatus and spacer are for dedicated use by one client and must not be shared.

A dry-powder inhaler (DPI) is inspiration driven, and as the name implies, it delivers dry powder directly into the client's lungs during an inhaled breath. One advantage of the DPI is that it doesn't require hand coordination, and thus it may be easier for some clients to use than the pMDI. However, a disadvantage is that the client must have a strong and quick inspiration in order for the dry medication particles to disperse. It is also important for the client not to exhale directly into the mouthpiece, and the device must be kept dry (Gardenhire et al., 2017).

For clients who cannot use a pMDI (e.g., young children or older adults) or those who need an alternative option for receiving inhaled medications, a nebulizer may be used. Nebulizers require a machine or a compressor in order to aerosolize the medication and turn the liquid into a mist. This is accomplished by using compressed air or oxygen flow. For some clients, such as those with chronic obstructive pulmonary disease (COPD), oxygen may be contraindicated, or it may only be used with caution. For more information on oxygen administration and safety, see Chapter 9.

Throughout the nebulizer procedure, the client should remain in a relaxed, upright position if not contraindicated and breathe normally through the mouthpiece or face mask until all the medication has dispensed. As with pMDIs, instruct the client to rinse his or her mouth out if corticosteroids are used and clean the equipment thoroughly (Gardenhire et al., 2017).

RECTAL AND VAGINAL ADMINISTRATION

The rectal and vaginal mucosa have a dense blood supply and a fairly rapid onset of action (usually about 10–15 minutes). Vaginal medications are often given as suppositories, but they can also be administered as gels, foams, creams, or rings (medication-embedded devices) (Le, 2018). The rectal route is appropriate for a variety of drugs, typically given by suppository. However, if a client is receiving radiation therapy or has neutropenia (low white blood cell count), rectal medications may be contraindicated due to the risk of rectal tears and infection. Additional contraindications include bleeding disorders and rectal fissures/fistulas.

Both the vaginal and rectal routes of administration require that the nurse apply clean disposable gloves and provide privacy to the client. Due to the sensitivity of these types of procedures, many facilities require a female nurse to be in attendance when vaginal or rectal medications are given to female clients. Some clients prefer a female nurse for this procedure. Check your facility policy, and if no policy exists, consider the wishes of your client.

APPLICATION OF THE NURSING PROCESS

Examples of Related ICNP Nursing Diagnoses, Expected Client Outcomes, and Nursing Interventions:

Nursing Diagnosis: Risk for impaired tissue integrity
Supporting Data: Client is receiving medications that can irritate the mucous membranes.
Expected Client Outcomes: The client will have no sign of impaired skin integrity as seen by:

- Mucous membranes pink and moist, without any signs of sores or lesions
- No evidence of redness, inflammation, or signs of infection of mucous membranes
- No evidence of excessive drainage, coughing, or irritation of mucous membranes.

Nursing Intervention Example: Monitor mucosa for any redness or irritation from medication.
Reference: International Classification for Nursing Practice. (n.d.). *eHealth & ICNP.* Retrieved from https://www.icn.ch/what-we-do/projects/ehealth-icnp.

CRITICAL CONCEPTS
Administering Mucous Membrane Applications

Accuracy (ACC)

Administration of mucous membrane applications is sensitive to the following variables:

Client-Related Factors

- Client's assessment, including level of consciousness and orientation
- Client's ability to hear and understand instructions regarding mucous membrane medications
- Client's ability to be positioned for mucous membrane medications (e.g., semi-Fowler, dorsal recumbent, left lateral positions)
- Client's mobility and ability to hold and use devices associated with mucous membrane medications (e.g., handheld inhalers and nebulizers)

Nurse-Related and System-Related Factors

- Adherence to rights of administration, safety checks, and standardized safety guidelines
- Proper storage and proper labeling of mucous membrane medications
- Technique used for processing orders, preparing and administering mucous membrane medications, and providing follow-up care and monitoring
- Proper use, handling, and assembly of equipment used for administering mucous membrane applications (e.g., inhaler and nebulizer equipment)

Client-Centered Care (CCC)

Respect for the client when administering mucous membrane applications is demonstrated by:
- promoting autonomy and ensuring that verbal consent is obtained
- providing privacy and ensuring comfort during sensitive procedures
- honoring cultural preferences and arranging an interpreter if necessary
- advocating for the client and family and explaining the procedures.

Infection Control (INF)

Healthcare-associated infection when administering mucous membrane applications is prevented by:
- preventing and reducing the transfer of microorganisms
- reducing the number of microorganisms.

Safety (SAF)

Safety measures when administering mucous membrane applications prevent harm and maintain a safe care environment, including:

- checking for allergies and contraindications and following safety checks and guidelines.

Communication (COM)

- Communication when administering mucous membrane applications exchanges information (oral, written, nonverbal, or electronic) between two or more people.
- Documentation records information in a permanent legal record.

Evaluation (EVAL)

When administering mucous membrane applications, evaluation of outcomes enables the nurse to determine the therapeutic response and safety of the care provided by:
- monitoring the therapeutic effect of the medication
- monitoring for side effects, adverse effects, interactions, or allergic reactions
- monitoring the client's breathing during administration of inhaled medications.

■ SKILL 11.3 Administering Sublingual or Buccal Medications

Medication cup
Clean gloves
Stethoscope and BP cuff, if needed

BEGINNING THE SKILL

1. **ACC** Review the order for:
   - name of sublingual or buccal medication and dosage
   - time intervals, frequency, and route of administration
   - special administration instructions for sublingual or buccal medication
   - purpose of administering medication (if PRN).
2. **ACC** Review the following (see Skill 11.1):
   - **SAF** client's allergies to medications or other substances
   - **SAF** indications and any contraindications for medications to be given
   - medical/surgical history, lab results, and clinical condition (particularly oral/facial)
   - medication history (to check for potential drug interactions)
   - appropriateness of sublingual or buccal medication for the client.
3. **INF** Perform hand hygiene.
4. **CCC** Introduce yourself to the client and family.
5. **SAF** Identify the client using at least two client identifiers.
6. **CCC** Provide privacy.
7. **ACC** Assess the client's level of consciousness and orientation to person, time, place, and situation. *Provides a baseline assessment of orientation before verbal consent is obtained.*

8. **ACC** Perform any client preassessments, which may include:
   - integrity of oral mucosa and any signs of lesions, sores, or areas of redness
   - level of pain or discomfort using a facility-approved pain assessment tool
   - vital signs if indicated and affected by medication (e.g., vasoactive drugs).
9. **CCC** Explain procedure and obtain verbal consent. *To provide client-centered care and prevent waste, consent should be obtained before preparing medications.*

PROCEDURE
Preparing the Sublingual and Buccal Medication

10. **SAF** Perform the **first safety checkpoint** when accessing the medication, and perform the **second safety checkpoint** when preparing the medication. Check the rights of administration, check the expiration date, and scan the bar code on the label if required (see Skill 11.1).
11. **ACC** If the sublingual or buccal medication is a prepackaged unit dose, leave packages in medication cup (unopened) and do not remove from wrappers until taken to bedside.
12. **ACC** If removing medication from a multidose bottle, pour the correct number of pills into the medication cup. (Note: Avoid directly touching the medication.)

Administering the Medication

13. **INF** Perform hand hygiene again upon entering the client's room.

14. **CCC** Maintain client privacy.
15. **SAF** Reverify the client's identity by using at least two client identifiers.
16. **SAF** Recheck the client's armband, and ask the client verbally if he or she has any allergies.
17. **SAF** Perform **third safety checkpoint** and review the medication with the client. Check the rights of administration again. *This facilitates client involvement.*
18. **CCC** Explain the purpose of each sublingual or buccal medication with the client as needed.
19. **INF** As each medication is verified, open medication packages (in the case of prepackaged unit doses) and drop in them in the medication cup without touching them. (Note: If required, scan the client's armband and the bar code on medication labels before opening packages.)
20. **SAF** Once all verifications and safety checks have been performed, place the client in an upright position (if not contraindicated) before administering sublingual or buccal medication. *Sitting the client in an upright position prevents choking if medication produces saliva as it is dissolving.* (Note: For clients who are receiving oral medications in addition to sublingual or buccal applications, administer oral medications and liquids *first* [Caple & Schub, 2016]).
21. **ACC** If the client is receiving a sublingual medication:
    a. Offer the client sips of liquid prior to administering the medication. *Provides moisture and facilitates comfort for clients who have a dry mouth.*
    b. Instruct the client to place the sublingual medication underneath the tongue and allow it to absorb until completely dissolved (Caple & Schub, 2016).

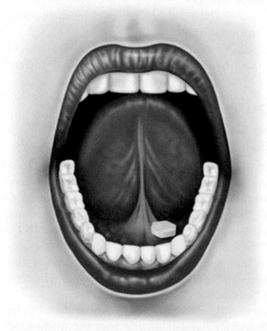

STEP 21B Place sublingual medication.

22. **ACC** If the client is receiving a buccal medication:
    a. Offer the client sips of liquid prior to administering medication. *Provides moisture and facilitates absorption for clients who have a dry mouth.*
    b. Instruct the client to place the buccal medication in the pocket between the cheek and gum, hold in place, and allow it to absorb until completely dissolved.

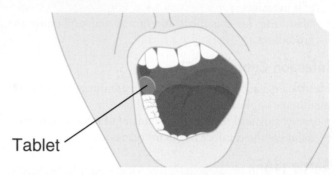

Tablet

STEP 22B Place buccal medication.

    c. Instruct the client to rotate medication sites between right and left cheeks if subsequent buccal medications are given. *Prevents mucosal irritation.*
23. **ACC** If the client is receiving a sublingual or buccal spray medication or is not able to self-administer the sublingual or buccal tablets:
    a. **INF** Perform hand hygiene and apply gloves.
    b. Assist with moistening areas where medication will be applied with water or saline. *Provides moisture and facilitates absorption for clients who have a dry mouth.*
    c. Gently spray or place sublingual or buccal medication at appropriate site.
    d. **INF** Remove gloves and perform hand hygiene again.
24. **ACC** If the client is receiving nitroglycerin sublingual medications, allow at least 5 minutes between medications, and obtain vital signs between doses. *Nitroglycerin can affect blood pressure, and waiting 5 minutes between doses allows the nurse to assess the full effect.*
25. **ACC** Instruct the client *not* to swallow or chew the sublingual or buccal medication (Caple & Schub, 2016). *Ensures that medication will be allowed to dissolve for proper absorption.*
26. **ACC** Remain with the client until the sublingual or buccal medication has dissolved. *Ensures that client has not discarded medication or had any difficulty with the medication.*
27. **SAF** If the facility has a **postadministration checkpoint,** review empty medication package labels again (if applicable) against the MAR or EMAR. If any errors occurred, notify the authorized healthcare provider immediately.
28. **EVAL** Monitor the client for any adverse or unexpected effects of the medication.

29. **CCC** If the client was given sublingual or buccal pain medication, monitor the client's pain level to assess relief. Notify the authorized healthcare provider if the medication did not relieve the client's pain.

FINISHING THE SKILL

30 **SAF** Ensure client safety and comfort. Ensure that the bed is in the lowest position, and verify that the client can identify and reach the nurse call system. *These safety measures reduce the risk of falls.*

31. **INF** Perform hand hygiene.

32. **EVAL** Monitor and evaluate the outcomes. Did the client respond to the medication as expected? Was the client's pain or angina relieved as expected? Did the client tolerate the procedure? Were the rights of administration followed (right client, drug, dose, route, time, and documentation)?

33. **COM** Document assessment findings, medication administration, and outcomes in the legal healthcare record:
   • name of medication given, exact time, date, dose, and dose given
   • pertinent postassessment data, such as vital signs or pain level
   • relief of angina (chest pain) if receiving sublingual nitroglycerin tablet
   • signature and initials of the clinician who administered the medication.

■ SKILL 11.4 Administering a Nasal Spray Medication

EQUIPMENT

Clean gloves
Tissues
Penlight, if needed
Cotton-tipped applicator or gauze, if needed
Nasal spray as prescribed at room temperature

BEGINNING THE SKILL

1. **ACC** Review the order for:
   • name of nasal medication and dosage
   • time intervals, frequency, and route of administration
   • special administration instructions (e.g., positioning)
   • purpose of administering medication (if PRN).

2. **ACC** Review the following:
   • **SAF** client's allergies to nasal medications or other substances
   • **SAF** indications and any contraindications for nasal medications to be given
   • medical/surgical history, lab results, and condition (particularly nasal or sinus)
   • medication history (to check for potential drug interactions)
   • appropriateness of nasal medication for the client.

3. **INF** Perform hand hygiene.

4. **CCC** Introduce yourself to the client and family.

5. **SAF** Identify the client using at least two client identifiers.

6. **CCC** Provide privacy.

7. **ACC** Assess the client's level of consciousness and orientation to person, time, place, and situation. *Provides a baseline assessment of orientation before verbal consent is obtained.*

8. **CCC** Explain the procedure and obtain verbal consent. *To provide client-centered care and prevent waste, consent should be obtained before preparing medications.*

9. **ACC** Perform any client preassessments, which may include:
   • integrity of oral mucosa and any signs of lesions, sores, or areas of redness
   • level of pain or discomfort of the nasal passages of the affected area.

PROCEDURE

Preparing the Nasal Spray Medication

10. **SAF** Perform the **first safety checkpoint** when accessing the nasal spray medication, and perform the **second safety checkpoint** when preparing the nasal spray medication. Check rights of administration, check expiration date, and scan the bar code on the label if required.

11. **CCC** Ensure that the nasal spray medication bottle has been at room temperature and per manufacturer recommendations. *Nasal medication that is too cold may cause client discomfort.*

Administering the Nasal Spray Medication

12. **INF** Perform hand hygiene again upon entering the client's room.

13. **SAF** Reverify the client's identity by using at least two client identifiers.

14. **SAF** Recheck the client's armband and ask the client verbally if he or she has any allergies.

15. **SAF** Apply gloves and place the client in the semi-Fowler (upright) position.

16. **ACC** Examine the client's nasal mucosa for lesions, severe irritation, obstructions, or excess mucus. Use penlight if necessary to visualize both nasal cavities. *Preassessment of the nares prevents complications related to nasal instillations (Richards & Heering, 2017).*

17. **ACC** If excessive mucus is present, use a cotton-tipped applicator to gently remove mucus or provide tissues and instruct the client to gently blow the nose. *Clearing excess mucus from the nasal cavities prior to instillation enhances absorption (Richards & Heering, 2017).*

18. **ACC** Ask the client if he or she is able to breathe through the nose. *Assesses patency of nose.*

19. **SAF** Perform **third safety checkpoint** and review the nasal medication with the client. Check rights of administration again. *This facilitates client involvement.* (Note: If required, scan the client's armband and the bar code on nasal medication label if available.)

20. **ACC** Administer the nasal spray per manufacturer recommendation. (Note: Client positioning and technique may vary depending on the specific nasal spray medication.)

    a. If recommended, gently shake spray bottle or container to ensure it is properly mixed.

    b. Remove cap from bottle or container and place it, inverted, on a clean, dry surface. *Maintains sterility of the cap between procedures.*

    c. Prime pump bottle by pumping into gauze pad if needed. *If pump bottle is being used for the first time, it may need to be primed (Richards & Heering, 2017).* (Note: Some nasal sprays, such as naloxone [Narcan], should *not* be primed prior to administration.)

    d. Position client per order or manufacturer recommendation. *The position of the client will vary depending on the purpose of the nasal medication and the intended area of treatment.*

    e. Place the gloved finger of your nondominant hand over the opposite nostril that will not receive the nasal medication, and ask the client to breathe in and out through the open nostril. *This verifies that the nostril receiving the medication is open and patent.*

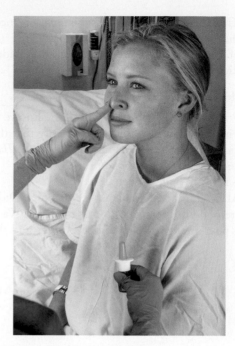

STEP 20E Check naris for patency.

    f. Using your dominant gloved hand, place the tip (or instruct client to place tip) of the container no more than 0.6 cm (¼ inch) away from the opening of the nostril without contaminating the tip of the container. Angle the tip toward the back of the client's head (or as ordered), and deliver the medication. Ask the client to breathe through nose as the medication is pumped or sprayed (Richards & Heering, 2017). (Note: Some manufacturers recommend inserting the spray tip further into the naris. Check the package insert.)

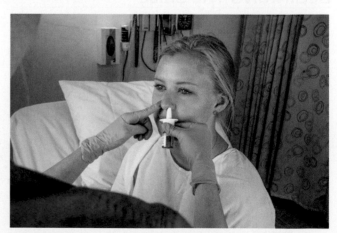

STEP 20F Position tip as directed.

21. **ACC If using naloxone (Narcan) nasal spray:**

    a. Remove nasal spray from box and peel back the tab to open spray.

    b. While supporting the client's head and neck, tilt the client's head back slightly, and gently insert the spray nozzle tip into the naris until your fingers touch the bottom of the client's nose. (Note: Your thumb should be on the plunger, and your fingers should be on either side of the spray nozzle.) *This position facilitates proper instillation of the nasal spray.* (Note: Use caution not to push the plunger until the nozzle is in the client's naris.)

c. Once the nozzle is safely in the naris, press the plunger with your thumb to administer the spray. Observe the client closely, obtain vital signs, and repeat dose in other naris if ordered and indicated. **WARNING:** This medication does not replace emergency medical care. Seek the appropriate emergency care for the client.

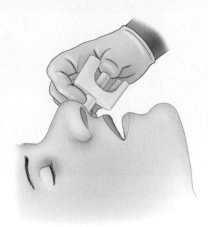

STEP 21C Insert nozzle for naloxone spray.

22. **CCC** Using a tissue or 4 × 4 gauze pad, clean excess medication or mucus around opening of the external naris or nares. *Facilitates client comfort and prevents skin irritation.*

23. **SAF** If the facility has a **postadministration checkpoint,** review the label of the nasal medication spray bottle again and compare it against the MAR or EMAR before returning it to storage. If any errors occurred, notify the authorized healthcare provider immediately.

24. **EVAL** Monitor the client for any adverse or unexpected effects of the nasal medication.

FINISHING THE SKILL

25. **SAF** Ensure client safety and comfort. Ensure that the bed is in the lowest position, and verify that the client can identify and reach the nurse call system. *These safety measures reduce the risk of falls.*

26. **INF** Perform hand hygiene.

27. **EVAL** Evaluate the outcomes. Did the client tolerate the procedure? Were the rights of administration followed (right client, drug, dose, route, time, and documentation)?

28. **COM** Document assessment findings, medication administration, and outcomes in the legal healthcare record:
    - name of nasal medication given, exact time, date, and dose given
    - which naris (right, left, or both) was used to administer medication
    - client's response to nasal medication administration
    - signature and initials of the clinician who administered the medication.

▪ SKILL 11.5 Administering Inhaled Medications

EQUIPMENT

pMDI and spacer, if ordered, or DPI
Clean gloves (if risk of exposure to body fluids)
Stethoscope and BP cuff, if needed

BEGINNING THE SKILL

1. **ACC** Review the order for:
   - type of inhaler (pMDI with or without spacer, or DPI)
   - name of medication to be given by inhaler
   - time intervals, dosage, route of administration, spacer
   - special administration instructions (e.g., positioning or priming inhaler)
   - purpose of administering inhaled medication (if PRN).

2. **ACC** Review the following:
   - **SAF** client's allergies to medications or other substances
   - **SAF** indications and any contraindications for inhaled medications to be given
   - appropriateness of inhaler for client
   - client's medical/surgical history, lab results, and condition (particularly respiratory)
   - client's medication history (to check for potential drug interactions).

3. **INF** Perform hand hygiene.

4. **CCC** Introduce yourself to the client and family.

5. **SAF** Identify the client using at least two client identifiers.

6. **CCC** Provide privacy, if needed.

7. **ACC** Assess the client's level of consciousness and orientation to person, time, place, and situation. *Provides a baseline assessment of orientation before verbal consent is obtained.*

8. **CCC** Explain the procedure and obtain verbal consent. *To provide client-centered care and prevent waste, consent should be obtained before preparing medications.*
9. **ACC** Perform client preassessments, including but not limited to the following:
   - character of respirations, work of breathing, and bilateral breath sounds
   - client's mobility and ability to manipulate and use the inhaler
   - vital signs if the client receiving medications with systemic effects.

PROCEDURE

Preparing the Inhaled Medication

10. **SAF** Perform the **first safety checkpoint** when accessing the inhaled medication, and perform the **second safety checkpoint** when preparing the inhaled medication. Check the rights of administration, check the expiration date, and scan the bar code on the label if required.
11. **ACC** Prepare and assemble the inhalers per manufacturer instructions.
12. **SAF** If the client is using a single-dose DPI, place the unopened medication (usually a capsule) in the medication cup and do not remove it from the wrapper until it is taken to client's bedside.

Administering the Inhaled Medication

13. **INF** Perform hand hygiene again upon entering the client's room.
14. **CCC** Maintain client privacy.
15. **SAF** Reverify the client's identity by using at least two client identifiers.
16. **SAF** Recheck the client's armband and ask the client verbally if he or she has any allergies.
17. **SAF** Perform **third safety checkpoint** and review the inhaled medications with the client. Check the rights of administration again. *This facilitates client involvement.* (Note: If required, scan the client's armband and the bar code on the inhaler label if available.)
18. **COM** Explain the purpose and demonstrate the use of the inhaler to the client as needed.
19. **SAF** Place the client in the semi-Fowler position if not contraindicated. *Helps lung expansion.*
20. **INF** Apply gloves if there is a risk of exposure to the client's body fluids.

If Client Is Using a Pressurized Metered-Dose Inhaler

21. **ACC** Hold the pMDI upright; shake thoroughly. *Shaking suspends the medication properly.* (Note: Some types of inhalers are breath actuated and do *not* require shaking or priming before use. Check manufacturer instructions carefully for specific variations before using the inhaler.)
22. **ACC** If needed, prime medication into the inhaler by pressing the inhaler button once. Priming the pMDI

once allows the inhaler medication to be up at the valve for administration.
23. **ACC** Remove the cap from the pMDI mouthpiece and place on a clean, dry surface.
24. **ACC** Ask the client to tilt the head/chin back slightly and exhale (breathe out) as much as possible.
25. **ACC** If the client is using a pMDI without a spacer, instruct the client to place the pMDI mouthpiece in the mouth and create a complete seal around the mouthpiece with his or her lips.

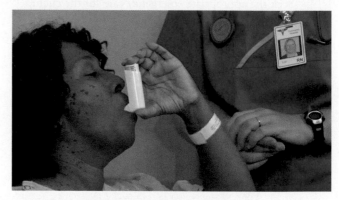

STEP 25 Using a pMDI without a spacer.

26. **ACC** If the client is using a pMDI with a spacer:
    a. Attach spacer to pMDI and ensure that it is secure.
    b. Instruct the client to place the spacer mouthpiece in the mouth and create a complete seal around the mouthpiece with his or her lips. *Facilitates medication delivery.*

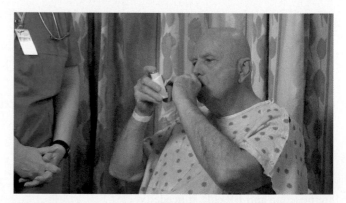

STEP 26B Using a pMDI with a spacer.

27. **ACC** If the client is using a spacer with a face mask, place the face mask securely over the client's nose and mouth and ensure that the mask has a good seal on the client's face. *Ensures medication won't leak.*
28. **ACC** While the pMDI is in place, instruct the client to inhale slowly (over 3–5 seconds) through the mouth and press the button on the pMDI for one "puff" as he or she is breathing in. (Note: Ensure that the client maintains a tight seal with the mouth around the mouthpiece during the breath.)

29. **ACC** Instruct the client to hold his or her breath for approximately 10 seconds after the puff. *Allows medication to distribute deeply in the client's lungs (Gardenhire et al., 2017).*

30. **ACC** After 10 seconds, the client may breathe out slowly through the nose or pursed lips.

31. **ACC** If the order calls for an additional dose, wait at least 1 minute between puffs. *Waiting at least 1 minute between puffs allows subsequent medication puffs to penetrate the lungs.*

32. **INF** If corticosteroids are used, instruct or assist the client in rinsing out the mouth directly after the procedure is complete. *Helps prevent possible yeast or fungal infections from medication.*

If Client Is Using a Dry-Powder Inhaler

33. **ACC** Instruct the client to hold the DPI securely and slide the lever per manufacturer instructions until the mouthpiece opens and locks in place. (Note: This may vary depending on the device.)

34. **ACC** Instruct the client to exhale as much as possible away from the DPI. *Exhaling directly into the DPI can cause increased humidity and affect the medication (Gardenhire et al., 2017).*

35. **ACC** Instruct the client to place his or her lips completely around the DPI mouthpiece and inhale quickly and deeply through the mouth, not the nose.

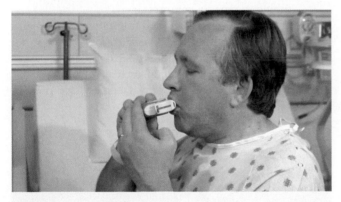

STEP 35 Using a DPI.

36. **ACC** While the DPI is still in place, instruct the client to hold his or her breath for approximately 10 seconds. *The facilitates retention of the medication and disbursement of the medication to the lungs.*

37. **ACC** Instruct the client to remove the device first and then breathe out. **WARNING:** Warn the client *not* to breathe out into the device. *The DPI must remain dry and free from humidity.*

38. **ACC** Slide the lever back in place to close the device per manufacturer instructions. *Sliding the lever releases a*

medication and prepares the next dose for inhalation (Gardenhire et al. 2017.)

39. **CCC** Assist the client to rinse the mouth if needed after the procedure. *Facilitates comfort.*

40. **ACC** Instruct the client to clean and dry the DPI after every use and to not allow the DPI to get wet. *If the DPI medication is allowed to get wet, it could become clumped and ineffective.*

41. **EVAL** Monitor the client for any adverse or unexpected effects of the inhaled medication.

42. **SAF** If the facility has a **postadministration checkpoint,** review the label of the MDI or DPI medication again and compare it against the MAR or EMAR before returning it to storage. If any errors occurred, notify the authorized healthcare provider immediately.

FINISHING THE SKILL

43. **INF** Remove gloves (if used) and perform hand hygiene.

44. **SAF** Ensure client safety and comfort. Ensure that the bed is in the lowest position, and verify that the client can identify and reach the nurse call system. *These safety measures reduce the risk of falls.*

45. **EVAL** Evaluate the outcomes. Was the client able to use the inhaler without difficulty? Are the client's lung sounds and respiratory effort improved after the use of the inhaler? Were the rights of administration followed (right client, drug, dose, route, time, and documentation)?

46. **COM** Document assessment findings, medication administration, and outcomes in the legal healthcare record:
    - type of inhaler used (e.g., pMDI with or without spacer, DPI)
    - name of medication given by inhaler, exact time, date, and dose given
    - pertinent postassessment, data such as vital signs (if affected by medication), lung sounds, respiratory effort, and use of accessory muscles
    - signature and initials of the clinician who administered the inhaled medication.

Follow-up Monitoring

47. **EVAL** Continue to monitor the client and ensure there are no adverse or delayed reactions to the inhaled medications. *Medication reactions may be immediate or delayed (Gardenhire et al., 2017).*

48. **EVAL** Ensure that the client is able to demonstrate proper use of the inhaler before discharge to home. *Proper use of the inhaler maximizes effectiveness and facilitates client safety in the home.*

■ SKILL 11.6 Administering Nebulized Medications

EQUIPMENT

Nebulizer medication as prescribed at room temperature
Nebulizer (disposable or dedicated for individual client use)
Nebulizer machine
Oxygen equipment (if oxygen used)
Clean gloves (if risk of exposure to body fluids)
Stethoscope and BP cuff, if needed

BEGINNING THE SKILL

1. **ACC** Review the order for:
   - name of medication to be given by nebulizer
   - time intervals, dosage, and route of administration
   - special administration instructions (e.g., positioning)
   - purpose of administering nebulizer medication (if PRN).
2. **ACC** Review the following:
   - **SAF** client's allergies to nebulizer medications or other substances
   - **SAF** indications and any contraindications for nebulizer medications to be given
   - appropriateness of nebulizer for client
   - client's medical/surgical history, lab results, and condition (particularly respiratory)
   - client's medication history (to check for potential drug interactions).
3. **INF** Perform hand hygiene.
4. **CCC** Introduce yourself to the client and family.
5. **SAF** Identify the client using at least two client identifiers.
6. **CCC** Provide privacy.
7. **ACC** Assess the client's level of consciousness and orientation to person, time, place, and situation. *Provides a baseline assessment of orientation before verbal consent is obtained.*
8. **CCC** Explain procedure and obtain verbal consent. *To provide client-centered care and prevent waste, consent should be obtained before preparing medications.*
9. **ACC** Perform client preassessments, including but not limited to the following:
   - character of respirations, work of breathing, and bilateral breath sounds
   - client's mobility and ability to hold and use nebulizer device
   - vital signs if the client is receiving medications with systemic effects.

PROCEDURE

Preparing the Medication for the Nebulizer

10. **SAF** Perform the **first safety checkpoint** when accessing the medication, and perform the **second safety checkpoint** when preparing the medication for the nebulizer. Check the rights of administration, check the expiration date, and scan the bar code on the label if required.

11. **SAF** If the medication for the nebulizer is provided in unit doses, leave the medication in the packaging until it is taken to the bedside and verified at the client's bedside. *Facilities safety and verification.*

Administering the Nebulizer Medication

12. **INF** Perform hand hygiene again upon entering the client's room.
13. **CCC** Maintain client privacy.
14. **SAF** Reverify the client's identity by using at least two client identifiers.
15. **SAF** Recheck the client's armband, and ask the client verbally if he or she has any allergies.
16. **SAF** Perform **third safety checkpoint** and review the medication with the client. Check rights of administration again. *This facilitates client involvement.* (Note: If required, scan the client's armband and the bar code on the medication label if available.)
17. **ACC** Prepare the equipment for the nebulizer procedure.
    a. Ensure that compressor machine is plugged in and functioning properly.
    b. Assemble mouthpiece or face mask, and connect tubing to port on compressor.
    c. If oxygen is ordered, attach tubing to nebulizer machine per manufacturer instructions. Set flow rate per orders (usually 6–8 liters per minute).
    d. Add medication to nebulizer reservoir; ensure that cap is secure. (Note: Many facilities have premeasured unit doses for nebulizers.)

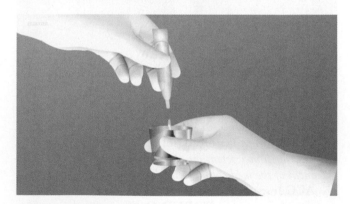

STEP 17D Add medication.

18. **SAF** Place the client in the semi-Fowler position if not contraindicated. *This position allows full inhalation effort and will increase the effectiveness of the nebulizer treatment.*
19. **INF** Apply gloves if there is a risk of exposure to the client's body fluids or mucous membranes.
20. **ACC** Turn on the nebulizer machine.

21. **ACC** Instruct the client to place his or her lips *firmly* around the mouthpiece of the nebulizer and breathe in and out normally. Ensure that the client maintains a tight seal around mouthpiece. (Note: The nebulizer machine should be delivering a continuous mist if working properly.)

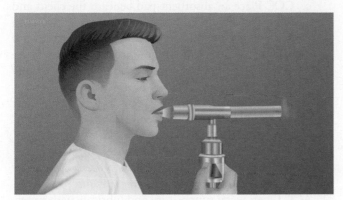

STEP 21 Assist with placement of the mouthpiece.

22. **ACC** If a face mask is used, ensure that the mask is securely fitted over the client's nose and mouth, and ensure that the tubing is attached to the compressor and oxygen (if used).
23. **EVAL** Monitor the client during the procedure; ensure that the nebulizer continues to produce a mist; and ensure that the client is breathing properly, without any signs of distress or discomfort.
24. **ACC** Ensure that all of the medication in the cap is being delivered. (Note: Some facilities may require that the medication cap be gently tapped to facilitate delivery of the medication.)
25. **ACC** After the medication has been delivered (usually about 10 minutes), turn off the machine.
26. **INF** If corticosteroids are used, instruct or assist the client to rinse out the mouth directly after the procedure is complete. *Helps prevent possible yeast or fungal infections from the medication.*
27. **SAF** If facility has a **postadministration checkpoint,** review the label of the nebulizer medication again and compare it against the MAR or EMAR. If any errors occurred, notify the authorized healthcare provider immediately.
28. **EVAL** Monitor the client for adverse or unexpected effects of the nebulizer medication. Obtain postprocedure vital signs if the client received nebulized medication with systemic effects.

FINISHING THE SKILL

29. **INF** Clean and rinse the client's nebulizer tubing and bottle and allow it to air dry. **WARNING:** Avoid using tap water. *Tap water may have harmful microorganisms.*
30. **INF** Remove gloves (if used) and perform hand hygiene.
31. **SAF** Ensure client safety and comfort. Ensure that the bed is in the lowest position, and verify that the client can identify and reach the nurse call system. *These safety measures reduce the risk of falls.*
32. **EVAL** Evaluate the outcomes. Did the client tolerate the nebulizer treatments? Are the client's breath sounds and respiratory effort improved after the nebulizer treatments? Were the rights of administration followed (right client, drug, dose, route, time, and documentation)?
33. **COM** Document assessment findings, medication administration, and outcomes in the legal healthcare record:
    * name of medication given by nebulizer, exact time, date, and dose given
    * client response to nebulizer medication administration
    * pertinent postassessment data, such as vital signs (if affected by medication), lungs sounds, respiratory effort, and use of accessory muscles
    * signature and initials of the clinician who administered the nebulizer medication.

■ SKILL 11.7 Administering a Rectal Suppository

EQUIPMENT

Clean gloves
Suppository
Water-soluble lubricant, tissues
Disposable absorbent pads and drape

BEGINNING THE SKILL

1. **ACC** Review the order for:
   * name of rectal suppository medication and dosage
   * time intervals and route of administration
   * special administration instructions (e.g., apex or base insertion)
   * purpose of administering medication (if PRN).
2. **ACC** Review the following:
   * **SAF** client's allergies to medications or other substances
   * **SAF** indications and any contraindications for medication to be given (Note: If clients have a low white blood cell [WBC] count or prolonged PT, PTT, or INR, the rectal route may be contraindicated because of risk of traumatizing the rectal mucosa.)
   * appropriateness of rectal medication for client

- client's medication history and medical-surgical history (particularly history of rectal surgery or disorders such as fissures or fistulas, neutropenia, or bleeding disorders).
3. **INF** Perform hand hygiene.
4. **CCC** Introduce yourself to the client and family.
5. **SAF** Identify the client using at least two client identifiers.
6. **CCC** Provide privacy, close the door and/or pull the curtain, and provide a drape.
7. **ACC** Assess the client's level of consciousness and orientation to person, time, place, and situation. *Provides a baseline assessment of orientation before verbal consent is obtained.*
8. **CCC** Explain the procedure and obtain verbal consent. *To provide client-centered care and prevent waste, consent should be obtained before preparing medications.*
9. **ACC** Perform client preassessments, including but not limited to the following:
   - level of pain or discomfort using a facility-approved tool
   - vital signs if client receiving medications with systemic effects.

PROCEDURE

Preparing the Rectal Suppository

10. **SAF** Perform the **first safety checkpoint** when accessing the rectal medication, and perform the **second safety checkpoint** when preparing the rectal medication. Check the rights of administration, check the expiration date, and scan the bar code on the label if required.
11. **ACC** Leave unopened suppository in medication package and do not remove from wrapper until taken to the bedside. *Allows identification check at bedside with suppository label.*

Administering the Rectal Suppository

12. **INF** Perform hand hygiene again upon entering the client's room.
13. **CCC** Maintain client privacy.
14. **CCC** If the client is in agreement, ask family members to leave during suppository administration.
15. **SAF** Reverify the client's identity by using at least two client identifiers.
16. **SAF** Recheck the client's armband, and ask the client verbally if he or she has any allergies.
17. **SAF** Perform **third safety checkpoint** and review the rectal medication with the client. Check the rights of administration again. *This facilitates client involvement.* (Note: If required, scan the client's armband and the bar code on the medication label if available.)
18. **CCC** Explain the purpose of the suppository medication to the client as needed.
19. **INF** Apply gloves.
20. **ACC** Prepare the client for the procedure.

a. Assist the client to the bathroom if needed *before* the suppository is inserted.
b. **SAF** Set up an ergonomically safe space. Raise the bed to a comfortable working height. *Setting up an ergonomically safe space prevents injury to the nurse and client.*
c. **CCC** Place an absorbent pad beneath the client and place the client in the left lateral position (lying on left side with top knee flexed and buttocks toward edge of bed). Provide pillow to the client to place between the knees if needed. *Provides comfort and proper alignment.*
d. Inspect the client's external rectal area to ensure there is no evidence of obstruction, irritation, or lesions. *These conditions could cause pain and trauma.*
e. **CCC** Drape the client with a sheet or towel to prevent exposure. *Draping the client properly protects the client's dignity and privacy during a sensitive procedure.*
21. **ACC** Open rectal suppository and lubricate with water-soluble lubricant. Avoid warming the suppository. *A water-soluble lubricant prevents rectal trauma as the suppository is inserted. Handling or holding the suppository can warm or soften it, which makes it difficult to insert.*
22. **ACC** Separate the buttocks and gently push the suppository base or apex into the rectum (depending on order/special instructions) with a gloved finger. Gently move the suppository past the external sphincter as long as there is no resistance. (Note: Suppositories should be inserted approximately 2.5 cm [1 inch] for adults and 1.27 cm [½ inch] for children.)

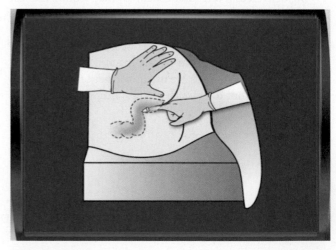

STEP 22 Place suppository.

23. **CCC** If resistance is met, ask the client to take slow, deep breaths as it is inserted. **WARNING:** Do *not* force the suppository into the client. *Slow breathing may help relax the client and facilitate insertion.*
24. **ACC** Ask the client to squeeze the buttocks together and remain in a lying-down position. *Remaining in a lying-down position facilitates retention and absorption of the medication.*
25. **CCC** Clean off any excess water-soluble lubricant with tissue. *Prevents skin irritation.*

26. **INF** Remove gloves and perform hand hygiene.
27. **SAF** Place the client's bed in the lowest position. If the facility has a **postadministration checkpoint,** review the empty suppository package against the MAR or EMAR. If any errors occurred, notify the authorized healthcare provider.
28. **EVAL** Monitor the client for any adverse or unexpected effects of the medication.
29. **CCC** If the client was given pain medication by suppository, monitor the client's pain level to assess relief. Notify the authorized healthcare provider if the medication did not relieve the client's pain.

FINISHING THE SKILL

30. **SAF** Ensure client safety and comfort. Ensure that the bed is in the lowest position, and verify that the client can identify and reach the nurse call system. *These safety measures reduce the risk of falls.*
31. **INF** Perform hand hygiene again.
32. **EVAL** Evaluate the outcomes. Did the client tolerate the procedure? Were the rights of administration followed (right client, drug, dose, route, time, and documentation)?
33. **COM** Document assessment findings, medication administration, and outcomes in the legal healthcare record:
    - name of suppository given, exact time, date, and dose given
    - pertinent postassessment data, such as vital signs or pain level
    - signature and initials of the clinician who administered the medication.

■ SKILL 11.8 Administering Vaginal Medications

EQUIPMENT

Clean gloves
Vaginal suppository (if ordered)
Disposable, prefilled vaginal applicator with gel or cream (if ordered)
Water-soluble lubricant, tissues
Disposable absorbent pad and drape
Sanitary napkin or pad, if needed

BEGINNING THE SKILL

1. **ACC** Review the order for:
   - name of vaginal medication and dosage
   - time intervals and route of administration
   - special administration instructions
   - purpose of administering vaginal medication (if PRN).
2. **ACC** Review the following:
   - **SAF** client's allergies to medications or other substances
   - **SAF** indications and any contraindications for vaginal medication to be given
   - appropriateness of vaginal medication for the client
   - client's medical/surgical history and any vaginal bleeding or disorders
   - client's medication history (to check for potential drug interactions)
3. **INF** Perform hand hygiene.
4. **CCC** Introduce yourself to the client and family.
5. **SAF** Identify the client using at least two client identifiers.
6. **CCC** Provide privacy, close the door and/or pull the curtain, and provide a drape.
7. **ACC** Assess the client's level of consciousness and orientation to person, time, place, and situation. *Provides a baseline assessment of orientation before verbal consent is obtained.*
8. **CCC** Explain the procedure and obtain verbal consent. *To provide client-centered care and prevent waste, consent should be obtained before preparing medications.*
9. **ACC** Perform client preassessments, including but not limited to the following:
   - level of pain or discomfort using a facility-approved tool
   - vital signs if the client is receiving medications with systemic effects.

PROCEDURE

Preparing the Vaginal Medication

10. **SAF** Perform the **first safety checkpoint** when accessing the vaginal medication, and perform the **second safety checkpoint** when preparing the vaginal medication. Check the rights of administration, check the expiration date, and scan the bar code on the label if required.
11. **ACC** Leave unopened vaginal medication in package and do not remove from wrapper until taken to the bedside. *Allows identification check at bedside with medication label.*

Administering the Vaginal Medication

12. **INF** Perform hand hygiene again upon entering the client's room.
13. **CCC** Maintain client privacy.
14. **CCC** If the client is in agreement, ask family members to leave during the vaginal administration. *This protects the client's dignity and privacy.*
15. **SAF** Reverify the client's identity by using at least two client identifiers.
16. **SAF** Recheck the client's armband, and ask the client verbally if he or she has any allergies.

17. **SAF** Perform **third safety checkpoint** and review the vaginal medication with the client. Check the rights of administration again. *This facilitates client involvement.* (Note: If required, scan the client's armband and the bar code on the medication label if available.)
18. **INF** Apply gloves.
19. **ACC** Prepare the client for the procedure.
    a. Assist the client to the bathroom if needed *before* the vaginal medication is inserted.
    b. **CCC** Ensure that a female staff member is present as required by facility policy.
    c. **SAF** Set up an ergonomically safe space. Raise the bed to a comfortable working height. *Setting up an ergonomically safe space prevents injury to the nurse and client.*
    d. **CCC** Place an absorbent pad beneath the client and assist the client to the dorsal recumbent position (client supine with knees bent, spread apart and to the sides) or the side-lying position. If the client is in the side-lying position, place pillow between knees for comfort/spinal support.
    e. **CCC** Ensure that the client remains properly draped to prevent exposure. *Draping the client properly helps protect the client's dignity and privacy during a sensitive procedure.*
20. **ACC** If administering a vaginal suppository, open package, remove suppository, and lubricate with water-soluble lubricant. Avoid warming the suppository. *A water-soluble lubricant prevents vaginal trauma. Handling or holding the suppository can warm or soften it.*
21. **ACC** If administering a vaginal gel/cream with an applicator, remove the applicator from the package, ensure that it is intact and without defects, and lubricate it with water-soluble lubricant.
22. **ACC** With your nondominant gloved hand, locate and separate the labia to locate the vaginal opening. Using your dominant hand, gently insert the lubricated suppository or applicator into the vaginal opening and then advance it approximately 5 cm (2 inches) toward the cervix. *Facilitates absorption.*
23. **ACC** If administering a gel/cream with an applicator, gently depress the plunger to deliver the medication after it has been advanced (Devesty & Balderrama, 2017).

24. **CCC** If resistance is met, ask the client to take slow, deep breaths as it is inserted. **WARNING:** Do *not* force the suppository or applicator into the client. *Slow breathing may help the client relax.*
25. **ACC** Instruct the client to remain in a lying-down position for at least 20 to 30 minutes and avoid sitting up. *Remaining in a lying-down position facilitates retention and absorption of the medication.*
26. **CCC** Clean off excess lubricant with tissue and offer pad if needed. *Sanitary pads protect the client's clothing if any leak occurs from the vaginal medication (Devesty & Balderrama, 2017).*
27. **INF** Dispose of equipment (e.g., applicator), remove gloves, and perform hand hygiene.
28. **SAF** Place the client's bed in the lowest position. If the facility has a **postadministration checkpoint,** review empty medication package against MAR or EMAR. If any errors occurred, notify authorized healthcare provider.
29. **EVAL** Monitor client for any adverse or unexpected effects of the vaginal medication.
30. **CCC** If the client was given vaginal pain medication, monitor the client's pain level to assess relief. Notify the authorized healthcare provider if the medication did not relieve the client's pain.

FINISHING THE SKILL

31. **SAF** Ensure client safety and comfort. Ensure that the bed is in the lowest position, and verify that the client can identify and reach the nurse call system. *These safety measures reduce the risk of falls.*
32. **INF** Perform hand hygiene again.
33. **EVAL** Evaluate the outcomes. Did the client tolerate the vaginal medication? Were the rights of administration followed (right client, drug, dose, route, time, and documentation)? Was the client's privacy and dignity protected during the procedure?
34. **COM** Document assessment findings, medication administration, and outcomes in the legal healthcare record:
    • name of vaginal medication given, exact time, date, and dose given
    • pertinent postassessment data, such as vaginal bleeding or irritation
    • signature and initials of the clinician who administered the medication.

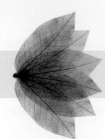

Administering Topical Medications

Topical medications include products that are administered on the skin, external surfaces, or body cavities. As with other nonoral drugs, topical medications avoid first-pass metabolism and the gastrointestinal system. Several variables can affect absorption through the skin, including the client's age, hydration, temperature, rate of blood flow, and skin integrity. For very young clients and older adults (who may have thin skin), absorption rates with topical medications may be somewhat unpredictable and erratic due to a variety of factors such as lack of adipose tissue.

The two major types of topical medications applied to the skin are (a) those intended for localized effects, such as dermatologic disorders, and (b) those intended for systemic effects, whereby the drugs are absorbed into the client's circulation for the treatment of pain and other conditions. In addition to accuracy and safety, one of the most important critical concepts when administering topical medications is health maintenance. For example, some topical medications can irritate the skin or disrupt skin integrity. Thus, it is important to properly prepare the client's skin and monitor for any reactions or disruptions of the skin. Because the client will often continue these treatment regimens at home, ensure that the client can accurately demonstrate the self-administration of topical medications.

TOPICAL MEDICATIONS FOR LOCALIZED EFFECT

Common types of topical medications used for localized effect include lotions, creams, gels, and ointments. When applying these topical medications, it is important to wear gloves and clean the skin thoroughly. Apply the medication with an applicator or a gloved finger in the same direction as the hair grows on the client's skin. Some facilities require that a transparent dressing be placed over the topical applications to facilitate absorption. This is particularly important for pediatric clients or clients who are restless and at risk of rubbing the medication off the skin.

TRANSDERMAL MEDICATIONS FOR SYSTEMIC EFFECT

Transdermal medications are increasingly being prescribed as commercially pre-prepared patches for systemic effects. Many of these products have an innovative mechanism for drug delivery and include a variety of medications, such as scopolamine and analgesics (e.g., fentanyl and buprenorphine patches). Each medication will have an FDA-approved package insert that contains information specific to that product, such as recommendations regarding optimal locations for applying the patches and any precaution notices. In general, transdermal patches should be applied to a central "core" location on the client, such as the chest, back, or abdomen, as opposed to distal extremities. Some medications also require an adequate amount of subcutaneous tissue for proper absorption to occur. Avoid bony areas or areas on the skin where there are open lesions, excessive hair, or signs of breakdown. Because absorption may occur slowly over many hours or days, monitor the client closely to ensure the patch remains in place.

EYE AND EAR MEDICATIONS

Topical medications that are administered in body cavities such as the eyes and ears are usually prescribed for localized effects, such as an infection. These products may be available OTC or be prescribed by the authorized healthcare provider. Eye medication is administered as eye drops or ointments, and ear medications are generally given as ear drops. If both are given, eye drops must be given before eye ointment. Both eye and ear medications need to be thoroughly shaken before being given and stored at room temperature.

When administering eye drops or ointments, position the client properly (usually with the head tilted back), and avoid touching the medication cap or the tip of the container to the client's eye. Eye irrigations may be indicated if the surface of the eye needs to be flushed to treat infections or for chemical burns and debris removal. The prescribed irrigation may be a medicated solution, or it could be normal saline or another type of fluid. If a smaller volume is prescribed (e.g., 30–60 mL), a syringe or commercial irrigator may be used. If a large volume of irrigation is ordered, an IV tubing setup with a bag of saline or other fluid is often used. Regardless of the type of method used, it is important to avoid cross-contamination of the unaffected eye during irrigation.

Irrigations of the ear are most often ordered to remove excessive ear wax or debris that does not respond to ear drops. More recent technology regarding irrigations of the ear involves electronic irrigators; these procedures are usually only performed by an advanced healthcare provider or specially trained nurse. For clients who have had recent ear surgery or who have a perforated eardrum or tubes in their ears, irrigation of the ear is contraindicated. As with eye irrigations, the solution should be at room temperature (not cold), and the client's head should be tilted toward the affected ear to facilitate flow by gravity. During the ear irrigation procedure, monitor the client closely for any sign of dizziness, pain, or distress. As with other topical medications, use sterile technique to prevent infection and maintain skin/tissue integrity.

APPLICATION OF THE NURSING PROCESS

Examples of Related ICNP Nursing Diagnoses, Expected Client Outcomes, and Nursing Interventions:

Nursing Diagnosis: Risk for cross-infection

Supporting Data: Client has an infection in one eye and is receiving topical medication in the affected eye.

Expected Client Outcomes: The client will have no sign of cross-infection, as seen by:

- Absence of signs and symptoms of infection in the unaffected eye
- Affected and unaffected eyes clear without signs of redness or drainage.

Nursing Intervention Example: Use sterile technique when administering topical medications.

Nursing Diagnosis: Risk for impaired skin integrity

Supporting Data: Client is receiving medications via transdermal patch.

Expected Client Outcomes:

- Absence of redness, lesions, or skin breakdown where topical medications are placed
- No subjective complaints by client of discomfort at transdermal medication site.

Nursing Intervention Example: Monitor skin for irritation, and rotate application sites.

Reference: International Classification for Nursing Practice. (n.d.). *eHealth & ICNP*. Retrieved from https://www.icn.ch/what-we-do/projects/ehealth-icnp.

CRITICAL CONCEPTS
Administering Topical Medications

Accuracy (ACC)

Administration of topical medications is sensitive to the following variables:

Client-Related Factors
- Client's assessment, including level of consciousness
- Client's ability to hear and understand instructions regarding topical medications
- Condition, integrity, and permeability of client's skin

Nurse- and System-Related Factors
- Proper storage and proper labeling of topical medications
- Proper site selection used for applying topical medications
- Technique used for processing orders, preparing and administering topical medications, and providing follow-up care and monitoring

- Proper use, handling, and assembly of equipment used for administering topical medications

Client-Centered Care (CCC)

Respect for the client when administering topical medications is demonstrated by:
- promoting autonomy and ensuring that verbal consent is obtained
- providing privacy and ensuring comfort when administering topical medications
- honoring cultural preferences and arranging an interpreter if necessary
- advocating for the client and family and explaining purpose of topical medications.

Infection Control (INF)

Healthcare-associated infection when administering topical medications is prevented by reducing the number and transfer of microorganisms.

Safety (SAF)

Safety measures when administering topical medications prevent harm and maintain a safe care environment, including:
- checking for allergies and contraindications and following safety checks and guidelines.

Communication (COM)

- Communication when administering topical medications exchanges information (verbal, nonverbal, written, or electronic) between two or more people.
- Collaboration with the client and client teaching facilitates effective administration of topical medications.
- Documentation records information in a permanent legal record.

Health Maintenance (HLTH)

Nursing is dedicated to the promotion of health and self-care abilities when administering topical medications by:
- protecting and caring for the client's skin before and after administering topical medications
- monitoring the client's skin for any sign of changes or breakdown.

Evaluation (EVAL)

When administering topical medications, evaluation of outcomes enables the nurse to determine the therapeutic response and safety of the care provided by:
- monitoring the therapeutic effect of the medication
- monitoring for side effects, adverse effects, interactions, or allergic reactions.

■ SKILL 11.9 Applying a Transdermal Patch

EQUIPMENT

Clean gloves
Tissue or washcloths and hypoallergenic tape, if needed
Transdermal patch (as prescribed)

BEGINNING THE SKILL

1. **ACC** Review the order for:
   - name of transdermal medication (generic) and dosage
   - time intervals, frequency, and route of administration
   - special administration instructions for transdermal patch
   - purpose of administering transdermal patch (if PRN).
2. **ACC** Review the following:
   - **SAF** client's allergies to medications or other substances
   - **SAF** indications and any contraindications for transdermal medication
   - appropriateness of transdermal medication for the client
   - client's lab results, medical/surgical history, and condition of the client's skin.
3. **INF** Perform hand hygiene.
4. **CCC** Introduce yourself to the client and family.
5. **SAF** Identify the client using at least two client identifiers.
6. **CCC** Provide privacy.
7. **ACC** Assess the client's level of consciousness and orientation to person, time, place, and situation. *Provides a baseline assessment of orientation before verbal consent is obtained.*
8. **CCC** Explain the procedure and obtain verbal consent. *To provide client-centered care and prevent waste, consent should be obtained before preparing medications.*
9. **ACC** Perform any client preassessments, including but not limited to the following:
   - skin condition and any signs of lesions, redness, broken skin, or irritated areas
   - level of pain or discomfort using a facility-approved pain assessment tool
   - vital signs if affected by the medication the client will be receiving.

PROCEDURE

Preparing the Transdermal Medication

10. **SAF** Perform the **first safety checkpoint** when accessing the transdermal medication, and perform the **second safety checkpoint** when preparing the transdermal medication. Check the rights of administration, check the expiration date, and scan the bar code on the label if required.
11. **SAF** Inspect the transdermal package to ensure the seal on the pouch is not damaged or compromised. Ensure that the patch is the correct dose and size. *This helps verify the integrity of the medication.*
12. **ACC** Leave transdermal medication in packaging and do not remove from wrapper or pouch until taken to the client's bedside. *Protects integrity of adhesive side of transdermal patch.*

Administering the Transdermal Medication

13. **INF** Perform hand hygiene again upon entering the client's room.
14. **CCC** Maintain client privacy.
15. **SAF** Reverify the client's identity by using at least two client identifiers.
16. **SAF** Recheck the client's armband, and ask the client verbally if he or she has any allergies.
17. **SAF** Perform **third safety checkpoint** and review the transdermal medication with the client. Check rights of administration again. *This facilitates client involvement.* (Note: If required, scan the client's armband and the bar code on the medication label if available.)
18. **ACC** Apply gloves and remove the previously administered transdermal patch (if present).
19. **ACC** Fold the patch over so that the adhesive sides stick together, and discard per policy. *Removing old patch prevents double-dosing the client when a new patch is applied.* (Note: If transdermal patch is a controlled substance or narcotic, another nurse may have to witness the disposal and sign as a witness. Follow facility protocol for disposal of medications.)
20. **ACC** After the old patch has been removed (if present), clean residue off the client's skin with tissue or a washcloth. Allow skin to air dry. *Removing the old patch and cleaning off residue prevent skin irritation and double dosing from previous patch if present.*

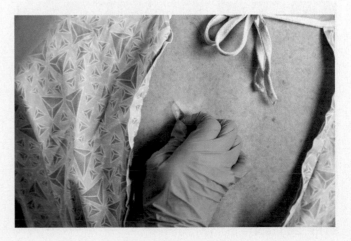

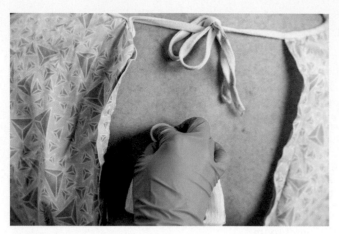

STEP 20 Remove the old patch and clean off residue.

21. **ACC** If gloves are contaminated from old patch, remove gloves, perform hand hygiene again, and apply new gloves. *Prevents residue from old patch from contaminating new patch.*

22. **HLTH** Assess the client's skin where the previous patch was applied for signs of breakdown or irritation. *Assessment allows the nurse to monitor the client's tolerance of the transdermal patch.*

23. **HLTH** Select site for the new transdermal medication patch based on manufacturer recommendations. Avoid the site where the previous patch was administered, and avoid areas of the skin with hair or any sign of lesions, irritation, or breakdown. *Rotating sites on the client's skin for the administration of transdermal medications prevents skin breakdown and loss of skin integrity.*

24. **ACC** After the new site is selected, clean the area (with water only) and pat dry. *Clean, dry skin will facilitate absorption of the transdermal medication and help keep the patch in place.*

25. **ACC** Open the new transdermal package and peel off the protective liner from the patch per manufacturer instructions. Avoid touching the sticky, adhesive side of the patch. *Touching the sticky side of the patch with your hands may reduce the effectiveness of adhesive.*

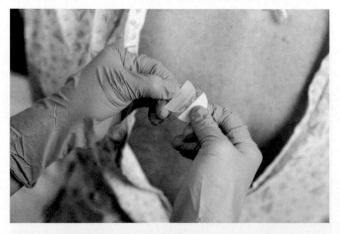

STEP 25 Prepare the new patch.

26. **ACC** Apply patch (sticky-side down) to the selected site and press down firmly for at least 30 seconds. Check edges around the patch to ensure the patch is secure. *Pressing down for at least 30 seconds facilitates adherence of the patch to the client's skin.*

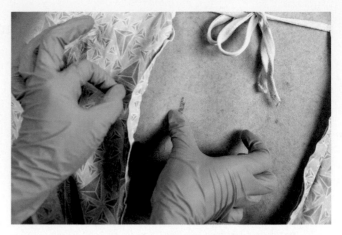

STEP 26 Apply the new patch and secure edges.

27. **ACC** If the edges of the patch are not sticking well, apply hypoallergenic tape (around the edges) per manufacturer instructions. *Creates seal and prevents patch from falling off.*

28. **ACC** Ensure that the transdermal patch is labeled with the time, date, and your initials. *Proper labeling of the patch facilitates communication between staff and prevents errors.*

29. **SAF** If the facility has a **postadministration checkpoint,** review transdermal package label against the MAR or EMAR. If any errors occurred, notify the authorized healthcare provider.

30. **EVAL** Monitor the client for any adverse or unexpected effects of the medication.

31. **EVAL** If the client was given transdermal pain medication, monitor the client's pain closely to assess relief of pain. Notify the authorized healthcare provider if the medication did not relieve the client's pain.

FINISHING THE SKILL

32. **INF** Remove gloves and perform hand hygiene.

33. **CCC** Ensure client safety and comfort. Ensure that the bed is in the lowest position, and verify that the client can identify and reach the nurse call system. *These safety measures reduce the risk of falls.*

34. **EVAL** Evaluate the outcomes. Is the client tolerating the transdermal patch? Were the rights of administration followed (right client, drug, dose, route, time, and documentation)?

35. **COM** Document assessment findings, medication administration, and outcomes in the legal healthcare record.
    - name of transdermal medication given, exact time, date, and dose given
    - pertinent postassessment data, such as vital signs or pain level
    - condition of the client's skin where transdermal medication has been placed
    - signature and initials of the clinician who administered the medication.

36. **EVAL** Provide follow-up monitoring of the client and ensure that the transdermal patch remains in place. *Transdermal patches can come off or lose adhesion of the backing over time.*

■ SKILL 11.10 Administering an Eye Medication (Drops or Ointment)

EQUIPMENT

Clean gloves
Tissues or washcloths
Eye drops or ointment as prescribed, at room temperature

BEGINNING THE SKILL

1. **ACC** Review the order for:
   - name of eye medication and dosage
   - time intervals and route of administration
   - special administration instructions
   - purpose of administering medication (if PRN)
   - specification of which eye (right or left) is to receive medication.
2. **ACC** Review the following:
   - **SAF** client's allergies to medications or other substances
   - **SAF** indications and any contraindications for eye medication
   - appropriateness of eye medication for client
   - client's medical/surgical history (particularly ophthalmic conditions).
3. **INF** Perform hand hygiene.
4. **CCC** Introduce yourself to the client and family.
5. **SAF** Identify the client using at least two client identifiers.
6. **CCC** Provide privacy.
7. **ACC** Assess the client's level of consciousness and orientation to person, time, place, and situation. *Provides a baseline assessment of orientation before verbal consent is obtained.*
8. **CCC** Explain the procedure and obtain verbal consent. *To provide client-centered care and prevent waste, consent should be obtained before preparing medications.*
9. **ACC** Perform any client preassessments, which may include:
   - condition of eyes and any signs of redness, drainage, or irritation
   - level of pain or discomfort in the affected eye or eyes.
10. **ACC** Assess the client for the presence of contact lenses. (Note: Depending on the medication, contacts may need to removed prior to receiving eye drops. Check with facility pharmacy or the authorized healthcare provider regarding specific medications.)

PROCEDURE

Preparing the Eye Medication

11. **SAF** Perform the **first safety checkpoint** when accessing the eye medication, and perform the **second safety checkpoint** when preparing the eye medication. Check the rights of administration, check the expiration date, and scan the bar code on the label if required. **WARNING:** Check the order (for first administration) and the MAR or EMAR for subsequent administrations to verify which eye or if both eyes will be receiving the eye medication.

12. **SAF** If the client wears contact lenses, ensure that the eye medication is free from preservatives. *Preservatives may increase the risk of corneal toxicity for these clients (Sharma, 2018a).*
13. **CCC** Ensure eye medication is at room temperature and gently shake or agitate the container or bottle (in the case of eye drops). *Cold eye medication can cause client pain or discomfort. Gently shaking container helps distribute medication and ensure that it is properly mixed.*

Administering the Eye Medication (Drops or Ointment)

14. **INF** Perform hand hygiene again upon entering the client's room.
15. **SAF** Reverify the client's identity by using at least two client identifiers.
16. **SAF** Recheck the client's armband and ask the client verbally if he or she has any allergies.
17. **SAF** Perform **third safety checkpoint** and review the eye medication with the client. Check the rights of administration again. *This facilitates client involvement.* (Note: If required, scan the client's armband and the bar code on the eye medication label if available.)
18. **SAF** Verify with the client which eye or if both eyes will be receiving the eye medication. *Validating the "correct eye" with the client at the bedside is another critical safety check.*
19. **ACC** After the correct eye has been verified, apply gloves and administer the eye medication. If the client is receiving eye drops and eye ointment, administer the eye drops first. *Instilling eye drops before eye ointment prevents washing ointment into the client's eyes. In addition, ointment waterproofs the eye (Sharma, 2018a). This could prevent proper absorption of drops.*
20. **SAF** Position the client in a supine position or semi-Fowler position if not contraindicated.
21. **ACC If the client is receiving eye drops:**
    a. Remove cap from container and place it (without touching inside) on clean, dry surface.
    b. Ask the client to tilt the head back and look upward (at a fixed point) toward the affected side. *This position may prevent the eye medication from running into the other eye.*
    c. With a gloved thumb or forefinger, gently pull down the client's lower eyelid to make a "pocket" for the eye drops. *This procedure exposes the client's lower conjunctival sac or inferior fornix behind the lower eyelid for the administration of eye drops.*
    d. Using your other gloved hand, invert the dropper and hold it no closer than 2 cm (3/4 inch) above the client's eye. *Prevents contamination of the eye and dropper.*
    e. Without touching the dispenser to the eye, allow *one* drop of medication to drop into the "pocket" of the lower or inferior fornix. Avoid placing the eye drop in the lacrimal gland or inner canthus. *Allowing only*

one drop at a time prevents overflow and loss of medication through nasolacrimal drainage (Sharma, 2018a).

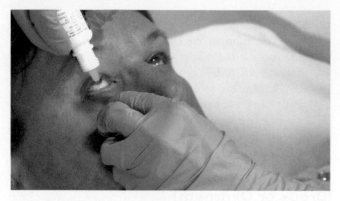

STEP 21E Instill one eye drop at a time.

    f. Instruct the client to close the eyes gently (without squeezing) for at least 60 seconds. *Increases absorption and prevents loss of medication (Sharma, 2018a).*

    g. If giving more than one drop, allow the client to close the eyes, and wait recommended time (usually at least 3–5 minutes) before the next drop. *Prevents loss of medication and maximizes absorption.* (Note: Manufacturer will have specific recommendations.)

    h. Replace cap on eye medication bottle without touching the inside of the cap.

    i. Clean excess medication off client using a clean tissue or cloth. Wipe eye from inner to outer canthus. *Prevents contamination of the lacrimal duct.*

22. **ACC If the client is receiving eye ointment:**

    a. Remove cap from tube and place it (without touching inside) on clean, dry surface.

    b. Ask the client to tilt the head back and look upward. *Positions client properly for ointment.*

    c. With gloved thumb or forefinger, gently pull down the client's lower eyelid.

    d. Without touching the ointment tube to the eye, squeeze out small ribbon (approximately 2 cm [¾ inch]) along the rim of the lower eyelid from the inner canthus to the outer canthus of the eye (Sharma, 2018a). (Note: Some facilities require ointment to be placed on a tissue and then applied by using an applicator or gloved finger.)

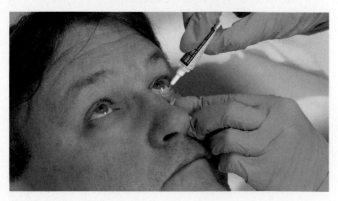

STEP 22D Apply eye ointment.

    e. Ask the client to blink the eye gently a few times and then close the eye for 3 to 5 minutes. *Facilitates distribution of ointment across the eye and facilitates absorption.*

    f. Clean excess ointment from the client's eye with a tissue or cloth. If ointment was placed in both eyes, use a different tissue for each eye. *Prevents cross-contamination.*

    g. Clean excess ointment off tube with tissue and replace cap.

23. **INF** If eye drops or ointment are ordered for the other eye, repeat the procedure. Use a different tissue to clean each eye. *Using different tissues for each eye prevents cross-contamination.*

24. **INF** If giving a different eye medication in the same eye, wait at least 3 to 5 minutes before instilling a different medication. *Prevents previous eye drop from not being absorbed.*

25. **SAF** If the facility has a **postadministration checkpoint,** review the eye medication label against the MAR or EMAR. If any errors occurred, notify the authorized healthcare provider.

26. **EVAL** Monitor the client for any adverse or unexpected effects of the eye medication.

FINISHING THE SKILL

27. **INF** Dispose of equipment per policy, remove gloves, and perform hand hygiene.

28. **SAF** Ensure client safety and comfort. Ensure that the bed is in the lowest position, and verify that the client can identify and reach the nurse call system. *These safety measures reduce the risk of falls.*

29. **EVAL** Evaluate the outcomes. Did the client tolerate the procedure? Were the rights of administration followed (right client, drug, dose, route, time, and documentation)?

30. **COM** Document assessment findings, medication administration, and outcomes in the legal healthcare record:

    • name of eye drop or ointment medication, exact time, date, and dose given

    • client response to eye medication, which eye or eyes received drops or ointment

    • signature and initials of the clinician who administered the eye drops or ointment.

31. **INF** As part of the client's follow-up care, or if the client will be self-administering eye drops or ointment, remind the client to use a separate tissue for each eye. *Using a separate tissue for each eye will prevent infection and cross-contamination of the eyes.*

■ SKILL 11.11 Irrigating the Eyes

EQUIPMENT

Clean gloves, personal protective equipment (PPE) if needed (e.g., face mask with splash shield)

Towels and/or disposable absorbent protective pads

Bath or kidney-shaped basin

Sterile eye irrigation solution at room temperature or warmed as prescribed

Sterile irrigation container with irrigation syringe

IV tubing and normal saline bag or other prescribed fluid

IV pole for IV setup and bag (if used)

BEGINNING THE SKILL

1. **ACC** Review the order for:
   - name and strength of solution for eye irrigation
   - time intervals, route of administration, and special administration instructions
   - purpose of administering irrigation (e.g., infection, foreign body)
   - specification of which eye (right or left) is to receive eye irrigation.

2. **ACC** Review the following:
   - **SAF** client's allergies to medications or other substances
   - **SAF** indications and any contraindications for eye irrigation (Note: Contraindications may include severe traumatic eye events, such as penetrating injuries or foreign objects.)
   - appropriateness of eye irrigation solution for the client
   - client's medical/surgical history (particularly ophthalmic conditions).

3. **INF** Perform hand hygiene.

4. **CCC** Introduce yourself to the client and family.

5. **SAF** Identify the client using at least two client identifiers (e.g., armband, bar code, verbal).

6. **CCC** Provide privacy.

7. **ACC** Assess the client's level of consciousness and orientation to person, time, place, and situation. *Provides a baseline assessment of orientation before verbal consent is obtained.*

8. **CCC** Explain procedure and obtain verbal consent. *To provide client-centered care and prevent waste, consent should be obtained before preparing medications.*

9. **ACC** Perform any client preassessments, which may include:
   - level of pain or discomfort in the affected eye or eyes
   - vision changes or loss of vision in the affected eye or eyes
   - condition of eyes and any signs of redness, drainage, or irritation.

PROCEDURE

Preparing the Eye Irrigation Solution

10. **SAF** Perform the **first safety checkpoint** when accessing the eye irrigation solution, and perform the **second safety checkpoint** when preparing the solution. Check the rights of administration, check the expiration date, and scan the bar code on the label if required. **WARNING:** Check the order (for first administration) and the MAR or EMAR for subsequent administrations to verify which eye or if both eyes will be receiving the eye irrigation. (Note: The solution and volume used for the eye irrigation will vary depending on the specific order and the client's condition.)

11. **SAF** Inspect the medication solution for any unusual cloudiness or particles.

12. **CCC** Ensure that the eye irrigation solution is at room temperature or warmed to a prescribed temperature (Sharma, 2018b). If the irrigation solution is warmed, a facility-approved warmer should be used. *Cold eye irrigation solution can cause client pain or discomfort.*

13. **SAF** Label the irrigation solution with the client's name, medication (if present), time and date.

Administering the Eye Irrigation

14. **INF** Perform hand hygiene again upon entering the client's room.

15. **SAF** Reverify the client's identity by using at least two client identifiers.

16. **SAF** Recheck the client's armband and ask the client verbally if he or she has any allergies.

17. **SAF** Perform the **third safety checkpoint** and review the eye irrigation solution with the client. Check the rights of administration again. *This facilitates client involvement.* (Note: If required, scan the client's armband and the bar code on the irrigation solution label if available.)

18. **SAF** Verify with the client which eye or if both eyes will be receiving the eye irrigation. *Validating the "correct eye" with the client at the bedside is another critical safety check.*

Setting up the Equipment

19. **ACC If the syringe method is used:**
   a. Remove lid from sterile irrigation solution, invert it, and place on table.
   b. Place sterile irrigation container on clean, dry surface at waist height.
   c. Pour the prescribed amount of irrigation solution (label-side up) into sterile container.
   d. Replace lid on container without touching the inside of the lid.

20. **ACC If the IV tubing method is used:**
   a. Obtain IV pole to hang IV bag or prescribed irrigation solution.
   b. Prepare and prime tubing with prescribed irrigation solution using sterile technique (see Chapter 12).

c. Keep distal end of IV tubing capped and sterile until ready for use.

Performing the Eye Irrigation

21. **INF** Apply clean gloves.
22. **INF** Apply face mask with a face shield if exposure to body fluids is expected. *A face mask with a shield will protect the nurse from unexpected splashing that may occur from the irrigation.*
23. **ACC** Position the client in a side-lying position or semi-Fowler position if not contraindicated. (Note: The client should lie toward the side of the affected eye for the irrigation procedure.)
24. **ACC** Place bath or kidney-shaped basin (with protective pads or towels under it) next to the client on the side of the client's affected eye. Provide additional protective pads or towels as needed. *Protects the client from irrigation fluid as it drains by gravity during the procedure.*
25. **INF** If the client has excess drainage on eyelids or eyelashes, clean gently with washcloth from inner to outer canthus. *Prevents debris from entering the client's eye during irrigation.*
26. **INF** Ask the client to keep the head turned toward the side of the affected eye. *Prevents cross-contamination and prevents irritant from flushing into the client's unaffected eye.*
27. **INF** If using the syringe method, insert sterile irrigator or syringe into irrigant solution and draw up irrigation fluid. Ensure that the tip of the irrigator or syringe remains sterile.
28. **INF** If using the IV tubing method, remove the distal cap and maintain the sterility of the distal end of the tubing. *Maintaining the sterility of the tubing prevents contamination and infection.*
29. **ACC** With your nondominant gloved hand, hold the eyelid open and gently pull down the lower lid to expose the lower conjunctival sac. *This facilitates irrigation in the proper location.*
30. **ACC** With your dominant hand, hold the syringe or distal end of the IV tubing no closer than 2.5 cm (1 inch) near eye, and *gently* administer irrigation from inner to outer canthus along the conjunctival sac. Avoid touching the eye or eyelid with the syringe tip or the distal end of the IV tubing. *Irrigating toward the conjunctival sac prevents injury to the cornea; irrigating from the inner to outer canthus without touching the eye prevents contamination.*

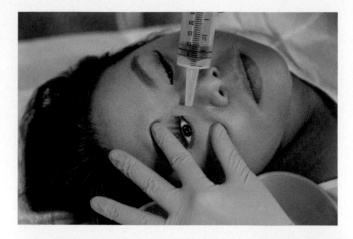

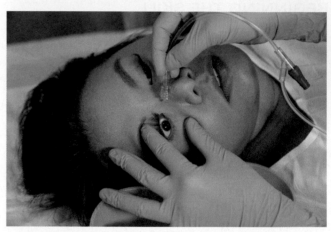

STEP 30 Position syringe or tubing for irrigation.

31. **ACC** Continue irrigation as prescribed and allow the irrigant to flow into the basin by gravity. Ask the client to look right and left with the eye (not turning the head) during irrigation. *Looking right and left maximizes irrigant flow across the eye surface and facilitates absorption.*
32. **EVAL** During the irrigation, monitor the client for any signs of distress, pain, or discomfort.
33. **CCC** At the end of the procedure or after 30 minutes of irrigation, ask the client to close his or her eyes for approximately 5 minutes. *Facilitates absorption and prevents run-off (Sharma, 2018b).*
34. **ACC** If eye irrigation is ordered for the other eye, repeat the procedure.
35. **INF** Clean excess irrigation fluid from the client's eye if needed. Use a different tissue to clean each eye. *Using different tissues for each eye prevents cross-contamination of the eyes.*
36. **ACC** If the client is receiving irrigation and eye ointment, perform irrigation first. Instilling *the irrigation before applying eye ointment prevents washing ointment into the client's eyes.*
37. **SAF** If the facility has a **postadministration checkpoint,** review the label on the irrigation solution against the MAR or EMAR. If any errors occurred, notify the authorized healthcare provider.

38. **EVAL** Monitor the client for any adverse or unexpected effects of the eye irrigation.

FINISHING THE SKILL

39. **INF** Dispose of equipment per policy, remove gloves, and perform hand hygiene.
40. **SAF** Ensure client safety and comfort. Ensure that the bed is in the lowest position, and verify that the client can identify and reach the nurse call system. *These safety measures reduce the risk of falls.*
41. **EVAL** Evaluate the outcomes. Did the client tolerate the procedure? Did the irrigation fluid improve the client's symptoms as expected? Were the rights of administration followed?
42. **COM** Document assessment findings, medication administration, and outcomes in the legal healthcare record:
    - which eye received eye medication
    - name of eye irrigation given, exact time, date, and volume given
    - temperature of irrigation solution if warmed (e.g., 37°C)
    - signature and initials of the clinician who administered the medication.

■ SKILL 11.12 Instilling Ear (Otic) Drops

EQUIPMENT

Tissues or washcloths
Clean gloves
Ear drops as prescribed at room temperature

BEGINNING THE SKILL

1. **ACC** Review the order for:
   - name and strength of solution for ear drops
   - time intervals, route of administration, and special administration instructions
   - purpose of administering medication (if PRN)
   - specification of which ear (right or left) is to receive ear drops.
2. **ACC** Review the following:
   - **SAF** client's allergies to medications or other substances
   - **SAF** indications and any contraindications for ear drops
   - appropriateness of ear drops (using medication rights)
   - client's medical/surgical history (particularly ear conditions).
3. **INF** Perform hand hygiene.
4. **CCC** Introduce yourself to the client and family.
5. **SAF** Identify the client using at least two client identifiers.
6. **CCC** Provide privacy.
7. **ACC** Assess client's level of consciousness and orientation to person, time, place, and situation. *Provides a baseline assessment of orientation before verbal consent is obtained.*
8. **CCC** Explain the procedure and obtain verbal consent. *To provide client-centered care and prevent waste, consent should be obtained before preparing medications.*
9. **ACC** Perform any client preassessments, including but not limited to the following:
   - condition of ears and any signs of redness, drainage, or irritation
   - level of pain or discomfort in the affected ear or ears
   - any hearing loss or "ringing" in the affected ear.

PROCEDURE

Preparing the Ear (Otic) Medication

10. **SAF** Perform the **first safety checkpoint** when accessing the ear (otic) medication, and perform the **second safety checkpoint** when preparing the ear medication. Check the rights of administration, check the expiration date, and scan the bar code on the label if required. **WARNING:** Check the order (for first administration) and the MAR or EMAR for subsequent administrations to verify which ear or if both ears will be receiving the ear medication.
11. **CCC** Ensure ear medication is at room temperature and gently shake or agitate the container or bottle (in the case of ear drops). (Note: To warm the medication, hold in your hand or gently roll the bottle between your hands for several minutes.) *Cold ear medication can cause client pain or discomfort. Gently shaking the container helps suspend and mix medication. (American Society of Health-System Pharmacists [ASHP], 2018).*

Administering the Ear (Otic) Medication

12. **INF** Perform hand hygiene again upon entering the client's room.
13. **SAF** Reverify the client's identity by using at least two client identifiers.
14. **SAF** Recheck the client's armband, and ask the client verbally if he or she has any allergies.
15. **SAF** Perform **third safety checkpoint** and review the ear (otic) medication with the client. Check rights of administration again. *This facilitates client involvement.* (Note: If required, scan client's armband and bar code on the ear medication label if available.)

16. **SAF** Verify with the client which ear or if both ears will be receiving the otic medication. *Validating the "correct ear" with the client at the bedside is another critical safety check.*

17. **ACC** After ear drops and "correct ear" are verified, apply gloves and perform the procedure. (Note: Some facilities may not require gloves if there is not a risk of exposure to body fluids.)

    a. Position the client in a lying-down position with the affected ear upward if not contraindicated. *This exposes the ear canal and facilities instillation of ear medication (ASHP, 2018).*

    b. Clean outer ear gently with warm washcloth and thoroughly pat dry. *Cleaning outer ear prevents debris from entering the client's ear when drops are instilled.*

    c. If not already done, gently agitate or shake container to suspend the medication.

    d. Remove cap from container and place it (without touching inside) on clean, dry surface.

    e. Inspect tip of dropper and ensure that it is not cracked or damaged.

    f. Ask the client to keep head in position while affected ear remains upward.

    g. Using your nondominant hand, pull pinna up and back for adults.

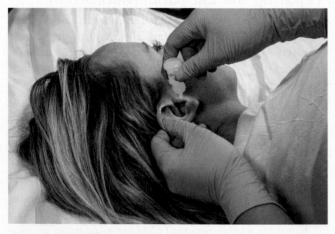

STEP 17G Pull pinna up and back for an adult client.

    h. For children less than 3 years of age, pull earlobe down and back. *Opening up and straightening the ear canal helps to optimize medication instillation.*

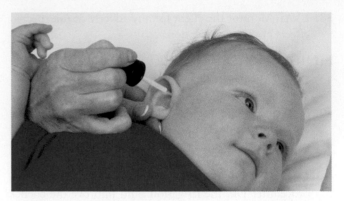

STEP 17H Pull earlobe down and back for a child. Wear clean gloves if there is a risk of exposure to body fluids.

    i. Using other gloved hand, squeeze medication into dropper and invert it. Without touching dropper to ear, instill number of ordered drops into ear.

    j. Instruct the client to keep the ear in place for at least 5 minutes before repositioning. *Keeping the ear in place helps retain the ear medication within the ear canal so that it can absorb properly.*

    k. Replace cap on ear medication bottle without touching the inside of the cap.

    l. Clean excess medication off the client's ear with a clean tissue or cloth.

18. **INF** If ear drops are ordered for the other ear, repeat the procedure. Use a different tissue to clean each ear. *Using different tissues for each ear prevents cross-contamination.*

19. **EVAL** Monitor the client for any adverse or unexpected effects of the ear irrigation.

FINISHING THE SKILL

20. **INF** Dispose of equipment per policy, remove gloves, and perform hand hygiene.

21. **CCC** Ensure client safety and comfort. Ensure that the bed is in the lowest position, and verify that the client can identify and reach the nurse call system. *These safety measures reduce the risk of falls.*

22. **EVAL** Evaluate the outcomes. Were the eardrops instilled successfully? Were the rights of administration followed (right client, drug, dose, route, time, and documentation)?

23. **COM** Document assessment findings, medication administration, and outcomes in the legal healthcare record.

    • name of ear drops given, exact time, date, and number of drops

    • which ear or ears (right, left, or both) received medication

    • signature and initials of the clinician who administered the medication.

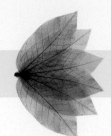

SECTION 5 Administering Parenteral Medications

Medications given by the parenteral route are administered and absorbed "outside of the gastrointestinal tract." For the purpose of this chapter, the parenteral routes that will be discussed are intradermal (ID), subcutaneous, and intramuscular (IM) injections. The intravenous (IV) route is discussed in Chapter 12. As with other nonoral routes, parenteral medications usually take effect more rapidly than enteral drugs, depending on the onset of action of the specific medication, the unique characteristics of the individual client, and other variables.

PREPARING EQUIPMENT FOR INJECTIONS

Before giving an injection, you must first select the most appropriate syringe and needle. Major categories of syringes include insulin syringes with markings in units, tuberculin syringes (1-mL syringes with 0.1-mL markings), and standard size syringes in different volumes. Examples of various syringes

are shown in Fig. 11.6. Needles come in a variety of sizes and lengths (Fig. 11.7). Needle length continues to be measured in inches by manufacturers. It is one of the very few aspects of medical care that has not converted to the metric system. Needle size is measured in gauge, which is a standardized unit of measure for metal wire. The smaller the number, the larger the gauge. For example, a 14-gauge needle is larger than an 18-gauge needle. The choice of an appropriate needle and syringe (which may be separate or preattached) varies and is based on (a) the route of administration ordered, (b) the type of medication being given, and (c) the client's size and muscle mass. If a medication is viscous (thick), a larger-gauge needle may be needed; conversely, if the medication is aqueous, a smaller-gauge needle may be indicated.

COMPONENTS OF A NEEDLE AND SYRINGE

The specific components of the needle and syringe are shown in Fig. 11.8. As the illustration depicts, specific components

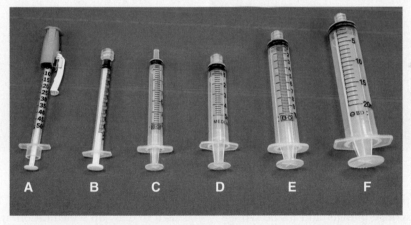

FIG. 11.6 Various syringe sizes. **A,** Insulin syringe. **B,** 1-mL tuberculin syringe. **C,** 3-mL syringe. **D,** 5-mL syringe. **E,** 10-mL syringe. **F,** 20-mL syringe.

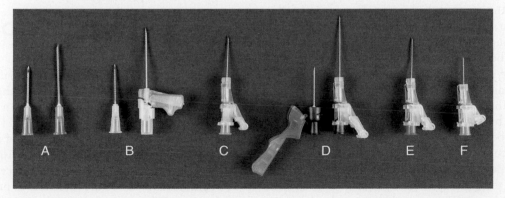

FIG. 11.7 Needles of various lengths and sizes. **A,** 18-gauge 1-inch and 18-gauge 1½-inch. **B,** 20-gauge 1-inch and 20-gauge 1½-inch. **C,** 21-gauge. **D,** 22-gauge 1-inch and 22-gauge 1½-inch. **E,** 23-gauge. **F,** 25-gauge.

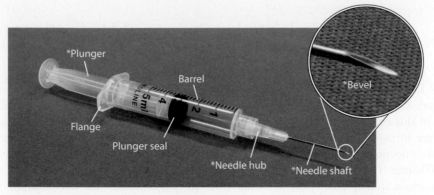

FIG. 11.8 Components of a needle and syringe. The components that must not be touched are noted with an *asterisk*.

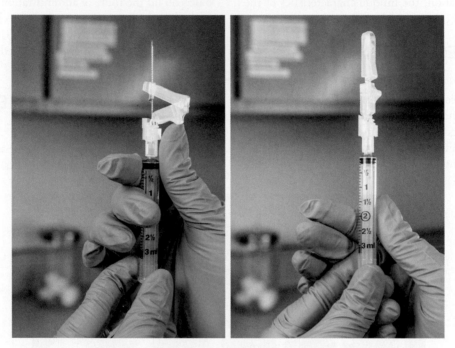

FIG. 11.9 Engaging the needle safety shield.

of the needle and syringe that must remain sterile and not be touched include (1) the syringe plunger and inside syringe barrel; (2) the Luer-Lok tip of the syringe that connects to the needle; and (3) the entire shaft of the needle, including the hub.

The bevel of the needle, which must also remain sterile, is the opening at the tip of the needle where the medication comes through (see Fig. 11.8). As discussed later in this chapter, the bevel of the needle remains "up" during the administration of intradermal injections.

After the medication is prepared, label the syringe per facility policy. The current National Patient Safety Goals (2019) provided by The Joint Commission recommend that medicines must be labeled in an area where supplies are set up. This is particularly important if there will be a delay in administration. Before the injection is given, some hospitals require that the needle be replaced with a fresh needle before administering the injection. However, the Advisory Committee on Immunization Practices (ACIP) of the CDC notes that needles only need to be replaced if they are

damaged or contaminated (CDC, 2019a). If a filter needle is used to draw up a medication, it must always be replaced before administration. When taking a prepared injection to the client, ensure that the cap is secure, and avoid placing the injection in your pocket.

USING SAFETY AND NEEDLELESS SYSTEMS

Both the CDC and the Occupational Safety and Health Administration (OSHA) recommend the use of safety needle shields and needleless systems. An example of the use of a safety shield is provided in Fig. 11.9. As shown in the example, hold the needle upright and away from your body, and use your gloved thumb to displace the shield over the needle until it "clicks" in place. This must be done immediately after the injection to prevent a needle-stick injury. For some safety needles (e.g., retractable needles), the device may be activated after the injection but before removing the needle from the client. In addition to safety needles and safety shields, needleless access devices or blunt cannulas can be used. Special safety adapters may also be used to withdraw medication from a vial or ampule.

PREPARING MEDICATIONS

Using a Vial

A vial is a small container (plastic or glass) that has a rubber stopper/septum on top for access. Although a new vial will have a protective cap, the manufacturer does *not* guarantee the sterility of the stopper. To prevent infection, it is important to "scrub the hub" of the vial's stopper/septum with an antiseptic wipe before penetration (even with a new vial).

The two major types of vials are single-dose vials (SDVs) and multidose vials (MDVs). SDVs (which have no preservatives) are used only once and then discarded after use, whereas MDVs can be used more than once for one client. However, once opened, MDVs must be discarded within 28 days (or sooner, per facility policy), and they must never be used past the expiration date (CDC, 2019b).

Some facilities now require that an MDV can only be used by one client and must be discarded within 24 hours. Furthermore, each time the vial is entered, a different syringe/needle must be used. According to the CDC and other authorities, the misuse of MDVs (e.g., using the same vial between clients, cross-contamination) has resulted in disease outbreaks and the transmission of potentially life-threatening infections such as hepatitis and meningitis. Thus, the use of SDVs is recommended if available. It is also important to remember that SDVs must never be stored for future use (CDC, 2019b).

Using an Ampule

An ampule is a glass container that contains a small volume of liquid medication (1–10 mL) and is designed for one-time use only. Ampules are often scored at the neck of the container, which can be "snapped" or broken (away from the nurse's body using a protective gauze pad) to access the medication (Caple, 2018). It is crucial to use a micron filter needle or straw to draw up the medication in order to prevent tiny glass particulates from entering the syringe. After drawing up the medication, replace the filter needle with a new needle before administering the medication.

Reconstituting a Medication in a Vial

When medications are only available in dry-powder form, they require reconstitution with a diluent for parenteral administration. Two of the most common types of diluents are sterile water for injection (SWFI) and normal saline for injection (NSFI). The manufacturer insert for each medication and the medication label will usually provide dilution

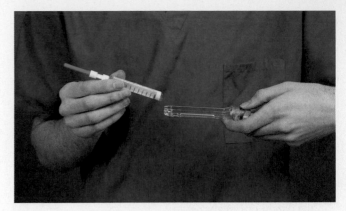

FIG. 11.10 Medication cartridge and prefilled syringe.

and reconstitution instructions for each medication. The diluents must be approved for this purpose.

The amount of medication to be given will depend on the concentration of the medication and dosage. Concentration refers to the specific amount of drug diluted within a specific amount of fluid (e.g., 250 mg/mL). After the medication is reconstituted and prepared, it is important to accurately label the vial and syringe. At a minimum, the label on the vial must contain the client's name, the name of the drug, the time of reconstitution, the time and route of administration, and the date after which the medication can no longer be used.

Using a Medication Cartridge

Some medications (in specific doses) may only be available as prefilled syringes that do not have a plunger. Therefore, the prefilled syringe must be placed within a medication cartridge in order to administer the medication (Fig. 11.10). When using these devices, review the manufacturer's guidelines closely for any specific directions. For example, enoxaparin sodium (Lovenox), which will be discussed shortly, may have a bubble within the prefilled syringe in order to avoid loss of the drug. This bubble is *not* to be removed before administering the medication.

ADMINISTERING INJECTIONS

Before any type of injection can be given, the nurse must find the appropriate site on the client. Depending on the type of injection and area of the body involved, specific anatomical landmarks must be used to find the optimal location. Avoid areas on the skin with bruising, scarring, redness, moles, or discoloration, and avoid areas where major nerves are located. Ask clients if they have areas of tenderness that need to be avoided or if they have preferences for injection sites. If clients are receiving multiple injections, rotate injection sites with each administration to avoid injury and scarring. Provide comfort measures and atraumatic care during injections, particularly for the pediatric population (Box 11.5).

BOX 11.5 Pediatric Considerations During Injections: Providing Atraumatic Care

Receiving any type of injection can be stressful, particularly for children. The nurse's skill and calm demeanor go a long way toward reducing a child's anxiety. Examples of evidence-based comfort measures for infants and children include the following (CDC, 2019a; WHO, 2015):
- Avoid language that will create anxiety, mistrust, or false reassurance.
- Encourage the parent to hold the child (3 years of age or younger) during the injection.
- Children older than 3 years of age should be seated in the parent or caregiver's lap.
- Encourage breastfeeding and sucking activity (for infants under 1 year of age), or provide sweet-tasting liquids or milk during the injection.
- Use tactile stimulation by gently stroking, or asking an assistant to stroke, the client's skin near the injection site for children 4 years of age and older.
- Use distraction techniques during the injection, such as encouraging the parent to read a book to the child or offering the child colorful toys or games.

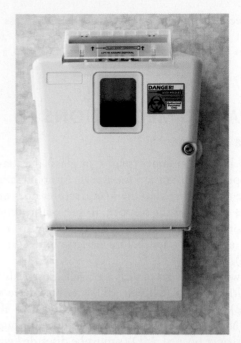

FIG. 11.11 Biohazard sharps box (wall unit).

Infection Control

As with other invasive procedures, use sterile technique when preparing and administering an injection. Cleanse the site thoroughly in a circular pattern with a facility approved antiseptic wipe, and then allow the site to completely dry without fanning it. Avoid contaminating or touching the site with your hand or nonsterile glove after it has been prepped.

Check your facility policy regarding the use of gloves. The CDC and OSHA do not require the use of gloves for administering vaccines unless there is a risk of exposure to body fluids. However, in an acute care facility, the client may be at increased risk for bleeding and require care immediately after the injection; which creates a need to apply gloves. If gloves are worn, discard the gloves and perform hand hygiene between clients (CDC, 2019a).

Sharps Safety

To prevent needle stick injury, ensure your own fingers are out of the way when you give the injection.

After administration of the injection, immediately dispose of the needle/syringe in a puncture-proof biohazard sharps box. It may be free-standing, but in many acute care areas, the biohazard box is a wall unit (Fig. 11.11). Identify the location of this box before the procedure. If activation of a safety needle is required, do this as soon as the needle is withdrawn or per manufacturer instructions. Avoid walking around with the needle and *never* re-cap the needle. Drop the needle/syringe as a unit into the biohazard box, and avoid placing your hand near the sharps in the box (Fig. 11.12).

ADMINISTERING INTRADERMAL INJECTIONS

Medications ordered by the intradermal (ID) route are injections given within the dermal layer of the skin. Intradermal

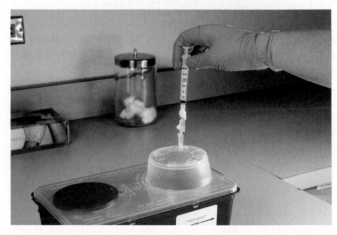

FIG. 11.12 Drop needle/syringe into biohazard box (needle first).

injections are typically used to test for localized antigen or allergic reactions. The dermal layer primarily has capillaries for absorption; therefore, the route of absorption is fairly slow. Because there are multiple nerves within the client's skin, ID injections can be somewhat uncomfortable.

Two of the most common types of testing performed using intradermal injections are the tuberculosis (TB) test (called Mantoux tuberculin skin test or purified protein derivative skin test [PPD]) and testing for specific allergies, whereby a small amount of the antigen or allergen is injected. For TB reactions, the site is usually checked 48 to 72 hours after injection and evaluated by using parameters. If the site is reddened, hardened, or indurated by a certain amount (usually 5 mm or more), the client may have been exposed to TB. However, a positive test does not always mean TB is currently active. Further medical testing is needed (Medline Plus, 2019).

When administering an intradermal injection, a 1-mL syringe (tuberculin syringe) is used with a needle size of ⅜ to ¾ inch long and 26 to 28 gauge. The maximum volume with

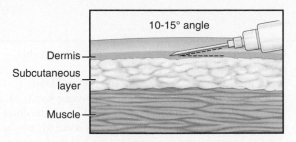

FIG. 11.13 Intradermal injection. Cross-sectional view of injection into intradermal tissue.

intradermals is usually 0.1 mL. The most common site is the inner aspect of the forearm. However, they may be given in the upper back, the back of arms, and the upper chest. The angle of injection can range from 5 to 15 degrees, with the bevel of the needle facing up (Fig. 11.13).

If the injection is properly within the dermal layer, a small wheal or bleb will form, which looks like a mosquito bite. Instruct the client not to rub the site (so that absorption remains slow). Some facilities require the nurse to circle the injection site with a waterproof marker for diagnostic purposes. It is also important to accurately document where the injection was given.

ADMINISTERING SUBCUTANEOUS INJECTIONS

Medication given by the subcutaneous route is injected into the subcutaneous or fatty tissue of the body (Fig. 11.14). Because the subcutaneous area has few blood vessels, the absorption rate is slower than that for intramuscular injections. Two common medications given by the subcutaneous route are insulin and heparin, which are also high-alert medications.

When administering subcutaneous injections, the size of the syringe is based on the volume of medication to be given (usually about 0.5 to 2 mL). Needle sizes commonly used are ⅜ to 1 inch long and 26 to 28 gauge. However, this may vary depending on the irritability of the medication and the amount of fatty tissue the client has. The maximum volume allowed is usually 2 mL for adults, whereas it is much smaller for children. Sites for these injections are commonly on the side and back of the arms, the tops of the thighs, and the abdomen (Fig. 11.15). The angle of insertion depends on the length of the needle, the medication being administered, and the amount of subcutaneous tissue the client has. These injections are often given at

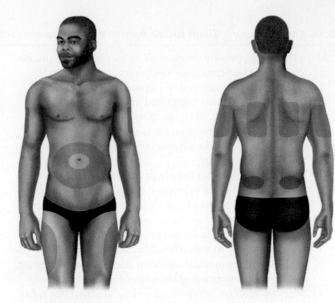

FIG. 11.15 Recommended sites for subcutaneous injections.

a 45-degree angle to avoid underlying muscle tissue. However, if the client has an adequate amount of subcutaneous tissue and the needle is short, a 90-degree angle may be acceptable because the needle will still be in the subcutaneous tissue. For some medications, the manufacturer may recommend using a 90-degree angle for subcutaneous injections.

In addition to insulin (to be discussed shortly) and heparin, a common subcutaneous injection is enoxaparin (Lovenox), which is an anticoagulant. After hospitalization, clients are frequently required to self-administer these subcutaneous injections at home. Thus, client teaching, follow-up, and return demonstrations are essential. Allowing practice time is also helpful. For more information about teaching clients how to self-administer subcutaneous injections, including enoxaparin (Lovenox), see Box 11.6 and Skill 11.17.

ADMINISTERING INTRAMUSCULAR INJECTIONS

Medications that are given by the IM route are injected into the muscles (at a 90-degree angle) below the dermal layer and subcutaneous tissue (Fig. 11.16). This area has more vasculature than intradermal or subcutaneous routes, so the absorption rate is usually more rapid. As with the subcutaneous

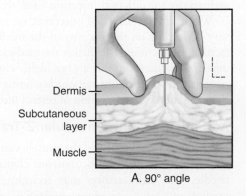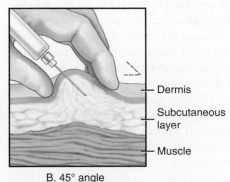

A. 90° angle   B. 45° angle

FIG. 11.14 Subcutaneous injection. Cross-sectional view of injection into subcutaneous tissue.

BOX 11.6 Teaching Client to Self-Administer Enoxaparin (Lovenox)

(Note: If available, provide an opportunity for the client to practice and demonstrate a subcutaneous injection on a practice model).

1. Wash hands and assemble equipment (sharps box, antiseptic wipes, and prescribed enoxaparin (Lovenox) prefilled syringe). Check the label on the enoxaparin (Lovenox) syringe to ensure it has the correct dosage. (Note: The prefilled enoxaparin (Lovenox) has a visible bubble in the syringe.)

2. **WARNING:** Instruct the client *not* to eject the visible air bubble out of the syringe. Explain to the client that this ensures all of the medicine is given with each injection. *If the bubble is ejected out of the syringe, the client may not receive the full enoxaparin (Lovenox) dose.*

3. Assist the client to a comfortable position that allows visualization of a potential injection site. *Facilitates accuracy and self-administration of the enoxaprin (Lovenox) dose.*

4. Select an injection site (preferably the abdomen) that is free from rashes, bruises, or scars and can be easily reached. If the client will receive recurring injections, instruct the client to rotate sites and give the injection at least 2.5 cm (1 inch) from the last injection site and at least 5 cm (2 inches) from the navel. *Prevents tissue damage or lipodystrophy.*

5. Instruct the client to clean the injection site with an antiseptic wipe and let it dry. After the site is cleaned, instruct the client to hold the syringe with the hand the client "writes with" (dominant hand) and the pull needle cover *straight* off with the nondominant hand. Instruct the client to avoid twisting the cover as it is being pulled off the needle. *Cleaning the injection site prevents infection. Twisting the needle cover could bend the needle.*

6. Instruct the client *not* to lay the syringe down at this point or contaminate the needle.

7. While pinching or "bunching up" the skin and tissue around the cleaned area with the nondominant hand, ask the client to hold the syringe "like a pencil" with the dominant hand. If the client demonstrates this correctly, ask the client to insert the entire needle into the bunched-up area.

8. While maintaining the bunched-up skin and tissue with his or her nondominant hand, the client should *slowly* press the plunger with the thumb or forefinger of his or her dominant hand until the entire injection is administered, including the air bubble. *Facilitates administration of the full dose.*

9. Instruct the client to "count to 10" and to maintain the "bunched-up" area until after the count.

10. After 10 seconds, the client should pull the needle straight out, point it away from him- or herself and others, and activate the safety shield by pushing firmly on the plunger rod until an audible click is heard. **WARNING:** Warn the client to *never* recap the needle. *Recapping the needle on a syringe increases the risk of a needle-stick injury.*

11. Instruct the client to "drop" the used syringe into a puncture-proof box, needle-side first.

12. Instruct the client to observe for leaking or bleeding from the site. Remind the client to apply gentle pressure if needed but not to massage site. *Massaging the site could increase bruising.*

13. Instruct the client to document the dose, time given, and injection site and to notify the authorized healthcare provider if the client has concerns or experiences unusual symptoms.

Reference: Sanofi U.S. LLC, 2018.

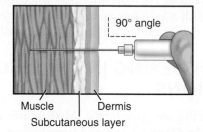

FIG. 11.16 Intramuscular injection. Cross-sectional view of injection into muscle tissue.

route, the IM route will have a systemic response. Two of the most commonly used sites for IM injection are the deltoid and vastus lateralis, although injections may also be given in the ventrogluteal site. Because of the risk of sciatic nerve damage, the dorsogluteal site is not recommended (Mann, 2016a). The vastus lateralis muscle is preferred for infants, neonates, and toddlers, and the deltoid muscle is preferred for children and adults who are 3 to 18 years old (CDC, 2019a). For more details on identifying IM injection sites, see Skill 11.18.

IM medications generally require a 1- to 3-mL syringe, depending on the volume given. The needle length for IM injection must be long enough to reach the muscle without affecting underlying nerves, vessels, or bone (CDC, 2019a). Some clients who are obese may need a longer needle (1.5 inch) to ensure the medication is injected within the muscle

and does not enter the subcutaneous tissue. In adults, the maximum volume allowed for IM injections depends on the size of the muscle. The deltoid muscle is smaller and will only allow up to 2 mL in an average-size adult, whereas the ventrogluteal site and the vastus lateralis muscle are larger muscles in the adult and may absorb more volume. In particular, the ventrogluteal site is also a good choice for deep IM or Z-track injections (Li, 2017). As with other injections, the gauge of the needle for IM injections should be determined by the viscosity of the drug. Viscous solutions usually require a larger-gauge needle than aqueous solutions. For a summary of key considerations when selecting the optimal needle and syringe size for different injection sites, see Box 11.7.

When administering IM injections, the rate of injection will vary depending on the viscosity of the medication and manufacturer instructions. The thicker the medication, the slower the injection. Medications that are not highly viscous, such as vaccinations, may be administered quickly. Some manufacturers still recommend the slow injection of certain medications.

Administering Intramuscular Z-Track Injections

Some medications given in the muscle can be painful if they seep back up into the subcutaneous channel created by the needle. The manufacturer may recommend giving certain medications known to cause irritation or staining (e.g., iron) by the Z-track method. This technique creates a seal and

BOX 11.7 Intramuscular (IM) Injections: Syringe, Needle, and Injection-Site Decision Making

---

KEY CONSIDERATIONS FOR IM INJECTIONS
- What is the age, size, and condition of the individual?
- What is the size and condition of the selected muscle for the injection?
- What is the volume and viscosity of the medication for injection?

VASTUS LATERALIS MUSCLE
- Preferred site for infants, neonates, and toddlers
- Alternative site for adolescents and adults if deltoid muscle cannot be used
- Neonates (first 28 days of life), and preterm infants: ⅝-inch, 22- to 25-gauge needle
- Infants and toddlers: 1-inch, 22- to 25-gauge needle
- Adults: 1- to 1½-inch, 22- to 25-gauge needle

DELTOID MUSCLE
- Preferred site for children age 3 to 18 years old
- Younger children: ⅝- to 1-inch needle
- Older children and adolescents: 1 inch needle
- Obese adolescents: 1½-inch needle to reach muscle tissue
- Adults (small), 60 kg (<130 lb): ⅝- to 1-inch needle
- Average-size adults: 1- to 1½-inch needle
- Obese adults: 1½-inch needle

VENTROGLUTEAL SITE
- Adults: 1- to 2-inch needle

Reference: Centers for Disease Control and Prevention, 2019a; Li, 2017.

allows the medication to stay deep in the muscle without tracking back into the subcutaneous tissue. For an illustration of the Z-track method, see Skill 11.18, step 28.

Risk Reduction Strategies When Giving Intramuscular Injections

Possible complications of IM injections may include local irritation, hematoma formation, or (more rarely) peripheral nerve injury and neuropathy (Li, 2017). The risk of complications can be reduced with excellent technique and proper identification of the injection site. Avoid inflamed or edematous areas and areas with scar tissue or lesions. It is also important to ensure that there is adequate muscle mass for clients who are frail or emaciated. Clients who have bleeding disorders or severe thrombocytopenia (low platelets), or those who are on certain medications, such as anticoagulants, may be at risk for hematoma formation. To prevent hematomas, hold firm pressure on the injection site for at least 2 minutes, but do *not* massage the area. In addition, a 23-gauge needle or finer should be used for clients with bleeding disorders (CDC, 2019a). Monitor the client closely to ensure there is no bleeding or seeping from the injection site.

Aspiration and Intramuscular Injections: Evidence-Based Practice Considerations

The issue of aspiration before an IM injection has been a matter of debate. The question is, "Do you need to aspirate or not before giving an IM injection?" The answer is that it depends on the situation, as well as the medication being administered. Because muscles have a rich blood supply, there may be a small risk of entering or passing through a vessel when administering IM injections. This can be determined by gently aspirating the syringe after the needle is inserted but before giving the injection. However, the CDC has advised that aspiration is not necessary for immunizations because there are no large vessels in the recommended vaccination sites. Moreover, most automatic-disposal (AD) syringes do not allow for aspiration (CDC, 2019a).

A study by Quatrara et al. (2016) supports the assertion that there is minimal risk of entry into a vessel when performing IM injections into the deltoid muscle of clients who are receiving vaccinations. In addition, a position paper by the World Health Organization (WHO) regarding strategies for reducing discomfort during vaccination notes that aspiration before IM vaccinations may cause unnecessary discomfort and is not recommended. The WHO guidelines are based on a systematic review of the literature and expert consensus on vaccinations.

Some authors have suggested that aspiration before IM injections should only be done for large molecule medications (e.g., antibiotics) or medications that have a high risk of causing severe reactions or anaphylaxis if administered intravenously. The expertise of the clinician, as well as the manufacturer guidelines, should be considered (Mann, 2016b).

Further research is needed regarding aspiration before IM injections. Check your facility policy and manufacturer guidelines for the specific medication. If aspiration is required, reduce discomfort by stabilizing the syringe with your nondominant hand to prevent needle and syringe movement. If a significant amount of blood comes back into the syringe, do not give the injection. Withdraw the needle and prepare another needle and syringe for injection.

ADMINISTERING INSULIN

Administration of insulin requires special considerations regarding equipment, preparation, and storage. Although insulin can be given IV, it is most often given by the subcutaneous route. Because insulin is ordered in units, it can only be administered in an insulin syringe designed for that purpose (Fig. 11.17). Select the size of the insulin syringe based on the dose needed. The needle size is usually ¼ inch to ½ inch in length and 28 to 31 gauge. Due to the potential for fatal errors, it is crucial to *never* use a regular tuberculin 1-mL syringe to administer insulin. Regarding storage, unopened insulin may be refrigerated until opened. Once opened, insulin is usually stored at a controlled room temperature. Mark the date of use on the vial, and note the expiration date, which is usually 28 days after it is opened. An example of an insulin vial is seen in Fig. 11.17.

Because most clients who receive insulin have diabetes, they may already have a routine they use for site rotation. If so, follow their rotation schedule. If not, rotate sites in a clockwise direction to avoid using the same site. This will prevent lipodystrophy, which is the process by which fat deposits may harden over time due to repeated injections (Becton

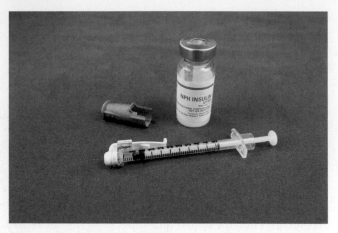

FIG. 11.17 Equipment used for administering insulin: Insulin vial and insulin syringe measured in units.

Dickenson [BD], 2015). Unless contraindicated, the abdomen is the preferred site for injections because absorption tends to be more reliable in that area. Repeated insulin injections should be spaced at least 2.5 cm (1 inch) apart and at least 5 cm (2 inches) away from the umbilicus (Slade, 2015).

Sometimes, two types of insulin will be ordered together (e.g. a short-acting insulin and an intermediate-acting insulin). If this is the case, the short-acting insulin will be drawn up first, and the intermediate-acting insulin will be drawn up last. For example, if regular insulin is ordered with NPH insulin, the regular is a faster-acting form, so it will be drawn up first. This prevents contamination of the short-acting insulin with the intermediate-acting insulin.

Check the manufacturer guidelines and facility policy closely before mixing insulin. Because there may be some intermediate-acting insulin products that are clear, it is not accurate to use the "clear then cloudy" terminology for drawing up two types of insulin medications, as was done in the past. In addition, there are some insulin products that must NOT be mixed.

Depending on the client, determination of their insulin dosages may be based on lab or fingerstick blood sugar (FSBS) results, or it may be guided by the client's carbohydrate, fat, and protein intake. Because insulin is considered to be a time-sensitive medication, clients who are on insulin need to receive their medication in a timely manner in order to prevent complications.

Subcutaneous Insulin Pumps

For clients who need an alternative to injections, insulin pump therapy (also referred to as continuous subcutaneous insulin infusion [CSII]) may be used. Most insulin pumps will be external. However, there are some devices that are fully implantable. For the external pump, the insulin is administered into the client's subcutaneous tissue through an insulin infusion device. As shown in Fig. 11.18A, the infusion device cannula or needle is inserted into the abdomen and held in place by an adhesive. This device is disposable and changed every 2 to 3 days. The programmable insulin pump (see Fig. 11.18B) is a battery-operated electronic device that has a microprocessor and dosing mechanisms (Woten & Heering, 2018). In some models, the

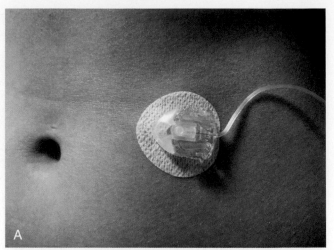

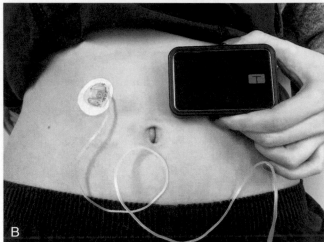

FIG. 11.18 External insulin pump. **A,** Insulin infusion device and cannula. **B,** Programmable insulin pump.

insulin pump may interface with a separate glucose sensor on the client that can help track and regulate glucose and insulin dosages. The insulin pump also contains a reservoir (which may be disposable) that stores the insulin cartridge. As shown in Fig. 11.18B, the flexible tubing provides a conduit from the client's insulin pump and cartridge to the infusion device.

The controls on the insulin pump allow for a constant amount of insulin to be administered (a basal rate) as well as for boluses (additional doses) to be self-administered by the client throughout the day. The client wears the pump around-the-clock and is thus able to maintain a steady state of insulin. If approved and ordered by the authorized healthcare provider, the client can remove the external pump for a short period of time (e.g., an hour) for showers or other activities.

If a hospitalized client has an external insulin pump, determine if the client plans to continue to use it. Depending on the client's medical diagnosis and individual needs, the client may have to revert back to injections during hospitalization per the orders of the authorized healthcare provider. Ensure that the pump is working properly and that the cannula remains intact. It is also important to continue to monitor the client for skin irritation and altered glucose levels (e.g., hypoglycemia, hyperglycemia).

Using Insulin Pens

A device that is being used with increasing frequency is an insulin pen. Insulin pens, which are about the size of a large marker, carry insulin in self-contained cartridges (Fig. 11.19). Some of the pens are reusable and have a replaceable cartridge, and some pens are disposable and discarded after a set number of doses is administered (BD, 2015). Check the manufacturer guidelines for specific instructions.

Because insulin pens are often used for self-injection, it is important to reinforce the procedure for use, as described in Box 11.8. As part of the procedure, the client should be reminded to follow manufacturer instructions for storage and usage. The National Alert Network (NAN) has issued a warning that clients must be reminded to remove both the outer cover of the pen as well as the inner cover that is on the needle. This is critical when using a standard needle at home because many standard needles have an inner needle shield. Several fatalities related to severe hyperglycemia have occurred due to the client failing to remove the inner needle shield before self-injection (NAN, 2017). Ensure that the client can demonstrate the use of the insulin pen, and provide follow-up monitoring to prevent potentially fatal errors.

SUMMARY

The critical concepts of accuracy, client-centered care, infection control, health maintenance, safety, communication, and evaluation are all applicable when administering parenteral medications. Because of the risk for injury, the critical concepts of safety and accuracy are particularly important. These critical concepts are also interrelated. For example, the risk of client injury is reduced and safety is enhanced if the anatomical landmarks for injections sites are accurately identified and the proper technique is used to perform parenteral injections. Using sterile technique and preventing infection will also prevent injury to the client.

APPLICATION OF THE NURSING PROCESS

Examples of Related ICNP Nursing Diagnoses, Expected Client Outcomes, and Nursing Interventions:
Nursing Diagnosis: Risk for injury

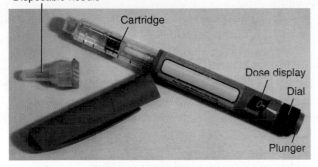

Disposable needle
Cartridge
Dose display
Dial
Plunger

FIG. 11.19 Insulin pen.

BOX 11.8 Client Teaching: Using an Insulin Pen

(Note: Instruct the client to perform the following steps, and encourage return demonstrations.)

1. Wash hands and assemble equipment (e.g., sharps box, wipes, antiseptic wipes, insulin pen).
2. Check the expiration date and client identifier on the label, and check to ensure the insulin pen contains the correct type of insulin. *These safety measures reduce the risk of medication errors.*
3. If the insulin suspension is cloudy, instruct the client to gently roll the insulin pen between the palms of his or her hands and invert or turn the pen upside down for 10 to 20 cycles. Do *not* shake the bottle. *Gentle rolling and inversion will resuspend the insulin.*
4. Wipe the end of the rubber seal cartridge head with an antiseptic wipe and wait until it dries. *These safety measures prevent infection.*
5. Attach a new needle to the end of the pen. Pull off the outer cover and set it aside. **Warn the client that the inner needle cover (if there is one) must also be removed.** *Failing to remove the inner cover prevents the insulin from being properly dispensed.*
6. Prime the pen per the manufacturer instructions. Instruct the client to confirm the flow by looking for a drop of insulin at the end of the pen. *Priming the pen helps to ensure accurate dosing.*
7. After the flow of insulin is confirmed, instruct the client to select the prescribed dose by adjusting the dial. *These safety measures facilitate accuracy.*
8. Select an injection site (usually the abdomen, or thigh if abdomen not acceptable). If the client does not have a rotation schedule, instruct the client to give the injection at least 2.5 cm (1 inch) away from the last injection site and at least 5 cm (2 inches) away from the navel. *This method prevents tissue damage or lipodystrophy.*
9. Instruct the client to clean the site with an antiseptic wipe and let it dry. After the site is cleaned, the client should insert the entire needle all the way into the skin or fat fold at the angle recommended by the manufacturer, press the plunger or button down until the entire dose is administered, and hold the needle in place for at least 10 seconds. (Note: A "pinch up" or fat fold may not be required for some insulin pens or shorter needles. Check the specific manufacturer guidelines.)
10. After 10 seconds, the client should remove the needle from the site and dispose of the needle according to the manufacturer's instructions. Remind the client *not* to massage the injection site. (Note: If the client is using a special safety or autoshield needle, follow the manufacturer instructions for activating the safety device.)
11. Instruct the client to record the dose and injection site in his or her diabetes log book.

References: Becton Dickenson, 2015; National Alert Network, 2017.

Expected Client Outcomes: The client will have no injury from parenteral medications, as seen by:
- absence of scarring, severe bruising, swelling, or lipodystrophy at injection sites
- absence of loss of function or signs and symptoms of nerve damage at injection site.

Nursing Intervention Example: Identify anatomical landmarks for injection sites.

Reference: International Classification for Nursing Practice. (n.d.). *eHealth & ICNP.* Retrieved from https://www.icn.ch/what-we-do/projects/ehealth-icnp.

CRITICAL CONCEPTS
Administering Parenteral Medications

Accuracy (ACC)

Administration of parenteral medications is sensitive to the following variables:

Client-Related Factors
- Client's assessment, including level of consciousness and orientation
- Client's ability to hear and understand instructions regarding injections
- Condition of client's skin (dermal layer), subcutaneous tissue, and musculature
- Client's age, weight, size of muscles, and presence of any muscle wasting.

Nurse-Related and System-Related Factors
- Adherence to approved safety guidelines (e.g., ISMP, The Joint Commission, FDA)
- Performing dosage calculation accurately when needed
- Proper storage, handling, and labeling of parenteral medications
- Correct identification of anatomical landmarks and appropriate selection of injection sites
- Technique used for processing orders, preparing and administering parenteral medications, and providing follow-up care and monitoring
- Proper use, selection, and assembly of equipment (e.g., syringes needle, ampules, vials).

Client-Centered Care (CCC)

Respect for the client when administering parenteral medications is demonstrated by:

- promoting autonomy and obtaining verbal consent before injections
- providing privacy and ensuring comfort during injections
- honoring cultural preferences and arranging an interpreter if needed
- advocating for the client and family and explaining injection procedures.

Infection Control (INF)

Healthcare-associated infection when administering parenteral medications is prevented by:
- preventing and reducing the transfer of microorganisms
- reducing the number of microorganisms.

Safety (SAF)

Safety measures when administering parenteral medications prevent harm and maintain a safe care environment, including:
- checking for allergies and contraindications and following safety checks and guidelines.

Communication (COM)

- Communication exchanges information (verbal, nonverbal, written, or electronic) between two or more people.
- Documentation records information in a permanent legal record.
- Collaboration with the client and other healthcare providers enhances care and client teaching.

Health Maintenance (HLTH)

Nursing is dedicated to the promotion of health and self-care abilities when administering parenteral medications by:
- protecting and caring for the client's skin and rotating sites for injections
- monitoring the client's skin for any sign of changes or breakdown at injection sites.

Evaluation (EVAL)

When administering parenteral medications, evaluation of outcomes enables the nurse to determine the therapeutic response and safety of the care provided by:
- monitoring the therapeutic effect of the medication
- monitoring for side effects, adverse effects, interactions, or allergic reactions.

▪ SKILL 11.13 Preparing a Medication From a Vial

EQUIPMENT

Medication vial
Antiseptic wipes
Syringe (size based on dose)
Safety needle (size based on type of injection)
Needleless access device and adapter for vial (if required)

BEGINNING THE SKILL

1. **ACC** Review the order for:
   - name, dosage, and strength of medication in vial for injection
   - time intervals, frequency, route of administration, any special instructions
   - purpose of administering medication

2. **ACC** Review the following:
   - **SAF** Client's allergies to medications or other substances
   - **SAF** Indications, contraindications, and appropriateness of medication for the client
   - Client's age, medical/surgical history, lab results, and medical condition
   - Medication history (to check for potential drug interactions).
3. **INF** Perform hand hygiene.
4. **CCC** Introduce yourself to the client and family.
5. **SAF** Identify the client using at least two client identifiers.
6. **CCC** Provide privacy.
7. **ACC** Assess the client's level of consciousness and orientation to person, time, place, and situation. *Provides a baseline assessment of orientation before verbal consent is obtained.*
8. **CCC** Explain the procedure and obtain verbal consent. *To provide client-centered care and prevent waste, consent should be obtained before preparing medications.*
9. **ACC** Perform additional client preassessments (e.g., vital signs, level of pain) as indicated.

PROCEDURE

Preparing the Medication From a Vial

10. **SAF** Perform the **first safety checkpoint** when accessing the medication, and initiate the **second safety checkpoint** when preparing the medication. Check the rights of administration, check the expiration date, and scan the bar code on the vial if required.
11. **SAF** Obtain a SDV for one-time, single client use if available. *SDVs are recommended to reduce the risk of contamination and unsafe practices.* (**WARNING:** Do not reuse a SDV or store for future use [CDC, 2019b]).
12. **SAF** If using an MDV, check facility policy and dedicate the vial for single client use if required. Label the vial with the date and client's name (CDC, 2019b). **WARNING:** Check the manufacturer recommendations. Some MDVs contain preservatives that should not be used for infants and neonates.
13. **SAF** Inspect the vial for any unusual cloudiness or particulates, and ensure that the label clearly shows the client's name, the date vial was opened, and the expiration date. If vial has expired or is past the safe-use date, discard the vial per policy and obtain a new vial. *Before using any vial, it is essential to know when it was opened to ensure that it has not exceeded the safe-use date.*
14. **ACC** Determine the volume of medication required for the order. Perform dosage calculations if necessary and double-check calculations.
15. **INF** Perform hand hygiene again.
16. **ACC** Assemble the equipment in the med-prep area, and prepare the medication. Continue the **second safety checkpoint** and check the rights of administration.

   a. **SAF** Place the vial on a clean, dry surface at an ergonomically safe working height.
   b. **INF** Remove the cap from the top of the vial. Cleanse the rubber stopper/septum firmly with an antiseptic wipe. *The manufacturer does not guarantee the sterility of rubber cap.*
   c. Open the syringe and needle package. Place the needle or needleless access device securely on the syringe without contaminating the needle, adapter, or syringe. Turn the syringe clockwise to tighten.

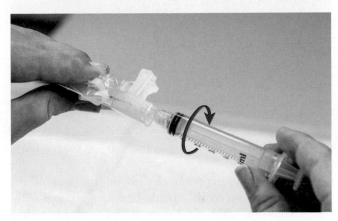

STEP 16C Attach the needle and syringe and ensure it is secure.

   d. Remove the cap from the needle or needleless access device by pulling it straight off and away from your hand. Place the cap on a clean, dry surface without contaminating it.

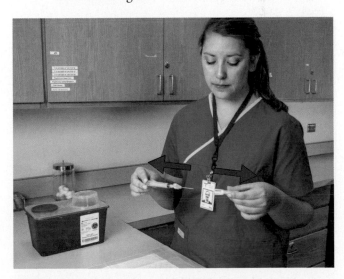

STEP 16D Pull the cap straight off the needle.

   e. Draw air back into the syringe in the amount that the dosage was calculated. For example, if 2 mL was calculated, pull 2 mL of air back into the syringe. Touch only the plunger tip when drawing back the plunger. *Touching the body of the plunger could contaminate the medication when the plunger is reinserted into syringe.*

f. Insert the needle or needleless access device into the vial. Inject air in syringe above the surface of the medication in the vial. *Prevents a vacuum from forming in the vial.*

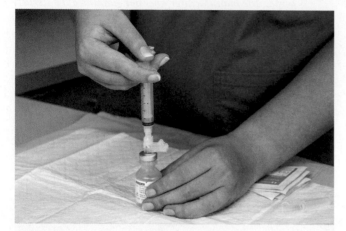

STEP 16F Insert the needle and inject air into vial.

g. While holding your thumb on the end of the plunger, invert the vial, hold it securely, and withdraw the calculated dose at eye level by pulling back on the syringe plunger tip. Ensure that tip of the needle or access device is below the surface of the fluid. *Holding the plunger tip after inverting the vial prevents the needle from displacing. Ensuring that the needle or access device remains below the surface of the medication prevents air from being drawn into the syringe.*

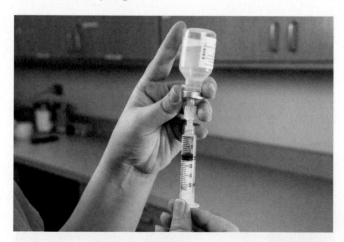

STEP 16G Withdraw the dose of medication at eye level.

h. While the vial is still inverted and the syringe is in the vial, remove any bubbles. (Note: Bubbles can be removed by using the plunger to pull down sharply enough to dislodge the bubbles, withdrawing some additional medication, and then pushing the air bubbles into the vial or by gently tapping the outer surface of the syringe with a fingernail or pen.) *Removing bubbles from the syringe is crucial to ensure that the correct dosage is given to the client.*

i. Adjust the volume of medication in the syringe to the volume calculated in Step 14. The ordered dose should be measured on the syringe scale at the top flat rim of the black plunger seal of the syringe (see Figure. 11.8). (Note: Do *not* remove the syringe from the vial and express medication into the air or trashcan. This wastes medication and risks splatter.)

j. Return the vial back to an upright position. *Pulling the needle and syringe or adapter out without returning the vial to an upright position can result in injury or medication spray from vacuum pressure.*

k. Remove the syringe and needle or adapter from the vial. Without contaminating the needle, safely scoop the cap on needle or needleless access device.

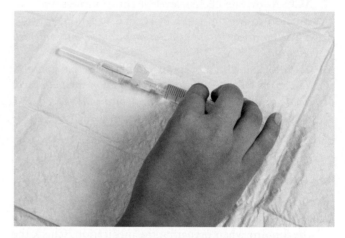

STEP 16K Use safe method to replace cap.

17. **SAF** Complete the **second safety checkpoint** and check the rights of administration again. Label the syringe per facility policy (e.g., client's name, medication, dose, route, date, time). Reverify the label on the syringe and medication ampule (if available) against the MAR or EMAR before taking the medication to the client's room. **WARNING:** Never prelabel a syringe before the medication is drawn up. *Prelabeling a syringe before the medication is drawn up may increase the risk of errors (ISMP, 2015).*

18. **SAF** Take the prepared and labeled medication to the client's bedside for the **third safety checkpoint** with the client. Ensure that the medication is given to the client as soon as possible. *Administering a prepared medication immediately reduces the risk of medication errors.*

FINISHING THE SKILL

19. **INF** Dispose of equipment used to prepare medication per policy. (Note: Many facilities require that SDVs must be disposed of immediately after opening and that MDVs must be disposed of within 24 hours after opening.)

20. **INF** Perform hand hygiene.

21. **EVAL** Evaluate the outcomes. Were infection control principles, safety checkpoints, and rights of administration followed? Was the medication prepared without contamination?

■ SKILL 11.14 Preparing a Medication From an Ampule

EQUIPMENT

Medication ampule (for one-time dose)
Filter needle or filter straw, puncture-proof sharps box
Antiseptic wipes and 2 × 2 or 4 × 4 gauze
Syringe (size based on dose)
Safety needle (size based on type of injection)
Clean gloves, per facility policy

BEGINNING THE SKILL

1. **ACC** Review the client's order for medication name, dosage, type, and route, and review the client's medical and surgical history (refer to Skill 11.13, steps 1 and 2).
2. **INF** Perform hand hygiene.
3. **CCC** Introduce yourself to the client and family.
4. **SAF** Identify the client using at least two client identifiers.
5. **CCC** Provide privacy.
6. **ACC** Assess the client's level of consciousness and orientation to person, time, place, and situation. *Provides a baseline assessment of orientation before verbal consent is obtained.*
7. **CCC** Explain the procedure and obtain verbal consent. *To provide client-centered care and prevent waste, consent should be obtained before preparing medications.*
8. **ACC** Perform additional client preassessments (e.g., vital signs, level of pain) as indicated.

PROCEDURE

Preparing the Medication From an Ampule

9. **SAF** Perform the **first safety checkpoint** when accessing the medication, and initiate the **second safety checkpoint** when preparing the medication. Check the rights of administration, check the expiration date, and scan the bar code (if present) on the medication if required.
10. **ACC** Inspect the ampule for any unusual cloudiness or particulates, and ensure that the label clearly shows the expiration date. If the ampule has expired or is past the safe-use date, discard per policy and obtain a new ampule. *Before using any ampule, it is essential to know that the medication has not expired.*
11. **ACC** Determine the volume of medication required for the order. Perform dosage calculations if necessary and double-check calculations.
12. **INF** Perform hand hygiene. If there will be a risk of exposure to body fluids or chemicals, apply gloves per facility policy.
13. **ACC** Assemble equipment in the med-prep area, and prepare the medication. Continue the **second safety checkpoint** and check the rights of administration.

a. **SAF** Place the ampule on a clean, dry surface at an ergonomically safe height.
b. **INF** Open up the syringe package and a filter needle or filter straw package. Maintain sterility of the syringe and needle.
c. **INF** Using sterile technique, attach the filter needle or straw to the syringe (see Skill 11.13). If using a filter straw, leave the tip in the sterile package until you are ready to draw up the medication. *This prevents contamination of the filter straw.*
d. Hold the ampule upright at eye level and ensure that the medication is clear and free of particulates, and ensure that the medication is in main body of the ampule (not above the neck). *Prevents loss of medication within the ampule head.*

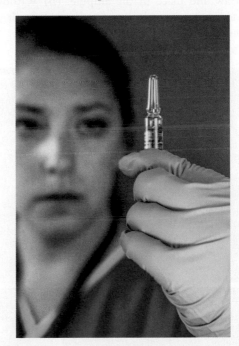

STEP 13D Inspect medication at eye level.

e. If there is medication above the neck of the ampule, use a brisk downward motion to displace the medication down into the ampule body. Avoid aggressive tapping.
f. **INF** Clean the neck of ampule with an antiseptic wipe. *Prevents contamination.*
g. **SAF** Using a gauze pad, snap the head of the ampule (away from your body) with your dominant hand, and discard the ampule head into a sharps box. *Breaking the head away from the nurse's body and hands, and using gauze protects the nurse from shard cuts.*

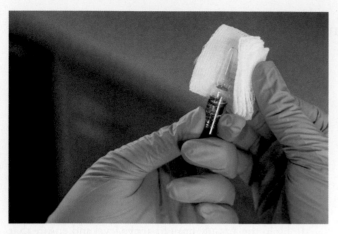

STEP 13G Use a protective gauze pad when snapping the head of the ampule.

h. (A) Insert the syringe with attached filter needle or straw and place in the ampule. (B) Withdraw the medication into the syringe. If needed, tilt the ampule to facilitate obtaining the medication.

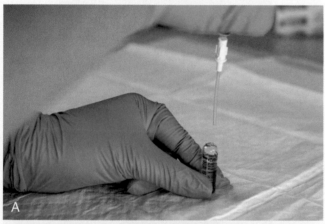

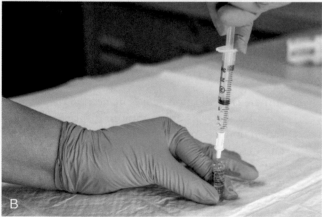

STEP 13H Withdraw medication using a filter straw.

i. Inspect the medication as it is withdrawn to ensure there are no glass shards in the medication. After removal of the medication, discard the ampule into a sharps box.

j. Activate the safety device on filter needle or remove the filter needle or straw, and replace it with a nonfilter needle or needleless device. Adjust the volume of medication in the syringe to the volume calculated in Step 11. Waste medication according to your facility policy. *Removing the filter needle prevents administration of glass shards into the client.* **WARNING:** Never give the client an injection with a filter needle in place.

k. Dispose of the filter needle or straw in a sharps box.

14. **SAF** Complete the **second safety checkpoint** and check the rights of administration again. Label the syringe per facility policy (e.g., client's name, medication, dose, route, date, time). Reverify the label on the syringe against the MAR or EMAR before taking the medication to the client's room. **WARNING:** Never prelabel a syringe before the medication is drawn up. *Prelabeling a syringe before the medication is drawn up may increase the risk of errors (ISMP, 2015).*

15. **SAF** Take the prepared and labeled medication to the client's bedside for the **third safety checkpoint** with the client. Ensure that the medication is given to the client as soon as possible. *Administering a prepared medication immediately reduces the risk of medication errors.*

FINISHING THE SKILL

16. **INF** Dispose of equipment per facility policy. (Note: Ampules are usually disposed of immediately in a puncture-proof sharps box after medication is obtained from the ampule.)

17. **INF** Remove gloves if worn and perform hand hygiene.

18. **EVAL** Evaluate the outcomes. *Was medication obtained from the ampule without difficulty?*

■ SKILL 11.15 Preparing a Medication That Requires Reconstitution

EQUIPMENT

Powdered medication vial

Diluent (e.g., sterile water for injection, normal saline for injection)

Puncture-proof sharps box

Antiseptic wipes

Syringe (size based on dose), safety needle (size based on type of injection)

Clean gloves, per facility policy

BEGINNING THE SKILL

1. **ACC** Review the client's order for medication name, dosage, type, and route, and review client's medical and surgical history (refer to Skill 11.13, steps 1 and 2).
2. **INF** Perform hand hygiene.
3. **CCC** Introduce yourself to the client and family.
4. **SAF** Identify the client using at least two client identifiers.
5. **CCC** Provide privacy.
6. **ACC** Assess the client's level of consciousness and orientation to person, time, place, and situation. *Provides a baseline assessment of orientation before verbal consent is obtained.*
7. **CCC** Explain the procedure and obtain verbal consent. *To provide client-centered care and prevent waste, consent should be obtained before preparing the medication.*
8. **ACC** Perform additional client preassessments (e.g., vital signs, level of pain) as indicated.

PROCEDURE

Preparing the Medication for Reconstitution

9. **SAF** Perform the **first safety checkpoint** when accessing the medication, and initiate the **second safety checkpoint** when preparing the medication. Check the rights of administration, check the expiration date, and scan the bar code on the medication vial if required.
10. **ACC** Inspect powdered medication within the vial for signs of unusual discoloration or contaminants in the medication. If the vial has expired, discard per facility policy and obtain a new vial. *Prevents unsafe medication practices (CDC, 2019b).*
11. **ACC** Review the medication package insert (provided by the manufacturer) and label for:
    - type of diluent required (e.g., sterile water or normal saline for injection in SDV)
    - amount of diluent required based on the concentration and dosage ordered
    - instructions for reconstituting, mixing, and storage of the medication, and instructions regarding the time frame of when medication must be discarded after reconstitution.

12. **ACC** Inspect the diluent vial for any unusual cloudiness or particulates, and ensure that the label clearly shows the expiration date. If the vial has expired or is past the safe-use date, discard per facility policy and obtain a new vial. *Before using any medication, it is essential to know that the medication has not expired.*
13. **ACC** Determine the volume of medication required for the order. Perform dosage calculations if necessary and double check calculations.
14. **INF** Perform hand hygiene again. If there will be risk of exposure to body fluids or chemicals, apply gloves per facility policy.
15. **ACC** Assemble equipment in the med-prep area, and prepare medication. Continue the **second safety checkpoint** and check the rights of administration.
    a. **SAF** Place both the powdered medication vial and the diluent vial on a clean, dry surface at an ergonomically safe height.

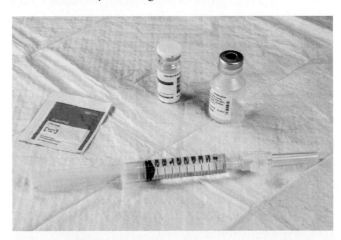

STEP 15A Prepare medication.

    b. **INF** Attach the sterile needle or needleless access device to the syringe. (Note: The optimal size of the syringe and needle will depend on the volume to be administered and the viscosity of the medication.)
    c. **INF** Remove caps from the medication vial and diluent vial and clean both rubber stoppers firmly with antiseptic wipes. Allow at least 10 seconds for both vials to dry. *The manufacturer does not guarantee the sterility of the stoppers of either vial.*
    d. **INF** Using sterile technique, withdraw the amount of diluent needed based on the dosage ordered and manufacturer instructions (see Skill 11.13).
    e. Inject diluent into powdered medication vial. Remove syringe from vial and safely scoop cap on needle or needleless access device (see Skill 11.13).

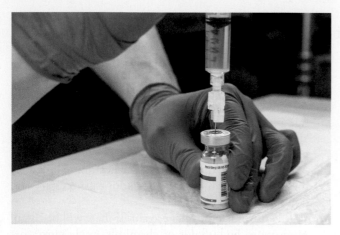

STEP 15E Inject diluent into the vial.

f. After the diluent has been injected into the medication vial, hold the vial and gently roll it between your hands per manufacturer instructions until the powdered medication is dissolved or suspended. (Note: Technique will vary for agitation of vials depending on the medication; some should not be shaken. Check the manufacturer insert for specific instructions.)

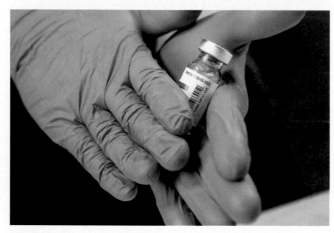

STEP 15F Gently roll vial.

g. Clean the stopper of the vial containing reconstituted medication again with an antiseptic wipe and allow to dry. *Provides an additional safeguard to prevent infection.*

h. Remove the cap from the syringe and draw up the ordered medication (see Skill 11.13).

16. **SAF** Complete the **second safety checkpoint** and check the rights of administration again. Label the syringe per facility policy (e.g., client's name, medication, dose, route, date, time). Reverify the label on the syringe and reconstituted medication vial (if available) against the MAR or EMAR before taking the medication to the client's room. **WARNING:** Never prelabel a syringe before the medication is drawn up. *Prelabeling a syringe before the medication is drawn up may increase the risk of errors.* (ISMP, 2015).

17. **SAF** Take the prepared and labeled medication to the client's bedside for the **third safety checkpoint** with the client. Ensure that the medication is given to the client as soon as possible. *Administering a prepared medication immediately reduces the risk of medication errors.*

FINISHING THE SKILL

18. **INF** Dispose of the equipment per facility policy. (Note: Many facilities require that the reconstituted medication vial be disposed of immediately after usage, depending on the stability of the reconstituted medication and the manufacturer instructions.)

19. **INF** Remove gloves if worn and perform hand hygiene.

20. **EVAL** Evaluate the outcomes. Did the reconstituted medication suspend properly as expected? Were the rights of administration followed? Was the medication labeled properly?

■ SKILL 11.16 Administering an Intradermal Injection

EQUIPMENT

Medication for injection (ampule, vial, or prefilled syringe)
Calculator (if needed for dosage calculation)
Clean gloves, per facility policy
Antiseptic wipes and gauze pads (if necessary)
Puncture-proof sharps box
Waterproof marker, if necessary
Syringe (1 mL) and needle (⅜–¾ inch, 26–28 gauge)

BEGINNING THE SKILL

1. **ACC** Review order for:
   • name of medication for injection and dosage
   • route of administration and special instructions

   • purpose of administering intradermal (e.g., TB skin test, allergy testing).

2. **ACC** Review the following:
   • client's allergies to medications or other substances
   • indications and any contraindications for intradermal medication
   • appropriateness of intradermal injection for the client (using medication rights)
   • medication history and history of previous intradermal injections and reactions
   • medical history (including history of positive TB skin tests and allergies).

3. **INF** Perform hand hygiene.
4. **CCC** Introduce yourself to the client and family.
5. **SAF** Identify the client using at least two client identifiers.
6. **CCC** Provide privacy.
7. **ACC** Assess the client's level of consciousness and orientation to person, time, place, and situation. *Provides a baseline assessment of orientation before verbal consent is obtained.*
8. **CCC** Explain the procedure and obtain verbal consent. *To provide client-centered care and prevent waste, consent should be obtained before preparing medications.*
9. **ACC** Perform client preassessments, including but not limited to the following:
   - condition of the skin in the area where the injection will be administered.

PROCEDURE

Preparing the Intradermal Medication

10. **SAF** If available, obtain a single-dose medication (ampule, vial, or prefilled syringe). *Single-dose medications are recommended if available (CDC, 2019b).*
11. **SAF** Perform the **first safety checkpoint** when accessing the medication, and initiate the **second safety checkpoint** when preparing the medication and injection. Check the rights of administration, check the expiration date, and scan the bar code on the medication if required.
12. **ACC** Perform dosage calculations if necessary and double-check calculations.
13. **ACC** Inspect intradermal medication (ampule, vial, or prefilled syringe) for unusual cloudiness or particulates. *Prevents administration of contaminated or unsafe medication.*
14. **ACC** Assemble equipment in the med-prep area, and prepare the intradermal injection. Continue the **second safety checkpoint** and check the rights of administration.
15. **ACC** If using a prefilled syringe for intradermal injection, ensure that safety needle and bar-code label (per facility policy) are secured on the syringe.
16. **ACC** If using a vial or ampule for intradermal injection:
    a. **SAF** Place the vial or ampule on a clean, dry surface at an ergonomically safe height.
    b. **INF** Cleanse the septum of vial (if used) vigorously with an antiseptic wipe and allow to dry.
    c. **INF** Using sterile technique, attach the needle to the syringe.
    d. Prepare and withdraw medication using the procedure shown in Skill 11.13 or 11.14.
17. **SAF** Complete the **second safety checkpoint** and check the rights of administration again before labeling the syringe. Label the syringe per facility policy (e.g., client's name, medication dose, route, date, time). Reverify the label on the syringe and medication vial (if available) against the MAR or EMAR before administering the intradermal injection. **WARNING:** Administer the

intradermal injection as soon as possible after preparation. *Immediate administration after preparation reduces the risk of medication errors.*

Administering the Intradermal Injection

18. **INF** Perform hand hygiene again upon entering the client's room.
19. **CCC** Maintain client privacy.
20. **SAF** Reverify the client's identity by using at least two client identifiers.
21. **SAF** Recheck the client's armband for allergies, and ask the client verbally if he or she has allergies.
22. **SAF** Perform the **third safety checkpoint** and review the medication with the client. Check the rights of administration again. *This facilitates client involvement.* (Note: If required, scan the client's armband and the bar code on the medication label if available.)
23. **ACC** After all safety checks are completed, apply gloves if required by facility policy and administer injection.
    a. Position the client in a comfortable position with the arm supported by a pillow or table.
    b. Select site for intradermal injection (usually on the inner aspect of forearm). Avoid sites of previous injections or areas that have bruising, broken skin, or lesions.
    c. Cleanse selected site with an antiseptic wipe by moving from the injection site outward in a circular pattern. *Moving outward in a circular pattern removes debris.*

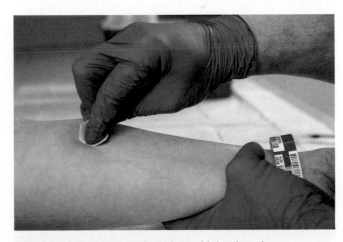

STEP 23C Prepare the intradermal injection site.

    d. Allow the site to dry completely. *Enhances antiseptic activity and prevents stinging at the site.*
    e. Remove the cap from the needle and stretch the skin taut with your nondominant hand. Avoid touching the site that has been prepped. *Prevents contamination of injection site.*
    f. Using your dominant hand, position the needle in a bevel-up position, and insert the needle into the skin at a 5- to 15-degree angle (almost parallel to the client's skin). *This angle facilitates entry into the dermal layer of the client's skin.*

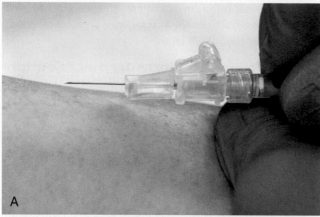

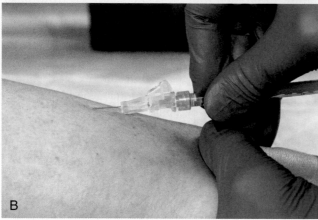

STEP 23F A, Position the needle bevel up. **B,** Insert the needle at a 10- to 15-degree angle.

g. Release skin and slowly inject the medication. Push the plunger with the thumb of your dominant hand while stabilizing the syringe with your nondominant hand. Look for a wheal formation. *A wheal verifies that the medication was given in the dermal layer.*

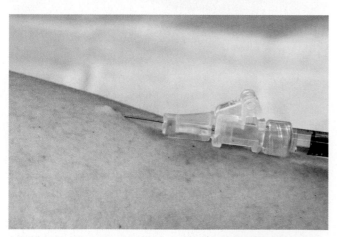

STEP 23G Inject medication and look for wheal.

h. After the injection is completed, remove the needle quickly and smoothly at the same point/angle it was inserted, and then activate the safety device on the needle guard. *Using a safety needle properly prevents injuries.* (Note: If using a special safety system or an automatic-disposable (AD) syringe, activate the mechanism and remove the syringe per the manufacturer recommendations.) **WARNING:** Do *not* massage the injection site.

i. Discard needle and syringe into puncture-proof sharps container.

24. **COM** If the injection is given for TB or allergy testing, circle the injection site with a waterproof marker per facility policy. *Facilitates identification of site for diagnostic purposes later.*

25. **COM** Instruct the client not to rub the arm at the injection site. *Rubbing the arm could alter the test.*

26. **SAF** If the facility has a **postadministration checkpoint,** review the used vial (if available) against the MAR or EMAR. If any errors occurred, notify the authorized healthcare provider immediately.

27. **EVAL** Monitor the client for any adverse or unexpected effects of the medication.

FINISHING THE SKILL

28. **INF** Remove gloves if worn and perform hand hygiene.

29. **SAF** Ensure client safety and comfort. Ensure that the bed is in the lowest position, and verify that the client can identify and reach the nurse call system. *These safety measures reduce the risk of falls.*

30. **EVAL** Evaluate the outcomes. *Did the client tolerate the injection without difficulty?*

31. **COM** Document assessment findings, medication administration, and outcomes in the legal healthcare record:

   • name of medication given, exact time, date, dose, and route

   • location of intradermal injection (e.g., right or left inner forearm)

   • appearance of injection site and presence of wheal or redness at site

   • signature and initials of the clinician who administered the medication.

▪ SKILL 11.17 Administering a Subcutaneous Injection

EQUIPMENT

Medication for injection (ampule, vial, or prefilled syringe)
Clean gloves, per facility policy
Antiseptic wipes
Bandage, 2 × 2 gauze pads, and hypoallergenic tape, if needed
Puncture-proof sharps box
Syringe (1–2 mL) and needle (⅜–1 inch, 26–28 gauge)

BEGINNING THE SKILL

1. **ACC** Review the order for:
   • name of medication for injection and dosage
   • route of administration and special instructions
   • purpose of administering subcutaneous injection.
2. **ACC** Review the following:
   • **SAF** client's allergies to medications or other substances
   • **SAF** indications and any contraindications for subcutaneous medication
   • appropriateness of subcutaneous medication for client (using medication rights)
   • client age and condition, lab results, medication history, and medical-surgical history.
3. **INF** Perform hand hygiene.
4. **CCC** Introduce yourself to the client and family.
5. **SAF** Identify the client using at least two client identifiers.
6. **CCC** Provide privacy.
7. **ACC** Assess the client's level of consciousness and orientation to person, time, place, and situation. *Provides a baseline assessment of orientation before verbal consent is obtained.*
8. **CCC** Explain the procedure and obtain verbal consent. *To provide client-centered care and prevent waste, consent should be obtained before preparing medications.*
9. **ACC** Perform client preassessments, including but not limited to the following:
   • condition and amount of subcutaneous tissue where injection will be administered
   • level of pain using a facility-approved pain tool if indicated.

PROCEDURE

Preparing the Subcutaneous Injection

10. **SAF** If available, use a single-dose medication (ampule, vial, or prefilled syringe). *SDVs and medications are recommended if available (CDC, 2019b).*
11. **SAF** Perform the **first safety checkpoint** when accessing the medication, and initiate the **second safety checkpoint** when preparing the medication and injection. Check the rights of administration, check the expiration date, and scan the bar code on the medication if required.

12. **ACC** Perform dosage calculations if necessary and double-check calculations.
13. **ACC** Inspect subcutaneous medication (ampule, vial, or prefilled syringe) for unusual cloudiness or particulates. *Prevents administration of contaminated or unsafe medication.*
14. **ACC** Assemble equipment in the med-prep area, and prepare subcutaneous injection. Continue the **second safety checkpoint** and check the rights of administration.
15. **ACC** If using a prefilled syringe for the subcutaneous injection, ensure that the safety needle and bar-code label (per facility policy) are secured on the syringe.
16. **ACC** If using a vial or ampule for subcutaneous injection:
    a. **SAF** Place the vial or ampule on a clean, dry surface at an ergonomically safe height.
    b. **INF** Cleanse the septum of the vial (if used) vigorously with an antiseptic wipe and allow to dry.
    c. **INF** Using sterile technique, attach the needle to the syringe. (Note: For subcutaneous injections, a needle size of ⅜ to 1 inch, 24 to 27 gauge, and a syringe size of 0.5 to 2 mL is used. If the client has limited subcutaneous tissue, a shorter needle may be needed.)
    d. Prepare and withdraw the medication using the procedure shown in Skill 11.13 or 11.14.
17. **SAF** Complete the **second safety checkpoint** and check the rights of administration again. Label the syringe per facility policy (e.g., client's name, medication dose, route, date, time). Reverify the label on the syringe and medication vial (if available) against the MAR or EMAR before administering the subcutaneous injection. **WARNING:** Administer the subcutaneous injection as soon as possible after preparation. *Immediate administration after preparation reduces the risk of medication errors.*

Administering the Subcutaneous Injection

18. **INF** Perform hand hygiene again upon entering the client's room.
19. **INF** Maintain client privacy.
20. **SAF** Reverify the client's identity by using at least two client identifiers.
21. **SAF** Recheck the client's armband for allergies, and ask the client verbally if he or she has allergies.
22. **SAF** Perform the **third safety checkpoint** and review the medication with the client. Check the rights of administration again. *This facilitates client involvement.* (Note: If required, scan the client's armband and bar code on the medication label if available.)

23. **ACC** After all safety checks have been completed, apply gloves if required by facility policy and administer the injection.

   a. Position the client in a comfortable position so that the injection site is easily accessible.

   b. Select site for subcutaneous injection (e.g., back of arm, abdomen). Avoid sites of previous injections or areas that have bruising, broken skin, scars, or lesions. If the client is receiving multiple injections, rotate sites. *Prevents trauma and tissue damage.*

   c. If giving medication in the abdomen, avoid the umbilicus by a 5-cm (2-inch) radius (Slade, 2015).

   d. Cleanse selected site with an antiseptic wipe by moving from the injection site outward in a circular pattern. Avoid touching the site where the injection will be given after it has been cleaned. *Moving outward in a circular pattern moves debris away from the site.*

   e. Allow site to dry. *Enhances antiseptic activity and prevents stinging at the site.*

   f. Remove cap from needle and set it aside. If required, pinch or bunch up the client's skin and subcutaneous tissue with your nondominant hand. Using your dominant hand, insert the needle into the client's subcutaneous tissue smoothly, quickly, and gently at a 45-degree angle. *This method helps ensure that the injection will enter the subcutaneous tissue and not the muscle. (CDC, 2019a)* (Note: Some manufacturers do not require pinching or bunching up of the skin. The angle of entry depends on the length of the needle, the manufacturer recommendation, and the amount of subcutaneous tissue the client has. If the client has adequate subcutaneous tissue and the needle is short enough to ensure entry into the client's subcutaneous tissue a 90-degree angle may be used.)

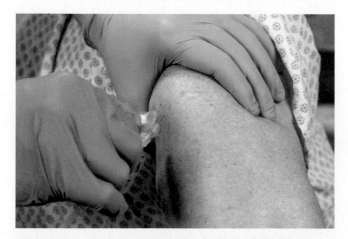

STEP 23F Approach the subcutaneous injection site.

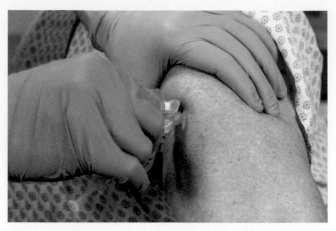

STEP 23F Insert the needle at a 45-degree angle.

   g. Using your dominant hand, inject the medication at an appropriate rate, depending on viscosity of the medication and the manufacturer recommendations. If needed, stabilize the syringe with your nondominant hand during the injection. *The rate of injection will vary depending on the viscosity of the medication. A higher viscosity will require slower injection. (Note: Aspiration before a subcutaneous injection is not necessary.)*

   h. If giving subcutaneous heparin, wait at least 10 seconds before withdrawing the medication. *Waiting at least 10 seconds may reduce bleeding and bruising (Slade, 2015).*

   i. After waiting the appropriate amount of time, remove the needle quickly/smoothly at the same point/angle it was inserted, and then activate the safety device on the needle guard. (Note: If using a special safety system or an automatic-disposable [AD] syringe, activate the device per manufacturer instructions. Apply gentle pressure to the injection site if needed.)

   WARNING: Do *not* massage site, particularly after subcutaneous heparin.

   j. Discard the needle and syringe into a puncture-proof sharps container.

   k. Place bandage or gauze pad with hypoallergenic tape on site if needed.

24. **SAF** If the facility has a **postadministration checkpoint,** review the used vial (if available) against the MAR or EMAR. If any errors occurred, notify the authorized healthcare provider.

25. **EVAL** Monitor the client for any adverse or unexpected effects of the medication. If the client received an anticoagulant, monitor the injection site closely for bleeding or bruising.

FINISHING THE SKILL

26. **INF** Remove gloves if worn and perform hand hygiene.

27. **SAF** Ensure client safety and comfort. Ensure that the bed is in the lowest position, and verify that the client can identify and reach the nurse call system. *These safety measures reduce the risk of falls.*

28. **EVAL** Evaluate the outcomes. *Did the client tolerate the injection? Is there minimal bruising at the injection site?*
29. **COM** Document assessment findings, medication administration, and outcomes in the legal healthcare record:
    - name of medication given, exact time, date, dose, and route
    - location of subcutaneous injection (e.g., left upper quadrant, abdomen)
    - signature and initials of the clinician who administered the medication.

Follow-up

30. **EVAL** Monitor the client for any redness, irritation, numbness, or other symptoms at the injection site. Instruct the client to report any difficulty with the injections after discharge.
31. **COM** If the client will be self-administering a subcutaneous medication such as enoxaparin (Lovenox), assess the client's orientation level and ability to perform the injection, and provide client/family teaching as described in Box 11.6.
32. **COM** Document the client education provided and the client's ability to perform the injection.

■ SKILL 11.18 Administering an Intramuscular Injection

Medication for IM injection (ampule, vial, or prefilled syringe)
Clean gloves, if required by facility policy
Antiseptic wipes
Bandage, 2 × 2 gauze pads, and hypoallergenic tape, if needed
Puncture-proof sharps box
Syringe and needle of correct size (refer to Box 11.7)

BEGINNING THE SKILL

1. **ACC** Review the order for:
   - name of medication for IM injection
   - dosage and any special instructions
   - purpose of administering IM injection.
2. **ACC** Review the following:
   - **SAF** client's allergies to medications or other substances
   - **SAF** indications and any contraindications for IM medication
   - appropriateness of IM medication for client (using medication rights)
   - age, condition, medical history (particularly muscle wasting or bleeding disorders)
   - medication history (to check for potential drug interactions)
   - recent lab work. **WARNING:** If client has low platelet count or coagulation disorders, notify authorized healthcare provider before administering IM injection.
3. **INF** Perform hand hygiene.
4. **CCC** Introduce yourself to the client and family.
5. **SAF** Identify the client using at least two client identifiers.
6. **CCC** Provide privacy.
7. **ACC** Assess the client's level of consciousness and orientation to person, time, place, and situation. *Provides*

a baseline assessment of orientation before verbal consent is obtained.
8. **CCC** Explain procedure and obtain verbal consent. *To provide client-centered care and prevent waste, consent should be obtained before preparing medications.*
9. **ACC** Perform client preassessments, which may include:
   - condition and amount of muscle mass in area where injection will be administered
   - vital signs if indicated and affected by medication (e.g., vasoactive drugs).

PROCEDURE

Preparing the IM Injection

10. **SAF** If available, obtain a single-dose medication (ampule, vial, or prefilled syringe). *Single-dose medications are recommended if available (CDC, 2019b).*
11. **SAF** Perform the **first safety checkpoint** when accessing the medication, and initiate the **second safety checkpoint** when preparing the medication and injection. Check the rights of administration, check the expiration date, and scan the bar code on the medication if required.
12. **ACC** Determine the volume of medication required for the order. Perform dosage calculations if necessary and double-check the calculations.
13. **ACC** Inspect IM medication (ampule, vial, or prefilled syringe) for unusual cloudiness or particulates. *Prevents administration of contaminated or unsafe medication.*
14. **ACC** Assemble equipment in the med-prep area, and prepare IM injection. Continue the **second safety checkpoint** and check rights of administration.
15. **ACC** If using a prefilled syringe for the IM injection, ensure that the safety needle and bar-code label (per facility policy) are secured on syringe.

16. **ACC** If using a vial or ampule for IM injection:
    a. Select appropriate needle and syringe based on the client's age, size, muscle tissue volume/viscosity of the medication, and injection site (see Box 11.7). (Note: If the client is frail, a shorter needle may be needed. If the client is obese, a longer needle, such as 1.5 inch, may be required to ensure entry into muscle instead of subcutaneous tissue.)
    b. **INF** Using sterile technique, attach needle to syringe.
    c. Withdraw medication using the procedure shown in Skill 11.13 or 11.14.
17. **SAF** Complete the **second safety checkpoint** and check the rights of administration again. Label the syringe per facility policy (e.g., client's name, medication dose, route, date, time). Reverify the label on the syringe and medication vial (if available) against the MAR or EMAR before administering the IM injection to the client. **WARNING:** Administer the IM injection as soon as possible after preparation. *Immediate administration after preparation reduces the risk of medication errors.*

Administering the Intramuscular Injection

18. **INF** Perform hand hygiene again upon entering the client's room.
19. **INF** Maintain client privacy.
20. **SAF** Reverify the client's identity by using at least two client identifiers.
21. **SAF** Recheck the client's armband for allergies, and ask the client verbally if he or she has allergies.
22. **SAF** Perform the **third safety checkpoint** and review the medication with the client. Check the rights of administration again. *This facilitates client involvement.* (Note: If required, scan the client's armband and the bar code on the medication label if available.)

Selecting the Site for the Intramuscular Injection

23. **ACC** After safety checks have been completed, apply gloves if required and select site for IM injection. Avoid sites of previous injections or areas that have bruising, broken skin, scars, or lesions. If the client is receiving multiple injections, rotate the injection sites. *Prevents tissue damage.* (Note: OSHA does not require the use of gloves when administering vaccines unless there is a risk of exposure to body fluids. Check facility policy [CDC, 2019a]).

Deltoid Injection Site

24. **ACC** Identify the deltoid injection site.
    a. Position the client in an upright sitting position and expose upper arm.
    b. Locate anatomical landmark of acromion process by palpating the top of the shoulder.

c. Identify deltoid injection site by dropping down approximately 3.5 to 5 cm (1½–2 inches) below acromion process near the middle of the largest part of the deltoid muscle.
    d. Using your thumb and forefingers, gently grasp the muscle to estimate location and mass.

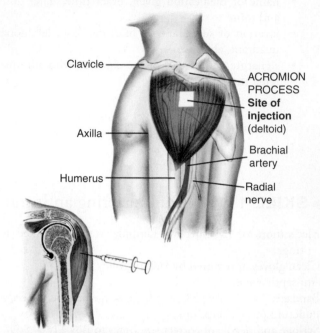

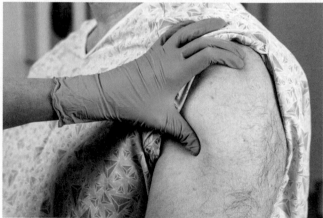

STEP 24 Deltoid injection site. Gently grasp the muscle to estimate location and size.

Vastus Lateralis Injection Site

25. **ACC** Identify the vastus lateralis injection site.
    a. Position the client in comfortable position with the thigh muscle exposed. Drape the client appropriately for privacy so that only the injection site is exposed.
    b. Locate the appropriate landmarks on the client's thigh. Place one handbreadth below the trochanter and one handbreadth above the knee.
    c. Visually divide the thigh into three lengthwise sections and identify the vastus lateralis site in the outer or mediolateral portion of the thigh.

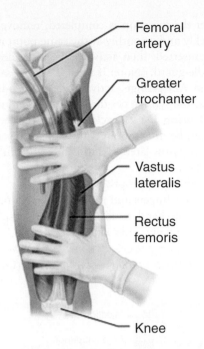

STEP 25 Vastus lateralis injection site.

Ventrogluteal Injection Site

26. **ACC** Identify the ventrogluteal injection site.
    a. Position the client in a side-lying position with a pillow between the knees for comfort and spinal support. Place the upper leg slightly in front of the lower leg, and flex the knee to facilitate muscle relaxation. Drape the client for privacy so that only the injection site is exposed.
    b. Locate anatomical landmark by placing an index finger on the anterior superior iliac spine (which is where the crest of the iliac bone curves toward the front of the body).
    c. Place palm of hand down on the client's greater trochanter, and then create a "V" by placing the middle finger approximately 5 cm (2 inches) away from the first finger.
    d. Identify ventrogluteal site as the center of the "V" in the largest part of the muscle.

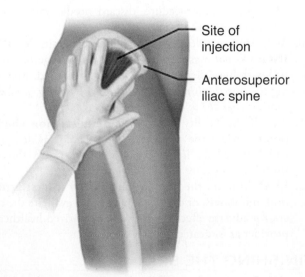

STEP 26 Ventrogluteal injection site.

Performing the IM Injection

27. **ACC** After the injection site has been identified and the client has been placed in the appropriate position, administer the IM injection.
    a. Cleanse the selected site with an antiseptic wipe by moving from the injection site outward in a circular pattern. Avoid touching the site where the injection will be given after it has been cleaned. *Moving outward in circular pattern moves debris away from the site.*
    b. Allow site to dry. *Enhances antiseptic activity and prevents stinging at the site.*
    c. Remove cap from needle and set it aside. Using your dominant hand, quickly but gently insert the needle into the largest part or "belly of the muscle" at a 90-degree angle. (Note: The insertion should be a smooth and steady motion.)

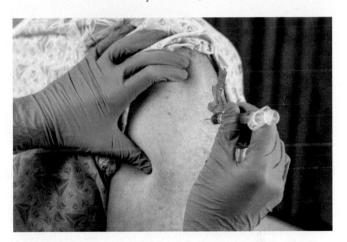

STEP 27C IM injection (deltoid). Insert needle at a 90-degree angle.

    d. If aspiration is indicated by policy or manufacturer recommendation, gently aspirate with your dominant hand while holding the syringe securely with your nondominant hand. Ensure there is no blood in the syringe. (Note: The CDC does not recommend aspiration when administering vaccinations. In addition, some AD syringes do not allow for aspiration. Check your facility policy.)
    e. Stabilize the syringe with your nondominant hand, and inject the medication by pushing the plunger with the thumb of your dominant hand. Inject at the appropriate rate, depending on the viscosity of the medication and any special instructions. (Note: Check the manufacturer recommendations.)

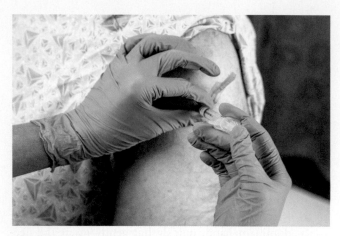

STEP 27E IM injection (deltoid). Stabilize syringe and inject medication.

f. After the injection is completed, remove the needle quickly and smoothly at the same point and angle it was inserted; then activate the safety device on the needle guard. (Note: If using a special safety system or an AD syringe, activate the mechanism and remove the syringe per the manufacturer guidelines.)

28. **ACC If using IM Z-track method:** (Note: This technique can be done in large muscles such as the ventrogluteal or vastus lateralis and is most helpful for irritating medications.)

   a. Identify the appropriate injection site.
   b. Use your fingers and the lateral aspect of your nondominant hand to displace skin and subcutaneous tissue laterally approximately 2.5 to 3.5 cm (1–1½ inches). *Using the Z-track method may prevent leakage of medication into subcutaneous tissues (Li, 2017).*

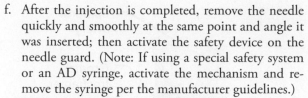

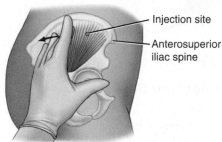

STEP 28A AND 28B Using the Z-track method. Identify the injection site (e.g. ventrogluteal) and displace the skin and tissue laterally.

c. While continuing to displace the tissue with your nondominant hand, administer the injection at a 90-degree angle with your dominant hand as described in step 27. (Note: The injection rate depends on the volume and viscosity of the medication. If aspiration prior to injection is required by your facility policy or manufacturer recommendations, use the aspiration procedure described in step 27d.)

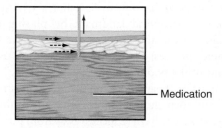

STEP 28D After Z-track injection, release the tissue as the needle is withdrawn to trap medication.

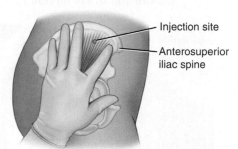

Insert needle at 90° angle

STEP 28C Administer the Z-track IM injection.

d. After the Z-track injection, release the displaced tissue at the same time the needle is withdrawn. *This method will help seal off the puncture track to prevent leaking of the medication out of the muscle tissue (Li, 2017).* (Note: If using a retractable safety needle, activate the device per manufacturer instructions.)

29. **ACC** After IM procedure, discard needle and syringe into puncture-proof sharps container.

30. **ACC** Apply gentle pressure to the injection site. **WARNING:** Do *not* massage the site. Place bandage or gauze pad with hypoallergenic tape on site if needed. *Massaging the injection site can cause bruising, seeping, and discomfort after IM and Z-track injections.*

31. **SAF** If the facility has a **postadministration checkpoint,** review the used vial (if available) against the MAR or EMAR. If any errors occurred, notify the authorized healthcare provider immediately.

32. **EVAL** Monitor the injection site for any redness, irritation, numbness, or other symptom, and evaluate the client for adverse effects. Notify the authorized healthcare provider as indicated.

FINISHING THE SKILL

33. **INF** Remove gloves if worn and perform hand hygiene.

34. **SAF** Ensure client safety and comfort. Ensure that the bed is in the lowest position, and verify that the client can identify and reach the nurse call system. *These safety measures reduce the risk of falls.*

35. **EVAL** Monitor the client and evaluate the outcomes. Did the client tolerate the IM injection without difficulty? Did the client experience any adverse effects?

36. **COM** Document assessment findings, medication administration, and outcomes in the legal healthcare record:
    - name of medication given, exact time, date, dose, and route
    - location of IM injection and site used (e.g., deltoid, vastus lateralis)
    - signature and initials of the clinician who administered the medication.

■ SKILL 11.19 Administering a Subcutaneous Insulin Injection

EQUIPMENT

Insulin (vials or prefilled syringe)
Clean gloves
Antiseptic wipes, puncture-proof sharps box
Bandage, 2 × 2 gauze pads, and hypoallergenic tape, if needed
Insulin syringe (with markings in units or half units)

BEGINNING THE SKILL

1. **ACC** Review the order for:
   - name and type of insulin medication
   - dosage with units spelled out (e.g., 6 units, not 6 u)
   - route and frequency of administration and any special instructions.

2. **ACC** Review the following:
   - **SAF** client's allergies to medications or other substances
   - appropriateness of insulin injection for the client (using medication rights)
   - client's medical history, type of diabetes, and history of insulin usage.

3. **INF** Perform hand hygiene.
4. **CCC** Introduce yourself to the client and family.
5. **SAF** Identify the client using at least two client identifiers.
6. **CCC** Provide privacy.
7. **ACC** Assess the client's level of consciousness and orientation to person, time, place, and situation. *Provides a baseline assessment of orientation before verbal consent is obtained.*
8. **CCC** Explain the procedure and obtain verbal consent. *To provide client-centered care and prevent waste, consent should be obtained before preparing medications.*
9. **ACC** Perform client preassessments, including but not limited to the following:
   - condition and amount of subcutaneous tissue in area where injection will be administered

- FSBS, if indicated.

PROCEDURE

Preparing the Insulin Injection

(Note: Insulin is usually refrigerated until used. Once opened it may be stored at controlled room temperature. Check manufacturer recommendations.)

10. **SAF** Perform the **first safety checkpoint** when accessing the insulin, and initiate the **second safety checkpoint** when preparing the subcutaneous insulin injection. Compare the MAR or EMAR with the order and label on the insulin vial or cartridge. Check the rights of administration, and check the client's name, type of insulin, expiration date, dosage, and any precautions. Scan the bar code on the label of the insulin vial if required. **WARNING:** Many facilities require that a client's multidose insulin vial be discarded within 28 days after being opened or used. Check the expiration date carefully. If in doubt, throw it out.

11. **ACC** Perform dosage calculations if necessary and double-check calculations.

12. **ACC** Inspect insulin vial or prefilled syringe for particulates or unexpected color. *Inspection prevents administration of contaminated or unsafe medication.*

13. **ACC** If the insulin is in a vial that needs to be suspended, roll the vial gently between the hands and agitate it until the crystals suspend. Avoid shaking the vial. *Shaking an insulin vial can create turbulence and air bubbles.*

14. **ACC** Assemble equipment in the med-prep area, and prepare the subcutaneous insulin injection. Continue the **second safety checkpoint** and check the rights of administration. **WARNING:** Use only insulin syringes measured in units to administer insulin.

15. **ACC** If using a prefilled syringe for the subcutaneous insulin injection, ensure that the safety needle and barcode label (per facility policy) are secured on the syringe.

16. **ACC** If using a vial for subcutaneous insulin injection:
    a. Place the vial on a clean, dry surface at an ergonomically safe height.

b. Cleanse the septum of the vial (if used) vigorously with an antiseptic wipe and allow to dry.

c. Using sterile technique, attach needle to syringe. (Note: For subcutaneous injections, a needle size of ⅜–1 inch, 24–27 gauge, and a syringe size of 0.5–2 mL are used. If the client has limited subcutaneous tissue, a shorter needle may be needed.)

d. Prepare and withdraw medication using the procedure shown in Skill 11.13.

Preparing an Injection With Two Types of Insulin

17. **ACC** If using two vials (short-acting insulin and intermediate-acting insulin) for the injection:

a. Verify that the two types of insulin are compatible with each other. **WARNING:** Check the manufacturer recommendations to ensure the two insulin products can be mixed. *Medications that are not compatible could cause biochemical and adverse reactions when mixed together. Some insulin products cannot be mixed with another insulin product.*

b. Draw up the short-acting insulin before the intermediate-acting insulin. *Drawing up the short-acting insulin first prevents contamination of the intermediate-acting insulin into the short-acting vial. Contamination of the short-acting insulin vial with intermediate-acting insulin could alter the pharmacological qualities of the short-acting insulin, such as onset of action.*

c. Arrange to have a second nurse witness the procedure. *Many facilities require a second nurse to witness the combining of high-alert, high-risk medicines such as insulin.*

d. Place both vials on a clean, dry surface at an ergonomically safe height.

e. Cleanse the rubber septum of both vials with separate antiseptic wipes and allow to dry.

f. Remove cap from insulin syringe needle with one motion. Set cap on clean, dry surface without contaminating the inside. *Maintains sterility of cap for insulin syringe.*

g. Determine the dosage of intermediate-acting insulin, pull back air into the insulin syringe in the amount of the dosage ordered, inject air into intermediate-acting insulin vial, and withdraw the needle. (Note: Ensure that the needle is above the surface of the intermediate-acting medication in the vial to avoid contamination of the insulin needle with the medication.)

h. Determine the dosage of short-acting insulin, pull back air into syringe in the amount of the short-acting dosage ordered, and inject air into short-acting insulin vial. Do not withdraw the needle.

i. While holding the needle securely in place, invert the vial of short-acting insulin, and withdraw the ordered dose. Return the vial to an upright position and remove the needle/syringe.

j. After drawing up the short-acting insulin, insert the needle/syringe into the intermediate-acting insulin, invert the vial while holding the needle securely in place, and withdraw the ordered dose of intermediate-acting insulin. Return the vial to an upright position and remove the needle from the vial. (Note: Use caution not to contaminate the insulin needle and not to contaminate either vial of insulin medication during the mixing procedure.)

k. Insert the syringe into the sterile cap by safe method per facility policy.

18. **SAF WARNING:** Verify dosage, order, and amount of insulin in syringe with a second nurse. *Insulin is a high-alert medication that requires independent checks.*

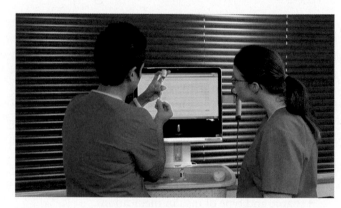

STEP 18 Verify the insulin with a second nurse.

19. **SAF** Complete the **second safety checkpoint,** and check the rights of administration again before labeling the syringe. Label the syringe per facility policy (e.g., client's name, medication dose, route, date, time). Reverify the label on the syringe and insulin vial (if available) against the MAR or EMAR before administering the insulin injection. **WARNING:** Administer the subcutaneous insulin injection as soon as possible after preparation. *Immediate administration after preparation reduces the risk of medication errors.*

Administering the Subcutaneous Insulin Injection

20. **INF** Perform hand hygiene again upon entering the client's room.

21. **INF** Maintain client privacy.

22. **SAF** Reverify the client's identity by using at least two client identifiers.

23. **SAF** Recheck the client's armband for allergies, and ask the client verbally if he or she has allergies.

24. **SAF** Perform the **third safety checkpoint** and review the insulin medication with the client. Check the rights of administration again. *This facilitates client involvement.* (Note: If required, scan the client's armband and the bar code on the medication label if available.)

25. **ACC** After safety checks have been completed, apply gloves, select the appropriate site, and administer the subcutaneous insulin injection as described in Skill 11.17.

26. **HLTH** Use the abdomen for insulin injections if not contraindicated, and ensure that injections are rotated to different sites (at least 2.5 cm [1 inch] apart) and are at least 5 cm (2 inches) away from the client's naval. *The abdomen is a good choice for injections because it allows for stable absorption. Rotation of injection sites prevents tissue damage (Slade, 2015).*

27. **SAF** If the facility has a **postadministration checkpoint,** review the insulin vial or vials against the MAR or EMAR. If any errors occurred, notify the authorized healthcare provider immediately.

28. **EVAL** Monitor the client's glucose and FSBS, and monitor the client for any adverse or unexpected effects of the insulin injection.

FINISHING THE SKILL

29. **INF** Remove gloves and perform hand hygiene.

30. **SAF** Ensure client safety and comfort. Ensure that the bed is in the lowest position, and verify that the client can identify and reach the nurse call system. *These safety measures reduce the risk of falls.*

31. **EVAL** Evaluate the outcomes. *Is the client's serum glucose or finger stick blood sugar levels within expected parameters? Is the client's skin near injection sites intact, without redness or irritation?*

32. **COM** Document assessment findings, medication administration, and outcomes in the legal healthcare record:
    - type or types of insulin given, exact time, date, dose, and route
    - location of insulin injection per site-rotation schedule
    - blood sugar measurements pre and post insulin administration, if available
    - signature and initials of the clinician who administered the medication.

Follow-up

33. **EVAL** Continue to monitor the client for any irritation or other symptoms at the injection site.

34. **COM** If the client will be using an insulin pen for self-administration, assess the client's orientation level and ability to perform injections, and provide client/family teaching as described in Box 11.8. Make appropriate referrals to the diabetic educator and other professionals as needed.

35. **COM** Document client education, client's ability to perform injections and any referrals made.

▪ SKILL 11.20 Caring for a Client With a Subcutaneous Insulin Pump (External)

EQUIPMENT

Clean gloves

Antiseptic wipes and sterile transparent dressing supplies, if needed

Bandage, 2 × 2 gauze pads, and hypoallergenic tape, if needed

Insulin pump supplies: insulin cartridge or prefilled syringe, sterile infusion set, if needed

BEGINNING THE SKILL

1. **ACC** Review the order for:
   - name and type of insulin medication
   - basal rate, bolus doses, and criteria for administering bolus doses
   - any special instructions
   - instructions allowing the client to self-manage insulin pump and doses.

2. **ACC** Review the following:
   - **SAF** client's allergies to medications or other substances
   - client's medical history, type of diabetes, and history of insulin use
   - client's age, condition, and medication history (to check for potential drug interactions)
   - recent lab work (especially chemistries with blood glucose levels).

3. **INF** Perform hand hygiene.

4. **CCC** Introduce yourself to the client and family.

5. **SAF** Identify the client using at least two client identifiers.

6. **CCC** Provide privacy.

7. **ACC** Assess the client for:
   a. skin integrity and any signs of breakdown, rashes, scars, or other skin conditions
   b. client's level of consciousness and understanding of insulin pump procedure
   c. client's ability to self-manage the pump if applicable.

8. **ACC** Perform client preassessments, including but not limited to the following:
   - condition and amount of subcutaneous tissue in the area where the injection will be administered
   - FSBS, if indicated.

9. **COM** If the client is self-managing his or her own insulin pump, instruct the client to notify the nurse or other healthcare provider of bolus doses and whether or not there is any difficulty with the pump. (Note: In some facilities, clients are responsible for self-managing their own pumps and bolus doses if they meet the criteria and for reporting this information back to the nursing staff.)

PROCEDURE

10. **INF** Perform hand hygiene again upon entering the client's room.
11. **ACC** Maintain client privacy.
12. **SAF** Recheck the client's identity using at least two client identifiers.
13. **SAF** Recheck the client's armband for allergies, and ask the client verbally if he or she has allergies.
14. **ACC** Apply gloves.
15. **ACC** Monitoring the client's insulin pump therapy:
    a. Ensure that the client's pump is intact and working properly.
    b. Ensure that the tubing and cannula are intact on the client and that the insulin reservoir is secure.
    c. Verify that insulin is infusing per the basal rate that is ordered by the authorized healthcare provider. Note any additional boluses the client has self-administered after meals.
16. **ACC** Caring for the client's skin and cannula site during therapy:
    a. Inspect the cannula site for any signs of redness, drainage, or irritation.
    b. Ensure that the sterile, transparent dressing on cannula is dry and intact.
    c. Ensure that cannula has not become dislodged and is not leaking.
    d. Assist the client with gently cleansing and/or redressing the cannula site as needed.
    e. If the cannula site is becoming irritated, assist the client to change the insertion site as needed. (Note: When rotating insertion sites, select a clean, dry site with adequate subcutaneous tissue per manufacturer recommendations. Avoid bony or scarred areas.)
17. **ACC** Replacing insulin cartridge and tubing for insulin pump:
    a. If ordered, assist the client as necessary with replacing the insulin cartridge and tubing.
    b. Check the insulin medication and orders, and perform **safety checks** per facility policy.

    c. Verify medication, dosage, and order with a second nurse per facility policy. *Insulin is a high-alert medication that requires double-checking with another clinician.*
    d. Scan the bar code on the insulin cartridge after verification as required by facility policy.
    e. Prime tubing and insert prefilled insulin syringe or reservoir into pump per manufacturer instructions. *Instructions will vary depending on the manufacturer.*

FINISHING THE SKILL

18. **INF** Remove gloves and perform hand hygiene.
19. **SAF** Ensure client safety and comfort. Ensure that the bed is in the lowest position, and verify that the client can identify and reach the nurse call system. *These safety measures reduce the risk of falls.*
20. **EVAL** Evaluate the outcomes. *Is the client's serum blood glucose well controlled?*
21. **COM** Document assessment findings, medication administration, and outcomes in the legal healthcare record:
    • type of pump and insulin, basal rate, and boluses given or self-administered
    • time and date of cannula tubing and insulin cartridge changes
    • location of cannula site, type/condition of dressing on site, skin condition.

Follow-up

22. **EVAL** Continue to monitor the client's glucose level and FSBS as needed, and continue to monitor the client for any signs of hyperglycemia or hypoglycemia.
23. **ACC** Ensure that the insertion site is rotated on a regular basis and that the tubing and insulin cartridge is changed at least every 72 hours per facility policy. *Changing the insertion sites and tubing on a regular basis prevents skin irritation and infection (Woten & Heering, 2018).*
24. **COM** Make referrals to diabetic educator, registered dietitian, and other professionals as needed. Document all referrals made. *Communication with other members of the healthcare team facilitates collaborative care.*

■ CASE STUDY

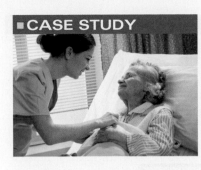

Sarah, a nurse who has recently graduated, is assigned to care for Mrs. Millie Campbell. Sarah has also been asked to care for Mrs. Millie Compton. Both clients are in their 80s. Mrs. Campbell has been admitted for problems related to diabetes, whereas Mrs. Compton is being treated for hypertension. Sarah notices that both of her clients have medications due at 8 AM. She is worried about getting behind, so she decides to obtain their medications from the ADS at the same time. Sarah reviews the original orders against the EMAR and then checks the EMAR against the medication labels. Because Mrs. Campbell's call light is going off, she goes to her room first. When Sarah enters the room, Mrs. Campbell is on the bedside commode and needs assistance with other matters. After assisting Mrs. Campbell, Sarah feels even more pressed for time. As Sarah begins to review each medication, Mrs. Campbell states, "Don't worry, honey. I have been taking these for a long time." Sarah then puts the meds in the cup, gives them to Mrs. Campbell, and leaves the room before Mrs. Campbell takes her pills.

Upon arriving at Mrs. Compton's bedside, Sarah notes that she needs to check her FSBS. When she says this aloud, Mrs. Compton expresses concern that she has never had problems with her blood sugar before. Quickly, Sarah looks at the medications and realizes she has given Mrs. Compton's pills to Mrs. Campbell and is about to give Mrs. Campbell's pills to Mrs. Compton! Because Sarah no longer has Mrs. Compton's pills, she returns to Mrs. Campbell's room. However, Mrs. Campbell has already taken all of the wrong pills, including Mrs. Compton's BP medication. Sarah initially feels unsure of what to do. However, she knows that the error must be reported to her charge nurse and authorized healthcare provider. Sarah also reviews Mrs. Campbell's records again and discovers she has a history of anxiety and a history of allergic reactions to one of Mrs. Compton's medications that she erroneously received.

Case Study Questions

1. What actions must Sarah immediately take because this medication error occurred?
2. Considering Mrs. Campbell's risk factors and the erroneous medications she received, what are the highest priorities regarding her care? What other interventions might help?
3. What are the safety checkpoints that Sarah skipped while going through the procedure of medication administration for Mrs. Campbell and Mrs. Compton? Which safety checks did Sarah do correctly? At what point could Sarah have possibly caught the error?
4. Are there other factors that contributed to the medication error? If so, what were the issues, and how could they have been handled?
5. How can Sarah be a role model for her co-workers and fellow new graduates, and how can these types of medication errors be prevented in the future?
6. **Application of QSEN Competencies:** One of the Quality and Safety Education for Nurses (QSEN) skills for Safety is to communicate concerns of potential hazards or errors to the healthcare team (Cronenwett et al., 2007) How did the competency of safety apply in this scenario? What could have been done differently?

■CONCEPT MAP

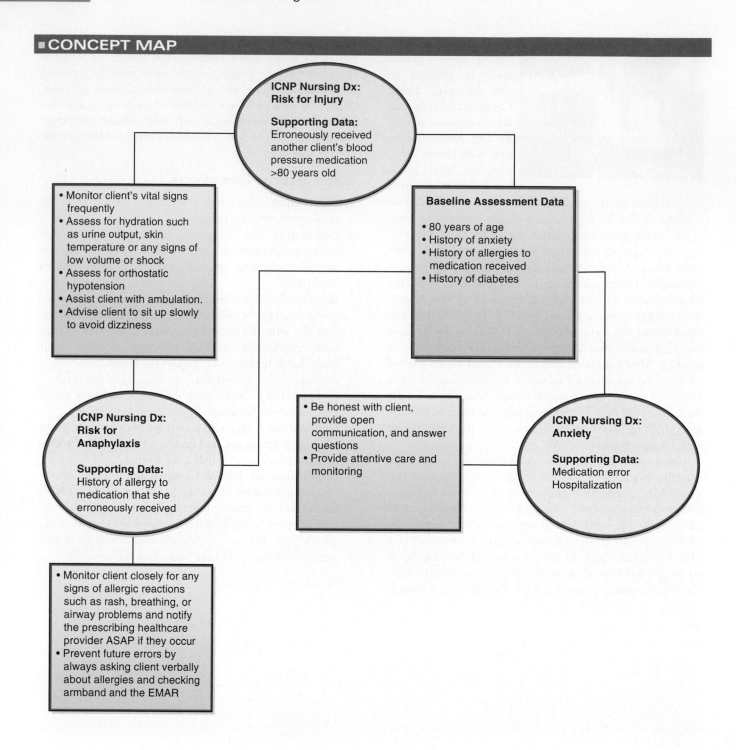

ICNP Nursing Dx: Risk for Injury

Supporting Data:
Erroneously received another client's blood pressure medication
>80 years old

- Monitor client's vital signs frequently
- Assess for hydration such as urine output, skin temperature or any signs of low volume or shock
- Assess for orthostatic hypotension
- Assist client with ambulation.
- Advise client to sit up slowly to avoid dizziness

Baseline Assessment Data

- 80 years of age
- History of anxiety
- History of allergies to medication received
- History of diabetes

ICNP Nursing Dx: Risk for Anaphylaxis

Supporting Data:
History of allergy to medication that she erroneously received

- Be honest with client, provide open communication, and answer questions
- Provide attentive care and monitoring

ICNP Nursing Dx: Anxiety

Supporting Data:
Medication error
Hospitalization

- Monitor client closely for any signs of allergic reactions such as rash, breathing, or airway problems and notify the prescribing healthcare provider ASAP if they occur
- Prevent future errors by always asking client verbally about allergies and checking armband and the EMAR

References

American Society of Health-System Pharmacists (ASHP). (2018). *Safe medication: Neomycin, polymyxin, and hydrocortisone otic.* Retrieved from http://www.safemedication.com/searchresults/DisplayDrug.aspx?id=a618030.

Becton Dickenson. (2015). *How to use an insulin pen.* Retrieved from http://www.bd.com/us/diabetes/page.aspx?cat=7001&id=7259.

Caple, C. (2018). Administration of medication: Withdrawing medication from an ampule. From *Nursing practice & skill.* Ipswich, MA: EBSCO Publishing. Retrieved from Cinahl Information Systems.

Caple, C., & Schub, T. (2016). Administration of medication: Oral, sublingual, and buccal. From *Nursing practice & skill.* Ipswich, MA: EBSCO Publishing. Retrieved from Cinahl Information Systems.

Centers for Disease Control and Prevention. (2018). *Medication safety program.* Retrieved from https://www.cdc.gov/medicationsafety/index.html.

Centers for Disease Control and Prevention. (2019a). Chapter 6: Vaccine administration. In J. Hamborsky, A. Kroger, & S. Wolfe (Eds.), *Epidemiology and prevention of vaccine-preventable diseases* (13th ed.). Washington, DC: Public Health Foundation.

Retrieved from. https://www.cdc.gov/vaccines/pubs/pinkbook/vac-admin.html.

Centers for Disease Control and Prevention. (2019b). *Injection safety. FAQs regarding safe practices for medical injections-background.* Retrieved from https://www.cdc.gov/injectionsafety/providers/provider_faqs.html.

Corrigan, M., Wilson, S. S., & Hampton, J. (2015). Safety and efficacy of intranasally administered medications in the emergency department and pre-hospital settings. *American Journal of Health-System Pharmacy, 72*(18), 1544–1554.

Cronenwett, L., Sherwood, G., Barnsteiner, J., Disch, J., Johnson, J., Mitchell, P., ... Warren, J. (2007). Quality and safety education for nurses. *Nursing Outlook, 55*(3), 122–131. Retrieved from http://qsen.org/competencies/pre-licensure-ksas/.

Devesty, G., & Balderrama, D. (2017). Administration of medication: Vaginal instillations. From *Nursing practice & skill.* Ipswich, MA: EBSCO Publishing. Retrieved from Cinahl Information Systems.

Dudek, S. G. (2017). *Nutrition essentials for nursing practice* (8th ed.). Philadelphia: Lippincott, Williams, & Wilkins.

Gardenhire, D. S., Burnett, D., Strickland, S., & Myers, T. R. (2017). *A guide to aerosol delivery devices for respiratory therapists* (4th ed.). American Association for Respiratory Care. Retrieved from http://www.aarc.org/wp-content/uploads/2015/04/aerosol_guide_rt.pdf.

International Classification for Nursing Practice. (n.d). *eHealth & ICNP.* Retrieved from https://www.icn.ch/what-we-do/projects/ehealth-icnp

Institute for Safe Medication Practices. (2015). *ISMP safe practice guidelines for adult IV push medications.* Retrieved from https://www.ismp.org/sites/default/files/attachments/2017-11/ISMP97-Guidelines-071415-3.%20FINAL.pdf.

Institute for Safe Medication Practices. (2016). Error alert: Administering drugs via feeding tube is prone to errors. *Pharmacy Today.* Retrieved from http://www.pharmacytoday.org/article/S1042-0991(16)30715-0/pdf.

Institute for Safe Medication Practices. (2017a). *ISMP's list of error-prone abbreviations, symbols, and dose designations.* Retrieved from https://www.ismp.org/recommendations/error-prone-abbreviations-list.

Institute for Safe Medication Practices. (2017b). *2018–2019 Targeted medication safety best practices for hospitals.* Retrieved from https://www.ismp.org/guidelines/best-practices-hospitals.

Institute for Safe Medication Practices. (2018a). *ISMP's list of high alert medications in acute care settings.* Retrieved from https://www.ismp.org/sites/default/files/attachments/2018-10/highAlert2018new-Oct2018-v1.pdf.

Institute for Safe Medication Practices. (2018b). *Oral dosage forms that should not be crushed.* Retrieved from https://www.ismp.org/recommendations/do-not-crush.

Institute for Safe Medication Practices. (2019). *ISMP's list of confused drug names.* Retrieved from http://www.ismp.org/Tools/confuseddrugnames.pdf.

The Joint Commission. (2018). *Facts about the official "Do not use" list of abbreviations.* Retrieved from file:///Users/iMac/Downloads/Do_Not_Use_List_9_14_18.pdf.

The Joint Commission. (2019). *National Patient Safety Goals,* 2019. Retrieved from https://www.jointcommission.org/standards_information/npsgs.aspx.

Le, J. (2018). Drug administration. *The Merck manual.* Retrieved from https://www.merckmanuals.com/en-ca/home/drugs/administration-and-kinetics-of-drugs/drug-administration.

Li, Y. (2017). *Injection (intramuscular).* [Evidence summary]. Retrieved from The Joanna Briggs Institute EBD Database, JBI@Ovid. JBI1139.

Mann, E. (2016a). *Injection (intramuscular): Clinician information.* [Evidence summary]. Retrieved from The Joanna Briggs Institute EBD Database, JBI@Ovid. JBI520.

Mann, E. (2016b). *Intramuscular injection: Aspiration.* Retrieved from The Joanna Briggs Institute EBD Database, JBI@Ovid. JBI10441.

Medication error: Court sees basis for liability, punitive damages. (2012). *Legal Eagle Eye Newsletter For The Nursing Profession.* Retrieved from http://www.nursinglaw.com.

Medline Plus. (2019). *PPD skin test.* Retrieved from https://medlineplus.gov/ency/article/003839.htm.

National Alert Network. (2017). *Severe hyperglycemia in patients incorrectly using insulin pens at home.* Retrieved from https://www.nccmerp.org/sites/default/files/nan-20171012.pdf.

Quatrara, B., Turner, M., Pitts, N., Parks, C., Murphy, F., & Conway, M. (2016). What is the likelihood of blood return using aspiration technique with intramuscular vaccine injection? *Annals of Nursing and Practice, 3*(5), 1058.

Richards, S., & Heering, H. (2017). Administration of medication: Nasal instillations. From *Nursing practice & skill.* Ipswich, MA: EBSCO Publishing. Retrieved from Cinahl Information Systems.

Sanofi U.S. LLC. (2018). *How to self-inject with Lovenox.* Retrieved from https://www.lovenox.com/patient-self-injection-video.

Sharma, L. (2018a). *Medication (ocular): Administration.* [Evidence summary]. Retrieved from The Joanna Briggs Institute EBD Database, JBI@Ovid. JBI220.

Sharma, L. (2018b). *Eye irrigation.* [Evidence summary]. Retrieved from The Joanna Briggs Institute EBD Database, JBI@Ovid. JBI1327.

Slade, S. (2015). *Injection (subcutaneous).* [Clinician information]. Retrieved from The Joanna Briggs Institute EBD Database, JBI@Ovid. JBI234.

U.S. Food and Drug Administration. (2016). *FDA drug safety communication: Important change to heparin container labels to clearly state the total drug strength.* Retrieved from https://www.fda.gov/drugs/drugsafety/ucm330695.htm.

U.S. Food and Drug Administration. (2018). *Disposal of unused medicines: What you should know.* Retrieved from https://www.fda.gov/drugs/resourcesforyou/consumers/buyingusingmedicinesafely/ensuringsafeuseofmedicine/safedisposalofmedicines/ucm186187.htm.

Woten, M., & Heering, H. (2018). Administration of medication: Using an insulin pump. From *Nursing practice & skill.* Ipswich, MA: EBSCO Publishing. Retrieved from Cinahl Information Systems.

World Health Organization. (2015, September). Reducing pain at the time of vaccination: WHO position paper. *Weekly Epidemiological Record.* Retrieved from https://www.who.int/wer/2015/wer9039.pdf?ua=1.

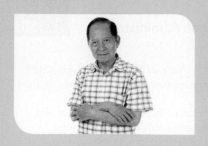
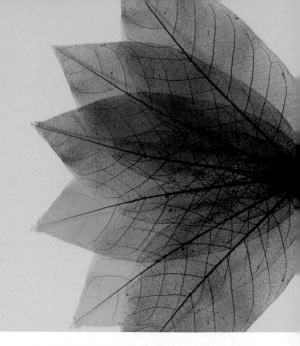

CHAPTER 12
Venous Access

"Memory is funny. Once you hit a vein, the problem is not how to remember but how to control the flow."

Tobias Wolff, American Author, 1989

LEARNING OBJECTIVES

By the end of this chapter, the reader will be able to:

1. Describe the method for selecting a vein for venipuncture or an intravenous (IV) line.
2. Demonstrate the technique for obtaining a venous specimen using a needle and syringe, a butterfly needle and syringe, a Vacutainer, and a butterfly needle with a Vacutainer.
3. Discuss strategies to ensure the accuracy of blood specimen collection.

4 Demonstrate the technique for initiating and dressing a peripheral intravenous (PIV) catheter using an over-the-needle catheter.

5 Demonstrate changing a transparent dressing on a PIV line.

6 Demonstrate discontinuing a PIV line.

7 Describe infection control strategies when initiating and maintaining a PIV line.

8 Describe the method for managing a saline lock.

9 Discuss the benefits and potential complications related to the management of IV fluids.

10 Demonstrate the correct technique to prepare and administer a primary PIV infusion line.

11 Demonstrate the correct technique to replace the IV fluids on an existing IV administration set.

12 Compare the management of IV fluids using an infusion pump versus gravity.

13 Discuss the benefits and potential complications of administering medications intravenously.

14 Demonstrate the correct technique to prepare and administer a secondary intermittent medication IV infusion line.

15 Demonstrate the correct technique to prepare and administer a medication via IV push.

16 Identify safety mechanisms used to prevent errors and harm when administering IV fluids and medications.

17 Identify the ABO and Rh compatibility system related to blood transfusions.

18 Discuss key nursing safety considerations related to blood administration.

19 Describe possible complications and the corresponding nursing interventions related to blood transfusions.

20 Demonstrate the administration of a blood transfusion.

TERMINOLOGY

Extravasation Inadvertent infiltration of a vesicant solution/medication into surrounding tissue.

Hemoconcentration An increase in cellular elements due to decrease in plasma volume.

Hemolysis The rupture of red blood cells.

Hypertonic solution A hyperosmotic solution with the solute concentration greater than the concentration inside a cell or physiological saline (0.9% NaCl solution).

Hypotonic solution A hypoosmotic solution with the solute concentration less than the concentration inside a cell or physiological saline (0.9% NaCl solution).

Infiltration Inadvertent administration of a nonvesicant solution/medication into surrounding tissue.

Isotonic solution An isosmotic solution that is equal to the concentration inside a cell or physiological saline (0.9% NaCl solution).

Sclerotic Thickening or hardening as a result of inflammation.

Vesicant An agent capable of causing blistering, tissue sloughing, or necrosis when it escapes from the intended vascular pathway into surrounding tissue.

ACRONYMS

BUN Blood urea nitrogen
CBC Complete blood count
INS Infusion Nurses Society
IVF Intravenous fluid
KVO Keep vein open
NSS Normal saline solution
PIV Peripheral intravenous line
PT Prothrombin time
PTT Partial thromboplastin time

The venous circulation drains blood from the capillaries and carries it to the heart. Veins carry blood under lower pressure than arteries. Veins will readily expand with more fluid volume and contract with less; thus, veins act as the blood reservoirs as well as the blood passageways to the heart. As veins get closer to the heart, they are larger vessels. See Fig. 12.1 for the major veins of the upper extremities. Veins and arteries often run in tandem in the extremities as well as to and from organs, such as the femoral artery and the femoral vein. However, the pattern of veins is unique to each person even more so than the pattern of arteries. For example, some individuals do not have a median cubital vein in their forearm.

Venous access is a critical aspect of providing medical care. By accessing a person's veins, a nurse can draw blood, instill fluids, administer medications, and administer lifesaving blood components. By accessing veins in the upper extremities to infuse medications, the medication is very quickly absorbed into the systemic circulation, and therefore the intravenous (IV) route has the most rapid-acting effect. The capacity of the venous system to expand allows IV fluids and blood components to be administered through venous access.

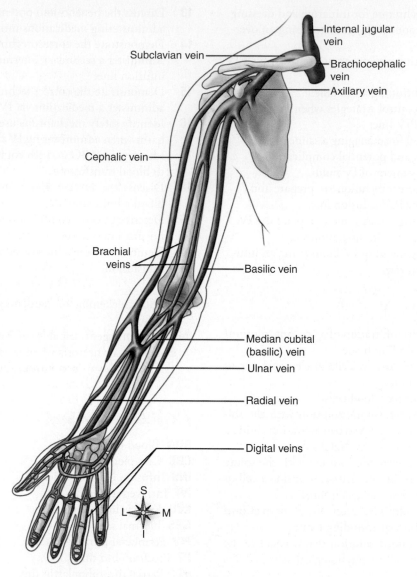

FIG. 12.1 Major veins of the upper extremities.

Labels on figure:
- Internal jugular vein
- Subclavian vein
- Brachiocephalic vein
- Axillary vein
- Cephalic vein
- Brachial veins
- Basilic vein
- Median cubital (basilic) vein
- Ulnar vein
- Radial vein
- Digital veins

SECTION 1   Collecting Venous Blood Specimens

Blood specimens are collected in health-care settings more frequently than other types of specimens, such as urine. Analysis of the blood specimen may be used to screen for, diagnose, rule out, or monitor a clinical problem; to determine a prognosis; or to monitor the effects or side effects of drug therapy. For certain medications, monitoring the peak and trough values is essential to ensure the levels are not so high as to be toxic and not so low as to be nontherapeutic. In some settings, the nurse caring for the client may draw the blood specimen. In other settings, a specialized nurse team or a phlebotomist draws the specimen.

ENSURING ACCURACY

Blood specimen collection requires specific measures to ensure the accuracy of the results. Accuracy is a critical concept for specimen collection. It is affected by multiple variables, including nurse-related variables, such as selecting the appropriate equipment, using the appropriate order of draw, and selecting an appropriate vein. Moreover, blood-related variables may affect the accuracy of the specimen collection, including hemolysis, hemoconcentration, and clotting.

Selecting Equipment

A variety of venipuncture equipment is available to nurses. Fig. 12.2 shows examples of the equipment described here. A simple needle and syringe may be sufficient if only one laboratory blood test is ordered. A Vacutainer collection system includes a double-headed needle and a plastic holder. One side of the double-headed needle is covered in soft plastic, and the other end has a cap and looks like a typical needle. The double-headed needle screws into the blood collection tube holder. The nurse pushes collection tubes onto the interior needle, negative pressure fills the tube to the appropriate amount, and then the nurse removes that tube and places a new tube as needed. When several blood tests are ordered, a Vacutainer system is helpful. A butterfly needle has plastic wings, allows for a low angle of entry, and is useful for small veins. Some types of venipuncture equipment allow the nurse to see a blood return, and some do not. Table 12.1 compares the advantages and disadvantages of venipuncture equipment.

Sequence of Specimen Collection (Order of Draw)

Analyses of blood specimens may be run on whole blood, serum, or plasma. Both serum and plasma are derived from whole blood from which the blood cells have been removed; however, in order to obtain plasma, the blood sample must be prevented from clotting. Various additives are used to obtain an optimal and accurate specimen. Blood collection tubes have tops of various colors that indicate the type of additive or lack of additive for that tube (Table 12.2). Nurses select the appropriate tube for the laboratory test ordered. When multiple laboratory tests are ordered, the nurse organizes the tubes according to the recommended sequence of specimen collection; this is called the order of draw, thereby preventing contamination from additives. Collection tubes without additives are usually drawn before additive tubes. Each facility may have specific recommendations for the order of draw; however, the order is generally as follows:

- Blood cultures are drawn first
- Red-top tube lab work (no additives)
- Blue-top tube lab work (sodium citrate)
- Green-top tube lab work (heparin additive)
- Lavender-top tubes (EDTA-K3 additive)
- Gray-top tubes (sodium fluoride oxalate)

Blood-Related Variables: Hemolysis, Hemoconcentration, and Clotting

A problem that commonly alters the accuracy of blood specimen analysis is hemolysis, the rupture of red blood cells

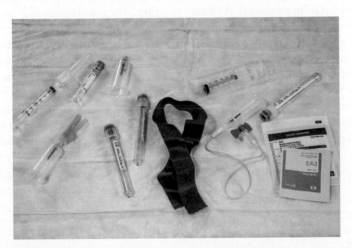

FIG. 12.2 Blood collection equipment. *Left of the tourniquet, clockwise:* Two red-top tubes, Vacutainer, needle and syringe, blue-top tube and transfer device. *Right of the tourniquet, clockwise:* Butterfly with a Vacutainer attached, syringe, red-top tube, gauze sponge, and antiseptic wipe.

TABLE 12.1 Comparing Blood Collection Equipment

Equipment	See a Flashback	Advantages	Disadvantages
Syringe/needle	Yes	Flashback	Can draw only a limited blood volume
Syringe/butterfly needle	Yes	Flashback Useful for small, fragile veins Can draw multiple syringes of blood	Takes time Slow process may allow blood to clot
Vacutainer	No	Can draw multiple lab tubes Rapid process	No flashback Vacuum exerts too much negative pressure on fragile veins
Vacutainer/ butterfly needle	Yes	Flashback Can draw multiple lab tubes Useful for small, fragile veins	Vacuum may exert too much negative pressure on fragile veins

(RBCs). Hemolysis can occur from drawing blood through a small-gauge needle or from shaking or otherwise roughly handling a specimen. Selection of the appropriate equipment and careful handling of the sample will reduce the risk of hemolysis.

Another common problem is hemoconcentration, the concentration of cellular elements resulting from a decrease in plasma. This can occur when a tourniquet is left in place for more than 60 seconds. For some types of specimens, the nurse does not want any clot formation in the blood sample. For example, if blood is not flowing easily through butterfly tubing, the blood may begin to clot in the line before reaching the additive. Selecting the best vein and appropriate equipment can minimize this potential problem.

SELECTING A VEIN

Venous blood samples are frequently obtained from any of the several large veins found in the antecubital fossa, including the basilic vein, cephalic vein, and median cubital vein (Fig. 12.3). Each person's venous pathway is unique to some extent, but each person has veins. Feel in the antecubital fossa for a vein that has a dense, rubbery texture and recoils when pressed. Feel the breadth and depth of the vein. Nurses select a vein that is palpable rather than one that is easily visible. Avoid veins with signs of repeated use, bruising, or poor skin integrity. Avoid arms with a peripheral intavenous (PIV) line. Never draw blood samples above or near an infusing IV line because the IV fluids can alter analysis results. Determine if the client has had an event or procedure that alters vascular patterns, such as the presence of an arteriovenous shunt, fistula, or graft used for dialysis, or has lymphedema or flaccidity following a stroke. Do not draw a blood sample in the same arm as a peripherally inserted central catheter (PICC). Listen to your client's suggestions for sites that have been successful and unsuccessful in the past. If your client has had frequent blood testing, he or she will often know a site that works well.

Often, people who are very sick, such as those in hospitals, do not have veins that are easily visible or palpable. Frequent blood specimen collection may leave scarring. Sclerotic medications can cause inflammation of the vein, resulting in thickening and hardening of the vein. For clients who do not have palpable veins in the antecubital fossa, the veins on the back of the hand or the forearm can be used. Avoid small superficial veins that are easily visible but do not have a dense, rubbery feeling. Do not attempt to access the veins on the inside of the wrist. These veins may be visible but are usually very small. In addition, both the radial artery and ulnar artery, as well as many nerve endings, are found there. Allow adequate time to find a vein with the best likelihood of success.

The only way to get better at feeling a vein is to practice. Nursing students need to practice feeling the veins of people of a variety of ages. Feel veins in children, adolescents, adults, and older adults to gain experience recognizing veins in many different people.

Encouraging a Vein to Dilate

Once you have selected a vein, the next step is to encourage the vein to dilate, thus making the inner lumen of the vein larger. There are several methods to encourage venous dilation. The most commonly used is a tourniquet. Tourniquets restrict blood return and cause the vein to swell. Tourniquets are applied only for a short time, not more than 60 seconds. Some client's veins do not tolerate the engorgement resulting from a tourniquet and will swell briefly and quickly collapse. On small veins, you can restrict blood return with your nondominant hand rather than using a tourniquet. Other methods of encouraging a vein to dilate are as follows:

- Gravity—holding an extremity below the heart helps to make the vein dilate.
- Muscular contractions, such as making a fist and releasing it, bring blood flow to the area and cause the veins to swell.

TABLE 12.2 Blood Collection Tubes

Color of Top	Additive	Purpose of Additive	Examples of the Laboratory Test
Purple	EDTA	Prevents blood from clotting	CBC Platelet count
Blue	Sodium citrate	Used when plasma is tested; prevents blood from clotting	PT, PTT
Gray	Sodium fluoride oxalate	Prevent glycolysis	Glucose Lactose tolerance Chemistry
Green	Heparin	Used when plasma is tested; prevents blood from clotting	Ammonia Carboxyhemoglobin Chemistry
Red	None	Used when serum is tested; allows sample to clot	Chemistry Bilirubin BUN Calcium
Red and black	None	Used to separate serum	Chemistry Serology

BUN, Blood urea nitrogen; *CBC,* complete blood count; *EDTA,* ethylenediamine tetraacetic acid; *PT,* prothrombin time; *PTT,* partial thromboplastin time.

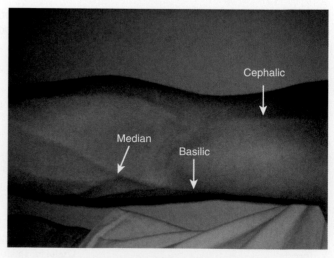

FIG. 12.3 Veins of the antecubital fossa.

- Warm compresses—heat brings blood flow to the area and causes vasodilation as well.
- Stroking or lightly tapping may help a vein to fill and will both encourage the dilation of the vein and enhance your assessment of the depth and breadth of the vein (Infusion Nurses Society [INS], 2016).

Cold, fear, and pain will encourage venous constriction. Thus, ensuring that the client is warm and reassured will facilitate venous access.

Preventing Problems

Venipuncture is a low-risk procedure. The most common problem is bruising at the site. The primary way to preventing bruising is to instruct the client to apply pressure on the site for 2 to 3 minutes. Not only does the wound need to form a clot, but more importantly, the vein needs pressure and time to form a clot. Frequently clients will check to see if their skin is still bleeding without understanding that they need to apply pressure until the vein has had time to form a clot. Discourage clients from bending the arm at the elbow because they cannot apply sufficient pressure on the vein in this position and, as a result, a hematoma may form.

Another potential problem, primarily for immune-compromised clients, is infection. Implementing infection control is the nursing intervention to prevent this problem. Cleansing the site and always using sterile equipment help to prevent the introduction of microbes. If an initial venipuncture attempt is not successful, and the needle touched or penetrated the skin, discard the needle and obtain a new sterile needle before making a second attempt.

APPLICATION OF THE NURSING PROCESS

Examples of Related International Classification for Nursing Practice (ICNP) Nursing Diagnoses, Expected Client Outcomes, and Nursing Interventions:

Nursing Diagnosis: Risk for injury

Supporting Data: Client is having blood specimen collection performed.

Expected Client Outcomes: Client will have no evidence of injury, such as:
- bruising at the specimen collection site.

Nursing Intervention Example: Apply pressure after specimen collection for 2 to 3 minutes. Apply pressure for 3 to 5 minutes if the client takes anticoagulants.

Reference: International Classification for Nursing Practice. (n.d.). *eHealth & ICNP*. Retrieved from https://www.icn.ch/what-we-do/projects/ehealth-icnp.

CRITICAL CONCEPTS
Collecting Venous Blood Specimens

Accuracy (ACC)

Venous blood specimen collection is subject to the following variables:

Client-Related Factors
- Client history, including age, allergies, medications, clinical status, and past procedures
- Client's veins, including size, characteristics, and integrity

Blood-Related Factors
- Hemolysis
- Hemoconcentration
- Clotting

Nurse-Related Factors
- Site of specimen collection
- Selection and use of equipment
- Use of sterile technique with blood cultures

Client-Centered Care (CCC)

When collecting venous blood specimens, respect for the client is demonstrated by:
- obtaining verbal consent and promoting autonomy
- explaining the procedure and arranging an interpreter if needed
- providing privacy and ensuring comfort
- answering questions before, during, and after collecting the blood specimen
- advocating for the client and family.

Infection Control (INF)

When collecting venous blood specimens, healthcare-associated infection is prevented by:
- containment of microorganisms
- preventing and reducing the transfer of microorganisms
- reducing the number of microorganisms.

Safety (SAF)

When collecting venous blood specimens, safety measures prevent harm and maintain a safe care environment, including:
- ensuring verification and documentation of the correct client and specimen.

Communication (COM)

- Communication exchanges information (oral, written, nonverbal, or electronic) between two or more people.
- Documentation records information in a permanent legal record.

Health Maintenance (HLTH)

When collecting venous blood specimens, nursing is dedicated to the promotion of health, including:
- protecting the client's skin integrity
- protecting vein wall integrity.

Evaluation (EVAL)

When collecting venous blood specimens, evaluation of outcomes enables the nurse to determine the efficacy of the care provided.

■ SKILL 12.1 Selecting a Vein

EQUIPMENT

Clean gloves, if there is a risk of exposure to body fluids
Warm compress
Tourniquet

BEGINNING THE SKILL

1. **SAF** Review the order. *Verifying the plan of care and medical history prevents injury to the client.*
2. **ACC** Review the following:
   - client's allergies, such as allergies to topical antimicrobials or latex
   - client's history related to procedures that alter vascular patterns, such as the presence of an arteriovenous shunt, fistula, or graft; lymphedema; or flaccidity following a stroke
   - client's medications, particularly medications that alter clotting time.
3. **INF** Perform hand hygiene.
4. **CCC** Introduce yourself to the client and family and explain that you are assessing the best site to draw blood. Ensure that the client gives verbal consent for the blood specimen collection. Listen to the client's suggestions and cautions.
5. **SAF** Identify the client using two identifiers.
6. **CCC** Provide privacy. Close the door, pull the curtain, and cover the client with a gown or blanket. *Chilling causes vasoconstriction.*
7. **INF** Apply gloves if there is a risk of exposure to body fluids. *If the skin is unbroken, there is little risk of exposure.*

PROCEDURE

8. **SAF** Set up an ergonomically safe space. If the client is in a bed, raise the bed to a comfortable working height and raise one side rail. *Setting up an ergonomically safe space prevents injury to the nurse and client.* If the client is seated, use the over-the-bed table to support the client's arms.
9. **ACC** Assess the following:
   - client's level of orientation and ability to follow instructions
   - presence of an IV line. *Do not draw venous blood samples above or near an infusing PIV line or in the same arm as a PICC because it may alter results, such as for a blood chemistry.*
10. **ACC** Inspect and palpate the client's veins in the antecubital area to determine size, pathway, and skin integrity. *Your assessment is to determine which vein has the best potential for obtaining a venous blood sample on the first try and has the fewest drawbacks.*
11. **ACC** Encourage vein dilation during your assessment through the following:
    - using gravity, keeping the site below heart level
    - muscular contractions, asking the client to squeeze and release his or her fist

- applying moist heat
- applying a tourniquet.

12. **ACC** To apply a tourniquet:
    a. Position the tourniquet behind the client's upper arm 5 to 10 cm (2–4 inches) above the selected vein.
    b. Place your thumbs close together on the tourniquet and stretch the tourniquet.

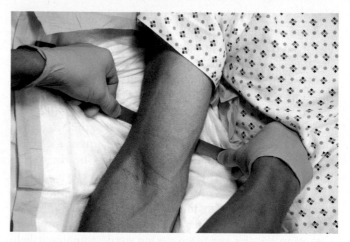

STEP 12B Stretch the tourniquet by placing your thumbs close together.

    c. Maintaining the tension in the tourniquet, bring the ends to the front of the client's arm. Transfer each tourniquet end to the opposite hand. Bring the end in your dominant hand to cross over the end in your nondominant hand. *Maintaining tension rather than pulling the tourniquet against the client's skin prevents pinching skin or pulling hair.*

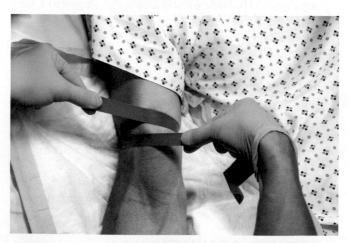

STEP 12C Change hands and cross the ends of the tourniquet.

    d. About 2 to 3 cm (about an inch) past the place where the two ends of the tourniquet cross each other, use a finger of your dominant hand to tuck a section of the tourniquet into the band of the tourniquet.

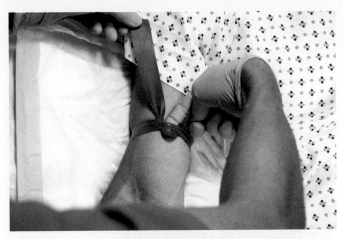

STEP 12D Tuck a section of the tourniquet into the band of the tourniquet.

e. The ends of the tourniquet should lie away from the venipuncture site. *This prevents the tourniquet from contaminating the cleaned area or getting in the way.*

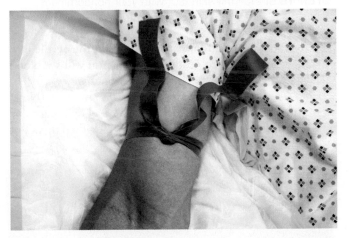

STEP 12E Place the tourniquet ends away from the site.

13. **ACC** Reassess the veins by feeling across the breadth of the vein and gently pressing on the vein to determine its recoil. *Veins are best selected by touch. Veins should have a dense, rubbery feel and spring back when pressed. Avoid thin superficial veins, veins that show signs of repeated access, and areas where the skin is in poor condition.*
14. **ACC** Select your vein of choice for venipuncture.
15. **CCC** Remove the tourniquet.

FINISHING THE SKILL

16. **SAF** Ensure client safety. Ensure that the bed is in the lowest position. Ensure the client can identify and reach the nurse call system. *These safety measures reduce the risk of falls.*
17. **CCC** Ensure client comfort. Provide reassurance and emotional support.
18. **INF** Perform hand hygiene.
19. **EVAL** Based on the assessment of the client's veins, select the appropriate equipment to proceed with Skill 12.2, Obtaining a Venous Blood Specimen.

■ SKILL 12.2 Obtaining Venous Blood Specimens

EQUIPMENT

Clean gloves
Antiseptic wipes
Tourniquet
Needle and syringe
Vacutainer assembly
Butterfly needle and syringe
Butterfly needle and Vacutainer
Laboratory vacuum blood collections tubes (see Table 12.2)
Cotton ball or gauze sponge
Disposable procedure pad

BEGINNING THE SKILL

1. **SAF** Review order. *Verifying the plan of care and medical history prevents injury to the client. Confirm your previous review of the following:*
   - client's allergies, such as allergies to topical antimicrobials or latex
   - client's history related to procedures that alter vascular patterns, such as the presence of an arteriovenous shunt, fistula, or graft; lymphedema; or flaccidity following a stroke
   - client's medications, particularly medications that alter clotting time.

2. **ACC** Determine and collect the color and number of laboratory vacuum collection tubes required to obtain the ordered laboratory tests.

3. **ACC** Select blood specimen collection equipment based on your assessment of the client's veins and the number of laboratory samples ordered. (Note: See Table 12.1 to review the advantages and disadvantages of various types of blood collection equipment.)

4. **INF** Perform hand hygiene.

5. **CCC** Introduce yourself to the client and family and explain the procedure.

6. **SAF** Identify the client using two identifiers. Recheck the client's allergies, such as allergies to topical antimicrobials or latex.

7. **CCC** Obtain verbal consent for the specimen collection. *Verbal consent supports the client's autonomy.*

8. **CCC** Provide privacy. Close the door, pull the curtain, and cover the client with a gown or blanket. *Chilling causes vasoconstriction.*

9. **INF** Apply clean gloves. Place a disposable procedure pad under the client's arm. *There is an inherent risk of exposure to blood when drawing a blood specimen. The disposable pad will contain any blood that may result from the specimen collection, thereby containing any blood-borne pathogens and protecting the surface from blood contamination.*

PROCEDURE

10. **SAF** Set up an ergonomically safe space. If the client is in a bed, raise the bed to a comfortable working height and raise one side rail. If the client is seated, use the over-the-bed table to support the client's arms. *Setting up an ergonomically safe space prevents injury to the nurse and client.*

11. **ACC** Prepare your work space and prepare your equipment. Determine the order of draw for the ordered blood tests. Set out the collection tubes in the order you will use them.

12. **INF** Return to the vein selected in the previous skill. Cleanse the selected site with an antiseptic wipe. If using isopropyl alcohol, cleanse by moving from the insertion site outward in a circular pattern. If using chlorhexidine, scrub in a back-and-forth pattern for 15 seconds. Do not touch the site after it has been cleaned. Allow the site to dry. *Allowing the site to dry enhances antiseptic activity and prevents stinging at the site.*

13. Apply the tourniquet again while the antiseptic is drying. See steps 12a to 12e in Skill 12.1.

Syringe/Needle

14. **ACC** Prepare the needle and syringe by attaching the needle to the syringe, ensuring a tight connection. Pull back the plunger of the syringe to break the seal, and then push the plunger in until almost all the air is out of the syringe. *Leaving a little room at the top of the syringe*

allows you to see blood enter the syringe. This is called the flashback.

15. **ACC** Remove the cap from the needle and set it aside. Position the needle bevel up. Stretch the skin taut with your nondominant hand.

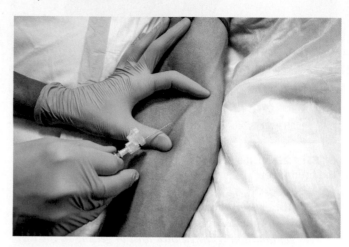

STEP 15 Stretch the skin taut with your nondominant hand.

16. **ACC** Using your dominant hand, insert the needle into the vein at a 30- to 45-degree angle. You will see blood enter the syringe. This is the flashback. *Your angle of entry is based on how deep or superficial the vein runs.* (Note: Entering the vein requires all of the bevel opening to be within the vein but not so far as to nick the far wall of the vein.)

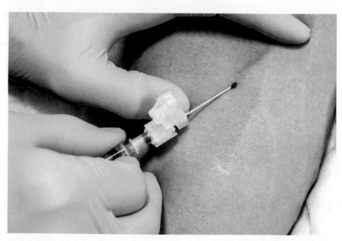

STEP 16 Insert the needle into the vein and you will see the flashback enter the syringe.

17. **SAF** Stabilize the syringe. Release the skin with your nondominant hand and pull back on the plunger until you have the required volume of blood in the syringe. *Stabilizing the syringe prevents the needle from moving in the vein, thereby preventing injury to the client and facilitating the blood draw.*

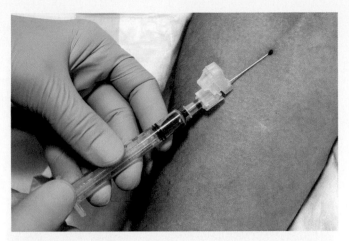

STEP 17 Pull back on the plunger.

18. **ACC** Release the tourniquet when blood is flowing into the syringe.
19. **CCC** Place a cotton ball or gauze lightly over the insertion site. Do not press firmly while the needle is in the vein. *Pressing on the needle could result in it nicking the vein.*

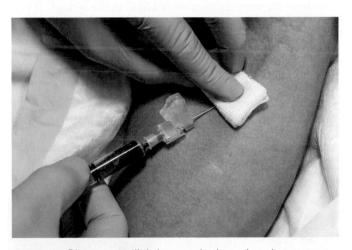

STEP 19 Place gauze lightly over the insertion site.

20. **HLTH** Remove the needle from the client's vein. Press the cotton ball or gauze more firmly over the insertion site. *Maintaining pressure over the insertion site prevents hematoma formation.*
21. **SAF** Activate the safety device on the needle guard. Discard the needle into a puncture-proof sharps container.
22. **HLTH** Place gauze pad with hypoallergenic tape on venipuncture site. Advise the client to maintain pressure over the venipuncture site for 2 to 3 minutes. *Pressure for 2 to 3 minutes is needed for the vein and wound to develop a clot.*
23. **SAF** Transfer blood into laboratory collection tubes using a needleless transfer device. Attach the syringe of blood to the transfer device, and then push the blood collection tube onto the needle (Occupational Safety and Health Administration [OSHA], 2015a).

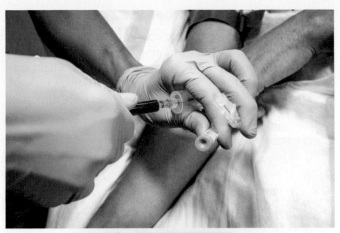

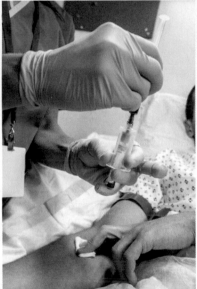

STEP 23 Transfer blood using a needleless transfer device.

24. **ACC** Gently invert laboratory collection tubes that contain additives to distribute the additive in the blood. Check with your laboratory if inversion is recommended. *There is evidence that mixing may not be necessary. Vigorous mixing is not recommended (Fernandez de Pinedo Perez, 2017).*

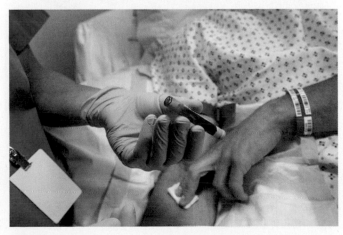

STEP 24 Gently invert laboratory collection tubes that contain additives.

Syringe/ Butterfly Needle

25. **ACC** Attach the syringe to the end of the butterfly needle tubing by twisting on the Luer-Lok hub of the syringe using sterile technique and ensuring a tight connection. Pull back the plunger of the syringe to break the seal, and then push the plunger in until almost all the air is out of the syringe.

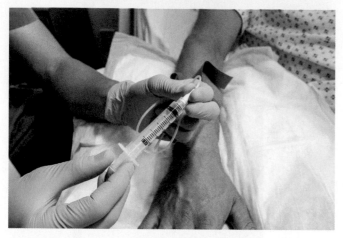

STEP 25 Attach the syringe to the end of the butterfly tubing.

26. **ACC** Remove the cap from the butterfly needle and set it aside. Some nurses prefer to fold the wings of the butterfly needle up and hold the wings positioned above the needle. Other nurses prefer to keep the wings horizontal. *A butterfly needle allows for variation in the angle of entry, including a lower angle of entry than a needle and syringe or Vacutainer.*

27. **ACC** Position the needle bevel up. Stretch the skin taut with your nondominant hand. Using your dominant hand, insert the needle into the vein at a 30- to 45-degree angle. You will see blood enter the tubing just after the butterfly needle. This is the flashback. *Entering the vein requires all of the bevel opening to be within the vein but not so far as to nick the far wall of the vein.*

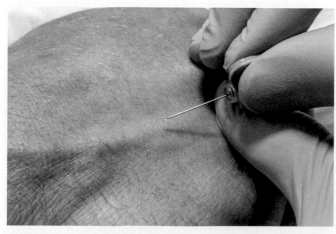

STEP 27 Position the needle bevel up. Stretch skin taut with your nondominant hand.

28. **ACC** Release the skin with your nondominant hand and stabilize the wings of the butterfly needle. Sometimes

nurses will secure the wings in position in the vein with tape.

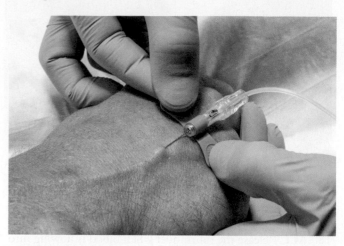

STEP 28 Stabilize the wings of the butterfly needle.

29. **ACC** Release the tourniquet as blood begins to enter the butterfly tubing.
30. **ACC** Pull back gently on the syringe plunger until you have the required volume of blood in the syringe. If you require more blood, detach the full syringe and attach a new syringe. *Pulling back the plunger too hard on a small vein can cause the vein to collapse.*
31. **CCC** Place a cotton ball or gauze lightly over the insertion site. Do not press firmly.
32. **HLTH** Remove the needle from the client's vein. Press the cotton ball or gauze more firmly over the insertion site.
33. **SAF** Activate the safety device on the butterfly needle guard. Discard the butterfly needle into a puncture-proof sharps container.

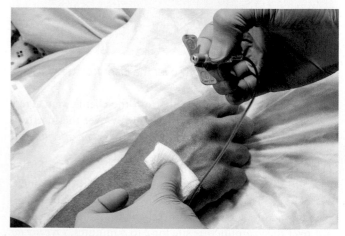

STEP 33 Activate the safety device on the butterfly needle guard.

34. **HLTH** Place gauze pad with hypoallergenic tape on venipuncture site. Advise the client to maintain pressure over the venipuncture site for 2 to 3 minutes. *Pressure for 2 to 3 minutes provides time for the vein and the skin to develop a clot.*
35. **SAF** Transfer blood into laboratory collection tubes using a needleless transfer device (OSHA, 2015a).

36. **ACC** Gently invert laboratory collection tubes that contain additives to distribute the additive in the blood. Check with your laboratory if inversion is recommended. *There is evidence showing that mixing may not be necessary. Vigorous mixing is not recommended (Fernandez de Pinedo Perez, 2017).*

Vacutainer

37. **ACC** Prepare the Vacutainer needle by attaching the Vacutainer holder to the two-sided needle using sterile technique. If the holder and needle are preassembled, ensure a tight connection and maintain sterile technique. Note the safety mechanism for your needle.

38. **ACC** Remove the cap from the needle and set it aside. Position the needle bevel up. Stretch the skin taut with your nondominant hand.

39. **ACC** Using your dominant hand, insert the needle into the vein at a 30- to 45-degree angle. You will *not* see blood. There is no flashback when using the Vacutainer system. *Entering the vein requires all of the bevel opening to be within the vein but not so far as to nick the far wall of the vein.*

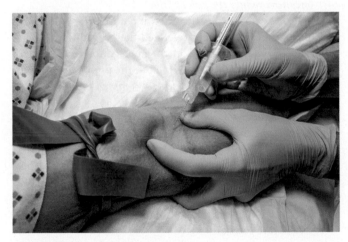

STEP 39 Insert the needle into the vein at a 30- to 45-degree angle.

40. **ACC** Stabilize the Vacutainer system. Pick up the first laboratory collection tube. Insert the tube into the holder and press it onto the Vacutainer needle. **WARNING:** You must hold the Vacutainer very still while pressing the laboratory collection tube. *Stabilization of the vacutainer will prevent needle movement in the vein.*

41. **ACC** Release the tourniquet as blood begins to enter the collection tube.

42. **ACC** Allow the laboratory collection tube to fill. When full, remove the laboratory collection tube while keeping the needle still in the vein. Apply a new laboratory collection tube for the next ordered lab. Repeat until all of the lab work is collected.

43. **CCC** Remove the last collection tube. Place a cotton ball or gauze lightly over the insertion site. Do not press firmly while the needle is in the vein. *Removing the last collection tube from the Vacutainer needle ensures that blood from the collection tube will not be released.*

44. **HLTH** Remove the needle from the client's vein. Press the cotton ball more firmly over the insertion site.

45. **SAF** Activate the safety device on the needle guard. Discard the Vacutainer system into a puncture-proof sharps container. (Note: OSHA [2015a] recommends discarding the needle and holder as a unit.)

46. **ACC** Gently invert laboratory collection tubes that contain additives to distribute the additive in the blood. Check with your laboratory if inversion is recommended. *There is evidence showing that mixing may not be necessary. Vigorous mixing is not recommended (Fernandez de Pinedo Perez, 2017).*

47. **HLTH** Place gauze pad with hypoallergenic tape on venipuncture site. Advise the client to maintain pressure over the venipuncture site for 2 to 3 minutes. *Pressure for 2 to 3 minutes provides time for the vein and the skin to develop a clot.*

Vacutainer/Butterfly Needle

48. **ACC** Attach the Vacutainer holder to the end of the butterfly tubing and ensure a tight seal.

49. **ACC** Remove the cap from the butterfly needle and set it aside. Position the butterfly wings. Fold the wings of the butterfly up and hold the wings positioned above the needle or keep the wings horizontal. *A butterfly needle allows for variation in the angle of entry, including a lower angle of entry than a needle and syringe or Vacutainer.* Position the needle bevel up. Stretch the skin taut with your nondominant hand.

50. **ACC** Using your dominant hand, insert the needle into the vein at a 15- to 30-degree angle. You will see blood enter the tubing just after the butterfly needle. This is the flashback. *Entering the vein requires all of the bevel opening to be within the vein but not so far as to nick the far wall of the vein.*

51. **ACC** Release the skin with your nondominant hand and stabilize the butterfly wings. Secure the butterfly wings in position in the vein with tape, as needed.

52. **ACC** Pick up the first laboratory collection tube. Insert the tube into the Vacutainer holder and press it onto the Vacutainer needle. (Note: With the butterfly Vacutainer system, the butterfly needle must be stabilized to prevent moving the needle in the vein. However, you do not have to worry about keeping the Vacutainer still as you insert and remove the laboratory collection tubes as you did with the Vacutainer system.)

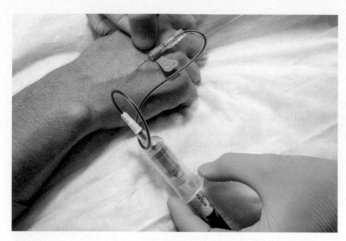

STEP 52 Insert the tube into the Vacutainer holder and press it onto the Vacutainer needle.

53. **ACC** Release the tourniquet as blood begins to enter the collection tube.
54. **ACC** Allow the laboratory collection tube to fill. When full, remove the laboratory collection tube and apply a new laboratory collection tube for the next ordered lab. Repeat until all of the lab work is collected.
55. **HLTH** Remove the needle from the client's vein. Press the cotton ball or gauze more firmly over the insertion site.

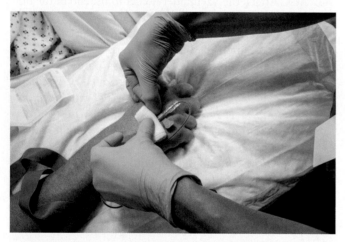

STEP 55 Remove the needle from the client's vein.

56. **SAF** Activate the safety device on the butterfly needle guard. Discard the butterfly needle into a puncture-proof sharps container.
57. **HLTH** Place gauze pad with hypoallergenic tape on venipuncture site. Advise the client to maintain pressure over the venipuncture site for 2 to 3 minutes. *Pressure for 2 to 3 minutes provides time for the vein and the skin to develop a clot.*
58. **SAF** Transfer blood into laboratory collection tubes using a needleless transfer device (OSHA, 2015a).
59. **ACC** Gently invert laboratory collection tubes that contain additives to distribute the additive in the blood. Check with your laboratory if inversion is recommended. *There is evidence showing that mixing may not be necessary. Vigorous mixing is not recommended (Fernandez de Pinedo Perez, 2017).*

FINISHING THE SKILL

60. **INF** Remove gloves and perform hand hygiene.
61. **SAF** Ensure client comfort and safety. Ensure that the bed is in the lowest position. Ensure the client can identify and reach the nurse call system. *These safety measures reduce the risk of falls.*
62. **EVAL** Evaluate the outcomes, including the blood sample and how the client tolerated the procedure.
63. **COM** Ensure the specimen label contains two client identifiers. Label the specimen in the presence of the client. *National safety guidelines recommend labeling specimens in the presence of the client.*
64. **COM** Document your initials and the date and time of blood specimen collection on the label, if agency policy.
65. **ACC** Transport to the laboratory per agency policy within the time limit. *Many institutions require transportation in a resealable plastic bag.*
66. **COM** Document date, time, and type of laboratory specimens collected and client outcomes in the legal healthcare record.

SECTION 2 Initiating, Dressing, and Discontinuing a Peripheral Intravenous Catheter

Vascular access may be an important part of a client's treatment regimen. An IV infusion may provide fluids when a client cannot drink sufficient fluid to remain hydrated or may provide IV medications. Initiating and safely maintaining a PIV requires attention to accuracy variables, such as anatomical landmarks and proper techniques, as well as infection control measures.

SELECTING A VEIN

Selecting a vein for a PIV infusion uses different criteria than selecting a vein for venipuncture. The objective is to select a site that will last for the full length of the prescribed fluid and or medication therapy. Collaboration with the client to mutually determine a site is preferred. A preinsertion assessment is a critical step to avoid venous access problems (Vizcarra et al., 2014).

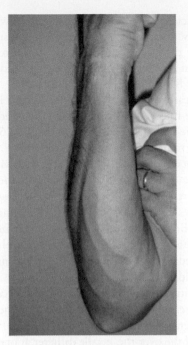

FIG. 12.4 Accessing veins on the forearm is advantageous because they are easily stabilized and do not interfere with joint movement. These veins are more often visible and palpable in men than in women.

Veins in any joint, including the antecubital fossa, are problematic for PIV infusion for several reasons, including the more superficial position of nerves and arteries at joints and the interrupted flow of IV fluid when the client flexes the joint. Common complications from using veins in a joint include infiltration and extravasation, nerve injury, and phlebitis and infection (Vizcarra et al., 2014).

PIV lines should be placed in an upper extremity. The ideal veins for a PIV are as follows:
- located distally
- not located over a joint
- at a site free of bruising or poor skin integrity
- straight
- lacking visible valves
- well stabilized in the connective tissue.

Veins frequently selected for PIV use in adults include the larger veins on the back of the hand, such as the basilic vein, and the cephalic vein just above the wrist. Accessing veins on the forearm is advantageous because the forearm is easily stabilized for minimal joint movement. These veins are more often visible and palpable in men than in women (Fig. 12.4). For infants, veins on the scalp or the upper and lower extremities may be selected (Centers for Disease Control and Prevention [CDC], 2015; INS, 2016). See Box 12.1 for details on using scalp veins for IV access.

The process of assessing a vein for a PIV line use is very similar to the assessment process for venipuncture. Inspect the client's hands and forearms using the methods to encourage venous dilation described for venipuncture in Skill 12.1, including the use of a tourniquet, muscular contractions, warm compress, and gravity. Listen to your client, and check the medical record to determine if the client has had an event

BOX 12.1 Lifespan Considerations: Using Scalp Veins for Venous Access in Infants

Infants have very small peripheral veins, and accessing those to insert a peripheral intravenous (PIV) line may be very difficult. In adults, the recommendation is to only use the upper extremities; however, in pediatrics, the lower extremities may be considered as well. In neonates and very young infants, veins in the upper and lower extremities may be accessed. Although seldom a first choice, scalp veins offer another option for very young infants, specifically the frontal posterior auricular and the superficial temporal veins. Advantages of the scalp veins include minimal subcutaneous fat over the vessel, lack of a flexible joint, and less movement than hands or feet. The lack of movement can make a scalp IV more stable than an IV in a hand.

When a scalp vein is selected, a rubber band is used as a tourniquet and is placed around the infant's head just above the eyes and ears to distend the scalp veins. Some of the infant's hair may need to be shaved in order to tape the IV securely. Seeing their infant with a scalp vein in place can be frightening for parents. Share with the parents the advantages of using the scalp and, if you must shave some of the infant's hair, save it to give to the parents.

or procedure that alters vascular patterns and prohibits venous access, such as the presence of an arteriovenous shunt, fistula, or graft used for dialysis; lymphedema; or flaccidity following a stroke. Feel the breadth, depth, and length of the vein. Veins have a dense, rubbery feel and recoil when pressed.

A vein-visualization assistive device may make finding a vein easier. The device may use transillumination, ultrasound, or near-infrared light to facilitate venous assessment. The use of vascular-visualization devices may be warranted after an initial attempt has failed or for clients with known difficult venous access. The use of a vein-visualization device is encouraged by the Intravenous Nurses Society (INS) and is an option for clients whose veins are difficult to palpate. The integration of vein-visualization technology has demonstrated shortened nursing time to initiate an IV line, improved first-time success rate, and improved client satisfaction (Kanipe, Shobe, Li, Kime, & Smith-Miller, 2018). Nurses must be competent in the use of vascular-visualization technology before attempting IV line insertion. Factors that impact nurses' ability to observe and palpate peripheral veins include the following:
- age—neonatal, pediatric, and geriatric
- skin tone and tattoos
- excessive hair
- history of IV drug use
- obesity
- diseases, such as diabetes
- courses of treatment and previous infusion therapy (INS, 2016).

Much of the initial research has been done in pediatric populations. However, the evidence on near-infrared (nIR) light technology does not show across-the-board improvement on first attempts. See Box 12.2 for further discussion of studies on nIR vein visualization.

BOX 12.2 **Lessons From the Evidence: Using Vein Visualization Devices With Children**

Obtaining venous access can be challenging in infants and children. Their veins are smaller and may be less visible under subcutaneous tissue than those of adults. Transillumination and ultrasound have been available for some time, but the newest tool is a near-infrared (nIR) light device. Many studies have been conducted, along with several systematic reviews and meta-analyses of those studies. The results are mixed. Park et al. conducted a comprehensive review of the literature screening 1310 studies. They identified 11 studies that were randomized controlled trials comparing peripheral intravenous (PIV) line initiation using nIR light and the traditional method of insertion. While the nIR light device did not have an impact on the failure rate at the first attempt, which was the primary outcome, the researchers noted that the risk of failure was lower in the NIR group than in the control group. This finding is consistent with a previous study showing that in children predicted to have difficult PIV initiation, the nIR light was helpful in reducing the risk of failure (Park et al., 2016).

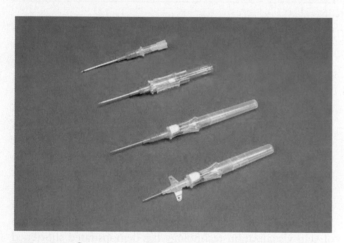

FIG. 12.5 Over-the-needle catheters in a variety of gauge sizes. Shown here are 18G green, 20G pink, 22G blue, and 24G yellow.

When selecting the best vein, keep in mind that a peripheral vein may not always be the best choice. Although venous access through a PIV is recommended if the antibiotic therapy will be less than 6 days, when it is determined that the client may require IV access for a longer period of time or past medication administration and illness have compromised the client's peripheral veins, then a midline catheter, PICC, or central venous catheter is preferred (CDC, 2015).

Using an Over-the-Needle Catheter

The primary equipment used to initiate a PIV line is an over-the-needle catheter. As shown in Fig. 12.5, over-the-catheter needles come in a variety of gauge sizes. The nurse selects the gauge to be used based on the size of the vein, the volume of fluid to be infused, the type and viscosity of medications to be infused, and the possibility of administering

blood products. Select the smallest gauge that will accommodate the prescribed fluids and medications, usually a 20- to 24-gauge. If there is a possibility of administering a blood product, then a 16- to 20-gauge catheter is needed to prevent hemolysis of RBCs (INS, 2016).

The soft catheter rests over the needle and is attached to a hub; some hubs have short wings. The needle is used to introduce the catheter into the vein (Fig. 12.6). Upon seeing a blood return in the flashback chamber, the device is advanced just enough to ensure the catheter is within the vein, and then the catheter is advanced without the needle. The angle of insertion is initially greater when accessing the vein, then decreases to almost parallel while threading the catheter in the vein. Box 12.3 shares an easy-to-visualize analogy for changing the angle of insertion. The use of steel needles (e.g., butterfly needles) is to be avoided for the administration of irritating fluids or medications (CDC, 2015).

Before initiating the PIV, assemble the necessary equipment for either a saline lock or IV fluids. A saline lock is made up of an extension set (a short piece of tubing) that attaches to the hub of the over-the-needle catheter at one end and has a needleless connector attached at the other. The equipment must be primed in order to insert into the IV catheter hub quickly once the IV catheter is threaded in the vein. The PIV catheter may be connected to an extension set or directly to the tubing of the primary line (administration set).

When initiating a PIV line, some facility policies may have the nurse inject 1% lidocaine or use a topical anesthetic, such as the numbing EMLA cream, to reduce discomfort. Initiating an IV line hurts more than venipuncture, so assess your client's degree of anxiety and level of cooperation before starting. Use the nonpharmacological comfort measures described in Chapter 7, such as distraction and guided imagery.

Preventing Infection

Infection prevention begins with hand hygiene and the use of clean gloves for personal protection. Any practice of not wearing gloves or removing a portion of a glove puts the nurse and client at risk.

Prior to inserting a PIV catheter, clean the skin at the insertion site with an approved antiseptic solution. Chlorhexidine gluconate in isopropyl alcohol has become the standard for skin preparation, except in infants less than 2 months of age; however, 70% alcohol or povidone-iodine may be used. The antiseptic solution must be allowed to dry before initiating insertion of the catheter (INS, 2016). The insertion site may not be touched after it has been cleaned unless the nurse puts on sterile gloves.

Placing a catheter into a vein creates a small wound and a potential opening for microorganisms to enter the body. The PIV dressing serves to protect the IV insertion site from microorganisms and still maintain easy visualization of the site to allow for frequent assessments. A transparent, semipermeable film dressing is placed over the insertion site. The dressing allows air exchange but prevents bacteria, viruses, and liquids from passing through the film barrier. If the IV site is not dry, a sterile gauze dressing may be placed over the site temporarily (CDC, 2015).

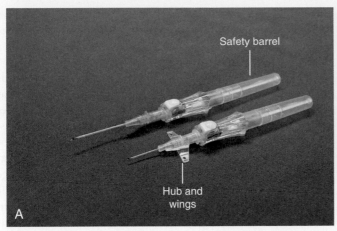
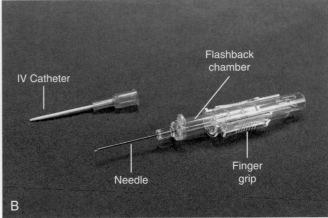

FIG. 12.6 Over-the-needle catheters have different types of safety devices. **A,** These have a white button that retracts the needle. **B,** With this type, the nurse slides the needle back into the clear plastic handle.

BOX 12.3 Lessons From Experience: Landing an Airplane Analogy

Caroline is a nursing student practicing initiating a peripheral intravenous (PIV) line in the skills lab. She comes to her instructor and states that she is having trouble understanding when to change the angle of entry when she is inserting the PIV line. She shares that she is nervous about piercing the skin and seeing blood.

Her instructor responds by sharing an analogy used in explaining PIV procedures to children. She feels that this analogy might help Caroline when she is starting a PIV line. "With children," she explains, "we might not say that we're going to put a needle into their vein. Instead, we might suggest that they think about the needle as an airplane. Our goal is to land the airplane on a runway, and their blue vein is our runway.

"So think about the client's vein as your runway. Think about your over-the-needle PIV catheter as your airplane. You need to adjust your angle of entry to get the airplane touching down on the runway, and then you need to drop your wheels (in other words, decrease your angle of entry) before you advance any further. Then, making sure your over-the-needle catheter is on the runway, separate the catheter from the needle and slide the catheter along the runway."

Caroline went back to the PIV mannequin and practiced "dropping her wheels" as soon as she saw a flashback. She quickly mastered decreasing her angle of entry and threading the catheter into the vein.

Antibiotic ointments are never placed over a PIV insertion site because evidence has demonstrated that the ointment does not prevent infection but, rather, provides an environment that supports fungal infections and antibiotic resistance. Once the transparent dressing is in place, do not allow the dressing to be immersed in water because this would allow microorganisms access to the insertion site. If clients with a PIV line are able to shower, the transparent dressing is covered with a waterproof barrier. Recommendations for changing PIV dressings state that any time the dressing is damp, loosened, or visibly soiled, the catheter site dressing is to be changed (CDC, 2015).

Stabilizing the Site During Insertion

When initiating a PIV, your nondominant hand will hold the skin taut and hold on to the vein. Holding the skin taut allows the needle to enter the skin smoothly and prevents the skin from bunching up. Some veins are fairly mobile; nurses refer to these as veins that roll. Envision the ropey veins on the back of an athletic person. Although they are easily visible, they are not tightly anchored in connective tissue. To be successful in inserting the over-the-needle catheter, you must use your nondominant hand to anchor the vein. Keep your thumb out of the way of the incoming catheter, and find a hold that allows you to achieve an angle of entry almost parallel to the skin. When initiating a PIV in an infant, a board is sometimes used, and the extremity is taped to the board. This stabilizes the vein during insertion and continues to prevent flexion at a joint.

Stabilizing the PIV

Once the dressing is in place, stabilize the PIV hub either with a catheter stabilization device or tape, and secure the IV tubing to prevent the catheter from moving within the vein or from being accidentally pulled out. Stabilization is essential to reduce movement at the catheter hub, which would irritate the vein, increasing the risk of phlebitis. The Infusion Nurses Society (INS) recommends the use of a stabilization device over tape (INS, 2016). Stabilization devices usually attach to the catheter hub and prevent movement that might kink the soft catheter. See Fig. 12.7 for one type of stabilization device. Ensure that the line and catheter cannot be easily disconnected or disengaged. As shown in Fig. 12.8, taping the tubing in a U-shape transfers the pressure changes of movement from the insertion site to the most distal point where the tape is secured.

Certain risk factors are known to contribute to losing a secure IV line and intact dressing. Tape does not adhere well to clients who are sweating or clammy, which is frequently seen with cardiovascular insufficiency. Children and confused clients often pick at dressings, sometimes without being aware they are doing so. When active clients rise and

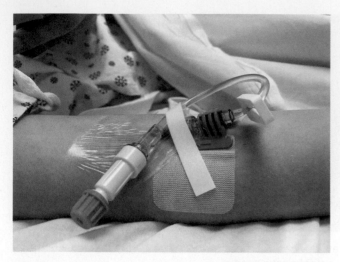

FIG. 12.7 A stabilization device secures the position of the catheter.

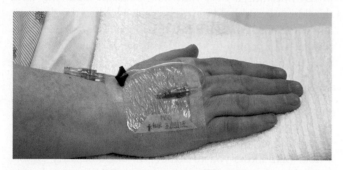

FIG. 12.8 Secure the tubing in a U-shape to prevent pulling on the catheter insertion site.

ambulate, the tubing, especially the Y-shaped medication port, may catch on the bed rails, or the weight of the tubing may pull the tape loose. Additionally, as clients stand, changes in venous pressure in a dependent hand or arm may cause blood return to back up into the tubing of the IV line. Unless the pressure is changed to flow fluid back into the vein and clear the catheter and tubing of blood, there is a risk of clot formation and IV line obstruction. The nurse who is aware of these risk factors can discuss with the client a plan of care to maintain a patent and secure PIV and can perform more frequent assessments, as discussed next.

Assessing an IV Site

When assessing the PIV site, the expected outcome is for the line to remain patent and secure and for the site to be free of infiltration, phlebitis, and local infection. Assess the site and the tape securing the IV line every hour in an intensive care setting or every 15 minutes during a blood transfusion. Many patent lines have been lost by not being adequately secured. Inspect and palpate the insertion site

through the transparent dressing to obtain an objective assessment. Ask the client if the site is tender for a subjective assessment. Tenderness is an early warning sign of a problematic IV line.

Assess the site for infiltration, the presence of IV fluids in the tissue around the vein. This may occur at any time as a result of a compromised vein, but the risk increases after changes in the pressure, volume, and type of infusing fluids. Nonvesicants are types of fluids and medications that are not irritating or damaging to the surrounding tissue. In contrast, vesicants are fluids and medications that can cause damage if they leak into the surrounding tissue. Infiltration of a vesicant is called extravasation. Irritants differ from vesicants in that they are irritating to the inside of the vein, whereas vesicants cause damage if they are outside of the vein. However, irritants such as sclerotic medications and fluids may increase the risk of infiltration.

The first sign of infiltration is often discomfort. Other signs of infiltration include swelling and blanching as IV fluid seeps into the surrounding tissue. The site may feel cool to the touch, due to the infusion of room-temperature IV fluid, which is significantly cooler than body temperature. Assess for dependent edema by comparing both hands and forearms bilaterally. Gravity will pull the fluid to the palm of the hand or posterior forearm, and without direct comparison, infiltration may go unrecognized. When infiltration is detected, the IV line must be discontinued.

Assess the site for phlebitis, which is inflammation of the vein. Signs of phlebitis include redness in streaks radiating from the vein, edema, and skin that is warmer to the touch. The area may be tender to the touch. When phlebitis is detected, the IV must be discontinued. In addition, assess for signs of infection. Look for discharge at the insertion site, redness, swelling, and tenderness.

Document each IV site assessment, noting the presence or absence of any signs of infiltration or phlebitis. Additionally, documenting the presence of blood return and the ease of flushing provides evidence that the nurse is checking the patency of the PIV. Careful documentation may be essential to defend against a charge of negligence (Box 12.4).

APPLICATION OF THE NURSING PROCESS

Examples of Related ICNP Nursing Diagnoses, Expected Client Outcomes, and Nursing Interventions:

Nursing Diagnosis: Risk for infection

Supporting Data: Potential for organism entry due to presence of an invasive line.

Expected Client Outcomes: The client will remain free from symptoms of infection while in the healthcare setting, as seen by:

- temperature and vital signs within established parameters

BOX 12.4 Lessons From the Courtroom: Nursing Documentation Provides Crucial Evidence

In 2010, a jury in a Florida circuit court found no negligence and awarded no damages to a woman who filed a $3.5 million lawsuit against a hospital. The client was a 46-year-old woman with chronic pancreatitis who was admitted and prescribed intravenous main medication, specifically Demerol and Phenergan. The nurses placed a peripheral intravenous (PIV) line in her left foot after unsuccessful attempts in an upper extremity. The nursing notes showed documentation that the PIV was assessed regularly. The next morning when the woman complained of pain in her foot, the PIV was discontinued. Unfortunately, the woman went on to develop gangrene in her foot, and the foot was amputated. However, because the nurses' careful documentation noted that the PIV line flushed easily and had a blood return, and that there was no redness or edema at the site throughout the time the PIV was infusing, the jury ruled there was no negligence by a hospital caregiver.

Note: In September of 2009, the U.S. Food and Drug Administration (FDA) began requiring a boxed warning for Phenergan (intravenous Promethazine) to communicate the risk for severe tissue injury, including gangrene, when administered intravenously.

Reference: IV Infiltration Alleged in Patient's Suit: Jury Sees No Negligence by Patient's Nurses, 2011.

- absence of heat, pain, redness, swelling, and unusual drainage at the IV insertion site.

Nursing Intervention Example: Use Standard Precautions, such as hand hygiene before each client encounter.

Nursing Diagnosis: Anxiety

Supporting Data: Client states, "I hate needles." Startles with each touch during vein assessment.

Expected Client Outcome: Client will relate increased psychological and physiological comfort, as seen by:
- describing own coping mechanisms
- identifying strategies to reduce anxiety

Nursing Intervention Example: Implement nonpharmacological comfort measures and pharmacological measures as prescribed.

Reference: International Classification for Nursing Practice. (n.d.). *eHealth & ICNP*. Retrieved from https://www.icn.ch/what-we-do/projects/ehealth-icnp.

CRITICAL CONCEPTS
Initiating a Peripheral Intravenous Line

Accuracy (ACC)

Initiating a PIV is subject to the following variables:

Client-Related Factors
- Client age, medical history, and clinical status, including allergies, medications, and past procedures
- Client's veins, including size, characteristics, and integrity

Nurse-Related Factors
- Site of PIV insertion
- Selection and use of equipment
- Preparation of equipment
- Use of sterile technique

Client-Centered Care (CCC)

When initiating a PIV line, respect for the client is demonstrated by:
- obtaining verbal consent and promoting autonomy, including site selection
- providing privacy and ensuring comfort, including the use of lidocaine, EMLA, or a vein visualizer
- answering questions before, during, and after initiating a PIV line
- explaining the procedure and arranging an interpreter if needed
- honoring cultural preferences, including right-hand/left-hand preferences
- advocating for the client and family.

Infection Control (INF)

When initiating a PIV, healthcare-associated infection is prevented by:
- containment of microorganisms
- preventing and reducing the transfer of microorganisms
- reducing the number of microorganisms
- preventing an environment conducive to microbial growth.

Safety (SAF)

When initiating a PIV line, safety measures prevent harm to the client. and maintain a safe care environment, including:
- verifying the correct client and the client allergies
- using a securement device or tape to maintain catheter position and patency.

Communication (COM)

- Communication exchanges information (oral, written, nonverbal, or electronic) between two or more people.
- Documentation records information in a permanent legal record.
- Collaboration with the client improves care when initiating a PIV line.

Health Maintenance (HLTH)

When initiating a PIV line, nursing is dedicated to the promotion of health, including:
- protecting the client's skin integrity
- protecting vein wall integrity.

Evaluation (EVAL)

When initiating a PIV line, evaluation of outcomes enables the nurse to determine the efficacy of the care provided.

▪ SKILL 12.3 Inserting and Dressing a Peripheral Intravenous Catheter

EQUIPMENT

Clean gloves
Antiseptic wipes
Tourniquet
Cotton ball or gauze sponge
Disposable procedure pad
Over-the-needle catheter
(10-mL) 0.9% Normal saline flush
Extension set
Needleless connector
Transparent dressing
Stabilization device, if available
Tape

BEGINNING THE SKILL

1. **SAF** Review the authorized healthcare provider's order and facility policy. Determine if IV fluids are ordered or the PIV will be put to a saline lock. *Verifying the plan of care prevents injury to the client.*
2. **INF** Perform hand hygiene.
3. **CCC** Introduce yourself to the client and family and explain the procedure. Explain that you are initially selecting a vein (see Skill 12.1) and will then be inserting a PIV line. Ensure the client has given verbal consent for the PIV insertions. Listen to the client's suggestions and cautions. Discuss options for procedural pain management, such as topical anesthetic or local anesthetic, if available in your agency.
4. **SAF** Identify the client using two identifiers.
5. **CCC** Provide privacy. Close the door and pull the curtain.

PROCEDURE
Assessing Veins

6. **SAF** Recheck the following by asking the client about:
   - client's allergies, such as allergies to topical antimicrobials or latex
   - client's history related to procedures that alter vascular patterns, such as the presence of an arteriovenous shunt, fistula, or graft; lymphedema; or flaccidity following a stroke
   - Client's medications, particularly medications that alter clotting time.
7. **SAF** Set up an ergonomically safe space. Use the over-the-bed table to support the client's arms, and pull up a seat to be at the client's level. Alternately, raise the bed to a comfortable working height and raise one side rail. *Setting up an ergonomically safe space prevents injury to the nurse and client.*
8. **INF** Place a disposable procedure pad under the client's forearm and hand. *The disposable pad will contain any blood that may result from the PIV insertion, thereby containing any blood-borne pathogens and protecting the surface from blood contamination.*

9. **ACC** Assess the client's vein using the procedure in Skill 12.1, and select your vein of choice for inserting a PIV. Use a vein-visualization assistive device, if available, for veins that are difficult to assess. Apply topical anesthetic, if ordered, and allow adequate time for the anesthetic to take effect.
10. **INF** Perform hand hygiene before leaving the room or collecting equipment.

Preparing for PIV Insertion

11. **ACC** Select over-the-needle catheter based on your assessment of the client's veins, IV rate, and medications ordered. *Catheter size should be the smallest gauge necessary to do the job.*
12. **INF** Perform hand hygiene before assembling equipment.
13. **ACC** Flush an extension tubing and needleless access cap, which can act as a saline lock, or connect to PIV line fluid as ordered. See Skill 12.7, Preparing a Primary Intravenous Line, if IV fluids are ordered.
    a. Open the sterile package of the extension tubing.
    b. Open the needleless connector and remove from the package.
    c. Remove the cap on the male adapter of the needleless connector, maintaining sterility.
    d. Remove the extension tubing from the package and remove the cap over the female adapter, keeping the opening sterile.
    e. Attach the needleless connector to the extension tubing.
    f. Scrub the hub of the needleless connector with alcohol and allow it to dry.
    g. Attach the 10-mL 0.9% normal saline flush to the needleless connector and flush saline through the extension tubing.

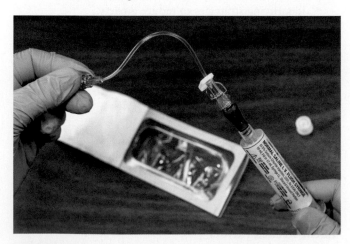

STEP 13G Flush an extension tubing and needleless connector.

h. Remove or loosen the cap at the other end of the extension tubing, the male adapter. Keep the end sterile by placing it back into the sterile packaging that it came in.

i. Place the extension set nearby so that you can see it easily in your peripheral vision.

Inserting the PIV Catheter

14. **INF** Apply gloves. *There is an inherent risk of exposure to blood.* Return to the vein selected. Cleanse the selected site with an antiseptic wipe for 15 seconds. Allow the site to air dry. **WARNING:** Do *not* touch the site after it has been cleaned unless you have applied sterile gloves and maintained sterility. (Note: If using chlorhexidine, scrub the site in a back-and-forth motion. If using isopropyl alcohol, cleanse by moving from the insertion site outward in a circular pattern.) *Allowing the site to dry enhances antiseptic activity and prevents stinging at the site.*

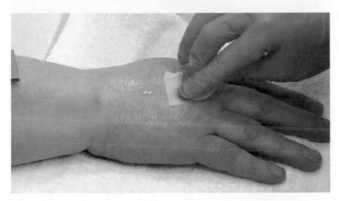

STEP 14 Cleanse selected site with an antiseptic wipe.

15. **CCC** Administer topical or local anesthetic, if ordered. (Note: If topical cream is ordered, it is applied and the appropriate amount of time must be allowed to pass. If local anesthetic is ordered, it is administered via the intradermal route, raising a wheal at the insertion site.)

16. **ACC** Apply the tourniquet (see Skill 12.1).

17. **ACC** Remove the cap from the needle and set it aside. Position the needle bevel up. (Note: Hold the catheter with your fingers above the catheter and not as a pencil.) With your nondominant hand, stretch the skin taut and anchor the selected vein below the identified insertion site.

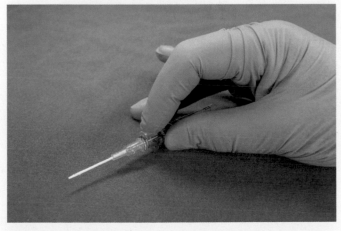

STEP 17 Hold the catheter with your fingers above the catheter and not like a pencil.

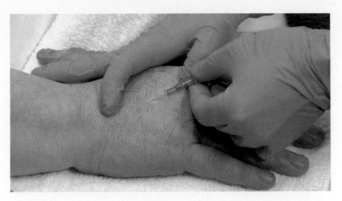

STEP 17 Stretch the skin taut and anchor the selected vein below the identified insertion site.

18. **ACC** Using your dominant hand, insert the needle into the vein at a 10- to 30-degree angle depending on the depth of the vein. *Deeper veins require a greater angle of entry; superficial veins require a smaller angle of entry.* If you are in the vein, you will see blood enter the catheter. This is the flashback. *Entering the vein requires all of the bevel opening to be within the vein, but do not advance so far as to nick the far wall of the vein.*

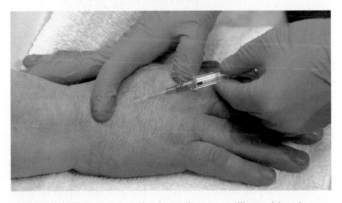

STEP 18 When you are in the vein, you will see blood enter the catheter.

19. **ACC** Decrease your angle of entry, and advance the needle just enough to ensure the catheter is within the vein. Hold the needle still and advance only the catheter along the path of the vein until the hub meets the skin.

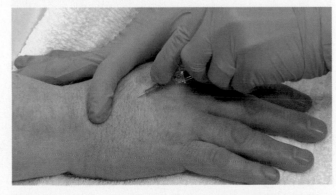

STEP 19 Advance only the catheter along the path of the vein.

20. **ACC** Hold the hub of the catheter, and do not allow the hub to move. Release the tourniquet. *The vein no longer needs to be dilated.*
21. **CCC** While keeping your eyes on the insertion site, locate the prefilled extension set or IV tubing. Do *not* take your eyes off the insertion site. Use your peripheral vision to locate your equipment.
22. **CCC** Place a finger over the vein above the IV insertion site and apply gentle pressure on the vein with your finger. *Gentle pressure will reduce the flow of blood while you disengage the needle from the catheter and will allow you to quickly insert the extension set with minimum blood flow.*
23. **SAF** Disengage the needle from the catheter hub and engage the needle safety mechanism. Do not allow the hub to twist or fold back. *Catheters are soft and flexible; once they have been bent, they will more easily kink.*

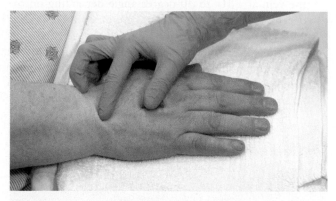

STEPS 22 AND 23 Apply gentle pressure on the vein with your finger. Remove the needle.

24. **ACC** Insert the prefilled extension set or IV tubing. Ensure the tourniquet has been released. Flush the tubing until all visible blood has been cleared from the line. As you flush, assess the site for any signs of infiltration. *Double checking that the tourniquet no longer blocks the flow of blood is important prior to adding flush solution to the vein.*

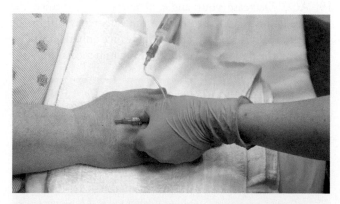

STEP 24 Flush the tubing until all visible blood has been cleared from the line.

Dressing the PIV Insertion Site

25. **ACC** Stabilize the catheter and tubing by applying a piece of tape across the tubing just below the catheter hub or applying a stabilization device. Add another piece of tape across the tubing to prevent the IV tubing from pulling on the insertion site.
26. **INF** If there is blood on the skin surrounding the insertion site, clean it off with an antiseptic wipe. *Blood supports bacterial growth, and the goal is to remain free from infection.*
27. **ACC** Open the transparent dressing package and remove the backing. Hold the dressing such that it does not stick to itself.
28. **INF** Apply the dressing over the insertion site, covering the colored catheter hub but not the junction of the hub and the extension set. Apply a stabilization device to the catheter hub, per facility policy.

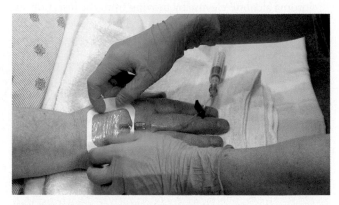

STEP 28 Apply the dressing over the insertion site and covering the colored catheter hub.

29. **SAF** Loop the tubing of the extension set or administration set and tape securely. *Taping the tubing prevents the weight of the IV administration tubing from moving the IV catheter within the vein or dislodging the IV catheter.*
30. **COM** Write the date, time, and your initials on the label found within the transparent dressing or on a piece of tape and apply it to the border of the transparent dressing.

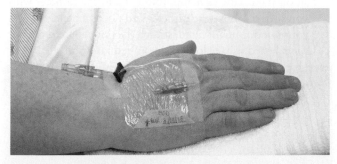

STEP 30 Write the date, time, and your initials on the label.

FINISHING THE SKILL

31. **INF** Dispose of the used supplies.
32. **INF** Remove gloves and perform hand hygiene.
33. **EVAL** Evaluate the outcomes, including how the client tolerated the procedure and the patency of the IV line.
34. **SAF** Ensure client safety. Ensure that the bed is in the lowest position. Ensure the client can identify and reach the nurse call system. *These safety measures reduce the risk of falls.*

35. **CCC** Ensure client comfort. Assist the client with positioning and rearrange bedding. Answer any questions the client may have about the PIV.
37. **COM** Document the care provided, including the gauge and length of the catheter, the site of the catheter, local anesthesia (if used), date and time of the insertion, fluids administered, client education provided and client outcomes.

■ SKILL 12.4 Changing a PIV Dressing

EQUIPMENT

Clean gloves
Antiseptic wipes
Cotton ball or gauze sponge
Disposable procedure pad
(10-mL) 0.9% Normal saline flush
Transparent dressing
Stabilization device, if available
Tape

BEGINNING THE SKILL

1. **INF** Identify the PIV dressing and stabilization device. Review agency policy for PIV dressing changes. Determine if the stabilization device should also be changed. *Damp, loosened, or soiled dressings must be changed. Dressing changes are recommended every 2 days for a gauze dressing and every 7 days for transparent dressings (CDC, 2015). Stabilization device manufacturers recommend changing the device every 7 days.*
2. **INF** Perform hand hygiene.
3. **CCC** Introduce yourself to the client and explain the procedure.
4. **SAF** Identify the client using two identifiers.
5. **CCC** Provide privacy. Close the door and pull the curtain.
6. **INF** Apply clean gloves. *There is an inherent risk of exposure to blood when dressing a PIV site.*

PROCEDURE

7. **SAF** Set up a workspace according to your hand dominance (right-handed on client's right side). *Setting up an ergonomically safe workspace prevents injury to the nurse and client.*
8. **INF** Place a disposable procedure pad under the client's forearm and hand. *The disposable pad will contain any blood that may result from the PIV, thereby containing any blood-borne pathogens and protecting the surface from blood contamination.*
9. **SAF** Holding the catheter hub securely, remove the old dressing by pulling it toward the insertion site. Discard

the dressing. *Pulling the dressing toward the insertion site reduces the risk of dislodging the catheter.* (Note: If removing the stabilization device, follow the manufacturer's recommendations. Some stabilization devices require the adhesive to be dissolved with isopropyl alcohol before removal.)

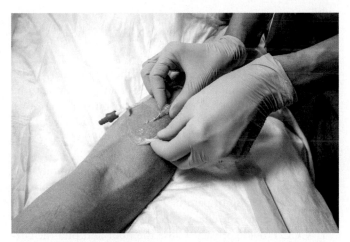

STEP 9 Hold the catheter hub and pull the dressing toward the insertion site.

10. **INF** Assess the insertion site for redness, swelling, drainage, or blood around the site. *Assessment is to detect signs and symptoms of infiltration, infection, or phlebitis. If present, then discontinue the IV.*
11. **INF** Cleanse selected site with an antiseptic wipe. Allow the site to air dry. Do not touch the site after it has been cleaned. If using chlorhexidine, scrub the site in a back-and-forth motion. If using isopropyl alcohol, cleanse by moving from the insertion site outward in a circular pattern.
12. **ACC** Continue to stabilize the catheter hub. If needed, apply a temporary piece of tape across the tubing just below the catheter hub.
13. Open the transparent dressing package and remove the backing. Hold the dressing such that it does not stick to itself.

14. **INF** Apply the dressing over the insertion site, covering the colored catheter hub but not the junction of the hub and the extension set.
15. **SAF** Loop the tubing of the extension set or administration set and tape securely. Remove any temporary tape. *Taping the tubing prevents the weight of the IV administration tubing from moving the IV catheter within the vein or dislodging the IV catheter.*
16. **COM** Write the date, time, and your initials on the label found within the transparent dressing or on a piece of tape and apply it to the border of the transparent dressing.

17. **INF** Dispose of the used supplies.
18. **INF** Remove gloves and perform hand hygiene.
19. **EVAL** Evaluate outcomes, including the patency of the IV line.
20. **SAF** Ensure client comfort and safety. Ensure that the bed is in the lowest position. Ensure client can identify and reach the nurse call system. *These safety measures reduce the risk of falls.*
21. **COM** Document the care provided, including assessment of the insertion site, date and time of dressing change, and client outcomes.

■ SKILL 12.5 Discontinuing a Peripheral Intravenous Catheter

EQUIPMENT

Clean gloves
Antiseptic wipes
Cotton ball or gauze sponge
Tape
Disposable procedure pad

BEGINNING THE SKILL

1. **SAF** Review the prescriptive healthcare provider's order and facility policy. Double-check that the PIV is to be discontinued and that there are no outstanding doses of IV medications to be given. *Verifying the plan of care prevents restarting a PIV if one is still required.*
2. **INF** Perform hand hygiene.
3. **CCC** Introduce yourself to the client and family and explain the procedure. Reassure the client that removing the catheter is not painful.
4. **SAF** Identify the client using two identifiers.
5. **CCC** Provide privacy. Close the door and pull the curtain.
6. **INF** Apply clean gloves. *There is an inherent risk of exposure to blood when removing a PIV catheter.*

PROCEDURE

7. **SAF** Set up a workspace according to your hand dominance (right-handed on client's right side). *Setting up an ergonomically safe workspace prevents injury to the nurse and client.*
8. **INF** Place a disposable procedure pad under the client's forearm and hand. *The disposable pad will contain any blood that may result from the PIV removal, thereby containing any blood-borne pathogens and protecting the surface from blood contamination.*
9. Remove tape securing the tubing.

10. **SAF** Remove old dressing by pulling it toward the insertion site. *Pulling the dressing toward the insertion site reduces the risk of dislodging the catheter before you have gauze over the site.*
11. **CCC** Place a cotton ball or gauze lightly over the insertion site.
12. **HLTH** Remove the catheter from the client's vein. Press the cotton ball or gauze more firmly over the insertion site.
13. **HLTH** Maintain pressure over the insertion site for 2 to 3 minutes. *Pressure for 2 to 3 minutes allows time for the vein and the wound to develop a clot.*
14. **SAF** Inspect the catheter to ensure that it is intact. *The catheter is fragile. Inspection ensures all of the catheter is removed.*

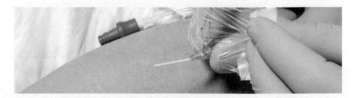

STEP 14 Inspect the catheter to ensure that it is intact.

15. **INF** Discard catheter according to facility policy.

FINISHING THE SKILL

16. **INF** Remove gloves and perform hand hygiene.
17. **SAF** Ensure client comfort and safety. Ensure that the bed is in the lowest position. Ensure the client can identify and reach the nurse call system. *These safety measures reduce the risk of falls.*
18. **EVAL** Evaluate outcomes.
19. **COM** Document date, time, catheter removal, whether it is intact, size of catheter, and client outcome.

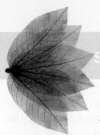

SECTION 3 Intravenous Fluids

A primary reason for establishing venous access is to provide intravenous fluids (IVFs). IVFs provide fluid volume and electrolytes. IVFs may supplement oral hydration or may be the sole source of fluids when an individual cannot maintain oral hydration. IVFs contain solutes such as dextrose and/or electrolytes such as sodium and potassium. Fluid and electrolyte balance is regulated by homeostatic mechanisms involving the kidneys, the hormones antidiuretic hormone (ADH) and aldosterone, and thirst.

MONITORING INTAKE AND OUTPUT

To monitor fluid and electrolyte balance when administering IVFs, nurses measure intake and output. Nurses compare fluid intake to output to evaluate the effectiveness of fluid therapy and to prevent the complications of fluid-volume overload, fluid-volume deficit, or electrolyte imbalance. Measuring intake and output is described in detail in Chapter 15. Healthy people can usually regulate fluid and electrolyte balance without difficulty, but individuals with complex health problems may not be able to compensate if they receive too much or too little fluid and electrolytes. When administering IVFs, carefully monitor the client's response, including output. Intake and output may be calculated hourly in critical situations or every 4 hours or every shift in less critical situations.

TYPES OF INTRAVENOUS FLUIDS

IVFs may be isotonic, hypotonic, or hypertonic. Isotonic fluids have a solute concentration similar to plasma. They are administered frequently because they do not result in a transfer of water or solute from the intravascular to extravascular space. They are commonly administered to expand the intravascular volume or as a vehicle for adding electrolytes or medication. An example of an isotonic fluid is normal saline solution (NSS), which is 0.9% NaCl. Review Table 12.3 for a comparison of common IVFs.

In addition to sodium chloride, another solute commonly found in IVFs is dextrose. PIV solutions may be dextrose 5% in water (D5W) or dextrose 10% in water (D10W). Dextrose concentrations higher than 10%, such as those found in total parenteral nutrition (TPN), are not usually administered via PIV because they are sclerotic to small peripheral veins. Dextrose solutions may also contain NaCl, such as dextrose 5% 0.45% NaCl (D5½NS [normal saline solution]). Hypertonic solutions are those with a higher solute concentration than plasma. However, although dextrose solutions are initially hypertonic, the dextrose is quickly drawn into cells and metabolized for energy. This uptake quickly reduces the solute concentration, and therefore there is little transfer of water into the vascular space. Hypotonic solutions have a lower solute concentration than plasma. They are not frequently administered because they draw water into the extravascular space.

In addition to NaCl and dextrose, several other solutes are added to IVFs. These include potassium chloride, calcium, and magnesium. When administering IVF with solutes, nurses carefully examine the IVF to ensure the solutes have not precipitated and there are no visible crystals within the solution prior to administration. When a high amount of solutes is required, a central line is preferred over a peripheral line (see Chapter 13).

TABLE 12.3 Common Intravenous (IV) Fluids

Tonicity of fluid	Solution	Impact	Used
Isotonic	0.9% NaCl in water Normal saline (NS)	Increases circulating volume	Dehydration Replace sodium Replace fluid loss
Isotonic	Lactated Ringer's Normal saline with electrolytes and buffers (LR)	Increases circulating volume Buffers pH	Blood loss Burns Gastrointestinal fluid loss
Isotonic	5% Dextrose in water (D5W)	Fluid volume without sodium	Hypernatremia Dehydration
Hypertonic → hypotonic	5% Dextrose in ½ Normal saline (D5½NS)	Provides calories and hydration	Daily maintenance
Hypotonic	0.45% NaCl in water (½ NS)	Increases fluids	Provide volume without dextrose
Hypertonic	5% Dextrose 0.9% NaCl in water D5NS	Adds calories, sodium, and chloride	Replace fluid with sodium and chloride
Hypertonic	10% dextrose in water D10W	Adds calories	Maintain blood sugar

INFECTION CONTROL

The concept of infection control is critical because another potential complication of IV therapy is the risk of infection. Infection may develop at the IV insertion site, develop in the IV catheter, or spread to the bloodstream. Although there has been much focus and research on central line bloodstream infections, current evidence suggests that PIV lines may also be introducing staphylococcal bloodstream infections, resulting in catheter-related blood-stream infections (CRBSIs). CRBSIs resulting from PIV are underevaluated. The volume of PIV use (over 330 million are sold each year in the United States) makes the need to reduce the risk of infection imperative (Zhang et al., 2016).

To prevent infection, nurses maintain the sterility of the IVF administration system. IVFs must always be sterile. Nurses check expiration dates and examine the fluid for any discoloration, leaks, or break in the integrity of the packaging prior to administration. Once the IVF is hung, sterility is maintained by thoroughly scrubbing any needleless connectors before connecting to the port. The "scrub the hub" protocol has been recommended for all ports with venous access, including PIV lines (The Joint Commission, 2013). Evidenced-based antiseptics for scrubbing access ports are chlorhexidine with alcohol or 70% isopropyl alcohol. The recommended action is to scrub in a twisting motion, as if juicing an orange, for about 15 seconds (The Joint Commission, 2013). The optimal timing of the scrub is debated because scrub times reported in the literature vary considerably from 5 to 60 seconds (INS, 2016). Allow the hub to air dry, and do not put it down or allow it to touch another object. Disinfectant impregnated caps are being used over PIV ports; in these instances, once the cap that was covering the port is removed, then the cap is discarded and, following access, the hub is re-covered with a new disinfectant cap. If the hub is accessed immediately after removing the cap, then the hub is not scrubbed. However, for each subsequent access of the hub a vigorous scrub is required (INS, 2016; Stango, Runyan, Stern, Macri, & Vacca, 2014).

SAFETY AND THE RIGHTS OF INTRAVENOUS FLUID ADMINISTRATION

IVFs are considered medications and must be ordered by the authorized healthcare provider. The order contains the date and time of the order, the client's name, the IV route, the type of intravenous fluid, the rate of administration, and the prescriber. The rate of administration of IVFs is given in milliliters per hour (mL/hr). The same five medication rights asked before the administration of a medication are required before the administration of IVFs, including an NS flush. The nurse must ask:

- Is this the right client?
- Is this the right IV fluid?
- Is this the right rate of infusion?
- Is this the right route?

- Is this the right time to administer?

As with medication administration, the sixth right is the "right documentation," which is done when the IVF is initiated and completed. Another similarity to medication administration is that client assessment, monitoring the client's response to the IV therapy, and documentation of the client response are an integral part of providing nursing care.

INTRAVENOUS FLUID ADMINISTRATION SETS

There are a variety of IVF containers and IV administration sets. IVFs usually come in IV bags; however, they may also come in plastic containers, and there are a few types that come in glass bottles (Fig. 12.9). All IV bags have two ports: one is the access port where the administration set spike is placed, and the other port allows medications to be added.

Various types of IV tubing, also called administration sets, are available, including those designed for specific types of IV pumps and those with varying numbers of medication ports. IV tubing can be classified as primary or secondary. Primary tubing is longer and offers medication ports. OSHA and the CDC recommend that these should be ports with needleless access in order to minimize occupational exposure to needles and blood-borne pathogens (OSHA, 2015b). Secondary tubing is shorter and designed to connect a secondary line to the primary line.

All IV tubing will have a spike that is inserted into the IVF container and a drip chamber, which is a hollow chamber that allows a space for air at the top and fluid at the bottom and has a predetermined drop-size opening (Fig. 12.10). The drip chamber helps to keep air out of the tubing and allows the nurse to see the rate of infusion. Some tubing has filters to prevent particles from flowing to the client. As shown in Fig. 12.11, macro-drop systems have larger drops and may have a drop factor of 10, 15, or 20 drops/mL. The

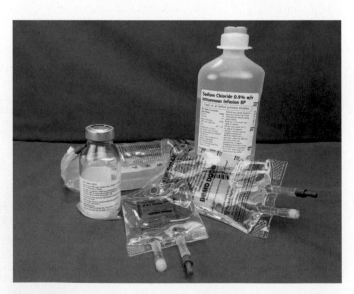

FIG. 12.9 Intravenous (IV) fluids may come in glass bottles *(left)*, plastic containers *(back)*, and bags of various sizes *(right and front)*.

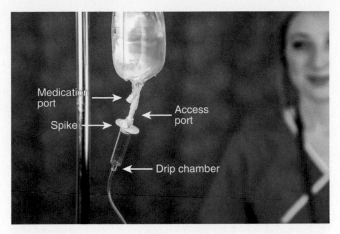

FIG. 12.10 Intravenous (IV) administration sets have a spike that inserts into the access port and a drip chamber.

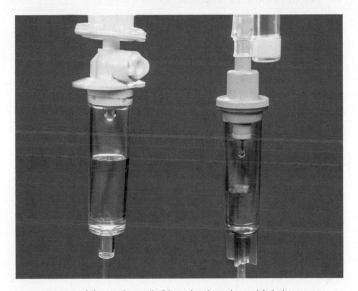

FIG. 12.11 Macrodrop *(left)* and microdrop *(right)*.

drop factor identifies how many drops it takes to fill 1 mL. Micro-drop systems produce very small drops and have a drop factor of 60 drop/mL (see Fig. 12.11).

The CDC offers specific guidelines concerning how often IV equipment is to be changed. The object is to maintain a sterile environment and to keep the cost of equipment and nursing time in mind as well. It is recommended that administration sets be replaced at least every 7 days but not more frequently than every 96 hours (4 days) as long as blood, blood products, or fat emulsions have not been infused in the set. Administration sets used for blood, blood products, or fat emulsions are to be replaced within 24 hours of initiating therapy. Needleless connectors are changed with the administration set (CDC, 2015).

PRIMING ADMINISTRATION SETS AND BUBBLE MANAGEMENT

Priming is the term for filling the IV tubing with fluid. When priming an administration set, the first objective is to have a solid column of fluid in the tubing without any

air bubbles. A second objective is to not waste medication or fluid. Bubbles are the bane of beginners, and with some experience it becomes easier to move fluid through tubing without trapping bubbles. It is important to keep in mind that air bubbles will rise in fluid. Trying to get air bubbles to move downward through fluid will only frustrate the student nurse. Therefore, position the tubing to allow the air to rise. There are several methods of moving air through fluid within IV tubing. Bubbles can be moved by tapping on the port or tubing. Allowing the fluid to move slowly while tapping will encourage the bubble to come away from the tubing wall and move with the fluid. If a segment of air is trapped in the IV tubing and it is too large to float through the fluid, then snapping the tubing smartly will break the air into smaller bubbles and allow them to float through the fluid. A third method of moving air is to displace the air by compressing the IV tubing. A situation where this is very helpful is when replacing an IV solution container that has run dry, but it is not yet time to change the IV tubing. In this instance, if there is air trapped in the tubing near the drip chamber, you can squeeze the tubing or wrap unrestricted tubing around your hand to displace the air upward into the drip chamber.

INFUSING FLUIDS

In most hospitals, IVFs are administered using an electronic IV pump that regulates the rate and volume of the IV infusion. Although various mechanisms are used in IV pumps to regulate the flow, pumps usually have several features in common. These include an alarm that sounds when the infusion is complete and when resistance to flow is sensed. Pumps have a number keypad that the nurse programs to indicate the rate per hour and the total volume to be infused.

IVF orders may be written in two different ways. One type of IV fluid order is written with the total volume (often of a liter fluid bag) over the hours to be infused, for example, 1000 mL NS/8 hours. In this instance, the nurse determines the rate (mL/hr) by dividing the volume by the number of hours (1000 mL/8 hr = 125 mL/hr). Other facilities may routinely order fluids with the rate per hour (mL/hr) indicated' for example, D5½NS at 25 mL/hr. If the total volume is not written in the order, then the pump is programmed based on the size of the IV bag that is hung. Adult medical/surgical areas usually use a liter bag of IVF (1000 mL).

The advantage of using an electronic IV pump is the ease of maintaining an accurate and constant flow rate; however, IV fluids are occasionally infused without a pump. For example, in outpatient surgery or on postpartum units, the need for IVFs is short term and the client population would not typically be adversely affected by an inadvertent bolus of fluid. Occasionally an IV may be ordered to run at KVO, or keep vein open. This would be the minimum amount that maintains the patency of the PIV (10-15 mL/hr depending upon facility policy). In addition, nurses should know how to calculate a drip rate in the event of a power outage. All hospitals have backup generators, but not all plugs are connected to those generators. In the event of a disaster/power outage, some hospitalized clients will need their fluids managed without

BOX 12.5 Using Drop Factors to Calculate IV Infusion by Gravity

The package of the intravenous (IV) tubing identifies the drop factor for that tubing.

MACRODROP

Macrodrop has three possible sizes: 10 gtts/mL, 15 gtts/mL, or 20 gtts/mL.

Macrodrop formula

mL per hour/60 minutes = mL/minute × your equipment drop factor (gtts/mL)

For example: An order for 120 mL/hr/60 = 2 mL/minute × 10 drop factor = 20 gtts/minute

Watching the drip chamber, this rate would be 10 gtts/30 seconds or about 5 gtts/15 seconds.

MICRODROP

Microdrop tubing has one size: 60 drops per 1 mL.

Microdrop tubing is more frequently used in pediatric populations or other situations were precise low volumes of infusion are needed.

Microdrop formula

mL per hour/60 minutes = mL/minute × drops per milliliter (drops/mL) = drops per minute

Note: One method of calculating this problem is to cancel out the 60 in the numerator and the 60 in the denominator.

For example, an order for 120 mL/hr/60 minutes = 2 mL/minute × 60 drop factor = 120 gtts/minutes

Watching the drip chamber, this rate would be 60 gtts/30 seconds or 30 gtts/15 seconds.

electricity. When an IV pump is not used, nurses calculate and manage the infusion rate by the drops per minute in the drip chamber. This requires knowing the drop factor (how many drops make up 1 mL) and regulating the drops per minute to achieve a specific mL/hour infusion. Use the formulas found in Box 12.5 to calculate the drops per minute.

APPLICATION OF THE NURSING PROCESS

Examples of Related ICNP Nursing Diagnoses, Expected Client Outcomes, and Nursing Interventions:

Nursing Diagnosis: Fluid Imbalance

Supporting Data: Potential for imbalanced fluid volume due to presence of IVF infusion.

Expected Client Outcomes: Client will demonstrate balanced fluid volume, as seen by:

- Vital signs remain within established parameters
- Urine output is greater than 0.5 ml/kg/hour
- The client is able to identify signs and symptoms of fluid-volume deficit (increased thirst, dry mucous

membranes, or poor skin turgor) or fluid-volume overload (bounding pulses, edema, shortness of breath).

Nursing Intervention Example: Measure, evaluate, and report intake and output.

Reference: International Classification for Nursing Practice. (n.d.). *eHealth & ICNP*. Retrieved from https://www.icn.ch/what-we-do/projects/ehealth-icnp.

CRITICAL CONCEPTS
Infusing Intravenous Fluids

Accuracy (ACC)

Accuracy when infusing IVFs is subject to the following variables:

- patency of the IV infusion.

Client-Related Factors

- Client age, medical history, and clinical status, including allergies, medications, and past procedures
- Client's veins, including size, characteristics, and integrity

Nurse-Related Factors

- Selection and use of equipment
- Preparation and technique used for the flush or IV infusion
- Use of sterile technique
- Assessment of insertion site for redness, swelling, drainage, or blood around the site
- Assessment of the client
- Technique used for processing orders

Client Centered Care (CCC)

When infusing IVFs, respect for the client is demonstrated by:

- obtaining verbal consent and promoting autonomy
- explaining the procedure, answering questions, and arranging an interpreter if needed
- providing privacy and ensuring comfort
- advocating for the client and family.

Infection Control (INF)

When infusing IVFs, healthcare-associated infection is prevented by:

- preventing and reducing the transfer of microorganisms
- reducing the number of microorganisms.

Safety (SAF)

When infusing IVFs, safety measures prevent harm and maintain a safe care environment, including:

- following all medication safety checks and guidelines
- labeling of IVF containers and tubing.

Communication (COM)

- Communication allows for exchanges of information (oral, written, nonverbal, or electronic) between two or more people.

- Documentation records information in a permanent legal record.

Health Maintenance (HLTH)

Nursing is dedicated to the promotion of health when infusing IVFs, including:
- maintaining circulation and fluid and electrolyte balance.

Evaluation (EVAL)

When infusing IVFs, evaluation of outcomes enables the nurse to determine the therapeutic response and safety of the care provided, including:
- evaluating the client's fluid status, vital signs, and lab values
- monitoring the infusion equipment and administration set to ensure a continuous infusion of fluid.

■ SKILL 12.6 Managing a Saline Lock

EQUIPMENT

Clean gloves
Antiseptic wipes
(10-mL) 0.9% Normal saline (NS) flush
Disinfectant cap

BEGINNING THE SKILL

1. **SAF** Review the authorized healthcare provider's order and facility policy. Perform **first safety checkpoint** when accessing the saline flush. Perform **second safety checkpoint** when preparing the saline flush. *Verifying medical orders prevents injury to the client.* Your review should include:
   a. type of fluid and volume
   b. route of administration
   c. time of administration and frequency
   d. pertinent client lab values.
2. **INF** Perform hand hygiene.
3. **CCC** Introduce yourself to the client and family and explain the procedure.
4. **SAF** Identify the client using two identifiers.
5. **CCC** Provide privacy. Close the door and pull the curtain.
6. **INF** Apply clean gloves. *There is an inherent risk of exposure to blood when maintaining venous access.*

PROCEDURE

7. **ACC** Assess the IV site for signs of infiltration or phlebitis using inspection and palpation.
8. **ACC** Unclamp the slide clamp on the extension set tubing (if slide clamp present).
9. **SAF** Perform **third safety checkpoint** with the client before administering the saline flush.
10. **ACC** Prepare the NS flush by removing all of the air in the syringe.
11. **INF** Remove the disinfectant cap, if present. If no cap is present, scrub the hub of the needleless connector for 5 to 60 seconds (or per agency policy). Allow the hub to air dry. Do not put down the hub, and do not touch the hub. *Holding the needleless connector maintains the cleanliness of the scrubbed end.*
12. **ACC** Attach the NS syringe to the hub of the needleless connector by pushing the syringe into the hub and ro-

tating the syringe while inserting. *This will Luer-Lok the syringe into place.*
13. **SAF** Aspirate gently to confirm blood return. (Note: In pediatric, neonatal, and other small-gauge catheters, the absence of a blood return may not be an indication that the catheter is not patent [Brown, 2017].)
14. **ACC** Flush the line with the prescribed amount of NS flush.

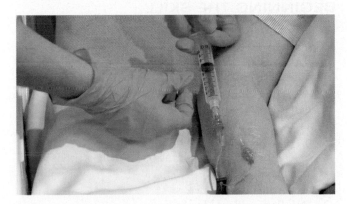

STEP 14 Flush the line with NS as ordered.

15. **ACC** While flushing, assess the site for ease of flush and signs of infiltration and ask the client if there is any discomfort with flushing the vein.
16. **ACC** Clamp the extension tubing using the slide clamp while completing the flush (if slide clamp present). Remove the syringe. Apply a new disinfectant cap.

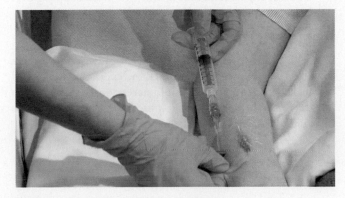

STEP 16 Clamp the extension tubing.

FINISHING THE SKILL

17. **INF** Dispose of the used supplies.
18. **INF** Remove gloves and perform hand hygiene.
19. **EVAL** Evaluate outcomes. Are there multiple indications the line is patent? Are there any indications of infiltration?
20. **SAF** Ensure client comfort and safety. Ensure that the bed is in the lowest position. Ensure the client can identify and reach the nurse call system. *These safety measures reduce the risk of falls.*
21. **COM** Document the assessment findings of the IV site, including the client's subjective report and ease of flushing. Document the volume of normal saline flushed and the date and time of the flush.

■ SKILL 12.7 Preparing a Primary Intravenous Infusion

EQUIPMENT

Clean gloves
IV fluid as prescribed by the authorized healthcare provider
Primary IV tubing
Antiseptic wipes
IV infusion pump

BEGINNING THE SKILL

1. **SAF** Review the healthcare provider's order and facility policy. Check each of the safety administration rights. Perform **first safety checkpoint** when accessing the IV fluids. Perform **second safety checkpoint** when preparing the IV fluids. *Verifying medical orders prevents injury to the client.* Your review should include:
   a. type of fluid and volume
   b. route of administration
   c. volume and rate of infusion, usually written in milliliters per hour
   d. pertinent lab values.
2. **INF** Perform hand hygiene.
3. **CCC** Introduce yourself to the client and explain the procedure.
4. **SAF** Identify the client using two identifiers.
5. **CCC** Provide privacy. Close the door or pull the curtain.
6. **INF** Apply gloves at the point when there is a risk of exposure to blood or chemicals. (Note: There is no risk of exposure to blood while you spike the IV bag and prime the tubing. When you access the PIV line, there is a risk of exposure to blood, and you should apply gloves before connecting the line to the IV site.)

PROCEDURE

7. **SAF** Open the IV solution cover if present and inspect the IV solution for clarity, color, expiration date, and leakage. Identify the IV fluid access port. *Most IV fluid bags have two ports. One is a medication port designed to insert medications, and one is the access port.*

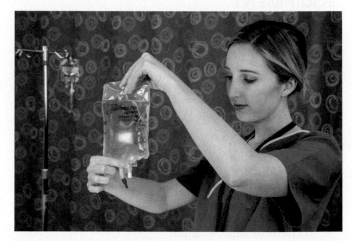

STEP 7 Inspect IV solution for clarity, color, expiration date, and leakage.

8. **SAF** Label the IV solution container with the client's name, type of IV solution, medications or electrolytes added (if any), date and time fluid is hung, and your initials. *Labeling IV fluid is a safety strategy.*
9. **ACC** Open the primary IV tubing package and close the primary tubing roller clamp. *If the clamp is not closed, you will not control the descent of the fluid.*

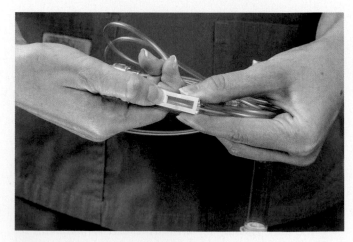

STEP 9 Close the primary tubing clamp.

10. **INF** Remove the cover from the access port of the IV fluid container and remove the protective sheath over the IV tubing spike. Maintain sterility of the port and insert the spike into the access port. *Maintains sterility of IV tubing and solution.*

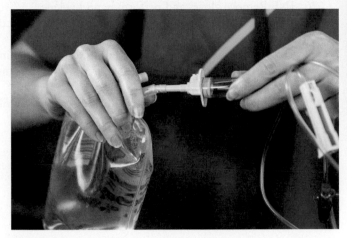

STEP 10 Insert the spike of the IV tubing into the IV solution access port.

11. **INF** If hanging an IV solution bag, hold in your non-dominant hand with the neck of the access port supported. With your dominant hand, insert the spike of the IV tubing into the IV solution access port by pushing while twisting in only one direction with about a quarter rotation. *Supporting the neck of an IV fluid bag prevents puncturing the IV bag.* (Note: If spiking a plastic container, place the container on a secure countertop.)

12. **ACC** Hang the IV container and fill the drip chamber until it is half full (or to the mark) by compressing and releasing the drip chamber. *Many drip chambers have a mark indicating the fill point. Compressing the drip chamber displaces air into the IV container and allows fluid to enter the drip chamber.*

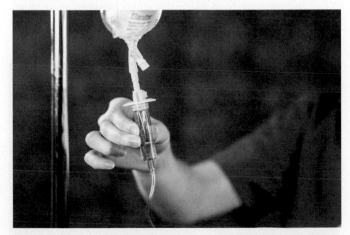

STEP 12 Compress and release the drip chamber until it is half full.

13. **ACC** Open the roller clamp and watch the descent of the fluid.

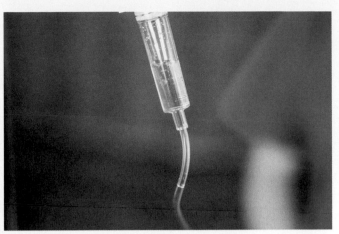

STEP 13 Open the roller clamp and watch the descent of the fluid.

14. **ACC** When you reach a medication port, slow the descent of the fluid, invert the port, and fill the medication port. You may need to tap on the port as the fluid is flowing to remove bubbles. Move the air bubble to the top of the column of fluid. *Removing air prevents the potential for air embolism.*

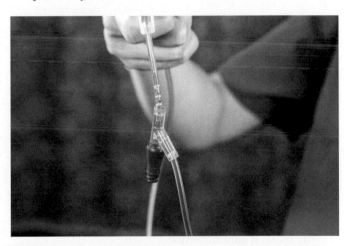

STEP 14 Ensure that the air is removed from the medication port.

15. **ACC** Use the roller clamp to regulate the rate of flow and continue the descent of fluid to the next medication port or IV pump cassette. Use the roller clamp to slow the rate of IV fluid and repeat the process of inverting the port or cassette, slowly advancing the fluid through the port, moving any bubbles out of the port with a combination of tapping and fluid movement.

16. **ACC** Open the roller clamp and continue priming to the end of the tubing.

17. **SAF** Close the roller clamp.

18. **SAF** Inspect the tubing for air bubbles.

19. **SAF** Perform **third safety checkpoint** with the client before administering. Label the administration set with the date of initiation, per agency policy.

20. **CCC** Place tubing in the IV pump, per manufacturer's recommendation.

21. **SAF** Trace the IV line from the insertion point on the client to the connection. *Tracing a line from the client's insertion site to the connection is a safety strategy to prevent misconnection errors.*
22. **INF** If the extension set has a disinfectant cap on the needleless connector, remove the cap and discard it. If the needleless connector does not have a cap, scrub the hub to the IV with isopropyl alcohol for 5 to 60 seconds (or according to facility policy).
23. **INF** Remove the cap on the distal end of the primary tubing and connect it to the needleless connector while avoiding contamination of either end. *Maintaining sterility reduces the risk of infection.*
24. **SAF** Initiate infusion at prescribed rate.

FINISHING THE SKILL

25. **CCC** Ensure client comfort and safety. Ensure that the bed is in the lowest position. Ensure the client can identify and reach the nurse call system. *These safety measures reduce the risk of falls.*
26. **INF** Remove gloves and perform hand hygiene.
27. **EVAL** Evaluate outcomes, including patency and security of the IV line.
28. **COM** Document IV site assessment findings and IV infusion, including solution, rate, patency of PIV line, and client outcomes.
29. **EVAL** Monitor IV site as fluid infuses for signs of infiltration or phlebitis and client reports of tenderness.

■ SKILL 12.8 Replacing Intravenous Infusion Fluid

EQUIPMENT

IV fluid, as prescribed by the authorized healthcare provider
Antiseptic wipes
IV infusion pump
Clean gloves

BEGINNING THE SKILL

1. **SAF** Review the healthcare provider's order and facility policy. Check each of the safety administration rights. Perform **first safety checkpoint** when accessing the IV fluids. Perform **second safety checkpoint** when preparing the IV fluids. Your review should include:
   a. type of fluid and volume
   b. route of administration
   c. volume and rate of infusion, usually written in milliliters per hour
   d. pertinent lab values.
   Verifying medical orders prevents injury to the client.
2. **INF** Perform hand hygiene.
3. **CCC** Introduce yourself to the client and explain the procedure.
4. **SAF** Identify the client using two identifiers.
5. **INF** Apply gloves at the point when there is a risk of exposure to blood or chemicals. (Note: There is no risk of exposure to blood while you spike the IV bag and prime the tubing. When you access the PIV line, there is a risk of exposure to blood, and you should apply gloves before touching connections to the IV site.)

PROCEDURE

6. **ACC** Assess the IV site for signs of infiltration or phlebitis using inspection and palpation.

7. **SAF** Open IV solution cover if present and inspect IV solution for clarity, color, expiration date, and leakage. Identify the IV fluid access port. *Most IV fluid bags have two ports. One is a medication port designed to insert medications, and one is the access port.*
8. **SAF** Label the IV solution container with the client's name, type of IV solution, medications or electrolytes added (if any), and date and time fluid is hung. Perform **third safety checkpoint** with the client before administering. Check the label on the tubing. *Labeling IVF is a safety strategy.*
9. **INF** Remove the empty IV fluid container from the IV pole. Invert the container and pull out the administration set spike. Maintain the sterility of the spike. One method is to place the spike between your third and fourth fingers. *This allows you to use your finger and thumb to remove the cover of the new IV bag access port.*

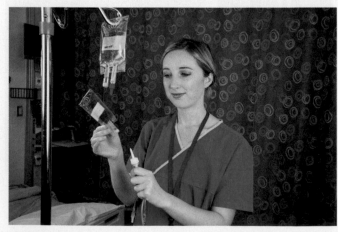

STEP 9 Pull out the administration set spike. Maintain the sterility of the spike.

10. Dispose of the empty bag. There may be a small amount of IV fluid remaining. Take measures to prevent it from spilling.
11. **INF** Remove the cover from the new IV fluid bag access port, maintaining the sterility of the port.
12. **INF** Hold the IV solution bag in your nondominant hand with the neck of the access port supported. With your dominant hand, insert the spike of IV tubing into the IV solution access port. *Supporting the neck of an IV fluid bag prevents puncturing the IV bag.* (Note: Alternatively, you may hang the solution container on an IV pole. If spiking a plastic container, place the container on a secure countertop.)

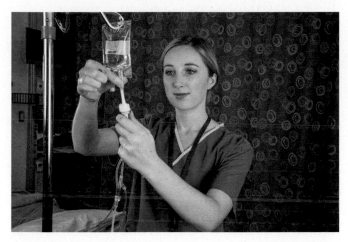

STEP 12 Support the neck of the access port and insert the spike.

13. **ACC** Hang the IV bag upright and squeeze the IV tubing drip chamber half full by compressing and releasing the drip chamber.
14. **ACC** Inspect the administration set tubing for air. Air below the drip chamber can be moved into the drip chamber. (Note: One method is to wrap unrestricted tubing around your hand to displace the air upward into the drip chamber.)

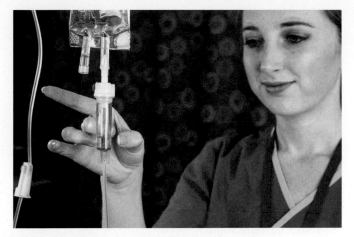

STEP 14 Inspect the administration set tubing for air.

15. **SAF** Trace the IV line from the insertion point on the client to the infusion pump. *Tracing a line from the client's insertion site to the equipment and fluid source prevents misconnection error.*
16. **SAF** Initiate infusion at prescribed rate. Ensure tubing is unclamped.

FINISHING THE SKILL

17. **INF** Dispose of the used supplies.
18. **INF** Remove gloves and perform hand hygiene.
19. **EVAL** Evaluate outcomes. Is the infusion flowing without difficulty? Does the client have any tenderness at the site? Are there any signs of infiltration or phlebitis?
20. **CCC** Ensure client comfort and safety. Ensure that the bed is in the lowest position. Ensure the client can identify and reach the nurse call system. *These safety measures reduce the risk of falls.*
21. **COM** Document assessment findings of the IV site, as well as the date, time, and type of IV fluid hung.
23. **EVAL** Monitor the IV site as fluid infusion begins for patency of the line and signs of infiltration.

SECTION 4   Administering Intravenous Medications

IV medications are administered through two methods. The first method is to administer the medication through a secondary medication IV bag that is "piggybacked" into the primary line. Often, a 50-mL bag of NS or sterile water is the diluent, and medication is added to the secondary bag. Antibiotics are very commonly administered in this manner. The medication IV bag is most commonly prepared by pharmacy, but in some instances the nurse may prepare it.

The second method is to administer the medication as an IV push, also called an IV bolus. IV push medications are drawn up in a syringe and may be slowly "pushed" by hand into the IV. IV push medications may also be administered using a syringe pump. Both methods of IV administration place the medication directly into the bloodstream, and the actions of the medication begin almost instantly.

ORDERS FOR INTRAVENOUS MEDICATIONS

Medications must be ordered by the authorized healthcare provider. The order contains the date and time of the order, the client's name, the IV route, the medication, the dose, the route of administration, and the prescriber. The five medication rights asked before the administration of any medication are required before the administration of an IV medication, including an NS flush. The nurse must ask:

- Is this the right client?
- Is this the right IV medication?
- Is this the right dose and frequency?
- Is this the right route?
- Is this the right time to administer?

Verifying the appropriateness of the order is a critical part of safely administering IV medications. Any concerns about the order should be discussed with the authorized healthcare provider or the pharmacist. Nurses are responsible for knowing their agency's policy for IV medication administration.

NURSING RESPONSIBILITIES

Nurses administering IV medications must be very knowledgeable about the medication given, because the effects will take place very rapidly. Nurses who administer IV medication or fluid must know its indications for therapy, side effects, potential adverse effects, and appropriate interventions to take before starting the infusion. Here are a few of the practice criteria identified by the INS (2016):

- Nurses are responsible for reviewing the order and checking the appropriateness of the order considering the client's age and health, as well as the dose, route, and rate of medication administration.
- Nurses are responsible for following the rights of medication administration.
- Nurses provide education to the client and family about the medication and any signs or symptoms to report.
- Nurses are responsible for evaluating and monitoring the effectiveness of the medication.
- Nurses are responsible for documenting client responses and nursing interventions and communicating related laboratory results to the client.

There are legal considerations related to IV medication administration. State nurse practice acts identify the scope of practice for registered nurses, licensed practical/vocational nurses, and medical assistants and may identify medications that nurses may not administer by IV push.

MEDICATION PREPARATION AND EQUIPMENT

Medication to be administered intravenously may come in a powder form and need to be reconstituted, in an ampule and need to be withdrawn from the ampule with a filter, or in a prefilled syringe. See Chapter 11 for specific instructions on

BOX 12.6 Setting Infusion Pumps for Medication Administration

Guidelines for medication administration are usually written in minutes; for example, "Administer over 30 minutes."

Pumps are programmed to run in milliliters per hour (mL/hr). The rate must be converted to the unit of measure that the pump uses. The pump will also be programed with the *Volume to be Infused,* which is the volume you have. So, in this instance, the *Volume to be Infused* is 50 mL. The pump will stop when 50 mL is infused

Medication volume/minutes to be administered × 60 minutes/1 hour = Medication rate mL/hr

The problem can be solved using many different methods:

Example Using the Desired Over Have Formula:

$$\frac{D}{H} \times V = \frac{60 \text{ minutes}}{30 \text{ minutes}} \times 50 \text{ mL} = 2 \times 50 \text{ mL} = 100 \text{ ml/hr}$$

Example Using the Ratio-Proportion Method:

50 mL medication/administered over 30 minutes × how many mL/60 minutes

$$\frac{50 \text{ mL}}{30 \text{ minutes}} \times \frac{X}{60 \text{ minutes}} = \frac{100 \text{ mL}}{60 \text{ minutes}}$$

drawing up medication. Next, check the compatibility of the medication to determine if the medication is compatible with the infusing IVF or other prescribed medications that will be given in the same line. The safest course is to flush with NS before and after medication administration. Determine the appropriate rate of administration. Consult the pharmacy or a pharmaceutical textbook because this information may not be written in the order. Electronic pumps with a pharmacy library will be programmed with the rate for specific medications (Box 12.6).

Intravenous Piggyback

The regulation of flow for the secondary line of an IV piggyback is dependent on the regulation of flow for the primary line. Three possible mechanisms are as follows:

- If the primary line is regulated by gravity flow, then the primary bag must be lowered and the secondary bag hung at a higher level during the infusion.
- When the primary line is on a pump and the secondary line connects to the primary line above the pump, and therefore only one line is regulated by the infusion pump, then the primary bag must be lowered and the secondary bag hung at a higher level during the infusion.
- If the primary line is on a pump with a separate infusion channel for the secondary (such as an A and B channel) and the secondary connects at the pump, then both bags are hung at the same level because gravity has no influence.

Many pumps have the option to back prime. This means using the fluid in the primary line to prime the tubing of the secondary line. The advantage is that there is no possibility of wasting medication. A disadvantage is that the medication reaches the client a little bit slower because the tubing is filled with primary fluid and not with medication. Back priming can be done using a pump or by gravity, but it has become more commonplace because of the ease of using it on a pump. When back priming, the secondary tubing is connected to the primary tubing before the drip chamber is filled. Once connected to the primary and the primary is inserted in the pump, open the roller clamp to the secondary line and hold down the back-prime button. The fluid will rise in the tubing up to the drip chamber. Release the back-prime button when the drip chamber is sufficiently full.

Intravenous Push

Follow medication administration guidelines to determine the appropriate preparation for the IV push medication. Dilution of some medications may be required by the manufacturer. Select the appropriate-size syringe for the prescribed dose, including the diluent, in order to draw up the medication without having the plunger fully extended. A syringe with the plunger fully extended is unwieldy and risks breaking sterility and losing medication. Select the appropriate diluent per the manufacturer's recommendations. Use a single-dose vial of diluent. Never use IVF solutions to prepare, dilute, or reconstitute medications. Never dilute a medication by drawing it up into a prefilled NSS flush syringe (INS,2016). Prepare the syringe in a clean, dry workspace immediately before administration. Preparing a syringe in advance of its use is not a safe practice. Always label the syringe with the name of the medication and dose, but do not prelabel an empty syringe (Institute for Safe Medication Practices [ISMP], 2015).

Just as with IV fluid administration, an important safety feature of the administration system is the use of needleless connector systems with a Luer-Lok to reduce the possibility of exposure to blood and blood-borne pathogens.

COMPLICATIONS OF INTRAVENOUS MEDICATION ADMINISTRATION

Administering medications via the IV route allows for the very rapid onset of therapeutic effect. However, medications may have side effects, adverse effects, or allergic reactions that will also manifest very quickly.

A potential complication of administering a medication is the possibility of an IV infiltrating while infusing a solution that is irritating to the vein and/or to the surrounding tissue. Extravasation is the unintentional infusion of a vesicant into the surrounding tissue. Some medications are so damaging to the surrounding tissue that extensive tissue damage may occur. Vancomycin (Vancocin) and phenytoin (Dilantin) are examples of vesicant medications. IV solutions can be vesicants as well. These include potassium chloride solutions and concentrated glucose solutions.

APPLICATION OF THE NURSING PROCESS

Examples of Related ICNP Nursing Diagnoses, Expected Client Outcomes, and Nursing Interventions:

Nursing Diagnosis: Risk for impaired tissue integrity

Supporting Data: Client has a vesicant medication or fluid prescribed.

Expected Client Outcomes: The client will be free of impaired tissue integrity, as seen by the following:
- skin that is warm, pink, and dry
- no complaints of tenderness, swelling, blanching, or redness at the IV insertion site

Nursing Intervention Examples: Frequent assessments of the IV site and administration with prescribed dilution and flush

Reference: International Classification for Nursing Practice. (n.d.). *eHealth & ICNP*. Retrieved from https://www.icn.ch/what-we-do/projects/ehealth-icnp.

CRITICAL CONCEPTS
Administering Intravenous Medications

Accuracy (ACC)

Accuracy when administering IV medications is subject to the following variables:
- patency of the IV infusion.

Client-Related Factors
- Client's age and medical history, including allergies, medications, and past procedures
- Client's veins, including size, characteristics, and integrity

Nurse-Related Factors
- Selection and use of equipment
- Preparation and technique used for the flush or IV infusion
- Use of sterile technique
- Assessment of insertion site for redness, swelling, drainage, or blood around the site
- Assessment of the client
- Technique used for processing orders

Client Centered Care (CCC)

When administering IV medications, respect for the client is demonstrated by:
- obtaining verbal consent and promoting autonomy
- providing privacy and ensuring comfort
- answering questions before, during, and after medication administration
- explaining the purpose of medication and arranging an interpreter if needed
- honoring cultural preferences, including the use of heparin derived from animal products
- advocating for the client and family.

Infection Control (INF)

When administering IV medications, healthcare-associated infection is prevented by:

- preventing and reducing the transfer of microorganisms
- reducing the number of microorganisms.

Safety (SAF)

When administering IV medications, safety measures prevent harm and maintain a safe care environment, including:

- following the rights of medication administration and medication safety checks and guidelines
- labeling IV medications and tubing.

Communication (COM)

- Communication allows for the exchange of information (oral, written, nonverbal, or electronic) between two or more people.

- Documentation records information in a permanent legal record.
- Collaboration with the pharmacy and other members of the healthcare team regarding preparation, compatibility, and administration of IV medications enhances safety.

Health Maintenance (HLTH)

When administering IV medications, nursing is dedicated to the promotion of health and self-care abilities.

Evaluation (EVAL)

When administering IV medications, evaluation of outcomes enables the nurse to determine the therapeutic response and safety of the care provided, including:

- monitoring the therapeutic effect of the medication
- monitoring for side effects, adverse effects, interactions, or allergic reactions

▪ SKILL 12.9 Administering Intermittent Intravenous Medication via Secondary Infusion

EQUIPMENT

Existing primary infusion with medication ports
Clean gloves
Medication administration record (MAR) or electronic medication administration record (EMAR)
IV medication in a secondary IV container
Secondary IV tubing
Antiseptic wipes
IV infusion pump

BEGINNING THE SKILL

1. **ACC** Review order for:
   - name and dosage of medication for infusion
   - diluent and volume of diluent
   - frequency, route of administration, and any special instructions
   - purpose of administering medication (if PRN).
     Verifying medical orders prevents injury to the client.
2. **COM** Consult with the client, pharmacist, or medical record to confirm the following:
   - client's allergies to medications or other substances
   - indications, contraindications, and appropriateness of medication
   - rate of administration (i.e., over how many minutes; consult pharmacy, pharmaceutical text, or electronic pump pharmacy library to determine the appropriate rate)
   - compatibility of medication with all infusing solutions
   - client's age, medical/surgical history, and clinical condition
   - medication history (to check for potential drug interactions)

   - recent lab work that would affect or be affected by the medication.
3. **INF** Perform hand hygiene. Apply gloves at the point when there is a risk of exposure to blood or chemicals.
4. **CCC** Introduce yourself to the client and explain the procedure.
5. **SAF** Identify the client using two identifiers. Ask the client to state his or her full name and date of birth.
6. **ACC** Perform additional client preassessments as indicated.

PROCEDURE

7. **SAF** Verify the client's consent to receive the medication before preparing the medication. Explain what the medication is and why it is prescribed. *To prevent waste, client consent must be obtained before medication is prepared.*
8. **SAF** Perform **first safety checkpoint** when accessing the medication. Compare the label on the medication to the EMAR or MAR or, if available, against original orders. Check each of the safety administration rights. Check label for medication name, dose, expiration date, and any precautions. *Before using any medication, it is essential to confirm that the medication has not expired.*
9. **SAF** Perform **second safety checkpoint** when preparing the medication. Compare the label on the medication to the EMAR or MAR. Check each of the safety administration rights a second time. (Note: If using bar-code technology, verify IV medication against MAR or EMAR, and scan bar code if indicated.)

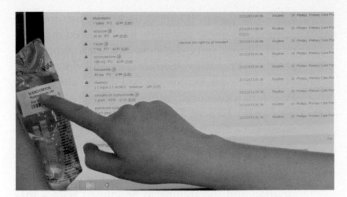

STEP 9 Perform second safety checkpoint by comparing MAR or EMAR with label on the IV medication.

10. **SAF** Inspect IV medication for clarity, color, and leakage.
11. **ACC** Open secondary IV tubing package and close secondary tubing roller clamp. **WARNING:** Closing the clamp is critical. *Forgetting to clamp the tubing may result in wasting medication and time spent removing trapped air in the tubing.*

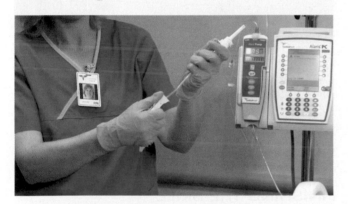

STEP 11 Close the secondary tubing roller clamp.

12. **INF** Remove the cover from the IV medication container access port and remove the protective sheath over the IV tubing spike. Be careful not to contaminate either the port or the spike. *Maintains sterility of IV tubing and solution.*
13. **ACC** Hold the secondary medication bag in your nondominant hand with the neck of the access port supported; then, with your dominant hand, insert the spike of IV tubing into the IV solution access port. (Note: If you are going to back prime the pump, skip to step 20.)
14. **ACC** Hold the IV medication container upright and squeeze the IV tubing drip chamber half full by compressing and releasing the drip chamber.
15. **ACC** Open the roller clamp and control the descent of the fluid. **WARNING:** Do not accidentally waste medication. (Note: There are no medication ports on secondary tubing, so the fluid will move very quickly.)
16. **ACC** Close the roller clamp when the medication reaches the end of the secondary tubing.
17. **SAF** Perform **third safety checkpoint** with the client before administering by checking the medication label

with client's ID band. Check each of the safety administration rights a third time. If using a bar-code system, scan the medication and the client now.

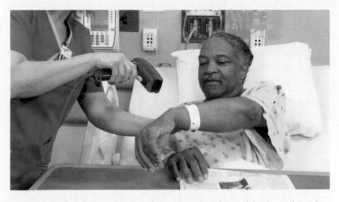

STEP 17 Perform third safety checkpoint with the client by checking the medication label against the client's ID band.

18. **INF** Perform hand hygiene and apply gloves. *Personal protective equipment (PPE) protects you from exposure to blood or chemicals.* (Note: There is not a risk of exposure to blood while you spike the IV bag and prime the tubing. There may be a risk of exposure to harmful chemicals, depending on the type of medication you are administering. There is always a risk of exposure to blood when you access the PIV line; therefore, you should apply gloves before you access the IV site.)
19. **ACC** Assess the patency of the IV line by assessing the IV site for signs of infiltration and checking for a blood return. Methods for checking a blood return include the following:
    (a) attaching an NSS flush syringe and checking ease of flush and blood return at the catheter hub with aspiration;
    (b) lowering the primary solution container and looking for blood return; or
    (c) pinching the primary tubing, thereby decreasing the IV solution flow, and checking for blood return. *Determining the patency of the IV line is critical before administering an IV medication.*
20. **INF** If the medication port has a disinfectant cap on the needleless connector, remove the cap and discard it. If the medication port does not have a cap, scrub the hub to the IV with isopropyl alcohol for 5 to 60 seconds (or according to facility policy). Allow the port to air dry. Do not put it down or touch it. *Holding the medication port maintains the cleanliness of the scrubbed end.*
21. **SAF** Trace the IV line from the insertion site to the medication port access. *Tracing a line from the client's insertion site to the connection is a safety strategy to prevent misconnection errors.*
22. **ACC If administering medication by gravity:**
    a. Remove the cap on the distal end of the secondary line and insert the secondary line into the medication port above the roller clamp, avoiding contamination of either end. If the medication port has a Luer-Lok,

push and twist to insert. *Maintaining sterility reduces the risk of infection.*

b. Hang the IV medication on the IV pole, and hang the primary IV solution container lower using the plastic hanger. *Lowering the primary IV solution allows the flow from the higher IV medication to exert more pressure and administer the IV medication. When the IV medication is fully administered (and no longer exerting pressure), the primary IV solution will continue to slowly administer.*

c. Open the roller clamp on the secondary line. (Note: The fluid does not yet begin to drip.)

d. Calculate the rate of administration based on the prescribed time for administration, and then calculate the drops/minute using the formula in Box 12.5.

e. Adjust the rate of administration using the roller clamp of the primary line to adjust the number of drops per minute in the drip chamber. Calculate the drops per 15 seconds to adjust the rate more easily.

23. **ACC If administering medication through a single-channel electronic pump:**

a. Remove the cap on the distal end of the secondary line and insert the secondary line into the primary line at the medication port above the electronic pump.

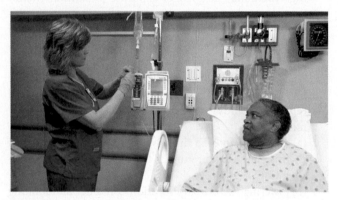

STEP 23A Insert the secondary line into the primary line at the medication port above the electronic pump.

b. Hang the IV medication on the IV pole, and hang the primary IV solution container lower using the plastic hanger. *Lowering the primary IV solution allows the flow from the higher IV medication to exert more pressure and administer the IV medication. When the IV medication is fully administered (and no longer exerting pressure), the primary IV solution will continue to slowly administer.*

c. Program the pump with the rate of administration based on the prescribed time for administration and the volume to be infused (rate = mL/hr; volume = size of the IVF container; see Box 12.6 for calculations to use in obtaining the mL/hr).

d. After the medication has infused, reprogram the pump with the rate of administration for the primary infusion.

24. **ACC If administering medication through a dual-channel electronic pump:**

a. Remove the cap on the distal end of the secondary line and insert the secondary line into the primary

line at the pump. (Note: If back priming, open the roller clamp of the secondary line and hold the back-prime button until the fluid fills the tubing completely and the drip chamber is half-filled.)

b. Hang the IV medication on the IV pole. The primary IV solution container continues to hang at the same level on the IV pole. The medication and the IV solution will be drawn into separate channels of the electronic pump, and the level of the bag does not matter.

c. Program the medication pump with the rate of administration based on the prescribed time for administration and the volume to be infused (rate = mL/hr; volume = size of the IVF container; see Box 12.6 for calculations to use in obtaining the mL/hr). Note that both the primary and the secondary infusions will be running simultaneously.

25. **SAF** Initiate medication infusion and observe the IV site and client response.

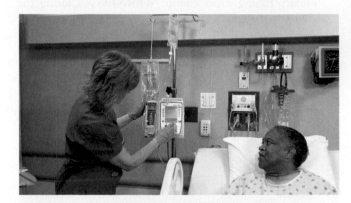

STEP 25 Initiate medication infusion at the prescribed rate

FINISHING THE SKILL

26. **INF** Dispose of the used supplies.

27. **INF** Remove gloves and perform hand hygiene.

28. **EVAL** Evaluate outcomes. As the infusion begins, monitor the IV site for patency of the line and signs of infiltration.

29. **CCC** Ensure client comfort and safety. Ensure that the bed is in the lowest position. Ensure the client can identify and reach the nurse call system. *These safety measures reduce the risk of falls.*

30. **COM** Document assessment findings of the IV site, medication administration, and client outcomes in the legal healthcare record, including:
    - name of medication given, exact time, date, dose, and route given
    - volume administered and rate
    - client response to IV medication and how the client tolerated the procedure
    - pertinent postassessment data, such as vital signs or pain level
    - signature and initials of the clinician who administered the medication.

32. **EVAL** Monitor the client for side effects, allergic reactions, or adverse reactions to the medication.

■ SKILL 12.10 Administering Intravenous Medication via Intravenous Push

EQUIPMENT

Existing primary infusion with medication ports or saline lock
Clean gloves
IV medication in a syringe
MAR or EMAR
Antiseptic wipes
Syringe (size based on dose)

BEGINNING THE SKILL

1. **ACC** Review the order for:
   - name and dosage of medication for injection
   - frequency, route of administration, and any special instructions
   - purpose of administering medication (if PRN) *Verifying medical orders prevents injury to the client.*

2. **ACC** Consult with the client, pharmacist, or medical record to confirm the following:
   - client's allergies to medications or other substances
   - indications, contraindications, and appropriateness of medication
   - client's age, medical/surgical history, and medical condition
   - medication history (to check for potential drug interactions)
   - recent lab work that would affect or be affected by the medication.

3. **ACC** Determine the compatibility of the medication with the infusing solution. Determine if medication needs to be diluted, the recommended diluent, and the recommended rate of infusion (i.e., over how many minutes). Consult pharmacy, a pharmaceutical text, or the electronic pump pharmacy library to determine compatibility and the appropriate rate.

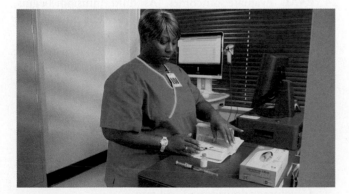

STEP 6 Determine the compatibility and the appropriate rate of administration.

4. **INF** Perform hand hygiene. Apply gloves at the point when there is a risk of exposure to blood or chemicals.

5. **CCC** Introduce yourself to the client and explain the procedure.

6. **SAF** Identify the client using at least two client identifiers. Ask the client to state his or her full name and date of birth.

7. **ACC** Perform additional client preassessments (e.g., vital signs, level of pain) as indicated for the medication.

PROCEDURE

8. **SAF** Verify the client's consent to receive the medication before preparing the medication. Explain what the medication is and why it is prescribed. *To prevent waste, client consent must be obtained* before *medication is prepared.*

9. **SAF** Perform **first safety checkpoint** when accessing the medication. Compare the label on the medication to the EMAR or MAR or, if available, against original orders. Check each of the safety administration rights. Check label for medication name, strength, expiration date, and any precautions. *Before using any medication, it is essential to confirm that the medication has not expired.*

10. **SAF** Perform **second safety checkpoint** when preparing the medication. Compare the label on the medication to the EMAR or MAR. Check each of the safety administration rights a second time. (Note: If using bar-code technology, verify IV medication against MAR or EMAR, and scan bar code if indicated.)

11. **ACC** Inspect medication solution for any unusual cloudiness or particulates.

12. **ACC** If medication is not in a ready-to-administer form, draw up the medication using sterile technique. (Note: The ISMP recommends IV push medications be provided in ready to administer form.) As necessary, reconstitute, dilute, or draw up medication using skills found in Chapter 11. Remove all air from the syringe. Perform dosage calculations as necessary. Double-check calculations.

13. **SAF** Label syringe with client's name, medication, time, date, and dosage per policy. *Labeling medication is a safety strategy.*

14. **SAF** Perform **third safety checkpoint** with the client before administering by checking the medication label with the client's ID band. Check each of the safety administration rights a third time. If using a bar-code system, scan the medication and client now.

15. **INF** Perform hand hygiene and apply gloves. *PPE protects you from exposure to blood or chemicals. There is not a risk of exposure to blood while you prepare the medication. There may be a risk of exposure to harmful chemicals, depending on the type of medication you are administering. There is always a risk of exposure to blood when you access the PIV; therefore, you should apply gloves before you access the IV site.*

16. **INF** If the medication port has a disinfectant cap on the needleless connector, remove the cap and discard it. If the medication port does not have a cap, scrub the hub to the IV with isopropyl alcohol for 5 to 60 seconds (or according to facility policy). Allow the medication port to air dry.

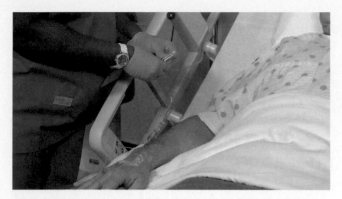

STEP 16 Scrub the medication port of the primary tubing with antiseptic.

17. **ACC** Assess the patency of the IV line by assessing the IV site for signs of infiltration and checking for a blood return. *Determining the patency of the IV line is critical before administering an IV medication.*
18. **SAF** Trace the IV line from the insertion site to the medication port access. *Tracing a line from the client's insertion site to the connection is a safety strategy to prevent misconnection errors.*
19. **ACC If a compatible IV solution is infusing:**
    a. Clamp the tubing above the medication port by folding the tubing on itself. *This prevents medication from going back up the tubing.*

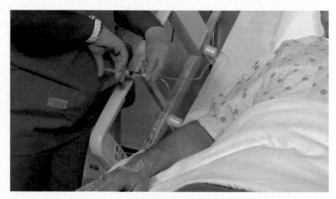

STEP 19A Clamp the tubing above the port before injecting the medication.

    b. Insert the medication syringe into the medication port, maintaining aseptic technique.
    c. Infuse the medication in small pushes per recommended rate. Remove medication syringe.
20. **ACC If accessing a saline lock:**
    a. Insert the NSS flush syringe into the access port of the saline lock, aspirate gently to check for blood return, and upon confirming blood return, inject NSS flush. Assess ease of flush and assess site with flushing. Remove flush syringe. *Flushing before administering IV push medication verifies IV patency and prevents extravasation.*
    b. Insert the medication syringe into the access port, maintaining aseptic technique. *Maintaining sterility reduces the risk of infection.*
    c. Infuse the medication in small pushes per recommended rate. Remove medication syringe.

    d. Insert the NSS flush syringe, maintaining aseptic technique and pushing the NSS flush into the medication port at the same rate the medication was pushed. Remove flush syringe. Apply a new disinfectant cap to the medication port if facility policy. *Flushing at the same rate administers the remaining medication in the tubing at the prescribed rate.*
21. **ACC If using a syringe pump and IV-compatible solution is infusing:**
    a. Attach microbore tubing to the syringe and prime the tubing.
    b. Insert the syringe into the syringe pump per manufacturer's instructions.

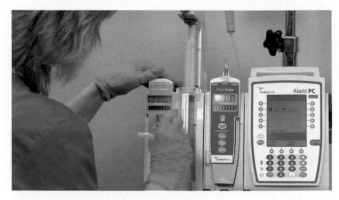

STEP 21B Insert the syringe into the syringe pump.

    c. Insert the distal end of the microbore tubing into the medication port.
    d. Set the rate for medication administration and start the syringe pump.

FINISHING THE SKILL

22. **INF** Dispose of the used supplies.
23. **INF** Remove gloves perform hand hygiene.
24. **EVAL** Evaluate outcomes. As fluid infusion begins, monitor the IV site for patency of the line and signs of infiltration.
25. **CCC** Ensure client comfort and safety. Ensure that the bed is in the lowest position. Ensure the client can identify and reach the nurse call system. *These safety measures reduce the risk of falls.*
26. **COM** Document assessment findings of the IV site, medication administration, and client outcomes in the legal healthcare record, including:
    - name of medication given, exact time, date, dose, and route given
    - volume administered and rate
    - client response to IV medication and how the client tolerated the procedure
    - pertinent postassessment data, such as vital signs or pain level
    - signature and initials of the clinician who administered the medication.
28. **EVAL** Monitor the client for side effects, allergic reactions, or adverse reactions to the medication.

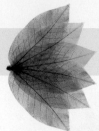

SECTION 5 Administering a Blood Transfusion

The administration of blood or blood products may be a routine or an emergent procedure. Because of the risks, blood transfusions must be ordered by the authorized healthcare provider, and there should be a clear indication for the transfusion. Some common indications include hemorrhage (blood loss) after surgery or trauma, anemia (low hemoglobin), and bleeding or clotting disorders. Blood transfusions may also be indicated for clients who have primary bone marrow disorders, such as myelodysplastic syndrome (MDS), leukemia, or aplastic anemia.

Blood transfusions may be particularly important if a client's hemoglobin is low. Most of the oxygen in our blood is bound to hemoglobin (Hgb) in the RBCs. An adequate circulating blood volume or Hgb is important for oxygen perfusion to the cardiac muscle and peripheral tissues. Therefore, clients who have anemia or clinical conditions that affect their Hgb may be at risk for developing cardiac, organ, or peripheral extremity ischemia. If this occurs, the client may develop chest pain and other symptoms (see Chapter 19). Nevertheless, the administration of blood transfusions should be used with caution, and the benefits of the transfusion must outweigh the risks. This is a procedure that cannot be delegated. Blood transfusions must be performed by a registered nurse (RN).

DIFFERENT TYPES OF BLOOD COMPONENTS

Blood consists of many different components, which can vary depending on the client's age, condition, and diet/nutritional health. The liquid component of blood primarily consists of plasma (about 55% of whole blood), and the solid component of blood primarily consists of RBCs (about 45% of whole blood) and white blood cells and platelets (<1% of whole blood). Although whole blood can be transfused, this is not a common practice due to the risk of circulatory overload. More often, whole blood is processed into components that are used to treat specific clinical needs (American Red Cross [ARC], 2018). Some of the most common components include packed red blood cells (PRBCs), platelets, fresh frozen plasma (FFP), and less commonly, cryoprecipitate AHF (antihemophilic factor). The major features and indications for these different components are described in Table 12.4.

TYPES OF BLOOD TRANSFUSIONS

Some common types of blood transfusions include random donor, directed donor, and autologous donor transfusions (Castillo et al., 2018). The random donor is a blood transfusion whereby the blood is obtained and stored in the blood bank until it is needed by the appropriate recipient. A directed donor is blood donated for a specific recipient. An autologous

TABLE 12.4 Selected Types of Blood Components

Blood Component	Features and Indications
Packed red blood cells (PRBCs)	• Increases oxygen-carrying capacity of the blood • Storage: Requires monitored refrigeration before use • Primarily indicated for anemia, blood loss, trauma, post-chemotherapy, and various primary bone marrow disorders
• Platelets	• Assists with clotting process by adhering to lining of vessels • Storage: *Do not refrigerate*: Platelets are stored at room temperature on constant agitation before use • Indicated for thrombocytopenia and clotting disorders
• Fresh frozen plasma (FFP)	• Contains albumin, fibrinogen, and globulins • Storage: Must be thawed prior to infusion • Indicated for coagulation disorders and certain procedures
• Cryoprecipitate antihemophilic factor (AHF)	• Contains fibrinogen and clotting factors (VIII and XIII) • Primarily indicated for hemophilia and von Willebrand disease

References: American Red Cross, 2018; Infusion Nurses Society, 2016.

transfusion, also called an auto-transfusion, is the collection of the client's own blood in order to reinfuse and replace volume to the client (Castillo et al., 2018). This type of transfusion is often used with clients who are having elective surgical procedures.

ABO COMPATIBILITY SYSTEM

Every individual has a blood type (A, B, AB, or O) that corresponds to the presence or absence of antigens. Antigens on the surface of the RBC can invoke an immune response. Antibodies are proteins found in the plasma that react to specific antigens on the RBC. If the client's blood is not compatible with the donor's blood, an antigen–antibody reaction may occur, which can cause agglutination (clumping) of the cells. This, in turn, can cause the client to have a severe or even a fatal reaction. Thus, the client's blood must be crossmatched with the donor's blood *before* the transfusion.

A description of the ABO compatibility system follows. Note that a client with type AB blood is a universal recipient, whereas a client with type O blood is a universal donor.

- **Type A**: Antigen A is present on the surface of the RBCs, and antibody B is present in the plasma. A client with this blood type may receive type A or O blood.
- **Type B**: Antigen B is present on the RBCs, and antibody A is present in the plasma. A client with this blood type may receive type B or O blood.

- **Type AB** (Universal Recipient): Antigens A and B are present on the RBCs, and no corresponding antibodies are present. The client may receive A, B, AB, or O blood.
- **Type O** (Universal Donor): Neither A nor B antigens are present on the RBCs, but both A and B antibodies are present in plasma. Clients may only receive blood from O blood donors, but they can be a donor for any blood type.

In addition to ABO compatibility, it is important to know the Rh type of the client's RBCs. A client who has the Rh antigen is Rh positive and can receive Rh-positive or Rh-negative blood. Clients who do not have the antigen are Rh negative and should only receive Rh-negative blood. In other words, if a client who is Rh-negative receives an Rh-positive blood transfusion, anti-RH antibodies can be produced and cause a reaction (Maitta, 2018).

SAFETY CONSIDERATIONS

Although administering blood is considered to be a life-saving and life-sustaining therapy, it is also a procedure with potential hazards. It is important to remember that blood is actually a liquid type of tissue transplant. Thus, careful consideration of key safety issues before, during, and after blood administration is a high priority. The client must also have a patent IV line. To prevent hemolysis, this requires a 16- to 20-gauge PIV or a central venous access device (CVAD) (see Chapter 13).

In an effort to improve blood administration safety, various entities, including the American Association of Blood Banks (AABB), the U.S. Food and Drug Administration (FDA), and other entities, have set forth guidelines for processing, storing, checking, and administering blood. The Joint Commission has implemented requirements for healthcare facilities related to transfusion policies to help ensure client safety and prevent errors. Unfortunately, some of the most common errors that occur are during the "preadministration phase" of blood therapy and relate to misidentification errors. Other errors that can occur include blood sampling errors for typing/crossmatching, incorrect recording of client details on the blood sample label or request form, and failing to do a two-person check at the bedside (Castillo et al., 2018).

Rights of Blood Administration

Just as with rights of medication administration, the rights of blood administration have evolved to address safety issues. At a minimum, nurses must verify three rights: right client, right blood, and right time. The complexity of transfusions has resulted in a comprehensive list that includes the following (Ontario Regional Blood Coordinating Network [ORBCON], 2015):

- **Right Client:** Use a two-person, independent identification process when the specimen is collected for typing, when the product is dispensed from the blood bank, and at the bedside before administration. Compare client information and unique identifier on blood bag against client information on armband. Include the client in the identification process as much as possible.
- **Right Reason:** What is the clinical indication for the transfusion? Verify that the indication for the blood is

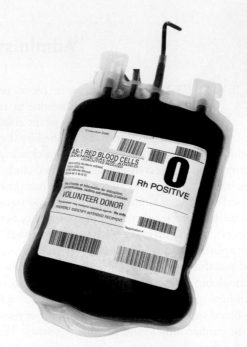

FIG. 12.12 Example of a unit of packed red blood cells (PRBCs). The label includes the blood type/Rh (e.g., type 0/Rh positive), any special preparation, the unit number (bar code), and the expiration date.

appropriate for the client's clinical status and condition. Have alternative options for blood been considered?

- **Right Blood:** Does the label on the product match the order? Based on clinical data (e.g., lab values), is the blood ordered appropriate for the client? Are special instructions correct? See Fig. 12.12.
- **Right Site:** Does the client have a patent IV line or CVAD that can be dedicated for the blood transfusion? Confirm this before calling for the blood from the blood bank. Is the IV line the appropriate size? Generally, an 18-gauge catheter is used. Use only 0.9 % NS with blood.
- **Right Time:** Start within 30 minutes of blood arriving on the unit. Start slowly (1–2 mL/minute). For PRBCs, the transfusion must not exceed 4 hours. Infuse as slow as medically indicated to avoid volume overload.
- **Right Dose:** Monitor the client's fluid-volume status. Is the client showing signs of circulatory overload, such as dyspnea or edema? If the client shows signs of circulatory overload, consider slowing down the rate of the transfusion per orders and within the required time limits.
- **Right Documentation:** Is the client's consent form on the chart? Was there a two-person identification check for pretransfusion checks? Are both electronic signatures on the transfusion form? Document vital signs before starting the transfusion, 15 minutes after starting, during the transfusion as indicated by policy, and at stop time. Document any unusual symptoms or signs of a reaction.
- **Right Response:** Did the transfusion have the desired outcome? Does the client have improved vital signs, improved oxygen-carrying capacity, or other indicators such as improved serum lab values (e.g., Hgb, hematocrit [Hct])?

EQUIPMENT USED FOR A BLOOD TRANSFUSION

When administering blood, it is important to obtain the appropriate equipment. For all blood products, only 0.9% NS can be used. Medications and other types of fluids (e.g., crystalloids and colloid solutions) are *not* compatible with blood and could cause hemolysis, clotting, and other reactions. Blood administration sets with built-in mesh filters (usually 170–260 micron) are also required. The filters are designed to prevent clots and debris from passing through to the client. In addition, the sets are usually nonvented to reduce the risk of contamination. Examples of blood and blood component administration sets include the following (Castillo et al., 2018; INS, 2016):

- Y-tubing blood administration set (with 170- to 260-micron filter): Y-tubing is commonly used for PRBCs, and it is usually primed with NS before the blood is given. One arm of the Y tubing is used for the NS bag, and the other arm is used for the blood. The set and filter should be changed after each unit or every 4 hours (INS, 2016). Many healthcare facilities limit an administration set to 2 units.
- Blood component set: This type of set usually has shorter tubing than other types. It may also have a built-in filter and is often used for certain blood components, such as platelets. Check facility policy regarding use.
- Straight blood administration set: Straight sets are for single use *only*, and they are used for only 1 unit, not multiple units, because of the risk of contamination. Thus, straight sets are not as commonly used as Y sets.
- Syringe/infusion set: These sets are designed to allow administration of blood in small and controlled doses, such as with neonatal and pediatric clients, by direct IV push. These sets may also be used for certain components (e.g., cryoprecipitate; factor products).

In some situations, special leukocyte-removal filters may be used if the blood is not leukocyte reduced. However, bedside reduction of leukocytes may cause low blood pressure or other serious complications, and it may not be as efficient as "pre-storage" leukocyte-reduced blood that is filtrated just after it is collected (INS, 2016). Many facilities are now routinely using leukocyte-reduced blood products for all clients.

Using an Infusion Pump for Blood Transfusions

Special blood administration infusion pumps for administering blood are becoming more common. They may be particularly helpful if the rate and volume must be regulated closely. However, pumps do not replace human observation. It is important to keep track of the volume infused and ensure that the client is receiving the blood at the appropriate rate. The pumps must be certified from the manufacturer as being safe for blood administration and without risk of hemolysis. In addition, the pumps must be maintained in good working order with a reliable alarm system (INS, 2016).

Using a Blood Warmer for Transfusions

Blood warmers are not routinely used for most adult transfusions. However, they may be indicated for clients who have clinically significant cold agglutinins or other conditions that create existing or potential hypothermia or for clients who will be receiving blood at a rapid rate. Blood warmers may be indicated for clients who have intraoperative hypothermia or for neonate and pediatric populations (INS, 2016).

When using a blood warmer, follow the manufacturer instructions, and only use a system that is cleared by the FDA. It is important to use a warmer that is equipped with a thermometer and alarm system. Alternatives for heating blood, such as microwaves, hot water baths, or other improvised methods, are not acceptable and should *never* be used due to the risk of hemolysis and client fatalities (INS, 2016).

PROCEDURE FOR ADMINISTERING A BLOOD TRANSFUSION

Regardless of the type of blood transfusion the client is receiving, all of the pre-transfusion procedures, assessments, and safety checks, including the rights of administration, must be conducted. As noted in the rights of administration, there must be documentation of client consent before the transfusion. In addition, the client should be allowed to ask questions before the procedure. These measures support autonomy and client-centered care.

During the transfusion, the client should be monitored closely at the bedside for any reactions. After the procedure, the client must continue to be monitored for at least 24 hours, depending on facility policy, due to the possibility of the client experiencing a delayed transfusion reaction.

Administering Packed Red Blood Cells

Among all of the blood products that can be given, PRBCs and platelets are two of the most common. The safety procedures and rights of administration are the same as for any blood product.

If the client is receiving PRBCs, a Y-tubing administration set must be used. Before the transfusion, the PRBCs must stay refrigerated in the blood bank at a temperature of 25°C to 35°C. Once the blood unit arrives, the transfusion should be started within 30 minutes and administered within 4 hours. Unless the client needs a massive blood transfusion for severe hemorrhage, it is not advised to obtain more than 1 unit at a time (INS, 2016; Maitta, 2018). The blood administration set used for PRBCs cannot be used for platelets; a new administration set must be obtained.

Administering Platelets

Platelets are now commonly ordered as single-donor platelets (SDPs), also known as an apheresis unit (Fig. 12.13). To administer platelets, blood component tubing that is appropriate for platelets must be used. Platelet and PRBC filters, particularly for leukocyte removal, use different technology

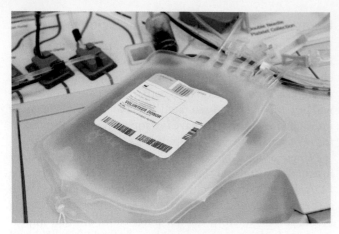

FIG. 12.13 Single-donor platelets (apheresis unit).

and may not be interchangeable (ClinLabNavigator [CLN], 2018). It is important to check with the blood bank and your facility policy about the specific product. In many facilities, the blood bank will send the appropriate tubing with the blood component to be administered at the time it is sent to the nursing unit.

Proper storage of platelets is also important. Unlike other blood transfusion products, platelets must remain at room temperature because refrigeration can damage platelets. As with PRBCs, the platelet transfusion must commence as soon as it arrives on the unit, and the transfusion should be started slowly in order to monitor for reactions. The infusion rate for platelets is usually 30 to 60 minutes, depending on the order, facility policy, and the client's condition.

Because platelets must be kept at room temperature, the potential for bacterial contamination and proliferation is higher than with other products (Maitta, 2018). If the client will be receiving both PRBCs and platelets, they should *not* be infused at the same time. Moreover, platelets should not be transfused through a set that was previously used for another blood product. If there will be any delay in transfusion once the pack arrives, it must be sent back to the lab and placed on the agitator/rocker. This is necessary in order to prevent the platelets from clumping.

POSSIBLE COMPLICATIONS

In most cases, the majority of blood transfusion reactions are mild and related to leukocyte (white blood cell) antigens present in the blood product. Symptoms may include urticaria (rash), pruritus (itching of the skin), low-grade temperature, mild shortness of breath, or joint/muscle aches. Many times, these symptoms can be managed by the authorized healthcare provider with the administration of diphenhydramine (Benadryl) or hydrocortisone (Solu-Cortef). Clients who have a history of allergy or those who are immunosuppressed may receive premedications to prevent anaphylactic reactions. These clients may also receive cytomegalovirus (CMV)-negative or irradiated blood. As mentioned previously, many facilities now only use leukocyte-reduced products.

TABLE 12.5 Examples of Serious Complications: Blood Transfusions

Complication	Characteristics
Transfusion-associated circulatory overload (TACO)	• May be caused by too high of volume or volume infused at a too-rapid rate. Clients with heart and kidney disease are at risk. • Symptoms may include dyspnea, respiratory distress, elevated central venous pressure (CVP), jugular venous distention (JVD), and other symptoms of heart failure.
Transfusion-related lung injury (TRALI)	• Respiratory distress and fluid overload that may be related to antibodies in donor blood. • May have evidence of hypoxemia and lung damage.
Acute hemolytic transfusion reactions (AHTR)	• May occur during, immediately after, or several hours after a client is given blood that is not compatible (e.g., wrong blood). • Client's body immediately begins to destroy the red blood cells, resulting in hemolysis. Symptoms may include (but are not limited to) back/flank pain, severe chills, fever, hematuria (blood in urine), hypotension, renal failure, and shock. • Hemolysis of cells could cause elevated potassium and other electrolyte problems due to release into the vascular space. This could lead to dysrhythmias and other complications.
Delayed hemolytic transfusion reaction (DHTR)	• May occur 24 hours after transfusion has ended. Symptoms may be similar to acute hemolytic reactions (AHTRs).

References: Food and Drug Administration, 2016; Infusion Nurses Society, 2016.

Severe adverse events are less common. According to the FDA, the incidence of severe reactions and/or fatalities is small relative to the number of transfusions given. Among the serious complications, transfusion-associated circulatory overload (TACO), transfusion-related lung injury (TRALI), and hemolytic reactions were the most common events reported in recent years that caused fatalities (FDA, 2016). However, other complications, such as anaphylaxis and microbial contamination, have occurred. For a more detailed description of the most common transfusion-related complications and reactions, see Table 12.5.

Procedure for Managing a Possible Transfusion Reaction

The procedure for managing a transfusion reaction is based on early recognition and timely interventions. If the client has a mild reaction (e.g., mild rash, itching, low-grade temperature, achy), slow or stop the transfusion depending on your facility policy, obtain vital signs, and call the authorized healthcare provider. It is important to perform a system-specific assessment to help determine the nature of the reaction.

If the client has a severe reaction, *stop* the transfusion immediately, call the authorized healthcare provider, and ensure that emergency equipment is available. If the client is in acute distress, stop the transfusion and call the emergency or rapid response team (RRT) as indicated.

BOX 12.7 System-Specific Assessment and Care for Clients Who Are Having a Possible Transfusion Reaction

Mild transfusion reactions may include (but are not limited to) urticaria, pruritus, low-grade temperature, or joint/muscle aches. Severe reactions are less common and may be manifested by a fever, tachycardia, chest pain, hypotension, respiratory distress, and severe anxiety (sec Table 12.5). If your client has a mild transfusion reaction, slow or stop the transfusion and notify the authorized healthcare provider. If your client has a severe reaction, *stop* the transfusion, provide emergency care if needed, notify the authorized healthcare provider, and follow facility protocol. Obtain vital signs and carefully assess your client using a system-specific approach. Assessment parameters include the following:

- Does your client have an elevated temperature? If so, how much?
- Are the client's vital signs significantly different from baseline?
- Is the client having chills, muscles aches, back pain, or chest pain?
- Does the client have heat or inflammation at the infusion site?
- **Skin:** Does the client have a rash, urticaria, itching, or edema (swelling)?
- **Nervous:** Does the client have tingling, numbness, or mental status changes?
- **Respiratory:** Does the client have dyspnea, wheezing, or coughing?
- **Gastrointestinal:** Does the client have nausea, vomiting, or cramping?
- **Cardiovascular:** Does the client have bounding pulses or clammy extremities?
- **Renal:** Does the client have changes in the color or volume of the urine? Does the urine appear dark or bloody? This may indicate the presence of hemoglobin (Hgb) in the urine.

In most facilities, the blood bank or the lab will have a specific protocol for how to manage the blood bag. Usually the blood bag will be saved and sealed in a secure container and sent to the lab for investigation. In addition, a urine specimen (first voided) and a blood specimen from the client may be collected. A transfusion reaction form must be completed. A reaction that is severe or life threatening is usually reported to the FDA.

It is important to understand that transfusion reactions can be immediate (during the transfusion) or delayed (several hours or days after the transfusion). Therefore, follow-up care and monitoring are essential after a transfusion. Meticulous documentation and communication are important. For a summary of assessment and care for clients who are having a possible transfusion reaction, see Box 12.7.

APPLICATION OF THE NURSING PROCESS

Examples of Related ICNP Nursing Diagnoses, Expected Client Outcomes, and Nursing Interventions:
Nursing Diagnoses: Risk for hypervolaemia (hypervolemia)

Supporting Data: Client has a history of cardiomyopathy and left ventricular failure.
Expected Client Outcomes: Client will have no signs of circulatory overload as demonstrated by:
- absence of shortness of breath
- breath sounds clear and equal bilaterally
- respirations regular and unlabored
- vital signs within expected parameters for the client

Nursing Intervention Examples: Avoid infusing blood rapidly. Use an FDA-approved infusion pump that is appropriate for blood transfusions. Monitor respiratory status.

Nursing Diagnoses: Risk for anaphylaxis
Supporting Data: Client has experienced allergic reactions in the past.
Expected Client Outcomes: The client will have no evidence of an anaphylaxis reaction as demonstrated by:
- vital signs (temperature, blood pressure, pulse, and respirations) at baseline and within expected parameters for the client
- absence of signs and symptoms of severe allergic reaction, such as swelling of the lips, tongue, pharynx, or airway, and absence of bronchospasm, laryngospasm, angioedema, or other reactions.

Nursing Intervention Examples: Monitor client's vital signs closely, administer premedications as ordered, and ensure that only leukocyte filters or leukocyte-reduced (washed) blood is used for transfusion as ordered.
Reference: International Classification for Nursing Practice. (n.d.). *eHealth & ICNP*. Retrieved from https://www.icn.ch/what-we-do/projects/ehealth-icnp.

CRITICAL CONCEPTS
Administering a Blood Transfusion

Accuracy (ACC)

When administering a blood transfusion, accuracy is affected by the following variables:
Client-Related Factors
- Client's assessment, including age, level of consciousness, and orientation
- Client's medical history
- Client's history of blood transfusions and previous reactions
- Client's veins, including size, characteristics, and integrity
- Client's understanding and ability to follow instructions related to transfusion
Nurse-Related Factors
- Proper selection and preparation of blood administration set and other equipment
- Proper technique for preparing, administering, and documenting blood transfusion
- Preparation of client and instructions regarding the blood transfusion

- Adherence to blood administration guidelines and facility policies

Equipment-Related Factors
- Proper functioning of infusion equipment and blood warmer when needed
- Proper functioning of blood administration equipment and micron filters

Client-Centered Care (CCC)

When administering a blood transfusion, respect for the client is demonstrated by:
- obtaining informed consent for the transfusion and promoting autonomy
- explaining the procedure and arranging an interpreter if needed
- providing culturally sensitive explanations
- answering questions before, during, and after transfusion
- ensuring comfort
- advocating for the client and family.

Infection Control (INF)

When administering a blood transfusion, healthcare-associated infection is prevented by:
- following guidelines for storage and administration time
- preventing and reducing the transfer of microorganisms

- reducing the number of microorganisms.

Safety (SAF)

When administering a blood transfusion, safety measures prevent harm and maintain a safe care environment, including:
- following blood administration safety checks and guidelines.

Communication (COM)

- Communication exchanges information (oral, written, nonverbal, or electronic) between two or more people.
- Collaboration with the blood bank and other members of the healthcare team enhances the effectiveness and safety of the blood transfusion
- Documentation records blood transfusion information in a permanent healthcare record.

Evaluation (EVAL)

When administering a blood transfusion, evaluation of outcomes enables the nurse to determine the therapeutic response and safety of the care provided, including:
- monitoring the therapeutic effect of the transfusion
- monitoring for adverse effects or allergic reactions.

■ SKILL 12.11 Administering Packed Red Blood Cells (PRBCs)

EQUIPMENT

Sterile Y-tubing administration set (Y set) with 170- to 260-micron/mesh filter

0.9% NS (250-mL bag)

Packed RBCs

(Note: Packed RBCs are stored in blood bank refrigerator until ready to use.)

IV catheter (16 to 20 gauge) or CVAD

Luer-Lok connector

Antiseptic wipes

Hypoallergenic tape

Clean gloves

Blood requisition form

Consent form

Blood identification bracelet

Protective eyewear (if splashing and exposure to body fluids is possible)

Stethoscope, blood pressure cuff, thermometer

Pump infusion set (if needed) (must be approved for blood administration)

Blood warmer if indicated (must be certified for blood administration)

BEGINNING THE SKILL

1. **ACC** Review the order. At a minimum, the order should state the following:
   a. type of transfusion
   b. number of units and duration of each transfusion (cannot exceed 4 hours)
   c. any special preparation or requirement (e.g., CMV negative, irradiated)
   d. whether a blood warmer will be required.
2. **ACC** Review medical/surgical history and history of any blood transfusions or reactions. *Assessing the client's history can help the nurse anticipate complications.*
3. **ACC** Ensure that the following have been completed:
   a. **COM** Blood bank has been notified of the order and number of units needed.
   b. **COM** Blood bank has received the transfusion request with required labels.
   c. **ACC** Appropriate blood sample has been drawn for the type and crossmatch.
   d. **SAF** Identification blood bracelet has been placed on the client with appropriate labels.
4. **INF** Perform hand hygiene.
5. **CCC** Introduce yourself to the client and family.

6. **SAF** Identify the client using two identifiers.
7. **CCC** Provide privacy and explain the procedure.

PROCEDURE

8. **ACC** Assess the client's level of consciousness and orientation to person, time, place, and situation. *Provides a baseline assessment of the client's cognitive level before transfusion.*
9. **CCC** Ensure that informed client consent has been obtained, and ensure that the client has received the following information:
   a. purpose and indication of transfusion
   b. risks, benefits, alternatives, and right to refuse blood transfusion.
   Clients need to be fully informed about procedure.
10. **CCC** Ensure that the client has an opportunity to ask questions before transfusion.
11. **ACC** Assess the client for the following:
    a. any known or suspected allergies, particularly to blood products
    b. presence of any rash or lesions on skin (pre-transfusion). *Provides baseline assessment for comparison in case a transfusion reaction occurs later.*
12. **ACC** Evaluate the client's IV line where blood will be infused and ensure there are no signs of infiltration or phlebitis. Ensure that catheter is appropriate size. *Appropriate IV access with a catheter that is 16 to 20 gauge is essential for safe transfusion and prevention of hemolysis.* (Note: If there is a risk of exposure to body fluids when assessing the IV line, apply gloves.)
13. **ACC** If the client does not have adequate IV access, then ensure that the appropriate IV line is placed *before* the unit of blood is obtained from the blood bank. *Administration of the blood must not be delayed more than 30 minutes once it arrives on the nursing unit.*
14. **SAF** If the client will be receiving any premedications, administer the medications approximately 30 minutes prior to blood administration to allow therapeutic effect. *Premedications can prevent transfusion reactions.*

Preparing the Blood Administration Set

15. **ACC** Prime the Y-tubing set with NS if required by policy.
    a. Ensure that the Y-tubing set has an appropriate filter (usually 170–260 micron).
    b. Obtain bag of 0.9% NS IV solution per order.
    c. Inspect NS solution for clarity, color, expiration, and leakage.
    d. Close all of the clamps on the tubing of the Y-tubing set.
    e. Using sterile technique, remove the cover from the NS solution bag access port, and remove the protective sheath that is over one of the tubing spikes of the Y-tubing set. Maintain the sterility of the NS port and the tubing spike.
    f. While supporting the neck of the NS access port with your nondominant hand,

use your dominant hand to insert one of the spikes of the Y-tubing set into the NS solution port. *Provides stability of bag/tubing.* (Note: Use precaution not to puncture the outside of the NS bag as the spike enters the IV solution.)
    g. Hang NS bag with the Y-tubing set on an IV pole. Open the clamp of one of the Y arms between the bag and the administration set drip chamber.
    h. Squeeze the drip chamber of the Y set until the level of the fluid is above the filter. *Prevents fracture (or lysis) of blood cells when blood is hung.*
    i. Keep the clamp on the other arm of the Y set closed. *This arm is where the blood will be hung later.*
    j. Remove the cap from the distal end of the tubing while maintaining the sterility of both the cap and the end of the tubing.
    k. Open the clamp below the drip chamber/filter. Slowly prime the remainder of the tubing to the end of the tubing. Close the clamp. *Priming slowly will reduce the chance of air bubbles due to lower velocity of flow.*
    l. Replace the cap on the end of the tubing and maintain the sterility of the administration set.
16. **ACC** If using an infusion pump for the administration of blood:
    a. Verify that the pump is approved for blood administration.
    b. Ensure that the pump is properly grounded and working properly.
    c. Prime the administration set and cassette per manufacturer's instructions.
17. **INF** Apply clean gloves.
18. **SAF** Before attaching the tubing to the client's IV, trace the IV line from the insertion point on the client to the infusion pump and NS bag. *Tracing a line from the client's IV insertion site to the fluid source prevents misconnection error.*
19. **SAF** Using sterile technique, attach Luer-Lok on the distal end of blood administration tubing that is primed with NS to the client's IV extension set. Ensure that the tubing is taped securely and looped to prevent tension. (Note: There is no need to add a needleless connector between the extension set and the blood administration set. A needleless connector can reduce flow rates with RBC administration (INS, 2016).) *Securing the tubing will prevent dislodgement of the client's IV.*
20. **ACC** Adjust NS flow rate to keep open rate, or whatever is ordered, until blood arrives. Monitor the client's IV site when the NS flow starts to ensure there is no sign of leaking or infiltration. *Ensures patency of IV line prior to transfusion.*
21. **INF** Remove gloves and perform hand hygiene.
22. **SAF** Label NS bag and tubing with appropriate information, including correct date and time. *Labeling prevents misidentification and wrong-client errors.*

Obtaining the Blood and Performing "Pre-Transfusion" Checks

23. **ACC** Obtain blood from blood bank when ready to administer. *PRBCs must be hung within 30 minutes of arrival to the nursing unit due to deterioration at room temperature.*
24. **SAF** When blood arrives, check blood with a second healthcare professional and match to client's information on the order, blood requisition, and other forms.
25. **SAF** Conduct a two-person "bedside check" with a second healthcare professional. Match the unit of blood with client's data at bedside, including:
    a. independent client identification checks
    b. client's name, date of birth, and gender
    c. client's unique ID number and other data on blood bracelet
    d. blood type (ABO, RH), blood unit number, donor number
    e. expiration of unit and expiration of crossmatch
    f. special requirements of blood (irradiated, CMV negative, etc.).

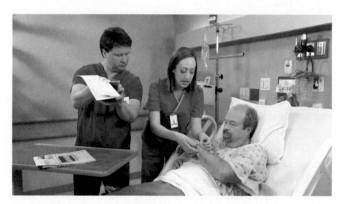

STEP 25 Conduct a two-person "bedside check."

26. **SAF** After blood is matched and verified at the bedside, both healthcare providers sign the client's electronic blood transfusion form. *Helps document that the safety checks were followed.* (Note: Electronic signatures are often used for the electronic health record.)
27. **ACC** Inspect blood carefully for unusual color, turbidity, or excessive bubbles, which could indicate contamination, or other unusual feature such as clots. Ensure that the blood bag is intact, without leaking around the seams. If leaking is visible, contact the blood bank.
28. **ACC** Obtain and record "pre-transfusion" vital signs and assessment (temperature, pulse, blood pressure, respirations, and oxygen saturation). Listen to the client's lungs and assess the client for discomfort. Assess for edema, dyspnea, or other signs of circulatory overload. *Baseline assessment will be used as a comparison during transfusion.*

Administering the Blood

29. **INF** Perform hand hygiene and apply clean gloves again.
30. **ACC** Remove the cover over the blood bag port and remove the protective sheath from the spike of the unused arm of the Y set.

31. **INF** Using sterile technique, carefully spike the Y tubing into the unit of blood and ensure that it is secure. **WARNING:** Be careful not to puncture through to the outside of the blood unit bag. If this occurs, the blood unit will have to be discarded due to contamination.

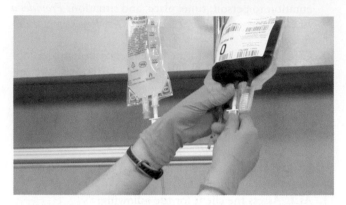

STEP 31 Spike the blood bag.

32. **ACC** Adjust clamps to allow blood to flow into the drip chamber. (Note: The clamp to the NS arm will be closed, and the clamp to the blood arm of the Y tubing and lower clamp will be open.)
33. **ACC** Ensure that the filter is completely covered with blood and that blood is dripping above the filter. *This will facilitate proper filtering and reduce the risk of lysing cells.*

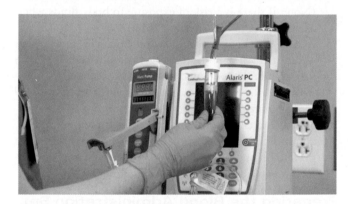

STEP 33 Ensure that blood is covering the filter.

34. **SAF** If a blood warmer is ordered, follow the manufacturer instructions and ensure that the warmer is approved for blood administration. **WARNING:** Do *not* use a microwave, hot water bath, or any other method of warming blood that is not an approved warmer. *Unauthorized warming devices can cause hemolysis of the cells, with fatal consequences (INS, 2016).*
35. **SAF** Before starting the transfusion, trace the tubing again from its point of origin (IV catheter) to the source (blood bag). *Tracing to the source prevents misconnection errors.*
36. **ACC** Begin the blood administration at a slow rate (for the first 15 minutes). *Starting blood at a slow rate will al-*

low the nurse to assess the client for any possible transfusion reactions.

37. **ACC** If a blood administration infusion pump is being used, start the infusion of blood per manufacturer guidelines and watch the client closely. Keep track of the amount of blood that is infusing into the client to make sure the pump is administering the blood as expected.

38. **ACC** Infuse blood over 1 to 4 hours per order. If the client becomes dyspneic or shows any signs of circulatory volume overload, reduce the rate of transfusion and contact the authorized healthcare provider immediately for further orders. **WARNING:** The total infusion time for PRBCs cannot exceed 4 hours.

39. **SAF** Remain with the client for at least the first 15 minutes. Repeat vital signs and compare to client's baseline, and assess the client for any unusual symptoms or complaints. *This allows the nurse to monitor and intervene quickly in the event of a transfusion reaction.*

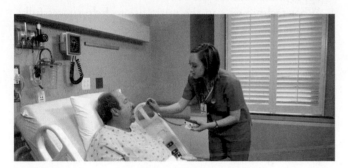

STEP 39 Repeat vital signs.

40. **SAF** Instruct the client to report any difficulty or unusual symptoms immediately.

41. **SAF** During the transfusion, continue to check vital signs every 15 minutes or per policy, and monitor the client's condition, including oxygen saturation, frequently.

42. **SAF** If the client has a change in vital signs, such as an elevated temperature, or any unusual symptoms, slow or stop the transfusion, depending on the policy, and notify the authorized healthcare provider. If the client has a severe reaction, *stop* the transfusion, notify the authorized healthcare provider, and follow the facility's acute transfusion reaction policy. (Note: For examples of serious transfusion reactions, see Table 12.5. For monitoring and care of a client who may have a transfusion reaction, see Box 12.7.)

43. **EVAL** Monitor transfusion, patency of the IV line, and the client's fluid status, including urine output.

44. **ACC** When the transfusion is complete, document the time that the transfusion ended and obtain posttransfusion vital signs. If subsequent PRBC transfusions will be administered, follow policy regarding how often the administration set is changed. **WARNING:** If the client needs to receive a platelet transfusion, do *not* administer them into the same Y-tubing set that was used for the PRBC transfusion. The remnants or debris from the PRBC transfusion could trap the platelets in the used filter.

45. **ACC** If required by policy, flush the line with a minimal volume of NS, or whatever is ordered by the authorized healthcare provider, to ensure the client receives blood.

46. **ACC** Discontinue the infusion and dispose of the equipment as required. (Note: Some facilities require that the blood bag not be disposed of in the event of a reaction. If the client has a suspected reaction, the blood bank may need the bag for investigation.) Resume IVF or convert the IV line to a saline lock per orders.

FINISHING THE SKILL

47. **INF** Remove gloves and perform hand hygiene.

48. **SAF** Ensure client comfort and safety. Ensure that the bed is in the lowest position. Ensure the client can identify and reach the nurse call system. *These safety measures reduce the risk of falls.*

49. **EVAL** Monitor and evaluate the outcomes. *Did the client tolerate the procedure? Are the client's clinical parameters and lab values (e.g., Hgb, Hct) improved after PRBCs transfusion?*

50. **COM** Document assessment findings, care given related to the transfusion, and outcomes in the legal healthcare record:
    - amount and type of blood transfused
    - indications for the use of PRBCs
    - total volume and time of transfusion initiation
    - time that transfusion ended
    - initials, signature, and credentials of clinicians
    - vital signs before, during, and after procedure.

51. **EVAL** Continue to monitor the client for at least 24 hours after the blood transfusion. Obtain vital signs 30 minutes after transfusion, and assess the client for any possible signs of delayed transfusion reactions. *Clients can have delayed transfusion reactions and complications that require immediate attention and interventions.*

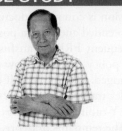

Mr. Jimmy Nguyen is a very thin 76-year-old Vietnamese American. He has been experiencing abdominal pain and weight loss for the last 6 months. He has sought medical care because he recently began vomiting contents that seemed to contain coffee grounds. Upon further questioning, Mr. Nguyen revealed that his stools have been very dark for several months. He is scheduled for a colonoscopy and given the instructions for the bowel prep to ensure his intestines are cleared and clean. The bowel prep consists of restricting his diet to clear liquids and taking a prescribed preparation that induces diarrhea, followed by drinking water to maintain hydration.

The morning of the colonoscopy, Mr. Nguyen is brought to the facility by his wife, who tells the nurse what a difficult evening they experienced as her husband had diarrhea most of the night. Upon assessing Mr. Nguyen, the nurse sees signs of dehydration. His lips are dry, his pulse is 86, and his blood pressure is 124/64. The skin on the back of his hands is loose, with poor skin turgor. In addition, Mr. Nguyen appears very tense. His lips are tight, and his body posture is almost rigid. When the nurse asks him how he is feeling, he states, "I have a bad feeling about this."

The nurse notes the medical orders include normal saline 100 mL/hr and an order to discontinue the IV line when the client is tolerating liquids well. After two attempts, the nurse places a PIV in Mr. Nguyen's hand and escorts him to the procedure room, where the sedation medication is administered via IV bolus. The procedure takes about 30 minutes, after which Mr. Nguyen is moved to the post-anesthesia care unit (PACU) and then to the admission unit to fully recover. As Mr. Nguyen becomes more alert, he also complains of nausea. He soon vomits a small amount of clear fluid.

Case Study Questions

1. Where would the nurse look to find veins suitable for this IV initiation?
2. What equipment does the nurse need to collect in order to start the IV line and IV fluids? What type of administration set would the nurse select?
3. What measures can the nurse use to help identify an appropriate vein for the PIV?
4. What techniques can the nurse use to help successfully initiate the PIV?
5. What measures can the nurse use to help Mr. Nguyen manage his anxiety?
6. When should the nurse discontinue the PIV?
7. **Application of QSEN Competencies:** One of the Quality and Safety Education for Nurses (QSEN) competencies for Evidence-Based Practice is to "describe reliable sources for locating evidence reports and clinical practice guidelines" (Cronenwett et al., 2007). Which nursing society is a well-known resource for vascular access clinical practice guidelines?

■CONCEPT MAP

ICNP Nursing Dx:
Impaired Fluid Volume

Supporting Data:
Negative balance of intake and output
Dry lips
NPO status and bowel prep

Accuracy and Evaluation

- Initiate PIV with 22-gauge catheter
- Use multiple methods to encourage dilation of the vein while assessing the vein for access
- Apply strategies to immobilize the vein during IV initiation
- Administer normal saline at 100 mL/hr
- Monitor urine output
- Monitor vital signs
- Monitor skin turgor and mucous membranes for signs of rehydration

Baseline Assessment Data

- 76-year-old thin male
- Lips dry
- Poor skin turgor
- Pulse 86
- BP 124/64
- History of dark stools, coffee ground vomit, and abdominal pain

ICNP Nursing Dx:
Anxiety

Supporting Data:
Increased pulse
Statement of having a "bad feeling"
Related to colonoscopy and findings

ICNP Nursing Dx:
Risk for Infection

Supporting Data:
Organism entry secondary to invasive lines

Client-Centered Care

- Speak slowly and calmly
- Stay with the client
- Support client's coping mechanisms
- Provide realistic reassurance

Infection Control

- Prep the skin before IV initiation for 30 seconds with antiseptic
- Allow the antiseptic to dry before initiating the IV
- Prepare the IV fluid administration set maintaining the sterility of all connections
- Stabilize the catheter hub and tubing to prevent movement

References

American Red Cross (ARC). (2018). *Blood components*. Retrieved from http://www.redcrossblood.org/learn-about-blood/blood-components.

Brown, T. L. (2017). Pediatric variations of nursing interventions. In *Wong's essentials of pediatric nursing* (10th ed., pp. 575–635). St. Louis, MO: Elsevier.

Castillo, B., Dasgupta, A., Klein, K., Tint, H., & Wahed, A. (2018). *Transfusion medicine for pathologists: A comprehensive review for board preparation, certification, and clinical practice*. Retrieved from https://www.vitalsource.com/za/products/transfusion-medicine-for-pathologists-brian-castillo-v9780128143148.

Centers for Disease Control and Prevention (CDC). (2015). *Guidelines for the prevention of intravascular catheter-related infections (2011)*. Retrieved from https://www.cdc.gov/infectioncontrol/guidelines/bsi/recommendations.html.

ClinLabNavigator (CLN). (2018). *Blood infusion*. Retrieved from http://www.clinlabnavigator.com/transfusion.html.

Cronenwett, L., Sherwood, G., Barnsteiner, J., Disch, J., Johnson, J., Mitchell, P., ... Warren, J. (2007). Quality and safety education for nurses. *Nursing Outlook, 55*(3), 122–131. Retrieved from http://qsen.org/competencies/pre-licensure-ksas/.

Fernandez de Pinedo Perez, V. (2017). *Blood specimen collection: Hemolysis prevention. [Evidence summary]*. Retrieved from The Joanna Briggs Institute EBD Database.

Food and Drug Administration (FDA). (2016). *Fatalities reported to FDA following blood collection and transfusion: Annual summary for fiscal year 2016*. Retrieved from https://www.fda.gov/downloads/BiologicsBloodVaccines/SafetyAvailability/ReportaProblem/TransfusionDonationFatalities/UCM598243.pdf.

Infusion Nurses Society (INS). (2016). Infusion therapy standards of practice. *Supplement to Journal of Infusion Nursing, 39*(1S), S1–S159.

Infusion Nurses Society (INS). (n.d.). *Mission and values*. Retrieved from https://www.ins1.org/about-us/.

Institute for Safe Medication Practices (ISMP). (2015). *ISMP Safe practice guidelines for adult IV push medications*. Retrieved from https://www.ismp.org/sites/default/files/attachments/2017-11/ISMP97-Guidelines-071415-3.%20FINAL.pdf.

International Classification for Nursing Practice (n.d.). *eHealth & ICNP*. Retrieved from https://www.icn.ch/what-we-do/projects/ehealth-icnp.

IV infiltration alleged in patient's suit: Jury sees no negligence by patient's nurses. (2011). *Legal Eagle Eye Newsletter for the Nursing Profession, 19*(1). Retrieved from http://www.nursinglaw.com/.

The Joint Commission. (2013). *Preventing central line–associated bloodstream infections: Useful tools, an international perspective*. Retrieved from http://www.jointcommission.org/CLABSIToolkit.

Kanipe, W., Shobe, K., Li, Y., Kime, M., & Smith-Miller, C. A. (2018). Evaluating the efficacy and use of vein visualization equipment among clinical nurses in an intermediate care environment. *Journal of Infusion Nursing, 41*(4), 253–258.

Maitta, R. (2018). *Clinical principles of transfusion medicine*. Retrieved from https://www.sciencedirect.com/book/9780323544580/clinical-principles-of-transfusion-medicine.

Occupational Safety and Health Administration (OSHA). (2015a). Disposal of contaminated needles and blood tube holders used for phlebotomy. In *Safety and health information bulletin* Retrieved from https://www.osha.gov/dts/shib/shib101503.html.

Occupational Safety and Health Administration (OSHA). (2015b). *Healthcare wide hazards: Needlestick/sharps injuries*. Retrieved from https://www.osha.gov/SLTC/etools/hospital/hazards/sharps/sharps.html.

Ontario Regional Blood Coordinating Network (ORBCON). (2015). *Bloody easy: Blood administration version 2: A handbook for health care professionals*. Retrieved from policyandorders.cw.bc.ca/resource-gallery/Documents/Transfusion%20Medicine/Bloody-Easy-Blood-Administration.pdf.

Park, J. M., Kim, M. J., Yim, H. W., Lee, W. C., Jeong, H., & Kim, N. J. (2016). Utility of near-infrared light devices for pediatric peripheral intravenous cannulation: a systematic review and meta-analysis. *European Journal of Pediatrics, 175*(12), 1975–1988.

Stango, C., Runyan, D., Stern, J., Macri, I., & Vacca, M. (2014). A successful approach to reducing bloodstream infections based on a disinfection device for intravenous needleless connector hub. *Journal of Infusion Nursing, 37*(6), 462–465.

Vizcarra, C., Cassutt, C., Corbitt, N., Richardson, D., Runde, D., & Stafford, K. (2014). Recommendations for improving safety practices with short peripheral catheters. *Journal of Infusion Nursing, 37*(2), 121–124.

Zhang, L., Cao, S., Marsh, N., et al. (2016). Infection risks associated with peripheral vascular catheters. *Journal of Infection Prevention, 17*(5), 207–213.

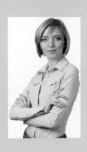

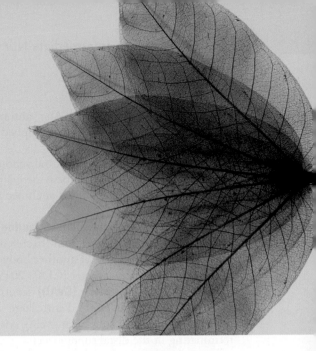

CHAPTER 13

Central Venous Access

"Eventually all things merge into one and a river runs through it." | **Norman Maclean, Author of**

A River Runs Through It

LEARNING OBJECTIVES

By the end of this chapter, the reader will be able to:

1 Describe the nurse's role during central venous access device (CVAD) catheter insertion, including preparation, client positioning and safety, and authorized healthcare provider assistance.

2 Perform the steps required to flush a CVAD catheter.

3 Demonstrate sterile technique while performing CVAD dressing changes.

4 Demonstrate sterile technique while performing needleless connector changes.

5 Collect blood samples from a CVAD and an implantable port.

6 Discuss proper procedures used to access, flush, infuse fluids, and deaccess via an implantable port.

7 Assemble equipment to infuse IV solutions, total parenteral nutrition (TPN), and lipids.

8 Perform the steps necessary to prime primary IV tubing and infuse IV solutions, TPN, and lipids via a central venous line.

9 Discuss the steps needed to safely administer IV solutions, TPN, and lipids via a central venous line.

10 Demonstrate the steps needed to discontinue a central venous catheter (CVC), specifically a peripherally inserted central catheter (PICC) and a triple-lumen catheter (TLC).

TERMINOLOGY

Antimicrobial disc (Biopatch) An antimicrobial disk (impregnated with chlorhexidine) applied at the central venous catheter insertion site.

Broviac catheter External-lying central venous access device that is tunneled under the subcutaneous tissue, inserted into the superior vena cava, and anchored with a Dacron cuff.

Central line associated bloodstream infection A laboratory-confirmed bloodstream infection (bacteremia) that is not secondary to an infection at another body site in a client with a central venous catheter (CDC, 2019).

Central venous access device (CVAD) Internal or external intravascular catheter inserted into large vessels (usually brachial, jugular, or subclavian vein) with catheter tip terminating in the distal superior vena cava; used for frequent and routine access to the vascular system.

Exit infection Presence of purulent drainage, with or without erythema, at the junction of the central venous catheter and the epidermis.

Groshong catheter External-lying tunneled central venous access device with a distal 3-way slit valve designed to reduce the risk of clot formation at the distal tip.

Hickman catheter A modification of the Broviac catheter with a thicker catheter wall and a wider catheter lumen; created to accommodate bone marrow transplantations.

Maximal sterile barrier Mask, cap, sterile gown, gloves, and full body drape.

Noncoring needle A specially designed percutaneous needle used to access implantable ports

Peripherally inserted central catheter (PICC) Single- or double-lumen external-lying catheter inserted into the cephalic or brachial vein in the antecubital fossa with the catheter tip terminating in the superior vena cava

Phlebostatic axis Anatomical point relative to right atrium, fourth intercostal space, and midaxillary line.

Pocket infection An infection involving the subcutaneous pocket containing the central venous access device.

Sutureless securement device (Stat-lock) A tape and sutureless alternative for the securement of PICC and other CVCs.

Triple-lumen catheter A short, external-lying catheter inserted into the internal jugular or subclavian vein with three separate lumens terminating into one catheter.

Tunneled catheter A central catheter that is inserted at one point, tunneled under the subcutaneous tissue, inserted into a distal central vein, and anchored with a Dacron cuff.

Valsalva maneuver The act of forcefully exhaling against a closed glottis to increase intrathoracic pressure.

ACRONYMS

CLABSI Central line–associated bloodstream infection
CVAD Central venous access device
CVC Central venous catheter
IV Intravenous
NS Normal saline
PICC Peripherally inserted central venous catheter
TPN Total parenteral nutrition
TLC Triple-lumen catheter
VTE Venous thromboembolism

SECTION 1 Caring for a Client With a CVAD

Central venous access devices (CVADs) have been used by healthcare professionals for more than 50 years (Gow, Tapper, & Hickman, 2017). A CVAD consists of a sterile polyurethane or soft silicone catheter that terminates in the distal superior vena cava, near the right atrium (Gow et al., 2017). It can be surgically inserted or inserted at the bedside.

CVADs are primarily inserted to ensure vascular access for IV infusions, such as chemotherapy, antibiotics, blood transfusions, or parenteral nutrition. Specifically, CVADs are inserted if a client has poor venous access, needs prolonged infusions, requires administration of sclerosing agents, or requires repeated blood draws.

Several factors influence the authorized healthcare provider's selection of the type of CVAD. These include, but are not limited to, the client's age, activity level, and comorbidities; duration of therapy; and characteristics of medication or solutions. Types of CVADs include (a) tunneled, internally inserted catheters; (b) nontunneled, externally inserted catheters; and (c) implanted, internally inserted venous access ports.

TUNNELED CATHETERS

Tunneled catheters are surgically inserted and secured into the subcutaneous tissue with a Dacron anchoring cuff (Fig. 13.1). This anchoring cuff serves to secure the catheter and reduce the migration of bacteria along the catheter (Harding, 2017). Although surgically inserted, these catheters exit the body at the chest wall and lie externally. They include Broviac, Groshong, or Hickman brands and are used for long-term infusion therapy, which may include the administration of chemotherapy; long-term medications, such as antibiotics; parenteral nutrition; or blood transfusions.

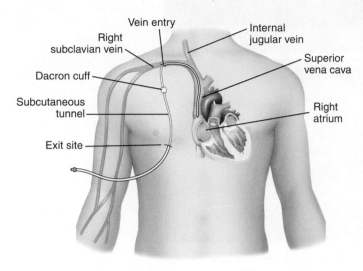

FIG. 13.1 Surgically inserted tunneled subclavian central venous access device (CVAD) with a Dacron anchoring cuff.

NONTUNNELED CATHETERS

Nontunneled catheters such as central venous catheters (CVCs) or peripherally inserted central catheters (PICCs) are inserted at the bedside. A CVC can be centrally inserted into the subclavian or internal jugular vein, whereas a PICC can be peripherally inserted into the basilic or cephalic vein located in the antecubital fossa (Fig. 13.2). A PICC is approximately 50 to 60 cm (approximately 20–23.5 inches) in length and may have a single, double, or triple-lumen catheter (Camp-Sorrell & Matey, 2017; Harding, 2017). Double-lumen PICCs are preferred because the dual lumens allow for simultaneous administration of medication that may be otherwise incompatible. PICC insertions cost less than CVC insertions and have a lower risk of complications; thus, there has been a steady increase in PICC insertions. Nurse-driven PICC teams, with the aid of portable ultrasound for vein identification, have allowed for accurate placement of a PICC at the client's bedside. In a medical emergency, a femoral catheter is sometimes inserted, but this site is highly discouraged due to an increased risk of thrombotic complications and central line–associated infection (Ge, Cavallazzi, Pan, Wang, & Wang, 2012). When a client has a PICC, blood pressure measurements and peripheral venous blood specimen collection should not be performed in the arm with the PICC (Camp-Sorrell & Matey, 2017).

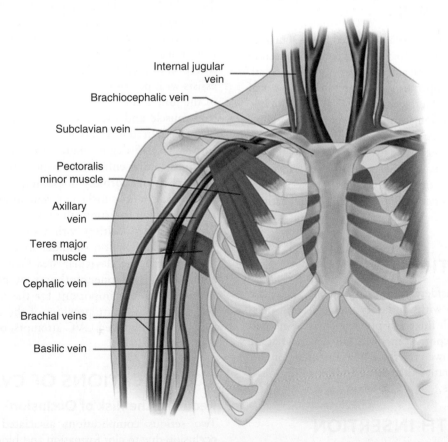

FIG. 13.2 Peripherally inserted central catheter (PICC) location in the brachial or cephalic veins.

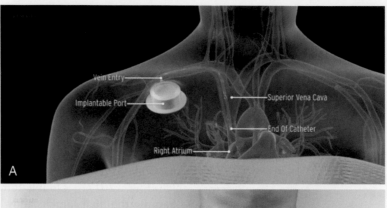

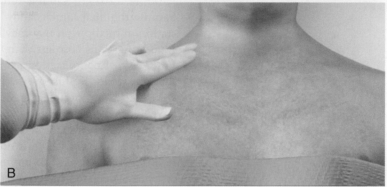

FIG. 13.3 An implantable port is placed surgically for long-term venous access **(A)** and is visible and palpable beneath the skin **(B)**.

IMPLANTED PORTS

Internal implanted ports are surgically inserted CVADs that are embedded under the skin (Fig. 13.3). These ports are placed in the subcutaneous pocket of the anterior chest wall (Port-a-cath or Mediport) or in the upper arm (Passport). They consist of two parts: the catheter and a reservoir. They are intermittently accessed and are used for long-term intravenous (IV) administration, antibiotic or chemotherapy administration, or frequent blood draws. Although they must be surgically inserted and removed, these ports have several advantages: they are low maintenance, have a low incidence of bloodstream infection, and allow for a less restrictive life (swimming and bathing permitted).

POWER-INJECTION CAPABLE

Some CVADs are considered power-injectable, and these devices are designed to withstand very high injection pressures. For example, high injection pressures may be needed with the instillation of contrast media. Only devices that are confirmed to be for power injection may be used for this purpose, and it is imperative that the client know this information about the device.

ASSISTING WITH INSERTION

At the bedside, the nurse assists the authorized healthcare provider during insertion of an external CVC. (Review Table 13.1 for a description of the types of CVCs.) After verifying informed consent has been obtained, and prior to insertion, the nurse assists the provider to identify key anatomical landmarks. For example, when considering the insertion of a CVC via the internal jugular vein, the nurse assists with positioning the client to optimize visualization of the junction between the heads of the sternocleidomastoid muscle and the clavicle. If tolerated, the client may be placed in the Trendelenburg position with the neck turned at a 45-degree angle away from the insertion site; this positioning enhances visualization of the jugular vein. If the client is morbidly obese, jugular vein insertion may not be safe, and subclavian vein insertion may be used. For subclavian insertion, the nurse places the client in the Trendelenburg position with a small, rolled towel placed between the client's shoulder blades; this positioning hyperextends the clavicular area (Yeager, 2017). To avoid complications of pneumothorax or nerve damage, prior to insertion, it is important for the nurse to inform the authorized healthcare provider of the client's medical history, previously failed CVC attempts, or skeletal anomalies (Ge et al., 2012).

COMPLICATIONS OF CVADs

Reducing the Risk of Occlusion

Two serious complications associated with CVADs are occlusion due to clot formation and bloodstream infections. The CVAD is a foreign body; therefore, over time, plasma proteins and fibrin adhere to and cover the catheter, thus

TABLE 13.1 Central Venous Access Device (CVAD) Overview

CVAD	Duration	Insertion Procedure	Flush When Not in Use	Blood Sample Discard Volume	Miscellaneous
Nontunneled catheters: Triple-lumen catheters	Short-term access; acute care setting	Placed by authorized healthcare provider at bedside or under fluoroscopy	Flush each lumen with 10 mL 0.9% NS every 12–24 hr or per facility policy.	Clamp all lumens not being used for blood sampling. Withdraw and discard 3–5 mL. Flush with 10–20 mL 0.9% NS after blood sampling.	May be placed in the subclavian or internal jugular vein. Removed at bedside. Accounts for the majority of CLABSI.
Nontunneled catheters: PICC and Power PICCs	Medium duration— several months	Placed by certified and trained RN at bedside with or without fluoroscopy	Flush each lumen with 10 mL 0.9% NS every 24 hours or per facility policy	Clamp all lumens not being used for blood sampling. Withdraw and discard 3–5 mL. Flush with 10–20 mL 0.9% NS after blood sampling.	ONLY Power PICCs (with purple hub) can be used for contrast infusions. Client needs to be taught to flush the catheter and change the needleless connector. Removed at bedside.
Tunneled catheters: Hickman, Groshong, and Broviac	Long-term access— can remain in place for years	Outpatient surgery to insert and remove Portion of catheter is exposed	Flush each lumen with 10 mL 0.9% NS every 24 hr or per facility policy	Withdraw and discard 3–5 mL. Flush with 10–20 mL 0.9% NS after blood sampling.	Client needs to be taught to flush the catheter and change the needleless connector. Lower rate of CLABSI than nontunneled.
Implanted ports: Power Ports, Medi-Ports, and PAS-Ports	Long-term access— can remain in place for years	Outpatient surgery to insert and remove No care required by the client	Flush with 10 mL prefilled 0.9% NS syringe. Followed with prefilled heparin syringe every 4–8 weeks by RN.	Withdraw and discard 3–5 mL. Flush with 10–20 mL 0.9% NS after blood sampling.	ONLY Power Port (has three bumps on septum) with a Power Port access needle can be used for contrast infusions. Lowest risk for CLABSI.

Adapted from The Joint Commission, 2013 and Camp-Sorrel & Matey, 2017.

promoting clot (thrombus) formation (Dal Molin et al., 2014). Additionally, clot formation may occur due to the crystallization of infusion solutions or drug-to-drug precipitants. The risk of thrombus formation is increased with femoral CVCs and is relatively low with subclavian CVADs (Ge et al., 2012).

Nursing care can reduce the risk of complications. In order to prevent clot formation, the nurse routinely flushes a CVAD. The patency of a CVAD is dependent on routine catheter flushing with sufficient solution, which creates turbulence and prevents clot formation within the catheter and at the distal tip. Accepted practices for flushing CVADs include:

- Routine flushing is with single-dose, preservative–free 0.9% normal saline (NS) before and after CVAD use.
- Flushing is performed with a 10-mL or larger syringe to prevent high-pressure surges that are possible with a small syringe.
- Flush with 10 to 20 mL of 0.9% NS after blood specimen collection.
- Clamp the lumen after the final flush to reduce the risk of occlusion and infection.
- Never force a flush (Camp-Sorrell & Matey, 2017; INS, 2016).

The most frequent flushing methods include positive pressure, pulsating, and continuous flushing, described as follows:

- A positive-pressure flush is performed as the nurse instills flush solution while clamping the catheter with a small amount of flushing solution remaining in the syringe. The combined action of the catheter being clamped, the flushing solution remaining in the syringe, and the immediate removal of the syringe from the catheter hub creates positive pressure to decrease blood return into the vascular device lumen (INS, 2016).
- Pulsating flushing (push-pause) is performed as the nurse instills flushing solution with a start–stop motion. Ten short pushes of 1 mL each are delivered to infuse a 10-mL flush. Push-pause or pulsating flush is the most effective at removing fibrin formations, but use of the pulsating flush may be device specific (Camp-Sorrell & Matey, 2017; INS, 2016).
- Continuous flushing is the infusion of flush solution with no breaks.

The type of needleless connector that is attached to the CVAD and the specific type of CVAD may have a manufacturer-recommended flush method. Therefore, it is important to refer to facility policy for a specific CVAD flush protocol.

An area of continued research is determining the optimal flushing solution, volume, and concentration (heparinized solution) for each CVAD (Box 13.1). Currently, there is not a definitive recommendation. However, the evidence shows that NS is comparable to heparin solutions for nonvalved

BOX 13.1 Lessons From the Evidence: Heparin Versus Saline for Central Venous Catheter Flushing

Routine central venous access device (CVAD) line flushing is needed before and after medication administration, blood transfusions, and blood draws and for routine CVAD care. Previously, to keep the catheter line patent, the catheter was routinely flushed with heparin (Randolph, Cook, Gonzales, & Andrew, 1998). However, bleeding and heparin-induced thrombocytopenia (HIT) have been identified as adverse effects of heparin flushing and have led clinicians and facilities to question the need for this routine care (Dal Molin et al., 2014; Mitchell, Anderson, Williams, & Umscheid, 2009). Heparin-induced thrombocytopenia can cause pulmonary emboli as well as thrombophlebitis.

Using the PICO format (P—problem, I—intervention, C—comparison, O—outcome), the clinical question is: When providing routine CVAD catheter care (P), does intermittent flushing with heparin (I) reduce the incidence of CVAD catheter occlusion (O) as compared to intermittent flushing with saline (C)?

After a thorough review of multiple research study findings, the recommendations are (a) there is an insufficient amount of scientific support on the effectiveness of heparin flushing to reduce the incidence of CVAD catheter occlusion; (b) there is no difference in catheter clotting, phlebitis, or duration of catheter life between saline and heparin flush; (c) there is no scientific evidence that heparin flushing reduces bloodstream infections; (d) flushing with heparin poses a risk for HIT; and (e) flushing CVAD catheters with saline may be a safer alternative for routine care than the previously used saline-heparin combination flush. These findings have resulted in a shift in policy for CVAD catheter flushing care. Previously performed CVAD routine flushing with heparin has been replaced with CVAD routine flushing with saline (Dal Molin et al., 2014; Harding, 2017; Mitchell et al., 2009).

vascular access devices (Camp-Sorrell & Matey, 2017). Many studies are demonstrating that flushing with NS has similar outcomes to flushing with heparinized solution, even in an implanted port (Camp-Sorrell & Matey, 2017). Nevertheless, heparinized solution may still be ordered.

Reducing the Risk of Infection

Central line–associated bloodstream infection is a very serious infection that results in prolonged hospital stays, increased costs, and the risk of death (Centers for Disease Control and Prevention [CDC], 2019). Nurses use evidence-based practices to reduce the introduction of organisms into the central access device (discussed in more depth shortly) and to assess and monitor the client for any signs of infection. The three main types of CVAD infections are (1) exit-site infection, (2) tunneled infection, and (3) central line–associated bloodstream infection (CLABSI). Collaborative efforts among members of the healthcare team to reduce CLABSI resulted in approximately a 50% reduction in this infection between 2008 and 2016 (CDC, 2017b).

Additionally, to reduce the risk for infection, nursing care is focused on assessing the insertion site for signs and symptoms of inflammation (erythema, tenderness, edema); performing routine dressing and cap changes; and performing cap changes when there is accumulated tape or blood debris on the needleless connectors. CVC dressings that become wet, soiled, or loose must be promptly changed. Routine dressing changes, usually every 7 days, should be done using sterile technique and involve cleansing the area with antiseptic solution and applying a transparent sterile dressing, a sutureless securement device, and an antimicrobial disc (CDC, 2017). When performing a routine CVC dressing change, a needleless access-cap change is usually included. Refer to facility policy for the recommended frequency of CVAD dressing changes and catheter needleless access-cap changes. See Box 13.2 for an example of why scissors are not used in a CVAD dressing change and why securement of the line is critical.

DRAWING BLOOD FROM A CVAD

One of the key advantages for a client with a CVAD is the ability to draw blood through the catheter, thus drastically reducing the number of client venipunctures. When a CVAD has multiple lumens, researchers recommend using the proximal lumen for blood sampling and IV fluid (IVF) therapy. The middle and distal lumens are reserved for medication administration and TPN (Camp-Sorrell & Matey, 2017). When drawing blood from a CVAD, it is important to withdraw sufficient blood to clear the catheter from the tip of the lumen to the needleless adapter or stopcock. This space is filled with blood diluted by flush solution. The precise volume for the client's CVAD device should be available in the information about that device, and three times this volume is the exact recommended amount to discard. A general guideline is that 3 to 5 mL is usually sufficient to clear the catheter of all flush solution for tunneled, nontunneled, and port catheters (Camp-Sorrell & Matey, 2017). It is not desirable to withdraw and discard more blood than this volume because blood-sparing techniques are considered a nursing practice standard of care (Camp-Sorrell & Matey, 2017). See Table 13.1 for discard volumes. If the nurse is drawing a blood culture, then the first 5 mL may be used for the blood culture to determine the organism. Some laboratory studies may be impacted by drawing through the CVAD, even when the line is flushed first and an adequate volume of discard has been withdrawn. Medications that adhere to the catheter wall (e.g., aminoglycosides, cyclosporine, gentamicin) and coagulation studies in catheters that have been heparinized have inconsistent results in studies. Drawing a blood sample from a peripheral vein may be necessary if results are suspect (Camp-Sorrell & Matey, 2017). The most commonly used method to draw blood from a CVAD is the syringe method. Some facilities are using systems that allow the withdrawn blood to be returned back to a client as a blood-sparing strategy, particularly with pediatric clients. Some facilities may use a Vacutainer system, which is very similar to that used in Skill 18.2.

BOX 13.2 Lessons From the Courtroom: A Groshong Catheter Dressing Change Gone Wrong

A client had a Groshong catheter inserted to receive long-term IV antibiotic therapy at home with home healthcare support. The home health nurse came to the client's house for a routine home healthcare visit. While assessing the Groshong catheter, the nurse began to perform a routine dressing change. During the dressing change, the nurse used scissors and inadvertently cut the catheter tube. Without realizing what she had done, the nurse left the client's home. The client's wife called the home health agency and requested the nurse return to the home. The nurse returned to the home and was witnessed, by a neighbor, pulling on the catheter, trying to apply tape over the cut in the tube, and attempting to flush the catheter with air. Unfortunately, the client's condition deteriorated, and the client was hospitalized. X-ray results indicated the catheter was lodged under the clavicle. The client died the next day (Newsletter, 2008).

This scenario highlights the need for a complete assessment of the site, dressing, and tubing after completing any CVAD-related care. Due to the risk of inadvertent cutting of the catheter, scissors are highly discouraged when flushing, changing the catheter hubs, or changing a client's CVAD dressing. The nurse in the scenario was responsible for assessing the Groshong catheter site dressing and tubing prior to completing her initial visit. During her follow-up visit, the nurse was attempting to manipulate the Groshong catheter herself and tape over the hole. Advancing or pulling back on a CVAD catheter is a violation of nurse's scope of practice. After a Groshong, or any CVAD catheter, is confirmed for placement by a chest x-ray, the catheter is to remain stationary and secured for placement in the distal one-third of the superior vena cava. The nurse in this situation should have immediately contacted the authorized healthcare provider.

Reference: Groshong Catheter, 2009.

CARE FOR A CLIENT WITH A SUBCUTANEOUS PORT: ACCESSING AND DEACCESSING

Caring for a client with a subcutaneous port requires slightly different techniques and equipment compared with the other CVADs. The reservoir only needs to be accessed if the port is going to be used for an infusion or blood draw. A port requires sterile technique while using a noncoring needle to access the reservoir, then applying a dressing. This access and the noncoring needle must be changed every 7 days. Once the client no longer requires medications, fluids, or blood draws, the nurse will flush with NS followed by heparin and remove the noncoring needle and dressing. If the port is not being utilized (no access is required), the port only needs to be flushed once every 4 to 6 weeks with NS and heparin.

DISCONTINUING A CVAD

When IV therapy is no longer needed, the CVAD is removed. Any assessment of a potential exit-site infection, tunneled infection, or CLABSI may require prompt CVAD removal. Externally placed, nontunneled CVADs can be removed safely at the bedside. While removing the catheter, have the client lie flat or in the Trendelenburg position and remove the catheter in the direction of the catheter insertion. If possible, to reduce the incidence of air emboli, instruct the client to perform the Valsalva maneuver during removal. Refer to facility policy for the management of suspected CLABSI and the specific protocol for CVAD removal. Tunneled anchored CVADs and implantable ports must be surgically removed in the operating room.

CRITICAL CONCEPTS AND CVADs

Infection Control

Through the past decade, much research has focused on reducing CLABSI (Camp-Sorrell & Matey, 2017). Best practices have emerged from the research, and toolkits are available for facility and unit adoption (AHRQ, 2018). Nurses implement infection control measures during the insertion of the catheter, during dressing changes, and with each access of the CVAD in order to reduce the introduction of organisms that may result in CLABSI.

Insertion Techniques

During insertion, the introduction of organisms may come from the client's skin or from a healthcare worker; therefore, interventions are aimed at blocking this transfer of organisms When inserting a CVAD, the "bundle" approach is recommended, which includes the following: good hand hygiene prior to insertion; sterile techniques, including sterile barrier precautions; proper use of chlorhexidine skin preparation for skin asepsis; and avoidance of the femoral site of insertion if possible. In addition, nontunneled central venous catheters should remain inserted for the shortest time possible. The nurse must ensure that maximal sterile barrier precautions are instituted and maintained throughout the insertion procedure of both centrally placed CVCs and PICCs (Fig. 13.4).

Hand Hygiene

The literature suggests hand hygiene as a critical step for safety and for preventing the transmission of transient organisms. According to the CDC guidelines and the Intravenous Nursing Society (INS) standards (CDC, 2015; INS, 2016), handwashing by all members of the healthcare team is critical to prevent infections on all central lines. All nurses must perform hand hygiene prior to any intervention on a CVAD.

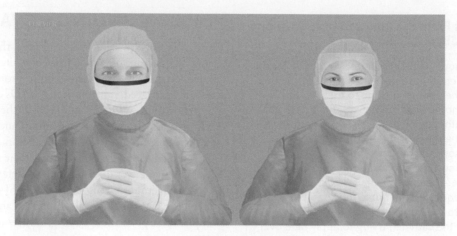

FIG. 13.4 Proper personal protective equipment (PPE) attire for the insertion of a central venous catheter (CVC).

BOX 13.3 Evidence-Based Practice: Needleless Connector Disinfection

The implementation of bundled best practice strategies during central venous catheter insertion has demonstrated a significant reduction in CLABSI (Association for Professionals in Infection Control and Epidemiology [APIC], 2015). Nevertheless, the longer the client has a CVAD, the greater the risk for CLABSI. Contamination through the catheter hub or needleless connector is considered to be the organism entry site in 50% of post-insertion infections (Moureau & Flynn, 2015).

However, what is the evidence for best practice during the maintenance of the CVAD? One important area of research is on the disinfection of needleless connectors. The types of needleless connectors have changed over the last decade and are currently a source of contamination, organism entry, and subsequent CLABSI. Research has been conducted to determine the proper length of time and solution to cleanse the needleless cap and/or hub. Moureau and Flynn (2015) conducted a systematic review of the literature on disinfection practices of catheter hubs, reviewing over 140 publications.

Healthcare team members need to consider the following: (1) the type of disinfectant to cleanse the hub, (2) the method of application (active scrub or passive cap), and (3) the duration of the scrub (if scrubbing).
- Although the 70% isopropyl alcohol wipe is the most commonly used disinfectant for connectors, more studies are needed to determine the optimal duration of scrubbing time. Reported scrub times of 5 to 60 seconds

demonstrated both effective and ineffective disinfection depending the design of the needleless connector (Moureau & Flynn, 2015).
- Alcoholic chlorhexidine (2% chlorhexidine in 70% isopropyl alcohol) is a superior disinfecting agent and has demonstrated effective disinfection with a 5- to 15-second scrub (Moureau & Flynn, 2015).
- Infections are drastically reduced when passive disinfectant caps are placed on access points to stop contamination.

The Infusion Society Nurses (2016) makes the following recommendations based upon this evidence:
- Acceptable disinfecting agents include 70% isopropyl alcohol, iodophors (e.g., povidone-iodine), or >0.5% chlorhexidine in alcohol solution.
- Scrub time and dry time depend upon the design of the needleless connector and the properties of the disinfecting agent.
- Use vigorous mechanical scrubbing methods for all needleless connectors, even those with antimicrobial properties.
- Use of passive disinfectant caps reduce contamination and CLABSI. Once a cap is removed, it is discarded and not replaced.
- Recommended: Use a vigorous 5- to 15-second scrub with each entry into the vascular access device, even after removing the disinfectant cap.

Dressing Changes

Another key time for the use of sterile technique is during assessment of the site and dressing changes. Chlorhexidine is the preferred solution for cleansing the skin. Studies report improved skin asepsis with chlorhexidine (Schiffer et al., 2013). For clients over the age of 18 with short-term, nontunneled CVADs, chlorhexidine-impregnated dressings are recommended. No recommendation is made for those younger than 18 except that chlorhexidine-impregnated dressings are *not* recommended for premature infants (CDC, 2017). The requirement for a chlorhexidine-impregnated dressing can be met by use of a chlorhexidine-impregnated sponge disc or a transparent dressing with a chlorhexidine-impregnated clear gel pad. Transparent dressing changes are recommended every 7 days or when the dressing becomes damp, loosened, or soiled. Gauze dressings are

changed every 2 days. Gauze dressings are used when the site is bleeding or oozing or if the client is diaphoretic and the transparent dressing will not adhere (CDC, 2015).

Tubing Changes

Continuous IV primary administration tubing sets only need to be changed every 72 to 96 hours. However, continuous infusions that enhance microbial growth (e.g., TPN, lipids, TPN with lipids) must be changed every 24 hours, including the fluid and the administration set. Intermittent infusion tubing or intermittent infusions that have primary tubing administration sets need to be changed every 24 hours.

As identified in Box 13.3, nursing research has examined infection control practices surrounding routine access

BOX 13.4 Home Care Considerations: Central Venous Access Devices

1. When do I need to flush my central venous access device (CVAD)?

If you have a *Hickman/Groshong*, flush it once every day or after each infusion with 10 mL of 0.9% NS.

If you have a *peripherally inserted central catheter* (*PICC*), flush it every day or after each infusion with 10 mL of 0.9% NS.

If you have an implanted port, you will need to schedule an appointment every 4 to 8 weeks with your authorized healthcare provider's office to have a registered nurse (RN) flush your implanted port.

2. Do I need to have a dressing on my CVAD?

If you have *Hickman/Groshong*, once the area around your catheter has healed, you do not need to wear any dressing.

If you have a *PICC,* your dressing will need to be changed weekly. An RN usually completes this dressing change.

If you have an *implanted port*, no dressing is needed if your port is not being used. A dressing is only required if your implanted port is being used to receive IVF intravenous (IV) fluids or medications.

3. What do I do if I can't flush my CVAD?

If you have a *Hickman/Groshong* catheter and you cannot flush it, try changing positions, such as lying down or sitting up, placing one arm over your head, or turning on your side, then attempt to flush your catheter. If you are still unable to flush your catheter, you should call your authorized healthcare provider.

If you have a *PICC* and you cannot flush it, try changing positions, such as lying down or sitting up, placing one arm

over your head, or turning on your side, then attempting to flush your catheter. If you are still unable to flush your catheter, you should call your authorized healthcare provider.

If you have an *implanted port* and your RN is unable to flush your implanted port, the nurse will ask you to change positions, and then your nurse will attempt to flush it.

4. When do I need to immediately call the doctor?

It is very important that you notify your authorized healthcare provider if you have a temperature greater than 101.5°F. It is also important look at the CVAD and call the authorized healthcare provider if you experience any unusual drainage, redness, swelling, or pain where the catheter enters your body.

5. What are some good safety habits?

Wash your hands before doing anything with your CVAD.

If you have a clamp on your catheter, always remember to clamp your line after flushing or changing your caps.

Do NOT attach any other type of clamp to your catheter; it could cause damage to the catheter.

Keep all your supplies for your CVAD in one special, dry, clean location.

Keep all hospital/outpatient center CVAD care instructions located with your supplies.

If you have any concerns, call your authorized healthcare provider's office and speak with the RN.

---

of the CVAD through the needleless connector. Scrubbing the hub or utilizing disinfectant caps are practices that have been implemented to reduce CLABSI. Many facilities are utilizing disinfectant caps over the hubs of all CVAD tubing.

Accuracy

The technique used to secure a CVAD affects the client's outcome in both maintaining the patency of the catheter and securing the correct anatomical placement of the catheter. The CDC guidelines recommend using a stabilizing device rather than sutures to secure a short-term CVC. A sutureless securement device reduces mechanical trauma at the insertion site, which results in reduced movement of the catheter and the resulting potential inflammation. In addition, it has been documented that a sutureless securement device reduces the risk of phlebitis and potential dislodgement of the CVAD (CDC, 2015).

Health Maintenance

The long-term nature of subcutaneous CVADs in particular suggests clients care for their CVADs independently at home. Clients with tunneled catheters are capable of having their CVADs in place for years. The type of CVAD will dictate the degree of health maintenance involved for the client.

If the client has a Hickman or a Groshong, the client will need to be taught how to flush the catheter on a daily basis while assessing the site. However, clients who have a port will need to return to the practitioner's office or medical facility to have the port flushed every 4 to 6 weeks if it is not being used. See Box 13.4 for exploration of client instructions for CVAD home care.

APPLICATION OF THE NURSING PROCESS

Examples of Related International Classification for Nursing Practice (ICNP) Nursing Diagnoses, Expected Client Outcomes, and Nursing Interventions:

Nursing Diagnosis: Risk for infection

Supporting Data: Client with a nontunneled central venous catheter.

Expected Client Outcomes: The client will remain free of infection, as seen by:

- lab work, particularly white blood cell (WBC) count within established parameters
- temperature and other vital signs at baseline and within established parameters
- absence of pain, purulent drainage, redness, swelling, or any sign of inflammation.

Nursing Intervention Example: Maintain strict sterile technique, scrub the hub with the appropriate solution for the recommended length of time, and allow it to dry.

Nursing Diagnosis: Impaired skin integrity
Supporting Data: Client with a nontunneled central venous catheter.
Expected Client Outcomes: The client will verbalize understanding of the following measures related to CVAD site skin integrity:
- reporting any pain or discomfort at CVAD insertion site
- self-care procedures related to CVAD care
- signs of impaired skin integrity.

Nursing Intervention Example: Maintain a clean, dry, and intact insertion-site dressing.
Reference: International Classification for Nursing Practice. (n.d.). *eHealth & ICNP.* Retrieved from https://www.icn.ch/what-we-do/projects/ehealth-icnp.

CRITICAL CONCEPTS
Caring for a Client With a CVAD

Accuracy (ACC)

Accuracy when managing central venous access devices is subject to the following variables:
Nurse-Related and System-Related Factors
- Assessment of client, including vital signs, level of discomfort, skin integrity, and lab values
- Assessment of insertion site for redness, swelling, drainage, or blood around the site
- Technique used for processing orders, monitoring the client, and providing follow-up care
- Appropriate flushing technique
- Technique used for equipment readiness, management, and securement of CVAD and subcutaneous ports
- Proper client positioning

Client-Centered Care (CCC)

Respect for the client when managing CVADs is demonstrated through:
- promoting autonomy and the client's right to make decisions related to the CVAD
- providing privacy and ensuring comfort
- answering questions that the client or family may have
- honoring cultural preferences

- advocating for the client and family.

Infection Control (INF)

When managing CVADs, healthcare-associated infection associated is prevented by:
- containment of microorganisms
- preventing and reducing the transfer of microorganisms
- reducing the number of microorganisms
- preventing an environment conducive to microbial growth.

Safety (SAF)

When managing CVADs, safety measures prevent harm and maintain a safe care environment, including:
- use of securement devices to maintain catheter position and patency
- use of proper clamping and flushing techniques
- proper labeling of lumens, tubing, and IVF containers.

Communication (COM)

- Communication allows for exchanges of information (oral, written, nonverbal, or electronic) between two or more people, including the nurse, client, family, and healthcare team.
- Documentation records information in a permanent legal record.
- Collaboration with the client is essential to achieve safe management of CVADs.

Health Maintenance (HLTH)

Nursing is dedicated to the promotion of health and self-care abilities related to managing CVADs, including:
- maintaining skin and tissue integrity of the CVC insertion site
- promoting the client's ability to provide self-care for the CVAD at home.

Evaluation (EVAL)

When managing CVADs, evaluation of outcomes enables the nurse to determine the efficacy of the care provided, including:
- monitoring the client for signs and symptoms of infection and or phlebitis
- monitoring the patency of the central line catheter
- the client's level of understanding of the homecare required for the CVAD.

■ SKILL 13.1 Assisting With Insertion

EQUIPMENT

Clean gloves
1 (10-mL) 0.9% NS flush per lumen
1 heparinized flush per lumen, as per facility policy
Central line kit
Extra pair of sterile gloves
Masks, if not included in kit

BEGINNING THE SKILL

1. **SAF** Review healthcare provider's order and facility policy. *Verifying the plan of care prevents injury to the client.*
2. **CCC** Verify that informed client consent has been obtained for insertion of a percutaneous central venous line. *To observe the client's right to autonomy and safety, obtaining consent is essential prior to insertion of a CVAD.*

3. **CCC** Introduce yourself to the client and family, if present.
4. **COM** Explain the procedure.
5. **INF** Perform hand hygiene.
6. **SAF** Identify the client using two identifiers.
7. **CCC** Provide privacy. Close the door or pull the curtain.

PROCEDURE

8. **SAF** Set up an ergonomically safe space. Raise the bed to a comfortable working height as per authorized healthcare provider preference. Raise one side rail. *Setting up an ergonomically safe space prevents injury to the nurse, authorized healthcare provider, and client.*
9. **ACC** Immediately prior to CVAD insertion, place the client in the Trendelenburg position for the insertion of a subclavian or internal jugular central line. For subclavian placement, a rolled towel placed between the client's shoulder blades is helpful (Yeager, 2017).

Positioning allows for enhanced anatomical visualization and reduced risk of air emboli.

10. **INF** Assist the authorized healthcare provider with his or her gown application. Enables the authorized healthcare provider to use maximal sterile barrier precautions per CDC recommendations.
11. **INF** The registered nurse (RN) and authorized healthcare provider each apply sterile gloves. *Maintaining sterility is vital to infection control when handling CVADs.*
12. **INF** Cleanse the client's skin with a >0.5% chlorhexidine preparation in a scrubbing motion for 30 seconds and allow to dry completely. *Cleaning with chlorhexidine is one of the evidence-based steps to prevent CLABSI. Cleansing prevents the introduction of microorganisms during insertion.*
13. **ACC** Assist the authorized healthcare provider during the insertion procedure by preparing the equipment: applying needleless connectors, flushing the catheter, and applying the sterile dressing after insertion with proper sterile technique.

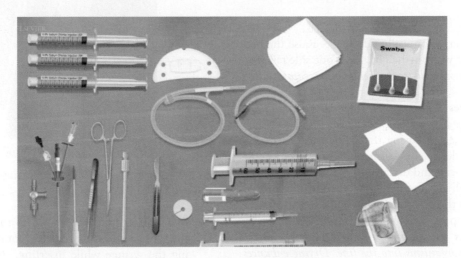

STEP 13 Prepare the equipment for catheter insertion.

14. **INF** Remove gloves and perform hand hygiene.
15. **ACC** Place the client in a supine position and prepare the client for a chest x-ray to confirm CVC placement. *Chest x-ray will confirm the location of the catheter tip.*

FINISHING THE SKILL

16. **CCC** Provide comfort measures for the client and assist the client with positioning.

17. **SAF** Ensure client safety. Place the bed in the lowest position. Ensure that the client can identify and reach the nurse call system. *These safety measures reduce the risk of injury from falls.*
18. **EVAL** Evaluate outcomes. Is the CVC well placed? Is the CVC patent? How did the client tolerate the procedure?
19. **COM** Document care, including date and site of insertion, length of catheter, confirmation of placement, blood return, and how the client tolerated the procedure.

■ SKILL 13.2 Flushing Central Venous Access Devices

EQUIPMENT

Clean gloves
1 (10-mL) 0.9% NS flush per lumen
1 heparinized flush per lumen, as per facility policy
2 chlorhexidine or 70% isopropyl alcohol wipes for each lumen
Disinfectant cap for each lumen

BEGINNING THE SKILL

1. **SAF** Review the healthcare provider's order or facility policy. *Verifying the plan of care prevents injury to the client.*
2. **CCC** Introduce yourself to the client and family.
3. **COM** Explain the procedure.
4. **INF** Perform hand hygiene.
5. **SAF** Identify the client using two identifiers.
6. **CCC** Provide privacy. Close the door or pull the curtain.

PROCEDURE

7. **SAF** Set up an ergonomically safe space. Raise the bed to a comfortable working height. Raise one side rail. *Setting up an ergonomically safe space prevents injury to the nurse and client.*
8. **INF** Apply gloves. *There is an inherent risk of contamination and exposure to blood when handling CVADs.*
9. Open the package enclosing the saline flush, if necessary. If the needleless connector hub has a disinfectant cap, remove the cap and discard it.
10. **INF** Mechanically scrub the needleless connector hub of the lumen with the chlorhexidine wipe for 5 to 15 seconds or 70% isopropyl alcohol wipe for 5 to 60 seconds. Allow to air dry. *Scrubbing the hub prevents the introduction of microorganisms into the line. Drying enhances bactericidal action (Moureau & Flynn, 2015).*

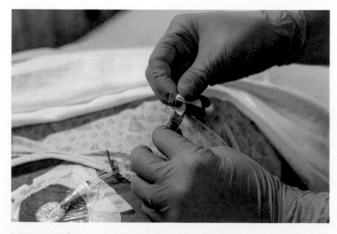

STEP 10 Scrub the needleless connector hub.

11. **SAF** Hold the NS flush (or heparinized solution) with the plunger side down and remove the cap from the end. *Minimizes risk for contamination and brings air to the top of the syringe.*

12. **SAF** Remove air from the syringe by pulling back on the plunger slightly to break the pressure seal, then push the plunger up to expel the air from the saline. *Pulling the plunger back helps control the flow of saline and removes air from syringe, reducing the risk of an air embolism.*
13. **SAF** Inspect the syringe to ensure all air has been removed.

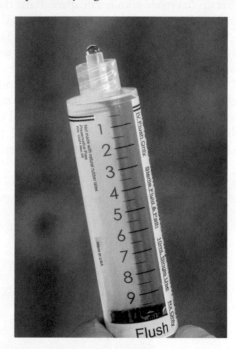

STEP 13 Inspect the syringe to ensure all air has been removed.

14. **ACC** Attach the NS syringe to the lumen by pushing the syringe into the needleless connector hub and rotating the syringe while inserting. *This will Luer-Lok the syringe into place.*
15. **ACC** Unclamp the lumen before flushing, if necessary.
16. **ACC** Pull back slightly on the plunger to assess for blood return. *Verifies patency of CVAD and prevents pushing a clot into the client.*

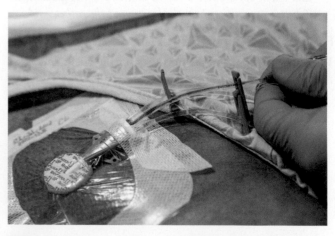

STEP 16 Pull back slightly on plunger to assess for blood return.

17. **ACC** Flush with 0.9% NS (or heparinized solution). Never inject saline against resistance. *Resistance may indicate venous thromboembolism (VTE).*

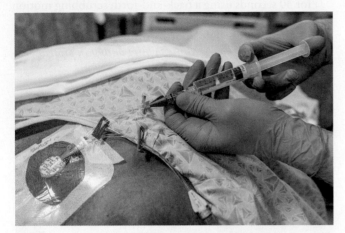

STEP 17 Flush with 0.9% NS.

18. **ACC** Clamp the lumen of the device and remove the syringe from the port of the lumen by rotating and pulling the syringe away from the port of the lumen.

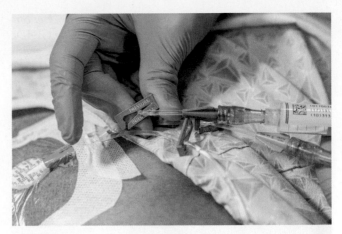

STEP 18 Clamp the lumen of the device.

19. **INF** Apply a new disinfectant cap to the hub.

FINISHING THE SKILL

20. **INF** Remove gloves and perform hand hygiene.
21. **EVAL** Evaluate outcomes, including the ease of flushing the CVC, line patency, and how the client tolerated the procedure.
22. **CCC** Provide comfort measures for the client.
23. **SAF** Ensure client safety. Place the bed in the lowest position. Ensure that the client can identify and reach the nurse call system. *These safety measures reduce the risk of injury from falls.*
24. **COM** Document the care provided, including ease of flushing, blood return, and how the client tolerated the procedure.

■ **SKILL 13.3** Changing the CVC or PICC Line Dressing

EQUIPMENT

Clean gloves
Sterile gloves, size appropriate
Central line dressing change kit (including chlorhexidine scrub and translucent dressing), as per facility policy
Mask, if not included in the kit
Mask for the client (if client unable to keep head turned away from the insertion site)
Sterile measuring tape
Antimicrobial disc (Biopatch) or dressing with a chlorhexidine gel pad
Sutureless securement device (Stat-Lock)

BEGINNING THE SKILL

1. **SAF** Review the healthcare provider's order or facility policy. *Verifying the plan of care prevents injury to the client.*

2. **CCC** Introduce yourself to the client and family.
3. **COM** Explain the procedure.
4. **INF** Perform hand hygiene.
5. **SAF** Identify the client using two identifiers.
6. **CCC** Provide privacy. Close the door and pull the curtain.

PROCEDURE

7. **SAF** Set up a workspace according to your hand dominance (e.g., right-handed RN on client's right side). *Setting up an ergonomically safe workspace prevents injury to the nurse and client.*
8. **INF** Put on your own mask and place a mask on the client. If the client cannot tolerate the mask, ask the client to turn his or her face away from the central line site. *Minimizes the risk for airborne microorganisms entering the CVC insertion site.*

9. **INF** Apply clean gloves. *There is an inherent risk of contamination and exposure to blood when handling CVADs.*

10. **SAF** Remove old dressing by pulling the dressing gently toward the insertion site. *Pulling the dressing toward the insertion site reduces the risk of dislodging the central line. With a PICC line, this involves pulling toward the axilla.* **WARNING:** Do not use scissors when removing the dressing. *Scissors or a sharp-edged clamp can damage or cut the catheter (Camp-Sorrell & Matey, 2017).*

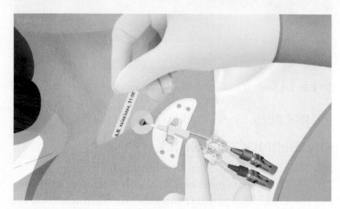

STEP 10 Remove the old dressing.

11. **INF** Remove the catheter-sutureless securement device per the manufacturer's instructions (some devices must be cleansed with alcohol to remove). *Minimizes the risk of dislodging the central line.*

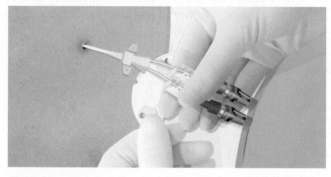

STEP 11 Remove the catheter sutureless securement device.

12. **INF** Discard old dressings and remove gloves appropriately (as per facility policy).

13. **ACC** Assess the insertion site for redness, swelling, drainage, or blood around the site. The assessment will be documented at the end of the procedure. *Accurate documentation of insertion-site skin is needed to note skin changes and to assess for signs and symptoms of infection and/or phlebitis.*

14. **INF** Perform hand hygiene.

15. **INF** Using sterile technique, open dressing change kit, antimicrobial disc, and sutureless securement device (as per facility policy).

16. **INF** Apply sterile gloves.

17. **INF** Activate the chlorhexidine scrub by pushing the two wings together and holding the applicator downward so that the chlorhexidine will fill the sponge pad on the end of the applicator.

18. **INF** Clean around the insertion site with chlorhexidine for 30 seconds using a back-and-forth scrubbing motion over a 6- to 8-cm square (1–1.5 sq. inch) area. Allow to air dry. Be careful not to dislodge the central line. *Drying allows chlorhexidine to bind with skin proteins, enhancing bactericidal action.*

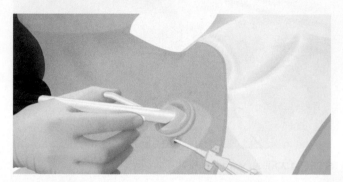

STEP 18 Clean around the insertion site.

19. **SAF** Apply the sutureless securement device and secure catheter, if applicable.

20. **INF** Apply antimicrobial disc to the insertion site, being careful not to dislodge the central line. *The use of an antimicrobial disc substantially reduces the risk of intravascular or exit-site bacterial colonization (Schifffer et al., 2013). (Note: Alternatively, apply a dressing with a chlorhexidine gel pad with a built-in securement device).*

21. **INF** Apply transparent dressing with the insertion site in the center of the dressing and easily visible through the dressing. *This allows easy visualization of the site.*

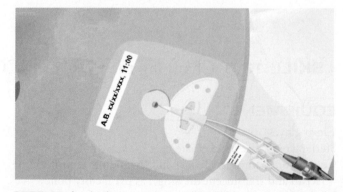

STEP 21 Apply the transparent dressing.

22. **COM** Use the label inside the kit to date, time, and initial the dressing change.

23. **SAF** For a PICC line dressing change: Measure the external length of the catheter and the circumference of the client's arm 10 cm (4 inches) above and below the antecubital fossa. *An increased arm circumference could indicate a VTE. These measurements are a safety strategy.*

FINISHING THE SKILL

24. **EVAL** Evaluate outcomes, including your assessment of the site and how the client tolerated the procedure.
25. **INF** Dispose of the used supplies.
26. **INF** Remove gloves and masks.
27. **INF** Perform hand hygiene.
28. **SAF** Ensure client safety. Place the bed in the lowest position. Ensure that the client can identify and reach the nurse call system. *These safety measures reduce the risk of injury from falls.*
29. **CCC** Provide comfort. Assist the client with positioning.
30. **COM** Document the care provided, including assessment of the insertion site, external length of catheter, circumference of the client's arm (if a PICC), and how the client tolerated the procedure.

■ SKILL 13.4 Changing the Needleless Connectors for a CVC/PICC Line

EQUIPMENT

Clean gloves
10-mL NS flush for each lumen
Needleless connectors (the same number as the number of lumens on the central/PICC line)
Disinfectant caps (the same number as the number of lumens on the central/PICC line)

BEGINNING THE SKILL

1. **SAF** Review the healthcare provider's order or facility policy. *Verifying the plan of care prevents injury to the client.*
2. **CCC** Introduce yourself to the client and family.
3. **COM** Explain the procedure.
4. **INF** Perform hand hygiene.
5. **SAF** Identify the client using two identifiers.
6. **CCC** Provide privacy. Close the door and pull the curtain.

PROCEDURE

7. **SAF** Set up an ergonomically safe space. Raise the bed to a comfortable working height. Raise one side rail. *Setting up an ergonomically safe space prevents injury to the nurse and client.*
8. **INF** Apply clean gloves.
9. **CCC** Open the packages containing the saline flush.
10. **SAF** Hold the saline flush with the plunger side down and remove the cap from the end. *Minimizes risk for contamination and brings air to the top of the syringe.*
11. **SAF** Remove air from the syringe by gently pulling back on the plunger slightly to break the pressure seal, then push the plunger up to expel the air from the saline. *Pulling the plunger back helps control the flow of saline and removes air and the risk for an air embolism.*
12. **SAF** Inspect the syringe to ensure all air has been removed.
13. **SAF** Attach the saline syringe to the new connector by pushing the syringe into the connector and rotating the syringe while inserting. *This will Luer-Lok the syringe into place.*
14. **SAF** Prime the connector by flushing with saline to expel the air from the connector. Leave the cover of the sterile tip of the connector in place until ready to use.

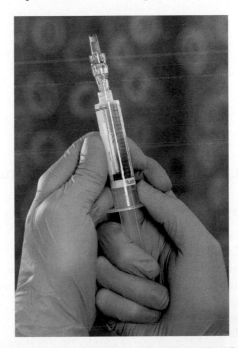

STEP 14 Prime the connector by flushing with saline.

15. **SAF** Remove the disinfectant cap (if applicable) on the first needleless connector.
16. **SAF** Clamp the catheter lumen (if applicable) and remove the old needleless connector. Remove the cover from the sterile tip of the new needleless connector and twist the new connector onto the lumen. *This action reduces the risk of air emboli.*
17. **SAF** Unclamp catheter lumen (if applicable).
18. **ACC** Flush the line with the remaining saline flush.

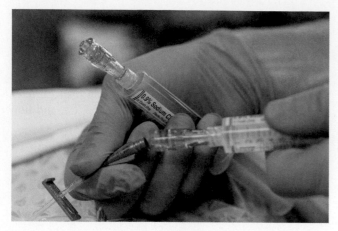

STEP 18 Flush the line with the remaining saline flush.

19. Repeat steps until all needleless connectors are changed.
20. **INF** Dispose of the old needleless connectors in a biohazard container.
21. **INF** Apply a disinfectant cap to each needleless connector.

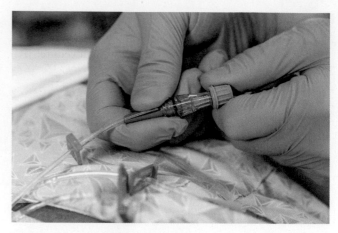

STEP 21 Apply a disinfectant cap.

FINISHING THE SKILL

22. **INF** Dispose of the used supplies.
23. **INF** Remove gloves.
24. **INF** Perform hand hygiene.
25. **CCC** Provide comfort. Assist the client with positioning.
26. **SAF** Ensure client comfort and safety. Place the bed in the lowest position. Ensure that the client can identify and reach the nurse call system. *These safety measures reduce the risk of injury from falls.*
27. **EVAL** Evaluate outcomes, including catheter patency and sterile technique.
28. **COM** Document needleless access-cap change, including ease of flushing.

■ SKILL 13.5 Collecting Blood Specimens/Blood Cultures

EQUIPMENT

Clean gloves
1 (10-mL) 0.9% NS flush per lumen
1 heparinized flush per lumen, as per facility policy
Chlorhexidine wipes or 70% isopropyl alcohol wipes for each lumen
Syringe method supplies:
    10-mL syringe for discard blood
    Appropriate syringe(s) for lab specimens
    Needleless transfer device
    Appropriate laboratory vacuum blood collection tubes
Disinfectant caps
Labels for tubes
Biohazard bag to transport blood specimen

BEGINNING THE SKILL

1. **SAF** Review the healthcare provider's order or facility policy. *Verifying the plan of care and medical history prevents injury to the client.*
2. **ACC** Determine the color and number of laboratory vacuum blood collection tubes required and the order of draw for the ordered blood tests. *Verifying the type of blood tubes and the order of draw facilitates the accuracy and timeliness of the laboratory work.*
3. **CCC** Introduce yourself to the client and family and explain the procedure.
4. **INF** Perform hand hygiene.
5. **SAF** Identify the client using two identifiers.
6. **CCC** Provide privacy. Close the door or pull the curtain.

PROCEDURE

7. **SAF** Set up an ergonomically safe space. Raise the bed to a comfortable working height. Raise one side rail. *Setting up an ergonomically safe space prevents injury to the nurse and client.*
8. **INF** Apply clean gloves. *There is an inherent risk of contamination and exposure to blood when handling CVADs.*
9. **ACC** Trace the line from the insertion point to the needleless connector hubs of each lumen. Identify which lumen is infusing fluids (if applicable). If there are multiple lumens, the proximal lumen is preferred for blood sampling. *Tracing a line from insertion to connection is a safety strategy.*

10. **ACC** Stop infusing fluids through all of the lumen(s) for at least 1 minute before drawing a blood specimen. Clamp all lumens not being used for the blood specimen collection. (Note: If the lumen was clamped and not infusing fluid, then patency of the line is established by flushing the lumen. Follow Skill 13.2, Steps 9 through 17). *Infusing fluids may alter the results of a blood specimen.*

11. Open up the package enclosing the saline flush.

12. **ACC** Clamp the lumen identified for blood sampling, if indicated. Remove the disinfectant cap, if applicable.

13. **INF** Mechanically scrub the needleless connector hub of the lumen with a chlorhexidine wipe for 5 to 15 seconds or a 70% isopropyl alcohol wipe for 5 to 60 seconds. *Cleaning prevents the introduction of microorganisms into the line (Moureau & Flynn, 2015).*

14. **INF** Allow to air dry. *Enhances bactericidal action.*

15. **ACC** Prepare the equipment for the blood specimen collection. Perform a syringe method blood draw.
    a. Attach empty 10-mL syringe.
    b. Open clamp.
    c. Aspirate 3 to 5 mL of blood as per facility policy for discard. If drawing blood cultures, this will be your blood culture; otherwise, discard appropriately in a biohazard container. *Blood sparing is a practice standard, and 3 to 5 mL is sufficient to clear the line of flush solution (Camp-Sorrell & Matey, 2017).*

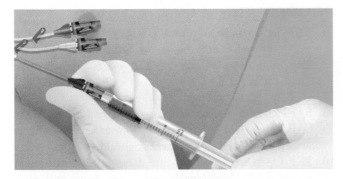

STEP 15C Withdraw and discard blood.

    d. Clamp the catheter.
    e. Attach a second empty 10-mL syringe to the needleless connector hub and open the clamp.
    f. Withdraw required amount of blood for all ordered lab tests.
    g. Clamp the catheter and remove the syringe.

16. **INF** Mechanically scrub the needleless connector hub of the lumen with a chlorhexidine wipe for 5 to 15 seconds or a 70% isopropyl alcohol wipe for 5 to 60 seconds. Allow to air dry. *Scrubbing the needleless connector hub prevents the introduction of microorganisms into the line. Drying enhances bactericidal action (Moureau & Flynn, 2015).*

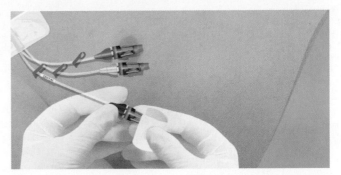

STEP 16 Scrub the needleless connector hub of the lumen.

17. **ACC** Attach 0.9% NS flush, open the clamp, and flush with 10 to 20 mL. Use the pulsating method if appropriate with the connector and device.

18. **ACC** Attach a heparinized syringe as per facility policy, or reestablish the IV infusion, if indicated. Change the needleless connector or apply a disinfectant cap as per facility policy if indicated.

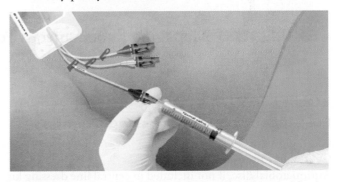

STEP 17 Attach a 0.9% NS flush, open the clamp, and flush.

19. **SAF** Attach a needleless transfer device to the syringe and transfer blood into laboratory collection tubes. *Using a needleless safety device prevents accidental needle sticks. (See Skill 12.2).*

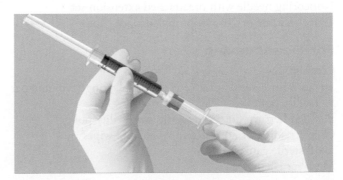

STEP 19 Attach the needleless transfer device to the syringe.

20. **COM** Ensure specimen label contains two client identifiers. Label specimen in the presence of the client. *National safety guidelines recommend labeling specimens in the presence of the client.*

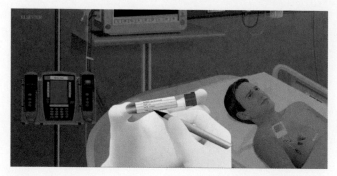

STEP 20 Ensure the specimen label contains two client identifiers.

21. **COM** Document your initials, date, and time of blood specimen collection on the label per facility policy. Place laboratory collection tubes in a biohazard bag. Many facilities require transportation in a plastic resealable biohazard bag.

22. **ACC** Transport blood specimens to the laboratory per facility policy within time limit.

FINISHING THE SKILL

23. **INF** Remove gloves and perform hand hygiene.
24. **CCC** Provide comfort measures for the client. Assist the client with positioning.
25. **SAF** Ensure client safety. Place the bed in the lowest position. Ensure that the client can identify and reach the nurse call system. *These safety measures reduce the risk of injury from falls.*
26. **EVAL** Evaluate outcomes, including ease of blood sampling and flushing. Were laboratory results within the expected ranges? *Coagulation studies and peaks/troughs of some antibiotics may be inaccurate when sampling through the CVAD.*
27. **COM** Document date, time, and type of laboratory specimens collected; CVAD flushing; ease of blood return; and how the client tolerated the procedure.

▪ SKILL 13.6 Managing Subcutaneous Ports: Accessing, Changing the Dressing, and Deaccessing

EQUIPMENT

For Accessing and Dressing Change

Clean gloves
Central line dressing change kit
Antimicrobial disc, if not included in central line dressing kit
Mask, if not included in dressing change kit
Second mask for client (if client unable to keep head turned away from the insertion site)
Sterile gloves
Needleless connector
10-mL sterile prefilled 0.9% NS syringe
Noncoring needle with preattached extension set
Chlorhexidine or 70% isopropyl alcohol wipes

For Deaccessing

Clean gloves
10- to 20-mL sterile prefilled 0.9% NS syringe (volume per facility policy)
Prefilled heparin flush syringe (as per facility policy)
Chlorhexidine or 70% isopropyl alcohol wipes
2 × 2 sterile gauze
Mask for client

BEGINNING THE SKILL

Accessing and Applying Dressing to the Subcutaneous Port

1. **SAF** Review the healthcare provider's order and facility policy. *Verifying the plan of care prevents injury to the client.*
2. **INF** Perform hand hygiene.
3. **SAF** Identify the client using two identifiers.

4. **CCC** Introduce yourself to the client and family and explain the procedure.
5. **CCC** Provide privacy. Close the door and pull the curtain.

PROCEDURE

6. **SAF** Set up an ergonomically safe space. Raise the bed to a comfortable working height. Raise one side rail. *Setting up an ergonomically safe space prevents injury to the nurse and client.*
7. **INF** Apply clean gloves.
8. **SAF** Palpate port septum and assess site; then remove gloves.
9. **SAF** Set up a workspace according to your hand dominance (e.g., right-handed RN on client's right side).
10. **INF** Open sterile central line dressing kit and prepare sterile field. Using sterile technique, open and place 0.9% NS syringe, needleless connector, noncoring needle with extension set attached, and antimicrobial disc onto sterile field.
11. **INF** Put on your own mask and either place a mask on the client or ask the client to turn his or her face away from the central line. *Minimizes the risk of airborne microorganisms entering the CVC insertion site.*
12. **INF** Apply sterile gloves.
13. **SAF** Using sterile technique, connect the needleless connector to the noncoring needle and extension set.
14. **ACC** Attach the 0.9% NS syringe to the needleless connector hub and prime extension set and noncoring needle. Return to sterile field.
15. **INF** Activate the chlorhexidine by pushing the two wings together and holding the applicator downward so that the chlorhexidine will fill the sponge pad on the end of the applicator.

16. **INF** Clean over previously palpated port septum with chlorhexidine for 30 seconds using a back-and-forth motion over a 6- to 8-cm square (1–1.5 sq. inches) area and allow to air dry. *Drying allows chlorhexidine to bind with skin proteins, enhancing bactericidal action.*

17. **SAF** Holding the noncoring needle in your nondominant hand, remove the needle cap using your dominant hand. Carefully, transfer the noncoring needle, without needle cap, to your dominant hand.

18. **SAF** With your nondominant hand, stabilize the port with the thumb and forefinger. Meanwhile, with your dominant hand, grasp the noncoring needle with extension set and NS syringe.

19. **COM** Instruct the client to hold his or her breath during insertion and to anticipate slight pressure upon insertion. *This instruction and warning helps to prevent the client from moving.*

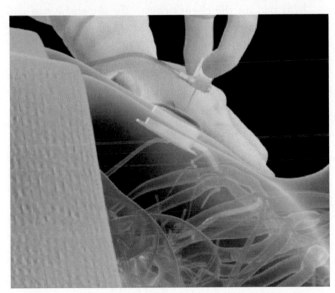

STEP 19 Instruct the client to hold his or her breath during insertion.

20. **ACC** Insert the noncoring needle into the center of the septum until the needle touches the bottom of the reservoir.

21. **SAF** Aspirate for blood return to confirm patency of port.

22. **SAF** Once blood return is observed, flush with the remaining 0.9% NS in a 10-mL syringe. *This reduces thrombus formation at the catheter tip.*

23. **SAF** Clamp the catheter once saline is infused. Remove syringe.

24. **INF** Place an antimicrobial disc at the insertion site of the noncoring needle. *The use of an antimicrobial disc substantially reduces the risk of intravascular or exit-site bacterial colonization (Schifffer et al., 2013).*

25. **INF** Apply transparent dressing over site; label dressing with date, time, and initials.

Deaccessing the Subcutaneous Port

26. **INF** Apply clean gloves and mask.

27. **INF** Cleanse the needleless connector hub with chlorhexidine wipe for 5 to 15 seconds or a 70% isopropyl alcohol wipe for 5 to 60 seconds. *Scrubbing the needleless connector hub prevents the introduction of microorganisms into the line. Drying enhances bactericidal action (Moureau & Flynn, 2015).*

28. **INF** Remove the disinfectant cap.

29. **ACC** Attach 0.9% NS syringe, open clamp, and flush using push-pause method.

30. **ACC** Remove syringe.

31. **INF** Cleanse the needleless connector hub of the lumen with a chlorhexidine wipe for 5 to 15 seconds or a 70% isopropyl alcohol wipe for 5 to 60 seconds. Allow to air dry. *Scrubbing the needleless connector hub prevents the introduction of microorganisms into the line. Drying enhances bactericidal action (Moureau & Flynn, 2015).*

32. **ACC** Attach prefilled heparinized solution syringe, open clamp, and flush using push/pause method.

33. **SAF** Remove old dressing by pulling the dressing toward the insertion site while stabilizing the noncoring needle with the thumb and forefinger of one hand. *Pulling the dressing toward the insertion site reduces the risk of dislodging the noncoring needle.*

34. **SAF** With your nondominant hand, stabilize the port with the thumb and forefinger, then grasp the noncoring needle with your dominant hand and withdraw the needle in a straight upward motion.

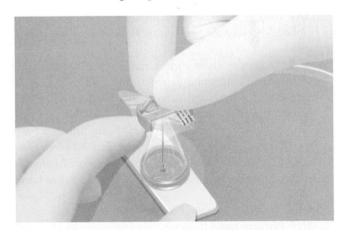

STEP 34 Withdraw the needle in a straight upward motion.

35. **INF** Discard the dressing as per facility policy. Discard the needle and extension set into a puncture-proof sharps container.

36. **EVAL** Evaluate the insertion site for redness, swelling, drainage, or blood around the site. Evaluate for any changes from your initial assessment. *You are looking for signs and symptoms of infection and/or phlebitis.*

FINISHING THE SKILL

37. **INF** Dispose of the used supplies.
38. **INF** Remove gloves and masks.
39. **INF** Perform hand hygiene.
40. **EVAL** Evaluate the outcomes. *Was the port easily accessed? Was the port patent? Did it aspirate and flush easily?*
41. **SAF** Ensure client safety. Place the bed in the lowest position. Ensure that the client can identify and reach the nurse call system. *These safety measures reduce the risk of injury from falls.*
42. **COM** Document attempts to access the port, patency of port with aspiration of blood, site assessment, dressing change, ease of deaccessing, and how the client tolerated the procedures.

■ SKILL 13.7 Discontinuing a Central Line

EQUIPMENT

Clean gloves
1 (10-mL) 0.9% NS flush per lumen
1 heparinized flush per lumen, as per facility policy
Central line sterile kit with supplies for removal
Central line dressing kit
Suture removal kit, if applicable
Extra pair of sterile gloves
Masks, if not included in the kit
Disposable absorbent pad

BEGINNING THE SKILL

1. **SAF** Review the healthcare provider's order and facility policy. *Verifying the plan of care prevents injury to the client.*
2. **SAF** Assess the client's most recent prothrombin time (PT), partial thromboplastin time (PTT), and/or international normalized ratio (INR) lab results for prolonged bleeding times. If PT, PTT, and INR are prolonged, notify the authorized healthcare provider prior to removal. *Bleeding is a possible complication of removing a CVC. If clotting factors are outside of normal limits, be prepared for extensive bleeding and the need for close monitoring.*
3. **CCC** Introduce yourself to the client and family.
4. **INF** Perform hand hygiene.
5. **SAF** Identify the client using two identifiers.
6. **COM** Explain the procedure to the client. Teach the client the procedure for the Valsalva maneuver.
7. **CCC** Provide privacy. Close the door or pull the curtain.

PROCEDURE

8. **SAF** Set up an ergonomically safe space. Raise the bed to a comfortable working height. Raise one side rail. *Setting up an ergonomically safe space prevents injury to the nurse and client.*
9. **ACC** Place the client in the Trendelenburg position for the removal of a subclavian or internal jugular central line. *Minimizes risk of air embolism.*
10. **INF** Apply clean gloves. Place a disposable absorbent pad on the client's chest. *The disposable pad will contain any blood that may result from discontinuing the central line, thereby containing any blood-borne pathogens.*
11. **INF** Put on your own mask and either place a mask on the client or ask the client to turn his or her face away from the central line. *Minimizes the risk of airborne microorganisms entering the CVC insertion site.*
12. **SAF** Clamp all catheter lumens.
13. **SAF** Remove old dressing by pulling the dressing toward the insertion site. *Pulling the dressing toward the insertion site reduces the risk of dislodging the central line.*
14. **SAF** Remove the sutureless securement device per the manufacturer's instructions. (Some devices must be cleansed with alcohol to remove them). *Minimizes the risk of dislodging the central line.*
15. **INF** Discard old dressing appropriately and remove gloves.
16. **ACC** Assess the site for redness, swelling, drainage, or blood around the site. If applicable, assess that sutures are intact. Make a mental note of how you will document these assessment findings.
17. **INF** Perform hand hygiene.
18. **INF** Using sterile technique, open central line dressing kit and suture removal kit, if needed.
19. **INF** Apply sterile gloves.
20. **INF** Activate the chlorhexidine scrub by pushing the two wings together and holding the applicator downward so that the chlorhexidine will fill the sponge pad on the end of the applicator.
21. **INF** Clean the insertion site with chlorhexidine for 30 seconds using a back-and-forth motion over a 6- to 8-cm square (1–1.5 sq. inches) area and allow to dry. Be careful not to dislodge the central line. *Drying allows chlorhexidine to bind with skin proteins, enhancing bactericidal action.*

22. **CCC** Clip and remove any sutures, if applicable.
23. **ACC** Instruct the client to perform the Valsalva maneuver while you remove the central line slowly and steadily in a continuous motion.

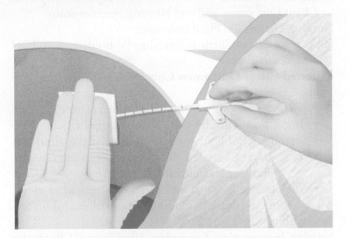

STEP 23 Remove the central line slowly and steadily.

24. **SAF** Immediately apply sterile 2 × 2 gauze to the insertion site, holding direct pressure for 5 minutes. Instruct the client to breathe normally. *Direct pressure ensures adequate clotting.*
25. **INF** Cover with an occlusive dressing, such as a petroleum jelly impregnated transparent dressing. *The dressing promotes clotting and minimizes the risk of infection.*

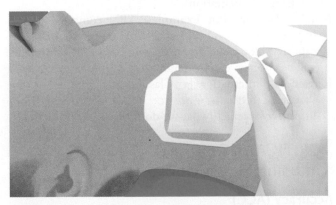

STEP 25 Cover with a petroleum jelly–impregnated transparent dressing.

26. **SAF** Inspect the catheter tip to ensure tip is intact. Measure the entire length of the catheter. Notify the authorized healthcare provider if the tip is not intact. *The catheter line and catheter tip may become fragmented and break off during removal.*

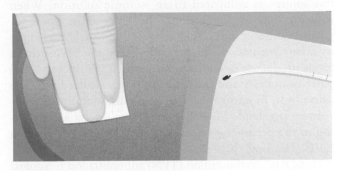

STEP 26 Inspect the catheter tip.
27. **INF** Remove gloves and perform hand hygiene.

FINISHING THE SKILL

28. **CCC** Provide comfort measures for the client and return the client to a supine position.
29. **SAF** Ensure client safety. Place the bed in the lowest position. Ensure that the the client can identify and reach the nurse call system. *These safety measures reduce the risk of injury from falls.*
30. **SAF** Instruct the client to minimize any activity for at least 1 hour after catheter removal. *Restricting activity will provide time for adequate coagulation at the removal site and prevent bleeding.*
31. **EVAL** Evaluate outcomes, including client anxiety versus relief at having the catheter removed.
32. **COM** Document insertion-site assessment; length of catheter; catheter tip intact; PTT, PT, and INR results; care provided; and how the client tolerated the procedure.
33. **EVAL** Monitor the site for any signs of bleeding or infection.

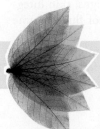

SECTION 2 Infusing Fluids With a CVAD

INFUSING FLUIDS

IVF therapy is prescribed to regulate intravascular fluid volume and manage electrolyte imbalances. Fluid therapy must be closely regulated based on the client's indicated fluid and electrolyte status. IV solutions are commonly referred to as crystalloid solutions because these solutions consist of water with dissolved inorganic and mineral solutes, with dextrose and sodium chloride being the most commonly used (Harding, 2017). These solutions and solutes are combined to form a hypotonic, isotonic, or hypertonic solution. Isotonic solutions contain a solution and solute mix to yield a concentration that is physiologically similar to plasma (0.9% NaCl concentration). Hypotonic solutions provide a greater level of water and less solutes as compared to an isotonic solution. When infusing hypotonic solutions, the nurse must assess for client manifestations of cellular swelling, such as changes in client mentation. Hypertonic solutions have greater levels of glucose or sodium ions, which will increase vascular osmolality and thus expand intravascular fluid. The nurse must monitor the client for manifestations of fluid-volume overload. Most hypertonic solutions are irritating to the peripheral vessels and must be given through a CVC (Harding, 2017).

Total parenteral nutrition (TPN) administration is required when clients are unable to ingest essential nutrients because of gastrointestinal problems such as surgery, malabsorption, or trauma. TPN is an IVF that combines varying percentages of glucose (10%–70%), lipids, amino acid, electrolytes, vitamins, and trace elements. The formula for TPN is prescribed by a healthcare provider and based on the client's nutritional needs. TPN is usually a hypertonic solution and requires a CVC for infusion.

Prior to administering TPN, the list of TPN components and additives must usually be verified by two licensed healthcare professionals (as per facility policy). Because TPN has a high glucose concentration, routine care associated with TPN administration includes blood sugar or urine glucose assessment performed every 6 hours. Additionally, the high glucose concentration can potentiate bacterial growth; therefore, clients who receive TPN are at an increased risk for CLABSI (Fonseca, Burgermaster, Larson & Seres, 2018). Because of this high risk, when infusing TPN, the tubing should remain a closed system throughout the prescribed administration time period, and the infusion time should not be interrupted; no other medications can be administered simultaneously through the TPN-designated lumen/port. Routine nursing care associated with TPN administration includes daily weights, strict intake and output measurements, and client assessment for signs and symptom of fluid-volume overload.

Lipid emulsion is a solution prepared as a 10% or 20% concentration of triglycerides, egg phospholipids, glycerol, and water. Lipids are given to provide a supplement of essential fatty acids (i.e., the omega-3 and omega-6 fatty acids), which cannot be synthesized by the body. Lipid emulsions can be combined with TPN or administered separately. A CVAD is usually inserted to support long-term TPN and lipid emulsion administration. If lipids are infusing alone, the rate is as follows:

- Lipid emulsions of 10% lipids are typically infused over at least 4 hours.
- Lipid emulsions of 20% lipids are typically infused over at least 6 hours.
- Lipids can hang for 12 hours.
- Lipids infusing with TPN can remain in place for 24 hours.

APPLICATION OF THE NURSING PROCESS

Examples of Related ICNP Nursing Diagnoses, Expected Client Outcomes, and and Nursing Interventions:

Nursing Diagnosis: Fluid imbalance

Supporting Data: Client is receiving IV fluids and/or TPN via a central line.

Expected Client Outcomes: Client will maintain fluid balance, as seen by:

- vital signs within established parameters for the client
- urine output greater than 0.5 mL/kg/hour
- the absence of signs and symptoms related to fluid-volume deficit (increased thirst, dry mucous membranes, poor skin turgor, tachycardia)
- the absence of signs and symptoms related to fluid-volume overload (bounding pulses, edema, shortness of breath).

Nursing Intervention Examples: Administer IV fluids per orders, and monitor hydration status.

Nursing Diagnosis: Electrolyte imbalance

Supporting Data: Client is receiving TPN via a central venous catheter.

Expected Client Outcomes: Client will maintain electrolyte balance, as seen by:

- the absence of signs and symptoms related to electrolyte imbalance (nausea, cramping, muscle weakness, or change in mentation).

Nursing Intervention Examples: TPN components will be checked by two licensed healthcare professionals, and capillary blood sugar and/or urine glucose assessments will be checked every 6 hours.

Reference: International Classification for Nursing Practice. (n.d.). *eHealth & ICNP*. Retrieved from https://www.icn.ch/what-we-do/projects/ehealth-icnp.

CRITICAL CONCEPTS
Infusing Fluids Through a CVAD

Accuracy (ACC)

Accuracy when infusing fluids through a CVAD is subject to the following variables:

Nurse-Related and System-Related Factors

- assessment of the client, including vital signs, skin integrity, urine output, lab values, and signs of fluid-volume overload or deficit
- technique used for processing orders, administering fluids, monitoring the client, and providing follow-up care
- preparation and technique used for the flush or IVF infusion
- selection and use of equipment
- use of strict sterile technique

Client-Centered Care (CCC)

Respect for the client when infusing through a CVAD is demonstrated through:

- promoting autonomy by verifying informed consent
- providing privacy and ensuring comfort

- answering questions that the client or family may have
- honoring cultural preferences
- advocating for the client and family.

Infection Control (INF)

When infusing through a CVAD, healthcare-associated infection is prevented by:
- containment of microorganisms
- preventing and reducing the transfer of microorganisms
- reducing the number of microorganisms.

Safety (SAF)

When managing CVADs, safety measures prevent harm and maintain a safe care environment, including:
- the consistent use of the rights of medication administration and medication safety checks and guidelines
- the proper labeling of lumens, tubing, and IVF containers.

Communication (COM)

- Communication allows for the exchange of information (oral, written, nonverbal, or electronic) between two or more people, including the nurse, client, family, and healthcare team.

- Documentation records information in a permanent legal record.
- Collaboration with the pharmacy, the client, and other members of the healthcare team is essential to achieve safe infusion of fluids and TPN and/or lipids through a CVAD.

Health Maintenance (HLTH)

Nursing is dedicated to the promotion of health and self-care abilities related to managing CVADs, including:
- maintaining circulation and fluid and electrolyte balance
- promoting the client's ability to provide self-care for the CVAD at home.

Evaluation (EVAL)

When managing CVADs, evaluation of outcomes enables the nurse to determine the efficacy of the care provided, including:
- signs and symptoms of fluid-volume overload or deficit
- patency of the central venous catheter.

▪ SKILL 13.8 Infusing IV Fluids

EQUIPMENT

Clean gloves
IVF, as prescribed by the authorized healthcare provider
Primary IV tubing
Chlorhexidine or 70% isopropyl alcohol wipes
10-mL prefilled 0.9% NS syringe
IV infusion pump

BEGINNING THE SKILL

1. **SAF** Review the healthcare provider's order and facility policy. Check each of the safety administration rights. Perform **first safety check** when accessing the medication. Perform **second safety check** when preparing the medication. Review should include the following:
   a. Type of fluid and volume
   b. Medications and dosage
   c. Route of administration
   d. Rate of infusion, usually written in mL/hour
   e. Pertinent lab values.
   Verifying medical orders prevents injury to the client.
2. **INF** Perform hand hygiene.
3. **CCC** Introduce yourself to the client and family and explain the procedure.
4. **SAF** Identify the client using two identifiers.
5. **CCC** Provide privacy. Close the door or pull the curtain.
6. **INF** Apply clean gloves. *There is an inherent risk of contamination and exposure to blood when handling CVADs.*

PROCEDURE

7. **ACC** Open primary IV tubing package and close primary tubing clamp.
8. **SAF** Open IVF container and inspect IV solution for clarity, color, expiration date, and leakage. Identify the IVF access port. *Most IVF bags have two ports. One is a medication port designed to insert medications, and one is the access port.*
9. **INF** Remove the cover from the IVF container access port and remove the protective sheath over IV tubing spike. Maintain the sterility of the port and spike. *Maintaining sterility reduces the risk of infection.*
10. **ACC** Hold the IVF container in your nondominant hand with the neck of the access port supported. With your dominant hand, insert the spike of the IV tubing into the IV solution access port.
11. **ACC** Hold the IVF container upright and squeeze the IV tubing drip chamber half-full by compressing and releasing the drip chamber.
12. **ACC** Open roller clamp and watch the descent of the fluid.
13. **ACC** When you reach a medication port, slow the descent of the fluid, invert the port, and slowly fill the medication port. You may need to tap on the port as the fluid is flowing to remove bubbles. Move the air bubble to the top of the column of fluid. *Removing air reduces the potential for air embolism.*

14. **ACC.** Close the roller clamp. Check tubing and ports to determine all air has been removed from the line. Place tubing in the IV pump, per facility policy. *Removing air reduces the potential for air embolism.*

15. **SAF** Perform **third safety check.** Ensure that the IVF label matches the client's ID band. Trace the line from the insertion point to the needleless connector hub. *Tracing a line from insertion to connection is a safety strategy to prevent misconnections.*

16. Remove the disinfectant cap, if present.

17. **INF** Mechanically scrub the client's needleless connector hub with a chlorhexidine wipe for 5 to 15 seconds or a 70% isopropyl alcohol wipe for 5 to 60 seconds. Allow to air dry. *Scrubbing the needleless connector hub prevents the introduction of microorganisms into the line. Drying enhances bactericidal action (Moureau & Flynn, 2015).*

18. **SAF** Attach 0.9% NS syringe to needleless cap. Open clamp on CVAD, if applicable.

19. **SAF** Aspirate CVAD to confirm blood return.

20. **SAF** Flush the CVAD using a continuous flushing method. Close clamp. Remove syringe. *Flushing establishes line patency and reduces the risk of clot formation. Clamping minimizes the risk for reflux at the catheter tip.*

21. **INF** Mechanically scrub the client's CVAD needleless connector hub with chlorhexidine wipe for 5 to 15 seconds or 70% isopropyl alcohol wipe for 5 to 60 seconds and allow to air dry. *Cleaning prevents the introduction of microorganisms into the line. Drying enhances bactericidal action (Moureau & Flynn, 2015).*

22. **INF** Remove the cap on the distal end of the primary tubing and connect the IV tubing to the CVAD needleless connector while avoiding contamination of either end. *Maintaining sterility reduces the risk of infection.*

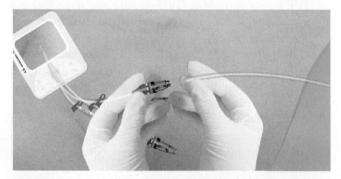

STEP 22 Connect the IV tubing to the CVAD needleless connector hub.

23. **SAF** Label the IVF container with the client's name, type of IVF, medications or electrolytes added (if any), date and time fluid is hung, and your initials. Label the tubing and lumen with appropriate information, including the correct date and time. *Labeling IVF is a safety strategy.*

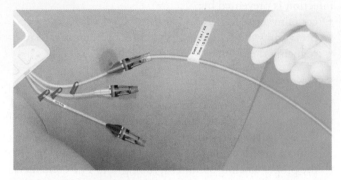

STEP 23 Label the lumen.

24. **ACC** Initiate infusion or medication at prescribed rate.

FINISHING THE SKILL

25. **SAF** Ensure client safety. Place the bed in the lowest position. Ensure that the client can identify and reach the nurse call system. *These safety measures reduce the risk of injury from falls.*

26. **INF** Remove gloves and discard. Perform hand hygiene.

27. **EVAL** Evaluate outcomes. *Is the solution infusing without difficulty and without any air in the line?*

28. **COM** Document IV infusion, including solution, rate, patency of CVAD, and how the client tolerated the infusion of fluids.

29. **EVAL** Monitor IV infusion, patency of CVAD, and client's fluid status, including urine output and vital signs.

■ SKILL 13.9 Initiating TPN and/or Lipids

EQUIPMENT

Clean gloves

TPN as prescribed by the authorized healthcare provider

Primary IV tubing with a 0.2-micron filter for nonlipid-containing solutions (filter is air eliminating and bacteria and particulate retentive)

Lipids and/or TPN with lipids as prescribed by the authorized healthcare provider

Primary IV tubing with a 1.2-micron filter that is particulate retentive and air eliminating for lipid infusions or 3-in-1 parenteral nutrition

Chlorhexidine or 70% alcohol wipes

10-mL prefilled 0.9% NS syringe

IV infusion pump

BEGINNING THE SKILL

1. **SAF** Perform **first safety check** when accessing the medication. Review the healthcare provider's order and facility policy, including the following:
   a. All additives in the TPN bag
   b. Route of administration
   c. Rate and possibly tapering rate at beginning or end of infusion
   d. Pertinent lab values: glucose, electrolytes, renal, and hepatic markers.

   No other medications can be administered simultaneously through the TPN-designated lumen/port. Verifying medical orders prevents injury to the client.

2. **SAF** Inspect TPN solution, lipids, and/or TPN with lipids for clarity, color, expiration date, and leakage.

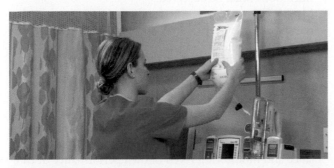

STEP 2 Inspect the TPN solution and/or lipids.

3. **SAF** Perform **second safety check** when preparing the medication for administration. A licensed healthcare professional(s) must independently review and confirm all TPN additives prior to administration, as per facility policy. *Minimizes risk of medication errors.*

4. **CCC** Introduce yourself to the client and family.

5. **COM** Explain the procedure and purpose of TPN to the client and family members present.

6. **INF** Perform hand hygiene.

7. **SAF** Identify the client using two identifiers.

8. **CCC** Provide privacy. Close the door or pull the curtain.

9. **INF** Apply clean gloves. *There is an inherent risk of contamination and exposure to blood when handling CVADs.*

PROCEDURE

10. **ACC** Open primary tubing with the appropriate filter and close tubing clamp.
    TPN only: 0.2-micron filter
    Lipids or TPN with lipids: 1.2-micron filter

11. **INF** Remove protective sheath over IV tubing port and TPN solution bag. Be careful not to contaminate either port. *Maintains sterility of IV tubing and TPN solution.*

12. **ACC** Hold the solution bag in your nondominant hand in an inverted position; then use your dominant hand to insert the spike of the IV tubing into the solution bag.

13. **ACC** Hold the solution upright and squeeze the IV tubing drip chamber half-full by compressing and releasing the drip chamber. Open the roller clamp, fill the filter by inverting it, and then continue priming the tubing. *Removing all air in the tubing prevents a potential air embolism.*

14. **SAF** Close the clamp.

15. **ACC** Place tubing in IV pump.

16. **SAF** Trace the line from the insertion point to the needleless connector hub. *Tracing a line from insertion to connection is a safety strategy to prevent misconnections.* Remove the disinfectant cap, if present.

17. **INF** Mechanically scrub the needleless connector hub of the lumen with a chlorhexidine wipe for 5 to 15 seconds or a 70% isopropyl alcohol wipe for 5 to 60 seconds. Allow to air dry. *Scrubbing the needleless connector hub prevents the introduction of microorganisms into the line. Drying enhances bactericidal action (Moureau & Flynn, 2015).*

18. **SAF** Attach 0.9% NS syringe. Open clamp on CVAD, if applicable.

19. **SAF** Aspirate CVAD to confirm blood return.

20. **SAF** Flush the CVAD using a continuous flushing method. Close clamp. *Flushing establishes line patency and reduces the risk of clot formation. Clamping minimizes the risk for reflux at the catheter tip.*

21. **ACC** Remove syringe.

22. **INF** Mechanically scrub the needleless connector hub of the lumen with a chlorhexidine wipe for 5 to 15 seconds or a 70% isopropyl alcohol wipe for 5 to 60 seconds. Allow to air dry. *Scrubbing the needleless connector hub prevents the introduction of microorganisms into the line. Drying enhances bactericidal action (Moureau & Flynn, 2015).*

23. **INF** Remove cap on distal end of TPN tubing and connect to CVAD needleless connector while avoiding contamination of either end. *Maintaining sterility reduces the risk of infection.*

24. **SAF** Perform **third safety check.** Ensure that the TPN label matches the client's ID band. Write the date and time of initiation on the label. Label TPN and lipid tubing and lumen with identifying information and the correct date and time.

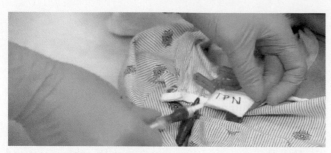

STEP 25 Label the lumen.

25. **SAF** Initiate the TPN infusion at the prescribed rate.

FINISHING THE SKILL

26. **SAF** Ensure client safety. Place the bed in the lowest position. Ensure that the client can identify and reach the nurse call system. *These safety measures reduce the risk of injury from falls.*

27. **INF** Remove gloves and discard. Perform hand hygiene.
28. **EVAL** Evaluate outcomes, including catheter patency and fluid infusion.
29. **COM** Document care, including TPN solution, rate, patency of CVAD, and how the client is tolerating the infusion.
30. **EVAL** Monitor TNP/lipid infusion, patency of CVAD, and client's electrolyte status, including vital signs and capillary glucose and/or urine glucose per authorized healthcare provider's orders.

■ **CASE STUDY**

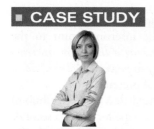

Ms. McGregor, a 39-year-old white, single, female executive with no children, was recently diagnosed with pancreatic cancer and is scheduled to receive intensive chemotherapy. She comes to the infusion center to receive her chemotherapy teaching and learns that she will also need to have a CVAD inserted. Sara, the infusion nurse, begins teaching Ms. McGregor about the CVAD her authorized healthcare provider has recommended for placement: left anterior chest wall subcutaneous port. Immediately, Ms. McGregor states she is terrified of needles and begins asking about alternative access selections.

One week later, Ms. McGregor is admitted to the hospital for surgical insertion of a double-lumen Hickman catheter into her left anterior chest wall. A chest x-ray confirms catheter tip placement in the distal superior vena cava. The authorized healthcare provider prescribes routine Hickman catheter care and her chemotherapy regimen. Ms. McGregor begins her 5-day infusion of chemotherapy.

On day 5 of her chemotherapy infusion, Ms. McGregor develops a fever of 102.5°F and erythema with purulent drainage at the insertion site of the Hickman catheter. The authorized healthcare provider orders blood cultures, culture and sensitivity of the drainage from the Hickman insertion site, and broad-spectrum antibiotics. Ms. McGregor responds to the antibiotic therapy, and her temperature returns to normal. The authorized healthcare provider orders TPN due to Ms. McGregor's nausea, vomiting, and low trending albumin and protein levels.

After 5 days of antibiotic therapy and TPN, Ms. McGregor is ready for discharge home. She has gained 2 pounds and will receive TPN at home. Her nurse completes all necessary discharge teaching, and coordinates home care with the case management nurse.

Case Study Questions

1. What must be included in the nurse's assessment of a Hickman catheter?
2. When admitted to a hospital, what is the routine care needed for a client with a Hickman catheter in regard to cap change, dressing change, and TPN infusion?
3. When infusing antibiotics and TPN, what nursing considerations must be observed?
4. Ms. McGregor is preparing for discharge. How does the nurse assess the client's level of readiness to care for her Hickman catheter at home?
5. What information should the nurse include in her discharge-teaching plan for a client receiving TPN at home?
6. **Application of QSEN Competencies:** One of the Quality and Safety Education for Nurses (QSEN) competencies on attitude for Safety states "Value vigilance and monitoring (even of own performance of care activities) by patients, families, and other members of the health care team" (Cronenwett et al., 2007). Discuss the level of vigilance Ms. McGregor will need to prevent CLABSI. What are some ways that the nurse could demonstrate the attitude of valuing vigilance and monitoring that will be needed by Ms. McGregor for her home care?

■ CONCEPT MAP

**ICNP Nursing Dx:
Risk for Infection
Supporting Data:**
Hickman catheter
temperature 102.5
degrees, erythema,
and drainage

Infection Control Measures

- Meticulous hand hygiene
- Adequate cleansing of skin
  with chlorhexidine
- Safe and accurate changing
  of cap
- Assessment of exit site
- Instruct client to report fever,
  erythema, drainage, or pain

Accuracy

- Have client demonstrate cap
  change
- Assess client's ability to safely
  flush catheter
- Have client verbalize rationale
  for good handwashing
  hygiene and safety use of
  clamps
- Have client verbalize normal
  color of exit site

Baseline Assessment Data

- 39-year-old female
- Newly diagnosed pancreatic
  cancer
- Surgery: Hickman catheter
  insertion
- Anxious regarding cancer
  diagnosis, chemotherapy,
  and new CVAD
- Fever 101.5 degrees
- Hickman exit site has
  erythema and purulent
  drainage

**ICNP Nursing Dx:
Lack of Knowledge of
Treatment Regime
Supporting Data:**
Client anxious
about newly inserted
Hickman catheter, TPN,
and chemotherapy

Health Maintenance

- Assess exit site of Hickman
- Flush with 0.9% normal saline
- Use only 10-mL syringes or
  larger
- Change needleless access
  cap weekly
- Assess for blood return prior
  to medication administration
- Ensure adequate at home
  supplies

Client-Centered Care

- Consult with authorized
  healthcare provider's office and
  TPN infusion company for
  necessary supplies
- Give client an information card
  for Hickman catheters
- Assess family involvement
  and suggest local cancer
  support group

Communication

- Assess client's readiness to
  learn CVAD self-care
- Involve client and family in
  Hickman catheter care
- Involve client in writing out
  flushing and cap change
  protocols
- Instruct client when to call the
  authorized healthcare provider

References

Agency for Healthcare Research and Quality (AHRQ). (2018). *Toolkit for reducing central line-associated blood stream infections*. Rockville, MD: Agency for Healthcare Research and Quality. Retrieved from http://www.ahrq.gov/professionals/education/curriculum-tools/clabsitools/index.html.

Association for Professionals in Infection Control and Epidemiology (APIC). (2015). *Guide to preventing central line-associated bloodstream infections*. Retrieved from https://apic.org/Resource_/TinyMceFileManager/2015/APIC_CLABSI_WEB.pdf.

Camp-Sorrell, D., & Matey, L. (2017). *Access device standards of practice for oncology nursing*. Pittsburgh, PA: Oncology Nursing Society.

Centers for Disease Control and Prevention (CDC). (2015). *Guidelines for the prevention of intravascular catheter-related infections (2011)*. Retrieved from https://www.cdc.gov/infectioncontrol/guidelines/bsi/index.html.

Centers for Disease Control and Prevention (CDC). (2017a). *Guidelines for the prevention of intravascular catheter-related infections, Updated recommendations on chlorhexidine-impregnated (C-I) dressings*. Retrieved from https://www.cdc.gov/infectioncontrol/guidelines/bsi/c-i-dressings/index.html.

Centers for Disease Control and Prevention (CDC). (2017b). *Data summary of HAIs in the US: Assessing progress 2006-2016*. Retrieved from https://www.cdc.gov/hai/data/archive/data-summary-assessing-progress.html.

Centers for Disease Control and Prevention (CDC). (2019). *Bloodstream infection event (central line–associated bloodstream infection and noncentral line associated bloodstream infection). [Device-associated module]*. Retrieved from https://www.cdc.gov/nhsn/pdfs/psc manual/4psc_clabscurrent.pdf.

Cronenwett, L., Sherwood, G., Barnsteiner, J., Disch, J., Johnson, J., Mitchell, P., ... Warren, J. (2007). Quality and safety education for nurses. *Nursing Outlook, 55*(3), 122–131. Retrieved from http://qsen.org/competencies/pre-licensure-ksas/.

Dal Molin, A., Allara, E., Montani, D., Milani, S., Frassati, C., Cossu, S., & Rasero, L. (2014). Flushing the central venous catheter: Is heparin necessary? *Journal of Vascular Access, 15*(4), 241–248.

Fonseca, G., Burgermaster, M., Larson, E., & Seres, D. S. (2018). The relationship between total parenteral nutrition and central line-associated bloodstream infections: 2009-2014. *Journal of Parenteral Enteral Nutrition, 42*(1), 171–175.

Ge, X., Cavallazzi, R., Li, C., Pan, S. M., Wang, Y. W., & Wang, F. L. (2012). Central venous access sites for the prevention of venous thrombosis, stenosis and infection. *The Cochrane Database of Systematic Reviews, 2012*(3) Art. No. CD004084. https://doi.org/10.1002/14651858.CD004084.pub3.

Gow, K., Tapper, D., & Hickman, R. (2017). Between the lines: The 50th anniversary of long-term central venous catheters. *The American Journal of Surgery, 213*, 837–848.

Harding, M. M. (2017). Fluid, electrolytes, and acid-base imbalances. In S. Lewis, L. Bucher, M. Heitkemper, & M. Harding (Eds.), *Medical-surgical nursing: Assessment and management of clinical problems* (10th ed.). St. Louis, MO: Elsevier.

Infusion Nurses Society (INS). (2016). Infusion therapy standards of practice. *Supplement to Journal of Infusion Nursing, 39*(1S), S1–S159.

International Classification for Nursing Practice. (n.d.). *eHealth & ICNP*. Retrieved from https://www.icn.ch/what-we-do/projects/ehealth-icnp.

The Joint Commission. (2013). *CLABSI toolkit—Preventing central line-associated bloodstream infections: Useful tools, an international perspective. Comparison of the major types of central venous catheters*. Retrieved from http://www.jointcommission.org/CLABSIToolkit.

Mitchell, M. D., Anderson, B. J., Williams, K., & Umscheid, C. A. (2009). Heparin flushing and other interventions to maintain patency of central venous catheters: A systematic review. *Journal of Advanced Nursing, 65*(10), 2007–2021.

Moureau, N. L., & Flynn, J. (2015). Disinfection of needleless connector hubs: Clinical evidence systematic review. *Nursing Research and Practice, 2015*. Article ID 796762. Retrieved from https://doi.org/10.1155/2015/796762.

Groshong catheter, & Patient's death tied to substandard nursing care. (2009, February). *Legal Eagle Eye Newsletter for the Nursing Profession*. Retrieved from http://www.nursinglaw.com/.

Randolph, A. G., Cook, D. J., Gonzales, C. A., & Andrew, M. (1998). Benefit of heparin in peripheral venous and arterial catheters: Systematic review and meta-analysis of randomised controlled trials. *BMJ, 316*(7136), 969–975.

Schiffer, C. A., Manqu, P. B., Wade, J. C., Camp-Sorrell, D., Cope, D. G., El-Rayes, B. F., & Levine, M. (2013). Central venous catheter care for the patient with cancer: American Society of Clinical Oncology clinical practice guideline. *Journal of Clinical Oncology, 31*(10), 1357–1370.

Yeager, S. (2017). Central venous catheter insertion (perform). In D. L. Weigand (Ed.), *AACN procedure manual for high acuity, progressive, and critical care* (7th ed.). St. Louis, MO: Elsevier.

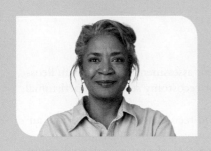

CHAPTER 14

Bowel Management

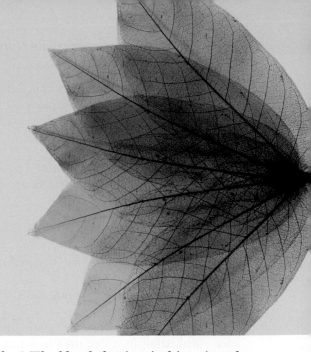

"Look at a patient lying long in bed. What a pathetic picture he makes! The blood clotting in his veins, the lime draining from his bones, the scybala stacking up in his colon … Teach us to live that we may dread unnecessary time in bed. Get people up and we may save our patients from an early grave."

Dr. Richard Asher (*The Dangers of Going to Bed*, 1947)

LEARNING OBJECTIVES

By the end of this chapter, the reader will be able to:

1. Discuss the rationale for client positioning during rectal procedures.
2. Perform digital rectal stimulation and evacuation.
3. Insert, secure, and remove a rectal tube.
4. Apply internal and external fecal management systems for continuous use.

5 Administer and record results from a cleansing enema, including the return flow technique.

6 Administer and record results from a commercially prepared enema.

7 Collect a stool specimen.

8 Provide instructions for obtaining a pinworm sample.

9 Collect stool specimen and test for occult blood.

10 Assess and document assessment findings of an ileostomy, colostomy, or cecostomy stoma and peristomal skin.

11 Empty, measure, and record effluent output from an ileostomy or colostomy.

12 Demonstrate the removal, cleansing, and application of a pouching system for a stoma.

13 Irrigate and document fecal return from a stoma site.

TERMINOLOGY

Chyme Semisolid mixture of food particles and digestive fluids.

Clostridium difficile An opportunistic, spore-forming, gram-positive bacillus.

Colonoscopy Fiberoptic flexible scope inserted rectally for visualization of colon; used to detect bowel disease, remove polyps, and biopsy colon tissue.

Constipation Decrease in normal frequency of bowel movements, resulting in difficult elimination of hard and dry stool.

Diarrhea Passage of at least three loose or liquid stools per day.

Hemoccult guaiac test Test done to detect fecal occult blood in stool specimen.

Effluent Fecal material eliminated from an intestinal stoma.

Fecal impaction Large, hard stool stuck in colon, usually due to long-term constipation.

Giardia Anaerobic protozoan parasite that causes diarrhea.

Hemorrhoids Internal or external engorgement of anal veins.

Malabsorption Impaired absorption of nutrients in the small intestine.

Melena Black tarry stools.

Ostomy Surgically formed artificial opening that brings the bowel or intestine to the outside, usually through the abdominal wall.

Peristomal Skin area around a stoma site.

Steatorrhea Greasy, frothy stool indicating malabsorption of fat.

Stoma Surgically created opening between a body passage or cavity and the body surface.

ACRONYMS

C. diff. *Clostridium difficile*
FIT Fecal immunochemical test
FMS Fecal management system
FOBT Fecal occult blood test
GI Gastrointestinal
IAD Incontinence-associated dermatitis
MASD Moisture-associated skin damage

The gastrointestinal (GI) tract begins at the mouth and ends at the anus (Fig. 14.1). The primary function of the GI tract is the digestion of ingested food into absorbable nutrients that will in turn be used for cellular metabolism. Initially, food is broken down in the mouth by enzymatic and mechanical activity. The bolus of food moves down the esophagus, via peristalsis, through the lower esophageal sphincter into the stomach. There, it undergoes further mechanical and chemical digestion and is mixed with fluid, forming a watery digestive "soup" called chyme.

From the stomach, chyme passes through the pyloric sphincter into the small intestine, the primary site of both digestion and absorption. Bile, synthesized by the liver and stored in the gallbladder, and digestive enzymes from the intestine and the pancreas are essential to the digestion of fats, carbohydrates, and proteins into absorbable nutrients. The three segments of the small intestine—the duodenum, jejunum, and ileum—contain many blood vessels and an inner lumen made up of circular folds lined with finger-like projections called villi, which are covered in even smaller microvilli. Together, these features provide a large surface area for the intestinal absorption of nutrients.

The remaining semiliquid indigestible fecal material passes through the ileocecal valve into the large intestine (or colon), where further fluid and electrolyte absorption occurs, leaving a semisolid fecal mass. This is propelled, via peristalsis or segmental colonic movement, up the ascending colon, across the transverse colon, and down the descending colon through to the sigmoid colon and rectum. When feces enter the rectum, sensory nerve endings are stimulated to promote defecation via the anal canal.

CHARACTERISTICS OF STOOL

Nurses assess stool characteristics and evaluate stool output. A feces specimen should be inspected for color, odor, consistency, and the presence of blood, fat, pus, or parasites. Generally speaking, feces are composed of water, undigested food particles, bile pigment, bacteria, minerals, and shed epithelial cells (McCance & Huether, 2019). The components of feces are contingent on a person's diet, intestinal health, and medication ingestion.

Normally, the color of stool is brown; however, there are many pathophysiological processes that can cause stool color

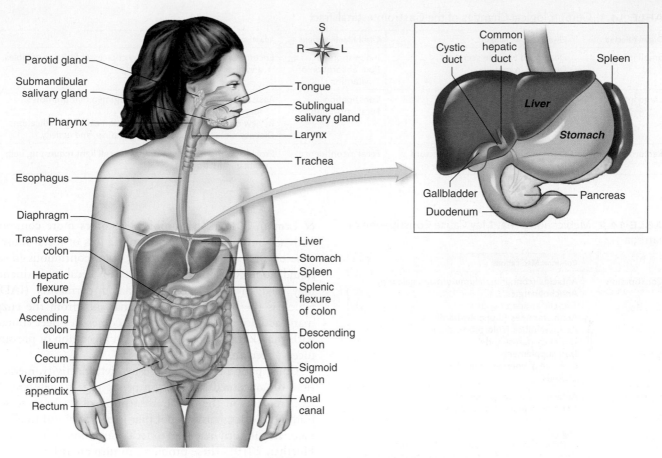

FIG. 14.1 Gastrointestinal tract organs.

changes. Melena, a dark, tar-colored stool, may indicate an upper GI bleed. Bright red blood in the stool may result from a lower GI bleed. If there is an obstruction in the biliary tract, stool may be grayish white in color. Greasy, yellow stool, called steatorrhea, occurs with malabsorption of fats. Melena and steatorrhea produce a characteristic odor due to the by-products of blood and fat (McCance & Huether, 2019).

Stool should be semiformed, large, and bulky. Stool that is hard and small or flat and long may indicate a problem with constipation, impaction, or bowel obstruction. If an inflammatory process is occurring in the bowel, stool may be slimy, with an increased mucus composition.

Communication between the nurse and client must be mutually respectful and collaborative. It is in the best interest of the nurse and client to establish open discussion about the client's bowel habits and regimens. Clients may feel uncomfortable discussing bowel regimens or bowel management programs with anyone. However, therapeutic and respectful discussions of common bowel habits and treatments may lead to future teaching opportunities between the nurse and client.

SECTION 1 Supporting Healthy Bowel Elimination

The purpose of developing a bowel regimen is to prevent constipation or incontinence. Bowel elimination patterns vary from person to person and range from three bowel movements per day to one bowel movement every 3 days. Factors influencing bowel elimination include, but are not limited to, the following:

- Age. The geriatric population may experience a decrease in peristalsis and muscle tone. Table 14.1 identifies some of the geriatric changes affecting bowel elimination.
- Diet. A high-residue diet moves through the colon more quickly than a low-residue diet.
- Physical activity. Increased activity promotes peristalsis.
- Fluid intake. Adequate hydration promotes elimination.

TABLE 14.1 Gerontological Changes of the Gastrointestinal Tract

Organ Affected	Physiological Changes	Client Manifestations	Adaptive Nursing Measures
Small intestine	Decreased enzyme secretion Decrease in motility	Indigestion Poor absorption of vitamins	Encourage client to select dietary choices of fruits, vegetables, and fiber.
Large intestine	Decrease in motility Longer transit time Decrease in defecation reflex	Constipation Fecal impaction	Assist client to establish a bowel regimen that promotes regular bowel evacuation. Review medication list for constipation-causing medications. Discuss dietary modifications, hydration, and activity.
Rectum and anus	Decrease in nerve supply to rectum Decrease in rectal muscle tone	Fecal incontinence	Provide prompt response to client's call light requesting help with elimination.

TABLE 14.2 Medications That May Cause Constipation or Diarrhea

	Common Medications
Constipation	Antacids (containing aluminum and calcium) Anticholinergics Tricyclic antidepressants Antihistamines (diphenhydramine) Antipsychotics (chlorpromazine) Diuretics (furosemide) Iron supplements Overuse of enemas or laxatives Opioids
Diarrhea	Antacids (with magnesium) Antibiotics and antimicrobials Methyldopa Digitalis Sorbitol-containing suspensions or elixirs Chemotherapy (5-fluorouracil, capecitabine, and irinotecan) Colchicine Lactulose

Adapted from Gallagher & Harding, 2017.

- Psychological factors. Stress and anxiety can increase or decrease peristalsis.
- Medications. Antacids, laxatives, antibiotics, and many other types of medications can influence bowel elimination. Table 14.2 identifies medications that may result in constipation and diarrhea.

BOWEL ELIMINATION PROBLEMS

The most common bowel elimination problems are diarrhea, characterized by watery loose stools, and constipation, which may lead to bowel obstruction. Acute diarrhea is usually associated with an infectious organism from contaminated food or water, such as the *Giardia* parasite; communicable diseases transmitted from person to person via the fecal-oral route, such as norovirus; or an opportunistic organism communicated to an immunocompromised client, such as *Clostridium difficile*. Osmotic diarrhea is usually due to the ingestion of large amounts of undigested carbohydrates, medications (stool softeners, laxatives), or poor digestion of dairy products in someone with lactase deficiency (Gallagher & Harding, 2017).

Frequent diarrhea may cause fecal incontinence, which is the involuntary loss of either solid or liquid stool (Robson

& Lembo, 2018). This problem becomes more common with age and usually happens from a loss of rectal muscle tone or anal sphincter control or from continuous loose, liquid stool (Robson & Lembo, 2018). Fecal incontinence may lead to incontinence-associated dermatitis (IAD), which is the breakdown of perianal skin from the enzymatic activity of the stool when it comes in direct contact with anal skin. IAD may lead to skin ulceration or pressure ulcers (Beeckman, 2017).

Constipation may be caused by diet, inactivity, medication, or continued suppression of the urge to defecate. As feces remains in the colon, absorption of water increases, leading to drier, harder stool that is more painful to eliminate. This in turn may lead to fecal impaction (McCance & Huether, 2019). These problems in turn are risk factors for hemorrhoids, which are dilated anal veins. Hemorrhoids are the main reason for rectal bleeding during defecation (Gallagher & Harding, 2017). It is important to note that abdominal cramping, a full rectum, and watery, foul-smelling stool could be due to a fecal impaction; therefore, do not treat what appears to be diarrhea with antidiarrheal medication.

To promote regular bowel function, the nurse needs to ensure a client's privacy and comfortable positioning. Because peristalsis is increased after a meal, this is the best time to provide bathroom assistance and promote bowel regularity. If the client's bowel regimen is disrupted and constipation or incontinence develops, the client may require assistance with bowel elimination, such as medications, enemas, or bowel diversions. A client who does not respond to stool softeners may need digital rectal stimulation or digital rectal evacuation for constipation. To maintain perianal skin integrity, fecal collection methods may be used to contain fecal incontinence.

Digital rectal stimulation and evacuation are invasive procedures that require an authorized healthcare provider's order. They are contraindicated for a client with a low platelet or white blood cell (WBC) count due to the possibility of bleeding or bacterial invasion. Either procedure may cause irritation to the rectal mucosa, bleeding, perforation, or infection. They also may stimulate a vagal response, resulting in an increase in parasympathetic stimulation prompting a vasovagal response: decreased heart rate and blood pressure. The nurse must check

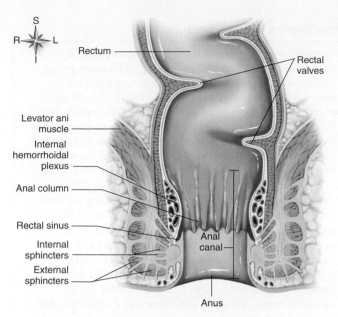

FIG. 14.2 Rectal and anal structures.

(Figure labels: S, R, L, I; Rectum; Rectal valves; Levator ani muscle; Internal hemorrhoidal plexus; Anal column; Rectal sinus; Internal sphincters; External sphincters; Anal canal; Anus)

the heart rate and blood pressure before the procedure to obtain baseline measurements and monitor the client throughout the procedure. During the procedure, if the client experiences lightheadedness or dizziness, an apical heart rate must be checked, and the procedure stopped. An oil retention enema may be administered prior to digital evacuation to soften the stool and facilitate ease of stool removal. Before performing either digital rectal stimulation or evacuation, the nurse ensures that his or her own fingernails are trimmed to prevent injury to the client. The nurse also needs a clear understanding of the anatomical structures of the anus and rectum before introducing objects into the rectum. Fig. 14.2 illustrates the anatomy of the rectum, including the internal and external sphincters.

A rectal tube requires an authorized healthcare provider's order and may be inserted for decompression of the bowel after any surgery that causes alterations in peristalsis or gas production or any surgery that involves the internal or external anal sphincter. The rectal tube is left in place for approximately 15 to 20 minutes to allow for the elimination of flatus. Frequent client position changes may improve decompression of the bowel by assisting with the passage and elimination of flatus.

A fecal management system (FMS) is used to divert and collect liquid or semiliquid stool. One method of collecting feces is an external pouch that is applied to the anus. A second method is an FMS that consists of a catheter tube secured in the rectal vault by a doughnut-shaped balloon at one end and a drainage bag at the other end. Insertion of an FMS may stimulate the vagal response discussed previously. Assessment of heart rate before, during (if the client complains of symptoms), and after is to reduce the risk of bradycardia resulting from vagal stimulation. An FMS requires an authorized healthcare provider's order. These systems are applied to minimize contact between stool and anal skin in

bedridden, immobilized, or incontinent clients and to prevent the spread of infection. Nurses spend a considerable amount of time attempting to keep the client clean and dry. Frequent linen changes may also be burdensome for the ill client. Skin protection and infection control are priority nursing considerations, and both the external pouch and an FMS assist in achieving these goals. The nurse must monitor the client for complications of FMS, including obstruction of the catheter, colonic or rectal ulceration, and rectal bleeding. Review the evidence supporting the appropriate use of FMS in Box 14.1.

APPLICATION OF THE NURSING PROCESS

Examples of Related International Classification for Nursing Practice (ICNP) Nursing Diagnoses, Expected Client Outcomes, and Nursing Interventions:

Nursing Diagnosis: Constipation

Supporting Data: Client reports the difficult elimination of hard and dry stool.

Expected Client Outcomes: Client will have reduced risk for constipation, as demonstrated by:
- fluid intake of 64 to 96 oz per day
- selection of dietary items that are high in fiber
- increase in activity level as tolerated.

Nursing Intervention Example: Promote bowel regularity and provide fluid for hydration.

Nursing Diagnosis: Diarrhea

Supporting Data: Client is experiencing three or more loose or liquid stools per day.

Expected Client Outcomes: Client will experience a soft formed bowel movement every 1 to 3 days.
- Client will identify the bulk-forming food groups.

Nursing Intervention Example: Provide education on bulk-forming foods and foods to avoid.

Reference: International Classification for Nursing Practice. (n.d.). *eHealth & ICNP*. Retrieved from https://www.icn.ch/what-we-do/projects/ehealth-icnp.

CRITICAL CONCEPTS
Supporting Healthy Bowel Elimination

Accuracy (ACC)

Accuracy in promoting bowel elimination is subject to the following variables:
- assessment of client, including vital signs, cooperation, mobility, level of abdominal discomfort, perianal skin integrity, and assessment of abdomen and stool
- proper client positioning
- identification of anatomical landmarks
- proper placement of fingers for digital stimulation or evacuation
- proper placement of rectal tube and fecal management system.

BOX 14.1 Lessons From the Evidence: Evidence on Fecal Incontinence Management

There continues to be much discussion about the most effective way to manage fecal incontinence in acute care and critical care settings. Internal rectal tubes (flare-tip rubber tube or urinary catheter with balloon inflated) continue to be used, without clear evidence to support the benefits or effectiveness of their use. The literature suggests that the first step to managing fecal incontinence is to assess the contributing risk factors and possible causes of diarrhea prior to implementing a fecal management system. A full assessment of the client's medical history and medications should be considered. Continued monitoring of the perianal skin while cleaning the skin with no-rinse bathing products and possible use of a wicking underpad is a more conservative approach to caring for fecal incontinence; avoid the use of diapers because they trap the feces against the skin.

If excessive diarrhea continues, a securely applied fecal management system effectively removes fecal liquid away from the perianal skin while protecting the internal rectal sphincter and internal mucosa. A study of the use of fecal management systems reported improvement in peri-genital skin integrity and normal rectal tissue, as per proctoscopy; moreover, healthcare providers reported ease with managing the system (Makic, VonRueden, Rauen, & Chadwick, 2011).

In another study conducted in the critical care setting, 59 clients with liquid fecal incontinence were randomized into one of three groups: bowel management system using a catheter, rectal/nasopharyngeal trumpet group, and usual-care group using barrier creams and an external fecal management pouch system. Clients were assessed for baseline perianal incontinence-associated dermatitis (IAD) and pressure ulcers prior to conducting the study. At baseline, the IAD scores (measured using the Incontinence-Associated Dermatitis and Severity Instrument) and the pressure ulcer assessment scores (measured using the National Pressure Ulcer Advisory Panel staging guidelines) did not differ among the three groups. However, over time, there was a statistically significant improvement in IAD scores in the usual-care group; the prevalence of pressure injury did not change among groups over time. Additionally, clinician satisfaction improved with the use of the bowel management system and the internal rectal/nasopharyngeal trumpet, and there was a reported cost savings when using the rectal/nasopharyngeal trumpet. Although the authors reported limitations to their study, specifically a low sample size and variability among the groups, with discontinuation of participation and some variability at baseline, there is a need to continue to evaluate the effectiveness of the use of internal and external fecal management systems in the critical care setting (Pittman, Beeson, Terry, Kessler, & Kirk, 2012).

Client-Centered Care (CCC)

Respect for the client when promoting bowel elimination is demonstrated by:
- promoting dignity and respecting client's autonomy
- providing privacy
- ensuring comfort and promoting relaxation
- honoring cultural preferences and arranging for an interpreter, if needed
- advocating for the client and family.

Infection Control (INF)

Healthcare-associated infections associated with bowel elimination are prevented by:
- containment of microorganisms
- preventing and reducing the transfer of microorganisms, such as GI pathogens
- reducing the number of microorganisms
- maintaining skin and tissue integrity in the perianal area.

Safety (SAF)

Safety measures when promoting bowel elimination prevent harm and provide a safe care environment, including:
- assessing and monitoring for bradycardia resulting from vagal stimulation.
- reducing the risk for injury by verifying identity and contraindications.

Communication (COM)

- Communication exchanges information (oral, written, nonverbal, or electronic) between two or more people.
- Collaboration with the client, client's family, and other healthcare professionals facilitates support of a healthy bowel regimen and effective teaching to ensure optimal outcomes.
- Documentation records information in a permanent legal record.

Health Maintenance (HLTH)

Nursing is dedicated to the promotion of health and self-care abilities related to bowel elimination, including:
- protecting the client's perianal skin integrity
- promoting the client's diet choices
- promoting the client's activity level to promote an optimal bowel regimen
- supporting health-seeking behaviors
- seeking community resources.

Evaluation (EVAL)

Evaluation of outcomes enables the nurse to determine the efficacy of the care provided, including:
- fecal or flatus output
- dietary choices to impact bowel management
- client's bowel management plan.

■ SKILL 14.1 Performing Digital Stimulation and Evacuation

EQUIPMENT

Clean gloves
Absorbent pad
Bedpan or bedside commode
Water-soluble lubricant
Washcloth or disposable wipe

BEGINNING THE SKILL

1. **SAF** Review the order. Review the client's history for contraindications (e.g. low platelet count, low WBC count).
2. **INF** Perform hand hygiene. Ensure your nails are trimmed.
3. **CCC** Introduce yourself to the client and family and explain the procedure and purpose of digital stimulation and evacuation. Ensure the client consents to the procedure.
4. **SAF** Identify the client using two identifiers.
5. **ACC** Determine the client's last bowel movement. Observe the abdomen for distention, listen for bowel sounds, and palpate the abdomen gently. *To establish a baseline assessment and monitor the effectiveness of the procedure.*
6. **SAF** Assess the client's heart rate and blood pressure for baseline measurements before rectal stimulation. *Parasympathetic stimulation may result in decreased heart rate and blood pressure.*
7. **INF** Apply clean gloves.
8. **CCC** Provide privacy: close the door and pull the curtain.

PROCEDURE

9. **SAF** Set up an ergonomically safe space. Place the head of the bed in the horizontal position, and position the client on the left side (Sims' position). *This position reduces the risk of perforation of the rectum, creating proper alignment with the normal anatomy of the bowel.* Raise the bed to a comfortable working height. Raise one side rail. *Setting up an ergonomically safe space prevents injury to the nurse and client.*
10. **SAF** Set up a workspace according to your hand dominance (e.g., right-handed on the client's right side). Place the bedpan close by. (Note: The client may need to be placed on the bedpan or bedside commode following digital stimulation, and stool is placed in the bedpan following evacuation.)
11. **CCC** Place the absorbent pad under the client.

Digital Stimulation

12. **CCC** Generously lubricate the gloved forefinger and middle finger on your dominant hand.
13. **ACC** Separate the buttocks and locate the anus. Visually inspect and palpate for hemorrhoids and observe for rectal bleeding. *If external hemorrhoids or rectal bleeding are present, stop the procedure. Notify the authorized*

healthcare provider to determine the course of action, and document assessment findings.

14. **ACC** Gently insert one lubricated finger into the rectum, 2.5 to 7 cm (1–3 inches), rotating the finger gently in a circular motion for 30 seconds or until the anal sphincter relaxes. *This stimulates a rectal contraction.*
15. **ACC** After providing stimulation, position the client on the toilet, bedside commode, or bedpan as tolerated. *Position the client to facilitate normal bowel elimination.*
16. **ACC** If no fecal return, the stimulation may be repeated in 20 minutes or digital evacuation may be performed. *Waiting allows the client a rest period.*

Digital Evacuation

17. **CCC** Generously lubricate the gloved forefinger and middle finger on your dominant hand.
18. **ACC** Separate the buttocks and locate the anus. Visually inspect and palpate for hemorrhoids and observe for rectal bleeding. *If external hemorrhoids or rectal bleeding are present, stop the procedure. Notify the authorized healthcare provider to determine the course of action, and document assessment findings.*
19. **ACC** Gently insert one lubricated finger into the rectum 2.5 to 7 cm (1–3 inches), rotating the finger around the stool.

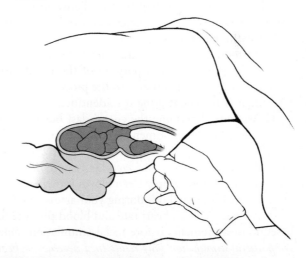

STEP 19 Rotate one finger around the stool.

20. **ACC** Begin to break the stool into pieces.
21. **ACC** Remove the stool as it breaks apart.
22. **INF** Place stool in the bedpan.
23. **CCC** Encourage the client to take slow, deep breaths throughout the procedure to relax the anal sphincter.
24. **SAF** Monitor the client's heart rate throughout the procedure. Stop the procedure if the client complains of lightheadedness or nausea or if the heart rate falls below

baseline. Monitor the client's heart rate and blood pressure until they return to baseline.

25. **EVAL** Allow for rest periods as needed.
26. **EVAL** Continue to remove stool in pieces as tolerated by the client.

FINISHING THE SKILL

27. **INF** Dispose of the used supplies.
28. **EVAL** Evaluate stool for color, consistency, and amount.
29. **HLTH** Clean the client's rectal area.
30. **INF** Remove gloves and perform hand hygiene.

31. **CCC** Provide comfort. Assist the client with positioning and rearrange bedding.
32. **SAF** Ensure client safety. Place the bed in the lowest position. Ensure that the client can identify and reach the nurse call system. *These safety measures reduce the risk of falls.*
33. **COM** Document date, time, characteristics, and amount of stool return and how the client tolerated the procedure in the legal healthcare record.
34. **COM** Provide follow-up care. Consult a registered dietitian to assist the client in selecting dietary items indicated for constipation.

■ SKILL 14.2 Inserting Rectal Tubes

EQUIPMENT

Clean gloves
Absorbent pad
Rectal tube
Tape
Water-soluble lubricant
Washcloth or disposable wipe

BEGINNING THE SKILL

1. **SAF** Review the order. Review the client's history for contraindications (e.g. low platelet or low WBC count).
2. **INF** Perform hand hygiene.
3. **CCC** Introduce yourself to the client and family and explain the procedure and purpose of the rectal tube. Ensure that the client consents to the procedure.
4. **SAF** Identify the client using two identifiers.
5. **ACC** Assess to determine the client's last bowel movement. Observe the abdomen for distention, listen for bowel sounds, and palpate the abdomen gently. *To establish a baseline assessment and monitor the effectiveness of the procedure.* (Note: Apply clean gloves if there is a risk of contact with body fluids during your assessment.)
6. **SAF** Assess the client's heart rate and blood pressure for baseline measurements before rectal stimulation. *Parasympathetic stimulation may result in a decrease in heart rate and blood pressure.*
7. **CCC** Provide privacy: close the door and pull the curtain.
8. **INF** Apply clean gloves, if not already applied.

PROCEDURE

9. **SAF** Set up an ergonomically safe space. Place the head of the bed in the horizontal position and position the client on the left side (Sims' position). *This position reduces the risk of perforation of the rectum, creating proper alignment with the normal anatomy of the bowel.* Raise the bed to a comfortable working height. Raise one side rail. *Setting up an ergonomically safe space prevents injury to the nurse and client*

10. **SAF** Set up a workspace according to your hand dominance (e.g., right-handed on the client's right side). Place the bedpan close by. *The client may need to be placed on the bedpan or bedside commode following the procedure.*
11. **CCC** Place the absorbent pad under the client.
12. **CCC** Lubricate the end of the rectal tubing with water-soluble lubricant if not prelubricated.
13. **ACC** Separate the buttocks and locate the anus. Visually inspect and palpate for hemorrhoids and observe for rectal bleeding. *If external hemorrhoids or rectal bleeding are present, stop the procedure. Notify the authorized healthcare provider to determine the course of action, and document assessment findings.*
14. **ACC** Insert the tube into the anus gently and advance approximately 7 to 10 cm (2–4 inches). *The tube should be inserted beyond the internal anal sphincter. Do not force the tube. It should insert easily.*

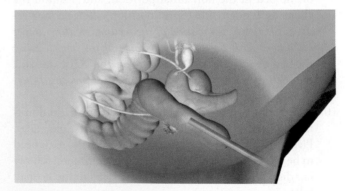

STEP 14 Advance the rectal tube approximately 7 to 10 cm (2–4 inches).

15. **CCC** Encourage the client to take slow, deep breaths throughout the procedure.
16. **ACC** Tape the tube to the client's buttock appropriately to prevent movement of the tube. Keep the tube in place for 15 to 20 minutes to allow flatulence to pass.

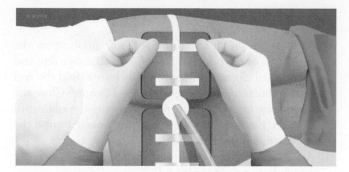

STEP 16 Tape the rectal tube appropriately.

17. **ACC** Encourage the client to move in the bed, if able. *Client movement promotes the passage and elimination of flatus.*
18. **ACC** Remove the tape and slowly remove the rectal tube.

FINISHING THE SKILL

19. **HLTH** Clean the client's rectal area.
20. **INF** Dispose of the used supplies.
21. **EVAL** Evaluate output of flatus for amount and stool, if present, for color, consistency, and amount.
22. **INF** Remove gloves and perform hand hygiene.
23. **CCC** Provide comfort. Assist the client with positioning and rearrange bedding.
24. **SAF** Ensure client safety. Place the bed in the lowest position. Ensure that the client can identify and reach the nurse call system. *These safety measures reduce the risk of falls.*
25. **COM** Document date, time, flatus return, and how the client tolerated the procedure in the legal healthcare record.

■ SKILL 14.3 Applying a Fecal Collection Pouch

EQUIPMENT

Clean gloves
Absorbent pad
Bandage scissors, if indicated
Fecal collection pouch
Urinary drainage bag, if liquid stool
Skin protectant
Washcloth or disposable wipes and water

BEGINNING THE SKILL

1. **SAF** Review order.
2. **INF** Perform hand hygiene.
3. **CCC** Introduce yourself to the client and family and explain the procedure and purpose of the fecal collection pouch. Ensure that the client consents to the procedure.
4. **SAF** Identify the client using two identifiers.
5. **CCC** Provide privacy: close the door and pull the curtain.
6. **INF** Apply clean gloves.

PROCEDURE

7. **SAF** Set up an ergonomically safe space. Place the head of the bed in the horizontal position and position the client on the left or right side (Sims' position). *This position exposes the rectum and perineum.* Raise the bed to a comfortable working height. Raise one side rail. *Setting up an ergonomically safe space prevents injury to the nurse and client.*
8. **SAF** Set up a workspace according to your hand dominance (right-handed on the client's right side).
9. **CCC** Place the absorbent pad under the client.
10. **ACC** Separate the buttocks and locate the anus. Assess the perianal area for skin breakdown. Visually inspect and palpate for hemorrhoids and observe for rectal bleeding. *If external hemorrhoids or rectal bleeding are present, stop the procedure. Notify the authorized healthcare provider to determine the course of action, and document assessment findings.*
11. **HLTH** Wash the perianal skin well with warm water. *The presence of emollients or residue from previous skin barrier adhesive will interfere with the adherence of the pouch.*
12. **SAF** If needed, trim perianal hair with bandage scissors prior to pouch application. **WARNING:** Do not shave the area. *Shaving can cause cuts in the skin and result in irritation or potential infection.*
13. **HLTH** Apply skin protectant and allow the area to dry. *Skin protectant will reduce the risk for incontinence-associated dermatitis (IAD) and potential infection.*
14. **ACC** If the precut opening is not slightly larger than the anus, trim the opening with scissors. *The opening on the pouch must allow for anal dilation during defecation.*
15. **ACC** Remove the backing from the adhesive pouch and fold the skin barrier lengthwise. Do not touch the adhesive with your fingers. *Folding the barrier allows the center to touch the skin first.*

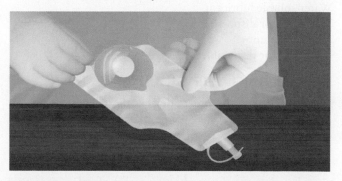

STEP 15 Remove the backing from the adhesive pouch.

16. **ACC** With your nondominant hand, separate the buttocks and apply the fecal pouch with your dominant hand, making sure to cover the anus.

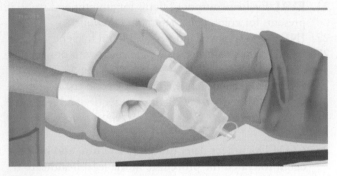

STEP 16 Separate the buttocks and apply the fecal pouch.

17. **ACC** Gently press and mold the adhesive around the anus and perineal area. *Pressing and molding warm the adhesive and improves adherence.* Release the buttocks.
18. **ACC** If the client is passing only liquid stool, attach a urinary drainage bag to the open end of a drainage tap of the fecal incontinence pouch.

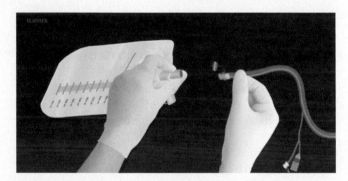

STEP 18 Attach a urinary drainage bag to the connector.

19. **ACC** Hang the drainage below the level of the bed to ensure gravity drainage.
20. **ACC** If the client is passing semisoft stools, trim the lower end of the pouch, removing the drainage tap, and apply a tail closure. To apply a tail closure, fold the end of the pouch over the edge of the tail closure. Close the tail closure by pressing the raised bar onto the edge until it clicks. Do not wrap the end of the pouch around the tail closure more than one time.
21. **ACC** Empty the pouch using the tail closure when the pouch becomes one-third full.
22. **HLTH** Clean the client's rectal area.

FINISHING THE SKILL

23. **INF** Dispose of the used supplies.
24. **EVAL** Evaluate output of stool for color, consistency, and amount.
25. **INF** Remove gloves and perform hand hygiene.
26. **CCC** Provide comfort. Assist the client with positioning and rearrange bedding.
27. **SAF** Ensure client safety. Place the bed in the lowest position. Ensure that the client can identify and reach the nurse call system. *These safety measures reduce the risk of falls.*
28. **COM** Document date, time, characteristics and amount of stool return, and how the client tolerated the procedure in the legal healthcare record.
29. **HLTH** Provide follow-up care by assisting the client in developing a diet that will promote a bowel regimen specific to the client's needs, such as hydration and electrolyte replacement for diarrhea.

■ SKILL 14.4 Setting Up a Fecal Management System

EQUIPMENT

Clean gloves
Absorbent pad
Fecal management system
Water-soluble lubricant
Washcloth or disposable wipe
Skin protectant
Washcloth or disposable wipes

BEGINNING THE SKILL

1. **SAF** Review the order. Review the client's history for contraindications (e.g., low platelet count, low WBC count).
2. **INF** Perform hand hygiene.
3. **CCC** Introduce yourself to the client and family and explain the procedure and purpose of the fecal management system. Ensure that the client consents to the procedure.

4. **SAF** Assess the client's heart rate and blood pressure to establish baseline measurements before rectal stimulation. *Parasympathetic stimulation may result in a decrease in heart rate and blood pressure.*
5. **SAF** Identify the client using two identifiers.
6. **CCC** Provide privacy: close the door and pull the curtain.
7. **INF** Apply clean gloves.

PROCEDURE

8. **SAF** Set up an ergonomically safe space. Place the head of the bed in the horizontal position and position the client on the left or right side (Sims' position). *This position exposes the rectum and perineum.* Raise the bed to a comfortable working height. Raise one side rail. *Setting up an ergonomically safe space prevents injury to the nurse and client.*

9. **SAF** Set up a workspace according to your hand dominance (e.g., right-handed on the client's right side).
10. **CCC** Place the absorbent pad under the client.
11. **ACC** Separate the buttocks and locate the anus. Visually inspect and palpate for hemorrhoids and observe for rectal bleeding. *If external hemorrhoids or rectal bleeding are present, stop the procedure. Notify the authorized healthcare provider to determine the course of action, and document assessment findings.*
12. **HLTH** Wash the perianal skin well with warm water. The presence of emollients or residue from previous skin barrier adhesive will interfere with the adherence of the pouch.
13. **ACC** Prepare and insert the fecal management system.
    a. If the balloon is inflated, aspirate air using a syringe attached to the inflation port.
    b. Remove the syringe and draw up 45 mL (or per manufacturer's instructions) of water or saline and connect the syringe to the inflation port. *Inflation ports are often marked with the maximum amount to be inflated, for example, 45 mL.*
    c. Lubricate the index finger of your dominant hand and insert your index finger into the identified finger pocket.

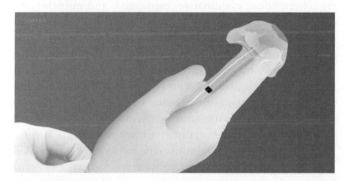

STEP 13C Insert index finger into the identified finger pocket.

    d. Lubricate the balloon end of the catheter and insert the balloon end well into the rectal vault, guiding the insertion with your index finger.

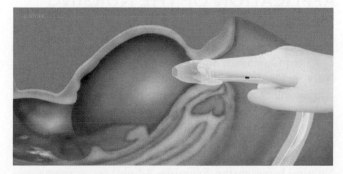

STEP 13D Insert the balloon end well into the rectal vault.

    e. Inflate the balloon. Your finger may stay in the rectum while the balloon is inflated, or you may remove it before the balloon is inflated.

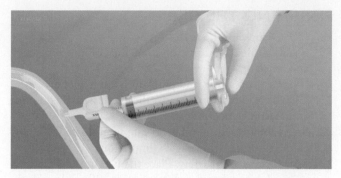

STEP 13E Inflate the balloon.

    f. **WARNING:** Do not inflate the balloon with more than 45 mL. Some systems may alert you when the optimal balloon inflation is reached. A minimum of 30 mL is usually required.
    g. Remove the syringe from the inflation port and tug gently on the catheter to ensure the balloon is securely positioned on the rectal floor.

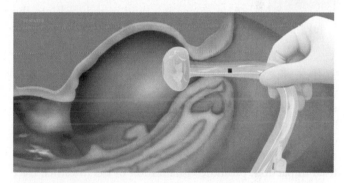

STEP 13G Tug gently on the catheter to ensure the balloon is securely positioned on the rectal floor.

14. **ACC** Place the catheter along the client's leg, avoiding kinks and obstruction.
15. **ACC** Note the position indicator line on the catheter relative to the anus. *Changes in the distance between the anus and the position indicator line indicate movement of the balloon, which may indicate a need for the balloon to be repositioned.*
16. **ACC** Hang the drainage bag below the level of the bed to ensure gravity drainage.

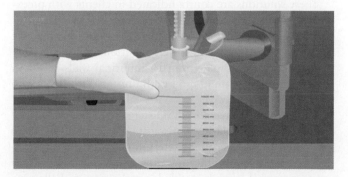

STEP 16 Hang the drainage bag below the level of the bed.

17. **HLTH** Clean the client's rectal area.

FINISHING THE SKILL

18. **INF** Dispose of the used supplies.
19. **EVAL** Evaluate output of stool for color, consistency, and amount.
20. **INF** Remove gloves and perform hand hygiene.
21. **CCC** Provide comfort. Assist the client with positioning and rearrange bedding.
22. **SAF** Obtain the client's heart rate to evaluate for bradycardia resulting from vagal stimulation.
23. **SAF** Ensure client safety. Place the bed in the lowest position. Ensure that the client can identify and reach the nurse call system. *These safety measures reduce the risk of falls.*
24. **INF** Perform hand hygiene.
25. **COM** Document date, time, characteristics and amount of stool return, and how the client tolerated the procedure in the legal healthcare record.
26. **HLTH** Provide follow-up care by assisting the client in developing a diet that will promote a bowel regimen specific to the client's needs, such as hydration and electrolyte replacement for diarrhea.

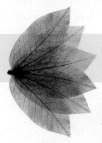

SECTION 2   Administering Enemas

An enema is a fluid introduced into the rectum to soften the stool, stimulate peristalsis, and promote elimination. An enema may also be administered to instill medication into the rectum. The authorized healthcare provider may prescribe any of three types of enemas: cleansing enemas, return-flow enemas, or retentions enemas.

Cleansing enemas may be administered using a disposable enema set or a commercially prepackaged enema. They are indicated to relieve constipation, break up and eliminate a fecal impaction, promote visualization of the intestinal tract during a procedure or exam, or assist with bowel regulation during a bowel training program (Robson & Lembro, 2018). Risks associated with enemas include leakage from the anus, minor cramps, bowel perforation, and sepsis (Niv, Grinberg, Dickman, Wasserberg, & Niv, 2013). Contraindications for enemas include low platelet count or low WBC count and rectal disorders. Cleansing enemas include large-volume enemas and small-volume enemas.

- Large-volume enemas (saline, tap water, or soapsuds) distend the colon, stimulate peristalsis, and soften the stool. Hypotonic solutions, such as tap-water–based solutions, cause electrolytes to diffuse from the body into the colon. These solutions are contraindicated in clients with preexisting fluid and electrolyte imbalances (Niv et al., 2013).
- Small-volume enemas use hypertonic solutions that are commercially prepared. These solutions stimulate peristalsis and draw fluid from the intestinal walls to soften the feces. They should not be administered to clients who are dehydrated.

Return-flow enemas are administered to relieve abdominal distention by stimulating peristalsis to eliminate intestinal gas. Using the skill sequence for administering a large-volume enema, a hypotonic or isotonic solution such as tap water or normal saline is instilled into the rectum. Following instillation, the container is lowered to allow the solution to return to the enema container. The process is then repeated several times until abdominal distention is relieved.

Retention enemas should be retained for a prescribed period of time. The most common types of retention enemas are oil-retention, carminative, medicated, and nutritive. An oil-retention enema is used to soften the stool. Carminative enemas are administered to relieve abdominal distention by removing intestinal gas. Medicated enemas are administered to instill prescribed medications into the colon, such as antibiotics or anthelminthic agents (drugs that are used to treat parasitic infections). Nutritive enemas are prescribed to provide hydration and nutrition to clients who are unable to take fluids or nutrition orally. If a retention enema is commercially prepared, it is administered following the same skill sequence for administering a commercially prepared enema but is retained for the prescribed amount of time. If a retention enema is not commercially prepared, it is administered using the same skill sequence for administering a cleansing enema but is retained for the prescribed amount of time. See Table 14.3 for more information about types of enemas.

APPLICATION OF THE NURSING PROCESS

Examples of Related ICNP Nursing Diagnoses, Expected Client Outcomes, and Nursing Interventions
Nursing Diagnosis: Impaired GI system processes
Supporting Data: Client reports an alteration in bowel elimination that is consistent with difficulty eliminating stool or no stool elimination for more than 3 to 5 days.
Expected Client Outcomes: Client will eliminate stool or gas after enema instillation.
Nursing Intervention Example: Administer an enema.
Reference: International Classification for Nursing Practice. (n.d.). *eHealth & ICNP.* Retrieved from https://www.icn.ch/what-we-do/projects/ehealth-icnp.

TABLE 14.3 Types of Enemas

Type of Enema	Amount of Fluid	Type of Solution	Suggested Retention Time
Large volume	500–1000 mL (adults) 100–250 mL (children)	Hypotonic—tap water Isotonic—normal saline	15–20 min
Small volume	70–120 mL (adults)	Hypertonic—prepackaged	5–10 min
Soapsuds	500–1000 mL (adults)	Isotonic—tap water + castile soap	15–20 min
Return flow	100–200 mL	Hypotonic—tap water Isotonic—saline	
Commercially prepared	230–250 mL	Hypertonic—oil	5–10 min
Retention	90–120 mL	Oil, carminative (magnesium or glycerin), medicated (antibiotics), nutritive	30 min

Adapted from Yoost & Crawford, 2016.

CRITICAL CONCEPTS
Administering Enemas

Accuracy (ACC)

Accuracy in administering enemas is subject to the following variables:
- assessment of client, including cooperation, mobility, level of abdominal discomfort, perianal skin integrity, and assessment of stool
- identification of anatomical landmarks
- proper client positioning
- proper placement of enema tip in rectum
- rate of flow of enema
- temperature of enema solution
- client's ability to tolerate the enema instillation and retain enema solution as prescribed.

Client-Centered Care (CCC)

When administering an enema, respect for the client is demonstrated by:
- promoting autonomy
- providing privacy
- ensuring comfort
- honoring cultural preferences
- advocating for the client and family
- arranging for an interpreter, if needed
- advocating for the client to self-administer commercially prepared enema, if appropriate.

Infection Control (INF)

When administering an enema, infection is prevented by:
- containment of microorganisms

- preventing and reducing the transfer of microorganisms
- reducing the number of microorganisms.

Safety (SAF)

Safety measures when administering an enema prevent harm and provide a safe care environment by reducing the risk of falls and ensuring a safe temperature of solution.

Communication (COM)

- Communication exchanges information (oral, written, nonverbal, or electronic) between two or more people.
- Documentation records information in a permanent legal record.
- Collaborating with the client and other healthcare professionals ensures proper use of enemas for bowel management.

Health Maintenance (HLTH)

Nursing is dedicated to the promotion of health and self-care abilities when caring for clients receiving an enema by:
- protecting the client's perianal skin integrity
- teaching the client lifestyle choices that will promote increased intestinal motility, thus reducing the client's risk for constipation
- supporting health-seeking behaviors.

Evaluation (EVAL)

Evaluation of outcomes enables the nurse to determine the efficacy of the care provided, including:
- fecal or flatus output.

■ SKILL 14.5 Administering a Cleansing Enema

EQUIPMENT

Clean gloves
Absorbent pad
Bedpan or bedside commode, if needed

Enema kit
Water-soluble lubricant
Washcloth or disposable wipe
Thermometer, if needed

BEGINNING THE SKILL

1. **SAF** Review the order.
2. **INF** Perform hand hygiene.
3. **CCC** Introduce yourself to the client and family and explain the procedure and purpose of the administration of an enema. Ensure the client consents to the procedure.
4. **SAF** Identify the client using two identifiers.
5. **ACC** Assess to determine the client's last bowel movement. Observe the abdomen for distention, listen for bowel sounds, and palpate the abdomen gently. *To establish a baseline assessment in order to later evaluate the effectiveness of the enema.* (Note: Apply clean gloves if there is a risk of exposure to body fluids during the assessment.)
6. **ACC** Assess the client's ability to cooperate and follow instructions. Determine the client's ability to retain the enema for the necessary period of time, as follows:
   The large-volume enema is usually retained for 15 to 20 minutes, if tolerable for the client.
   The small-volume enema is usually retained for 5 to 10 minutes.
   The soapsuds enema is usually retained for 15 to 20 minutes.
7. **INF** Apply clean gloves, if not already applied.
8. **CCC** Provide privacy: close the door and pull the curtain.

PROCEDURE

9. **SAF** Set up an ergonomically safe space. Place the head of the bed in the horizontal position and position the client on the left side (Sims' position). *This position reduces the risk of perforation of the rectum, creating proper alignment with the normal anatomy of the bowel.* Raise the bed to a comfortable working height. Raise one side rail. *Setting up an ergonomically safe space prevents injury to the nurse and client.*
10. **SAF** Set up a workspace according to your hand dominance (e.g., right-handed on the client's right side). Place the bedpan close by. *The client may need to be placed on the bedpan or bedside commode following the procedure.*
11. **CCC** Place the absorbent pad under the client.
12. **SAF** Fill the enema bag with prescribed solution. Warm the solution using warm tap water. The appropriate temperature is just under body temperature, approximately 33° to 37° C (92° to 98° F) (Mitchell, 2019). **WARNING:** Do not microwave the solution. *Hot solution can cause bowel damage. Cold solution can cause abdominal cramping.*
13. **ACC** Hang the filled enema bag from the intravenous (IV) pole, with the clamp closed.

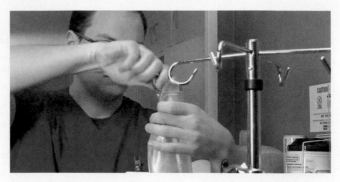

STEP 13 Hang the enema bag from the IV pole.

14. **ACC** Open the clamp slowly, allowing the solution to prime the tubing. *Allowing air into the bowel will cause cramping.*

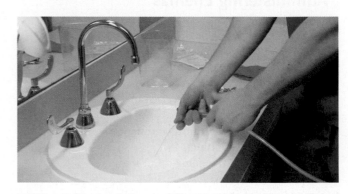

STEP 14 Allow solution to prime the tubing.

15. **ACC** Separate the buttocks and locate the anus. Visually inspect and palpate for hemorrhoids and observe for rectal bleeding. *If external hemorrhoids or rectal bleeding is present, stop the procedure. Notify the authorized healthcare provider to determine the course of action, and document assessment findings.*
16. **CCC** Lubricate the end of the enema tubing with water-soluble lubricant if not prelubricated. *Lubricating the end of the tubing will ease insertion and decrease discomfort.*
17. **ACC** Insert the tube into the anus gently and advance approximately 7 to 10 cm (2–4 inches) toward the umbilicus. *Do not force the tube; it should insert easily.*
18. **ACC** To begin instillation, remove the enema bag from the IV pole and lower the bag to the level of the client's hip, and then unclamp the tubing. *The level of the bag determines the speed of the flow. A rapid rate of flow may cause cramping and an intense urge to defecate.*

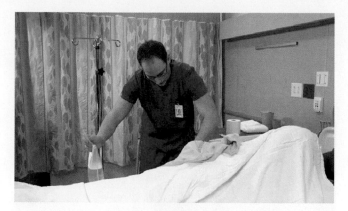

STEP 18 Lower the bag, then unclamp the tubing.

19. **ACC** Slowly raise the enema bag approximately 30 to 45 cm (12–18 inches) to increase the gravitational flow of the solution into the bowel.

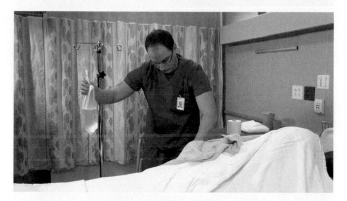

STEP 19 Raise the enema bag approximately 30 to 45 cm (12–18 inches).

20. **EVAL** Communicate with the client throughout enema instillation, monitoring the client's ability to tolerate instillation and retention of enema solution as prescribed.
21. **CCC** Continuously monitor the client for discomfort. If the client complains of cramping, the bag may be lowered to slow the flow of the solution.
22. **ACC** After the correct amount of solution has been instilled or when the client cannot tolerate any more fluid (client complains of abdominal cramping), clamp and remove the tubing.

23. **ACC** For a return-flow enema, do not remove the tubing. Lower the enema bag to allow the solution to return to the bag. This process of instilling solution and return flow can be repeated several times until the client indicates relief of distention. After the client indicates relief, clamp and remove tubing. *If the solution becomes thick before the client indicates relief, clamp and remove the tubing, dispose of the bag and solution, and begin with new supplies.*
24. **HLTH** Clean the client's rectal area.
25. **ACC** Instruct the client to try to wait to use the bedpan, bedside commode, or bathroom until the prescribed amount of time. **WARNING:** If you leave the room, ensure the client can identify and reach the nurse call system. Retention times are as follows:
    Large-volume enema: 15 to 20 minutes
    Small-volume enema: 5 to 10 minutes
    Soapsuds enema: 15 to 20 minutes
26. **INF** Dispose of the used supplies. Remove gloves and perform hand hygiene.
27. **SAF** After the prescribed amount of enema retention time, perform hand hygiene; apply gloves; and assist the client onto the bedpan, to the bedside commode, or to the bathroom as tolerated.

FINISHING THE SKILL

28. **EVAL** Once the enema is expelled, evaluate stool for color, consistency, and amount.
29. **HLTH** Assist the client to clean the perianal skin.
30. **INF** Assist the client to perform hand hygiene. Remove your gloves and perform hand hygiene.
31. **SAF** Assist the client back to the bed. Ensure client safety. Ensure that the bed is in the lowest position. Ensure that the client can identify and reach the nurse call system. *These safety measures reduce the risk of falls.*
32. **CCC** Provide comfort. Assist the client with positioning and rearrange bedding.
33. **COM** Document date, time, how the client tolerated the procedure, and the characteristics and amount of fecal return in the legal healthcare record.
34. **HLTH** If the enema was ordered for constipation, follow up by providing a consultation with a nutritionist to assist the client in selecting dietary items high in fiber.

■ SKILL 14.6 Administering a Commercially Prepared Enema

EQUIPMENT

Clean gloves
Absorbent pad
Bedpan or bedside commode
Prepackaged enema
Water-soluble lubricant
Washcloth or disposable wipe

BEGINNING THE SKILL

1 **SAF** Review the order.
2. **INF** Perform hand hygiene. Apply clean gloves if there is a risk of exposure to body fluids during your assessment.
3. **CCC** Introduce yourself to the client and family and explain the procedure and purpose of administration of an enema. Ensure the client consents to the procedure.

4. **SAF** Identify the client using two identifiers.
5. **ACC** Assess to determine the client's last bowel movement. Observe the abdomen for distention, listen for bowel sounds, and palpate the abdomen gently. *To establish a baseline assessment to monitor the effectiveness of the enema.*
6. **COM** Assess the client's ability to cooperate and follow instructions. Retention of the enema is 5 to 10 minutes. *Your assessment is to determine the client's ability to retain the enema.*
7. **INF** Apply clean gloves, if not already applied.
8. **CCC** Provide privacy: close the door and pull the curtain.

PROCEDURE

9. **SAF** Set up an ergonomically safe space. Place the head of the bed in the horizontal position and position the client of the left side (Sims' position). *This position reduces the risk of perforation of the rectum, creating proper alignment with the normal anatomy of the bowel.* Raise the bed to a comfortable working height. Raise one side rail. *Setting up an ergonomically safe space prevents injury to the nurse and client.*
10. **SAF** Set up a workspace according to your hand dominance (e.g., right-handed on the client's right side). Have the bedpan close by. *The client may need to be placed on the bedpan or bedside commode following the procedure.*
11. **CCC** Place the absorbent pad under the client.
12. **SAF** Warm the solution using warm tap water. The appropriate temperature is just under body temperature, approximately 33° to 37° C (92° to 98° F) (Mitchell, 2019). **WARNING:** Do not microwave the solution. *Hot solution can cause bowel damage. Cold solution can cause abdominal cramping.*
13. **ACC** Open the prepackaged enema and remove the plastic cap on the end of the container.

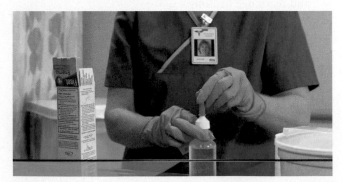

STEP 13 Remove the plastic cap.

14. **ACC** Separate the buttocks and locate the anus. Visually inspect and palpate for hemorrhoids and observe for rectal bleeding. *If external hemorrhoids or rectal bleeding are present, stop the procedure. Notify the authorized healthcare provider to determine the course of action, and document assessment findings.*

15. **CCC** Apply water-soluble lubricant to the end of the enema tip. *The end comes prelubricated; however, extra lubrication will ease insertions and decrease discomfort for the client.*
16. **ACC** Tilt the enema and insert the tip completely into the anus gently toward the umbilicus. *Do not force the tip; it should insert easily.*

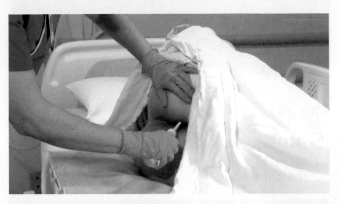

STEP 16 Tilt the enema toward the umbilicus.

17. **ACC** To begin instillation, gently roll and squeeze the container to instill all of the solution.

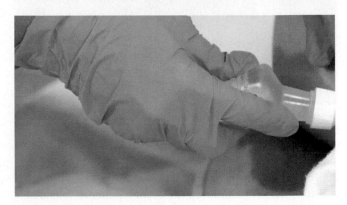

STEP 17 Squeeze the container to instill all of the solution.

18. **CCC** Continuously monitor the client for discomfort. If the client complains of cramping, stop the instillation and encourage slow, deep breaths until the client is ready to continue.
19. **ACC** After the correct amount of solution is instilled or the client cannot hold any more fluid, remove the enema tip from the rectum.
20. **HLTH** Clean the client's rectal area and cover the client.
21. **ACC** Instruct the client to hold the enema for 5 to 10 minutes.
22. **SAF WARNING:** If you leave the room, ensure the client can identify and reach the nurse call system.
23. **INF** Dispose of the used supplies. Remove gloves and perform hand hygiene.
24. **SAF** After the appropriate amount of retention time, perform hand hygiene; apply gloves; and assist the client onto the bedpan, to the bedside commode, or to the bathroom as tolerated.

FINISHING THE SKILL

25. **EVAL** Once the enema is expelled, evaluate stool for color, consistency, and amount.
26. **HLTH** Assist the client to clean the perianal skin.
27. **INF** Assist the client to perform hand hygiene. Remove your gloves and perform hand hygiene.
28. **SAF** Assist the client back to the bed. Ensure client safety. Ensure that the bed is in the lowest position. Ensure that the client can identify and reach the nurse call system. *These safety measures reduce the risk of falls.*
29. **CCC** Provide comfort. Assist the client with positioning and rearrange bedding
30. **COM** Document date, time, how the client tolerated the procedure, and the characteristics and amount of fecal return in the legal healthcare record.

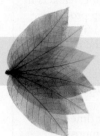

SECTION 3 Collecting Specimens

Stool specimens are obtained to test for infection, bowel function, blood, or parasites. Persons experiencing acute diarrhea will frequently have a stool specimen ordered because acute diarrhea can be a result of infection or an osmotic, motility, or secretory bowel problem (Gallagher & Harding, 2017). *C. diff.*, which is prevalent in healthcare facilities today, releases a toxin that is readily identified by a specific toxin assay technique.

Infections occur despite the GI tract's protection against endogenous and exogenous infections. The acidic environment of the stomach is hostile to most bacteria, and the circular folds, villi, and microvilli of the small intestine provide a large protective mucosal lining that defends against pathogenic invasion. Furthermore, the GI tract produces antibodies and enzymes that assist in infection control. The small intestine has a low concentration of aerobic organisms. The colon's normal flora consists of healthful anaerobic organisms; however, antibiotics may deplete this normal, protective flora and promote the proliferation of antibiotic-resistant strains of harmful bacteria, such as *C. diff.* (Gallagher & Harding, 2017).

If an infection is diagnosed, nurses play a pivotal role in infection control for clients, primarily through performing and teaching the client proper hand hygiene, especially prior to eating and after elimination. Proper disposal of stool, as well as strict contact precautions, are imperative when a client has a communicable GI tract infection. Pathogenic microorganisms may cause colon inflammation and severe secretory diarrhea; therefore, strict hand hygiene, gown, and gloving must be enforced. It is vital that the nurse implement evidence-based practices when caring for the client with communicable diseases of the GI tract.

Stool samples may be analyzed in the laboratory or at the bedside as per facility policy. An adequate stool sample size is approximately 2.5 cm (1 inch) of solid stool or 20 to 30 mL (1 oz) of liquid stool. Gather the sample from two different areas of the stool and include any blood, mucus, or purulent drainage in the specimen. Stool specimens should be collected before taking any antibiotics, antidiarrhea compounds, barium, bismuth, or mineral oil. Assess for interfering factors for some types of stool tests. For example, menstruation can interfere with testing stool for blood. Instruct the client to void before collecting the stool specimen in order to prevent contamination of the specimen with urine and to keep toilet paper out of the stool sample. The stool container must be clean and dry. All stool contains microorganisms; therefore, handle stool samples in a manner that contains and prevents the transfer of microorganisms.

An example of stool testing that may be done at the bedside by the nurse is testing for fecal occult blood. Fecal occult blood indicates GI bleeding. Occult blood is not visible to the naked eye. Bright red blood visible in a stool sample usually indicates rectal or anal irritation or the presence of irritated hemorrhoids. There are two types of fecal occult blood tests (FOBTs) using a cardboard collection slide and reagent drops. A guaiac test checks for the presence of hemoglobin. There are several interfering factors with guaiac tests, including intake of vitamin C, ingestion of foods rich in peroxidase, and ingestion of animal hemoglobin, such as large amounts of red meat, and anticoagulant use prior to obtaining stool specimen for occult blood. Another type of testing for fecal occult blood is a fecal immunochemical test (FIT), which also can be performed at the bedside with a cardboard collection slide and reagent drops. This type of testing is as sensitive as guaiac testing but is not impacted by diet or drugs. A positive occult blood result usually indicates gastrointestinal bleeding. However, both types of fecal occult blood testing will react to menstrual blood or blood from rectal irritation, resulting in a false positive.

Gastrointestinal bleeding can be a sign of colorectal cancer because tumors bleed easily. The U.S. Preventive Services Task Force (USPSTF, 2019) recommends colorectal cancer screening for men and women aged 50 to 75 using high-sensitivity FOBT annually. Additional screening is also recommended with sigmoidoscopy at 5-year intervals and colonoscopy at 10-year intervals. For annual FOBT screening, nurses may instruct clients to apply stool to the testing cards at home and then bring the cards to a lab or healthcare provider for testing. In addition to screening for colorectal cancer, it is important for nurses to obtain a thorough health history, noting any medications that may place a client at risk for GI bleeding.

Parasitic infections are also tested by stool samples. Giardiasis is a common parasitic infection that is more common in children than adults and most frequently reported in children 1 to 4 years of age. The *Giardia* parasite attaches itself to the lining of the small intestine, where it disrupts the body's absorption of fats and carbohydrates, resulting in diarrhea (CDC, 2015). Another common childhood infection found in the intestine is a parasitic pinworm infection, which affects millions of people each year. Nurses may instruct parents on specimen collection and on pinworm tape tests to be collected in the home. If stool specimen reveals a parasite or helminth infection, the nurse should explain to the client the social obligation to communicate results to family members in the house and, if the client is a child, the playmates of the child. Box 14.2 provides instructions for pinworm collection.

Nurses may consult the laboratory regarding collecting and testing a stool specimen in order to provide information for the client and family about the number of specimens that will be needed and determine the optimal collection technique and timing of transport.

APPLICATION OF THE NURSING PROCESS

Examples of Related ICNP Nursing Diagnoses, Expected Client Outcomes, and Nursing Interventions:

Nursing Diagnosis: Fluid imbalance

Supporting data: Diarrhea; blood in stool

Expected Client Outcomes: Client will experience a decrease in episodes of diarrhea, as demonstrated by:

- report of soft, formed bowel movements
- adherence to medication regimen prescribed to treat the identified microorganism
- clean and intact perianal skin
- fluid and electrolyte balance.

Nursing Intervention Example: Collect a stool specimen.

Reference: International Classification for Nursing Practice. (n.d.). *eHealth & ICNP*. Retrieved from https://www.icn.ch/what-we-do/projects/ehealth-icnp.

CRITICAL CONCEPTS
Collecting Specimens

Accuracy (ACC)

Accuracy in collecting stool specimens is subject to the following variables:

- client assessment, including menstruation, intake of vitamin C, foods rich in peroxidase, and anticoagulant use prior to obtaining stool specimen for occult blood
- following manufacturer's directions for specimen collection
- separation of urine from stool
- size of sample.

Client-Centered Care (CCC)

When collecting stool specimens, respect for the client is demonstrated by:

- promoting autonomy if client prefers to obtain his or her own stool specimen

---

BOX 14.2 Home Care Considerations: Providing Instructions for Obtaining a Pinworm Specimen

EQUIPMENT
Specimen label
Clean gloves
Pinwheel paddle and tube
Flashlight

PROCEDURE

- Introduce yourself to the client and family and explain the purpose of stool specimen collection. If testing for pinworms in a child, involve the parents or caretakers in the procedure, and explain the step-by-step process.
- Instruct the parents or caregivers in the importance of handwashing. Provide or encourage the parents or caregivers to wear gloves when observing and applying the adhesive tape or pinworm paddle. *Pinworm eggs are microscopic and can survive on surfaces for 2 to 3 weeks.*
- Instruct parents or caregivers that the best time to observe for pinworms is first thing in the morning before bathing or voiding. Use a flashlight to visualize the anus and surrounding areas. Spread the buttocks to visualize the anus. Observe for any worms that are visible to the naked eye. *Adult pinworms are sometimes visible to the naked eye around the anal area.*
- Instruct parents or caregivers to apply the pinworm paddle before the child goes to bed or first thing in the morning. *While the infected person sleeps, the adult pinworms lay their eggs around the anus, causing unrelenting itching at the anal opening. When the client scratches the anal area, the pinworm's eggs are transferred to the client's fingers and then to various surfaces (Centers for Disease Control and Prevention [CDC], 2013).*
- To collect the specimen:
  - Hold the paddle by the cap and remove it from the tube.
  - Spread the buttocks and apply the sticky side of the paddle to several areas around the anal opening.
  - Return the paddle to the tube for transport to a lab.
  - Label the specimen with the client's name and the date and time of specimen collection.

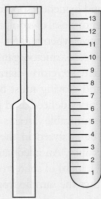

- Instruct parents and caregivers regarding where and when to bring the specimen.

- providing privacy for client and assistance if needed
- arranging for an interpreter, if needed
- honoring cultural preferences regarding this potentially embarrassing procedure and the client's beliefs about cleanliness.

Infection Control (INF)

When collecting stool and parasite specimens, client infection and healthcare-associated infections are prevented by:
- containment of microorganisms and parasites
- preventing and reducing the transfer of microorganisms and parasites
- reducing the number of microorganisms.

Safety (SAF)

Safety measures when collecting stool specimens prevent harm and provide a safe care environment.

Communication (COM)

- Communication exchanges information (oral, written, nonverbal, or electronic) between two or more people.

- Collaborating with the client and other healthcare professionals facilitates proper collection techniques.
- Documentation records information in a permanent legal record.

Health Maintenance (HLTH)

Nursing is dedicated to the promotion of bowel health and self-care abilities during stool specimen collection by:
- teaching the client lifestyle choices, such as hand hygiene and food safety measures, that will reduce the client's risk for GI infections
- supporting health-seeking behaviors, such as educating the client on the importance of medication adherence and on the importance of further testing.

Evaluation (EVAL)

Evaluation of outcomes enables the nurse to determine the efficacy of the care provided.

▪ SKILL 14.7 Collecting a Stool Specimen

EQUIPMENT

Sterile specimen container or formalin transport vial
Specimen label
Clean gloves
Tongue depressor
Bedpan or toilet "hat"

BEGINNING THE SKILL

1. **SAF** Review the order.
2. **CCC** Introduce yourself to the client and family and explain the procedure and purpose of collecting a stool specimen.
3. **SAF** Identify the client using two identifiers.
4. **CCC** Provide privacy to discuss the stool specimen.
5. **COM** Let the client and family know if multiple stool specimens will be collected over several days. Ensure that the client and family understand and will collaborate with the procedure. *When testing for bacteria or parasites and ova, up to three stool specimens over a 1- to 3-day period may be collected because a single specimen can give a negative result.*
6. **INF** Perform hand hygiene and apply clean gloves.

PROCEDURE

7. **ACC** Determine the appropriate container for the type of test and whether the test will be done by the nurse or in the lab.
8. **SAF** Assist the client to the bathroom or bedside commode if able. Otherwise, place the client on the bedpan.
9. **ACC** Instruct the client to void before collecting the stool specimen.
10. **ACC** Place a toilet "hat" in the back of the commode to collect the stool. This allows the urine to fall into the commode and the stool into the container.

11. **ACC** Instruct the client to defecate into the toilet hat. Instruct the client not to contaminate the specimen with urine or toilet paper and to notify you when there is stool in the toilet hat.
12. **CCC** Ensure privacy when defecating. Close the door and pull the curtain.
13. **INF** After the client has stooled, assist the client to perform thorough hand hygiene before assisting the client back to bed. (Note: If you leave the area, remove your gloves, perform hand hygiene, and reapply gloves before contact with the client's hands or stool.)
14. **ACC** Take a sample from two separate areas of the stool with a tongue depressor. *If one area is watery or bloody, choose one sample from that area.*

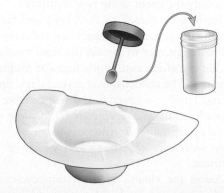

STEP 14 Take a sample from two separate areas of the stool.

15. **ACC** Place the sample into the stool transport vial or specimen container with the sterile tongue depressor, and dispose of the blade as per facility policy. Ensure the specimen container lid is tightly closed. Follow stool transport vial instructions regarding shaking the vial.

Stool transport vials for bacterial pathogens, including for C. diff., may need to be shaken well.

16. **INF** Dispose of the remaining stool in the toilet. Rinse out the toilet hat, or bedpan if used, with cool water. Dispose of the water in the toilet. Store the toilet hat or bedpan per facility policy. *Rinsing reduces the odor of urine and growth of microorganisms.*

FINISHING THE SKILL

17. **INF** Remove gloves and perform hand hygiene.
18. **SAF** Ensure client safety and comfort. Place the bed in the lowest position. Verify that the client can identify and reach the nurse call system. *These safety measures reduce the risk of falls.*
19. **HLTH** Encourage the client to perform thorough hand hygiene after using the toilet and before eating. *Nursing encourages healthy infection control practices to reduce the risk of GI infection.*

20. **COM** Document date and time of stool specimen collection on the label, as per facility policy. Ensure that the specimen label contains two client identifiers. Secure the label to the specimen cup. *The specimen cup is labeled rather than the lid because the lid can be easily separated from the specimen.*
21. **ACC** Transport to the laboratory per agency policy within the time limit or place in a refrigerator. *Many facilities require transportation in a plastic resealing biohazard bag. Depending on the type of laboratory testing ordered, the specimen may need to go to the laboratory immediately or may need to be refrigerated to ensure the accuracy of laboratory results.*
22. **COM** Document assessment of stool characteristics, care given, date and time of specimen collection, and how the client tolerated the procedure in the legal healthcare record.

■ SKILL 14.8 Obtaining a Stool Specimen for Occult Blood

EQUIPMENT

Sterile specimen container or fecal occult blood slide
Developer/buffer solution
Specimen label
Clean gloves
Tongue depressor
Bedpan or toilet "hat"

BEGINNING THE SKILL

1. **SAF** Review the order. Determine facility policy on bedside or laboratory testing for fecal occult blood. Determine the type of fecal occult blood slide available.
2. **INF** Perform hand hygiene.
3. **SAF** Identify the client using two identifiers.
4. **CCC** Introduce yourself to the client and family and explain the purpose of stool specimen collection.
5. **CCC** Provide privacy to discuss the stool specimen.
6. **COM** Let the client and family know if multiple stool specimens will be collected over several days. Ensure the client and family understand and will collaborate with the procedure. *When screening for GI bleeding related to colorectal cancer, testing is recommended over a minimum of 3 days because a single sample may miss bleeding that is intermittent.*
7. **ACC** Assess the client's menstruation cycle, if applicable. Assess recent intake of nonsteroidal antiinflammatory drugs (NSAIDs), vitamin C supplements, citrus fruits, and red meat. *Any blood, such as menstrual blood or bleeding hemorrhoids, may result in a false-positive result. Ingestion of drugs that can result in GI bleeding, peroxidase-rich foods, vitamin C, and animal hemoglobin*

(more than 8 oz of red meat) may result in a false-positive result when using the guaiac test. The fecal immunochemical test is not affected by diet or drugs. Communicate your assessment findings to the healthcare provider to determine if testing for fecal occult blood should be rescheduled.
8. **INF** Apply clean gloves.

PROCEDURE

9. **CCC** Assist the client to the bathroom or bedside commode if able. Otherwise, place the client on the bedpan.
10. **ACC** Instruct the client to void before collecting the stool specimen, if needed.
11. **ACC** Place a clean container in the back of the commode to collect the stool. *This allows the urine to fall into the commode and the stool into the container.*
12. **ACC** Instruct the client to defecate into the container.
13. **ACC** Ensure the specimen is not contaminated with urine or toilet paper.
14. **ACC** Take a sample from two separate areas of the stool. Observe for blood in the stool. If blood is visible in the stool, it may be from hemorrhoids or an anal fissure and not from the intestinal tract. If the lab performs the test, go to step 28.

If Using a Fecal Guaiac Test Slide

15. **AAC** If the test is to be done at the bedside, open the specimen side of the slide.
16. **ACC** Use the tongue depressor to smear a thin layer stool on the window of the slide. Repeat from a separate area of the sample and smear onto the other window of the slide.

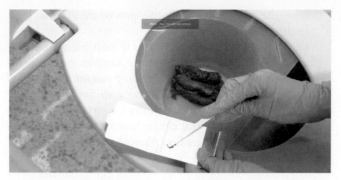

STEP 16 Smear a thin layer of stool on the window of the slide.

17. **ACC** Close the slide and turn the slide over to open the opposite side of the slide.

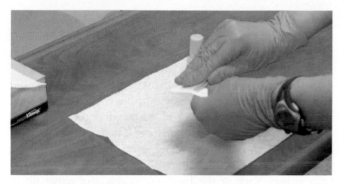

STEP 17 Open the opposite side of the slide.

18. **ACC** Drop 1 to 2 drops of developer solution on the opposite side of where the stool was placed.

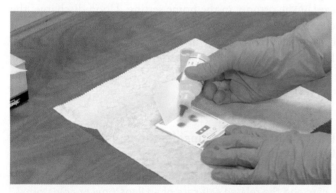

STEP 18 Drop 1 to 2 drops of developer solution.

19. **ACC** Follow package directions for reading results. *Blue indicates a positive result.*

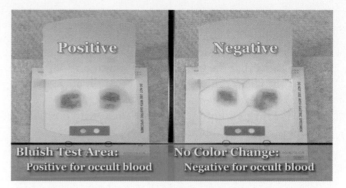

STEP 19 If the area turns blue, it is a positive result.

20. **INF** Dispose of slide as per facility policy

If Using a Fecal Immunochemical Test (FIT) Slide

21. **ACC** If the test is to be done at the bedside, open the specimen side of the slide so that it can lie flat.
22. **ACC** Remove the sample tab from the back of the card by lifting it up from the bottom and pulling it off.
23. **ACC** Use the tab to place a small amount of stool on top of the sample pad, and place the tab blue side down in the slide.
24. **ACC** Add three free-falling drops of the buffer solution to the center of the sample pad.
25. **ACC** Keeping the slide flat on a surface, close the collection slide. Keep the slide flat and wait 5 minutes.
26. **ACC** Read the test results as follows:
    The test is positive for fecal occult blood if there is any trace of pink in the test window.
    The test is negative for fecal occult blood if only the control line is visible and there is no trace of pink in the test line area.
    The test is invalid if the control line does not appear. If this occurs, the test should be repeated.
27. **INF** Dispose of slide as per facility policy. *The collection slide contains fecal matter.*

If the Lab Performs Fecal Occult Blood Testing

28. **INF** If the lab performs the procedure, place the stool in the specimen container with a sterile tongue depressor or facility-specific collection tool. Dispose of collection tool as per facility policy. Replace the lid of the specimen cup. *Stool is a potentially infectious material.*
29. **COM** Ensure specimen label contains two client identifiers. Document date and time of stool specimen collection on the label as per facility policy. Secure the label to the specimen cup. *The specimen cup is labeled rather than the lid because the lid can be easily separated from the specimen.*
30. **ACC** Transport to the laboratory per facility policy within the time limit or place in a refrigerator. *Many facilities require transportation in a plastic resealing biohazard bag. Depending on the type of laboratory testing ordered, the specimen may need to go to the laboratory immediately or may need to be refrigerated to ensure the accuracy of laboratory results.*

FINISHING THE SKILL

31. **INF** Remove gloves and perform hand hygiene.
32. **SAF** Assist the client back to the bed. Ensure client safety. Ensure that the bed is in the lowest position. Ensure that the client can identify and reach the nurse call system. *These safety measures reduce the risk of falls.*
33. **CCC** Provide comfort. Assist the client with positioning and rearrange bedding.
34. **COM** Document assessment of stool characteristics, care given, date and time of specimen collection, and how the client tolerated the procedure in the legal healthcare record.
35. **COM** Follow up with the client if multiple stool specimens have been ordered to verify samples were provided. *When screening for GI bleeding related to colorectal cancer, testing is recommended over a minimum of 3 days.*
36. **HLTH** Instruct the client on the importance of regular screening for colorectal cancer and follow-up based on the stool specimen results. *Nursing supports health-seeking behaviors.*

SECTION 4 Caring for a Client With a Bowel Diversion

An ostomy is a surgical procedure in which an opening is created on the abdomen, usually to allow for the elimination of either urine or feces. Clients with bowel disease may require an ileostomy, colostomy, or cecostomy, all of which allow for a diversion of bowel contents through a stoma (ostomy site). In North America, there are approximately 1 million people living with an ostomy. Additionally, there are approximately 100,000 new ostomy sites surgically created every year (UOAA, 2017) .

The fecal waste excreted from the stoma site is referred to as the effluent. The consistency of the effluent is contingent on the anatomical placement of the stoma as well as the client's food and fluid intake. Because there is no sphincter control at the stoma, a pouching device must always be worn over the stoma site.

The purpose of routinely assessing the stoma of a client with an ileostomy, colostomy, or cecostomy is to ensure adequate blood circulation to the stoma site. A healthy stoma site will be slightly edematous, red, shiny, and moist. Signs of ineffective tissue perfusion to the stoma site include gray, brown, or black stoma discoloration. Stoma discoloration may indicate tissue ischemia and should be reported to the surgeon or authorized healthcare provider immediately. Stomas can be flush with the skin or protruding. Accurate documentation of the anatomical location of the stoma, as well as the stoma's color, shape, and size, is a part of the nurse's assessment. The skin around the stoma, called the peristomal skin, should be dry and intact. The nurse frequently assesses the effluent from the stoma and documents the amount, color, and consistency. As the nurse assesses and cares for the stoma site, it is important to also assess the client's understanding of stoma care and the client's emotional reaction to the stoma.

The emotional response that follows surgery is expected. However, clients recovering from ostomy surgery may react with a wide range of emotions, from disbelief to shock and grief or relief. These responses may be influenced by the client's age and occupation, the type and severity of the disease that prompted the surgery, and the client's cultural beliefs about cleanliness. Due to the stoma formation and effluent collection system, body image is often a priority nursing consideration when caring for a client who has a stoma. Box 14.3 describes cultural considerations for the Islamic faith.

Stoma and ostomy care instruction should begin prior to surgery and continue throughout the entire hospital stay. While performing stoma care in the hospital, the nurse must assess the client's readiness to learn self-care. To enhance client learning about ostomy care, assess the client's learning style, and make educational materials available through multiple venues, such as the Internet, videos, and paper documents. Schedule a consultation with a registered dietitian to teach the client dietary considerations, some of which are identified in Table 14.4. Support from a family member or a support group may help ensure a smooth transition to self-care of the ostomy in the home setting. Upon discharge, the client should know how to contact a support group and an ostomy nurse, or follow-up home care should be arranged. Box 14.4 identifies national ostomy support groups.

BOX 14.3 Cultural Considerations: Islamic Faith and Ostomy Care

Clients practicing the Islamic faith may be averse to stoma care and the related self-care of an ileostomy or colostomy. Muslims adhere to strict rules of cleanliness: impurities, such as feces, are viewed as a barrier to religious practices. For this reason, surgeons have been encouraged to place stomas on the left side of the abdomen to ensure a greater level of fecal containment and regulation. Additionally, Muslims are asked to clean with the left hand after defecation; left-sided stomas are more accessible for left-handed cleaning. Muslims are also encouraged to sleep on their right side; therefore, a left-sided stoma would not pose any restrictions. The literature suggests that Muslim clients would prefer stoma placement on the left side of the abdomen to address the aforementioned considerations (Iqbal, Zaman, & Bowley, 2013).

CARE OF THE STOMA AND PERISTOMAL SKIN

Peristomal moisture-associated skin damage (MASD) is a very common complication clients complain of after the surgical creation of a colostomy or ileostomy (Salvadalena, 2016). MASD is formally defined as "inflammation and erosion of skin due to prolonged exposure to various sources of moisture, including urine, stool, perspiration, wound exudate, mucus, or saliva" (Young, 2017). Prevention of MASD and impending peristomal skin breakdown is accomplished through continuous assessment of the ostomy site for moisture, erythema, maceration, and blister formation; accurate pouching of the stoma; appropriate peristomal skin care; and prevention of pouch leakage. To protect the peristomal skin, the adhesive device should routinely be changed every 3 to 4 days or twice a week. If leakage occurs around the adhesive device, the device must be changed (Piras & Hurley, 2011). Table 14.5 compares considerations in caring for the peristomal site.

When pouching the stoma, appropriate sizing of the adhesive device is imperative to protect the peristomal skin from the effluent. When choosing the type of pouching system, consider the contour of the abdomen, anatomical location of the stoma, and type of stoma. For example, a one-piece precut system may be better for clients with poor vision or dexterity. The two-piece system stays in place for a longer time and may decrease injury to the peristomal skin.

To prevent leakage, the drainable pouch should be emptied when the bag is one-third full. A nondrainable pouch should be emptied when it is one-half full. Change the pouch and adhesive device between meals, when the client will have less effluent. After removal of the pouch and adhesive device, assess the peristomal skin for MASD and skin breakdown, clean the peristomal skin with tap water, and ensure the skin is dry before application of the new adhesive device.

Make sure the new adhesive device completely adheres to the peristomal skin. The device must be cut to fit appropriately (no more than 3 mm [⅛ inch] larger than the stoma). Stoma paste may be used as a barrier to protect any peristomal skin that is not covered by the adhesive device. The paste also helps to create a seal and prevent leakage of the effluent onto the skin. Peristomal skin preparation wipes or sprays help the adhesive device adhere to the skin.

Although colostomies and ileostomies are both abdominal stomas that eliminate stool, they differ in the consistency and amount of effluent eliminated from the stoma; this is due to the anatomical placement of the stoma. Colostomies may need to be irrigated to stimulate peristalsis, prevent or treat constipation, or regulate effluent output. Regulation

TABLE 14.4 Dietary Considerations With an Ileostomy and Colostomy

Foods That Promote Gas Formation	Foods That Cause Odor	Foods That May Cause Obstruction
Beans, cabbage, and onions Milk and cheese Foods high in fat Beer and carbonated beverages Cauliflower and cucumbers	Eggs Fish Garlic and onions Asparagus, broccoli, and cabbage Alcohol Baked beans Strong cheese	Nuts and seeds Popcorn Raw vegetables, especially corn (whole kernel) and celery Foods with skins, (apple peel) dried fruits Oranges, pineapple, coconut

Modified from: Goldberg, 2016.

BOX 14.4 Ostomy Support Groups

Crohn's and Colitis Foundation of America (CCFA): http://www.ccfa.org/

Intestinal Disease Education and Awareness Society: http://weneedideas.ca/

Hollister Incorporated: http://www.hollister.com/us/

Lance Armstrong Foundation: http://www.livestrong.org/

United Ostomy Association of America: http://www.ostomy.org/

Wound, Ostomy and Continence Nurses Society: http://www.wocn.org/

TABLE 14.5 Peristomal Skin Care Considerations

Type	Considerations	Nursing Measures
Ileostomy	Difficulty changing pouching system with continuous effluent	Placement of drainage pad or absorbent wick Possible cardboard tube application (Heale, 2013)

Ileostomy or colostomy	Thinning skin of older adults
	Scarring around stoma site and skinfolds may affect appliance adherence.
	Continuous sweating in the summer months may affect appliance adherence.
	Frequent appliance changes can strip away protective epidermal skin layer.
	Assess client for considerations that may lead to poor stoma care adherence:
	  client living alone
	  client avoids assistance
	  frequent exposure to water
	  lack of access to appliance products.
		Remove flange with silicone-based remover.
		Avoid oil- and alcohol-based adhesives and removers.
		Change appliance when leakage is detected.
		Compare peristomal skin to surrounding abdominal skin.
		Clean peristomal area thoroughly.
		With help from a professional, establish routine protocol for ostomy care.
		Teaching points:
		Do not microwave appliance to soften backing.
		Do not reinforce appliance when leaking—change appliance.
		Do not leave pouch off to expose skin area to air for drying.

References: Gray, Colwell, Doughty, Goldberg, Hoeflok, Manson, & Rao, 2013; Young, 2017.

of colostomy effluent can occur with descending or sigmoid colostomies because the distal stomas have greater water absorption, and the effluent becomes more formed like normal stool.

In contrast, ileostomies generally have a steady flow of liquid effluent through the stoma. They are thus never irrigated. It is very important to maintain peristomal skin integrity in the client with an ileostomy because of the copious proteolytic enzymatic effluent. Because the effluent is liquid, the client is also at an increased risk of dehydration.

During the postoperative period, the registered nurse must assess for stoma and peristomal skin integrity, ensure proper fitting of the pouching system, and evaluate the client's readiness to learn and psychological adjustment to the new stoma and pouching system. Finally, the registered nurse is responsible for conducting client and family teaching of ostomy care. However, assistive personnel may empty and record the effluent output per facility policy.

IRRIGATING A COLOSTOMY

Clients with a sigmoid or descending colostomy have the option of managing their stool output using irrigation. Colostomy irrigation is instilling tap water into the stoma and then allowing the tap water to come back out, expelling any stool that was present in the colon in the process. Although performing a colostomy irrigation may take up to an hour, many people prefer controlling the stool output and therefore not having any stool in a pouch. With colostomy irrigation, the client may wear only a stoma cap between irrigations to manage flatulence and mucus. Colostomy irrigation may be performed every day or every other day (Carmel, 2016).

CECOSTOMY

The purpose of a cecostomy is to administer irrigation solution to promote fecal elimination or decompress the distal colon in an emergency situation. In children, a cecostomy tube (C-tube) is surgically inserted into the cecum so the client can instill solution to irrigate and empty the bowel, via the anus, while sitting on the toilet. This procedure was developed in the 1990s to treat unresolved constipation resulting from disease processes that alter emptying of the large intestine, such as myelomeningocele, anorectal malformations, and Hirschsprung disease (Sockett, 2013).

To achieve a routine bowel elimination program, the child sits on the toilet while the instilled solution flushes the large intestine. The C-tube is flushed daily to maintain patency. If the C-tube becomes clogged, the client may experience leakage around the tube insertion site. The C-tube has a button on the end, at the abdominal skin level, to close the system. To maintain skin integrity, the nurse should clean around the C-tube insertion site with warm water and allow the area to dry thoroughly. Table 14.6 shows pediatric lifespan considerations, including considerations for cecostomy.

TABLE 14.6 Pediatric Considerations in Ostomy Care

	Pediatric Considerations	Nursing Measures
Infant and toddler	Severe fecal incontinence is usually diagnosed in toddler years. The client may have an anorectal malformation or childhood gastrointestinal disease process causing fecal incontinence.	Need for involved parent teaching and support if child has a cecostomy tube inserted. C-tubes must be replaced annually. Parental assessment of C-tube insertion site for infection and overgrowth is necessary. Dietary and irrigation adjustments are needed to provide client-centered care. Client growth and development warrant ongoing adjustment for parents to transition youth to care for C-tube.
Preschool and school age	With socialization, children are exposed to communicable intestinal diseases, such as *Giardiasis* and pinworms.	When collecting a stool specimen from an infant, line the back half of the diaper with plastic wrap. If child experiences continuous diarrhea or anal itching, obtain a stool sample, or observe for pinworm activity while the child sleeps.
12–18 years	Physical changes cause intense feelings regarding body image. Physical development leads to introspection and physical comparisons to peer group. Physical appearance is highly valued. Intimacy and sexual exploration may occur. Need for autonomy—client should begin to assume care of ostomy. Chronic disease may slow the maturation process.	Recognize that client and family are a unique unit. When talking with client, consider all respectfully expressed feelings from client. Listen more than you speak. Certain phrases will help facilitate client–nurse communication—for example, "Other teens have shared with me that ... Is that something you are wondering about?" Including client in decisions related to ostomy care: set up appliance change schedule. Role-play social situations client may experience to help with socialization. Facilitate ostomy peer-to-peer support. Share websites for social networking: Intestinal Disease Education and Awareness Society Crohn's and Colitis Foundation of America (CCFA) My Child Has an Ostomy United Ostomy Association Children's Hospital of Boston Reach Out for Youth With Ileitis and Colitis, Inc. The Pediatric Ostomy Care Best Practices for Clinicians

References: Mohr, 2012; Sockett, 2013.

APPLICATION OF THE NURSING PROCESS

Examples of Related ICNP Nursing Diagnoses, Expected Client Outcomes, and Nursing Interventions:

Nursing Diagnosis: Risk for imbalanced fluid volume

Supporting Data: Client has a recent ileostomy.

Expected Client Outcomes: Client will maintain hydration, as demonstrated by:

- intake of 64 to 96 ounces per day, if not contraindicated
- vital signs within the established parameters
- urine output greater than 0.5 mL/kg/hour
- verbalized understanding of relationship between fluid loss from ileostomy effluent and need for hydration
- balanced oral intake as related to effluent
- measurement of effluent on a daily basis and regulation of fluid intake accordingly
- verbalization of the need to weigh and record weight daily.

Nursing Intervention Example: Instruct the client, and the client's family if appropriate, on the knowledge and skills needed to maintain balanced fluid volume.

Reference: International Classification for Nursing Practice. (n.d.). *eHealth & ICNP.* Retrieved from https://www.icn.ch/what-we-do/projects/ehealth-icnp.

CRITICAL CONCEPTS
Caring for a Client With a Bowel Diversion

Accuracy (ACC)

Accuracy in caring for a client with a bowel diversion is subject to the following variables:

- proper client positioning
- identification of anatomical landmarks of stoma site
- assessment of abdomen, peristomal skin, stoma site, and pouching system
- assessment and measurement of effluent output to ensure balanced hydration status
- preparation and placement of catheter in colostomy stoma for irrigation.

Client-Centered Care (CCC)

Respect for the client when caring for a client with a bowel diversion is demonstrated by:

- promoting client autonomy and self-esteem by assessing client's readiness to learn ostomy care

- ensuring privacy and confidentiality when assisting client in maintaining a position conducive to pouching or irrigating an ostomy
- honoring cultural preferences for sensitive aspects of ostomy care
- arranging for an interpreter, if needed
- assessing client's readiness for family involvement with stoma care.

Infection Control (INF)

When caring for a client with a bowel diversion, client infection and healthcare-associated infections are prevented by:

- containment of microorganisms and effluent
- preventing and reducing the transfer of microorganisms
- reducing the number of microorganisms
- maintaining peristomal skin integrity

Safety (SAF)

When caring for a client with a bowel diversion, safety measures prevent harm and provide a safe care environment.

Communication (COM)

- Communication exchanges information (oral, written, nonverbal, or electronic) between two or more people.
- Collaborating with the client and other healthcare providers is essential to achieve proper care for a client with a bowel diversion.
- Documentation records information in a permanent legal record.

Health Maintenance (HLTH)

Nursing care when caring for a client with a bowel diversion is dedicated to the promotion of health and self-care abilities, including:

- assessing the client's readiness to learn self-care of the ostomy site
- assisting the client with self-care of the ostomy site
- ensuring a proper return demonstration of self-care procedures for ostomy care
- protecting the client's peristomal skin area
- assessing the client's knowledge of dietary items to avoid with his or her respective ostomy site (see Table 14.5)
- securing contact information for a local ostomy support group.

Evaluation (EVAL)

Evaluation of outcomes enables the nurse to determine the efficacy of the care provided.

■ SKILL 14.9 Pouching a Stoma

EQUIPMENT

Clean gloves
Absorbent pad
Collection container: bedpan, urinal, or graduated cylinder
Washcloth
Scissors with a pointed end

Ostomy measuring guide
Tissue or toilet paper
New pouch, skin barrier, and adhesive
Pouch closure device, such as a clamp
Stoma paste (optional)
Skin preparation

BEGINNING THE SKILL

1. **SAF** Review the order.
2. **INF** Perform hand hygiene.
3. **CCC** Introduce yourself to the client and explain the procedure and purpose for pouching the stoma. Ensure that the client gives verbal consent for the procedure.
4. **SAF** Identify the client using two identifiers.
5. **CCC** Provide privacy: close the door and pull the curtain.
6. **INF** Apply clean gloves.
7. **ACC** Assess the stoma site. Observe for leakage. Observe the abdomen for distention, listen for bowel sounds, and palpate the abdomen gently. *To establish a baseline assessment.*

PROCEDURE

8. **SAF** Set up an ergonomically safe space. Raise the bed to a comfortable working height. Raise one side rail. Set up a workspace according to where the stoma is located. Stand on the side of the bed closest to the stoma. *Setting up an ergonomically safe space prevents injury to the nurse and client.*
9. **ACC** Place the head of the bed in the horizontal position and position the client supine so that no skinfolds occur along the line of the stoma. *Skinfolds could allow the effluent to leak.*
10. **CCC** Place the absorbent pad under the stoma site.
11. **ACC** Determine the type of system, one piece or two pieces. Have the supplies close by.
12. **AAC** If the pouch is drainable, remove the pouch, then remove the clamp and empty the effluent into the collection container. *Save the clamp for reuse.* (Note: Not all pouches are drainable.)

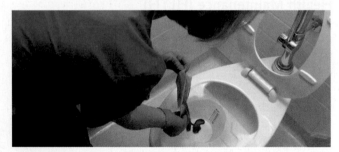

STEP 12. Empty the effluent into the collection container.

13. **AAC** Remove the adhesive appliance with one hand, beginning at the edge and proceeding in toward the stoma. At the same time, use the other hand to hold tension on the skin in the opposite direction of the pull.

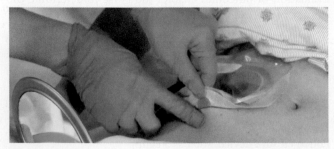

STEP 13 Apply tension on the skin, pushing away from the appliance.

14. **INF** Dispose of the old pouch and adhesive appliance as per facility policy. Instruct the client to dispose of effluent in the toilet when providing self-care at home.
15. **HLTH** Assess the stoma and the peristomal skin for MASD and potential breakdown.
16. **HLTH** Cleanse the stoma and surrounding skin with warm water. Allow the area to dry. *Using soap on the peristomal skin is not recommended because it is too drying.*
17. **ACC** Measure the size of the stoma using the stoma measuring guide or a previously used cut template or by measuring the stoma from side to side to approximate the stoma circumference.

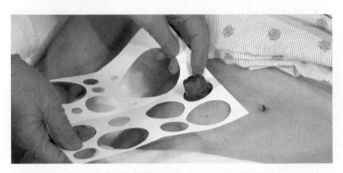

STEP 17 Use the stoma measuring guide to identify the size of the stoma.

18. **INF** Place a clean 4 × 4 or washcloth over the stoma while preparing the appliance to prevent effluent from leaking onto the skin.
19. **INF** Remove gloves and wash hands.
20. **ACC** Trace the size of the opening onto the back of the new adhesive appliance.

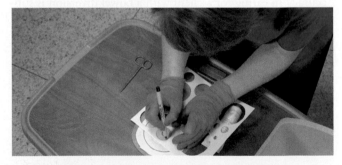

STEP 20 Trace the size and shape of the measured opening.

21. **ACC** Cut the opening approximately 1.5 to 3 mm (1/16 to 1/8 inch) larger than the measured opening.

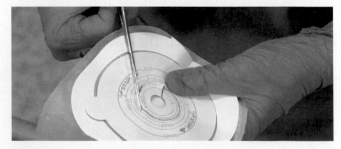

STEP 21 Cut the opening approximately 1.5 to 3 mm (1/16-1/8 inch) larger than the measured opening.

22. **INF** Apply clean gloves.
23. **ACC** Remove the 4 × 4 or washcloth.
24. **HLTH** Apply ostomy skin care protectants or paste at this time and allow to dry.

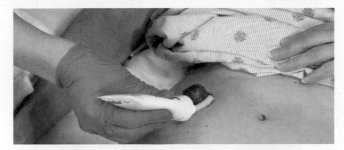

STEP 24 Apply ostomy skin care protectants or paste.

25. **ACC** Peel the paper off the back of the adhesive appliance.
26. **ACC** Center the appliance over the stoma and press down gently. Ask the client to tighten the abdominal muscles or push out against your pressing motion.
27. **ACC** Hold the appliance for 30 to 60 seconds to activate the adhesive.

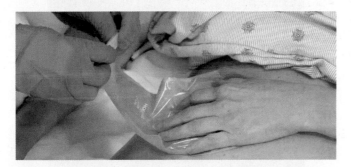

STEP 27 Hold the appliance to activate the adhesive.

28. **ACC** When the appliance is sealed, attach the bag following the manufacturer's instructions.
- If using a one-piece pouch, make sure the bag is pointed toward the client's feet. *To assist with emptying the pouch.*

- If using a two-piece system, place the adhesive appliance on first.
- For an open-ended pouch, fold the end of the pouch over the clamp and close the clamp, listening for a "click" to ensure it is secure.

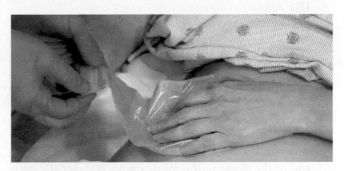

STEP 28 Close the end of the bag with clip or Velcro closure.

FINISHING THE SKILL

29. **INF** Dispose of the used supplies.
30. **INF** Remove gloves and perform hand hygiene.
31. **SAF** Ensure client safety and comfort. Place the bed in the lowest position. Verify that the client can identify and reach the nurse call system. *These safety measures reduce the risk of falls.*
32. **COM** Document date, time of procedure, stoma site characteristics, peristomal skin area, effluent characteristics and amount, client education provided, and how the client tolerated the procedure in the legal healthcare record.
33. **COM** Provide follow-up care by educating the client to monitor for leaking around the appliance and report any leakage immediately.
34. **HLTH** Encourage the client to participate in ostomy care. Observe the client demonstrate self-care before discharge.

■ SKILL 14.10 Irrigating an Ostomy

EQUIPMENT

Clean gloves
Washcloth
Ostomy irrigation system
Stoma cone
Irrigation sleeve
Water-soluble lubricant
New pouch or stoma cap

BEGINNING THE SKILL

1. **SAF** Review the order.
2. **INF** Perform hand hygiene.
3. **CCC** Introduce yourself to the client and explain the purpose of irrigating the stoma. Use this opportunity to educate the client and family members, if appropriate, concerning the need for and procedure involved in routine irrigation for a bowel training regime.

4. **SAF** Identify the client using two identifiers.
5. **ACC** Assess the stoma site. Observe for leakage. Observe the abdomen for distention, listen for bowel sounds, and palpate the abdomen gently. *To establish a baseline assessment.*
6. **INF** Apply clean gloves.
7. **CCC** Provide privacy; close the door and pull the curtain.

PROCEDURE

8. **SAF** If the client is mobile, assist the client to the bedside commode or toilet for the ostomy irrigation procedure. Ensure proper footwear for the client when getting out of bed to perform colostomy irrigation. Have the client sit on the toilet or bedside commode. Place the end of the sleeve in the toilet. *Proper footwear is a safety measure to reduce the risk of falls.*
9. **SAF** If the client is in the bed, set up an ergonomically safe space. Raise the bed to a comfortable working height. Raise one side rail. Place the head of bed in the horizontal position and position the client supine to flatten out any skin folds occurring along the line of the stoma. Set up a workspace according to where the stoma is located. Stand on the side of the bed closest to the stoma. Have the supplies close by.
10. **CCC** Place the absorbent pad under the stoma site.
11. **ACC** Determine the type of system, one piece or two pieces.
12. **INF** If the pouch is drainable, remove the clamp and empty the effluent into the toilet, bedside commode, or collection container. *Save the clamp for reuse.* (Note: Not all pouches are drainable.)
13. **ACC** If it is a one-piece system, remove the pouch and adhesive device. Remove the adhesive appliance with one hand, beginning at the top and proceeding in a downward direction. At the same time, use the other hand to hold tension on the skin in the opposite direction of the pull. If it is a two-piece system, remove the pouch.
14. **INF** Dispose of the old pouch (two-piece system), or dispose of the pouch and adhesive appliance (one-piece system), as per facility policy.
15. **HLTH** Assess the stoma and the peristomal skin for MASD and potential breakdown.
16. **ACC** Attach the irrigation sleeve to the adhesive device or secure the belt. *A one-piece sleeve requires a belt to create a watertight seal.* With a two-piece system, attach the irrigator sleeve to the adhesive device.
17. **SAF** Fill the bag with 500 to 1000 mL of lukewarm water (38°C–40° C [100°F–105°F]). **WARNING:** Do not microwave the solution. *Hot solution can cause bowel damage. Cold solution can cause abdominal cramping.*

18. **ACC** Hang the bag from the IV pole with the clamp closed.
19. **AAC** Open the clamp slowly, allowing the solution to prime the tubing. *Allowing air into the bowel will cause cramping.*
20. **ACC** Open the top of the irrigator sleeve.
21. **ACC** Through the opened top of the irrigator sleeve, place the lubricated irrigator cone into the stoma. *Lubricating the cone of the irrigation system will ease insertion and decrease discomfort.*

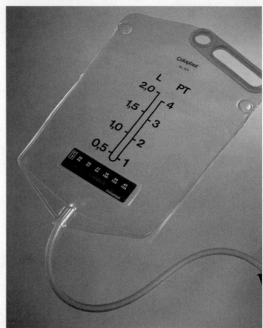

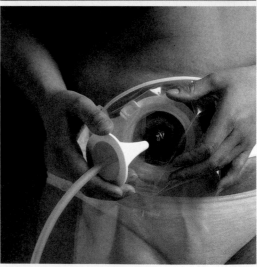

STEP 21 Place the lubricated irrigator cone into the stoma.

22. **ACC** Hold the cone in place with one hand and open the clamp of the irrigation system to begin the flow.

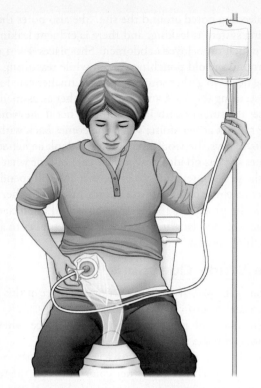

STEP 22 Hold the cone in place with one hand, and open the clamp of the irrigation system to begin the flow.

23. **ACC** To begin the instillation, remove the bag from the IV pole and lower to the level of the client's hip, and then unclamp the tubing. *The level of the bag determines the speed of the flow.*

24. **AAC** Slowly raise the bag to approximately 30 to 45 cm (12–18 inches) above the stoma to slowly increase the gravitational flow into the intestines.

25. **CCC** Continuously monitor the client for discomfort. If the client complains of cramping, the bag may be lowered to slow the flow of the solution.

26. **AAC** After the correct amount of solution is instilled, clamp the tubing, remove the cone, and close the top of the irrigation sleeve. (Note: The results [solution and stool] will flow out of the stoma, down the sleeve, and into the toilet.)

27. **ACC** When the bowel is empty (contents will be the color of light tea and contain no solid residue), remove the irrigator sleeve and set aside. *It may take 30 to 45 minutes for the bowel to empty.*

28. **ACC** To reapply the ostomy pouch, center the appliance over the stoma and press down gently. *Hold the appliance for 30 to 60 seconds to activate the adhesive.*

29. **ACC** When the appliance is sealed, attach the bag following the manufacturer's instructions.

• If using a one-piece pouch, make sure the bag is pointed toward the client's feet.

• If using a two-piece system, place the adhesive appliance on first.

• For an open-ended pouch, fold the end of the pouch over the clamp and close the clamp, listening for a "click" to ensure that it is secure.

FINISHING THE SKILL

30. **INF** Dispose of the used supplies.

31. **INF** Remove gloves and perform hand hygiene.

32. **SAF** Assist the client back to the bed if client has been on a toilet or commode chair. Ensure client safety. Ensure that the bed is in the lowest position. Ensure that the client can identify and reach the nurse call system. *These safety measures reduce the risk of falls.*

33. **CCC** Provide comfort. Assist the client with positioning and rearrange bedding.

34. **COM** Document date, time of procedure, client education provided, how the client tolerated the procedure, and characteristics and amount of return in the legal healthcare record.

Follow-up

35. **COM** Educate the client concerning routine irrigation for a bowel training regime.

36. **HLTH** Facilitate the client's connection with an ostomy support group (see Box 14.4).

37. **HLTH** Consult a registered dietitian to assist the client in selecting recommended dietary items (see Table 14.5).

38. **HLTH** Observe the client perform a return demonstration of irrigating the ostomy.

■CASE STUDY

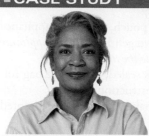

Joyce Harris, a 68-year-old African American female, presents to her healthcare provider with complaints of feeling bloated and constipated for the past 6 weeks. Joyce reports that she sometimes goes for 5 days without having a bowel movement. Until 2 months ago, Joyce has had regular bowel movements once a day. Presently, Joyce reports that her stool is hard and that she sometimes sees blood in the toilet and on the toilet paper. She also reports occasional pain (5/10) in the left upper quadrant (LUQ) and left lower quadrant (LLQ) of her abdomen. The healthcare provider orders blood work, stool for occult blood, and a colonoscopy.

After the colonoscopy is completed, Joyce meets with the healthcare provider to discuss the results from her procedure. A 4.5-cm tumor was noted at the junction between the descending and sigmoid colon; a tissue biopsy was obtained during the procedure. Seven days later, the pathology report showed a poorly differentiated adenocarcinoma of the colon. Resection surgery is scheduled with the possible creation of a sigmoid colostomy.

One month later, Joyce has surgery to resect her sigmoid colon tumor. The tumor was resected from the descending and sigmoid colon, but there was extensive penetration through the colon wall throughout the mesentery and into the peritoneal membrane; abdominal lymph nodes were biopsied during surgery. A colostomy was created, and Joyce is returned to the surgical floor following colon resection with the creation of descending colostomy.

Sue is the nurse caring for Joyce on her fourth day after colon resection with the creation of a left-sided, mid-abdominal descending colostomy. During report, she is told that Joyce will be discharged tomorrow and that the nurses have been assuming full care of the colostomy. It is reported that Joyce has refused to even look at her stoma site and has not been receptive to any teaching. Sue obtains morning vital signs and conducts a morning assessment. Upon assessment of the stoma, she notes a swollen, red stoma with some bleeding noted around the site. She also notes that the pouching system is leaking, and there is effluent leaking out of the pouch onto Joyce's abdomen. She places 4 × 4 gauze pads around the old pouching system while reassuring Joyce that she needs to gather some supplies to further care for her. While securing the 4 × 4 and completing her assessment, she discusses the surgery with Joyce and asks her if she would be willing to look at her stoma when she comes back with supplies. Joyce says she would be willing to look at her stoma, but states she has no idea how to take care of it or what to do when she gets home. Sue tells Joyce that she will spend time with her teaching her about stoma care and helping her work through the procedure. Joyce says she would appreciate the help and calls her daughter on the phone to ask her to attend the teaching session.

Case Study Questions

1. What is the priority nursing action for Joyce at this time? What are the critical assessments?
2. What care will the nurse provide for Joyce when she returns with the supplies?
3. Why do you think Joyce was receptive to the nurse's request to teach her about her colostomy and the related care?
4. **Application of QSEN Competencies:** One of the Quality and Safety Education for Nurses (QSEN) skills for Patient-Centered Care (which we call client-centered care) is to "Provide care with sensitivity and respect for the diversity of human experience" (Cronenwett et al., 2007). Can the nurse providing care for Joyce Harris know exactly what she is experiencing? How can the nurse demonstrate sensitivity and respect for Joyce's experience?
5. List the components of the teaching plan for Joyce to assume care of her colostomy.
6. What is the priority teaching point for Joyce? What are the critical assessments?
7. Discuss the rationale for colostomy irrigation. Do you think Joyce will need to do colostomy irrigations? If so, why?
8. Can any of Joyce's immediate care be delegated to assistive personnel?

■ CONCEPT MAP

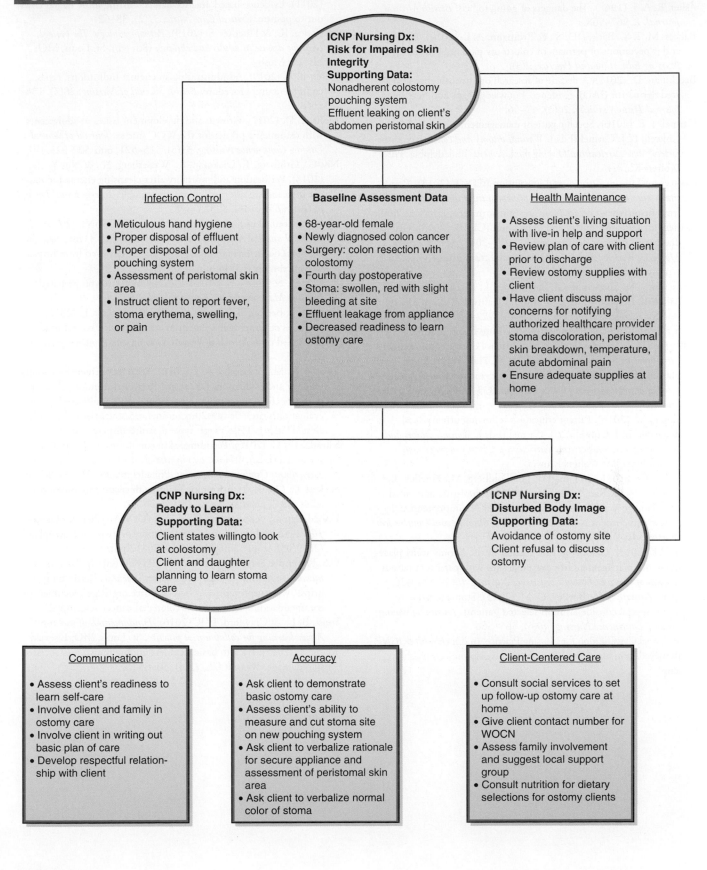

ICNP Nursing Dx:
Risk for Impaired Skin Integrity
Supporting Data:
Nonadherent colostomy pouching system
Effluent leaking on client's abdomen peristomal skin

Infection Control

- Meticulous hand hygiene
- Proper disposal of effluent
- Proper disposal of old pouching system
- Assessment of peristomal skin area
- Instruct client to report fever, stoma erythema, swelling, or pain

Baseline Assessment Data

- 68-year-old female
- Newly diagnosed colon cancer
- Surgery: colon resection with colostomy
- Fourth day postoperative
- Stoma: swollen, red with slight bleeding at site
- Effluent leakage from appliance
- Decreased readiness to learn ostomy care

Health Maintenance

- Assess client's living situation with live-in help and support
- Review plan of care with client prior to discharge
- Review ostomy supplies with client
- Have client discuss major concerns for notifying authorized healthcare provider stoma discoloration, peristomal skin breakdown, temperature, acute abdominal pain
- Ensure adequate supplies at home

ICNP Nursing Dx:
Ready to Learn
Supporting Data:
Client states willingto look at colostomy
Client and daughter planning to learn stoma care

ICNP Nursing Dx:
Disturbed Body Image
Supporting Data:
Avoidance of ostomy site
Client refusal to discuss ostomy

Communication

- Assess client's readiness to learn self-care
- Involve client and family in ostomy care
- Involve client in writing out basic plan of care
- Develop respectful relationship with client

Accuracy

- Ask client to demonstrate basic ostomy care
- Assess client's ability to measure and cut stoma site on new pouching system
- Ask client to verbalize rationale for secure appliance and assessment of peristomal skin area
- Ask client to verbalize normal color of stoma

Client-Centered Care

- Consult social services to set up follow-up ostomy care at home
- Give client contact number for WOCN
- Assess family involvement and suggest local support group
- Consult nutrition for dietary selections for ostomy clients

References

Asher, R. A. J. (1947). The dangers of going to bed. *British Medical Journal, 2*, 967–968.

Backes, M. T. S., Backes, D. S., & Erdmann, A. L. (2012). Feelings and expectations of permanent colostomy patients. *Journal of Nursing Education and Practice, 2*(3).

Beeckman, D. (2017). A decade of research on incontinence-associated dermatitis (IAD): Evidence, knowledge gaps and next steps. *Journal Tissue Viability, 26*(1), 47–56.

Carmel, J. E. (2016). Specific patient management issues. In J. Colwell, & J. Carmel (Eds.), *Wound, ostomy and continence nurses society™ core curriculum: Ostomy management*. Philadelphia, PA: Wolters Kluwer.

Centers for Disease Control and Prevention (CDC). (2013). *Parasites—enterobiasis (also known as pinworm infection)*. Retrieved from http://www.cdc.gov/parasites/pinworm/gen_info/faqs.html.

Centers for Disease Control and Prevention (CDC). (2015). Giardiasis surveillance—United States, 2011–2012. *Morbidity and Mortality Weekly Report, 64*(3). Retrieved from https://www.cdc.gov/mmwr/pdf/ss/ss6403.pdf.

Cronenwett, L., Sherwood, G., Barnsteiner, J., Disch, J., Johnson, J., Mitchell, P., ... & Warren, J. (2007). Quality and safety education for nurses. *Nursing Outlook, 55*(3), 122–131. Retrieved from http://qsen.org/competencies/pre-licensure-ksas/.

Gallagher, D. L., & Harding, M. M. (2017). Lower gastrointestinal problems. In S. Lewis, L. Bucher, M. M. Heikemper, & M. Harding (Eds.), *Medical-surgical nursing: Assessment and management of clinical problems* (10th ed.) (pp. 833–853). St. Louis, MO: Elsevier.

Goldberg, M. (2016). Patient education following urinary/fecal diversion. In J. Colwell, & J. Carmel (Eds.), *Wound, ostomy and continence nurses society core curriculum: Ostomy management*. Philadelphia PA: Wolters Kluwer.

Gray, M., Colwell, J. C., Doughty, D., Goldberg, M., Hoeflok, J., Manson, A., & Rao, S. (2013). Peristomal moisture-associated skin damage in adults with fecal ostomies: A comprehensive review and consensus. *Journal of Wound, Ostomy, and Continence Nursing, 40*(4), 389–399.

Heale, M. (2013). Cardboard tube technique for ostomy wafer placement and management of peristomal skin with persistent output. *Journal of Wound Ostomy Continence Nursing, 40*(4), 424–426.

Iqbal, F., Zaman, S., & Bowley, D. M. (2013). Stoma location requires special consideration in selected patients. *Journal of Wound Ostomy Continence Nursing, 40*(6), 565–566.

International Classification for Nursing Practice. (n.d.). *eHealth & ICNP*. Retrieved from https://www.icn.ch/what-we-do/projects/ehealth-icnp.

Makic, M. B. F., VonRueden, K. T., Rauen, C. A., & Chadwick, J. (2011). Evidence-based practice habits: Putting more sacred cows out to pasture. *Critical Care Nurse, 31*(2), 38–62.

McCance, K., & Huether, S. (2019). *Pathophysiology: The biologic basis for disease in adults and children* (8th ed.). St. Louis, MO: Elsevier Mosby.

Mitchell, A. (2019). Administrating an enema: Indications, types, equipment and procedure. *British Journal of Nursing, 28*(3). 154-156.

Mohr, L. D. (2012). Growth and development issues in adolescents with ostomies: a primer for the WOC nurses. *Journal of Wound Ostomy Continence Nursing, 39*(5), 515–521, quiz 522-523.

Niv, G., Grinberg, T., Dickman, R., Wasserberg, N., & Niv, Y. (2013). Perforation and mortality after cleansing enema for acute constipation are not rare but are preventable. *International Journal of General Medicine, 6*, 323–328.

National Council of State Boards of Nursing (NCSBN). (2019). *NCSBN and the American Nurses Association (ANA) issue new Joint National Guidelines for nursing delegation*. Retrieved from https://www.ncsbn.org/13546.htm.

Piras, S. E., & Hurley, S. (2011). Ostomy care: Are you prepared? *Nursing Made Incredibly Easy, 9*(5), 46–48.

Pittman, J., Beeson, T., Terry, C., Kessler, W., & Kirk, L. (2012). Methods of bowel management in critical care: A randomized controlled trial. *Journal of Wound, Ostomy, and Continence Nursing, 39*(6), 633–639.

Robson, K. M., & Lembo, A. J. (2018). Fecal incontinence in adults: etiology and evaluation. *UpToDate*. Retrieved from http://www.uptodate.com/contents/fecal-incontinence-in-adults-etiology-and-evaluation?search=fecal%20incontinence&source=search_result&selectedTitle=1~150&usage_type=default&display_rank=1.

Salvadalena, G. (2016). Peristomal skin conditions. In J. Colwell, & J. Carmel (Eds.), *Wound, ostomy and continence nurses society™ core curriculum: Ostomy management*. Philadelphia PA: Wolters Kluwer.

Sockett, C. (2013). Transitioning youth with cecostomy tubes to adult care. *Canadian Nurse, 109*(3), 20–21.

United Ostomy Associations of America (UOAA). (2017). *Ostomy 101*. Retrieved from https://www.ostomy.org/wp-content/uploads/2019/03/ostomy_infographic_20170812.pdf.

U.S. Preventive Services Task Force (USPSTF). (2019). *Final recommendation statement: Colorectal cancer: Screening*. Retrieved from https://www.uspreventiveservicestaskforce.org/Page/Document/RecommendationStatementFinal/colorectal-cancer-screening2.

Yoost, B. L., & Crawford, L. R. (2016). *Fundamentals of nursing: Active learning for collaborative practice*. St. Louis, MO: Elsevier.

Young, T. (2017). Back to basics: Understanding moisture-associated skin damage. *Wounds UK, 13*(4), 56–65.

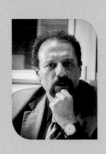

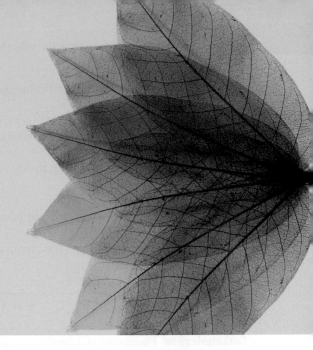

CHAPTER 15

Urine Elimination

"All that is gold does not glitter." | **J. R. R. Tolkien (*The Lord of the Rings*, 1954)**

LEARNING OBJECTIVES

By the end of this chapter, the reader will be able to:

1 Measure and record intake and urine output.

2 Measure a specific gravity.

617

3 Measure chemical properties of urine by dipstick analysis.
4 Measure urine volume with a bladder scanner.
5 Obtain a urine specimen from a closed urinary drainage system.
6 Obtain a urine specimen using the clean-catch method.
7 Obtain a 24-hour urine specimen.
8 Obtain a bagged urine specimen from an infant or child.
9 Insert and remove a straight catheter in a male client.

10 Insert and remove a straight catheter in a female client.
11 Insert an indwelling Foley catheter in a male client.
12 Insert an indwelling Foley catheter in a female client.
13 Remove an indwelling catheter.
14 Provide nursing care to male and female clients with indwelling catheters.
15 Perform intermittent closed bladder irrigation.
16 Perform continuous closed bladder irrigation.
17 Provide suprapubic catheter care.
18 Change a noncontinent ileal conduit pouch and wafer.
19 Catheterize and irrigate a urostomy.

TERMINOLOGY

Anuria Lack of urine production.
Bacteriuria Bacteria in the urine.
Catheterization Placement of a sterile tube (catheter) into a vessel or body cavity.
Continent Ability to maintain sphincter control of either urine or feces.
Dehydration Condition resulting from loss of body fluid when output of fluid is greater than intake of fluid.
Distention Swelling in size due to increased volume in an organ or vessel.
Diuresis Increased production of urine.
Dysuria Painful urination.
Foley catheter An indwelling urinary catheter with a balloon that is inflated in the bladder, keeping the catheter in place.
Genitourinary Having to do with the genitals and urinary systems.
Glycosuria Glucose present in urine.
Hematuria Blood present in urine.
Hydrometer Instrument used to measure specific gravity.
Incontinence Inability to maintain sphincter control of either urine or feces.
Indwelling catheter A catheter that is inserted into the bladder and remains in the bladder. The most common indwelling catheter is the Foley catheter.
Irrigation Rinsing or flushing with fluids; may refer to equipment, such as a catheter (urinary), or a cavity or canal of the human body, such as bladder irrigation.
Micturition Voiding or emptying the bladder.
Nocturia Increased production of urine at night.
Noncontinent A stoma without sphincter control of either urine or feces.
Oliguria Decreased production of urine.
Patency State of being open.

Polyuria Increased production of urine.
Pyuria Pus present in urine.
Renal Related to the kidneys.
Sediment The substance that settles at the bottom of a liquid.
Specific gravity The ratio of the weight of a volume compared with an equal volume of water used to determine the concentrations of substances in an aqueous solution (specific gravity of water = 1.000).
Stoma An artificial opening (from the Greek *stoma*, meaning "mouth").
Suprapubic aspiration Aspiration of urine by inserting a needle through the lower abdominal wall into the bladder.
Urethra The canal through which urine from the bladder flows to the outside of the body.
Urinary diversion Alternate method of discharging urine created by surgical intervention.
Urinary tract infection An infection of the urinary tract, including the kidneys, ureters, bladder, and urethra, most commonly the lower urinary system, bladder, and urethra.

ACRONYMS

ADH Antidiuretic hormone
BPH Benign prostatic hyperplasia
CA-ASB Catheter-associated asymptomatic bacteriuria
CAUTI (or CA-UTI) Catheter-associated urinary tract infection
HICPAC Healthcare Infection Control Practices Advisory Committee
I&O Intake and output
IDSA Infectious Diseases Society of America
SP GR Specific gravity
UTI Urinary tract infection

Urine elimination focuses on skills related to the urinary system. Nurses assess the characteristics of urine and urine production, measure urine, collect urine specimens, and assist clients in managing urine elimination. As shown in Fig. 15.1, urine is produced by the kidneys, carried to the bladder through the ureters, and stored in the bladder until discharged out of the body past two sphincters through the urethra.

URINE ELIMINATION

The bladder is the reservoir for urine and consists of a muscular meshwork of three layers of smooth muscle. It can expand to hold between 700 and 1000 mL of urine, although damage occurs to the lining and vasculature of the bladder with excessive distention. The average volume of urine that results in a full

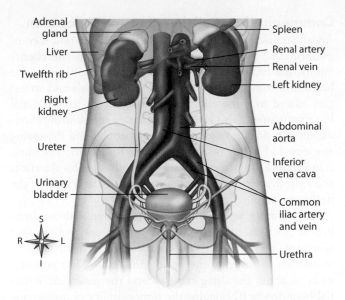

Adrenal gland
Liver
Twelfth rib
Right kidney
Ureter
Urinary bladder
Spleen
Renal artery
Renal vein
Left kidney
Abdominal aorta
Inferior vena cava
Common iliac artery and vein
Urethra

FIG. 15.1 Urine is produced by the kidneys, carried to the bladder through the ureters, and stored in the bladder until discharged out of the body past two sphincters through the urethra.

TABLE 15.1 Terms and Etiologies for Altered Urine Output

Terms	Definition	Etiologies
Dysuria	Painful urination	Inflammation Trauma Infection
Polyuria	Increased urine output without increased fluid intake >2500–3000 mL/24 hours	Untreated diabetes insipidus Hyperglycemia Diuretics, caffeine, and alcohol
Oliguria	Decreased urine output <500 mL/24 hours	Dehydration
Anuria	No urine output <100 mL in 24 hours	Kidney failure
Urgency	Inability to delay voiding voluntarily	Inflammation Infection Psychological stress Incompetent urethral sphincter
Frequency Overactive bladder	Voiding at frequent intervals	Urinary tract infection Pregnancy
Nocturia	Voiding during sleeping hours	Congestive heart failure Benign hypertrophic prostate Pregnancy Consuming caffeine and alcohol before sleep
Glycosuria	Glucose in urine	Diabetes mellitus
Hematuria Gross hematuria—visible Occult hematuria—not visible	Blood in urine	Urinary tract infection Urinary tract tumors Renal calculi Poisoning Trauma
Pyuria	Pus in urine	Urinary tract infection

bladder and the need to void is between 250 and 450 mL, with an average of about 300 mL. When the bladder is empty, the bladder lining falls into folds. The urethra has a flat, ribbon-like shape except when distended with urine while voiding.

Urine has specific characteristics. The color reflects the dilution of the urine: very dilute urine may be a very pale yellow, and very concentrated urine may be dark amber. Specific gravity is a measure of the concentration of particles in the urine, as compared to pure water. The normal specific gravity of urine is a range of 1.005 for very dilute urine to 1.030 for very concentrated urine. Specific gravity is an easy, noninvasive means of measuring hydration. Urine is usually sterile, unless an infection is present. Once urine leaves the body, it does not remain sterile for long. Urine has a distinct odor; however, infection and medications can alter this.

Urine production is vital to healthy body functioning. Measuring hourly urine output enables a rapid determination of impaired urinary elimination. Urine output is an easily measured parameter that reflects aspects of the body's status, including fluid status from hydration to dehydration. The production of urine also reflects perfusion of the kidneys and circulating blood volume; thus, measuring urine output is an indirect means of evaluating whether the cardiovascular system is effectively circulating blood and perfusing the kidneys. Urine output may be altered by many factors, including hormones, medications, pregnancy, and surgery. See Table 15.1 for terms describing urine output and potential etiologies. For example, urine output is directly affected by fluctuations in antidiuretic hormone (ADH), the hormone that controls water reabsorption. Trauma, pain, anesthesia, and opioid drugs increase ADH production, thereby decreasing urine output. Caffeinated beverages, alcohol, and cold temperatures decrease ADH productions and thereby increase urine production, resulting in diuresis.

Impaired Urine Elimination

Urine elimination may be impaired by both acute and progressive changes. Stroke often results in impaired elimination. Estimates are that 33% to 60% of people who recently experienced a stroke and are in an acute care setting and 15% of those at 6 months to 1 year still have signs of impaired urine elimination (Carter, 2018). Other diseases, such as Parkinson disease and multiple sclerosis, are also accompanied by problems with urine elimination. Neurologic conditions such as spinal cord injury and traumatic brain injury result in impaired patterns of elimination. Progressive changes, such as an enlarged prostate, can produce a urinary obstruction that may decrease the volume of urine output for each void, resulting in the need for more frequent voiding. Other types of altered urinary elimination are surgical interventions that change the route by which urine is discharged from the body and dialysis, a procedure that substitutes for the lost filtration capabilities of diseased kidneys.

Infection Control

One of the most important critical concepts related to urine elimination is infection control. The mucous membrane lining the urinary tract is continuous from the urethra to the kidneys and poses no barrier to ascending bacteria. This creates a risk factor for a urinary tract infection (UTI). An additional UTI risk factor for women is that they have a short urethra, averaging 4 cm (1.5 inches) in length. In contrast, the average length of the male urethra is 20 cm (about 8 inches). Nurses prevent the introduction of microorganisms into the urinary tract, thereby helping to prevent UTIs, which are the most frequent type of healthcare-associated infection. UTIs represent a painful burden to the client, as well as additional cost, time of treatment, and length of hospital stay. Nurses use infection control strategies and principles, as well as evidence-based care protocols, to prevent UTIs.

Communication: Collaboration and Delegation

Another critical concept related to urine elimination is communication. The nurse, the client, and often the client's family, the healthcare provider, and other members of the healthcare team must collaborate, sharing goals and strategies related to urine elimination in order to have optimal health outcomes. This is not always easy because urine elimination is a private matter for many people, and discussing any aspect of it may be uncomfortable for clients. The nurse is in a unique and trusted role to be an advocate for the client and help the client understand the language and goals of the healthcare team.

Furthermore, several aspects of care related to urine elimination, such as measuring urine output and collecting a specimen, may be delegated by the registered nurse (RN) to another member of the healthcare team. Clear communication about the delegated task and the results are essential because the RN retains the responsibility to oversee the intervention and outcomes.

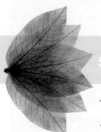

SECTION 1 Collecting Urine Measurements and Specimens

Nurses monitor the client's intake of fluid and output of urine, measure the volume of urine in the bladder, and collect urine specimens for analysis.

ASSESSING PRODUCTION AND VOLUME OF URINE

The rate of urine production provides valuable information about kidney function. It is assessed by measuring and recording the client's fluid intake (oral and intravenous) and his or her urine output (I&O). I&O may be monitored as closely as hourly measurements or at the end of the nursing shift. A comparison of the two measurements can reveal information about the client's fluid balance.

The use of a bladder scanner allows nurses to measure urine within the bladder. A variety of conditions exist where the assessment of the volume of urine in the client's bladder allows healthcare professionals to diagnose a problem or determine the appropriate intervention. Clients may be unable to void or deny the need to void following an epidural. In this instance, measurements may be taken to determine if catheterization is necessary. Measurements are also taken to determine if the client is retaining urine after voiding, referred to as *postvoid residual* urine volume. Table 15.2 shows how measurements of postvoid residual volume can indicate a voiding dysfunction. There are some

limitations to what a bladder scanner can detect via ultrasound. It cannot distinguish urine from other fluids and will measure any fluid that has accumulated in the suprapubic region, including fluid from ascites, a hematoma, or lymphocele. Moreover, it cannot measure a volume greater than 999 mL.

COLLECTING SPECIMENS

Urine specimens are collected by a variety of methods based on the age and medical condition of the client and the type of specimen to be collected. Noninvasive methods for specimen collection include the clean-catch method for adults and a bagged collection from an infant or child. These methods have a greater probability of specimen contamination (from microorganisms on the skin) than invasive methods, such as intermittent catheterization performed by a nurse or suprapubic aspiration

TABLE 15.2 Postresidual Volume Measurements

mL of Urine	Implications
<30–50 mL	Acceptable
50–100 mL	Further evaluation necessary
>200–300 mL	Possible bladder or urethra disorder
>300 mL	Significant urinary retention

Adapted from Asimakopoulos et al., 2016.

performed by an authorized healthcare provider. If the client has an indwelling transurethral catheter, a specimen can be collected from the sampling port but not from the urine collection bag because contamination is likely. See Box 15.1 for an example of a specimen collection error with a bad outcome. The time of day at which the nurse collects a urine specimen varies according to the type of laboratory test. For example, when screening for protein and nitrates, obtaining a specimen from the first void of the morning is helpful because the urine is more concentrated. Timed specimens, such as the 24-hour urine specimen, allow for the analysis of excreted substances over one day. This is particularly helpful if the substance excreted varies over the 24-hour period. The term *random specimen* means the time of day is not important for that laboratory test.

The accuracy of laboratory urine testing can be augmented or negated by the method of specimen collection. A *urine culture* is frequently ordered to diagnose a UTI. Urine culture results are negated if the specimen is contaminated. If at 24 hours the culture has a sufficient number of colony-forming units of one pathogen, then a UTI is likely. If multiple pathogens form, the specimen is most likely contaminated. For children between the ages of 2 months and 2 years, the American Academy of Pediatrics (2016) recommends that a urine specimen for culture be obtained by transurethral catheterization or suprapubic aspiration because the culture of a specimen collected in a pediatric bag is not reliable.

Urinalysis

Urinalysis is another frequently performed laboratory test. Urinalysis screens for a wide range of problems through a physical, chemical, and microscopic examination of urine. See Table 15.3 for information about the components of a urinalysis. For accurate urinalysis, urine samples must be fresh. Refrigeration is often required if the specimen is not immediately delivered to the laboratory. Check with the healthcare facility's laboratory for timing guidelines.

The measurement of the chemical properties of urine is not always done in a laboratory. Nurses may analyze urine at the point of contact. For example, specific gravity is easily measured in the client's bathroom. There are three methods available to nurses. A refractometer is a handheld optical device that requires only a few drops of urine placed on the prism platform. It is then held up to the light, and the nurse reads the specific gravity on a visible scale (Fig. 15.2). A hydrometer consists of two pieces; one is a cylindrical stem with a scale at the top and a weighted bulb at the base, and the second piece is a tall cylindrical container. Urine is poured into the cylindrical container, and the bulb is lowered until it floats. A scale inside the stem allows the nurse to measure where the surface of the urine reaches on the scale.

Another measurement nurses perform at the point of contact is a dipstick analysis of urine for specific gravity analysis, pH, and measurement of compounds, including glucose, protein, ketones, bilirubin, nitrites, and leucocyte esterase. Dipstick analysis is reliable for detecting diabetes mellitus and for ruling out albuminuria (Nguyen, 2017). Dipstick analysis provides very rapid results and has been found very reliable for glucose, nitrites, and blood (Zamanzad, 2009). Dipstick analysis is sometimes used as a screening tool. However, caution must be taken in interpreting results. A positive reagent strip does not always mean a positive urine culture, especially with older adults (Nguyen, 2017). Dipstick analysis is easily performed in an outpatient setting as a screening tool or at home to monitor health status or to evaluate the impact of a therapeutic regime. Performing a dipstick analysis may be delegated to assistive personnel. The RN is responsible for reporting any abnormal results to the healthcare provider. The accuracy of dipstick analysis is dependent on the viability of the reagent test strips. Check the expiration date on the bottle, and always put the lid on securely because the strips react to light and oxygen.

To perform a dipstick analysis of urine:

- Dip reagent strip into a fresh, clean sample of urine, ensuring the reagent pads are covered with urine.
- Check your watch and count the appropriate number of seconds for each of the compounds as identified on the reagent strip label.

BOX 15.1 Lessons From the Courtroom: Urine Sample Collection Error Leads to Misdiagnosis of Renal Bleeding

In a lawsuit in Delaware in 2003, the Superior Court of Delaware upheld a jury verdict in the client's favor for $570,000. In this case, the client visited an emergency room with flank pain and kidney-related complaints. A computed tomography (CT) scan without contrast and a urinalysis were ordered. The intention was for the urinalysis specimen to be obtained by straight catheterization to prevent contamination, but that was not specified. Instead, the nurses collected the specimen by clean catch. The lab analysis showed blood in the urine; however, the authorized healthcare provider, upon learning the sample was obtained via clean catch, assumed the blood was from contamination and not from the kidney. The client was released. When she returned to the emergency room 2 days later, the authorized healthcare provider determined that she had a blood clot in her kidney. In the subsequent surgery, it was determined that the kidney could not be saved, and it was removed.

The jury apportioned the damages as follows: 40% against the hospital for the nurses' negligence and 60% against the authorized healthcare provider for misdiagnosing the client's condition based on the error in urine sample collection by the nurses. This court case illustrates the importance of interprofessional communication to ensure the best care for the client.

Reference: Urine Sample: Misdiagnosis of Renal Bleeding Tied to Nurses' Negligence, 2006.

TABLE 15.3 Urinalysis

Component of Urinalysis	Normal Results	Abnormal Results	Potential Disorders
Color	Clear, pale yellow	Cloudiness, discolored	
pH	4.5–8	<4.5 or >8	Persistent alkalinity or extreme acidity indicates an increased risk of kidney stones.
Specific gravity	1.005	1.030	Elevated—dehydration Very dilute—diabetes insipidus (a pituitary disorder), use of diuretics, chronic renal failure, and excessive water intake
Glucose	Negative for glucose or <130 mg/dL	Positive for glucose	Diabetes mellitus or kidney disease
Ketones (metabolites of fatty acids)	Negative for ketones	Small: <20 mg/dL Moderate: 30–40 mg/dL Large: >80 mg/dL	Diabetes mellitus Persistent diarrhea or fasting
Blood	Negative for hematuria <3 red blood cells (RBCs)	Positive for hematuria	Urinary tract infection, kidney stones, prostatitis, a cancerous process, anticoagulant use, or recent vigorous exercise (e.g., contact sports, marathon running)
Protein	<150 mg/dL		Chronic kidney disease due to damage to the kidney
Nitrite	Negative for nitrites	Positive for nitrites	Urinary tract infection
Leukocyte esterase	Negative for leukocytes	Positive for leukocytes	Urinary tract infection
Bilirubin and urobilirubin	Negative for bilirubin Small amount of urobilirubin (0.5–1 mg/dL)		Liver disorders Hemolytic anemia

Adapted from Lerma & Slivka, 2015.

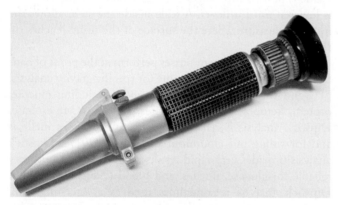

FIG. 15.2 To read a specific gravity with a refractometer, place drops of urine on the prism platform and hold the refractometer up to the light to see the measurement on the scale.

- Hold the reagent strip alongside the bottle and compare the colors of the pads on the reagent strip to the color chart on the reagent strip bottle label.
- Discard the reagent strip and record the results (Fig. 15.3).

APPLICATION OF THE NURSING PROCESS

Examples of Related International Classification for Nursing Practice (ICNP) Nursing Diagnoses, Expected Client Outcomes, and Nursing Interventions:

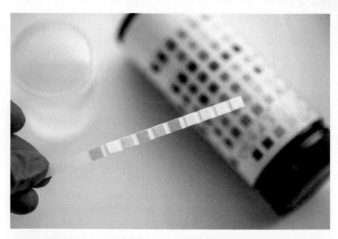

FIG. 15.3 To determine dipstick analysis, hold the reagent strip alongside the bottle and compare the colors of the pads on the reagent strip to the color chart on the reagent strip bottle label.

Nursing Diagnosis: Impaired fluid volume

Expected Client Outcomes: The client will demonstrate an adequate fluid volume, as demonstrated by clear yellow urine with a specific gravity (SP GR) of 1.005 to 1.010.

Nursing Intervention Example: Measure urine output and specific gravity.

Reference: International Classification for Nursing Practice. (n.d.). *eHealth & ICNP.* Retrieved from https://www.icn.ch/what-we-do/projects/ehealth-icnp.

CRITICAL CONCEPTS
Obtaining Urine Measurements and Specimens

Accuracy (ACC)

Urine measurement is subject to the following variables:
- size of the container
- height of the container when reading the volume
- color perception
- lighting
- appropriate entering of client's sex when programming a bladder scanner
- appropriate angle of image when using a bladder scanner
- understanding of procedure by client and family.

Urine specimen collection is subject to the following variables:
- time lapsed from collection
- use of sterile technique
- temperature
- time of voiding
- understanding of procedure by client and family.

Client-Centered Care (CCC)

When measuring urine and collecting urine specimens, respect for the client is demonstrated by:
- promoting autonomy
- providing privacy
- ensuring comfort
- honoring cultural preferences
- arranging for an interpreter, if needed
- advocating for the client and family.

Infection Control (INF)

When measuring urine and collecting urine specimens, healthcare-associated infection is prevented by:

- containment of microorganisms
- preventing and reducing the transfer of microorganisms
- reducing the number of microorganisms.

Safety (SAF)

When measuring urine and collecting urine specimens, safety measures, such as placing the bed in the lowest position, provide a safe care environment and prevent harm to the client.

Communication (COM)

- Communication exchanges information (oral, written, nonverbal, or electronic) between two or more people.
- Documentation records information in a permanent legal record.
- Collaboration with the client, client's family, and members of the healthcare team is essential to obtain accurate urine measurements and to collect uncontaminated urine specimens.
- Delegation of tasks related to obtaining urine measurements and specimens requires clear communication of the task and the outcome.

Health Maintenance (HLTH)

Nursing is dedicated to the promotion of health and self-care abilities when collecting urine specimens, including:
- protecting the client's skin integrity when collecting urine specimens.

Evaluation (EVAL)

Evaluation of outcomes enables the nurse to determine the efficacy and accuracy of the care when measuring urine and collecting urine specimens.

■ SKILL 15.1 Measuring and Recording Intake and Output

EQUIPMENT

Graduated cylinder
Toilet urine "hat" or "nun's cap" (urine measuring device for the toilet)
Antiseptic wipe
Clean gloves
Bedpan or urinal

BEGINNING THE SKILL

1. **INF** Perform hand hygiene.
2. **CCC** Introduce yourself to the client and explain the purpose of keeping an accurate measurement of intake and urine output. Provide privacy, if needed.
3. **SAF** Identify the client using two identifiers.
4. **COM** Determine if the client is voiding or has a transurethral catheter.

PROCEDURE

If Client Is Voiding

5. **ACC** Assess the client's ability to cooperate and follow instructions. If the client is able to cooperate, instruct the client to save all urine and void into either a urinal, bedpan, or toilet "hat."
6. **COM** Instruct the client not to put toilet paper in with the urine.
7. **COM** Instruct the client to try to keep bowel movements and urine separate.

If Client Has a Foley Catheter and Urine Collection Bag

8. **INF** Perform hand hygiene and apply gloves.
9. **INF** If emptying a urine collection bag, ensure drainage collection bag remains below the client's bladder at all time. *Gravity moves the urine to the collection bag; raising the collection bag above the level of the bladder could result in the transfer of urine and microorganisms into the client's bladder.*
10. **INF** Remove the spigot from where it is secured on the drainage bag and unclamp the spigot. Pour urine into a calibrated measuring container, preventing the spigot from touching the calibrated measuring container.

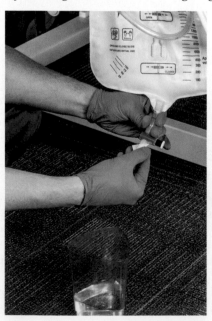

STEP 10 Pour urine into a calibrated measuring container.

11. **INF** Clean the spigot with an antiseptic wipe. Secure the spigot back on the drainage bag. *Cleaning prevents the transfer of microorganisms into the drainage bag.*

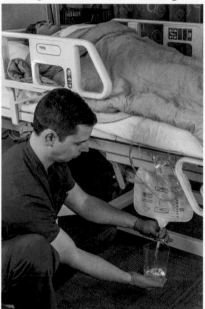

STEP 11 Clean the spigot with an antiseptic wipe.

12. **ACC** Measure the volume of urine. Assess the characteristics of the urine, including color, clarity, and odor. If using a clear graduated cylinder, measure the volume at eye level. *Reading above or below eye level will alter the measurement reading.*

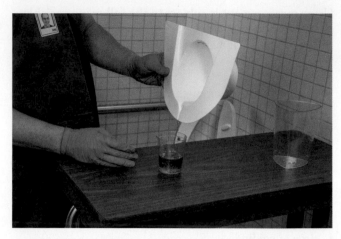

STEP 12 Pour urine into a calibrated measuring container appropriate for the volume.

13. **INF** Pour out the urine in the toilet. Rinse out the measuring container, and urinal or bedpan if used, with cool water. Dispose of the water in the toilet. Store the measuring container, bedpan, or urinal per facility policy. *Rinsing reduces the odor of urine and the growth of microorganisms.*

FINISHING THE SKILL

14. **INF** Remove gloves and perform hand hygiene.
15. **SAF** Ensure client safety and comfort. Ensure that the bed is in the lowest position. Ensure that the client can identify and reach the nurse call system. *These safety measures reduce the risk of injury from falls.*
16. **COM** Document urine volume and time of measure in the I&O record.
17. **COM** Calculate and document urine output totals for each shift and 24-hour totals per facility policy.
18. **EVAL** Evaluate output and compare to fluid intake. *Minimum urine output for an adult is 0.5 mL/kg/hour. Urine output is normally approximately equal to fluid intake. Urine output of less than 0.5 mL/kg/hour and significant differences in fluid intake and urine output should be communicated to the authorized healthcare provider.*

■ SKILL 15.2 Measuring Urine Volume With a Portable Bladder Scanner

EQUIPMENT

Bladder scanner
Ultrasound gel
Clean gloves
Manufacturer's recommended antiseptic agent and wipe
Washcloth or disposable wipe to remove gel

BEGINNING THE SKILL

1. **SAF** Review the order.
2. **INF** Perform hand hygiene
3. **CCC** Introduce yourself to the client and explain the purpose of measuring urine volume in the client's bladder.
4. **SAF** Identify the client using two identifiers.
5. **INF** Apply clean gloves.
6. **ACC** Assess to determine if the client's bladder is full. Ask the client when he or she last emptied the bladder. Palpate gently, moving down from the umbilicus, to determine if the top edge of the bladder is easily palpable.
7. **ACC** Instruct the client to void if measuring a postvoid residual urine volume.
8. **CCC** Provide privacy; close the door and pull the curtain.

PROCEDURE

9 **SAF** Set up an ergonomically safe space. Raise the bed to a comfortable working height. Raise one side rail. *Setting up an ergonomically safe space prevents injury to the nurse and client.*
10. **SAF** Set up a workspace according to your hand dominance; that is, if you are right-handed, stand on the client's right side.
11. **INF** Clean the scanner head with manufacturer-recommended antiseptic agent.
12. Turn on the bladder scanner.
13. Press the scan button.
14. **ACC** Select the appropriate gender. (Note: Some models of scanner require the nurse to select male gender if the client is female but has had a hysterectomy and no longer has a uterus.)

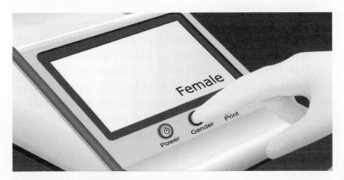

STEP 14 Select the appropriate gender.

15. **ACC** Place the ultrasound gel midline about 3 to 5 cm (1–1½ inches) above the symphysis pubis.

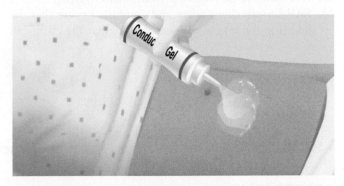

STEP 15 Place ultrasound gel above the symphysis pubis.

16. **ACC** Position the scanner head on the gel with the head pointed toward the client's head or coccyx according to the manufacturer's instructions. Aim the scanner toward the bladder and press the scan button.

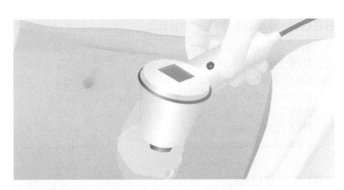

STEP 16 Position the scanner head on the gel.

17. **EVAL** Check the image to ensure that the bladder is centered in the image.

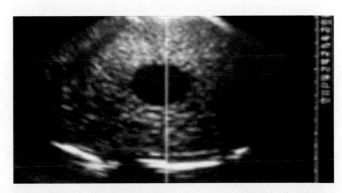

STEP 17 Verify that the bladder is centered in the image

18. **EVAL** Reposition the scanner head and rescan as needed until the bladder is centered in the image.
19. Press the done button.

20. **CCC** Remove the gel from the client's abdomen.
21. **INF** Clean the scanner head with manufacturer-recommended antiseptic agent.

FINISHING THE SKILL

22. **INF** Remove gloves and perform hand hygiene.
23. **SAF** Ensure client safety and comfort. Ensure that the bed is in the lowest position. Ensure that the client can identify and reach the nurse call system. *These safety measures reduce the risk of injury from falls.*
24. **EVAL** Evaluate urine volume and compare to previous measurements.
25. **COM** Document date, time, and bladder volume measurement in the legal healthcare record.

■ SKILL 15.3 Obtaining a Urine Specimen From a Closed Urinary Drainage System

EQUIPMENT

Luer-Lok syringe or syringe with needleless blunt cannula
Sterile specimen container
Specimen label
Clean gloves
Antiseptic wipe

BEGINNING THE SKILL

1. **SAF** Review the order.
2. **INF** Perform hand hygiene.
3. **CCC** Introduce yourself to the client and explain the purpose of obtaining a urine specimen.
4. **SAF** Identify the client using two identifiers.
5. **INF** Apply clean gloves.
6. **CCC** Provide privacy. Close the door; pull the curtain.

PROCEDURE

7. **ACC** Expose the drainage tube and aspiration port.
8. **SAF** Clamp or bend the drainage tubing distal to the port per facility policy until enough urine has collected for the specimen. **WARNING:** Do not allow the tubing to remain clamped for more than 30 minutes. (Note: Some facilities may not allow clamping of the tubing due to the risk of bladder distention.)

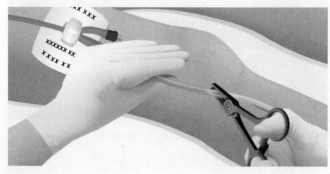

STEP 8 Clamp the drainage tubing until enough urine has collected for the specimen.

9. **INF** Clean the port with an antiseptic wipe for 15 seconds and allow to air dry. *Cleaning prevents the transfer of microorganisms into the specimen.*
10. **ACC** Insert Luer-Lok syringe by pushing and rotating the syringe into the port, or insert a needleless cannula into the aspiration port. Slowly aspirate sufficient urine for the specimen. *The brand of Foley catheter will determine the type of access device needed to access urine through the access port. Your facility laboratory can recommend the volume of urine needed for the specimen.*

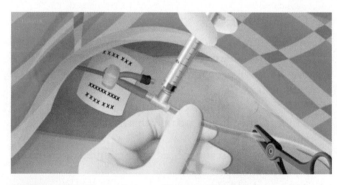

STEP 10 Slowly aspirate sufficient urine for the specimen.

11. **INF** Remove the Luer-Lok syringe or needleless cannula and ensure the sterility of the syringe tip. *Ensuring the sterility of the specimen is necessary to ensure the accuracy of laboratory results.*
12. **SAF** Unclamp or unbend the drainage tubing. Ensure urine is flowing to the drainage collection bag. *Blockage of the urine flow may result in bladder distention.*
13. **INF** Open the specimen cup, maintain the sterility of the interior and lid interior, and slowly inject the urine specimen into the specimen cup. *Ensuring the sterility of the specimen is necessary to ensure the accuracy of laboratory results. Forceful injection may cause the urine to splash out of the cup.*

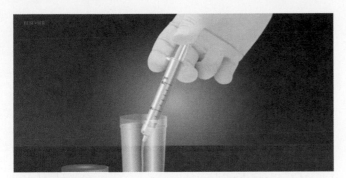

STEP 13 Maintain the sterility of the specimen cup interior.

14. **INF** Replace the lid of the specimen cup to maintain sterility.
15. **COM** Ensure the specimen label contains two client identifiers. Label in the presence of the client. Secure label to the specimen cup. *The specimen cup, rather than the lid, is labeled because the lid can easily be separated from the specimen. National safety guidelines recommend labeling specimens in the presence of the client.*
16. **COM** Document date and time of urine specimen collection on the label, if facility policy.
17. **INF** Prepare the specimen for transport. *Many institutions require transportation in a plastic resealable biohazard bag. Depending on the type of laboratory testing ordered, the specimen may need to go to the laboratory im-*

mediately, may need to go on ice, or may need to be refrigerated in order to ensure the accuracy of laboratory results.

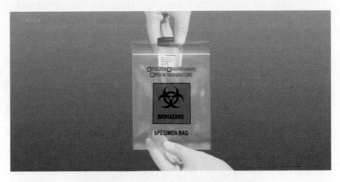

STEP 17 Transport in a plastic resealable bag.

FINISHING THE SKILL

18. **INF** Remove gloves and perform hand hygiene.
19. **SAF** Ensure client safety and comfort. Ensure that the bed is in the lowest position. Ensure that the client can identify and reach the nurse call system. *These safety measures reduce the risk of injury from falls.*
20. **ACC** Transport to the laboratory per facility policy within the time limit, or place in a refrigerator.
21. **COM** Document assessment of urine characteristics, care given, and date and time of specimen collection in the legal healthcare record.

■ SKILL 15.4 Obtaining a Urine Specimen Using the Clean-Catch Method

EQUIPMENT

Soap and water or hygienic wipes
Specimen cup
Clean gloves
Bedpan or urinal
Bedside commode or toilet with toilet urine "hat"
Specimen label

BEGINNING THE SKILL

1. **SAF** Review the order.
2. **INF** Perform hand hygiene.
3. **CCC** Introduce yourself to the client and explain the purpose of obtaining a clean-catch specimen. Ensure that the client consents to the procedure.
4. **SAF** Identify the client using two identifiers.
5. **INF** Apply clean gloves.

PROCEDURE

6. **ACC** Assess the client's ability to assist. If the client is able to obtain the specimen independently, give clear instructions. If the client is not reliably able to obtain the specimen without contamination, provide assistance.
7. **INF** Instruct or assist the client to wash his or her hands. *Handwashing helps to prevent the transfer of microorganisms to the specimen.*
8. **SAF** Position the client on a bedpan or commode chair or show the client to the toilet. *The assessment in Step 6 helps to determine the safest location for the client.*
9. **INF** Instruct or assist the client to clean the urinary meatus.
   a. For a female, separate the labia and wipe from front to back using a moist hygienic wipe. Make only one

pass from front to back with each wipe. Wipe three times, using a new wipe each time. First wipe to one side of the urinary meatus, then to the other side, and then pass the third wipe directly over the urinary meatus.

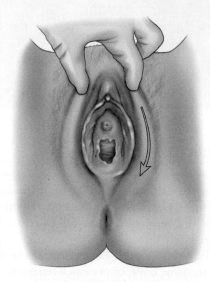

STEP 9A Wipe from front to back using a moist hygienic wipe.

b. For an uncircumcised male, retract the foreskin and wipe with a moist hygienic wipe in a circular motion starting from the urinary meatus and then wiping outward around the head of the penis. *Clean from cleanest to dirtiest area.*

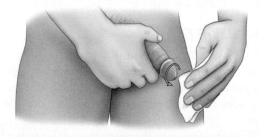

STEP 9B Wipe in a circular motion, starting from the urinary meatus.

c. For a circumcised male, wipe with a moist hygienic wipe in a circular motion starting from the urinary meatus and then wiping outward around the head of the penis. *Clean from cleanest to dirtiest area.*

10. **ACC** Instruct the client to start to void and then stop the flow of urine, if he or she is able. *Collecting a specimen midstream flushes out microorganisms and ensures a fresh specimen of urine.*

11. **ACC** Instruct the client to void into the specimen cup. If the client is unable to stop and start the flow of urine, instruct the client to pass the specimen cup into the stream of urine. *Collecting a specimen midstream flushes out microorganisms and ensures a fresh specimen of urine.*

12. **ACC** Place the lid on the specimen cup. *Quickly placing the lid reduces the risk of contamination of the urine specimen. Ensuring the sterility of the specimen is necessary to ensure the accuracy of laboratory results.*

13. **INF** Wipe off the outside of the specimen cup. *The outside of the specimen cup is easily contaminated with urine.*

14. Remove the bedpan or assist the client off the commode chair.

15. **CCC** Provide perineal care, as needed. Return the foreskin to its original position, as needed.

16. **COM** Ensure that the specimen label contains two client identifiers. Label in the presence of the client. Secure label to the specimen cup. *The specimen cup, rather than the lid, is labeled because the lid can easily be separated from the specimen. National safety guidelines recommend labeling specimens in the presence of the client.*

17. **COM** Document date and time of urine specimen collection on the label, per facility policy.

18. **INF** Prepare the specimen for transport. *Many institutions require transportation in a plastic resealable biohazard bag. Depending on the type of laboratory testing ordered, the specimen may need to go to the laboratory immediately, may need to go on ice, or may need to be refrigerated in order to ensure the accuracy of laboratory results.*

FINISHING THE SKILL

19. **INF** Remove gloves and perform hand hygiene.

20. **SAF** Ensure client safety and comfort. Ensure that the bed is in the lowest position. Ensure that the client can identify and reach the nurse call system. *These safety measures reduce the risk of injury from falls.*

21. **ACC** Transport to the laboratory per facility policy within the time limit, or place in a refrigerator.

22. **COM** Document assessment of urine characteristics, care given, client outcome, and date and time of specimen collection in the legal healthcare record.

▪ SKILL 15.5 Obtaining a 24-Hour Urine Specimen

EQUIPMENT

Urine specimen container (may contain preservative)
Sign stating "24-hour urine specimen in progress"
Clean gloves
Bedpan or urinal
Bedside commode or toilet with toilet urine "hat"
Specimen label
Container with ice large enough to hold the urine specimen
   container

BEGINNING THE SKILL

1. **SAF** Review the order.
2. **INF** Perform hand hygiene.
3. **CCC** Introduce yourself to the client and explain the purpose of obtaining a 24-hour urine specimen.
4. **SAF** Identify the client using two identifiers.
5. **INF** Apply clean gloves if there is a risk of exposure to body fluids.

PROCEDURE

6. **ACC** Assess the client's ability to cooperate and follow instructions to save all urine. If the client is able to cooperate, provide client instructions. Ensure that the client consents to the procedure. If the client cannot reliably assist, provide assistance.
7. **COM** Instruct the client not to put toilet paper in with the urine.
8. **COM** Instruct the client to try to keep bowel movements and urine separate.
9. **COM** Instruct the client to empty his or her bladder and then discard this urine. If I&O is ordered, measure the volume before discarding urine.
10. **ACC** All urine from this point forward is collected and placed in the 24-hour specimen. *Ensuring the accurate collection time of the specimen is necessary to ensure the accuracy of laboratory results.*

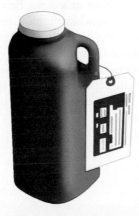

STEP 10 Place all urine in the 24-hour specimen collection container.

11. **ACC** If the specimen is to be kept on ice, ensure there is sufficient ice to keep the specimen cold and that the specimen collection container remains in the ice. *Ensuring the temperature of the specimen is necessary to ensure the accuracy of laboratory results.*
12. **ACC** Immediately before the 24-hour urine collection is complete, instruct the client to empty his or her bladder and place this specimen in the urine collection container. *Ensuring the accurate collection time of the specimen is necessary to ensure the accuracy of laboratory results.*
13. **COM** Ensure the specimen label contains two client identifiers. Label in the presence of the client. Secure the label to the specimen container. *The specimen container is labeled rather than the lid because the lid can be easily separated from the specimen. National safety guidelines recommend labeling specimens in the presence of the client.*
14. **COM** Document the date and time of urine specimen collection on the label, per facility policy.
15. **INF** Prepare the specimen for transport. *Many institutions require transportation in a plastic resealable biohazard bag. Call the laboratory to determine how this container is to be transported.*

FINISHING THE SKILL

16. **INF** Remove gloves, if applied. Perform hand hygiene.
17. **SAF** Ensure client safety and comfort. Ensure that the bed is in the lowest position. Ensure that the client can identify and reach the nurse call system. *These safety measures reduce the risk of injury from falls.*
18. **ACC** Transport to the laboratory per facility policy within the time limit, or place in a refrigerator. *Depending on the type of laboratory testing ordered, the specimen may need to go to the laboratory immediately or may need to be refrigerated in order to ensure the accuracy of laboratory results.*
19. **COM** Document assessment of urine characteristics, care given, and date and time of specimen collection completion in the legal healthcare record.

■ SKILL 15.6 Obtaining a Bagged Urine Specimen From an Infant or Child

EQUIPMENT

Sterile self-adhesive pediatric urine collection bag
Basin of warm water, hypoallergenic soap, washcloth, and towel
Absorbent pad
Gloves

BEGINNING THE SKILL

1. **INF** Perform hand hygiene.
2. **CCC** Introduce yourself to the client and parent, if present.
3. **COM** Explain the purpose of obtaining a urine specimen.
4. **SAF** Identify the client using two identifiers.
5. **INF** Apply clean gloves.
6. **CCC** Provide privacy; close the door and pull the curtain.

PROCEDURE

7. **SAF** Set up an ergonomically safe space. Raise the bed to a comfortable working height. Ensure the infant or child cannot fall off the surface. *Setting up an ergonomically safe space prevents injury to the nurse and client.*
8. **SAF** Set up a workspace according to your hand dominance; that is, if you are right-handed, stand on the client's right side.
9. **CCC** Find a caregiver to help hold the infant/child's legs.
10. **CCC** Place a disposable absorbent pad under the infant/child's buttocks.
11. **INF** Wash, rinse, and dry the genitals.
    a. **For a male**, position supine, with the legs slightly apart. Wash, rinse, and dry the penis, scrotum, and perineal area, washing the scrotum first, then from the tip of the penis to the base, and wipe the rectal area last.
    b. **For a female**, position supine with feet apart, knees flexed, and hips externally rotated.
       Wash and rinse, wiping from front to back, cleaning between the labia. Use a different section of the washcloth for each stroke. Wipe the rectal area last. *Clean from cleanest to dirtiest area.*
12. **ACC** If using soap, rinse carefully.
13. **ACC** Dry thoroughly in all skinfolds. *If the skin is not completely dry, the adhesive will not stick.*
14. **INF** Wipe with an antiseptic agent, per facility policy. Allow to dry completely. *If the skin is not completely dry, the adhesive will not stick.*

15. **CCC** Ask a caregiver to hold the infant/child's legs gently open.
16. **ACC** Apply the urine collection bag.
    a. **For a male,** keeping the paper backing on the adhesive, position the collection bag over the penis and scrotum. Remove the lower half of the paper backing and apply the adhesive to the perineum. Apply upward and outward. Then remove the top half of the paper backing and apply the adhesive smoothly on the skin. *Any wrinkles will allow urine to leak.*

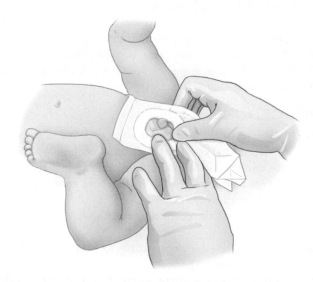

STEP 16A Applying the urine collection bag on a male infant.

    b. **For a female,** remove only the lower half of the paper backing covering the adhesive. *It is easier to secure the adhesive one section at a time.* Bend the backing so that the center touches the skin first. Apply the adhesive first on the perineum (bridge of skin between the rectum and the genitals). Apply the adhesive upward and outward from the perineum. Remove the top half of the paper backing and apply the adhesive smoothly on the outer labia. *Any wrinkles will allow urine to leak.*

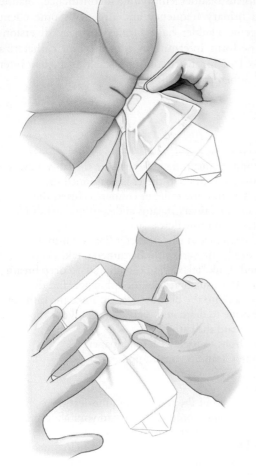

STEP 16B Applying the urine collection bag on a female infant.

17. **CCC** Place a diaper or underwear on the infant/child.
18. **EVAL** Check frequently to see if the infant/child has voided.
19. **ACC** When there is urine in the collection bag, remove the collection bag. Determine whether a caregiver is needed to restrain the infant/child's legs to safely remove the collection bag without spilling urine.
20. **INF** Perform hand hygiene and apply gloves.

21. **HLTH** Gently remove the adhesive, working from front to back. *An infant's skin is very delicate. Gentle removal helps to protect skin integrity.*
22. **ACC** Pour urine into a sterile specimen cup using clean technique. *Ensuring the lack of contamination of the specimen is necessary to ensure the accuracy of laboratory results.*
23. **ACC** Place the lid on the specimen cup. *Quickly placing the lid reduces the risk of contamination of the urine specimen.*
24. **HLTH** Cleanse the perineal area and assess for skin irritation from the adhesive. *An infant's skin is very delicate. Assess the integrity of the skin. Cleansing helps to protect skin integrity.*
25. **COM** Ensure the specimen label contains two client identifiers. Label in the presence of the client. Secure the label to the specimen cup. *The specimen cup, rather than the lid, is labeled because the lid can easily be separated from the specimen. National safety guidelines recommend labeling specimens in the presence of the client.*
26. **COM** Document date and time of urine specimen collection on the label, per facility policy.
27. **INF** Prepare the specimen for transport. *Many institutions require transportation in a plastic resealable biohazard bag. Depending on the type of laboratory testing ordered, the specimen may need to go to the laboratory immediately, may need to go on ice, or may need to be refrigerated in order to ensure the accuracy of laboratory results.*

FINISHING THE SKILL

28. **INF** Remove gloves and perform hand hygiene.
29. **SAF** Ensure client safety.
30. **CCC** Provide comfort, such as swaddling an infant or returning a child to his or her parent.
31. **ACC** Transport to the laboratory per facility policy within the time limit, or place in a refrigerator. *Many institutions require transportation in a plastic resealable bag. Depending on the type of laboratory testing ordered, the specimen may need to go to the laboratory immediately or may need to be refrigerated in order to ensure the accuracy of laboratory results.*
32. **COM** Document assessment of urine characteristics, care given, client outcome, and date and time of specimen collection completion in the legal healthcare record.

SECTION 2 Urine Elimination With a Transurethral Catheter

Voiding (or *micturition*) is a voluntary act involving contraction of the bladder muscles and relaxation of the urethra. When clients cannot void, an elimination strategy is to place a *transurethral catheter* through the opening of the urethral meatus through the urethra into the bladder in order to drain urine from the bladder. There are two methods of catheterization:

- **Intermittent catheterization** is when the catheter is placed, urine is drained from the bladder, and the catheter is promptly removed. This is also called straight catheterization.
- **Indwelling catheterization** most commonly uses a Foley catheter, named after Dr. Frederic Foley, who first designed it. The catheter is placed into the bladder, and a small balloon is inflated to maintain its position. Urine then drains continuously.

Individuals may be unable to void for a wide variety of reasons. Short-term reasons, such as surgery, anesthesia, or spinal or regional blocks, may temporarily impede voiding. Long-term reasons include neurologic conditions that affect the motor neurons of the bladder, such as spinal cord injury and traumatic brain injury. These injuries result in an altered pattern of elimination called *neurogenic bladder*. Problems associated with neurogenic bladder include urinary retention, incomplete bladder emptying, incontinence, bladder spasms, and urinary frequency and urgency. Some clients with neurogenic bladder have surgical urinary diversions, but others perform intermittent transurethral catheterization. See Box 15.2 for instructions on teaching a client intermittent self-catheterization.

BOX 15.2 Home Care Considerations: Intermittent Self-Catheterization

Nurses teaching people to perform transurethral self-catheterization must ensure that the client has a clear understanding of urinary tract anatomy. Women in particular may need help identifying the urethral meatus.

All clients need to be taught to wash their hands thoroughly prior to and after the procedure and to use clean equipment. In the home environment, clients are not exposed to the kinds of microorganisms present in the healthcare environment; moreover, because they catheterize themselves, they are not at risk from transferred microorganisms. Thus, most clients at home can use clean technique for self-catheterization. However, clients who are immunocompromised should be taught to use sterile technique.

Clients also need to be taught to self-catheterize about every 4 to 6 hours to prevent the bladder from becoming overdistended. Regular drainage also prevents infection and injury to the upper urinary tract.

The equipment needed at home includes a urinary catheter, water-soluble lubricant, soap and water to clean the urethra, and a hand mirror for females. When catheterization is repeatedly performed, it is very important to use the smallest size French catheter that reaches the bladder in order to prevent irritation and injury to the urethra. Best practice does not recommend reusing single-use catheters. Nevertheless, some clients use a variety of methods to clean and reuse catheters, including washing with soap and water, boiling, microwave sterilization, and soaking in an antiseptic solution (Newman & Willson, 2011).

Where to perform catheterization at home depends on the mobility of the person. If the client is able to sit on the toilet to catheterize, then all liquids can drain directly into the toilet. Sometimes men prefer to stand in front of the toilet. If clients are not able to move to the bathroom, then a container is needed to collect both urine and soapy water, and a towel or disposable absorbent pad might be prudent to catch drips.

Instructions for teaching clients to self-catheterize at home are as follows:

FOR FEMALES
- Wash hands. Set out the catheter, lubricant, and mirror.
- Wash and rinse the urethra with soap and water or personal hygiene toilettes. Wipe from front to back over the urethral opening, always using a new section of the washcloth or wipe. Wash hands again.
- Use a mirror to find the urethral opening.
- Lubricate the catheter tip. Do not touch the tip.

- Use your nondominant hand to separate the labia. Check that the distal end of the catheter is positioned such that urine will flow into the toilet or container. Insert the catheter into the urinary meatus and continue to advance the catheter until urine flows.
- If you feel resistance at the sphincter (i.e., no urine), maintain steady pressure with the catheter, take deep breaths, and think "relax." You can also take a deep breath and cough. This usually relaxes the sphincter, and the catheter passes into the bladder. Do not force the catheter.
- Allow the urine to drain and then slowly pull out the catheter. Discard the catheter.
- Wipe from front to back with toilet paper.
- Wash hands. Clean up your equipment.

FOR MALES
- Wash hands. Set out the catheter and lubricant.
- Holding your penis pointing up toward your abdomen, wash and rinse the urethral meatus with soap and water or personal hygiene toilettes. If you are not circumcised, retract the foreskin and wash the urethral meatus. Wash hands again.
- Lubricate the catheter tip, rotating the catheter to spread the lubricant around the surface of the catheter for several inches.
- Check that the distal end of the catheter is positioned such that urine will flow into the toilet or container, and then insert the catheter into the urinary meatus and continue to advance the catheter until urine flows.
- You may feel resistance where the urethra passes the prostate and/or at the sphincter just before the bladder. If you feel resistance before entering the bladder and seeing urine, rotate the catheter and gently tug your penis away from your body. Rotating the catheter allows it to find the path of least resistance, and tugging the penis straightens the urethral passage. Another technique is to maintain steady pressure with the catheter, take deep breaths, and think "relax." You can also take a deep breath and cough. This usually relaxes the sphincter, and the catheter passes into the bladder. Do not force the catheter.
- Allow the urine to drain and then slowly pull out the catheter. Discard the catheter.
- Wash hands. Clean up your equipment.

In conclusion, home self-catheterization can become a part of the client's daily routine. Clients will also need to know whom to call for advice and troubleshooting and where to go if they find that they cannot pass the catheter or they have symptoms of a urinary tract infection.

TYPES OF TRANSURETHRAL CATHETERS

As shown in Fig. 15.4, many types and sizes of transurethral catheters are available. Catheters may be made of latex, silicone, or polyvinyl chloride. They can be coated with silver alloy or impregnated with antimicrobial agents. Most catheter tips are straight; however, a Coudé catheter has a curved tip and is sometimes used when catheter insertion is difficult, such as with an enlarged prostate or urethral strictures. Coudé-tip catheters are available in a variety of sizes and may be intermittent or indwelling.

Catheter sizes are measured by the diameter of the lumen, using the French scale. Typical sizes range from a small diameter, 8 Fr for infants, to a 14 Fr or 16 Fr for adults, but much larger sizes are sometimes used. Transurethral catheters may be single lumen, double lumen, or triple lumen (Fig. 15.5).

- **Single-lumen catheters** are used for intermittent catheterization.
- **Double-lumen catheters**, such as a Foley catheter, have two separate lumens that do not communicate. One lumen extends from the distal to the proximal end to drain urine, and another lumen extends from the distal end to the balloon. When an indwelling catheter is placed in a bladder, the balloon is filled with sterile water from the designated balloon port in order to keep the catheter in place. To remove the catheter, a syringe is attached to the balloon port, the sterile water is aspirated out, and the balloon is emptied.
- **Triple-lumen catheters** have a lumen for urine drainage, a lumen for balloon inflation and deflation, and an additional lumen to permit closed bladder irrigation.

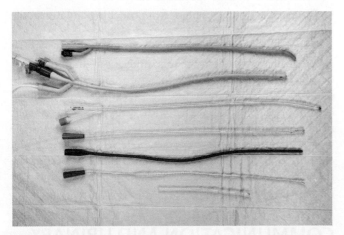

FIG. 15.4 There are many types and sizes of transurethral catheters. *From the top:* 16 Fr indwelling catheter with a Coude tip; 16 Fr triple-lumen catheter; 14 Fr silicone Indwelling catheter; PVC straight catheter; 14 Fr red rubber straight catheter; 8 Fr PCV catheter with a Coude tip; and self-cath for a female.

INFECTION CONTROL WITH URINARY CATHETERS

Intermittent catheterization is performed using sterile technique in the acute care setting and using clean technique in a nonacute setting, such as at home. Intermittent catheterization has a much lower risk of infection than the placement of an indwelling Foley catheter.

The insertion of an indwelling Foley catheter is accompanied by the risk of acquiring a catheter-associated urinary tract infection (CAUTI). CAUTIs are the fourth most common healthcare-associated infection and are associated with increased morbidity, mortality, and cost and length of stay (Centers for Disease Control and Prevention [CDC], 2019). In an effort to reduce CAUTI, the Healthcare Infection Control Practices Advisory Committee (HICPAC) has reviewed extensive literature and established current recommendations, including indications for and against the use of indwelling Foley catheters (Box 15.3).

The greatest risk factor for CAUTI is how long clients remain catheterized. For every day a client has an indwelling catheter, the risk of getting CAUTI increases by 3% to 7%. The United States has made progress in decreasing the rate of CAUTI, but CAUTI represented more than 12% of infections reported by hospitals (CDC, 2019). To meet the criteria of acute care CAUTI, the client must have had an indwelling catheter for more than 2 days, be symptomatic with at least one sign of infection such as fever or tenderness, and have a urine culture with no more than two species or organisms with $>10^5$ CFU/mL (CDC, 2019). In long-term care facilities, residents typically have longer durations of catheterization and subsequently higher rates of bacteriuria, which may not result in overt signs of infection.

The recommendation of HICPAC and the Infectious Diseases Society of America (IDSA) is two-fold: to reduce the use and duration of indwelling catheters and to prevent CAUTI. In order to prevent infection, nurses need to understand the sources and routes of entry of microorganisms. Sources of microorganisms include endogenous microorganisms from the client's own meatus, rectum, or vaginal areas and exogenous microorganisms from healthcare workers' hands or equipment. Microorganisms can ascend the catheter and enter the bladder from both the outside and inside of the catheter. Treating these microorganisms is not a simple task. Pathogens often create microcolonies on the catheter surface, develop antimicrobial resistance, develop from a single microorganism to polymicrobic, and eventually develop into a mature biofilm. A biofilm is a complex microcolony structure adhering to a surface. Biofilms can colonize the bladder and change urine pH, resulting in an increased incidence of encrustations and catheter blockage.

Nurses can be instrumental in preventing CAUTI by following current evidence-based practices. CDC-recommended nursing actions to prevent CAUTI include the following:

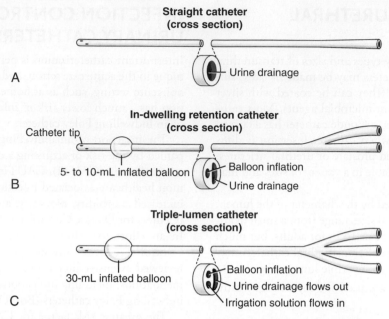

**Straight catheter
(cross section)**

A — Urine drainage

**In-dwelling retention catheter
(cross section)**

Catheter tip

5- to 10-mL inflated balloon

B — Balloon inflation
Urine drainage

**Triple-lumen catheter
(cross section)**

30-mL inflated balloon

C — Balloon inflation
Urine drainage flows out
Irrigation solution flows in

FIG. 15.5 Transurethral catheters may be single lumen (A), double lumen (B), or triple lumen (C).

BOX 15.3 Indications for Indwelling Catheter Use

EXAMPLES OF APPROPRIATE INDICATIONS FOR INDWELLING URETHRAL CATHETER USE
- Clients with acute urinary retention or bladder outlet obstruction
- Need for accurate measurements of urinary output in critically ill clients
- Perioperative use for selected surgical procedures:
  - Clients undergoing urologic surgery or other surgery on contiguous structures of the genitourinary tract
  - Anticipated prolonged duration of surgery (catheters inserted for this reason should be removed in the post-anesthesia care unit [PACU])
  - Clients anticipated to receive large-volume infusions or diuretics during surgery
  - Need for intraoperative monitoring of urinary output
- To assist in healing of open sacral or perineal wounds in incontinent clients
- Client requires prolonged immobilization (e.g., potentially unstable thoracic or lumbar spine, multiple traumatic injuries such as pelvic fractures)
- To improve comfort for end-of-life care if needed

EXAMPLES OF INAPPROPRIATE USES OF INDWELLING CATHETERS
- As a substitute for nursing care of the client or resident with incontinence
- As a means of obtaining urine for culture or other diagnostic tests when the client can voluntarily void
- For prolonged postoperative duration without appropriate indications (e.g., structural repair of urethra or contiguous structures, prolonged effect of epidural anesthesia, etc.)

Reference: Centers for Disease Control and Prevention, 2015a.

- Maintain a closed drainage system and use drainage collection systems with preconnected, sealed catheter tubing junctions. *Opening the drainage system allows microorganisms to enter and ascend the catheter.*
- Use Standard Precautions during any manipulation of the catheter or drainage collection system.
- Prevent kinking of the catheter or collecting tubing in order to maintain an unobstructed flow of urine.
- Keep the drainage bag below the level of the bladder at all times.
- Empty the collection bag at regular intervals using a clean collection container specific to each client.
- Prevent the drainage spigot from touching any nonsterile container (CDC, 2015b).

To avoid injury to the urethral mucosa, nurses use the smallest-diameter catheter that is sufficient to drain the bladder and keep catheters secured to prevent movement and subsequent urethral irritation. In the past, catheter care included cleaning the periurethral area with antiseptics. The current recommendation is routine cleansing with plain disposable wipes. Plain disposable wipes are preferred for periurethral cleaning over chlorhexidine gluconate (CHG) wipes for the prevention of CAUTI (Strouse, 2015). Routine catheter or urine drainage bag changes are also not recommended.

COMMUNICATION AND URINARY CATHETERS

A key nursing concept related to managing transurethral catheterization is communication, both with the client and with other members of the healthcare team. Nurses are in an instrumental position to communicate the presence of an indwelling catheter and the number of days it has been in place. Implementation of automated catheter reminders and "stop orders" (when an order has a set expiration date) have resulted in significantly fewer CAUTIs (Meddings et al., 2014). An example of an automated reminder could be a pop-up in the electronic medical record (EMR).

PROVIDING CLIENT-CENTERED CARE TO SPECIFIC POPULATIONS

Nurses provide client-centered care when inserting transurethral catheters. Urinary catheterization is unpleasant and perhaps uncomfortable for most people, but it should not be traumatic. In order to provide atraumatic care, nurses must adapt their nursing care for the insertion and removal of urinary catheters to the experiences and age of the client. For example, catheterization for a client who has experienced sexual assault can be traumatic. Reports of the pain experience during transurethral catheterization suggest that discomfort varies based on gender and age, with men reporting more discomfort than women and younger individuals reporting more discomfort than older people. Trauma to the epithelium of the urethra can be painful and increase the risk of infection. Generous lubricant on the catheter for female clients helps to reduce trauma or irritation. Generous lubricant instilled directly into the urethra for male clients dilates and coats the urethra. Slow instillation of 10 mL/10 seconds is recommended over rapid instillation (Tzortzis, Gravas, Melekos & dela Rosette, 2009). Nurses need to be knowledgeable of the current evidence related to procedural pain management during catheterization. See Box 15.4 for a description of research on pain management related to transurethral catheterization in men, women, and children. Collaborate with the client and the authorized healthcare provider to develop a plan of care.

Many older women find it difficult and painful to flex and rotate their hips and legs. The position strains the hip ligaments and muscles. One nursing intervention is to provide support for each leg. Place rolled towels or bath blankets or pillows under and outside the thigh to support the leg. An alternative would be to assist the client into the Sims' position. Box 15.5 describes catheterizing an older woman. For older men, the challenge may be an enlarged prostate. Collaborating with the urologist to obtain a prescription for lidocaine gel lubricant may be an alternative. See the Case Study at the end of this chapter for further discussion of strategies for clients with an enlarged prostate.

For teenagers, the invasion of privacy during an age of heightened embarrassment is difficult. Ask the client if he or she would like to have a second person present for support. A caregiver or family member attends to the teenager by distracting, soothing, and keeping a hand on the client's open knee as a reminder to keep the knee still. Teenage girls may have "nervous legs"; that is, as you touch their inner thighs or labia, the knees slam shut almost involuntarily. Teenagers may also like to listen to music as a distraction during the procedure. Allowing them to use an electronic device and earbuds to "tune out" the experience may help them cope with the invasion of privacy.

Providing client-centered care includes ensuring the client understands the procedure before the event and has the ability to select a nurse of the same gender. Individuals may have cultural, religious, or personal reasons for preferring a same-gender nurse. Courts have upheld that it is not gender-based discrimination to allow a same-gender caregiver when care involves intimate personal privacy. Individuals should also be allowed to determine if they wish a family member to be with them or not. A clear understanding of the procedure and the use of relaxation and distraction strategies helps to decrease anxiety in clients of all ages.

Catheterization and Young Children

Catheterizing children can be very challenging. Toddlers and preschoolers are cognitively unable to understand why the procedure is necessary. Developmentally, their focus has been on toilet-training, and this creates a mind-set that this catheterization must be related, usually as a punishment. Let the child know that catheterization is not a punishment and that the child did nothing to cause this to happen. Furthermore, it is not always possible to distinguish between pain, fear, and anxiety in this age group. The term *distress* best describes the young child's response. Unfortunately, urinary tract infections are not uncommon in young girls in this age group.

Effective nonpharmacological strategies to prepare children for catheterization include as much play exposure as possible, for instance, dolls with catheters, practicing the positioning before catheterization, and age-appropriate relaxation techniques and distraction strategies, such as blowing on a pinwheel or blowing out a birthday candle. Large medical centers may have access to a child-life therapist to assist with the procedure. Sucrose is often used to manage pain in newborns and infants; however, a study examining the effectiveness of sucrose on pain with bladder catheterization in infants less than 90 days found no difference between the intervention group and the control group (Wente, 2013).

There are also several pharmacological interventions to reduce children's distress. An analysis of the research examining the efficacy of lidocaine gel for reducing discomfort in children demonstrated no reduction in discomfort for those less than 4 years old and the need to further study those 4 to 11 years of age (Chau et al., 2017). The conclusions of the meta-analysis were that nonpharmacological strategies were more desirable than lidocaine gel. It is interesting to note that in Israel, it is the standard of care to provide mild sedation to children receiving transurethral bladder catheterization, and research there demonstrated a reduction in contaminated specimens when the child received a sedative (Shavit, Feraru, Miron, & Weiser, 2014). Nitrous oxide is also identified as a possible pharmacologic intervention to reduce distress for an invasive procedure (Brown, Hart, Chastain, Schneeweiss, & McGrath, 2009).

BOX 15.4 Lessons From the Evidence: Intraurethral Lidocaine

How does nursing establish evidence-based practice when the evidence is not clear? Several research studies have been conducted examining the effectiveness of decreasing discomfort associated with urinary catheterization by inserting lidocaine gel into the urethra before insertion of the catheter. However, the intervention, use of 2% lidocaine lubricant, was not consistently administered in the studies, and the results were quite different. At this time, current best practice is evolving and is based primarily on the practitioner's preference (Tzortzis, Gravas, Melekos, & de la Rosette, 2009). What is the lesson you can take away from the research studies described here?

MEN

In a 2004 study by Siderias, Guadio, and Singer, the intervention group of men received an intraurethral injection of 2% lidocaine gel 15 minutes before the catheter was inserted, and the control group received water-soluble lubricant. The study demonstrated significantly less pain in the men in the group pretreated with lidocaine gel. This research has been cited frequently, and many facilities have adopted the use of 2% lidocaine for male clients. However, when a similar study was conducted in Australia, the wait time was 2 minutes between 2% lidocaine injection and catheterization. This study found little decrease in pain (Garbutt, McD Taylor, Lee, & Augello, 2008). A 10-minute wait period is the current recommendation (Aygin & Usta, 2017).

WOMEN

In 2004, Tanabe et al. compared the reported pain during transurethral catheterization for women given an injection of 2% lidocaine gel versus a water-soluble lubricant. Half of the women were catheterized with an 8-Fr straight catheter and half with a 16-Fr indwelling catheter. In this study, the lubricants were administered only 1 minute before the catheter was inserted. Women reported a low level of pain regardless of the type and size of the catheter and the type

of lubricant used. The authors note that a primary limitation of this study was the short length of time between the injection of lidocaine gel and the insertion of the catheter. This research continues to be frequently cited as proof that urinary catheterization is not painful for women.

In 2015, a study examined the difference in pain level when 2% lidocaine was injected into the female urethra versus placed on the distal end of the catheter. The process of injecting the lidocaine gel was rated as causing more discomfort and is not recommended for women (Stav et al., 2015).

Contrary to the previous two studies, a study in Singapore found that women did find pain relief with 2% lidocaine gel; however, the length of time before catheterization was not specified (Chan et al., 2014).

CHILDREN

Lidocaine analgesia was tested in 80 children between 0 and 3 years of age who required transurethral bladder catheterization to determine the presence of a urinary tract infection. In this study, 2% lidocaine was inserted into the urethra using a blunt-tip Uro-Jet applicator. The amount of gel was determined by infant weight. After a 5-minute wait, the child was catheterized. They found no significant difference between the intervention group and the control group (Uspal et al., 2018).

SUMMARY

Determining evidence-based care is not always straightforward when the variables within the studies and the outcomes of the studies are not congruent. Aygin and Usta (2017) describe a clear review of the literature describing seven published articles on the effect of lubricant use in catheterization of men and women, including the size of catheter used, the type of lubricant, and the time allotted before catheterization.

BLADDER IRRIGATION

In specific circumstances, it is recommended to irrigate the bladder through an indwelling urinary catheter. Bladder irrigation involves introducing fluid into the bladder and then removing the fluid. Irrigation can be performed intermittently with a bolus amount put in and drained out or continuously with a steady infusion into and out of the bladder. When irrigation is performed via a closed urinary drainage system, it is termed *closed bladder irrigation*. Irrigation can be performed with a triple-lumen catheter or through the port in the drainage tubing. The triple-lumen catheter has a third port at the distal end of the catheter that leads to an opening at the proximal end. Whenever bladder irrigation is anticipated, a triple-lumen catheter is usually placed. When the client has a double-lumen catheter but the need arises to irrigate the catheter or bladder, then the drainage tubing can be clamped and fluid instilled through the port in the tubing

into the bladder. If the urinary drainage system is opened and fluid is injected through the distal port of the catheter, it is termed *open bladder irrigation*. The open method is not recommended for bladder irrigation because it is a portal for microorganisms.

Routine bladder irrigation is not recommended for the prevention of CAUTI by the CDC, the European Association of Urology, HICPAC, and IDSA (Lo et al., 2014). Review of research on irrigation with antimicrobials or normal saline for clients with long-term indwelling catheters showed no significant difference in CAUTI (CDC, 2015b). The exception is surgical clients having genitourinary surgery, such as transurethral surgery or prostatectomy, and with this population, bladder irrigation with antiseptics has shown less catheter-associated bacteriuria (Hooton et al., 2010).

Although routine bladder irrigation to prevent bacteriuria is not recommended, bladder irrigation is used to maintain the patency of the catheter. For example, bladder irrigation

BOX 15.5 Expect the Unexpected: Visualizing the Urethral Meatus

Lindy Johnson is in her last semester of nursing school. She is in a 3-to-11 clinical on a surgical floor and is providing care for Mrs. Telma Garcia Perez, a 77-year-old client who had a hysterectomy the day before. Mrs. Garcia Perez's reproductive history shows that she has six grown children and also had two preterm infants who did not survive.

Her vital signs are stable, and she is getting out of bed slowly. Her indwelling Foley catheter was removed this morning approximately 24 hours after her surgery. Lindy realizes that Mrs. Garcia Perez has not voided and reports this information to the primary nurse. Together they assess the client and find that she has a full palpable bladder and rates her pain as a 5 on a scale of 0 to 10. At noon, her pain rating had been a 3. They assist Mrs. Garcia Perez to the bathroom and try pouring tap water over her perineum, but she is unable to void. The primary nurse encourages Lindy to call the surgeon. Lindy reports using the situation-background-assessment-recommendation (SBAR) technique.

The healthcare provider writes an order for a bladder scan; if more than 400 mL is present in the bladder, the order is to perform a straight catheterization. Lindy programs the bladder scanner using the "female" setting. Then she remembers that if the uterus has been removed, she should use the "male" setting. Using the male setting, she obtains a result of 435 mL.

Lindy assists Mrs. Garcia Perez into a supine position with her hips adducted. Initially, this is uncomfortable for Mrs. Garcia Perez, but Lindy places rolled bath towels under Mrs. Garcia Perez's thighs to help support her legs. Lindy opens the straight catheter kit and sets up her sterile field. She tells Mrs. Garcia Perez that she is going to clean the area and that it will feel wet and cold. Her nondominant hand is holding the labia open. As Lindy passes the swab over the pelvic floor, she is not certain she is visualizing the urethral meatus. She picks up the urinary catheter and puts gentle pressure just above the vagina, the catheter slides in, and she advances the catheter, looking for urine return. There is no urine return. Puzzled, Lindy looks up at the primary nurse. The nurse says, "Leave that one in place. I'm opening another catheter. Now, with your dominant hand, press the labia open a little wider and lift your hand just a little." Lindy opens the labia wider and lifts her hand toward Mrs. Garcia Perez's symphysis pubis. Now she sees what she believes to be the urethral meatus and tries again with a new catheter. This time as she advances the catheter, urine immediately begins to flow.

Mrs. Garcia Perez states she is much more comfortable and declines any medication. After leaving the room, Lindy asks the primary nurse, "Was the first catheter in the vagina?"

"Yes," the nurse replies. "If you accidentally catheterize the vagina, leave that catheter in place to give you a landmark. You know the urethral meatus is above the vagina, and that will help you. Lifting the labia just a little toward the symphysis pubis helps to visualize the urinary meatus, especially with older women. You did a good job."

with normal saline is effective in clients undergoing bladder surgery to reduce blockage from clots and to reduce infection. If bladder irrigation is performed to prevent obstruction of the catheter, then continuous closed irrigation is recommended (CDC, 2015b). Bladder irrigation is also used in the detection and treatment of bladder malignancies and to prevent the formation of bladder stones. Occasionally a catheter may be placed for the sole purpose of instilling medication into the bladder. In that procedure, adherence to sterile technique is critical to prevent the introduction of microorganisms. Medications are injected slowly to prevent irritation of the bladder mucosa.

APPLICATION OF THE NURSING PROCESS

Examples of Related ICNP Nursing Diagnoses, Expected Client Outcomes, and Nursing Interventions:

Nursing Diagnosis: Risk for infection

Supporting Data: Presence of a transurethral catheter

Expected Client Outcomes: The client will not demonstrate any signs of a catheter-associated urinary tract infection, such as fever or tenderness, while the catheter is in place or within 48 hours of removal.

Nursing Intervention Example: Insert catheter using strict aseptic technique.

Reference: International Classification for Nursing Practice. (n.d.). *eHealth & ICNP*. Retrieved from https://www.icn.ch/what-we-do/projects/ehealth-icnp.

CRITICAL CONCEPTS
Urine Elimination with a Transurethral Catheter

Accuracy (ACC)

Accuracy in urine elimination with a transurethral catheter is subject to the following variables:

- assessment of client, including cooperation, mobility, level of discomfort, characteristics of urine, and volume of urine output
- identification of anatomical landmarks
- preparation and placement of the catheter in the bladder
- placement of urine, tubing, and drainage collection bag
- type of catheter and patency of catheter
- preparation and administration of bladder irrigant.

Client-Centered Care (CCC)

When caring for a client with a transurethral catheter, respect for the client is demonstrated by:

- promoting and respecting the client's autonomy
- providing privacy
- ensuring comfort and promoting relaxation
- honoring cultural preferences

- arranging for an interpreter, if needed.
- advocating for the client and family.

Infection Control (INF)

When caring for a client with a transurethral catheter, urinary tract infection is prevented by:
- containment of microorganisms
- preventing and reducing the transfer of microorganisms
- reducing the number of microorganisms
- preventing an environment conducive to microbial growth.

Safety (SAF)

When caring for a client with a transurethral catheter, safety measures provide a safe care environment and prevent harm to the client, including:
- following proper technique for urinary catheter maintenance.

When irrigating a transurethral catheter, safety measures provide a safe care environment and prevent harm to the client, including:
- proper labeling of urinary irrigation tubing and irrigant fluid containers
- using the rights of medication administration and following safety checks and guidelines for bladder irrigants.

Communication (COM)

- Communication exchanges information (oral, written, nonverbal, or electronic) between two or more people.
- Documentation records information in a permanent legal record.
- Collaboration with the client and other members of the healthcare team regarding the insertion, removal, and irrigation of a transurethral catheter enhances safety and decreases the risk of infection.

Health Maintenance (HLTH)

When caring for a client with a transurethral catheter, nursing is dedicated to the promotion of health and self-care abilities, including:
- protecting the client's skin integrity
- preventing irritation, injury, or infection of the urinary tract.

Evaluation (EVAL)

When caring for the client with a transurethral catheter, evaluation of outcomes enables the nurse to determine the efficacy, adherence to sterile technique, and safety of the care provided.

■ SKILL 15.7 Inserting and Removing a Straight Catheter in a Female Client

EQUIPMENT

Straight catheter kit (containing straight catheter, sterile gloves, lubricant, urine collection container, and cleansing swabs or cotton balls and antiseptic solution)
Straight catheter (if not in the kit)
Water-soluble lubricant (if not in the kit)
Antiseptic swabs or forceps, cotton balls, and antiseptic solution (if not in the kit)
Sterile specimen container, if specimen is ordered
Washcloth/basin/water or hygienic wipes
Clean gloves
Sheet or bath blanket
Absorbent pad
Additional light source (e.g., gooseneck lamp, flashlight)

BEGINNING THE SKILL

1. **SAF** Review the order.
2. **INF** Perform hand hygiene.
3. **CCC** Introduce yourself to the client and explain the purpose and procedure for performing a straight catheterization. Ensure that the client consents to the procedure.
4. **SAF** Identify the client using two identifiers.

5. **SAF** Determine if the client has any pertinent allergies, such as iodine or latex. *Antiseptic solution may be betadine, and the catheter may be latex.*
6. **CCC** Provide privacy; close the door and pull the curtain.
7. **INF** Apply gloves.

PROCEDURE

8. **SAF** Set up an ergonomically safe space. Raise the bed to a comfortable working height. Raise one side rail. Set up a workspace according to your hand dominance; that is, if you are right-handed, stand on the client's right side. *Setting up an ergonomically safe space prevents injury to the nurse and client.*
9. **INF** Set up a work triangle: sterile field, client, and trash receptacle. *Preparing your work area with a trash receptacle helps to maintain sterile technique.*
10. **ACC** Assess the client's degree of cooperation, degree of mobility, and discomfort. *Your assessment is to determine the extent to which the client can cooperate during the procedure and tolerate positioning. You may need to find a colleague or family member to assist you with this procedure.*
11. **ACC** Assess urine output.

Position the Client for Catheterization

12. Fold the top bedding to the bottom of the bed.
13. **ACC** Position a woman supine with the feet apart, knees flexed, and hips externally rotated. If this position strains the hip joints, position pillows under the knees. *This frog-leg position allows for visualization of the urinary meatus. Supporting the legs may prevent discomfort and strain on the hip joints.*
14. **CCC** If this position is not tolerable, the Sims position may be used (see Skill 1.6).
15. **CCC** Cover the client from the waist to the neck. One method of covering a woman in a supine position is to position a bath blanket with one corner pointed to her neck, the two lateral corners wrapped around her legs, and the last corner folded back to expose the perineum. *Covering the client from the waist up or as described previously provides privacy and prevents chilling. Clients feel much less exposed if they are partially covered.*

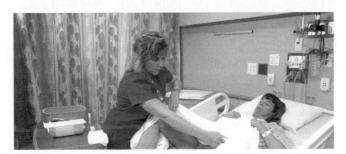

STEP 15 Cover the client from the waist to the neck.

16. **CCC** Place a disposable absorbent pad under the client's buttocks. *Disposable absorbent pads prevent spillage on the client's sheets.*
17. **INF** Perform periurethral cleaning if this is your facility's policy. *Further research is needed on the necessity and the type of solution used for periurethral cleaning prior to catheterization (CDC, 2015b).*
18. **INF** Remove gloves and perform hand hygiene.
19. **ACC** Position additional lighting source to help visualize the urinary meatus.

Prepare the Straight Catheter Kit

20. **INF** Open the straight catheter kit on a clean over-the-bed table. If additional supplies are needed, create a sterile field, and add supplies using sterile technique.
21. **INF** Drape the client. Paper drapes may be placed before you put on sterile gloves if the drapes are only touched on the outer 2.5-cm (1-inch) border. Place the square drape without a window between the client's thighs just under the buttocks. Place the fenestrated drape, the one with a diamond-shaped window, over the perineal area, exposing the labia. *Use of a drape is proper technique for urinary catheter insertion. Draping may be a factor in reducing the rate of infection (Barbadoro et al., 2015; CDC, 2015b).*

22. **INF** Apply sterile gloves. (Note: Alternatively, apply sterile gloves and then place drapes as described previously, but do not allow your sterile gloves to become contaminated. Hold the corners of the drape between your thumb and forefinger with the thumb superior; rotate your hands, cuffing them in the sterile drape.)

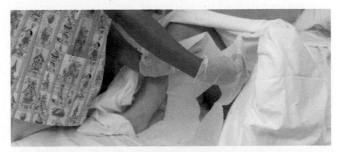

STEP 22 Hold the corners of the drape between your thumb and forefinger with the thumb superior.

23. **HLTH** Open the lubricant and place the catheter tip into the lubricant package or squeeze lubricant onto a sterile surface. *Adequate lubrication helps to prevent irritation or injury to the urethra (Aygin & Usta, 2017).*
24. **INF** Open the package of antiseptic swabs or open and pour the antiseptic solution over cotton balls, depending on the contents of the kit.
25. **ACC** If a urine specimen is ordered, remove the lid of the sterile specimen container. Protect the sterility of the inside of the lid. *Ensuring the sterility of the specimen is necessary to ensure the accuracy of laboratory results.*
26. **INF** Place the urine collection container between the client's legs. To move the container, press your thumb and forefinger against the inner walls of the container to lift and move it. *Touching only the inside of the container maintains the sterility of your gloves.* If the client is uncooperative, maintain your container on the over-the-bed table and position the table as close as possible. (Note: Your decision may impact the sterility of your procedure.)

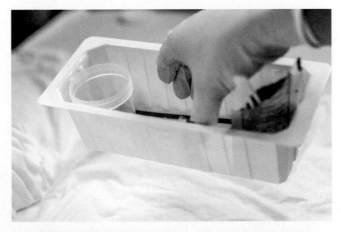

STEP 26 Place the urine collection container between the client's legs.

Clean the Urinary Meatus

(Note: Your nondominant hand will expose the urinary meatus, becoming nonsterile, and your dominant hand will remain sterile.)

27. **ACC** With your nondominant hand, spread the inner labia to reveal the urethral meatus. This hand will continue to hold the labia open until the catheter is inserted. *Spread the labia to visualize the anatomical landmarks, including the clitoris, urethral meatus, and vagina.*

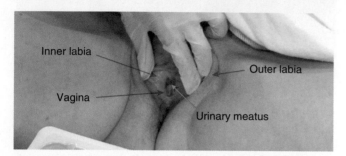

STEP 27 Spread the labia to reveal the urinary meatus.

28. **ACC** Observe carefully for the exact position of the urethral meatus as you pass over the opening with a swab or cotton ball. *Gentle pressure from the swab or cotton ball may make visualization of the urethral meatus easier.*
29. **INF** With your dominant hand, use either antiseptic swab or forceps holding an antiseptic-soaked cotton ball and wipe from above the clitoris toward the rectum (front to back) to one side of the urinary meatus. *Clean from cleanest to dirtiest area.*
30. **INF** Discard the soiled antiseptic swab or cotton ball without passing over the sterile field. *Sterile fields are three-dimensional, and nonsterile items do not cross over the sterile field.*
31. **INF** Wipe from above the clitoris toward the rectum on the other side of the urinary meatus and discard the cotton ball. Clean from cleanest to dirtiest area.
32. **INF** Wipe the third pass directly over the urinary meatus. Always use a new swab or cotton ball each time you wipe.

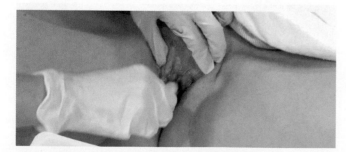

STEP 32 Wipe from above the clitoris toward the rectum.

Insert the Catheter

33. **HLTH** Pick up the catheter. Ensure the tip is well lubricated, and ensure the distal opening of the catheter is in the urine collection tray. If a specimen is to be collected, place the distal end in the specimen container. *Adequate lubrication helps to prevent irritation or injury to the urethra (Aygin & Usta, 2017).*

34. **INF** Hold the catheter 5.0 to 7.5 cm (2–3 inches) from the proximal tip and insert it into the urethra. Slide the catheter through your fingers such that your fingers do not come into contact with the client's skin. *Not touching the client's skin maintains the sterility of your gloved fingers and the catheter.*

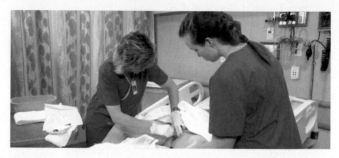

STEP 34 Insert the straight catheter into the urethra.

35. **ACC** Advance the catheter until urine flows.
36. **ACC** If you meet slight resistance, instruct the patient to take a deep breath and blow out slowly through pursed lips. You may also rotate the catheter. *Rotating the catheter allows it to find the path of least resistance. Blowing through pursed lips creates a gentle bearing down which helps relax the sphincter.* **WARNING:** Do not force the catheter.
37. **ACC** When urine is flowing, release the labia with your nondominant hand and hold the catheter securely. Allow the urine to drain until it stops. If you are collecting a specimen, you may need to move the distal end of the catheter from the specimen container when it is full and collect the remainder of the urine in the drainage container.

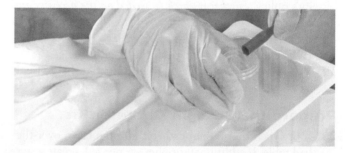

STEP 37 Hold the catheter securely while urine is flowing.

38. **ACC** When the urine flow stops, gently pull out the catheter.
39. **ACC** Remove the container from between the client's legs and place on a secure surface, such as the over-the-bed table. Remove the drapes and discard into the trash.
40. **ACC** If collecting a specimen, secure the specimen container and close the lid tightly. Ensuring the sterility of the specimen is necessary to ensure the accuracy of laboratory results.

41. **ACC** If measuring urine output, note the volume of urine in the specimen container and collection container. Assess the characteristics of the urine.
42. **INF** Dispose of urine in the toilet.
43. **HLTH** Clean the perineal area with warm water and a washcloth to remove the antiseptic solution. Wipe from front to back and using a different section of the washcloth for each stroke. *Antiseptic solution can irritate the periurethral skin. Cleansing helps to protect skin integrity.*
44. **CCC** Remove the disposable absorbent pad from under the client's buttocks.
45. **INF** Remove gloves and perform hand hygiene.
46. **CCC** Assist the client into a comfortable position and return the top bedding to cover the client.
47. **SAF** Place the bed in the lowest position. *These safety measures reduce the risk of falls.*
48. **INF** Apply clean gloves. *If the specimen cup has urine on it, you are protecting yourself from body fluids.*
49. **COM** Ensure the specimen label contains two client identifiers. Label in the presence of the client. Secure the label to the specimen cup. *The specimen cup, rather than the lid, is labeled because the lid can easily be separated*

from the specimen. National safety guidelines recommend labeling specimens in the presence of the client.
50. **COM** Document the date and time of urine specimen collection on the label, if facility policy.
51. **INF** Clean the surface of the over-the-bed table with your facility's disinfectant cleanser.

FINISHING THE SKILL

52. **INF** Remove gloves and perform hand hygiene.
53. **SAF** Ensure client safety and comfort. Ensure the client can identify and reach the nurse call system.
54. **ACC** If a specimen was ordered, transport to the laboratory per facility policy within the time limit or place in a refrigerator. *Many institutions require transportation in a plastic resealable bag. Depending on the type of laboratory testing ordered, the specimen may need to go to the laboratory immediately, may need to be put on ice, or may need to be refrigerated in order to ensure the accuracy of laboratory results.*
55. **COM** Document assessment of urine characteristics, volume of urine output, care given, date and time of specimen collection, and client outcome in the legal healthcare record.

■ SKILL 15.8 Inserting and Removing a Straight Catheter in a Male Client

EQUIPMENT

Straight catheter kit (containing straight catheter, sterile gloves, lubricant, urine collection container, and cleansing swabs or cotton balls and antiseptic solution)
Straight catheter (if not in the kit)
Water-soluble lubricant (if not in the kit)
Water-soluble 2% lidocaine hydrochloride jelly in a syringe, if ordered
Antiseptic swabs or forceps, cotton balls, and antiseptic solution (if not in the kit)
Sterile specimen container, if specimen is ordered
Washcloth/basin/water or hygienic wipes
Clean gloves
Sheet or bath blanket
Absorbent pad

BEGINNING THE SKILL

1. **SAF** Review the order.
2. **INF** Perform hand hygiene.
3. **CCC** Introduce yourself to the client and explain the purpose and procedure for performing a straight catheterization. Ensure that the client consents to the procedure.
4. **SAF** Identify the client using two identifiers.

5. **SAF** Determine if the client has any pertinent allergies, such as iodine or latex. *Antiseptic solution may be betadine, and the catheter may be latex.*
6. **CCC** Provide privacy; close the door and pull the curtain.
7. **INF** Apply gloves.

PROCEDURE

8. **SAF** Set up an ergonomically safe space. Raise the bed to a comfortable working height. Raise one side rail. Set up a workspace according to your hand dominance; that is, if you are right-handed, stand on the client's right side. *Setting up an ergonomically safe space prevents injury to the nurse and client.*
9. **INF** Set up a work triangle: sterile field, client, and trash receptacle. *Preparing your work area with a trash receptacle helps to maintain sterile technique.*
10. **ACC** Assess the client's degree of cooperation, mobility, and level of discomfort. *Your assessment is to determine the extent to which the client can cooperate during the procedure and tolerate positioning. You may need to find a colleague or family member to assist you with this procedure.*
11. **ACC** Assess urine output.

Position the Client for Catheterization

12. Fold the top bedding to the bottom of the bed.
13. **ACC** Position a man supine or in the Fowler position with the knees flexed and the thighs abducted.
14. **CCC** Use the top bedding to cover the client's legs and a bath blanket to cover the torso. *Covering the client prevents chilling and provides privacy. Clients feel much less exposed if they are partially covered.*
15. **CCC** Place a disposable absorbent pad under the client's buttocks. *Disposable absorbent pads prevent spillage on the client's sheets.*
16. **INF** Perform periurethral cleaning if this is your facility policy. *Further research is needed on the necessity and the type of solution used for periurethral cleaning prior to catheterization (CDC, 2015b).*
17. **INF** Remove gloves and perform hand hygiene.

Prepare the Straight Catheter Kit

18. **INF** Open the straight catheter kit on a clean over-the-bed table. If additional supplies are needed, add supplies using sterile technique. If 2% lidocaine hydrochloride jelly has been ordered, add the syringe to the kit.
19. **INF** Drape the client. Paper drapes may be placed before you put on sterile gloves if the drapes are only touched on the outer 2.5-cm (1-inch) border. Place the square drape without a window between the client's thighs just under the buttocks. Place the fenestrated drape, one with a diamond-shaped window, over the perineal area, exposing the penis. *Use of a drape is proper technique for urinary catheter insertion. Draping may be a factor in reducing the rate of infection (Barbadoro et al., 2015; CDC, 2015b).*
20. **INF** Apply sterile gloves. (Note: Alternatively, apply sterile gloves and then place drapes as described previously, but do not allow your sterile gloves to become contaminated. Hold the corners of the drape between your thumb and forefinger with the thumb superior; rotate your hands, cuffing them in the sterile drape.)
21. **HLTH** If not using lubricant jelly in a syringe, open the lubricant and squeeze out the lubricant on a sterile surface. *Adequate lubrication helps to prevent irritation or injury to the urethra (Aygin & Usta, 2017).*
22. **INF** Open the package of antiseptic swabs or open and pour the antiseptic solution over cotton balls.
23. **ACC** If a urine specimen is ordered, remove the lid of the sterile specimen container. Protect the sterility of the inside of the lid. *Ensuring the sterility of the specimen is necessary to ensure the accuracy of laboratory results.*
24. **INF** Place the urine collection container between the client's legs. To move the container, press your thumb and forefinger against the inner walls of the container to lift and move it. *Touching only the inside of the container maintains the sterility of your gloves.*

Clean the Urinary Meatus

(Note: Your nondominant hand will hold the penis, becoming nonsterile, and your dominant hand will remain sterile.)

25. **ACC** Hold the penis in your nondominant hand, and if the client is uncircumcised, retract the foreskin. This hand will continue to hold the penis until the catheter is inserted.
26. **INF** With your dominant hand, use either the antiseptic swab or forceps holding an antiseptic-soaked cotton ball to wipe in a circular motion, starting from the urethral meatus and then wiping outward around the head of the penis. *Clean from cleanest to dirtiest area.*

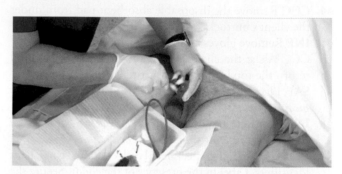

STEP 26 Wipe in a circular motion, starting from the urethral meatus.

27. **INF** Discard the soiled antiseptic swab or cotton ball without passing over the sterile field. *Sterile fields are three-dimensional, and nonsterile items do not cross over the sterile field.*
28. **INF** Clean from the urethral meatus, wiping outward around the head of the penis with the antiseptic solution two more times. Always use a new swab or cotton ball each time you wipe. *Do not allow the dirty swab or cotton ball to return to a cleaned area because that would contaminate the area.*

Insert the Catheter

29. **HLTH** Insert the tip of the syringe into the urethral meatus and slowly inject 5 to 10 mL of water-soluble lubricant or water-soluble 2% lidocaine hydrochloride jelly. If a syringe of lubricant is not available, generously lubricate the catheter tip 13 to 18 cm (5–7 inches). *Instillation of lubricant dilates the urethra, coats the urethra, and facilitates insertion of the catheter. Adequate lubrication helps to prevent irritation or injury to the urethra. Use of 2% lidocaine has shown to decrease discomfort in men (Aygin & Usta, 2017).*
30. **ACC** Pick up the catheter and ensure the distal opening of the catheter is in the urine collection tray. If a specimen is to be collected, place the distal end in the specimen container.
31. **ACC** Hold the penis perpendicular to the client's legs and gently stretch the penis upward, straightening the urethra.
32. **INF** Hold the catheter about 8 cm (3 inches) from the proximal tip and insert it into the urethra. Slide the catheter through your fingers such that your fingers do not

come into contact with the client's skin. *Not touching the client's skin keeps your gloved fingers and the catheter sterile.*

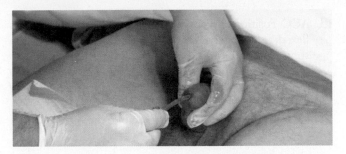

STEP 32 Insert the straight catheter into the urethra.

33. **ACC** Advance the catheter until urine flows, which in the male is about 20 cm (8 inches) but may be longer.
34. **ACC** If you meet slight resistance, instruct the patient to take a deep breath and blow out slowly through pursed lips. You may also rotate the catheter. *Rotating the catheter allows it to find the path of least resistance. Blowing through pursed lips creates a gentle bearing down which helps relax the sphincter.* **WARNING:** Do not force the catheter.
35. **ACC** Once urine is flowing, release the penis and hold the catheter securely at the meatus. If you are collecting a specimen, you may need to move the distal end of the catheter from the specimen container when it is full and collect the remainder of the urine in the drainage container.

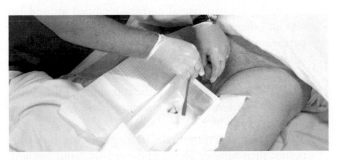

STEP 35 Hold the catheter securely until urine stops flowing.

36. **ACC** When urine stops flowing, gently pull out the catheter.
37. **ACC** Remove the container from between the client's legs and place on a secure surface, such as the over-the-bed table. Remove the drapes and discard into the trash.
38. **ACC** If collecting a specimen, secure the specimen container and close the lid tightly. *Ensuring the sterility of the*

specimen is necessary to ensure the accuracy of laboratory results.

39. **ACC** If measuring urine output, note the volume of urine in the specimen container and collection container.
40. **INF** Dispose of urine in the toilet.
41. **HLTH** Clean the penis with warm water and a washcloth to remove the antiseptic solution. *Antiseptic solution can irritate the periurethral skin. Cleansing helps to protect skin integrity.*
42. **CCC** Remove the disposable absorbent pad from under the client's buttocks.
43. **INF** Remove gloves and perform hand hygiene.
44. **CCC** Assist the client into a comfortable position and return the top bedding to cover the client.
45. **SAF** Place the bed in the lowest position and lower the side rail. *These safety measures reduce the risk of falls.*
46. **INF** Apply gloves. *If the specimen cup has urine on it, you are protecting yourself from body fluids.*
47. **COM** Ensure the specimen label contains two client identifiers. Label in the presence of the client. Secure the label to the specimen cup. *The specimen cup, rather than the lid, is labeled because the lid can easily be separated from the specimen. National safety guidelines recommend labeling specimens in the presence of the client.*
48. **COM** Document the date and time of urine specimen collection on the label, if facility policy.
49. **INF** Clean the surface of the over-the-bed table with your facility's disinfectant cleanser.

FINISHING THE SKILL

50. **INF** Remove gloves and perform hand hygiene.
51. **SAF** Ensure client safety and comfort. Ensure the client can identify and reach the nurse call system.
52. **ACC** If a specimen was ordered, transport to the laboratory per facility policy within the time limit or place in a refrigerator. *Many institutions require transportation in a plastic resealable bag. Depending on the type of laboratory testing ordered, the specimen may need to go to the laboratory immediately or may need to be refrigerated in order to ensure the accuracy of laboratory results.*
53. **COM** Document assessment of urine characteristics, volume of urine output, care given, date and time of specimen collection, and client outcome in the legal healthcare record.

■ SKILL 15.9 Inserting an Indwelling Foley Catheter in a Female Client

EQUIPMENT

Indwelling Foley catheter kit (containing indwelling Foley catheter, sterile gloves, lubricant and cleansing swabs or cotton balls and antiseptic solution)

Sterile gloves (if not in the kit)

Water-soluble lubricant (if not in the kit)

Antiseptic swabs or forceps, cotton balls, and antiseptic solution (if not in the kit)

Urine drainage collection bag and tubing with preconnected, sealed junctions

Tape or catheter securement device

Washcloth/basin/water or hygienic wipes

Clean gloves

Sheet or bath blanket

Absorbent pad

Additional light source (e.g., gooseneck lamp, flashlight)

BEGINNING THE SKILL

1. **SAF** Review the order.
2. **INF** Perform hand hygiene.
3. **CCC** Introduce yourself to the client and explain the purpose and procedure for inserting an indwelling catheter. Ensure that the client consents to the procedure.
4. **SAF** Identify the client using two identifiers.
5. **SAF** Determine if the client has any pertinent allergies, such as iodine or latex. *Antiseptic solution may be betadine, and the catheter may be latex.*
6. **CCC** Provide privacy; close the door and pull the curtain.
7. **INF** Apply gloves.

PROCEDURE

8. **SAF** Set up an ergonomically safe space. Raise the bed to a comfortable working height. Raise one side rail. Set up a workspace according to your hand dominance; that is, if you are right-handed, stand on the client's right side. *Setting up an ergonomically safe space prevents injury to the nurse and client.*
9. **INF** Set up a work triangle: sterile field, client, and trash receptacle. *If the client has the potential to move abruptly, do not set up your sterile field on the bed; use an over-the-bed table. Preparing your work area with a trash receptacle helps to maintain sterile technique.*
10. **ACC** Assess the client's degree of cooperation, degree of mobility, and discomfort. *Your assessment is to determine the extent to which the client can cooperate during the procedure and tolerate positioning. You may need to find a colleague or family member to assist you with this procedure.*
11. **ACC** Assess urine output. Palpate for bladder distension if there has been no recent output.

Position the Client for Catheterization

12. Fold the top bedding to the bottom of the bed.

13. **ACC** Position a woman supine with feet apart, knees flexed, and hips externally rotated. If this position strains the hip joints, position pillows under the knees. *This frog-leg position allows for visualization of the urinary meatus. Supporting the legs may prevent discomfort and strain on the hip joints.*
14. **CCC** If this position is not tolerable, the Sims position may be used (see Skill 1.6).

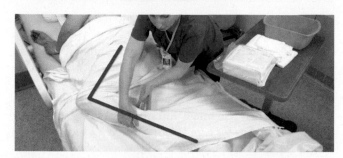

STEP 14 The Sims position is an alternative to the dorsal recumbent position.

15. **CCC** Cover the client from the waist to neck. One method of covering a woman in a supine position is to position a bath blanket with one corner pointed to her neck, the two lateral corners wrapped around her legs and then the last corner folded back to expose the perineum. *Covering the client from the waist up or as described above provides privacy and prevents chilling. Clients feel much less exposed if they are partially covered*
16. **CCC** Place a disposable absorbent pad under the client's buttocks. *Disposable pads prevent spillage on the client's sheets.*
17. **INF** Perform periurethral cleaning, if this is facility policy, then remove gloves and perform hand hygiene. (Note: Some kits come with perineal wipes. If wipes are in the kit, perform periurethral cleaning at Step 22.) *Further research is needed on the necessity and the type of solution used for periurethral cleaning prior to catheterization (CDC, 2015b).*
18. **ACC** Position additional lighting to help visualize the urinary meatus. *Identifying correct landmarks is critical for accurate catheter placement.*

Prepare the Indwelling Foley Kit

19. **INF** If the catheter pack has an outer wrapper, you may choose to use it for a trash receptacle. Peel open the outer wrapper, cuff the top, and place at the client's hip. Set up a work triangle: sterile field, client, trash receptacle.
20. **INF** Position the pack with the top flap of the wrapper set to open away from you on a clean over-the-bed table (see Skill 10.1).
21. **INF** Open the flaps (1) away from you, (2) right, and (3) left, and lastly, grasp the final flap and pull toward you (see Skill 10.1).

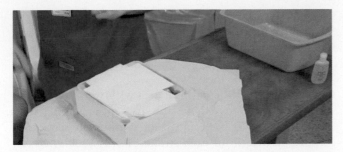

STEP 21 Open the first flap away from you.

22. Inspect the catheter kit. (Note: Some kits come with perineal wipes. If wipes are in the kit, apply clean gloves, perform perineal care, and then remove gloves and perform hand hygiene. Many indwelling catheter kits have two tiers, with the catheter insertion supplies in the top tier and the urine drainage collection bag, tubing, and catheter with preconnected, sealed junctions in the bottom tier.)
23. **INF** If additional supplies are needed, create a sterile field, and add supplies using sterile technique.
24. **INF** Drape the client. Paper drapes may be placed before you put on sterile gloves if the drapes are only touched on the outer 2.5-cm (1-inch) border with *clean* hands. Pluck the drape from the catheter kit. Place the square drape without a window between the client's thighs just under the buttocks. Place the fenestrated drape, one with a diamond-shaped window, over the perineal area, exposing the labia. *Draping may be a factor in reducing the rate of infection (Barbadoro et al., 2015; CDC, 2015b).*
25. **INF** Apply sterile gloves. (Note: Alternatively, apply sterile gloves and then place drapes as described previously, but do not allow your sterile gloves to become contaminated. Hold the corners of the drape between your thumb and forefinger with the thumb superior; rotate your hands, cuffing them in the sterile drape.)
26. **ACC** If the client is fully cooperative, move the top tier or sterile catheter tray between the client's legs. If the client is uncooperative, maintain your container on the over-the-bed table and position the table as close to the client as possible.

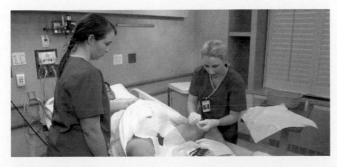

STEP 26 Position the catheter tray between the client's legs and prepare the tray.

27. **INF** Move the box with the bottom tier with the catheter, tubing, and drainage collection bag just below the sterile field between the client's legs. To move the box and maintain the sterility of your gloves, keep your gloved fingers on the inside of the box and press outward on the walls (see Skill 15.7, Step 26).
28. **HLTH** Open the lubricant and squeeze lubricant onto a sterile surface. *Adequate lubrication helps to prevent irritation or injury to the urethra (Aygin & Usta, 2017).*
29. **INF** Open the package of antiseptic swabs or open and pour the antiseptic solution over the cotton balls, depending on the contents of the kit.
30. **ACC** Attach the syringe of sterile water to the balloon port of the catheter. *Attaching the syringe in advance allows you to inject the sterile water and inflate the balloon with one hand later when the catheter is in the bladder.*
31. **ACC** Open the perforated plastic cover of the Foley catheter and position the catheter on the sterile tray. *The catheter is attached to the drainage tubing and has the syringe of sterile water attached. It is unwieldy and tends to move, so position it carefully to ensure the sterility of the procedure.*

Clean the Urinary Meatus

(Note: Your nondominant hand will expose the urinary meatus, becoming nonsterile, and your dominant hand will remain sterile.)

32. **ACC** With your nondominant hand, spread the labia to reveal the urinary meatus. This hand will continue to hold the labia open until the catheter is inserted.

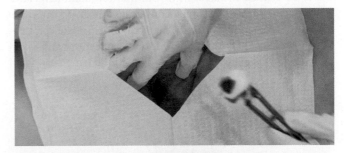

STEP 32 With your nondominant hand, spread the labia to reveal the urinary meatus.

33. **ACC** As you pass over the urinary meatus, look carefully for the exact position of the opening. *Gentle pressure from the swab or cotton ball may make visualization of the opening easier.*
34. **INF** With your dominant hand, use either the antiseptic swab or forceps holding an antiseptic-soaked cotton ball, wipe from above the clitoris toward the rectum (front to back) to one side of the urinary meatus. *Clean from cleanest to dirtiest area.*

35. **INF** Discard the soiled antiseptic swab or cotton ball without passing over the sterile field. *Sterile fields are three-dimensional, and nonsterile items do not cross over the sterile field.*
36. **INF** Wipe from above the clitoris toward the rectum on the other side of the urinary meatus and discard the cotton ball. *Clean from cleanest to dirtiest area.*
37. **INF** Wipe the third pass directly over the urinary meatus. Always use a new swab or cotton ball each time you wipe. *Do not allow the dirty swab or cotton ball to return to a cleaned area because that would contaminate the area.*

Insert the Catheter

38. **HLTH** Pick up the catheter. Lubricate the tip 4 to 5 cm (1–2 inches) and ensure the attached drainage tubing has enough slack to allow you to insert the catheter. *Adequate lubrication helps to prevent irritation or injury to the urethra (Aygin & Usta, 2017).*
39. **INF** Hold the catheter 5 to 7.5 cm (2–3 inches) from the proximal tip and insert it into the urethra. Slide the catheter through your fingers such that your fingers do not come into contact with the client's skin. *Not touching the client's skin keeps your gloved fingers and the catheter sterile.*
40. **ACC** Advance the catheter until you see urine flowing in the drainage tubing.
41. **ACC** If you meet slight resistance, instruct the patient to take a deep breath and blow out slowly through pursed lips. You may also rotate the catheter. *Rotating the catheter allows it to find the path of least resistance. Blowing through pursed lips creates a gentle bearing down which helps relax the sphincter.* **WARNING:** Do not force the catheter.
42. **ACC** Once urine is flowing, advance the catheter an additional 4 to 5 cm (1–2 inches). *Advancing the catheter ensures the balloon is completely in the bladder when you inflate it.*
43. **ACC** Release the labia with your nondominant hand and hold the catheter securely. Your dominant hand can then inject the sterile water in the syringe to inflate the balloon. (Note: If you are comfortable injecting with your nondominant hand, you do not need to change hands.)

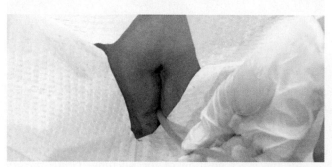

STEP 43 Release the labia with your nondominant hand and hold the catheter securely.

44. **ACC** Gently tug the catheter in order to position the balloon into the neck of the bladder.
45. **INF** Remove the top and bottom tiers of the catheter kit and discard into the trash. Remove the drapes and discard into the trash.
46. **HLTH** Clean the perineal area with warm water and a washcloth to remove the antiseptic, wiping only from front to back and using a different section of the washcloth for each stroke. *Antiseptic solution can irritate the periurethral skin. Cleansing helps to protect skin integrity.*
47. **CCC** Remove the disposable absorbent pad from under the client's buttocks.
48. **HLTH** Secure the catheter to the client's thigh. Facilities have a variety of devices to secure catheters. If a specific device is not available, the tubing can be taped to the thigh. *Preventing movement helps to prevent irritation of the urethra.*
49. **SAF** Secure the urine drainage bag to the bed frame. *If you secure the bag to any moving parts of the bed, it may accidentally place tension on the catheter when moved.*

FINISHING THE SKILL

50. **INF** Remove gloves and perform hand hygiene.
51. **CCC** Ensure client comfort. Assist the client into a comfortable position and return the top bedding to cover the client.
52. **SAF** Ensure client safety. Place the bed in the lowest position. Ensure that the client can identify and reach the nurse call system. *This safety measure reduces the risk of falls.*
53. **INF** Apply gloves.
54. **ACC** Assess urine output.
55. **INF** Clean the surface of the over-the-bed table with your facility's antiseptic. Remove gloves and perform hand hygiene.
56. **COM** Document assessment of urine characteristics, volume of urine output, size of catheter inserted, care given, and client outcome in the legal healthcare record.

■ SKILL 15.10 Inserting an Indwelling Foley Catheter in a Male Client

EQUIPMENT

Indwelling Foley catheter kit (containing indwelling Foley catheter, sterile gloves, lubricant and cleansing swabs or cotton balls and antiseptic solution)

Sterile gloves (if not in the kit)

Water-soluble lubricant in a syringe (if not in the kit)

Water-soluble 2% lidocaine hydrochloride jelly in a syringe, if ordered

Antiseptic swabs or forceps, cotton balls, and antiseptic solution (if not in the kit)

Urine drainage collection bag and tubing with pre-connected, sealed junctions

Tape or catheter holder

Washcloth/basin/water or hygienic wipes

Clean gloves

Sheet or bath blanket

Absorbent pad

BEGINNING THE SKILL

1. **SAF** Review the order.
2. **INF** Perform hand hygiene.
3. **CCC** Introduce yourself to the client and explain the purpose and procedure for inserting an indwelling catheter. Ensure that the client consents to the procedure.
4. **SAF** Identify the client using two identifiers.
5. **SAF** Determine if the client has any pertinent allergies, such as iodine or latex. *Antiseptic solution may be betadine, and the catheter may be latex.*
6. **CCC** Provide privacy; close the door and pull the curtain.

PROCEDURE

7. **INF** Apply gloves.
8. **SAF** Set up an ergonomically safe space. Raise the bed to a comfortable working height. Raise one side rail. Set up a workspace according to your hand dominance; that is, if you are right-handed, stand on the client's right side. *Setting up an ergonomically safe space prevents injury to the nurse and client.*
9. **INF** Set up a work triangle: sterile field, client, trash receptacle. *If the client has the potential to move abruptly, do not set up your sterile field on the bed; use an over-the-bed table. Preparing your work area with a trash receptacle helps to maintain sterile technique.*
10. **ACC** Assess the client's degree of cooperation, degree of mobility, and discomfort. *Your assessment is to determine the extent to which the client can cooperate during the procedure and tolerate positioning. You may need to find a colleague or family member to assist you with this procedure.*
11. **ACC** Assess urine output. Palpate for bladder distension if there has been no recent output.

Position the Client for Catheterization

12. **ACC** Position a man supine or in the Fowler position with the knees flexed and thighs abducted.
13. **CCC** Use the top bedding to cover the client's legs and a bath blanket to cover the torso. *Covering the client prevents chilling and provides privacy.*
14. **INF** Place a disposable absorbent pad under the client's buttocks. *Disposable pads prevent spillage on the client's sheets.*
15. **INF** Perform periurethral cleaning, if this is facility policy, then remove gloves and perform hand hygiene. (Note: Some kits come with perineal wipes. If wipes are in the kit, perform periurethral cleaning at Step 22.) *Further research is needed on the necessity and the type of solution used for periurethral cleaning prior to catheterization (CDC, 2015b).*

Prepare the Indwelling Foley Kit

16. **INF** If the catheter kit pack has an outer wrapper, you may choose to use it for a trash receptacle. Peel open the outer wrapper, cuff the top and place at the client's hip. Set up a work triangle: sterile field, client, trash receptacle.

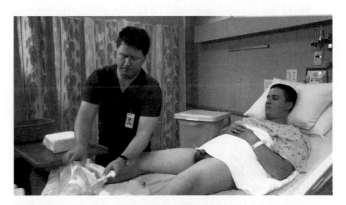

STEP 16 Identify a trash receptacle.

17. **INF** Position the pack with the top flap of the wrapper set to open away from you on a clean over-the-bed table (see Skill 10.1).
18. **INF** Open the flaps (1) away from you, (2) right, and (3) left, and lastly, grasp the final flap and pull toward you.
19. Inspect the catheter kit pack. (Note: Some kits come with perineal wipes. If wipes are in the kit, apply clean gloves, perform perineal care, and then remove gloves and perform hand hygiene. It may have two tiers with the catheter insertion supplies in the top tier and the urine drainage collection bag, tubing, and catheter with preconnected, sealed junctions in the bottom tier.)

20. **INF** If additional supplies are needed, add supplies using sterile technique. If 2% lidocaine hydrochloride jelly has been ordered, add the syringe to the kit.

21. **INF** Drape the client. Paper drapes may be placed before you put on sterile gloves if the drapes are only touched on the outer 2.5-cm (1-inch) border with *clean* hands. Pluck the drape from the catheter kit. Place the square drape without a window over the client's thighs. Place the fenestrated drape, one with a diamond-shaped window, over the penis. *Draping may be a factor in reducing the rate of infection (Barbadoro et al., 2015; CDC, 2015b).*

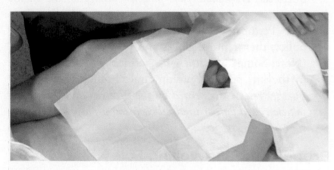

STEP 21 Drape the client.

22. **INF** Apply sterile gloves. Alternatively, apply sterile gloves and then place drapes as described previously, but do *not* allow your sterile gloves to become contaminated. Hold the corners of the drape between your thumb and forefinger with the thumb superior; rotate your hands, cuffing them in the sterile drape.

23. **ACC** If the client is fully cooperative, move the top tier or sterile catheter tray between the client's legs. To move the tray and maintain the sterility of your gloves, keep your gloved fingers on the inside of the tray and press outward on the tray walls. If the client is uncooperative, maintain your container on the over-the-bed table and position the table as close to the client as possible.

24. **INF** Move the box with the bottom tier with the catheter, tubing, and drainage collection bag just below the sterile field between the client's legs. To move the box, keep your gloved fingers on the inside of the box and press outward on the walls.

25. **HLTH** If not using lubricant jelly in a syringe, open the lubricant and squeeze lubricant onto a sterile tray surface. *Adequate lubrication helps to prevent irritation or injury to the urethra (Aygin & Usta, 2017).*

26. **INF** Open the package of antiseptic swabs or open and pour the antiseptic solution over cotton balls, depending on the contents of the kit.

27. **ACC** Attach the syringe of sterile water to the balloon port of the catheter. *Attaching the syringe in advance allows you to inject the sterile water and inflate the balloon with one hand later when the catheter is in the bladder.*

28. **ACC** Open the perforated plastic cover of the Foley catheter and position the catheter on the sterile tray. *The catheter is attached to the drainage tubing and has the syringe of sterile water attached. It is unwieldy and tends*

to move, so position it carefully to ensure the sterility of the procedure.

Clean the Urinary Meatus

(Note: Your nondominant hand will expose the urinary meatus, becoming nonsterile, and your dominant hand will remain sterile.)

29. **ACC** Hold the penis in your nondominant hand, and if the client is uncircumcised, retract the foreskin. This hand will continue to hold the penis until the catheter is inserted.

30. **INF** With your dominant hand, use either the antiseptic swab or forceps holding an antiseptic-soaked cotton ball to wipe in a circular motion starting from the urethral meatus and then wiping outward around the head of the penis. *Clean from cleanest to dirtiest area.*

31. **INF** Discard the soiled antiseptic swab or cotton ball without passing over the sterile field. *Sterile fields are three-dimensional, and nonsterile items do not cross over the sterile field.*

32. **INF** Clean from the urethral meatus, wiping outward around the head of the penis with the antiseptic solution two more times. Always use a new swab or cotton ball each time you wipe. **WARNING:** Do not allow the dirty swab or cotton ball to return to a cleaned area because that would contaminate the area.

Insert the Catheter

33. **HLTH** Insert the tip of the syringe into the urethral meatus and slowly inject 5 to 10 mL of water-soluble lubricant or water-soluble 2% lidocaine hydrochloride jelly. If a syringe of lubricant is not available, generously lubricate the catheter tip 13 to 18 cm (5–7 inches). *Instillation of lubricant dilates the urethra, coats the urethra, and facilitates insertion of the catheter. Adequate lubrication helps to prevent irritation or injury to the urethra. The use of 2% lidocaine has been shown to significantly decrease discomfort (Aygin &Usta, 2017).*

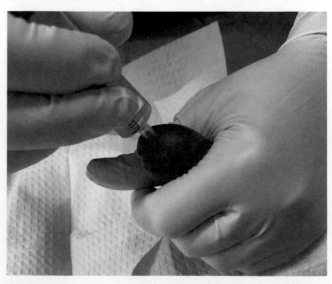

STEP 33 Slowly inject 5 to 10 mL of water-soluble lubricant.

34. **INF** Pick up the catheter and ensure the attached drainage tubing has enough slack to allow you to insert the catheter and maintain the sterility of the catheter.

35. **ACC** Hold the penis perpendicular to the client's legs and gently stretch the penis upward, straightening the urethra.

36. **INF** Hold the catheter about 8 cm (3 inches) from the proximal tip and insert it into the urethra. Slide the catheter through your fingers such that your fingers do not come into contact with the client's skin. *Not touching the client's skin maintains the sterility of your gloved fingers and the catheter.*

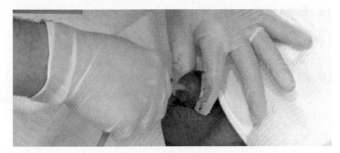

STEP 36 Insert the catheter into the urethra.

37. **ACC** Advance the catheter until you see urine flowing in the drainage tubing, which in the male may be between 20 and 30 cm (8–12 inches).

38. **ACC** If you meet slight resistance, do not force the catheter. Instruct the client to take a deep breath and blow out slowly through pursed lips. You may also rotate the catheter. *Rotating the catheter allows it to find the path of least resistance. Blowing through pursed lips creates a gentle bearing down, which helps relax the sphincter.*

39. **ACC** Once urine is flowing, advance the catheter 4 to 5 cm (1–2 inches) to the bifurcation of the ports. *Advancing the catheter ensures the balloon is completely in the bladder when you inflate it. Some urologists prefer the catheter to be inserted up to the balloon port.*

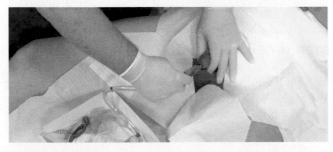

STEP 39 Advance the catheter up to the bifurcation of the ports.

40. **ACC** Release the penis with your nondominant hand and hold the catheter securely. Your dominant hand can then inject the sterile water in the syringe to inflate the balloon. *If you are comfortable injecting with your nondominant hand, you do not need to change hands.*

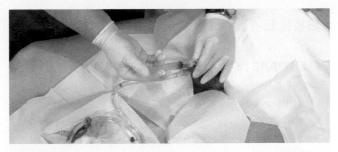

STEP 40 Inject the sterile water in the syringe to inflate the balloon.

41. **ACC** Gently tug the catheter in order to position the balloon into the neck of the bladder.

42. **INF** Remove the top and bottom tiers of the catheter kit and discard into the trash. Remove the drapes and discard into the trash.

43. **HLTH** Clean the penis with warm water and a washcloth to remove the antiseptic. *Antiseptic solution can irritate the periurethral skin. Cleansing helps to protect skin integrity.*

44. **CCC** Remove the disposable absorbent pad from under the client's buttocks.

45. **HLTH** Secure the catheter to the client's thigh or abdomen. (Note: Facilities have a variety of devices to secure catheters. If a specific device is not available, the tubing can be taped to the thigh.) *Preventing movement helps to prevent irritation of the urethra.*

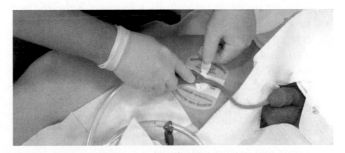

STEP 45 Secure the catheter to the client's thigh.

46. **SAF** Secure the urine drainage bag to the bed frame. *If you secure the bag to any moving parts of the bed, it may accidentally place tension on the catheter when moved.*

FINISHING THE SKILL

47. **INF** Remove gloves and perform hand hygiene.

48. **CCC** Ensure client comfort Assist the client into a comfortable position and return the top bedding to cover the client.

49. **SAF** Ensure client safety. Place the bed in the lowest position. Ensure that the client can identify and reach the nurse call system. *These safety measures reduce the risk of falls.*

51. **ACC** Apply gloves and assess urine output.

52. **INF** Clean the surface of the over-the-bed table with your facility's antiseptic. Remove gloves and perform hand hygiene.

53. **COM** Document assessment of urine characteristics, volume of urine output, size of catheter inserted, care given, and client outcome in the legal healthcare record.

■ **SKILL 15.11** Removing an Indwelling Foley Catheter

EQUIPMENT

Clean gloves
10-mL Luer-Lok syringe, or larger as indicated on the balloon port
Graduated cylinder
Absorbent pad
Washcloth/basin/water or hygienic wipes
Paper towel

BEGINNING THE SKILL

1. **SAF** Review the order.
2. **INF** Perform hand hygiene.
3. **CCC** Introduce yourself to the client and explain the purpose and procedure for removing an indwelling catheter. Ensure that the client consents to the procedure.
4. **SAF** Identify the client using two identifiers.
5. **CCC** Provide privacy; close the door and pull the curtain.
6. **INF** Apply gloves.

PROCEDURE

7. **SAF** Set up an ergonomically safe space. Raise the bed to a comfortable working height. Raise one side rail. *Setting up an ergonomically safe space prevents injury to the nurse and client.*
8. **SAF** Set up a workspace according to your hand dominance, right-handed on the client's right side.
9. **SAF** Assess the client's degree of cooperation, degree of mobility, and discomfort. *Your assessment is to determine the extent to which the client can cooperate during the procedure and tolerate positioning.*
10. **ACC** Position the client.
    a. **For a man,** position supine or in the Fowler position with the knees flexed and thighs abducted. Use the top bedding to cover the client's legs and a bath blanket to cover the torso. *Covering the client prevents chilling and provides privacy.*
    b. **For a woman,** fold the top bedding to the bottom of the bed. Position supine with the feet apart, knees flexed, and hips externally rotated. If this position strains the hips joints, position pillows under the knees. Drape a bath blanket over the woman, with one corner pointed to her neck, the two lateral corners wrapped around her legs, and then the last corner folded back to expose the perineum. *The frog-leg position allows for visualization of the urinary meatus. Supporting the legs may prevent discomfort and strain on the hip joints.*
    c. If the woman cannot tolerate supine positioning, the Sims position may be used.
11. **CCC** Place a disposable absorbent pad under the client's buttocks. *Disposable pads prevent spillage on the client's sheets.*
12. **ACC** Release the catheter tubing from any device used to secure the catheter and remove the catheter holder.
13. **ACC** Move any urine in the drainage bag tubing into the drainage bag. Empty the drainage bag.
14. **EVAL** Measure and record the urine output. Assess urine characteristics.
15. **ACC** Assess the urethral meatus for signs of irritation or infection (e.g., redness, drainage).
16. **ACC** Examine the catheter and confirm the balloon size. Attach the 10-mL Luer-Lok syringe to the balloon port and gently aspirate the fluid from the balloon. *Most indwelling Foley catheters have markings indicating the balloon volume. Most balloons are inflated with 10 mL of sterile water, but larger balloons do exist. Rapid aspiration of the balloon may collapse the lumen to the balloon.*

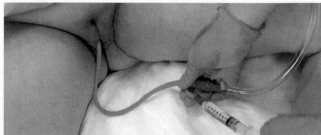
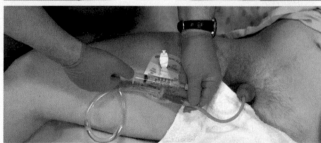

STEP 16 Gently aspirate the fluid from the balloon.

17. **SAF** Gently tug on the catheter to ensure it is moving freely. **WARNING:** Do not remove the catheter forcefully if it is not moving freely. *Attempting to remove the catheter if it is not moving freely will result in urethral damage.*
18. **EVAL** Confirm you have aspirated the volume indicated on the balloon port. *Significant injury to the urethra can occur if the balloon is not completely deflated.*
19. **ACC** Pinch the catheter near the urethral meatus and pull it out of the urethra.

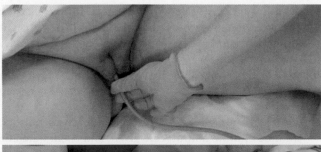

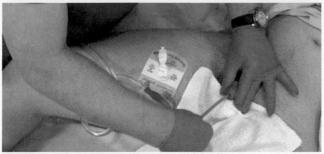

STEP 19 Pull the catheter out of the urethra.

20. **INF** Place the catheter in a disposable absorbent pad for disposal.
21. **INF** Remove the drainage bag from the bed frame and place the urinary catheter/drainage bag system into the proper receptacle per facility policy.

FINISHING THE SKILL

22. **INF** Remove gloves and perform hand hygiene.
25. **CCC** Ensure client comfort. Assist the client into a comfortable position and return the top bedding to cover the client.
26. **SAF** Ensure client safety. Place the bed in the lowest position. Ensure that the client can identify and reach the nurse call system. *These safety measures reduce the risk of falls.*
28. **HLTH** Encourage fluid intake. Provide the client with fresh ice water or other liquids. *Fluid intake helps to keep urine dilute and prevent encrustations.*
29. **COM** Document urine characteristics, volume of urine output, assessment of urethral meatus, size of catheter removed, care given, and outcomes in the legal healthcare record.

■ SKILL 15.12 Managing an Indwelling Foley Catheter

EQUIPMENT

Clean gloves

BEGINNING THE SKILL

1. **INF** Perform hand hygiene.
2. **CCC** Introduce yourself to the client and explain the purpose of managing an indwelling Foley catheter.
3. **SAF** Identify the client using two identifiers.
4. **SAF** Determine if the client has any pertinent allergies, such as iodine or latex. *Antiseptic solution may be betadine, and the catheter may be latex.*
5. **CCC** Provide privacy; close the door and pull the curtain.
6. **INF** Apply gloves.

PROCEDURE

7. **ACC** Maintain an unobstructed flow of urine by keeping the catheter and tubing free from kinks.
8. **ACC** Keep the urine collection back below the level of the bladder at all times.
9. **SAF** Hang the collection bag from the bed frame and not from any moveable part of the bed. *Hanging the collection bag on a moveable part such as the side rail may result in inadvertent pulling and trauma to the urethral meatus and bladder neck.*

10. **INF** Clean the catheter insertion site and periurethral area with routine bathing. Do not clean with antiseptics.
11. **HLTH** Remove any catheter holder used to secure the client's catheter per facility protocol. Assess the skin. If there are signs of irritation, resecure the catheter on the other leg.

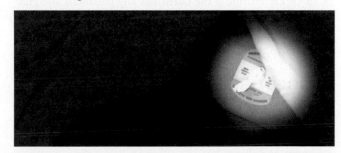

STEP 11 Assess the skin around the securing device.

12. **INF** Use client-specific, labeled, calibrated measuring containers to measure urine from the drainage collection bag. Do not share measuring containers between clients.
13. **INF** Do not allow the urine drainage bag spigot to touch the calibrated measuring container when draining urine.
14. **HLTH** Empty the urine drainage bag when it is one-half to two-thirds full or every 3 to 6 hours. *Emptying*

the bag prevents unnecessary tension on the catheter and subsequent irritation or injury to the urethra.

15. **ACC** If obtaining a urine specimen, use sterile technique and access the urine from the drainage tubing port.
16. **ACC** Assess urine output according to facility protocol.
17. **ACC** Assess urine characteristics, including color, clarity, and odor.

FINISHING THE SKILL

18. **INF** Remove gloves and perform hand hygiene.

19. **SAF** Ensure client safety and comfort. Ensure that the bed is in the lowest position and verify that the client can identify and reach the nurse call system. *These safety measures reduce the risk of falls.*
20. **HLTH** Encourage fluid intake. Provide the client with fresh ice water or other liquids. *Fluid intake helps to keep urine dilute and prevent encrustations.*
21. **COM** Document assessment of urine characteristics, volume of urine output, care given, and client outcome in the legal healthcare record.

■ SKILL 15.13 Performing Intermittent Closed Bladder Irrigation

EQUIPMENT

Clean gloves
Bottle of sterile normal saline solution
Sterile graduated cylinder
Antiseptic wipe
60-mL Luer-Lok syringe (and needleless cannula), depending on the type of system used
Absorbent pad
Clamp

BEGINNING THE SKILL

1. **SAF** Review the order.
2. **INF** Perform hand hygiene.
3. **CCC** Introduce yourself to the client and explain the purpose and procedure for intermittent bladder irrigation. Ensure that the client consents to the procedure.
4. **SAF** Identify the client using two identifiers.
5. **SAF** Determine if the client has any pertinent allergies.
6. **CCC** Provide privacy; close the door and pull the curtain.
7. **INF** Apply clean gloves.

PROCEDURE

8. **SAF** Set up an ergonomically safe space. Raise the bed to a comfortable working height. Raise one side rail. *Setting up an ergonomically safe space prevents injury to the nurse and client.*
9. **SAF** Set up a workspace according to your hand dominance, right-handed on the client's right side.
10. **SAF** Assess the client's degree of cooperation and discomfort. *Your assessment is to determine the client's pain level prior to irrigation and compare to the pain level after irrigation and assess the extent to which the client can cooperate during the procedure.*
11. **ACC** Assess the type of catheter in place. *If the client has a double-lumen or two-way catheter, the irrigant will be instilled through the port in the tubing. If the client has a triple-lumen or three-way catheter, the irrigant can be instilled through the third lumen.*

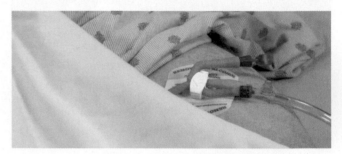

STEP 11 Assess the type of catheter in place.

12. **ACC** Assess the patency of the urinary catheter by inspecting the urine output. Empty the urine drainage bag.
13. **ACC** Assess to determine if the client's bladder is full. Palpate gently, moving down from the umbilicus, to determine if the top edge of the bladder is easily palpable. (Note: The authorized healthcare provider may also order a bladder volume measurement using a bladder scanner.)
14. **ACC** Assist the client into a comfortable position that allows access to the distal end of the Foley catheter tubing. *The semi-Fowler position with the knees bent and thighs slightly separated is appropriate for male and female clients.*
15. **CCC** Use the top bedding to cover the client's legs and a bath blanket to cover the torso. *Covering the client prevents chilling and provides privacy.*
16. **CCC** Place a disposable absorbent pad under the injection port of the urinary catheter tubing. *Disposable absorbent pads help to prevent the bed linens from becoming wet and soiled.*
17. **SAF** Perform medication safety checks for the irrigant, including expiration date, and six rights. Determine if the irrigant is to be immediately released from the bladder or instilled for a specific amount of time. *Bladder irrigant is injected into the body and therefore is a medication.* (See discussion of medication administration in Chapter 11.)
18. **ACC** Pour irrigant into a sterile graduated container. A typical volume is 30 to 60 mL. Pour a little more than ordered into the container.
19. **ACC** Aspirate prescribed volume of irrigant in a 60-mL Toomey syringe if a triple-lumen catheter is in place or a Luer-Lok syringe if a double-lumen catheter is in place.

Maintain the sterility of the tip. If using a needleless cannula, attach the cannula using sterile technique.

20. **SAF** Clamp the drainage tubing distal to the port per facility policy.

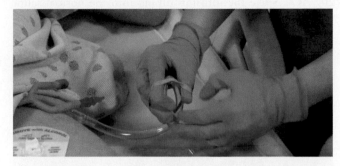

STEP 20 Clamp the drainage tubing distal to the port per facility policy.

21. **INF** Clean the designated port with an antiseptic wipe and allow to air dry. *Cleaning prevents the transfer of microorganisms into the bladder.*
22. **ACC** If a triple-lumen catheter is in place, remove the sterile cap and insert the sterile tip of the Toomey syringe into the designated port. If a double-lumen catheter is in place, insert the Luer-Lok syringe by pushing the syringe into the port and rotating, or insert a needleless cannula into the aspiration port.
23. **ACC** Slowly inject the irrigant into the bladder. *Rapid injection may be uncomfortable for the client and may trigger bladder spasms.*

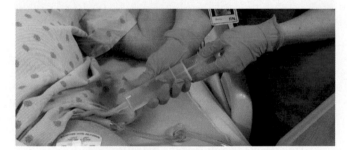

STEP 23 Slowly inject the irrigant into the bladder.

24. **ACC** Release the clamp on the drainage tubing after the prescribed time and observe the drainage tubing for urine output. Determine if a second flush of irrigant is ordered. *Know your facility protocol on the length of time urinary tubing can be clamped. Facilities may have specific time limits due to the risk of bladder distention.*
25. **INF** Remove the irrigant syringe. If a triple-lumen catheter is in place, place a new sterile cap on the third lumen.
26. **INF** Empty the urine collection bag. Do not allow the spigot to touch the calibrated measuring container. *This prevents the transfer of microorganisms into the drainage bag.*
27. **ACC** Assess the volume of urine output. Subtract the volume of irrigant and record the urine output.
28. **ACC** Assess the characteristics of the urine, including sediment or clots that may obstruct the urinary drainage system.
29. **CCC** Remove the irrigant container, 60-mL Luer-Lok syringe, absorbent pad, and all other unnecessary items from the client's bed and discard into the trash.

FINISHING THE SKILL

30. **INF** Remove gloves and perform hand hygiene.
31. **CCC** Ensure client comfort. Assist the client into a comfortable position and return the top bedding to cover the client.
32. **SAF** Ensure client safety. Ensure that the bed is in the lowest position. Verify that the client can identify and reach the nurse call system. *These safety measures reduce the risk of falls.*
33. **COM** Document assessment findings, including urine output and characteristic of output before and after the irrigation, type and volume of irrigant administered, care given, and outcomes in the legal healthcare record.
35. **EVAL** Monitor the urine output the drainage collection bag to assess the patency of the urinary catheter.
36. **EVAL** Monitor client discomfort.

■ SKILL 15.14 Performing Continuous Closed Bladder Irrigation

EQUIPMENT

Clean gloves
Sterile normal saline irrigation bags (1000-mL solution bag, or larger 3000- to 4000-mL irrigation solution bags may be used)
Fluid administration set
Additives for solution, if ordered
Sterile graduated cylinder
4 × 4 sterile gauze drain
Intravenous (IV) pole
Labels

BEGINNING THE SKILL

1. **SAF** Review the order. Determine if the authorized healthcare provider's order or facility protocol is for a single solution set or if a primary and secondary set is used. *Often two bags are hung with a Y-connector so that when one bag finishes, the second bag begins to infuse, much like the IV piggyback setup.*
2. **INF** Perform hand hygiene.
3. **CCC** Introduce yourself to the client and explain the purpose and procedure for continuous bladder irrigation. *Continuous bladder irrigation may have been set up*

following surgery. When the client is awake and aware following surgery, you can explain the purpose of the bladder irrigation.

4. **SAF** Identify the client using two identifiers.
5. **SAF** Determine if the client has any pertinent allergies.
6. **CCC** Provide privacy; close the door and pull the curtain.
7. **INF** Apply gloves.

PROCEDURE

8. **SAF** Set up an ergonomically safe space. Raise the bed to a comfortable working height. Raise one side rail. *Setting up an ergonomically safe space prevents injury to the nurse and client.*
9. **SAF** Set up a workspace according to your hand dominance, right-handed on the client's right side.
10. **SAF** Assess the client's degree of cooperation and discomfort. *Your assessment is to determine the client's level of discomfort prior to irrigation and compare it to the pain level after irrigation and also to assess the extent to which the client can cooperate during the procedure.*
11. **ACC** Assess the patency of the urinary catheter by inspecting the urine output. Empty the urine drainage bag. If there is no urine output, the irrigant solution is not instilled into the bladder until it can be determined that the catheter is patent.
12. **ACC** Assess to determine if the client's bladder is full. Palpate gently, moving down from the umbilicus, to determine if the top edge of the bladder is easily palpable. *The authorized healthcare provider may also order a bladder volume measurement using a bladder scanner.* **WARNING:** Bladder irrigation should not be performed if the indwelling Foley catheter is not draining urine. If the catheter was obstructed and irrigant was injected into the bladder, the bladder would become distended and potentially injured.
13. **ACC** Assist the client into a comfortable position that allows access to the distal end of the Foley catheter tubing. *The semi-Fowler position with the knees bent and thighs slightly separated is appropriate for male and female clients.*
14. **CCC** Use the top bedding to cover the client's legs and a bath blanket to cover the torso. *Covering the client prevents chilling and provides privacy.*
15. **CCC** Place a disposable absorbent pad under the distal end of the urinary catheter tubing. *Disposable absorbents pads help to prevent the bed linens from becoming wet and soiled.*
16. **SAF** Perform safety medication checks for the irrigant, including expiration date and six rights. *Bladder irrigant is injected into the body and therefore is a medication.* (See discussion of medication administration in Chapter 11.)
17. **ACC** Inject additives into the irrigant, if ordered. Ensure there are no incompatibilities between the additives and the irrigant.
18. **SAF** Label the normal saline solutions bags "For Bladder Irrigation Only—Not for IV use." **WARNING:** Labeling the bag helps to prevent confusion between bladder irrigant solutions and IV solutions. In some facilities, the protocol may also include labeling the tubing. *Labeling irrigant is a safety strategy to prevent misconnection errors.*

19. **ACC** Close the roller clamp on the infusion tubing.
20. **ACC** Spike the infusion tubing into the normal saline solution bag (or bags if using a dual system), using sterile technique.

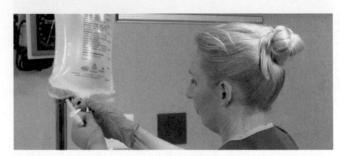

STEP 20 Spike the infusion tubing into the irrigant solution bag.

21. **ACC** Squeeze the drip chamber until it is one-third to one-half full if the system has a drip chamber.

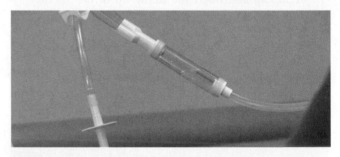

STEP 21 Squeeze the drip chamber until it is one-third to one-half full.

22. **ACC** Open the roller clamp and allow the solution to flow through the tubing in order to prime the infusion set tubing. When the air is removed, close the roller clamp. *Removing air from the tubing prevents air from entering the bladder during the irrigation.*
23. **ACC** Hang the solution bags on an IV pole.
24. **INF** Clean the irrigation port with an antiseptic wipe and allow to air dry. *Cleaning prevents the transfer of microorganisms into the bladder.*
25. **ACC** Connect the irrigation tubing into the irrigation port using sterile technique. If the port plug is difficult to remove, use a sterile gauze sponge to grasp it.

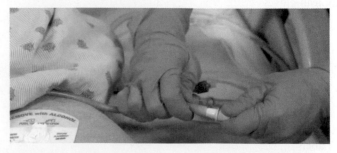

STEP 25 Connect the irrigation tubing into the irrigation port.

26. **ACC** Open the roller clamp to the primary irrigant and adjust the rate of irrigant infusion per orders.
27. **EVAL** Monitor the output in the drainage collection bag in order to evaluate the patency of the urinary catheter and to note the characteristics of the output. *The output includes urine and irrigant and potentially blood, tissue, sediment, and clots. The color of the output will be between clear and bright red blood, depending on the degree of hematuria. Assess for clots that may obstruct the urinary drainage system.*
28. **ACC** Empty the drainage collection bag per order or protocol and measure the volume of output. Subtract the volume of infused irrigant and record the urine output.
29. **CCC** Remove any unnecessary items from the client's bed and discard into the trash.

FINISHING THE SKILL

30. **INF** Remove gloves and perform hand hygiene.
31. **CCC** Ensure client comfort. Assist the client into a comfortable position and return the top bedding to cover the client.
32. **SAF** Ensure client safety. Place the bed in the lowest position. Verify that the client can identify and reach the nurse call system. *These safety measures reduce the risk of falls.*

34. **COM** Document assessment findings, care given, and outcomes in the legal healthcare record, including urine volume, color, and characteristics.
35. **EVAL** Continue to monitor urine output by measuring the output in the drainage collection bag, subtracting the volume of infused irrigant, and recording the urine output in order to assess the patency of the urinary catheter. Note the characteristics of the output. (Note: Perform hand hygiene and apply gloves each time you touch the catheter or drainage bag. Perform hand hygiene each time you remove gloves.)

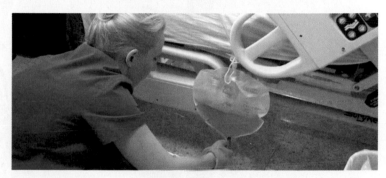

STEP 35 Monitor the output to assess catheter patency.

36. **EVAL** Monitor client discomfort.

SECTION 3   Urine Elimination With a Urinary Diversion

Although medical, nonoperative interventions are the first choice to manage urine elimination, sometimes people have conditions that require surgical intervention. Several types of surgical procedures can assist with urine elimination.

SUPRAPUBIC CATHETER

A *suprapubic catheter* is a catheter draining the bladder through a cystostomy, a surgically created opening through the abdominal wall into the bladder. The surgeon places a suprapubic catheter through the abdominal and bladder musculature into the bladder (Fig. 15.6).

If the individual's bladder is intact and functional but urethral injury, disease, or infection creates a contraindication for a transurethral catheter, a suprapubic catheter is an alternative. Indications include an acute event such as severe trauma with pelvic fracture and urethral disruption or, more commonly, urethral obstructions such as urethral strictures or prostatic hyperplasia. A suprapubic catheter provides a long-term urine elimination solution for clients with neurogenic bladder. Clients have fewer urinary tract infections

with a suprapubic catheter than with an indwelling catheter because the insertion site is much further from perineal microorganisms, as well as fewer complications associated with transurethral catheters such as urethritis (Cohen & Lakin, 2016).

Urine elimination for a client with a suprapubic catheter is similar to that of a client with an indwelling Foley catheter. The catheter drains into a drainage collection bag, usually a leg bag in the daytime. In the night, a suprapubic catheter is usually secured to a larger drainage collection bag that holds a larger volume and does not have to be emptied until morning. Key elements of care include maintaining an unobstructed flow of urine into the drainage collection system, using Standard Precautions during any manipulation of the catheter, keeping the drainage bag below the level of the bladder, and emptying the collection bag at regular intervals.

In the postoperative period, the cystostomy site is cleaned using sterile technique, but once the cystostomy site has healed, the site is cleaned with soap and water, usually in the daily bath. Some clients prefer to cover the site with gauze; others leave off the gauze. Cystostomy site care for clients immediately after the surgical procedure includes site

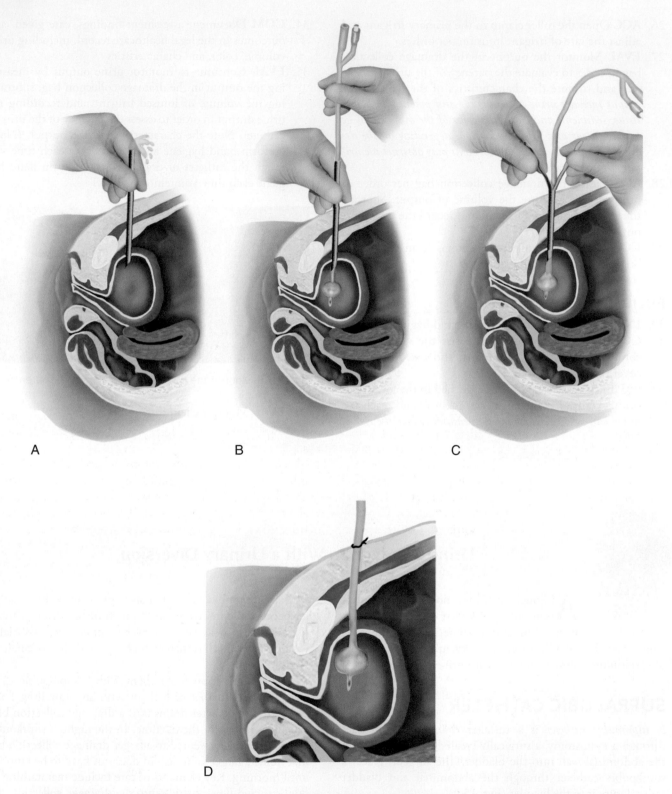

A

B

C

D

FIG. 15.6 A suprapubic catheter passes through the abdominal and bladder musculature into the bladder.

cleaning, site assessment, and dressing changes according to the authorized healthcare provider's orders and facility policy. In addition, nurses assess the characteristics of the urine and volume of urine output.

Complications of a suprapubic catheter are dislodgment and obstruction from sediment. If the catheter comes out shortly after it was surgically inserted, the muscles of the bladder and abdomen close over the opening, and it is very

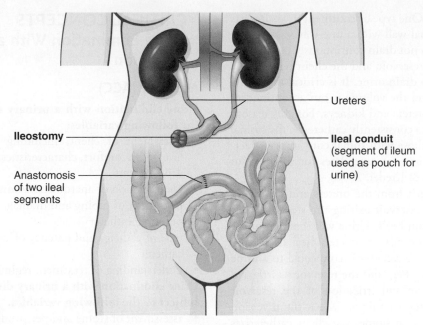

FIG. 15.7 In an ileal conduit urinary diversion, the ureters are attached to one end of a segment of ileum, and the other end is brought out of the abdominal wall and rolled back to form a stoma.

difficult to reinsert and may require surgical reintroduction of the catheter. If the catheter comes out after the client is discharged home, the client should seek immediate medical attention to replace the catheter. After 4 to 6 weeks, which allows time for the tract to the bladder to heal, the catheter is changed monthly (Cohen & Lakin, 2016). Sediment is also a complication of suprapubic catheters. Interventions to prevent catheter obstruction from sediment include drinking plenty of liquids to keep urine dilute, placing a larger French catheter, and monitoring the urine output to respond to a sediment obstruction.

URINARY DIVERSIONS

If the individual's bladder can no longer serve as the urine reservoir, but the kidneys and ureters are healthy and produce urine, a surgical diversion is an option to eliminate urine. The most common reason for a person to have a urinary diversion is bladder cancer and the subsequent need to remove the bladder. Occasionally individuals with spinal cord injury or a congenital anomaly may also need a urinary diversion (Costa & Kreder, 2016). Two basic types of diversion are performed. The most common is a noncontinent urinary diversion, in which the urine drains continuously as the kidneys produce it. Continent urinary diversions, in which the client must actively assist with the urine elimination, have more complications and are less common.

Noncontinent Urinary Diversion

A cutaneous ureterostomy is the simplest form of noncontinent urinary diversion but is seldom performed, except sometimes in pediatrics as a temporary measure before further surgery. In the procedure, the ureters are directly attached to the skin of the abdominal wall. The client has two stoma appliances to capture the draining urine. This type has no bowel segment involved (Costa & Kreder, 2016).

The typical noncontinent diversion is the ileal conduit urinary diversion, in which a segment of bowel, usually a portion of the ileum, is removed with the blood supply intact. The ureters are attached to one end, and the other end is brought out of the abdominal wall and rolled back to form a stoma (Fig. 15.7). The stoma should be moist, red, round, and raised above the skin level. Because the stoma is created from intestine, it is very vascular and can bleed easily; it also continues to produce mucus. A stoma has no nerve endings and therefore no sensation. The ileum creates a channel for the urine to drain. The client will use a stoma appliance to capture the draining urine.

Care for a person with a noncontinent urinary diversion is similar to any other ostomy care. The stoma appliance is emptied regularly to prevent urinary reflux back into the higher urinary tract, which could result in a urinary tract infection. The stoma and skin around the stoma are kept clean and intact to prevent infection and leakage. Care of the stoma in the postoperative period may be performed by the nurse using sterile technique. However, as the client heals, care of the stoma and infection prevention is performed by the client, and when the diversion has healed, clean technique is used. However, if an uncontaminated urine specimen is needed from a client with a noncontinent urinary diversion, the correct technique is to catheterize the ileal loop using sterile technique.

Continent Urinary Diversion

Several types of surgical procedures result in a continent urinary diversion. A segment of bowel, often the ileum, is used to create a reservoir for the urine. The surgeon refashions the tubular shape of the bowel into a spherical shape that has a greater volume capacity. One type of continent diversion has a stoma on the abdominal wall with a one-way valve as the insertion site. Urine does not drain continuously but collects in the surgically created reservoir, and the client periodically catheterizes the stoma to drain urine. It is critical that urine never accumulates beyond the volume it can accommodate and backs up into the ureters and kidneys. For this reason, clients who are not able to consistently catheterize the stoma, such as the very old or those with spinal cord injury affecting hand coordination, are not candidates for this type of urinary diversion (Costa & Kreder, 2016).

After the surgery, stents from the ureters and a catheter from the newly formed reservoir exiting the stoma are left in place until the diversion heals. Urine will drain from the catheter until the reservoir has completely healed. During this postoperative time, the catheter is connected to a urine collection container or leg bag, and the reservoir is irrigated regularly. Care of the site and irrigation of the reservoir are performed using sterile technique. When the diversion is healed and the client is at home, the client catheterizes and irrigates the reservoir and cleans the stoma using clean technique.

A second type of continent diversion is the orthotopic neobladder. *Orthotopic* means "in the same place," and *neobladder* means "new bladder." This diversion may be created for clients who have a healthy urethra and urethra sphincter but must have the bladder removed. A surgically created bladder substitute is made from bowel and attached to the urethra. The urethral sphincter holds the urine in, but without the musculature of the bladder contracting to expel urine, the client must use the abdominal musculature to squeeze the neobladder and pass urine. Some clients cannot express all of the urine and must perform transurethral intermittent catheterization. The frequency of catheterization will vary from once or twice a day to every 2 to 3 hours, depending on the person. The advantage for clients is that they do not have a stoma or any external signs of their urinary diversion (United Ostomy Associations of America [UOAA], 2019).

APPLICATION OF THE NURSING PROCESS

Examples of Related ICNP Nursing Diagnoses, Expected Client Outcomes, and Nursing Interventions:

Nursing Diagnosis: Lack of knowledge of treatment regimen

Supporting Data: Presence of a urinary diversion

Expected Client Outcomes: Client will achieve moderate knowledge of treatment regimen, as demonstrated by caring for the appliance by the date of discharge.

Nursing Intervention Example: Demonstrate and ask the client to do a return demonstration of the care for the appliance.

Reference: International Classification for Nursing Practice. (n.d.). *eHealth & ICNP.* Retrieved from https://www.icn.ch/what-we-do/projects/ehealth-icnp.

CRITICAL CONCEPTS
Urine Elimination With a Urinary Diversion

Accuracy (ACC)

Urine elimination with a urinary diversion is subject to the following variables:
- assessment of client, including cooperation, mobility, level of discomfort, characteristics of urine and volume of urine output
- identification of anatomical landmarks
- placement of tubing and drainage collection bag for a suprapubic catheter
- type of catheter and patency of catheter for a suprapubic catheter
- understanding of treatment regimen by client and family.

Urine elimination with a urinary diversion with a stoma is subject to the following variables:
- assessment of stoma and peristomal skin
- preparation of peristomal skin
- preparation and placement of stoma wafer
- preparation and placement of a urostomy catheter
- preparation and administration of urostomy irrigant.

Client-Centered Care (CCC)

When assisting a client with a urinary diversion, respect for the client is demonstrated by:
- promoting and respecting the client's autonomy
- providing privacy and ensuring comfort
- answering questions that the client or family may have
- honoring cultural preferences
- arranging for an interpreter, if needed
- advocating for the client and family.

Infection Control (INF)

When assisting a client with a urinary diversion, healthcare-associated infection and client infection is prevented by:
- containment of microorganisms
- preventing and reducing the transfer of microorganisms
- reducing the number of microorganisms.

Safety (SAF)

Safety measures when assisting a client with a urinary diversion prevent harm to the client and provide a safe care environment, including:
- verifying client allergies and the plan of care.

Communication (COM)

- Communication exchanges information (oral, written, nonverbal, or electronic) between two or more people.
- Documentation records information in a permanent legal record.
- Collaboration with the client, client's family, and members of the healthcare team is essential for the client with

a urinary diversion to maintain client autonomy and to implement an effective plan of care.

Health Maintenance (HLTH)

Nursing is dedicated to the promotion of health and abilities when assisting with urine elimination for the client with a urinary diversion, including:
* protecting the client's peristomal skin integrity

* preventing irritation, inflammation, and infection of the urinary tract
* protecting the mucosal integrity of the client's stoma.

Evaluation (EVAL)

Evaluation of outcomes enables the nurse to determine the efficacy of the care provided when assisting with urine elimination for the client with a urinary diversion.

▪ SKILL 15.15 Providing Suprapubic Catheter Care

EQUIPMENT

Clean gloves
Cotton-tipped applicators, if providing postoperative care
Sterile cleansing solution as ordered, if providing postoperative care

BEGINNING THE SKILL

1. **INF** Perform hand hygiene.
2. **INF** Apply gloves. *The CDC recommends the use of Standard Precautions during any manipulation of the catheter or urine drainage collection system.*
3. **CCC** Introduce yourself to the client and explain the purpose of managing a suprapubic catheter.
4. **SAF** Identify the client using two identifiers.
5. **SAF** Determine if the client has any pertinent allergies, such as latex.
6. **CCC** Provide privacy; close the door and pull the curtain.

PROCEDURE

Caring for a Client With a Suprapubic Catheter

7. **ACC** Maintain an unobstructed flow of urine by keeping the catheter and tubing free from kinks.
8. **ACC** Keep the urine collection bag below the level of the bladder at all times.
9. **SAF** Hang the collection bag from the bed frame and not from any moveable part of the bed. *Hanging the collection bag on a moveable part such as the side rail may result in inadvertent pulling and trauma to the urethral meatus and bladder neck.*
10. **INF** Do not place the urine collection bag on the floor.

Cleaning the Cystostomy Site

11. **INF** Remove the dressing around the suprapubic catheter. Note any drainage on the dressing.
12. **INF** In the immediate postoperative period, clean the cystostomy site with sterile cotton-tipped applicators and sterile solution as ordered. If the cystostomy site is healed, clean the cystostomy catheter insertion site with routine bathing. Do not clean with antiseptics.

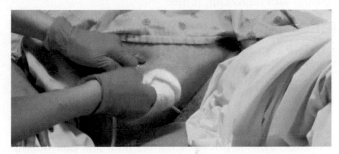

STEP 12 If the cystostomy site is healed, clean the catheter insertion site with routine bathing.

13. **INF** Apply a drain sponge around the catheter and secure the sponge with tape. Label the dressing with date, time, and initials. *Do not cut a gauze drainage sponge because it will unravel and shed small threads of cotton.*

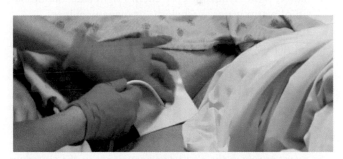

STEP 13 Apply a drain sponge dressing around the catheter.

FINISHING THE SKILL

14. **INF** Remove gloves and perform hand hygiene.
15. **SAF** Ensure client safety. Ensure that the bed is in the lowest position. *The lowest bed position reduces the risk of injury from falls.*
16. **CCC** Ensure client comfort. Ensure that the client can identify and reach the nurse call system.
17. **HLTH** Encourage fluid intake. Provide the client with fresh ice water or other liquids. *Fluid intake helps to keep urine dilute and prevent encrustations.*
18. **COM** Document assessment of urine characteristics, volume of urine output, assessment of suprapubic site, care given, and outcomes in the legal healthcare record.
19. **EVAL** Follow up and reassess the dressing and the client's urine output within your shift.

■ **SKILL 15.16** Changing a Stoma Appliance on an Ileal Conduit

EQUIPMENT

Two pairs of clean gloves
Graduated cylinder
Washcloth/basin/water or hygienic wipes
Absorbent pad
4 × 4 sterile gauze drain
Ostomy appliance
Stoma measuring guide
Scissors (sharp, curved scissors are ideal)
Topical skin protectant, if used

BEGINNING THE SKILL

1. **INF** Perform hand hygiene.
2. **CCC** Introduce yourself to the client and explain the procedure and purpose for changing the stoma appliance.
3. **SAF** Identify the client using two identifiers.
4. **SAF** Determine if the client has any pertinent allergies.
5. **CCC** Provide privacy; close the door and pull the curtain.
6. **SAF** Set up an ergonomically safe space. Raise the bed to a comfortable working height. Raise one side rail. *Setting up an ergonomically safe space prevents injury to the nurse and client.*
7. **SAF** Set up a workspace according to your hand dominance, right-handed on the client's right side. Set up basin of warm water, washcloth, or hygienic wipes.
8. **INF** Apply clean gloves. *The CDC recommends the use of Standard Precautions during any manipulation of a urine drainage collection system.*

PROCEDURE

9. **COM** Assess the client's knowledge related to the care of an ileal conduit urinary diversion, particularly changing the stoma appliance. *Your assessment is to determine the extent to which the client can participate in the procedure and to determine any knowledge deficiencies.*
10. **ACC** Assess the client's activity level, cognitive function, degree of mobility, and discomfort. *Your assessment is to determine the extent to which the client can participate in the procedure.*
11. **ACC** Position the client for the appliance change. If the client is able to participate in the appliance change, position the client sitting up comfortably. If the client is unable to participate in the appliance change, position the client supine.
12. **CCC** Use the top bedding to cover the client's legs and raise the client's gown to expose the urinary stoma and appliance. *Covering the client prevents chilling and provides privacy.*
13. **CCC** Place a disposable absorbent pad under the client. *The ileal conduit drains urine continuously. Position the*

pad so that it will catch draining urine from the stoma or inadvertent spills when removing the stoma appliance.

14. **ACC** Empty the urine drainage pouch into a calibrated measuring container. Match the measuring container to the volume. *Small volumes cannot be accurately measured in a graduated cylinder; use a calibrated specimen cup.*

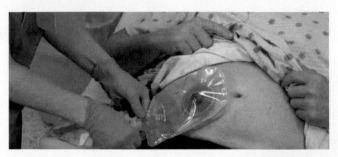

STEP 14 Empty the urine into a measuring container.

15. **ACC** Place the container on a flat, even surface and measure the volume of urine at eye level. Assess the characteristics of the urine, including color, clarity, and odor. *Reading above or below eye level will alter the measurement reading.*
16. **INF** Dispose of urine and rinse out the measuring container. *Rinsing reduces the odor of urine and the growth of microorganisms.*
17. **INF** Remove gloves and perform hand hygiene.
18. **INF** Apply clean gloves. *The CDC recommends the use of Standard Precautions during any manipulation of a urine drainage collection system.*
19. **HLTH** Gently remove the stoma wafer from the skin by pushing the skin down (not pulling the wafer up) and working systematically around the circumference of the wafer. Use adhesive removal wipes or gauze saturated with warm water to help remove the wafer. *Gentle wafer removal and cleansing help to protect skin integrity.*

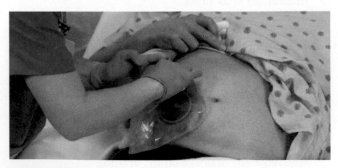

STEP 19 Gently remove the stoma wafer from the skin by pushing the skin down.

20. **INF** Dispose of the wafer. Dispose of the bag, if appropriate. *In the acute care setting, the bag is usually disposable. In home care, the bag may be washed and reused.*

21. **ACC** Assess the stoma and the surrounding skin. (Note: The stoma should be moist, red, round, and raised above the skin level. The skin should be free of irritation.)

22. **ACC** Roll a 4 × 4 gauze sponge to create a wick, or use a tampon. Insert the gauze or tampon into the stoma to absorb urine while cleaning the skin and applying the stoma appliance. *A noncontinent ileal urinary device produces urine as the kidneys produce urine, and the client cannot control urine elimination.*

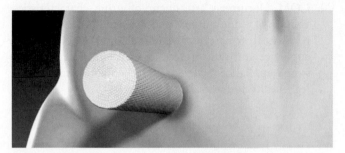

STEP 22 Insert the gauze or tampon into the stoma to absorb urine.

23. **HLTH** Clean the stoma and skin surrounding the stoma with warm water or an approved ostomy skin cleanser. Do not use soap or rubbing alcohol. Do not use ordinary moist wipes because the perfume and other ingredients may cause allergic reactions. *Both soap and rubbing alcohol are drying, and soap residue may prevent the new appliance from adhering well. Appropriate cleansing helps to protect skin and stoma mucosa integrity.*

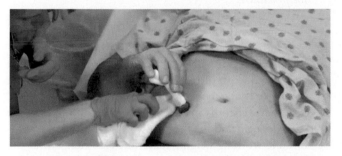

STEP 23 Clean the stoma and skin surrounding the stoma.

24. **HLTH** Pat dry with cotton gauze. *Appropriate drying helps to protect skin integrity.*

25. **HLTH** Allow the skin around the stoma to dry completely. Apply a liquid skin barrier film that creates a waterproof barrier. (Note: The liquid skin barrier dries, creating a transparent coating on the skin [Thayer, Rozenboom, & Baranoski, 2016]). *Skin protectant helps protect skin integrity.*

26. **ACC** Use the stoma measuring guide to determine the size and shape of the opening of the new appliance wafer. Identify the size of the stoma opening that fits over the stoma, leaving about a 0.3-cm (1/8-inch) gap, and does not touch the stoma. Trace that size opening onto the back of the stoma wafer. *If the stoma wafer is too large, the peristomal skin will be in contact with urine and become irritated.*

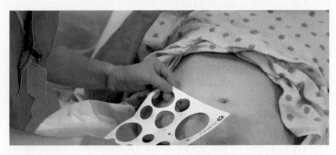

STEP 26 Determine the size and shape of the stoma.

27. **ACC** Cut the opening of the stoma wafer with sharp scissors, adjusting the opening to fit the shape of the client's stoma. *The stoma does not have innervation and therefore does not have sensation. If the stoma wafer is not the correct size and puts pressure on the stoma, the client may not feel the pressure, and the stoma will develop a break in the integrity of the mucosa.*

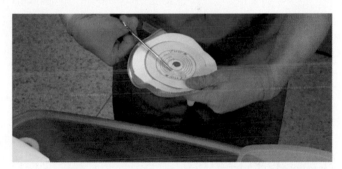

STEP 27 Cut the opening of the stoma wafer to fit the stoma.

28. **ACC** Place the clamp on the bottom of the appliance pouch. *Pressing the appliance wafer in place may elicit urine drainage from the stoma. If the clamp is not in place, the urine will leak out of the pouch.*

29. Remove the 4 × 4 gauze wick or tampon.

30. **HLTH** Ensure the skin is dry and place the appliance wafer over the stoma.

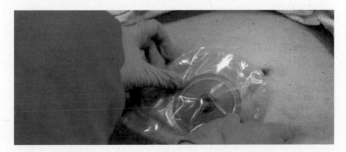

STEP 30 Place the appliance wafer over the stoma.

31. **ACC** Position the wafer and pouch so that urine drains toward the client's feet if the client is mobile. If the client is bedbound, the pouch may be more comfortable filling to the client's side.

32. **EVAL** Check that the wafer is not touching the stoma and that there is not a gap larger than 0.3 cm (1/8 inch) where the skin is exposed to urine. *If the stoma wafer is too large, the peristomal skin will be in contact with urine and become irritated. If the stoma wafer is not the correct size and puts pressure on the stoma, the client will not feel the pressure, and the stoma will develop a break in the integrity of the mucosa.*

33. **CCC** Remove the disposable absorbent pad from under the client and place in trash receptacle.

34. Clean up the work area.

FINISHING THE SKILL

35. **INF** Remove gloves.
36. **INF** Perform hand hygiene.
37. **CCC** Assist the client into a comfortable position and return the top bedding to cover the client.
38. **SAF** Place the bed in the lowest position. *The lowest bed position reduces the risk of injury from falls.*
39. **CCC** Ensure client comfort. Ensure that the client can identify and reach the nurse call system.
40. **COM** Document assessment of urine characteristics, volume of urine output, and assessment of stoma and peristomal skin; care given, including type of stoma appliance and skin protectant used and date and time stoma appliance changed; and client outcomes in the legal healthcare record.

■ SKILL 15.17 Catheterizing and Irrigating a Continent Urostomy

EQUIPMENT

Straight catheter (or straight catheter kit containing sterile gloves and cleansing wipes)
Sterile gloves (if not in the kit)
Water-soluble lubricant (if not in the kit)
Clean gloves
Personal protective equipment (PPE) (face shield and gown)
Absorbent pad
Graduated cylinder
Stoma cleanser, if ordered
4 × 4 sterile gauze drain
Tape
Urine collection container, if toilet is not used
Irrigation tray (containing catch basin, irrigation solution container, 60-mL irrigating piston, syringe with a catheter tip, and waterproof drape)
Sterile normal saline solution bottle

BEGINNING THE SKILL

1. **INF** Perform hand hygiene.
2. **INF** Apply clean gloves.
3. **CCC** Introduce yourself to the client and explain the purpose of catheterizing and irrigating the continent urostomy.
4. **SAF** Identify the client using two identifiers.
5. **SAF** Determine if the client has any pertinent allergies, such as latex.
6. **CCC** Provide privacy; close the door and pull the curtain.

PROCEDURE

7. **COM** Assess the client's knowledge related to catheterizing and irrigating the continent urostomy and client preferences. *Your assessment is to determine the extent to which the client can participate in the procedure, client preferences, and any knowledge deficiencies.*

8. **ACC** Assess the client's activity level, cognitive function, degree of mobility, and discomfort. *Your assessment is to determine the extent to which the client can participate in the procedure.*

9. **ACC** Position the client for catheterizing and irrigating the continent urostomy. If the client is able to participate in catheterizing and irrigating the continent urostomy, position the client in the bathroom sitting on or near the toilet. If the client is unable to participate in the appliance change, position the client supine.

10. **SAF** If the client is in bed, set up an ergonomically safe space for you and for the client. Raise the bed to a comfortable working height. Raise one side rail. Lower the head of the bed to the extent tolerated by the client. *Setting up an ergonomically safe space prevents injury to the nurse and client.*

10. **CCC** Use the top bedding to cover the client's legs and raise the client's gown to expose the continent urostomy. *Covering the client prevents chilling and provides privacy.*

11. **CCC** Place a disposable absorbent pad under the client. Position the pad so that it will catch urine from the stoma or inadvertent spills during catheterization and irrigation.

12. **ACC** Remove the stoma covering and clean any visible mucus from the stoma.

13. **ACC** Assess the stoma and surrounding skin. *The stoma should be moist, red, round, and raised above the skin level. The skin should be free of irritation.*

14. **INF** Put on face shield, if irrigating the urostomy. *Piston syringes do not provide consistent pressure and may squirt.*
15. **INF** If using sterile technique in an acute care setting, remove clean gloves and perform hand hygiene.
16. **INF** Open the catheter kit on a clean surface. If additional supplies are needed, create a sterile field, and add supplies using sterile technique.
17. **ACC** If irrigating the continent urostomy, draw up 30 to 60 mL of normal saline solution in a piston syringe, maintaining the sterility of the syringe tip.
18. **INF** Apply sterile gloves.
19. **INF** Open catheter package, maintaining the sterility of the catheter.
20. **CCC** Open the lubricant. Lubricate the tip of the catheter. *Lubricant will ease the insertion of the catheter through the stoma.*
21. **ACC** Ensure the distal opening of the catheter is in the urine collection tray.
22. **ACC** Gently insert the catheter into the reservoir until urine flows.
23. **ACC** If you meet slight resistance, do not force the catheter. You may also rotate the catheter; this allows the catheter to find the path of least resistance.
24. **ACC** Instruct the client to take a deep breath and blow out slowly through pursed lips. *Blowing through pursed lips creates a gentle bearing down, which helps empty the reservoir.*
25. **ACC** Instruct the client to turn slightly to facilitate emptying the reservoir.
26. **ACC** When the urine has drained out, assess the volume and characteristics of the urine.
27. **ACC** Hold the catheter in position in the reservoir and attach the piston syringe with normal saline solution to the distal end of the catheter.
28. **ACC** Gently inject the normal saline through the catheter into the reservoir.
29. **ACC** Disconnect the syringe and allow the normal saline solution to flow out.
30. **ACC** If mucus is observed, draw up 30 to 60 mL of normal saline solution in the piston syringe and repeat the irrigation process until the solution runs clear.
31. Remove the piston syringe and catheter.
32. **HLTH** Clean the stoma according to the authorized healthcare provider orders or facility policy or client preference. *In the postoperative period, the surgeon may prescribe an antimicrobial. In the home setting, mild soap and water is recommended (Wound, Ostomy and Continence Nurses Society, 2018).*
33. **CCC** Apply stoma covering per client's preference.
34. **CCC** Remove the disposable absorbent pad from under the client and place in trash receptacle.
35. Clean up the work area.

FINISHING THE SKILL

36. **INF** Remove gloves and perform hand hygiene.
37. **CCC** Assist the client into a comfortable position and return the top bedding to cover the client.
38. **SAF** Place the bed in the lowest position. *The lowest bed position reduces the risk of injury from falls.*
39. **SAF** Ensure client safety and comfort. Ensure that the client can identify and reach the nurse call system.
40. **COM** Document the following in the legal healthcare record:
    * assessment of urine characteristics
    * volume of urine output
    * assessment of stoma and peristomal skin
    * mucous output rinsed out with irrigation
    * care given, including date and time of catheterization and irrigation
    * client outcomes.

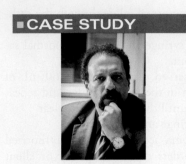

■ CASE STUDY

Mr. Huessin Tehrani is a 62-year-old professional. He has had increased urinary frequency for a few months and is now waking up two to three times a night to urinate. One day he becomes aware that he is very uncomfortable with a full bladder, but he is unable to void. He realizes that he has not voided for at least 8 hours. He talks with his wife, and they go to the emergency department of their local hospital.

At the emergency department, Mr. Tehrani requests a same-gender caregiver. Although he was born in the United States, when asked where his family is from, he answers Persia. He is a practicing Muslim. Tom is a registered nurse in the emergency department that shift. He takes a set of vital signs and performs an assessment of Mr. Tehrani. Mr. Tehrani's vital signs are as follows: temperature 98.8°F, pulse 86, respirations 18, and blood pressure 142/92. He rates his pain as a 6 on a scale of 0 to 10.

Tom assesses that Mr. Tehrani has a palpable distended bladder. The authorized healthcare provider orders a bedside bladder scan with ultrasound. Tom performs the scan, and it reads 800 mL of urine. The authorized healthcare provider diagnoses Mr. Tehrani with benign prostatic hyperplasia (BPH) and orders placement of an indwelling Foley catheter to empty the bladder. Tom has lots of experience passing urinary catheters, and he is able to place an indwelling catheter in Mr. Tehrani. Later that day, Mr. Tehrani leaves the emergency department with the indwelling Foley catheter attached to a leg bag, a prescription for a medication called tamsulosin, and a referral to a urologist. The urologist is able to see him 3 days later and removes the indwelling Foley catheter.

Within the next 6 months, Mr. Tehrani has had to return to the emergency department three times because of an inability to void with a distended bladder. He discusses surgery with his urologist, and a transurethral resection of the prostate (TURP) is scheduled. Mr. Tehrani is admitted to the hospital for the surgery. He is told that a triple-lumen catheter will be placed in surgery and left in place for 2 or 3 days following surgery. After surgery, he has continuous saline irrigation to prevent clot formation and maintain the patency of the catheter. On the third postoperative day, Mr. Tehrani's catheter is removed. Unfortunately, 6 hours later, he has been unable to void, and an indwelling Foley catheter is placed.

Case Study Questions

1. Considering Mr. Tehrani's medical history and signs and symptoms on admission to the emergency department, what is the top priority regarding his care?
2. Does the nursing staff in the emergency department have any obligation to assign a same-gender nurse to provide care for Mr. Tehrani? Can a healthcare facility make a policy excluding opposite-sex caregivers?
3. Before inserting the indwelling catheter, what information should Tom share with Mr. and Mrs. Tehrani? What other client-centered care strategies might Tom use?
4. What strategies can Tom use to manipulate the catheter past Mr. Tehrani's enlarged prostate?
5. How will clot formation be prevented from obstructing the urinary catheter in the immediate postoperative period?
6. Why did Mr. Tehrani experience postoperative urinary retention?
7. What is Mr. Tehrani's risk of acquiring a CAUTI? What evidence-based nursing strategies will help minimize the risk of CAUTI?
8. **Application of QSEN Competencies:** One of the Quality and Safety Education for Nurses (QSEN) skill competencies within Quality Improvement is to "Identify gaps between local and best practice" (Cronenwett et al., 2007). Where can outcome information that reflects differences between local and best practice on CAUTI be found?

■ CONCEPT MAP

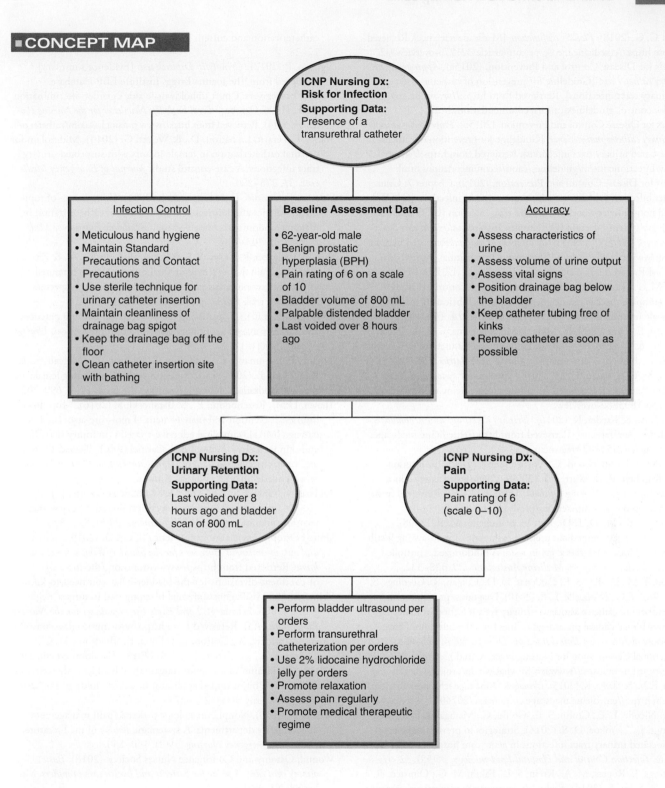

ICNP Nursing Dx:
Risk for Infection
Supporting Data:
Presence of a
transurethral catheter

Infection Control

- Meticulous hand hygiene
- Maintain Standard Precautions and Contact Precautions
- Use sterile technique for urinary catheter insertion
- Maintain cleanliness of drainage bag spigot
- Keep the drainage bag off the floor
- Clean catheter insertion site with bathing

Baseline Assessment Data

- 62-year-old male
- Benign prostatic hyperplasia (BPH)
- Pain rating of 6 on a scale of 10
- Bladder volume of 800 mL
- Palpable distended bladder
- Last voided over 8 hours ago

Accuracy

- Assess characteristics of urine
- Assess volume of urine output
- Assess vital signs
- Position drainage bag below the bladder
- Keep catheter tubing free of kinks
- Remove catheter as soon as possible

ICNP Nursing Dx:
Urinary Retention
Supporting Data:
Last voided over 8 hours ago and bladder scan of 800 mL

ICNP Nursing Dx:
Pain
Supporting Data:
Pain rating of 6 (scale 0–10)

- Perform bladder ultrasound per orders
- Perform transurethral catheterization per orders
- Use 2% lidocaine hydrochloride jelly per orders
- Promote relaxation
- Assess pain regularly
- Promote medical therapeutic regime

References

American Academy of Pediatrics. (2016). Reaffirmation of AAP clinical practice guideline: The Diagnosis and management of the initial urinary tract infection in febrile infants and young children 2–24 months of age. [Clinical practice guideline]. *Pediatrics, 138*(6), 1–5.

Asimakopoulos, A. D., De Nunzio, C., Kocjancic, E., Tubaro, A., Rosier, P. F., & Finazzi-Agrò, E. (2016). Measurement of post-void residual urine. *Neurourology and Urodynamics, 35*(1), 55–57.

Aygin, A., & Usta, E. (2017). The effect of lubricants used in indwelling bladder catheterization through urethra on procedure-related pain: a literature review. *International Journal of Clinical and Experimental Medicine, 10*(2), 1995–2005.

Barbadoro, P., Labricciosa, F. M., Recanatini, C., Gori, G., Tirabassi, F., Martini, E., & Prospero, E. (2015). Catheter-associated urinary tract infection: Role of the setting of catheter insertion. *American Journal of Infection Control, 43*(7), 707–710.

Brown, S. C., Hart, G., Chastain, D. P., Schneeweiss, S., & McGrath, P. A. (2009). Reducing distress for children during invasive procedures: Randomized clinical trial of effectiveness of the PediSedate®. *Pediatric Anesthesia, 19*(8), 725–731.

Carter, G. G. (2018). *Bladder dysfunction.* [Medscape reference]. Retrieved from https://emedicine.medscape.com/article/321273-overview#a2.

Centers for Disease Control and Prevention. (2015a). *Appropriate urinary catheter use.* [Guideline for prevention of catheter-associated urinary tract infections]. Retrieved from https://www.cdc.gov/infectioncontrol/guidelines/cauti/recommendations.html.

Centers for Disease Control and Prevention. (2015b). *Proper techniques for urinary catheter maintenance.* [Guideline for prevention of catheter-associated urinary tract infections]. Retrieved from https://www.cdc.gov/infectioncontrol/guidelines/cauti/recommendations.html.

Centers for Disease Control and Prevention. (2019). Chapter 7: Urinary tract infection (catheter associated urinary tract infections [CAUTI] and non-catheter-associated urinary tract infection [UTI] and other urinary system infection [USI] events. In *National Healthcare Safety Network (NHSN) patient safety component manual* Retrieved from https://www.cdc.gov/nhsn/pdfs/pscmanual/pcsmanual_current.pdf.

Chan, M.F., Tan, H.Y., Lian, X., Ng, L.Y., Ang, L.L., Lim LH, Ng, W.M., … Taylor, B.J. (2014). A randomized controlled study to compare the 2% lignocaine and aqueous lubricating gels for female urethral catheterization. *Pain Practice, 14,* 140–145.

Chau, M. E., Firaza, P. N. B., Ming, J. M., Silangcruz, J. M. A., Braga, L. H., & Lorenzo, A. J. (2017). Lidocaine gel for urethral catheterization in children: A meta-analysis. *Journal of Pediatrics, 190,* 207–214.

Cohen, S. A., & Lakin, C. M. (2016). *Suprapubic cystostomy.* [Medscape reference]. Retrieved from https://emedicine.medscape.com/article/1893882-overview.

Costa, J. A., & Kreder, K. (2016). *Urinary diversions and neobladders.* [Medscape reference]. Retrieved from http://emedicine.medscape.com/article/451882-treatment.

Cronenwett, L., Sherwood, G., Barnsteiner, J., Disch, J., Johnson, J., Mitchell, P., … Warren, J. (2007). Quality and safety education for nurses. *Nursing Outlook, 55*(3), 122–131. Retrieved from http://qsen.org/competencies/pre-licensure-ksas/.

Garbutt, R. B., Mc D, T. D., Lee, V., & Augello, M. R. (2008). Delayed versus immediate urethral catheterization following instillation of local anaesthetic gel in men: A randomized, controlled clinical trial. *Emergency Medicine Australasia, 20,* 328–332.

Hooton, T. M., Bradley, S. F., Cardenas, D. D., Colgan, R., Geerlings, S. E., Rice, J. C., & Nicolle, L. E. (2010). Diagnosis, prevention, and treatment of catheter-associated urinary tract infection in adults: 2009 International clinical practice guidelines from the Infectious Diseases Society of America. *Clinical Infectious Diseases, 50*(5), 625–663.

International Classification for Nursing Practice. (n.d.). *eHealth & ICNP.* Retrieved from https://www.icn.ch/what-we-do/projects/ehealth-icnp.

Lerma, E. V., & Slivka, K. (2015). *Urinalysis.* [Medscape reference]. Retrieved from https://emedicine.medscape.com/article/2074001-overview#a1.

Lo, E., Nicolle, L. E., Coffin, S. E., Gould, C., Maragakis, L. L., Meddings, J., … Yokoe, D. S. (2014). Strategies to prevent catheter-associated urinary tract infections in acute care hospitals: 2014 Update. *Infection Control and Hospital Epidemiology, 35*(52), 32–47.

Meddings, J., Rogers, M. A., Krein, S. L., Fakih, M. G., Olmsted, R. N., & Saint, S. (2014). Reducing unnecessary urinary catheter use and other strategies to prevent catheter-associated urinary tract infection: An integrative review. *BMJ Quality & Safety, 23,* 277–289.

Newman, D. K., & Willson, M. M. (2011). Review of intermittent catheterization and current best practices. *Urologic Nursing, 31*(1), 12–28.

Nguyen, P. (2017). *Urinalysis: Dipstick test.* [Evidence summary]. Retrieved from The Joanna Briggs Institute EBP Database.

Same-sex caregivers: Court upholds male aide's gender discrimination claim. (1996, October). *Legal Eagle Eye Newsletter for the Nursing Profession, 14*(4), Retrieved from http://www.nursinglaw.com/catheter.pdf.

Shavit, I., Feraru, L., Miron, D., & Weiser, G. (2014). Midazolam for urethral catheterization in female infants with suspected urinary tract infections: A case-control study. *Journal of Emergency Medicine, 31,* 278–280.

Siderias, J., Guadio, F., & Singer, A. J. (2004). Comparison of topical anesthetics and lubricants prior to urethral catheterization in males: a randomized controlled trial. *Academic Emergency Medicine, 11*(6), 703–706.

Stav, K., Ohlgisser, R., Siegel, Y. I., Beberashvili, I., Padoa, A., & Zisman, A. (2015). Pain during female urethral catheterization: Intraurethral lubricant injection versus catheter tip lubrication—A prospective randomized trial. *Journal of Urology, 194*(4), 1018–1021.

Strouse, A. C. (2015). Appraising the literature on bathing practices and catheter-associated urinary tract infection prevention. *Urologic Nursing, 35*(1), 11–17.

Tanabe, P., Steinmann, R., Anderson, J., Johnson, D., Metcalf, S., & Ring-Hurn, E. (2004). Factors affecting pain scores during female urethral catheterization. *Academic Emergency Medicine, 11*(6), 699–702.

Thayer, D.M., Rozenboom, B., & Baranoski, S. (2016). "Top-down" injuries: Prevention and management of moisture-associated skin damage (MASD), medical adhesive-related skin injury (MARSI), and skin tears. In J. Colwell & J. Carmel (Eds.), *Wound, Ostomy and Continence Nurses Society™ Core Curriculum: Ostomy Management.* Philadelphia PA: Wolters Kluwer.

Tzortzis, V., Gravas, S., Melekos, M. M., & de la Rosette, J. J. (2009). Intraurethral lubricants: a critical literature review and recommendations. *Journal of Endourology, 23*(5), 821–826.

United Ostomy Associations of America (UOAA). (2019). *The ins and outs of continent diversions for the bladder: What you need to know.* Retrieved from https://www.ostomy.org/the-ins-outs-of-continent-diversions-for-the-bladder-what-you-need-to-know/.

Urine sample: Misdiagnosis of renal bleeding tied to nurses' negligence. (2006, February). *Legal Eagle Eye Newsletter for the Nursing Profession, 14*(4), Retrieved from http://www.nursinglaw.com/#U.

Uspal, N., Strelitz, B., Gritton, J., Follmer, K., Bradford, M. C., Colton, T. L., … Merguerian, P. A. (2018). Randomized clinical trial of lidocaine analgesia for transurethral bladder catheterization delivered via blunt tipped applicator in young children. *Pediatric Emergency Care, 34*(4), 273–279.

Wente, S. (2013). Nonpharmacologic pediatric pain management in emergency departments: A systematic review of the literature. *Journal of Emergency Nursing, 39*(2), 140–150.

Wound, Ostomy and Continence Nurses Society. (2018). *Basic ostomy skin care: A guide for patients and health care providers.* Mt. Laurel, NJ: Author.

Zamanzad, B. (2009). Accuracy of dipstick urinalysis as a screening method for detection of glucose, protein, nitrites and blood. *Eastern Mediterranean Health Journal, 15*(5), 1323.

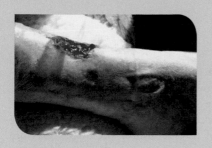

CHAPTER 16
Wound Care

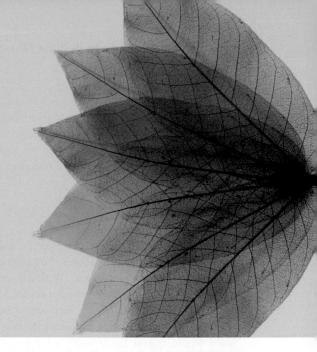

"Children show scars like medals. Lovers use them as secrets to reveal. A scar is what happens when the word is made flesh." | **Leonard Cohen, Author of *The Favorite Game* (1963)**

LEARNING OBJECTIVES

By the end of this chapter, the reader will be able to:

1. Describe types and classifications of wounds.
2. Discuss the effects of having a wound on the client, family, and healthcare system.
3. Identify the reasons a careful skin and wound assessment is necessary.
4. Describe the elements of a wound assessment.
5. Remove a dressing, clean a wound, and apply a new wound dressing.
6. Perform a wound culture.

7. Identify types of wound drains and perform wound drain care.
8. Identify categories of common dressings.
9. Compare types of debridement.
10. Describe the implications of pressure, venous, and diabetic wounds.
11. Apply a compression dressing, Ace wrap, or Unna boot
12. Perform a foot examination, including a monofilament test and an ankle-brachial index (ABI).

667

TERMINOLOGY

Arterial ulcer Caused by peripheral arterial disease; a non–pressure-related disruption or blockage of the arterial blood flow to an area causes tissue necrosis; commonly occurs on the tips and tops of the toes, top of the foot, or distal to the medial malleolus (Centers for Medicare and Medicaid Services [CMS], 2017).

Dehiscence A surgical complication in which a wound ruptures along the surgical suture line.

Diabetic ulcer Caused by the neuropathic and small blood vessel complications of diabetes. Requires a diagnosis of diabetes. Diabetic foot ulcers typically occur over the plantar (bottom) surface of the foot on load-bearing areas, such as the ball of the foot. Ulcers are usually deep, with necrotic tissue, moderate amounts of exudate, and callused would edges. The wounds are regular in shape, and the wound edges are even, with a punched-out appearance. These wounds typically are not painful (CMS, 2017).

Epithelial tissue New skin that is light pink and shiny (even in persons with darkly pigmented skin).

Eschar Dead or devitalized tissue that is hard or soft in texture; usually black, brown, or tan in color; and may appear scab-like and firmly adherent to the base of the wound and often the sides/edges of the wound (CMS, 2017).

Granulation tissue Pink or red tissue with a "cobblestone" or bumpy appearance and a moist, granular appearance; bleeds easily when injured (CMS, 2017).

Moisture-associated skin damage Skin damage caused by moisture from any source (rather than pressure).

Pressure injury Localized damage to the skin and/or underlying tissue, usually over a bony prominence or related to a medical or other device. The injury can present as intact skin or an open ulcer and may be painful. The injury occurs as a result of intense and/or prolonged pressure or pressure in combination with shear (National Pressure Injury Advisory Panel [NPIAP], 2016).

Skin tear Results when shearing, friction, or trauma to the skin causes a separation of the skin layers.

Slough Nonviable yellow, tan, gray, green, or brown tissue; usually moist; can be soft, stringy, and mucinous in texture and may be adherent to the base of the wound or present in clumps throughout the wound bed (CMS, 2017).

Venous ulcer Caused by peripheral venous disease; most commonly occurs proximal to the medial or lateral malleolus, above the inner or outer ankle, or on the lower-calf area of the leg (previously known as "stasis ulcer"); an open lesion of the skin and subcutaneous tissue of the lower leg, usually occurring in the pretibial area of the lower leg or above the medial ankle (CMS, 2017).

ACRONYMS

ABI Ankle-brachial index (ABI)
JP drain Jackson-Pratt drain
MASD Moisture-associated skin damage
NPWT Negative-pressure wound therapy
PVA Polyvinyl alcohol
TIME Tissue, infection, moisture, edges

SECTION 1 Providing Wound Care

Careful wound assessment is a critical step in developing a wound care plan. Different wound types have different etiologies, so before care can be planned, it is important to determine the type and/or cause of the wound (Baranoski & Ayello, 2015). Some wounds have mixed etiologies as the result of comorbid conditions such as diabetes and poor lower-extremity vascular status. Determining the type of wound may involve collaboration between multiple medical specialties and extensive medical tests.

WOUND TYPES

A wound may be planned (surgical), traumatic or accidental (fall, skin tear), a result of illness (vascular, neuropathic) or pressure-related injury (pressure injury), or associated with moisture (moisture- or incontinence-associated skin damage). It may also be an unusual wound (snake or insect bite) or the result of an allergic reaction. Partial-thickness wounds extend through the epidermis and into, but not through, the dermis. Partial-thickness wounds heal mainly by reepithelialization. Full-thickness wounds extend through the epidermis and dermis. These wounds may involve subcutaneous tissue, muscle, and possibly bone. Full-thickness wounds heal by filling with granulation tissue, scar formation, and reepithelialization from the wound edges. Wounds heal by primary, secondary, and delayed primary intention.

Primary-intention healing takes place in surgical wounds that are repaired or superficial wounds with no tissue loss and that involve the epidermis only. Examples of superficial wounds include first-degree burns and stage I and II pressure injuries. Primary healing occurs through reepithelialization (i.e., the outer layer of skin grows closed). Cells grow in from the wound margin and out from epithelial cells lining the hair follicles and glands. These wounds heal in an orderly, predictable manner and are usually healed in 4 to 14 days, with minimal scarring (Fig. 16.1).

Secondary-intention healing occurs when a wound has some amount of tissue loss. Examples would be full-thickness (stage III and IV) pressure injuries. Healing occurs through the formation of granulation tissue and reepithelialization (mostly from the wound edges). The edges of these wounds cannot be easily pulled together. Wounds that heal through secondary intention can be either partial- or full-thickness wounds. Full-thickness wounds may involve subcutaneous tissue, muscle, and possibly bone. Wounds that heal by secondary intention take longer to heal, result in scar formation, and have a higher rate of complications than wounds that heal by primary intention (Fig. 16.2).

Delayed primary intention occurs when primary closure is delayed or a wound is deliberately left open to allow edema or infection to resolve or exudate (debris) to be removed before the wound is closed. Wounds healed by delayed primary intention form more scar tissue than wounds closed through primary intention but less than wounds that heal by secondary intention.

The underlying cause of the wound must be known in order to plan a healing strategy. For example, in arterial wounds, vascular bypass grafting restores circulation and allows healing. However, in wounds that have both arterial and vascular compromise, this isn't possible, so healing these wounds is difficult. Wounds often result from a combination of factors. Table 16.1 describes the different types of wounds.

Anatomical location helps identify the type of wound. For example, vascular ulcers are often on the legs, and neuropathic (diabetic) wounds are frequently found on the feet. Pressure injuries usually occur over bony prominences in the lower two-thirds of the body (sacrum/coccyx, trochanter, ischial tuberosity, ankle, and heel). However, other areas at risk may include the elbows, ears, scapula, and the back of the head. Pressure injuries are localized injuries to the skin and underlying tissue, usually over a bony prominence as a result of pressure or pressure in combination with friction and shear (NPIAP, 2016). Pressure injuries are also called decubitus ulcers, bedsores, pressure sores, or pressure ulcers. Pressure injury is discussed in more detail in Section 3 of this chapter.

THE IMPACT OF WOUNDS

Wounds cause pain and suffering for the client, are expensive for the healthcare system, and can lead to serious even life-ending complications. For example, pressure injuries are estimated to affect 2.5 million persons a year, with the majority being persons over age 65 (Agency for Healthcare Research Quality [AHRQ], 2011; Russo, Steiner, & Spector, 2008). As a result, Medicare is the biggest payer of pressure-injury care. The average cost to heal a wound has been found to be between $3900 and $9300 (Fife & Carter, 2012).

Consequently, it is important for healthcare providers to know how to correctly identify and care for a client who has developed a wound. Unfortunately, nurses may receive little updated wound education in their undergraduate education, and even experienced nurses were found to score a "C" on a standardized pressure ulcer knowledge test (Pieper & Zulkowski, 2014; Zulkowski, Capezuti, Ayello, & Sibbald, 2015). The registered nurse is responsible for wound assessment and dressing changes. Aspects of wound care that may be delegated include emptying and measuring a closed wound drainage collection system. However, the registered nurse is responsible for the assessment of the site and drainage.

CLIENT CONSIDERATIONS

The ideal expected client outcome is to prevent or to heal all wounds. However, this may not be possible, even with the best evidence-based care. Client factors affect the ability of

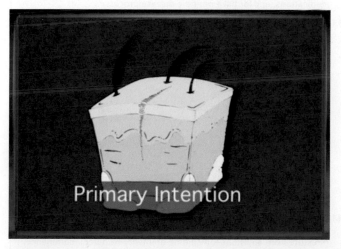

FIG. 16.1 In primary intention, the edges of the wound are closed.

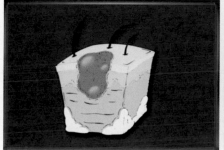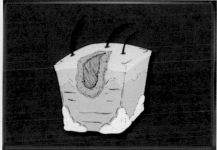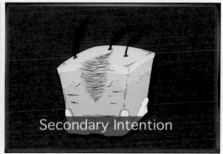

FIG. 16.2 In seconardy intention, granulation tissue forms and the edges of the wound contract more slowly.

TABLE 16.1 Types of Common Wounds

Vascular Ulcers

A vascular or lower-limb ulcer is an open lesion caused by poor circulation to the lower extremities. These ulcers are classified as arterial, venous, or mixed in origin. They occur because of inadequate circulation in the lower extremities (legs and feet). Medical conditions such as peripheral vascular disease or diabetes are often present.

Venous Ulcers

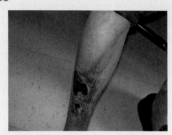

Venous ulcers are the most common ulcers of the lower leg. Persons with venous ulcers often have lower-leg edema and a history of previous phlebitis and tired or aching legs. These wounds may occur after a minor traumatic event, such as bumping the leg. Most venous ulcers are located on the medial malleolus (gaiter region), and the skin surrounding the wound is hyperpigmented.

Arterial Ulcers

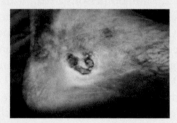

Peripheral vascular occlusive disease, which often presents as intermittent claudication, can also lead to slow-to-heal wounds. Many of the risk factors are similar to those for coronary artery disease. As with venous ulcers, the direct cause of an arterial ulcer is often a minor bump or bruise. Arterial ulcers often have a "punched-out" appearance, and there are signs of impaired tissue perfusion, such as pale skin and diminished or absent pedal pulses.

Diabetic Ulcers

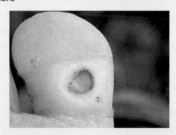

The term *diabetic ulcers* is frequently used to describe ulcers that occur at the head of the metatarsal or bottom of the feet in persons with diabetes mellitus. The direct cause of these ulcers is often pressure. Peripheral neuropathy, structural foot deformities, or limited range of motion in the foot may increase pressure and contribute to the development of these ulcers. People with neuropathy may also step on a sharp object. Because they have no feeling in their feet, these wounds can become very large before they are noticed.

Mixed Etiology

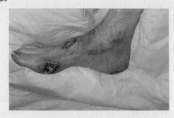

Some wounds have mixed etiology. There may be both venous and arterial components to the wound, and pressure may have also contributed from improperly fitting footwear.

Skin Tear

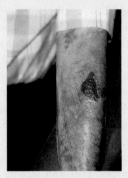

A traumatic injury caused by friction and/or shear of the skin that causes the epidermis and dermis to separate. People who are more likely to develop skin tears include those who use corticosteroids for an extended period, are of an advanced age, are immobile, have dry skin or are dehydrated, do not have adequate nutritional intake, take multiple medications, and/or have multiple disease processes.

Moisture-Associated Skin Damage (MASD)

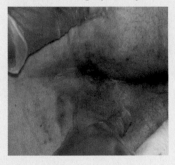

MASD (sometimes referred to as *perineal dermatitis, diaper rash,* or *incontinence-associated dermatitis*) is damage to the skin caused by moisture from any source, including drainage/exudate, incontinence, and perspiration. An inflammation develops on the skin in the perineal area, on and/or between the buttocks, in the skinfolds, and down the inner thighs.

a wound to heal. Chronic conditions, such as diabetes and peripheral vascular disease, as well as age, tissue oxygenation, medication, and immune status, affect healing. Wounds that fail to heal may become chronic.

Cultural Considerations

The client's culture must also be considered when developing wound care strategies. For example, some dressings contain beef or pork ingredients that are prohibited in some religious practices (Boyer, 2013). In the Muslim faith, wound care that interferes with praying and fasting is considered to adversely affect a person's quality of life. Other faiths have dietary restrictions, and many variations exist within cultures and religions, and they can vary by gender as well.

Home Care Considerations

Home care considerations are needed when developing wound care strategies or strategies to prevent a wound. For older individuals, hitting a leg on the edge of a table may result in a vascular wound, or tripping over a rug or pet can result in a fall and fracture. Preparations for going home with wound care may also require social service and/or occupational therapy interventions. Some older people do not have adequate food or the ability to prepare their own meals. Adequate nutrition is integral to tissue healing. Transportation may be an issue that affects access to healthy nutrition as well as access to medical appointments. Older homes may only have a bathroom on an upper level that is difficult for older adults to access, making wound care in the home more difficult.

WOUND ASSESSMENT

A complete wound assessment is important, regardless of the cause of the wound. The location should be documented accurately, the size determined in a consistent manner, and the wound description and surrounding skin documented. If there is a dressing in place, this should be noted each shift, and the wound description should be accurately and completely documented at every dressing change. The amount of healing, change, or deterioration/nonhealing of the wound should be recorded as well. If the wound is a pressure injury, then the stage of the pressure injury is also noted. After noting the location and size of the wound, examine the following four areas, represented by the acronym TIME: (1) the tissue in the wound, (2) signs of infection or potential of the wound to develop infection, (3) the amount and characteristics of moisture in the wound, and (4) the wound edges and surrounding skin. Box 16.1 offers more detail on these four areas.

Wounds must be cleansed prior to assessment. Some dressing may leave residue in the wound, and this must be removed for adequate tissue assessment. In addition, some dressings have an odor when the cover dressing is removed that may be mistaken for wound odor that could indicate infection. Wounds may be cleaned with a commercial wound cleanser, prepackaged normal saline, or even water that is suitable for drinking. The advantage of commercial wound cleansers is that they have ingredients to prevent contamination and can't be sprayed with too much force that would damage fragile wound tissue.

No more than 15 psi is recommended for cleansing (National Pressure Ulcer Advisory Panel [NPAUP], European Pressure Ulcer Advisory Panel [EPUAP], & Pan Pacific Pressure Injury Alliance [PPPIA], 2014). Wound cleansing should be a gentle procedure. Forceful irrigation will damage the fragile new tissue and should be only used as a debridement procedure. For example, cleaning a wound using a 35-mL syringe with a 19-gauge intravenous (IV) catheter tip would result in a pressure of approximately 8 psi and therefore would be appropriate for cleaning (NPUAP et al., 2014). To prevent cross-contamination, all cleansers should be left in the room once taken there, and the client's name and the date should be labeled on the bottle.

WOUND CARE

Wound care encompasses multiple procedures. It includes assessment of the wound, removing old dressings, cleaning the wound, removing sutures or staples, dressing the wound, and documentation of the wound characteristics. The initial steps in all wound care include obtaining supplies, handwashing, and gloving (Zulkowski, 2013). *Hands are always washed and sanitized when entering or leaving a client's room.* You may do dressing changes and wound assessment alone or have a second person to help. Supplies for dressing changes may either be stored in a designated container that is kept in the client's room or brought into the room at the time of the dressing change. Surplus items always remain in the room. Often, it is not necessary to use sterile gloves for a dressing change. Unless the dressing change is for a recent surgical wound, it is most likely a clean procedure (Doughty & McNichol, 2016). However, the principles of infection control are critical. Organisms such as *Clostridium difficile* (*C. diff.*) and methicillin-resistant *Staphylococcus aureus* (MRSA) can live on a dry surface in a client's room for 3 to 4 months (Claro, Daniels, & Humphreys, 2014; Gehemmo, Louvel, Nouvellon, Caillard, & Pestel-Caron, 2009). In addition, a type of yeast called *Candida auris* that is known to cause hospital-associated infections can live on surfaces for at least 7 days (Piedrahita et al., 2017). If strict adherence to handwashing and disposal of client materials is not adhered to, these organisms can be easily spread to another client.

The goal during wound care is to protect the client from environmental bacteria. This includes what has been left in the room and what people coming into the room bring with them. In the past, dressing changes were done as a sterile procedure. This is not always necessary because the bacteria found on a person's skin cannot be removed and will reenter the wound immediately. However, the wound must be protected from environmental bacteria by ensuring the supplies used for wound care are not contaminated.

If either staples or sutures are present, they need care, including cleansing and assessment of the incision and surrounding skin. Proper cleansing and assessment of healing should be documented to ensure the wound is pulling together before the staples or sutures are removed. Assessment of the incision during staple or suture removal is important to prevent dehiscence of the wound. When staples or sutures are removed, wound closure strips, sometimes called butterfly

BOX 16.1 Wound TIME: Tissue, Infection, Moisture, and Edges

(T) Tissue: Assess the wound bed itself for the presence of granulation tissue, fibrin slough, and necrotic tissue and epithelium. Amount and type of exudate, as well as odor, should also be assessed. Surrounding skin should also be examined.

Predominate tissue in ulcer: The type of tissue present in an ulcer indicates if healing or deterioration is taking place. Noting the percentage of each type of tissue (necrotic, granulation, or epithelial) present in the wound helps guide care and facilitates evaluating progress.

Epithelial tissue is light pink and shiny (even in people with darkly pigmented skin) and can be seen in the center and edges of partial-thickness wounds. In full-thickness wounds, new epithelium advances from the edges of the wound only. It is important not to confuse the leading edge of the new epithelium with maceration of the surrounding skin.

Healthy granulation tissue that is necessary for repairing the injured dermis is **red** and has a "cobblestone" appearance. Because granulation tissue contains many new blood vessels, it bleeds easily when injured.

When a wound begins to heal, the granulation tissue may appear **pink.** If granulation tissue is well established and turns pink, dull, or dusky, the wound is not healing well.

Necrotic tissue can appear yellow, white, gray, or **black. Black** necrotic tissue is often referred to as eschar. It is unusually dry and adherent to the wound bed. Necrotic tissue that appears gray, white, or yellow is more hydrated. The latter is often referred to as fibrinous slough because it mainly contains dead fibrinous tissue. Necrotic tissue delays wound healing and may increase the risk of infection.

Skin tissue surrounding wound: The tissue surrounding the wound should be examined for color, feel, temperature, edema, and induration. Note if the skin is intact or open, weepy or moist. Redness of the surrounding tissue might indicate unrelieved pressure, a reaction to the topical agents or dressings used, or an infection. If infection is suspected (see following item for other signs of infection), the client's authorized healthcare provider should be notified.

(I) Infection: Any open area in the skin can allow bacteria to penetrate, and an infection can result. Even if a wound is not currently infected, there is still the potential for future infection. Continuous monitoring is important.

Temperature: A feeling of warmth in the area surrounding the wound may indicate the presence of infection. Conversely, skin that is extremely cool to the touch may not have adequate blood flow to provide needed nutrients and oxygen to the skin. Signs of infection include increased wound temperature or client temperature, reddening of the wound margins, edema, increased pain, pus, increased or change in color of exudates (drainage), odor, discoloration of granulation tissue, further wound breakdown, or lack of progress toward healing.

Odor: Wound odor is difficult to assess consistently, and all wounds that have been covered with a dressing for a few days emit an odor. Some dressings may also cause an odor. As a rule, this odor disappears as soon as the soiled dressing is discarded. However, it is still important to describe the presence or absence of wound odor because a sudden increase in the amount or a change in wound odor is indicative of a change in the wound status and may potentially indicate that infection is present.

(M) Moisture: The amount of moisture or drainage is an important consideration for how well the wound is healing and what type of dressing or treatment may be needed.

Exudate/drainage: Wound exudate, amount, and type can provide important information about the status of the wound. Exudate amounts are usually large when there is edema of the surrounding tissues, during the inflammatory phase of the healing process, and when the body is breaking down necrotic tissue. Hence, as healing progresses, the amount of exudate should diminish.

Amount may be described as none (tissue is dry), scant (tissue is moist), small (tissues are wet), moderate (tissues are saturated and dressing needs to be changed frequently), or large (tissues are saturated and drainage can be freely expressed).

Color and consistency may be described as serous, sanguineous, serosanguineous, or purulent.

(E) Edges: Wound edges should be examined and documented. Descriptive adjectives include indistinct/diffuse, attached or not attached, rolled under, hyperkeratosis, and fibrotic tissue. Evaluate the epithelial edges for continuity. Local trauma may cause new epithelial tissue to erode. In some wounds, the edges must be removed (debrided) before healing can begin.

Tunneling (undermining or sinus tract): The tissue around the wound must be carefully assessed for the presence of tunneling, undermining, or sinus tracts. If tunneling is present, the tip of a sterile, cotton-tipped applicator should be used under the wound edge to determine the distance and direction of tunneling. The measurement technique is then the same as with depth.

Undermining: A passageway of tissue destruction under the skin surface that has an opening at the skin level from the edge of the wound.

closures or Steri-strips, may be applied over the incision to temporarily provide additional support and reinforce the area.

Another consideration is whether your goal for healing is curative or palliative. Not all wounds will heal, for example, because of overall illness, circulation, or impending death. The determination of how aggressively to treat a wound should be made as part of a team decision that includes the client and family. If the decision is for palliative care, then the goal is to treat the client's most bothersome symptoms, such as pain, odor, or excessive drainage. The same dressing might be used as for curative care, but the goal is different.

Gloving

Knowing the type of gloves (sterile or clean) that is required and when and how to change gloves is an important aspect of wound care. The goal is to protect the client from organisms brought into the room or to protect the wound from organisms that have contaminated the room (Sergent et al., 2012). Therefore, as stated before, hand hygiene is always performed when entering and leaving a client's room. Bacteria, viruses, fungi, and mites are present on everyone's skin. Some of these microorganisms are beneficial to the host and may actually have a role in developing immunity in the skin's T cells so that the body can react against more virulent strains of the colonizing organism (Grice & Segre, 2011). Most other organisms on the skin are not harmful to the person (Grice & Segre, 2011). In adults, bacteria colonization is present on normal intact skin and rarely results in the development of an infection. The types and amounts of bacteria remain relatively constant over time, in part because the skin has an acid (pH <5) mantle. Fetal skin is sterile in utero, and colonization begins immediately after birth. Individuals have different flora density and types on different body regions. Therefore, if the client has dressings to be changed on multiple body areas (e.g., forearm, sacrum, heel), gloves should be changed when performing dressing applications on different body regions.

COLLECTING WOUND SPECIMENS

Culturing wounds is controversial. Bacteria is present on everyone's skin and is present in the wound. As a result, what is cultured is usually the person's normal bacteria. However, if that bacteria is present in high concentrations, if biofilms develop, or if the wound has virulent bacteria in it, healing will be delayed, and the wound will become chronic. Think of a person's infection potential as the number and virulence of bacteria moderated by the person's immune functioning. A person with poor immune functioning will develop an infection with fewer numbers and/or less virulent bacteria than a person whose immune system is functioning well.

Wound culturing may be done by swab, biopsy, or needle aspiration. Specimens collected by needle aspiration or biopsy require advanced training to perform. Nurses assist authorized healthcare providers with these types of specimen collection.

- **Tissue biopsy:** A piece of viable tissue is removed with a scalpel or punch biopsy instrument. The sample should not be taken from necrotic tissue.

- **Needle aspiration:** Exudate is collected by inserting a 22-gauge needle into various locations within the wound and withdrawing fluid into a 10-mL syringe.

Nurses collect swab cultures from wounds. Swab cultures obtain only surface organisms from the exudate but are the easiest to perform. It is appropriate to monitor the number of organisms in the wound. Culture samples are sent to the lab in a tube with a growth medium.

Some labs have separate tubes for anaerobic (bacteria that do not require the presence of oxygen) and aerobic (bacteria that grow in the presence of oxygen) organisms. Aerobic organisms are usually found in wounds close to the skin surface, whereas anaerobic organisms are usually found in deeper wounds or abscesses.

MANAGING COMPLEX WOUNDS

A balanced, moist environment is necessary for wound healing. This environment facilitates cellular growth and collagen proliferation. Too much moisture can impair healing and damage the periwound skin. If the environment is too dry, cells cannot migrate across the wound bed. In addition, the pH of the wound bed is important (Zulkowski, 2013). Normal skin is acidic, and this pH may prevent opportunistic organisms from proliferating on the skin or in a wound (Frank et al., 2009; Power, Moore, & O'Connor, 2017). However, chronic or deep wounds are more alkaline, and healing is impaired. Chronic wounds are most often stalled in the inflammatory phase. This results in extended redness and edema surrounding the wound and increased exudate. Chronic wounds tend to have a low level of tissue oxygen, which, in addition to being more alkaline, can facilitate the growth of bacteria. Chronic wounds are more likely to be colonized with multiple species of aerobic and anaerobic bacteria and have a greater potential for biofilm formation than acute wounds (James et al., 2008).

Biofilms are complex microbial communities made up of microorganisms (bacteria and fungi). These microorganisms synthesize and secrete a protective exopolymeric matrix (EPM) of polysaccharides, proteins, and bacterial DNA that attaches the biofilm firmly to a living or nonliving surface. Biofilm can only be removed from a wound by debridement (Rajpaul, 2015).

Debriding Wounds

It is necessary to remove necrotic or devitalized tissue for healing to occur, but there has to be adequate underlying vascularity of the wound bed (NPUAP et al., 2014). The presence of necrotic tissue impedes reepithelialization of the wound bed and may mask underlying issues, including abscess and infection. Necrotic tissue can be black or brown and thick and leathery. It can also be moist and yellow, green, tan, or gray. The method used to debride the necrotic tissue depends on the client's condition and the location of the wound. For example, heel wounds are not usually debrided unless there is adequate vascularization in the limb. Debridement methods include surgical/sharps, autolytic, enzymatic, biologic, ultrasound, and mechanical (Baranoski & Ayello, 2015; Beheshti, Shafigh, Parsa, & Zangivand, 2014; NPUAP et al., 2014). The nurse's role depends on the type of debridement used. For example, for sharps debridement, the nurse's role is to get the client ready for surgery. The nurse's role for enzymatic debridement is to apply enzymatic ointment to the wound. Check your facility's policies. More information on each type of debridement is as follows:

- **Surgical sharps:** Sharps debridement is a surgical procedure that uses scissors, scalpels, and other sharp instruments to cut away or remove necrotic tissue. It is most often carried out in the operating room but can sometimes be done in the clinic or bedside setting. It is the fastest way to debride a wound, but the person's anesthetic risk due to other medical issues means it is not useful for everyone.
- **Autolytic:** Autolytic debridement uses moisture from the wound to soften and remove dead tissue. This is often done using dressings that promote a moist environment, such as film, hydrogel, or honey alginate. It is a slower but nonsurgical process.
- **Enzymatic:** Chemical enzymes are used to soften and remove dead tissue. The product must be placed on the tissue to be removed, and hard tissue must be cross-hatched to improve effectiveness. A cover dressing is used to absorb the moisture from liquefying dead tissue.
- **Biologic:** Biologic debridement, also known as larval or maggot therapy, is the intentional introduction (by a healthcare practitioner) of live, disinfected maggots (fly larvae) raised in special facilities into nonhealing skin and soft tissue wounds. This therapy is designed to selectively clean out only the necrotic tissue within a wound and promote wound healing. The number of maggots needed depends on the size of the wound and how much debridement is needed. Maggots are contained in the wound dressing and must have air-permeable covers to survive. They are changed every 2 days. Only medical-grade maggots (raised in controlled conditions) should be used.
- **Ultrasound mist therapy:** Low-energy ultrasonic waves are used on the wound bed using a mist spray (Beheshti et al., 2014). This washes out the dead tissue as it is removed and does not harm the "healthy" tissue. This procedure requires multiple treatments.
- **Mechanical debridement:** Mechanical debridement most often uses hydrotherapy, such as directed wound irrigation. This can be jet-therapy, which uses sterile water directed at the wound bed under high pressure to remove the dead tissue. Baths with whirlpool water flow should not be used to manage wounds because a whirlpool will not selectively target the tissue to be removed and can damage all tissue. Wet-to-dry dressings also mechanically debride the wound, but this is nonselective, removing both dead and healthy tissue, and is not recommended.

DRESSING SELECTION AND APPLICATION

Modern dressings are designed to optimize the healing environment in the wound. Wet-to-dry or wet-to-moist dressings are not evidence-based treatments for wound healing (NPUAP et al., 2014). Many dressings are combination dressings, and it is important to know the characteristics of all the products in the

dressing. Typically, wounds have a primary dressing that covers the wound and then a secondary dressing to hold it in place, help manage exudate, and provide protection to the wound. The majority of dressings used as the secondary (cover) dressing have adhesive borders. If tape has to be used to secure the dressing, be sure it is appropriate for the skin and will not tear the skin when removed. Pull tape gently from the edges toward the dressing, and if the area has hair, try to pull gently in the direction of hair growth. Never pull the dressing off too quickly. You may damage the new granulation tissue and delay healing.

Primary Intention Incisional Wounds

The technique for wound care and dressing application may vary based on the wound type. Ideally, the sterile occlusive dressing that was applied following surgery remains clean, dry, and intact for the first 48 hours. The purpose of the dressing is to prevent microorganisms from entering the surgical site and protect the site while reepithelization takes place. Surgical facilities are very concerned with preventing surgical site infections (SSIs) because these are healthcare-associated infections, and insurance or Medicare/Medicaid does not cover the costs. Industry has been responsive to that concern, and new occlusive dressing products are available that prevent bacteria from entering the surgical site. If the initial surgical dressing becomes soiled and needs to be changed before epithelialization is complete, then sterile supplies and sterile technique are recommended for the dressing change (Brindle & Creehan, 2016). Once epithelial resurfacing is complete, which usually occurs within 48 to 72 hours, then the dressing may be removed, and the client may shower. However, if the client has impaired healing and the incision is not resurfacing, sterile technique is used to redress the incision with a primary layer that promotes reepithelization (Brindle & Creehan, 2016).

Secondary Intention Wounds

Secondary-intention wounds have to heal from the bottom up so that an abscess does not form. The dressing material is designed to absorb exudate and keep the wound moist. For example, a wound with a large amount of exudate needs a dressing to absorb moisture, whereas one with little exudate may need a dressing to add moisture. If a wound is deep or tunnels under the skin, the dressing material will need to fill the void. Depending on the wound characteristics, different materials may be used, which can include negative-pressure wound therapy (NPWT), as discussed in the section on wound drains and Skill 16.6.

Wound Dressing Products

Although the wound nurse, nurse practitioner, or authorized healthcare provider usually orders the dressing, it is important for all nurses to know the characteristics of each type of dressing and how to correctly apply it. Selection is based on the wound size, type, location, and TIME (tissue, infection, moisture, edges) principles. Focus on the type of dressing rather than the trade name. Different dressing manufacturers have different-sounding names for their products, but the dressings fit into a category. It's important to know the category so that accurate information can

TABLE 16.2 Wound Dressing Categories

Dressing Category	Definition	Considerations
Transparent film	Polyurethane and polyethylene membrane film coated with a layer of hypoallergenic acrylic adhesive. Moisture vapor transmission rates (MVTRs) vary.	Often used as a secondary dressing because it is transparent and protects from outside bacteria entering the wound. Used as a primary dressing when there is little exudate but the wound needs protection, such as in a skin tear. Do not stretch to apply. There should not be any wrinkles in the film dressing when applied.
Hydrocolloid	Gelatin, pectin, and carboxymethylcellulose in a polyisobutylene adhesive base with polyurethane or film backing. Hydrophilic colloid particles bound to polyurethane foam.	Cut to fit in the wound. Use the warmth of your hand to help mold it to a contoured area. These dressings may have an odor during a dressing change. Used for wounds with moderate exudate.
Hydrogel	Water- or glycerin-based, nonadherent, cross-linked polymer. May or may not be supported by a fabric net, high water content, varying amounts of gel-forming material (glycerin, co-polymer, water, propylene glycol, humectant).	This dressing adds moisture to a wound. It may be used in combination with other dressings, such as silver or honey.
Foam	Inert material that is hydrophilic and nonadherent; modified polyurethane foam	May be used as a cover dressing or to pad the wound. As a primary dressing, absorbs moderate to large amounts of exudate. May have antibacterial properties.
Calcium Alginate	Calcium sodium salts of alginic acid (naturally occurring polymer in seaweed). Nonwoven composite of fibers from a cellulose-like polysaccharide that acts via an ion-exchange mechanism, absorbing serous fluid or exudate and forming a hydrophilic gel that conforms to the shape of the wound.	Cut to shape of wound. Never pack in wound because this needs to gel as it absorbs exudate. Never wet to apply, but when removing from wound, if alginate dressing appears dry and fibrous, then wet with normal saline to remove. Used for wounds with large amounts of exudate.
Silver	Topical silver has broad-spectrum antimicrobial activity that has been shown to be effective against many antibiotic-resistant wound pathogens.	Found in a variety of composite dressings or as a powder.
Iodine	Iodine is another metal that can be used in various forms of dressings to address inflamed or infected wounds.	Found in a variety of composite dressings.
Honey	Use or addition of Manuka honey as a part of a variety of composite dressings. Manuka honey provides a hypertonic environment thought to assist with microbial control.	May be in composite dressings, including hydrogel, calcium alginate, and hydrocolloid, and as a liquid. Honey alginate may be used on dry wounds or eschar.

Note: Use TIME principles to determine the best primary and/or secondary dressing.

be transferred between facilities that use different manufacturers' products. Table 16.2 identifies wound dressing categories and their uses. In addition, new dressings and products are constantly being developed, so the nurse must stay current. All nurses need a basic understanding of how to care for a wound and how to examine the current evidence for best practice.

APPLICATION OF THE NURSING PROCESS

Examples of Related International Classification for Nursing Practice (ICNP) Nursing Diagnoses, Expected Client Outcomes, and Nursing Interventions:

Nursing Diagnosis: Impaired tissue integrity
Supporting Data: Presence of a partial-thickness wound
Expected Client Outcomes: Client will have wound healing, as demonstrated by decreasing wound size and increasing granulation tissue.
Nursing Intervention Example: Apply a dressing that provides a moist wound-healing environment, allows absorption of exudate, and fills any dead space.
Reference: International Classification for Nursing Practice. (n.d.). *eHealth & ICNP*. Retrieved from https://www.icn.ch/what-we-do/projects/ehealth-icnp.

CRITICAL CONCEPTS
Providing Wound Care

Accuracy (ACC)

Providing wound care is subject to the following variables:
- assessment of the client, including level of discomfort
- assessment of the wound, including dimensions, tissue present in wound, exudate, wound odor, wound's margins/edges, and tissue surrounding wound
- time lapsed during collection or following specimen collection
- use of sterile technique when obtaining cultures
- understanding of the procedure by the client and family.

Client-Centered Care (CCC)

When providing wound care, respect for the client is demonstrated by:
- obtaining verbal consent
- promoting autonomy
- providing privacy and ensuring comfort
- answering questions before, during, and after wound care
- honoring cultural preferences
- arranging for an interpreter, if needed
- advocating for the client and family.

Infection Control (INF)

When providing wound care, healthcare-associated and client infections are prevented by:
- containment of microorganisms
- preventing and reducing the transfer of microorganisms
- reducing the number of microorganisms
- preventing an environment conducive to microbial growth.

Safety (SAF)

When providing wound care, safety measures prevent harm to the client and provide a safe care environment, including:
- verifying the plan of care, allergies, and current medications.

Communication (COM)

- Communication exchanges information (oral, written, nonverbal, or electronic) between two or more people.

- Documentation records information in a permanent legal record.
- Collaboration between the nurse, the client, the client's family, and members of the healthcare team is essential for effective wound care.

Health Maintenance (HLTH)

When providing wound care, nursing is dedicated to the promotion of health, including:
- Protecting the client's periwound skin integrity and new granulation or scar tissue.

Evaluation (EVAL)

When providing wound care, evaluation of outcomes enables the nurse to determine the efficacy of the care provided.

■ SKILL 16.1 Dressing Change for a Primary-Intention Wound

EQUIPMENT

Clean gloves
Normal saline or wound cleanser
Disposable tape measure
Sterile cotton swab
Gauze pads or nonadherent pads
Supplies necessary for primary and secondary dressing, based on authorized healthcare provider order
Tape as needed

BEGINNING THE SKILL

1. **SAF** Review the authorized healthcare provider's order and facility policy. *Verifying the plan of care prevents injury to the client.*
2. **INF** Perform hand hygiene.
3. **CCC** Introduce yourself to the client and family and explain each step of the procedure. Ensure the client gives verbal consent for the procedure.
4. **SAF** Identify the client using two identifiers.
5. **CCC** Provide privacy. Close the door and pull the curtain.

PROCEDURE

6. **SAF** Set up an ergonomically safe space. If the client is in a bed, raise the bed to a comfortable working height and raise one side rail. *Setting up an ergonomically safe space prevents injury to the nurse and client.*
7. **SAF** Set up a workspace according to your hand dominance and the wound location as the room space allows. You can set up your workspace facing the client's head or turn around and face the client's feet in order to meet your needs. Set up a work area and trash receptacle.

8. **INF** Apply clean gloves. *There is an inherent risk of exposure to you and the client when changing a dressing.* (Note: If additional supplies are needed, you must remove your gloves and wash your hands to exit the room. When you return to the room, perform hand hygiene and reapply gloves.)
9. **SAF** Review the following:
   - client's allergies, such as allergies to topical antimicrobials or latex
   - client's medications, particularly medications that alter clotting time.
10. **ACC** Assess the following:
    - client's level of orientation and ability to follow instructions
    - client's pain level using a consistent facility-approved pain tool.
    If the client is disoriented, obtain assistance for the dressing change. If the client is experiencing pain, medicate the client and wait for the medication to take effect before changing the dressing.
11. **CCC** Position the client for the dressing change, exposing only the area that has the dressing. (Note: If the client is soiled in the body area of the dressing to be changed, cleanse the client, remove gloves, perform hand hygiene, and reapply clean gloves.)
12. **INF** To remove the dressing, first loosen the adhesive border or tape. Pull the adhesive border or tape parallel to the skin and in the direction of the wound. Remove the dressing one layer at a time. Remove the secondary dressing first, and then remove the inner layer and discard into the appropriate receptacle/bag per facility policy and procedure.

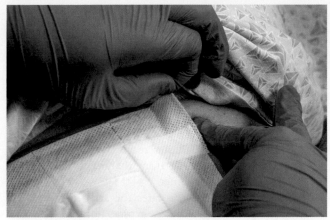

STEP 12 Pull the border of the dressing toward the wound.

13. **INF** Remove gloves, perform hand hygiene, and reapply clean gloves.
14. **INF** Cleanse and dry periwound and wound bed with the prescribed solution. Spray on wound cleanser. If the client is on his or her side, spray top to bottom. *The goal is to wash debris away from the wound.*
15. **HLTH** Gently pat the wound dry with a gauze pad. Using a new pad, dry the surrounding skin from the wound edge to the outer areas.

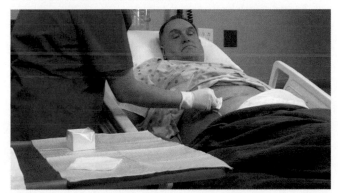

STEP 15 After cleaning, dry the surrounding skin.

16. **ACC** Assess the wound and surrounding tissue after cleansing, including location, length, width, depth, and TIME (tissue, infection [or potential for infection], moisture, wound edges and peri-skin condition). Use the measuring tape to measure the length of the incision. If the wound is closed, there is no depth or width. Review Box 16.1.
17. **ACC** Determine if the incision is to be left open to the air or if a new dressing is to be applied. Determine if the new dressing should be applied using sterile or clean technique.

If Using Sterile Technique and Sterile Dressings

(Note: For the first 48 to 72 postoperative hours, sterile dressings and sterile technique are recommended. Postoperative incisions healing by delayed primary closure should also be cared for with sterile technique and sterile dressings.)

   a. **INF** Open all packages of the primary dressing. Keep the dressing material on the package, maintaining the sterility of the dressing.

   b. **INF** Open the package of secondary dressing material. Keep the dressing material on the package, maintaining the sterility of the dressing.

   c. **INF** Apply sterile gloves if indicated. Otherwise, apply clean gloves.

   d. **INF** Pinch primary dressing on the top to carry it over to the client and apply to the incision. *Pinching the primary dressing allows the nurse to place the dressing without touching the client's skin.*

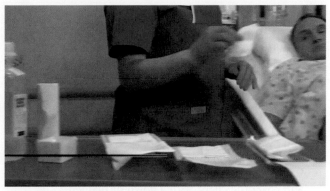

STEP 17D Pinch the primary dressing on the top.

   e. Apply as much dressing as is needed to cover and protect the incision. (Sterile gauze or a nonadherent dressing is commonly used.)

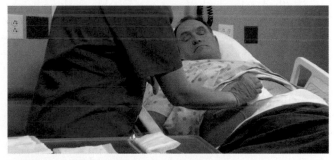

STEP 17E Cover with the dressing as ordered.

18. **ACC** Cover with a secondary dressing and secure. (Note: Secondary dressings may have an adhesive border, so tape may not be necessary.) If tape is used to secure the wound, apply it around the border of the secondary dressing. Be sure the tape will not damage the skin upon removal and that it is not so tight that circulation is compromised. *This is especially important with compression dressings because they apply pressure.*
19. **INF** Properly dispose of used supplies and soiled dressings according to facility policy. Remove gloves and perform hand hygiene.

FINISHING THE SKILL

20. **CCC** Ensure client comfort. Assist the client with repositioning. Provide reassurance and emotional support.
21. **SAF** Ensure client safety. Place the bed in the lowest position. Ensure the that client can identify and reach the nurse call system. *These safety measures reduce the risk of falls.*
22. **INF** Perform hand hygiene.
23. **EVAL** Evaluate outcomes, including reassessing the client's pain level.

24. **COM** Document assessment findings, date and time of the dressing change, care given, how the client tolerated the procedure, and outcomes in the legal healthcare record.

25. **COM** Notify the authorized healthcare provider if the wound has signs of infection or any significant change.

■ SKILL 16.2 Collecting Wound Specimens

EQUIPMENT

Clean gloves
Culture swab/tubes
Sterile normal saline or wound cleanser

BEGINNING THE SKILL

1. **INF** Perform hand hygiene.
2. **CCC** Introduce yourself to the client and family and explain the procedure. Ensure the client gives verbal consent for the procedure.
3. **SAF** Identify the client using two identifiers.
4. **CCC** Provide privacy. Close the door, pull the curtain, and cover the client with a gown or blanket.

PROCEDURE

5. **SAF** Review the order. *Verifying the plan of care and medical history prevents injury to the client.*
6. **SAF** Set up an ergonomically safe space. If the client is in a bed, raise the bed to a comfortable working height and raise one side rail. *Setting up an ergonomically safe space prevents injury to the nurse and client.*
7. **SAF** Set up a workspace according to your hand dominance and the wound location as the room space allows. You can set up your workspace facing the client's head or turn around and face the client's feet in order to meet your needs. Set up a work area and trash receptacle.
8. **INF** Perform hand hygiene and apply clean gloves. (Note: If additional supplies are needed, you must remove your gloves and wash your hands to exit the room. When you return to the room, perform hand hygiene and reapply gloves.)
9. **ACC** Assess the following:
   • client's level of orientation and ability to follow instructions
   • client's pain level using a consistent facility-approved pain tool.
   Your assessment is to determine the extent to which the client can cooperate during the procedure. You may need to find a colleague to assist you with this procedure. If the client is experiencing pain, medicate the client and wait for the medication to take effect before obtaining the culture.
10. **CCC** Position the client for the dressing change, exposing only the area that has the dressing.

Obtaining a Swab Culture Specimen

11. **INF** Remove dressing and cleanse the wound. (Note: For an accurate specimen, you must have fresh exudate from the wound, and the sample must be from viable tissue [not necrotic].)
12. **ACC** Moisten the cotton swab with normal saline prior to swabbing the wound. Then use either the Z-stroke or Levine method for collecting the swab.

• The Z-stroke technique rotates the swab between the fingers, swabbing from margin to margin in a 10-point zigzag manner.
• The Levine method rotates the swab over a 1-cm² area with enough force to express fluid.

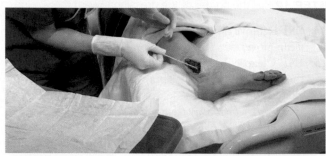

STEP 12 The Levine swab method rotates the swab over a 1-cm² (<0.5-inch²) area.

13. **ACC** Place the swab in the correct culture tube, label it, and send it to the lab.

Assisting With Obtaining an Aspiration or Biopsy Specimen

14. **ACC** Assist the authorized healthcare provider as needed.
15. **ACC** Place the biopsy in the correct culture tube, label it, and send it to the lab. Ensure that the specimen label contains two client identifiers. Label the specimen in the presence of the client. *National safety guidelines recommend labeling specimens in the presence of the client.*
16. **INF** Properly dispose of the used supplies in the appropriate receptacle and according to facility policy. Remove gloves and perform hand hygiene.

FINISHING THE SKILL

17. **INF** Reapply the dressing using sterile or clean technique as appropriate. Remove gloves and perform hand hygiene.
18. **CCC** Provide comfort. Assist the client with positioning.
19. **SAF** Ensure client safety. Place the bed in the lowest position. Ensure that the client can identify and reach the nurse call system. *These safety measures reduce the risk of falls.*
20. **INF** Perform hand hygiene.
21. **EVAL** Evaluate outcomes, including evaluating the client's pain level.
22. **COM** Document assessment findings, care given, and outcomes in the legal healthcare record, including:
   • wound assessment finding
   • date and time of specimen collection
   • type of laboratory specimen collection
   • how the client tolerated the procedure.
23. **ACC** Transport to the laboratory per facility policy within the time limit. Many institutions require transportation in a plastic resealable bag.

■ SKILL 16.3 Removing Sutures and Staples

EQUIPMENT

Clean gloves
Suture- or staple-removal package
Sterile normal saline or wound cleanser
Cotton-tipped applicators or 4 × 4 gauze sponges

BEGINNING THE SKILL

1. **INF** Perform hand hygiene.
2. **CCC** Introduce yourself to the client and family and explain the procedure. Ensure the client gives verbal consent for the procedure.
3. **SAF** Identify the client using two identifiers.
4. **CCC** Provide privacy. Close the door, pull the curtain, and cover the client with a gown or blanket.

PROCEDURE

5. **SAF** Review the order. *Verifying the plan of care and medical history prevents injury to the client.*
6. **SAF** Review the following:
   - client's allergies, such as allergies to topical antimicrobials or latex
   - client's medications, particularly medications that alter clotting time
   - client's pain level using a consistent facility-approved pain tool
   - client's risk factors for delayed healing.
7. **ACC** Assess the client's ability to follow instructions and discomfort.
8. **SAF** Set up an ergonomically safe space. If the client is in a bed, raise the bed to a comfortable working height and raise one side rail. *Setting up an ergonomically safe space prevents injury to the nurse and client.*
9. **SAF** Set up a workspace according to your hand dominance and the wound location. Set up a work area and trash receptacle.
10. **INF** Perform hand hygiene and apply clean gloves.
11. **CCC** Position the client for suture or staple removal, exposing only the area needed.
12. **INF** Remove any dressing and discard into the appropriate receptacle/bag per facility policy and procedure.
13. **INF** Cleanse incision and surrounding area with normal saline and dry. Assess incision site and surrounding tissue after cleansing for signs of infection or inadequate healing. If dried blood or exudate is present on the staples or suture, use a moistened sterile cotton swab to remove as much as possible. (Note: A warm washcloth can help loosen debris.) *Removing dried blood or exudate reduces the risk of an environment conducive to microbial growth.*
14. **SAF** Alternating staples or sutures are removed first to prevent any dehiscence. **WARNING:** If the wound begins to dehisce, do not remove any more sutures or staples. Stop the procedure and notify the authorized healthcare provider.

Staples

15. **ACC** Slip the end of the staple remover under the center of the staple.

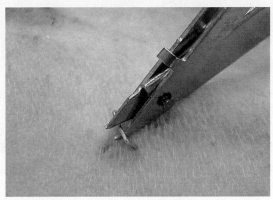

STEP 15 Slip the end of the staple remover under the center of the staple.

16. **ACC** Squeeze the handle. The staple can be gently lifted out of the skin, first one side, then the other.

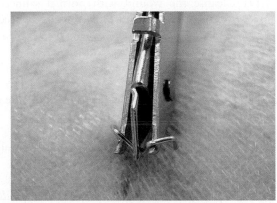

STEP 16 Squeeze the handle. The staple can be gently lifted out of the skin.

Sutures

17. **ACC** Use sterile tweezers to pull the suture away from the skin by the knot.

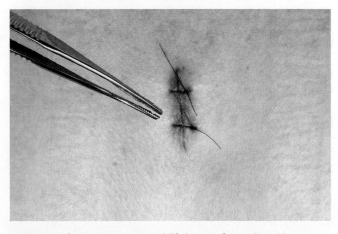

STEP 17 Grasp the knot and lift it way from the skin.

18. **ACC** Slip the scissor blade with the curved notch under the suture knot and snip.

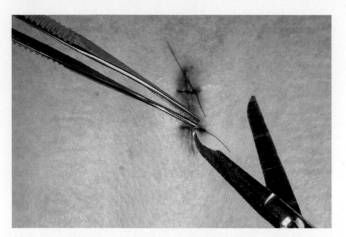

STEP 18 Slip the scissor blade with the curved notch under the suture knot and snip.

19. **ACC** Use the tweezers to gently pull the suture from the incision. (Note: Be sure *not* to pull the knot end or the section of the suture that has been positioned across the incision through the skin.)
20. **HLTH** Cleanse the wound with normal saline, dry thoroughly, and place wound closure strips as needed. *Wound closure strips serve to approximate the wound edges and minimize tension on the new scar tissue.*
    a. Remove the smaller backing strip.
    b. Lift off one closure strip.
    c. Start in the middle of the wound and apply the closure strip on one side of the wound.
    d. Ensure the wound is well approximated.
    e. Apply the closure strip to the other side. Press firmly in place.
    f. Apply additional closure strips approximately 3 mm (⅛ inch) apart. *Leaving space between the strips allows for visualization of the wound.*
21. **INF** Properly dispose of used supplies and soiled dressings according to facility policy. Remove gloves and perform hand hygiene.

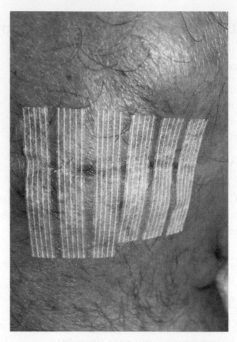

STEP 20F Place wound closure strips as needed.

FINISHING THE SKILL

22. **COM** Provide comfort. Assist the client with repositioning.
23. **SAF** Ensure client safety. Place the bed in the lowest position. Ensure that the client can identify and reach the nurse call system. *These safety measures reduce the risk of falls.*
24. **INF** Perform hand hygiene.
25. **EVAL** Evaluate outcomes, including evaluating the client's pain level.
26. **COM** Document assessment of the incision; date and time of the suture or staple removal; care given, such as application of closure strips; how the client tolerated the procedure; and outcomes in the legal healthcare record.
27. **COM** Notify authorized healthcare provider if the wound is dehiscing.

■ SKILL 16.4 Dressing a Partial- or Full-Thickness Wound

Clean gloves
Gown and mouth, nose, and eye protection, if there is a risk of spray during wound cleaning
Normal saline/wound cleanser
4 × 4 gauze sponges
Skin barrier prep pads
Small trash bag
Bandage scissors
Dressings

BEGINNING THE SKILL

1. **SAF** Review the order and facility policy. *Verifying the plan of care prevents injury to the client.*
2. **INF** Perform hand hygiene.
3. **CCC** Introduce yourself to the client and family and explain the procedure. Ensure the client gives verbal consent for the procedure.
4. **SAF** Identify the client using two identifiers.
5. **CCC** Provide privacy. Close the door and pull the curtain.

PROCEDURE

6. **ACC** Assess the following:
   - client's level of orientation and ability to follow instructions
   - client's pain level using a consistent facility-approved pain tool.

   If the client is disoriented, obtain assistance for the dressing change. If the client is experiencing pain, medicate the client and wait for the medication to take effect before changing the dressing.

7. **SAF** Set up an ergonomically safe space. Raise the bed to a comfortable working height and raise the opposite side rail. *Setting up an ergonomically safe space prevents injury to the nurse and client.*

8. **SAF** Set up a workspace according to your hand dominance. You can set up your workspace facing the client's head or turn around and face the client's feet in order to meet your needs. Set up the work area and trash receptacle.

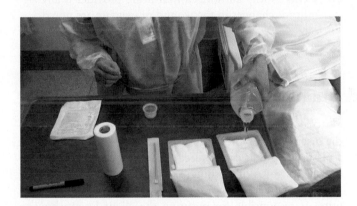

STEP 8 Set up work area and trash receptacle.

9. **INF** Perform hand hygiene. Apply clean gloves. Apply a gown to prevent soiling your clothing, and apply mouth, nose, and eye protection, such as a face shield, if there is a risk of spray during wound cleaning. *There is an inherent risk of exposure when cleaning and changing a dressing.* (Note: If additional supplies are needed, you must remove your gloves and wash your hands to exit the room. When you return to the room, perform hand hygiene and reapply gloves.)

10. **CCC** Position the client for the dressing change, exposing only the area that has the dressing. (Note: If the client is soiled in the body area of the dressing to be changed, cleanse the client, remove gloves, perform hand hygiene, and reapply clean gloves.)

11. **INF** If a dressing is present, remove the dressing gently and discard in the appropriate receptacle/bag per facility policy.

12. **INF** Remove gloves, perform hand hygiene, and reapply clean gloves.

13. **INF** Cleanse the wound and surrounding tissue with wound cleanser or normal saline. Spray on wound cleanser or rinse with normal saline. If the client is on

his or her side, spray top to bottom. *The idea is to wash debris away from the wound.*

14. **HLTH** Gently pat wound dry with a gauze pad. Using a new pad, dry the surrounding skin from the wound edge to the outer areas.

15. **ACC** After cleansing, assess the wound characteristics and the amount of tunneling or undermining with a moistened sterile cotton applicator.

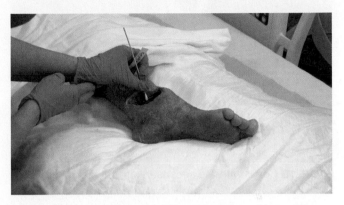

STEP 15 Assess the wound characteristics with a moistened sterile cotton applicator.

16. **HLTH** Prior to placing the new dressing, wipe skin barrier prep on the surrounding skin, going 2.5 to 5 cm (1–2 inches) out from the edge of the wound. *This protects the surrounding skin from exudate.*

17. **ACC** If the dressing is to be placed into the wound without overlapping the edges or is to be placed into an area with tunneling or undermining, you will need to cut the new primary dressing to size.

18. **HLTH** Gently place the primary dressing into the wound area. It should fill the space but not press on the wound bed. Use a sterile cotton applicator to gently push the material into the tunneled area. *The dressing absorbs exudate and protects granulation tissue.*

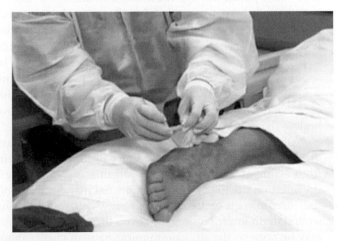

STEP 18 Gently put the primary dressing into the wound area with a cotton applicator.

19. **ACC** Cover with the secondary dressing and secure. Write the date and time of the dressing change on a

piece of tape and place it on the dressing. (Note: Secondary dressings may have an adhesive border, so tape might not be necessary.) If tape is used, be sure it will not damage the skin upon removal or is not so tight that circulation is compromised. *This is especially important with compression dressings because they apply pressure.*

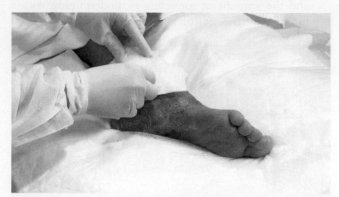

STEP 19 Cover with the secondary dressing and secure.

20. **INF** Properly dispose of used supplies and soiled dressings according to facility policy. Remove gloves and perform hand hygiene.

FINISHING THE SKILL

21. **CCC** Provide comfort. Assist the client with repositioning.
22. **SAF** Ensure client safety. Place the bed in the lowest position. Ensure that the client can identify and reach the nurse call system. *These safety measures reduce the risk of falls.*
23. **INF** Perform hand hygiene.
24. **EVAL** Evaluate outcomes, including evaluating the client's pain level.
25. **COM** Document assessment, including wound assessment, exudate amount and type of dressing used for wound care and/or packing, care given, how the client tolerated the procedure, and outcomes, in the legal healthcare record.
26. **COM** Notify authorized healthcare provider if any significant changes in the wound or exudate are noted.

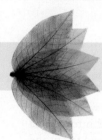

SECTION 2 Managing Wound Drainage

DRAINS AND NEGATIVE-PRESSURE WOUND THERAPY

Drains and suction devices are used to promote healing at the wound site. A drain may be inserted into or near a wound after a surgical procedure is completed when it is anticipated that fluid will collect in the closed area and delay healing. The other tube end is passed through the incision or through a separate opening called a stab wound. Tubes that are to be connected to suction or have a built-in reservoir are sutured to the skin. It is important that you know the type of drain or tube in use so that patency and placement can be accurately assessed. In addition to the drains used in surgical sites, negative-pressure wound therapy (NPWT) is used to manage wounds with excessive drainage or with full-thickness wounds to improve healing (Baranoski & Ayello, 2015; Khanh-Dao Le, 2017).

Nurses caring for clients with drains need to be aware of infection control measures in order to prevent the drain from acting as a vehicle for microorganisms. Nurses assess the insertion site for signs of infection and may clean around the insertion site with normal saline when ordered. The wound drain insertion site may have a dressing applied, or it may be open to the air. Communicating with clients about the expected changes in drainage volume and appearance reassures the client that healing is progressing as expected. Communication may also prevent misunderstandings, such as the example found in Box 16.2. When a client has a drain, the drain needs to be secured in order to prevent pulling on

the insertion site. The Jackson-Pratt (JP) and Hemovac have a plastic loop that can be used to safety pin the reservoir to the client's gown or clothing, as shown in Fig. 16.3.

Clients often go home with a drain still in place, and the nurse is responsible for ensuring the client knows how to empty and support the reservoir; identify signs of infection; and incorporate the drain into activities of daily living, such as bathing.

Penrose Drain

The Penrose drain is made of flexible, soft rubber. The Penrose drain is an open drainage system placed during a surgical procedure to prevent the buildup of fluid. The Penrose drain draws any fluid, such as pus or blood, along its surfaces by capillary action and gravity. The external end of the Penrose drain may exit through the incision or through a stab wound adjacent to the surgical incision. The drain may be secured to the skin with a suture or it may have a large safety pin or tab outside the wound to maintain its position and prevent it from slipping into the incision. As the wound heals, the Penrose drain is sometimes slowly pulled out of the wound to help facilitate healing. It is often shortened by 2 to 4 cm (3/4–1.5 inches) each day until it falls out. This is called advancing the Penrose. Drainage from a Penrose is not contained. The Penrose dressing absorbs the drainage that is produced. Therefore, the nurse assesses the drainage production and builds a dressing tailored to the amount of drainage. A drawback to an open drainage system is that organisms may enter the wound.

BOX 16.2 Lessons From Experience: Do-It-Yourself (DIY) Wound Drain Care

Steve is an experienced nurse on a busy orthopedic floor, and he is precepting Cody, a junior nursing student. Steve had been off over the weekend and was meeting his assigned clients for the first time. He learned at the change-of-shift report that Mr. Johnson had knee surgery 2 days earlier. He had a Jackson-Pratt drain and a small dressing around the drain. When they walked into the client's room, it was obvious that Mr. Johnson's wife was upset with him. "Tell the nurses what you did!" his wife said. Mr. Johnson told Steve that he had become concerned because there was not much drainage in his "grenade" drain, and he thought it was clogged up. So he popped off the grenade and sucked on the tubing. He didn't think he got the clog out because there still wasn't any drainage in the "grenade."

Steve explained to Mr. Johnson that the internal end of his drain tube was placed very near the knee joint, so by putting his mouth on the tubing, he may have introduced bacteria to the knee. He also explained that it was expected that the amount of drainage coming from his knee would decrease over time following the surgery. Steve explained that he would need to notify the surgeon about sucking on the tube and see if additional antibiotics would be prescribed.

When Steve and Cody left the room, Cody asked, "How can you anticipate that someone would suck on the drain tube?" Steve replied that this was the first time for him. But perhaps if Mr. Johnson had known that his care providers were anticipating a decrease in drainage and had heard how important it was to keep the tubing clean, he might not have taken matters into his own hands and sucked on the drainage tube. Letting your clients know the signs of healing in addition to the signs of infection allows them to celebrate each step in the healing process.

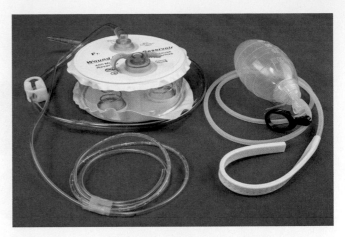

FIG. 16.4 Wound drains: Hemovac *(left)* and JP drain *(right)*.

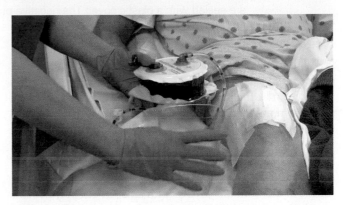

FIG. 16.5 A Hemovac holds more drainage than a Jackson-Pratt (JP) drain.

Jackson-Pratt or Hemovac Drain

As shown in Fig. 16.4, both the JP and Hemovac drains are closed drainage systems that provide low suction to a collection reservoir. These drains are placed in the operating room. Regularly compressing these devices creates the negative pressure. A JP is drain has an oval, grenade-shaped reservoir. JP drains can collect about 100 to 200 mL of drainage in 24 hours. The drain's reservoir or "bulb" should be concave or flat and not fully inflated. If it is fully inflated after emptying, it is not providing negative pressure to evacuate drainage. The proper technique for compressing a JP drain to create negative pressure is to squeeze the sides of the reservoir together (Carruthers, Eisemann, Lamp, & Kocak, 2013). Compressing the reservoir from bottom to the top creates little to no measurable negative pressure (Carruthers et al., 2013).

A Hemovac (Fig. 16.5) is a round drain with springs inside that are compressed to establish suction. A Hemovac can collect up to 500 mL of fluid in 24 hours. Nurses empty and compress these devices. Assessment and measurement of drainage are essential for the appropriate and safe removal of the drains (Kasbekar, Davies, Upile, Ho, & Roland, 2016). Dressings may be placed around the insertion site for these drains, or they may be open to the air. Nurses assess the drain insertion site for any signs of infection.

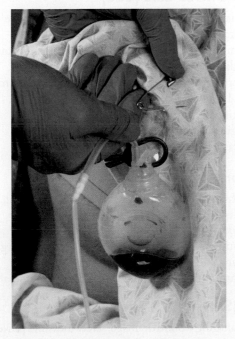

FIG. 16.3 Secure the Jackson-Pratt (JP) drain to clothing.

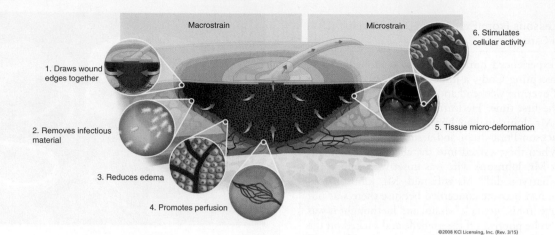

Macrostrain

Microstrain

1. Draws wound edges together

2. Removes infectious material

3. Reduces edema

4. Promotes perfusion

5. Tissue micro-deformation

6. Stimulates cellular activity

©2008 KCI Licensing, Inc. (Rev. 3/15)

FIG. 16.6 When using negative-pressure wound therapy (NPWT), the surface of the wound is covered with an open-cell polyurethane or polyvinyl alcohol (PVA) foam. The wound and dressing are sealed with a plastic cover. The negative-pressure environment promotes wound healing.

Negative-Pressure Wound Therapy

NPWT is commonly used for full-thickness wounds that require contraction and granulation tissue formation. Full-thickness wounds can be the result of a pressure injury or venous ulcer, a surgical wound that dehisces, or trauma. NPWT is the application of a controlled level of subatmospheric pressure to a wound at 50 to 175 mm Hg suction; suction may be either intermittent or continuous and will be ordered by the authorized healthcare provider. As shown in Fig. 16.6, the entire interior surface of the wound is covered with an open-cell polyurethane or polyvinyl alcohol (PVA) foam or other dressing. The dressing material is cut to fit the size and shape of the wound. However, the material should never be cut over the wound to prevent any pieces from falling into the wound. The wound and dressing are sealed with a plastic cover. The suction effect is generated by a portable programmable pump. The result is a negative-pressure environment that promotes wound healing by removing drainage and enhancing circulation and thus promoting granulation formation (Brindle & Creehan, 2016).

APPLICATION OF THE NURSING PROCESS

Examples of Related ICNP Nursing Diagnoses, Expected Client Outcomes, and Nursing Interventions:

Nursing Diagnosis: Risk for infection

Supporting Data: Site for organism invasion secondary to wound drains

Expected Client Outcomes: The client will remain free from symptoms of infection while in the healthcare setting, as demonstrated by:

- absence of heat, pain, redness, swelling, and unusual drainage at the wound drain site
- temperature and vital signs within established parameters.
- no reports of increased weakness and fatigue
- white blood cell (WBC) and differential counts within established parameters for the client.

Nursing Intervention Example: Assess, clean with normal saline, and apply a gauze dressing to the insertion site if ordered.

Reference: International Classification for Nursing Practice. (n.d.). *eHealth & ICNP.* Retrieved from https://www.icn.ch/what-we-do/projects/ehealth-icnp.

CRITICAL CONCEPTS
Managing Wound Drainage

Accuracy (ACC)

Managing wound drainage is subject to the following variables:

- assessment of client, including level of discomfort
- assessment of the drainage
- assessment of the periwound skin and any exudate
- understanding of procedure by client and family.

Client-Centered Care (CCC)

When managing wound drainage, respect for the client is demonstrated by:

- obtaining verbal consent and promoting autonomy
- providing privacy and ensuring comfort
- answering questions before, during, and after managing wound drainage
- honoring cultural preferences
- arranging for an interpreter, if needed
- advocating for the client and family.

Infection Control (INF)

When managing wound drainage, healthcare-associated and client infections are prevented by:

- containment of microorganisms
- preventing and reducing the transfer of microorganisms
- reducing the number of microorganisms
- preventing an environment conducive to microbial growth.

Safety (SAF)

When managing wound drainage, safety measures prevent harm to the client and provide a safe care environment, including:

- verifying contraindications for NPWT.

Communication (COM)

- Communication exchanges information (oral, written, nonverbal, or electronic) between two or more people.
- Collaboration with the client and other healthcare professionals facilitates managing wound drainage.
- Documentation records information in a permanent legal record.

Health Maintenance (HLTH)

When managing wound drainage, nursing is dedicated to the promotion of health and self-care abilities, including:
- protecting the client's periwound skin integrity, wound bed, and new granulation tissue.

Evaluation (EVAL)

When managing wound drainage, evaluation of outcomes enables the nurse to determine the efficacy of the care provided.

■ SKILL 16.5 Managing a Penrose Drain

EQUIPMENT

4 × 4 gauze or drain sponges or other absorbent dressing
Cover dressing or pad
Tape
Sterile scissors
Clean gloves
Sterile safety pin, if needed
Sterile cotton-tipped applicator
Wound cleanser or normal saline
Small trash bag
Measuring device

BEGINNING THE SKILL

1. **SAF** Review the authorized healthcare provider's order and facility policy. *Verifying the plan of care prevents injury to the client.*
2. **INF** Perform hand hygiene.
3. **CCC** Introduce yourself to the client and family and explain the procedure. Ensure the client gives verbal consent for the procedure.
4. **SAF** Identify the client using two identifiers.
5. **CCC** Provide privacy. Close the door and pull the curtain.

PROCEDURE

6. **SAF** Set up an ergonomically safe space. Raise the bed to a comfortable working height and raise the opposite side rail. *Setting up an ergonomically safe space prevents injury to the nurse and client.*
7. **SAF** Set up a workspace according to your hand dominance. Set up the work area and trash receptacle.
8. **INF** Perform hand hygiene and apply clean gloves. *There is an inherent risk of exposure when managing wound drainage.* (Note: If additional supplies are needed, you must remove your gloves and wash your hands to exit the room. When you return to the room, perform hand hygiene and reapply gloves.)
9. **ACC** Review the following:
    - client's level of orientation and ability to follow instructions
    - client's pain level using a consistent facility-approved pain tool.
10. **CCC** Carefully remove the old dressing, taking care not to pull out the drain. Loosen tape and pull toward the drain insertion site, never away from the insertion site. Loosen tape with normal saline or an adhesive removal pad if it does not come off easily.
11. **ACC** Assess exudate characteristics and amount on dressing, and then dispose of dressing according to facility policy.
12. **INF** Remove gloves if soiled, perform hand hygiene, and reapply gloves. (Note: One method of containing a soiled dressing is to remove a glove, turning it inside out, with the soiled dressing remaining in the glove.)

Advancing the Penrose Drain

13. **ACC** Advance the drain the ordered amount with a dressing forceps or hemostat. Place the safety pin at the new position next to the incision. Then cut the excess drain with sterile surgical or bandage scissors.
14. **SAF** Be sure the safety pin on the drain is securely fastened to prevent client injury.
15. **EVAL** Evaluate the skin at the drain insertion site. Note any redness or maceration.
16. **INF** Cleanse surrounding tissue with wound cleanser or normal saline using a cotton-tipped applicator.
17. **SAF** Gently dry surrounding skin with 4 × 4 gauze and/or cotton swab, being careful not to dislodge the drain.
18. **ACC** Place 4 × 4 gaze pad or a more absorbent dressing, such as an ABD pad, under and over the drain and secure with tape.

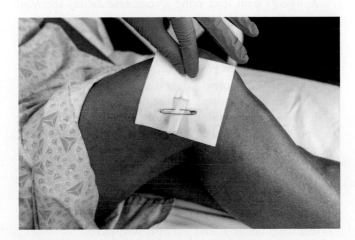

STEP 18 Place drain sponges under the drain.

19. **INF** Properly dispose of used supplies and soiled dressings according to facility policy. Remove gloves and perform hand hygiene.

FINISHING THE SKILL

20. **CCC** Ensure client comfort. Reposition client and bedding.
21. **SAF** Ensure client safety. Place the bed in the lowest position and lower the side rail. Ensure that the client can identify and reach the nurse call system. *These safety measures reduce the risk of falls.*

23. **INF** Perform hand hygiene.
23. **EVAL** Evaluate outcomes, including evaluating the client's pain level.
24. **COM** Document assessment findings, including exudate amount and characteristics, dressings, care given, how the client tolerated the procedure, and outcomes in the legal healthcare record.
25. **COM** Notify authorized healthcare provider if significant changes in the wound drainage are noted. Instruct the client on signs of infection.

■ SKILL 16.6 Emptying a Jackson-Pratt (JP) Drain or Hemovac

EQUIPMENT

Clean gloves
4 × 4 gauze or drain sponge
Tape
Sterile cotton-tipped applicator
Wound cleanser or normal saline
Measuring device (graduated cylinder or specimen cup)

BEGINNING THE SKILL

1. **SAF** Review the authorized healthcare provider's order and facility policy. *Verifying the plan of care prevents injury to the client.*
2. **INF** Perform hand hygiene.
3. **CCC** Introduce yourself to the client and family and explain the procedure. Ensure the client gives verbal consent for the procedure.
4. **SAF** Identify the client using two identifiers.
5. **CCC** Provide privacy. Close the door and pull the curtain.

PROCEDURE

6. **ACC** Review the following:
   - client's level of orientation and ability to follow instructions
   - client's pain level using a consistent facility-approved pain tool.
7. **SAF** Set up ergonomically safe space. Raise the bed to a comfortable working height and raise the opposite side rail. *Setting up an ergonomically safe space prevents injury to the nurse and client.*
8. **SAF** Set up a workspace according to your hand dominance and the wound location. Set up the work area and trash receptacle. (Note: If additional supplies are needed, you must remove your gloves and wash your hands to exit the room. When you return to the room, perform hand hygiene and reapply gloves.)
9. **INF** Perform hand hygiene and apply clean gloves. *There is an inherent risk of exposure when managing wound drainage. Gloves protect you from body fluids.*

10. **CCC** Expose the wound drainage device, but arrange the covers to maintain the client's privacy.

Jackson-Pratt Drain

11. **ACC** Open the port at the top of the reservoir.

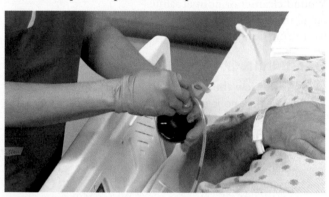

STEP 11 Open the reservoir port.

12. **ACC** Empty the JP into an appropriately sized measuring device and record the amount and characteristics of drainage. *A small amount of drainage should be measured in a small measuring device.*

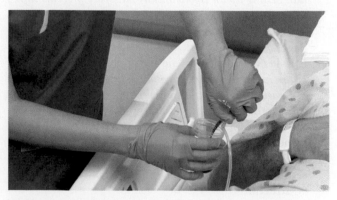

STEP 12 Empty the drainage into a measuring device.

13. **INF** Wipe the opening and plug with an antiseptic wipe. *Cleaning the opening reduces the transmission of microorganisms.*

14. **ACC** To reestablish negative pressure for the JP bulb, gently compress the bulb from side to side until flat and place the plug in the port. Slowly release your grip.

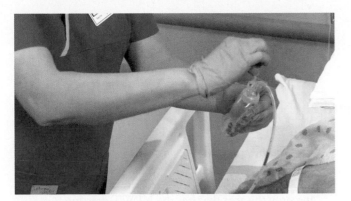

STEP 14 Gently compress the device and insert the plug.

15. **ACC** If the JP drain has a dressing, gently remove the old dressing. Assess the periwound skin and any exudate.

16. **INF** If cleaning around the drain insertion site is ordered, clean around the tube with sterile normal saline and a sterile cotton-tipped applicator.

17. **INF** If a dressing change is ordered, place drain sponge or folded gauze sponge 4 × 4 around the insertion site and secure with tape. (Note: Do not cut gauze sponges because they will readily shed fibers if cut.)

Hemovac Drain

18. **ACC** Empty the Hemovac into an appropriately sized measuring device and record the amount and characteristics of drainage. *A small amount of drainage should be measured in a small measuring device.*

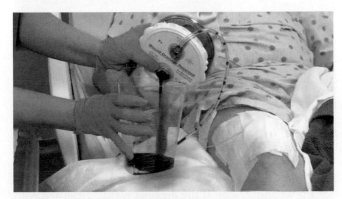

STEP 18 Empty the Hemovac into an appropriately sized measuring device.

19. **INF** Wipe the opening and plug with an antiseptic wipe. *Cleaning the opening reduces the transmission of microorganisms.*

20. **ACC** To reestablish negative pressure for the Hemovac, press the device flat to compress the springs and place the plug in the air hole. Slowly release your grip.

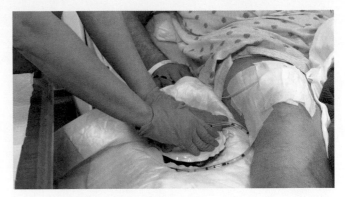

STEP 20 Press the device flat to compress the springs, and place the plug in the port.

21. **ACC** If the Hemovac drain insertion site has a dressing, gently remove the old dressing. Assess the periwound skin and any exudate.

22. **INF** If cleaning around drain tube insertion site is ordered, clean around the tube with sterile normal saline and a sterile cotton-tipped applicator.

23. **ACC** If a dressing change is ordered, place drain sponge around the insertion site and secure with tape. (Note: Do not cut gauze sponges because they will readily shed fibers if cut.)

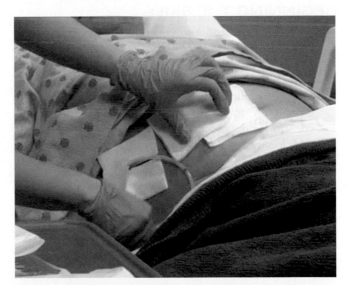

STEP 23 Place drain sponge around insertion site and secure with tape.

24. **INF** Properly dispose of used supplies and soiled dressings according to facility policy. Remove gloves and perform hand hygiene.

FINISHING THE SKILL

25. **CCC** Ensure client comfort. Reposition client and bedding.

26. **SAF** Ensure client safety. Ensure that the bed is in the lowest position. Ensure that the client can identify and reach the nurse call system. *These safety measures reduce the risk of falls.*

27. **INF** Perform hand hygiene.

28. **EVAL** Evaluate outcomes, including evaluating the client's pain level.
29. **COM** Document assessment findings in the legal healthcare record, including:
    - drainage amount, color, and characteristics
    - assessment of the drain tube insertion site
    - exudate amount and characteristics, if present around the drain tube
    - dressings and care given
    - how the client tolerated the procedure and outcomes.
30. **COM** Notify the authorized healthcare provider if significant changes in the wound or exudate are noted. Instruct the client on signs of infection and anticipated changes in drainage.

■ SKILL 16.7 Negative-Pressure Wound Therapy (NPWT)

EQUIPMENT

Clean gloves
NPWT kit
Normal saline or wound cleanser
4 × 4 gauze sponge
Skin barrier prep pads
Small biohazard trash bag
Bandage scissors
New vacuum-assisted closure (VAC) drainage canister, if needed

BEGINNING THE SKILL

1. **SAF** Review the authorized healthcare provider's order and facility policy. *Verifying the plan of care prevents injury to the client.*
2. **INF** Perform hand hygiene.
3. **CCC** Introduce yourself to the client and family and explain the procedure. Ensure the client gives verbal consent for the procedure.
4. **SAF** Identify the client using two identifiers.
5. **CCC** Provide privacy. Close the door and pull the curtain.

PROCEDURE

6. **ACC** Assess the following:
    - client's level of orientation and ability to follow instructions
    - client's pain level using a consistent facility-approved pain tool
    - client's medications, particularly medications that alter clotting time
    - client's lab work, specifically clotting factors.
7. **SAF** Set up an ergonomically safe space. Raise the bed to a comfortable working height and raise the opposite side rail. *Setting up an ergonomically safe space prevents injury to the nurse and client.*
8. **SAF** Set up a workspace according to your hand dominance. Set up work area and trash receptacle. (Note: If additional supplies are needed, you must remove your gloves and wash your hands to exit the room. When you return to the room, perform hand hygiene and reapply gloves.)
9. **INF** Perform hand hygiene. Apply clean gloves. *There is an inherent risk of exposure when managing wound drain-age. This helps prevent the introduction of bacteria into the wound.*
10. **CCC** Position client for NPWT dressing change, exposing only the area that has the NPWT dressing.
11. **SAF WARNING:** NPWT should not be used with clients who have coagulopathy issues because excessive bleeding can occur. (Note: NPWT is also contraindicated on exposed vital organs unless covered by protective mesh, inadequately debrided wounds, untreated osteomyelitis, malignancy, or allergy to any components.)
12. **ACC** Close clamps on tubing. Disconnect and drain tubing. Turn off NPWT equipment. Remove the transparent dressing, taking care to gently pull the dressing laterally (not vertically), and discard the dressing and old tubing. (Note: Gently lift, rather than pull, the dressing cover off the skin. If necessary, wipe the edge of the dressing with adhesive remover as it is removed.)

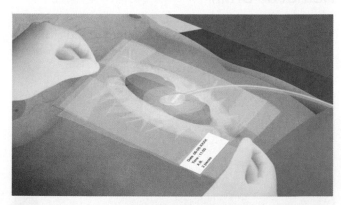

STEP 12 To remove the transparent dressing, pull laterally, not vertically.

13. **INF** Gently remove foam or other dressing from inside the wound. (Note: If the dressing is stuck, moisten with normal saline to loosen.) Dispose of saturated sponges in a biohazard bag.
14. **INF** Remove gloves, perform hand hygiene, and apply clean gloves.
15. **CCC** Cleanse the wound and surrounding tissue with wound cleanser or normal saline. Gently dry skin with 4 × 4 gauze sponges.

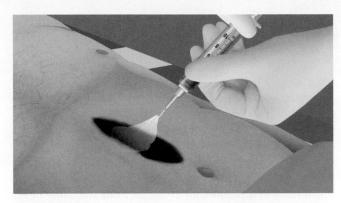

STEP 15 Cleanse the wound and surrounding tissue with wound cleanser or normal saline.

16. **ACC** Assess the wound and surrounding tissue.
17. **HLTH** Apply skin barrier prep on the surrounding skin, going 2.5 to 5 cm (1–2 inches) out from the edge of the wound. *Skin prep helps to protect the surrounding skin integrity.*

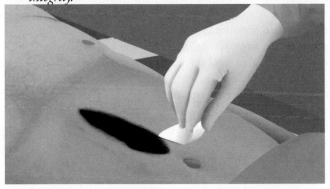

STEP 17 Apply skin barrier prep on surrounding skin.

18. **ACC** Cut the foam sponge or other dressing appropriate for the NPWT brand to fit the size and shape of the wound. If more than one piece is used, they must be touching or overlap. **WARNING:** Do not cut any of the dressing materials over the wound itself to prevent particles from falling into the wound. Note how many pieces of foam or other dressing material are used in the wound.

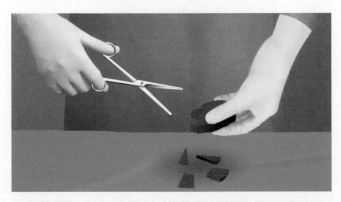

STEP 18 Cut the foam sponge to fit the size and shape of the wound.

19. **CCC** Gently place the foam or dressing into the wound cavity, covering the wound base and extending into any tunneling or undermining. **WARNING:** If tendons, nerves, or blood vessels are exposed in the wound, they must be protected. Place protective dressing as ordered over them prior to placing the foam sponge or dressing.

20. **ACC** Select the correct size of covering, or trim the plastic covering to be large enough to cover the wound and maintain an airtight seal. It should extend past the wound about 2 cm ($\frac{3}{4}$ of an inch) to the surrounding skin. Place this cover dressing over the wound.

21. **ACC** Cut a hole about the size of a quarter in the outer plastic covering over the foam and attach the suction end of the tubing by removing the backing. Be sure the plastic covering adheres securely. Then attach the new tubing to the NPWT unit. (Note: If the canister of drainage needs to be changed, do this now.)

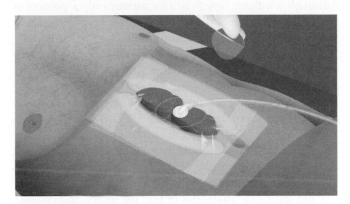

STEP 21 Cut a hole about the size of a quarter in the outer plastic covering over the foam and attach the suction.

22. **ACC** Unclamp tubing and start machine. Check machine settings to ensure proper suction amount. Foam should be sucked into the wound.
23. **INF** Properly dispose of used supplies and soiled dressings in a biohazard bag and remove from the room according to facility policy. Remove gloves and perform hand hygiene.

FINISHING THE SKILL

24. **CCC** Ensure client comfort. Reposition client and bedding.
25. **SAF** Ensure client safety. Ensure that the bed is in the lowest position. Ensure that the client can identify and reach the nurse call system. *These safety measures reduce the risk of falls.*
26. **INF** Perform hand hygiene.
27. **EVAL** Evaluate outcomes, including evaluating the client's pain level and how the client tolerated the procedure.
28. **COM** Document assessment findings, wound care given, and outcomes in the legal healthcare record. Include the following:
    - exudate amount and characteristics found in VAC canister
    - amount/number and type of dressings in wound.
29. **COM** Notify the authorized healthcare provider if significant changes in the wound or exudate are noted.

SECTION 3 Preventing and Treating Pressure Injury and Venous and Diabetic Ulcers

The skin is the largest organ and reflects the health of all other organs, such as the heart, lungs, liver, and kidneys. Therefore, as other organs fail, so can the skin. In 2014, wounds or wound-related infections affected nearly 15% (8.2 million) of Medicare beneficiaries. In addition, wound care is costly (Nussbaum et al., 2018). Total Medicare annual spending for all wound types was estimated to be $28.1 billion (low-range estimate) to $31.7 billion (midrange estimate) but possibly as high as $96.8 billion for 2014 (Nussbaum et al., 2018). Although Medicare beneficiaries represent only a portion of the total population of the United States, it is quite clear that chronic wounds are a prevalent problem.

It is important for the nurse to observe and document all clients' skin because in some cases, clients may not be aware of any alterations in their skin. For example, some clients may lack the flexibility to fully examine the bottom of their feet and may have decreased sensation due to comorbidities. This means a skin assessment (head to toe) and risk assessment should be completed for every client. Facilities may use a standardized skin risk assessment tool, such as the Braden Scale, which is described in more detail in Chapter 2. Good communication, including for test and screening results, risk of pressure injury, and presence of abnormalities, needs to be maintained among all healthcare providers. In addition, the appropriate documentation must be completed in a timely manner. Fig. 16.7 diagrams an algorithm for assessment and potential care planning.

PRESSURE INJURY

Pressure injuries (also called pressure ulcers/sores, bedsores, and decubitus ulcers) are localized damage to the skin and/or underlying tissue, usually over a bony prominence or related to a medical or other device. The injury occurs as a result of intense and/or prolonged pressure or pressure in combination with friction and shear (NPIAP, 2016). Pressure injuries usually occur over bony prominences in the lower two-thirds of the body, such as the sacrum/coccyx, trochanter, ischial tuberosity, ankle, and heel. Other at-risk areas may include the elbows, ears, scapula, and the back of the head. Medical device–related pressure injuries (MDRIs) are localized injuries to the skin or mucous membrane as a result of pressure from a device, such as an endotracheal tube, feeding tube, or nasal cannula. The ability of the individual's tissue to tolerate pressure and shear may be affected by microclimate, nutrition, perfusion, comorbidities, and the condition of the soft tissue (NPIAP, 2016). Annually, 2.5 million people in the United States will develop a pressure injury, and 60,000 will die of related complications (Sullivan & Schoelles, 2013). However, the implementation of evidence-based prevention and treatment strategies can effectively reduce the rate of development of injuries and/or complications.

Staging or classifying a pressure injury identifies the depth of the wound and the tissues involved. Pressure injuries may be partial (stage I or II) or full thickness (stage III or IV). Table 16.3 defines pressure injuries by stage. The staging system was developed to help standardize the initial assessment of pressure injuries and facilitate communication between healthcare providers. The severity of a pressure injury ranges from reddening of the skin to severe, deep craters that extend down to bone and muscle.

Although locations, risk factors, and care considerations for pressure injuries vary across the lifespan, as shown in Table 16.4, in an acute-care facility, any pressure injury that develops is considered facility acquired. Therefore, it is important for nurses in any setting to document accurately to show that care planning has been appropriate. Client factors, including age, comorbid conditions, inadequate circulation, poor nutritional status, incontinence, and immobility, increase the risk, and pressure injuries may develop quickly. Box 16.3 describes the importance of developing a plan of care, implementing the plan, and documenting the plan.

All pressure injuries may not be preventable. In long-term care facilities an unavoidable pressure ulcer is defined as a pressure ulcer that developed even though the facility had evaluated the resident's clinical condition and pressure injury risk factors. In addition, the facility defined and implemented interventions that were consistent with resident needs, goals, and recognized standards of practice; monitored and evaluated the impact of the interventions; and revised the approaches as appropriate (CMS, 2017; Schmitt et al., 2017). More research is needed in the area of unavoidable pressure injuries. Box 16.4 describes research related to healthcare unit characteristics and pressure injury.

VENOUS ULCERS

Venous leg ulcers affect an estimated 600,000 Americans each year and cost the healthcare system between $1.5 and $3.5 billion (Hankin, Knispel, Lopes, Bronstone, & Maus, 2012). Up to 1% of adults will have a leg ulcer at some time, with the majority being venous in origin (Nelson & Bell-Syer, 2014). This percentage increases with age. Venous ulcers are caused by high pressure in the veins as a result of blockage or weakness of the valves in the veins of the leg. Prevention and treatment of venous ulcers are aimed at reducing the pressure, either by removing/repairing the veins or by applying compression bandages/stockings to reduce the pressure in the veins (Nelson & Bell-Syer, 2014). The majority of venous ulcers heal with compression bandages; however, ulcers frequently recur. To prevent recurrence, clinical guidelines recommend continued compression, usually in the form of hosiery (tights, stockings, socks), after an ulcer heals (Nelson & Bell-Syer, 2014).

SKIN AND WOUND
ASSESSMENT AND CARE PLANNING

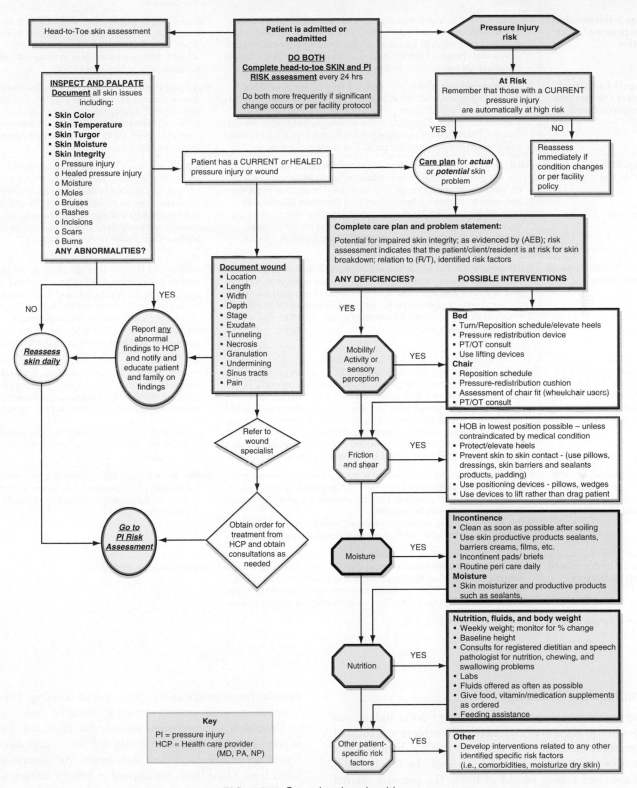

FIG. 16.7 Care-planning algorithm.

TABLE 16.3 Pressure Injury Stages

	Definition	Further Description
Stage I: Nonblanchable erythema of intact skin	Intact skin with a localized area of nonblanchable erythema, which may appear differently in darkly pigmented skin. Presence of blanchable erythema or changes in sensation, temperature, or firmness may precede visual changes. Color changes do not include purple or maroon discoloration; these may indicate deep-tissue pressure injury.	The area may be painful, firm, and soft. May be warmer or cooler compared to adjacent tissue. Stage I may be difficult to detect in individuals with dark skin tones. May indicate "at-risk" persons (a heralding sign of risk).
Stage II: Partial-thickness skin loss with exposed dermis	Partial-thickness loss of skin with exposed dermis. The wound bed is viable, pink or red, and moist, and may also present as an intact or ruptured serum-filled blister. Adipose tissue (fat) and deeper tissues are not visible. Granulation tissue, slough, and eschar are not present. These injuries commonly result from adverse microclimate and shear in the skin over the pelvis and shear in the heel.	This stage should not be used to describe moisture-associated skin damage (MASD), including incontinence-associated dermatitis (IAD), intertriginous dermatitis (ITD), medical adhesive–related skin injury (MARSI), or traumatic wounds (e.g., skin tears, burns, abrasions).
Stage III: Full-thickness skin loss	Full-thickness loss of skin, in which adipose tissue (fat) is visible in the ulcer, and granulation tissue and epibole (rolled wound edges) are often present. Slough and/or eschar may be visible. The depth of tissue damage varies by anatomical location; areas of significant adiposity can develop deep wounds. Undermining and tunneling may occur. Fascia, muscle, tendon, ligament, cartilage, and/or bone are not exposed. If slough or eschar obscures the extent of tissue, loss this is an unstageable pressure injury.	The depth of a stage III pressure injury varies by anatomical location. The bridge of the nose, ear, occiput, and malleolus do not have subcutaneous tissue, and stage III injuries can be shallow. In contrast, areas of significant adiposity can develop extremely deep stage II injuries. Bone/tendon is not visible or directly palpable.
Stage IV: Full-thickness skin and tissue loss	Full-thickness skin and tissue loss with exposed or directly palpable fascia, muscle, tendon, ligament, cartilage, or bone in the ulcer. Slough and/or eschar may be visible. Epibole (rolled edges), undermining, and/or tunneling often occur. Depth varies by anatomical location. If slough or eschar obscures the extent of tissue loss, this is an unstageable pressure injury.	The depth of a stage IV pressure injury varies by anatomical location. The bridge of the nose, occiput, and malleolus do not have subcutaneous tissue, and these ulcers can be shallow. Stage IV ulcers can extend into muscle and/or supporting structures (e.g., fascia, tendon, joint capsule), making osteomyelitis possible. Exposed bone/tendon is visible or directly palpable.
Deep-tissue pressure injury: Persistent nonblanchable deep-red, maroon, or purple discoloration	Intact or nonintact skin with localized area of persistent; nonblanchable; deep-red, maroon, or purple discoloration or epidermal separation revealing a dark wound bed or blood-filled blister. Pain and temperature change often precede skin color changes. Discoloration may appear differently in darkly pigmented skin. This injury results from intense and/or prolonged pressure and shear forces at the bone–muscle interface. The wound may evolve rapidly to reveal the actual extent of tissue injury or may resolve without tissue loss.	If necrotic tissue, subcutaneous tissue, granulation tissue, fascia, muscle, or other underlying structures are visible, this indicates a full-thickness pressure injury (unstageable, stage III, or stage IV). Do not use deep-tissue pressure injury to describe vascular, traumatic, neuropathic, or dermatologic conditions.
Unstageable pressure injury: Obscured full-thickness skin and tissue loss	Full-thickness skin and tissue loss in which the extent of tissue damage within the ulcer cannot be confirmed because it is obscured by slough or eschar. If slough or eschar is removed, a stage III or stage IV pressure injury will be revealed. Stable eschar (i.e., dry, adherent, and intact, without erythema or fluctuance) on an ischemic limb or the heel(s) should not be softened or removed.	Stable (dry, adherent, intact without erythema or fluctuance) eschar on the heels serves as "the body's natural (biological) cover" and should not be removed.
Medical device–related pressure injury	Medical device–related pressure injuries result from the use of devices designed and applied for diagnostic or therapeutic purposes. The resultant pressure injury generally conforms to the pattern or shape of the device. The injury should be staged using the staging system.	This describes an etiology.

Reference: National Pressure Injury Advisory Panel (NPIAP), 2016.

Compression Dressings

Compression dressings are used to treat edema and venous congestion in the lower extremities. To achieve a graduated compression gradient, one needs to apply a bandage at a consistent tension, and the bandage should be able to retain its shape over a long period of time. The pressure exerted on a limb is directly related to the number of layers one applies and to the circumference of the limb and width of the bandage. The more layers, the higher the tension and pressure. The smaller the limb and narrower the bandage, the higher the pressure. Compression dressings are available in short-stretch and long-stretch versions. Others, such as multilayered or total-contact casting, are applied by advanced medical practitioners and require special training. For diabetic foot wounds, contact casting is primarily used.

Short-stretch compression, inelastic bandages, also known as short-stretch bandages, have minimal stretch and can only extend up to 30% to 70% of their length. An example is the Unna boot. Unna boots are disposable inelastic bandages that have zinc or calamine paste components that may decrease pruritus and dry stasis dermatitis lesions and help soothe discomfort. One can apply the Unna boot directly over the wound bed or over another primary wound dressing. Long-stretch compression bandages have high elasticity and are able to stretch up to several times their length. They accommodate the shape of the leg and sustain high pressures during both ambulation and relaxation.

TABLE 16.4 Pressure Injury Across the Lifespan

Age	Location	Risk Factors	Care Considerations
Newborn	Usually found on the back of the head or heel Usually related to medical devices	Skin texture immaturity and endotracheal (ET) intubation	Use appropriate risk assessment tool for age. Provide nutritional assessment and support. Support surface should be age and need appropriate. Reposition the head when sedated and/or ventilated. Elevate the heels.
Pediatric	Around medical devices, back of the head; sites vary as child growth increases	Decreased mobility, moisture, tissue profusion, pyrexia, and low serum albumin	
Adult	Sacrum/coccyx and heels and around medical devices	Clients who have a spinal cord injury, are in critical care/intensive care unit (ICU), have comorbid conditions, are heavily sedated, or have diabetes are at high risk.	Perform risk assessment and associated care planning and head-to-toe skin assessment on admission. Turn and reposition according to guidelines. Provide nutritional assessment and support.
Older adult	Sacrum/coccyx and heels and around medical devices	Same as adult; also, clients who have a hip fracture, peripheral vascular disease, or immobility issues	Same as adult but may also need speech consult for swallowing ability
Palliative	Usually sacrum/coccyx and heels May also include trochanter, head, elbows, and around medical devices	Skin failure at life's end or Kennedy terminal ulcers are common. The skin is the largest organ and reflects what is happening in the body. As the kidneys, heart, lungs, or liver begin to fail, so does the skin.	Education of the client and family on what to expect is critical. Care is based on risk and pain control. Wound care is based on the needs of the client, such as pain, odor, and excessive exudate. The same treatments or dressings may be used as in curative care, but healing is not the goal.

Reference: National Pressure Injury Advisory Panel (NPIAP), 2016.

BOX 16.3 Lessons From Experience

The legal standard maintains that nurses must provide care equivalent to that of a wound nurse in the absence of a wound nurse. This means that all nurses must have basic wound knowledge and "do no harm" to the client. Documentation is the best defense in any legal proceedings. Lawsuits usually take years to go to court, and remediation efforts are tried first. As a lawsuit progresses, the nurse can be subpoenaed for a deposition. A deposition is taking the nurse's statement under oath. However, the nurse may not remember the client, and all the nurse can rely on is what he or she documented. As a wound "expert," this author was an expert witness and asked to review the medical records and say if the facility was at fault for the pressure ulcer. The expert witness does not know the people involved, so all that is available is the medical record. At times, the expert witness will show that the nurse did turn/reposition the client by counting where it was documented, when the client was in physical therapy, and so forth. The better the documentation, the easier an issue is to defend.

Here is an example similar to many cases in which this author was called to be an expert witness:

Mrs. Smith was an 87-year-old female who was admitted to a long-term care residence for physical therapy after she fell at home and fractured her hip. The family brought a lawsuit against the facility after her death, stating that Mrs. Smith was neglected and that the staff at the residence did not provide appropriate care to her. Additionally, the family lawsuit alleged that there was a failure to decide how to treat the wound, whether with curative or palliative care. The lawsuit alleged that because of the negligence of the long-term care residence, the wound developed into a stage IV open wound, became infected with methicillin-resistant *Staphylococcus aureus* (MRSA) and osteomyelitis, and did not heal or show significant improvement from the time it developed until the time Mrs. Smith died almost a year later.

Mrs. Smith was a high-risk client for pressure ulcer development on the Braden Scale. The long-term care residence was therefore required to treat her with high-risk protocols in relation to a potential pressure ulcer. The lack of documented care planning for her needs meant that this was a preventable pressure ulcer by Centers for Medicare and Medicaid standards (CMS, 2017). The long-term care residence also needed to use physical interventions and measures such as appropriate chair cushions and the use of an appropriate specialty bed. Mrs. Smith also had urinary and bowel problems that required the staff to change her briefs frequently to keep her clean and dry.

This author as the expert witness for the plaintiff found the following in a review of the medical record:

- Mrs. Smith's pressure ulcer began to develop in June of 2015.
- Changes of briefs and turning and repositioning were not documented on a regular basis.
- The pressure ulcer continued to develop, but Mrs. Smith was not seen until July 12, when the staff consulted with an authorized healthcare provider.
- On August 2, Mrs. Smith was referred to the wound clinic, and she was seen on August 9.
- Mrs. Smith's open wound became infected with MRSA, and she subsequently developed osteomyelitis

All of the nurses who took care of Mrs. Smith were deposed and may have had to testify if the case had not been settled out of court. Keep in mind that lawsuits such as these may take years to settle or go to trial, and even when the nurses are no longer working at that care facility, they will have to testify and can be included as a defendant in the lawsuit.

In summary, nurses are required to meet standards of care for pressure injury assessment and care, standards set in this case by the Centers for Medicare and Medicaid Services for the long-term care resident (CMS, 2017). Assessment, care, and communication with other members of the healthcare team must be documented in the legal healthcare record.

BOX 16.4 Lessons From the Evidence

Preventing pressure ulcers is a problem for all levels of medical care. As a result, studies have addressed the problem in a variety of ways, including hospital characteristics (e.g., staffing).

This study used data from 789 medical-surgical units in 215 hospitals to examine the effect of unit/client characteristics, nurse workload, nurse expertise, and hospital pressure ulcer preventative clinical processes of care on unit-level hospital-acquired pressure ulcer (HAPU) development. Fewer HAPUs were predicted by a combination of unit/client characteristics (shorter length of stay, fewer at-risk clients, fewer male clients), registered nurse (RN) workload (more hours of care, greater client turnover), RN expertise (more years of experience, fewer contract staff hours), and processes of care (more completed risk assessments). The study concluded that RN workload, nurse expertise, and processes of care (risk assessment/interventions) are significant predictors that may be addressed to reduce HAPU. Client risk factors could not be changed, but other variables, such as staffing, were modifiable and could be changed/improved upon. This study was conducted at facilities using quality benchmarking, which were typically larger academic settings, thus limiting the generalizability of the findings.

Reference: Aydin, Donaldson, & Stotts, 2015.

PREVENTING DIABETIC ULCERS

Diabetes affects over 346 million persons worldwide. A person with diabetes has a 15% to 25% lifetime chance of developing a foot ulcer and a 50% to 70% ulcer recurrence rate over the ensuing 5 years (Ayello, Sibbald, Ostrow, & Smart, 2012). For clients with diabetes, a foot ulcer precedes nontraumatic lower-limb amputation in over 80% of cases (Woo, Botros, Kuhnke, Evans, & Alavi, 2013). Therefore, careful examination of the lower leg and foot should be done as part of routine care at each doctor's visit for anyone with a history of diabetes (Woo et al., 2013). This includes examination of the skin, hair, and nails; notation of presence and severity of calluses and/or edema; assessment of temperature, muscle strength, and pedal pulse; observation for foot deformities; monofilament testing; and assessment of the ankle-brachial index (ABI) (Varnado, 2016).

The monofilament test is a noninvasive and inexpensive method of looking at sensation in the foot and can be done by the nurse at the bedside. A nylon monofilament designed to give way under 10 g of pressure is applied to 4 to 10 sites on the foot to test for sensation (Varnado, 2016). A client who is unable to sense the monofilament at one or more of the test sites is considered at high risk of ulceration because of the loss of protective sensation and should receive education on foot protection and daily foot inspection (Varnado, 2016). Nursing supports the client's goals toward healing, as explored in Box 16.5.

The ABI result is used to predict the severity of peripheral arterial disease (PAD). This test is done by measuring blood pressure at the ankle and in the arm while a person is at rest. It can also be done following exercise because a slight drop in the ABI with exercise, even if the ABI is normal at rest, may indicate PAD. The ABI is also noninvasive and can be done by nurses at the beside. Box 16.6 shows how to interpret the ABI results.

BOX 16.5 Lessons From Experience

Treating a client with a wound involves not only physical care but also emotional care for both the client and family. Education is critical. People are afraid of what will happen and if they will ever heal. For example, several years ago, a slightly disheveled, older gentleman named Sam came to the clinic. He explained that he had a wound on his great toe and that he thought the wound clinic (60 miles away from where he lived) was not treating it correctly and was "dissing" his concerns. I had him come in, sit down, and take off his shoes. I cleaned his toe.

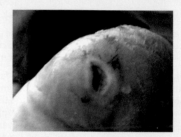

When you look at the toe, it is obvious that he has a diabetic wound that has been present for a while. I questioned him about his medical issue, and he admitted that he hadn't controlled his diabetes very well. He went on to say that sometimes he slept in his car, but right now, he was staying at his mother's and was taking care of her. He said he needed to be able to walk.

I used my cell phone to take a picture of the wound on the bottom of the toe. I showed it to him and explained what I saw and why it had happened. He probably had some osteomyelitis (infection of the bone) at that point, but because of his diabetic neuropathy, he couldn't feel the pain but realized his shoes didn't fit anymore. I talked to him about how his diet and control of his diabetes would help him get better. We discussed palliative versus curative care, and he said he just wanted to be able to walk around and had no interest in being off his feet for healing or having more tests. I put a dressing on his toe and showed him how to change it every other day. I also called my friend at a satellite clinic from his large one and asked her to see him. I explained the situation to her, and we set an appointment. She had the wound staff from the first clinic contact me so that I could explain his concerns.

Sam called several times and made more of an effort to take care of himself. However, the long-term prognosis for his foot was a nonhealing wound and possibly toe amputation. Although I would have preferred aggressive treatment and testing, I supported Sam's decision and helped him have what he considered quality of life.

BOX 16.6 Interpreting Ankle-Brachial Index (ABI) Results

A diagnosis of diabetes mellitus may influence the reliability of the results.

The American Heart Association ABI interpretation levels are as follows:

>1.3:	Noncompressible arteries
1.00 to 1.29:	Normal
0.91 to 0.99:	Borderline (equivocal)
0.41 to 0.90:	Mild to moderate peripheral arterial disease (PAD)
00.00 to 0.40:	Severe PAD

ABI values may be falsely elevated in clients with diabetes.

APPLICATION OF THE NURSING PROCESS

Examples of Related ICNP Nursing Diagnoses, Expected Client Outcomes, and Nursing Interventions:

Nursing Diagnosis: Risk for diabetic foot ulcer

Supporting Data: History of diabetes and diabetic neuropathy

Expected Client Outcomes: The client will participate in daily foot checks, will wear shoes to protect skin integrity, and will describe preventive measures.

Nursing Intervention Example: Perform a foot examination and monofilament testing.

Reference: International Classification for Nursing Practice. (n.d.). *eHealth & ICNP*. Retrieved from https://www.icn.ch/what-we-do/projects/ehealth-icnp.

CRITICAL CONCEPTS
Preventing and Treating Pressure Injury and Venous and Diabetic Ulcers

Accuracy (ACC)

Preventing and treating pressure injuries and ulcers are subject to the following variables:
- assessment of client, including skin integrity, peripheral sensation, and ABI
- assessment of the wound (TIME)
- selection of compression dressing material
- direction and pattern of compression dressing application
- results of monofilament testing
- understanding of procedure and teaching to client and family.

Client-Centered Care (CCC)

When preventing and treating pressure injuries and ulcers, respect for the client is demonstrated by:
- obtaining verbal consent and promoting autonomy
- providing privacy and ensuring comfort
- answering questions before, during, and after providing care
- honoring cultural preferences
- arranging for an interpreter, if needed
- advocating for the client and family.

Infection Control (INF)

When preventing and treating pressure injuries and ulcers, healthcare-associated and client infections are prevented by:
- containment of microorganisms
- preventing and reducing the transfer of microorganisms
- preventing an environment conducive to microbial growth.

Safety (SAF)

When preventing and treating pressure injuries and ulcers, safety measures prevent harm to the client and provide a safe care environment.

Communication (COM)

- Communication exchanges information (oral, written, nonverbal, or electronic) between two or more people.
- Collaboration with the client, client's family, and other health care providers is essential to prevent and treat pressure injuries and ulcers.
- Documentation records information in a permanent legal record.

Health Maintenance (HLTH)

When preventing and treating pressure injuries and ulcers, nursing is dedicated to the promotion of health and self-care abilities, including:
- protecting the client's skin integrity
- promoting self-care behaviors
- teaching the client and family about risk factors and prevention.

Evaluation (EVAL)

When preventing and treating pressure injuries and ulcers, evaluation of outcomes enables the nurse to determine the efficacy of the care provided.

■ SKILL 16.8 Applying Compression Dressings or Unna Boot

EQUIPMENT

Ace wraps or compression/Unna boot kit
Normal saline/wound cleanser
4 × 4 gauze
Clean gloves
Disposable tape measure

BEGINNING THE SKILL

1. **SAF** Review the authorized healthcare provider's order and facility policy. *Verifying the plan of care prevents injury to the client.*

2. **INF** Perform hand hygiene.
3. **CCC** Introduce yourself to the client and family and explain the procedure.
4. **SAF** Identify the client using two identifiers.
5. **CCC** Provide privacy. Close the door and pull the curtain.

PROCEDURE

6. **ACC** Assess the following:
   - client's level of orientation and ability to follow instructions

- client's pain level using a consistent facility-approved pain tool.

7. **SAF** Set up ergonomically safe space. Raise the bed to a comfortable working height and raise the opposite side rail. *Setting up an ergonomically safe space prevents injury to the nurse and client.*

8. **SAF** Set up a workspace according to your hand dominance and which leg you are wrapping. Set up the work area and trash receptacle.

9. **INF** Perform hand hygiene and apply clean gloves. *This helps prevent the introduction of bacteria into the wound.* (Note: If additional supplies are needed, you must remove your gloves and wash your hands to exit the room. When you return to the room, perform hand hygiene and reapply gloves.)

10. **ACC** Carefully remove old compression dressing and any dressing in the client's leg. Discard if heavily soiled. (Note: Some Ace bandages may be washed and reused by the same client when dry.) **WARNING:** An authorized healthcare provider should remove any contact cast with a specially designed saw.

11. **ACC** Assess any exudate present on the dressing or Ace bandage.

12. **EVAL** Evaluate the skin under the compression wrap or Unna boot. Note redness or maceration.

13. **HLTH** Cleanse leg and foot tissue with wound cleanser or normal saline and gently dry skin with 4 × 4 gauze. As you provide care, teach the client about risk factors and prevention strategies.

Ace Wrap or Elastic Bandage Application

14. **ACC** Start the wrap on the top of the foot above the toes and circle the foot twice. Then circle around the ankle and heel in an X pattern. (Note: The order may specify that you need to leave the toes and heel open.)

15. **ACC** Wrap in a spiral pattern up the leg, overlapping each turn 50% and continuing up the leg to about 2.5 cm (1 inch) below the knee. (Note: If the order is thigh height, use an X pattern around the knee and continue up to the mid-thigh.)

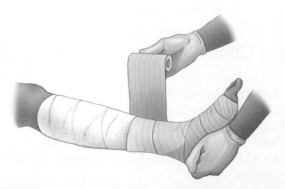

STEP 15 Apply the bandage in a spiral pattern with a 50% overlap.

16. **ACC** If two or more rolls are used, overlap the beginning of the next roll about 5 cm (2 inches) of the previous one, wrap around once to secure, and continue up the leg.

17. **SAF** Secure the end with the metal clips covered with tape or with tape alone. *The tape will prevent the clamps from coming off or the client being cut by the clamp.*

18. **SAF** Check the toes frequently for discoloration, which may indicate that the wrap is too tight, and tell the client to immediately report any change in the pain intensity in the extremity.

Unna Boot or Two- or Three-Layer Compression Bandages

19. **ACC** Position the foot at a right angle to the leg.

20. **ACC** Wrap the medicated gauze or padding firmly but not tightly around the client's foot, being sure to cover the heel. Continue up the leg in a spiral pattern, overlapping each turn 50% and continuing up the leg to about 2.5 cm (1 inch) below the knee.

21. **SAF** Smooth out wrinkles to prevent areas of pressure under the compression wrap.

22. **ACC** Apply an Ace bandage or other nonelastic cover as the final layer. (Note: A Coban or other 10-cm (4-inch) cohesive-type wrap is most commonly used.)

23. **INF** Properly dispose of used supplies and soiled dressings in a biohazard bag and remove from room according to facility policy. Remove gloves and perform hand hygiene.

FINISHING THE SKILL

24. **CCC** Ensure client comfort. Reposition client and bedding.

25. **SAF** Ensure client safety. Ensure that the bed is in the lowest position. Ensure that the client can identify and reach the nurse call system. *These safety measures reduce the risk of falls.*

26. **INF** Perform hand hygiene.

27. **EVAL** Evaluate outcomes, including reassessing the client's pain level.

28. **COM** Document procedure, assessment of lower extremity, exudate amount and characteristics, client's pain before and after the procedure, dressing or ointment used, care given, client education provided, how the client tolerated the procedure, and outcomes in the legal healthcare record.

29. **COM** Notify the authorized healthcare provider if significant changes in the wound, pain, or exudate are noted.

■ SKILL 16.9 Foot Examination and Monofilament Testing

EQUIPMENT

Clean gloves
Hand mirror
Monofilament

BEGINNING THE SKILL

1. **SAF** Review the authorized healthcare provider's order and facility policy. *Verifying the plan of care prevents injury to the client*
2. **SAF** Identify the client using two identifiers.
3. **CCC** Introduce yourself to the client and family and explain the procedure.
4. **CCC** Provide privacy. Close the door and pull the curtain.

PROCEDURE

5. **ACC** Review the following:
   - client's level of orientation and ability to follow instructions
   - client's pain level using a consistent facility-approved pain tool.
6. **SAF** Set up an ergonomically safe space. Raise the bed to a comfortable working height and raise the opposite side rail. The client may be supine or sitting for the foot exam. *Setting up an ergonomically safe space prevents injury to the nurse and client.*
7. **SAF** Set up a workspace according to your hand dominance. If appropriate, set up the work area and trash receptacle.
8. **INF** Perform hand hygiene. Apply clean gloves. (Note: If additional supplies are needed, you must remove your gloves and wash your hands to exit the room. When you return to the room, perform hand hygiene and reapply gloves.)
9. **HLTH** As you do these examinations, teach the client to report any worsening symptoms, including pain, and remind the client never to walk barefooted. Teach the client how to check the feet at home. (Note: A hand mirror on the bathroom floor allows for easy visualization of each foot.)
10. **ACC** Carefully remove any dressing and inspect the client's feet for broken skin, blisters, swelling, or redness. Be sure to look between the toes. *This means taking any stockings or socks off.*
11. **ACC** Check pedal pulses on both feet. Mark the pulse with a pen. *Marking the spot where you found the pulse with a pen will be helpful when measuring the ABI.*

Perform Monofilament Testing (Semmes–Weinstein Test)

12. **ACC** Touch the monofilament wire to the client's skin on the arm or hand to demonstrate what the touch feels like and instruct the client to respond "Yes" each time he or she feels the pressure of the monofilament on the foot during the exam. Have the client close his or her eyes and keep the toes pointing straight up during the exam.
13. **ACC** Hold the monofilament perpendicular to the client's foot. Press it against the foot, increasing the pressure until the monofilament bends into a C shape. Hold the

monofilament in place for about 1 second. (Note: The client should sense the monofilament by the time it bows.)

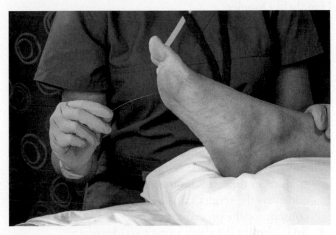

STEP 13 Press the monofilament against the client's foot.

14. **ACC** Locations for testing: On both feet, use the first, third, and fifth metatarsal heads and plantar surface of the distal hallux and third toe (see diagram). Avoid callused areas. Record response on foot screening form with "+" for yes and "−" for no.

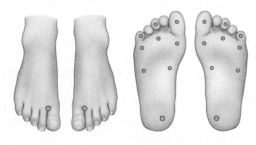

STEP 14 Locations for monofilament testing.

15. **INF** Properly dispose of used supplies and soiled dressings according to facility policy.

FINISHING THE SKILL

16. **INF** Remove gloves and perform hand hygiene.
17. **CCC** Ensure client comfort. Reposition client and bedding.
18. **SAF** Ensure client safety. Ensure that the bed is in the lowest position. Ensure the client can identify and reach the nurse call system. *These safety measures reduce the risk of falls.*
19. **EVAL** Evaluate outcomes, including reassessing the client's pain level, how the client tolerated the procedure, and the client's understanding of the procedure.
20. **CCC** Answer any client questions.
21. **COM** Document the assessment of foot, monofilament results by foot (right or left), any care given, education provided, and how the client tolerated the procedure in the legal healthcare record.
22. **COM** Notify authorized healthcare provider if significant changes in the foot assessment are noted.

■ SKILL 16.10 Measuring the Ankle-Brachial Index (ABI)

EQUIPMENT

Blood pressure (BP) cuffs in various sizes
Handheld Doppler
Transducer gel
Clean gloves, if there is a risk of exposure to body fluids

BEGINNING THE SKILL

1. **SAF** Review the authorized healthcare provider's order and facility policy. *Verifying the plan of care prevents injury to the client.*
2. **INF** Perform hand hygiene.
3. **CCC** Introduce yourself to the client and family and explain the procedure. (Note: Be sure the client has not smoked in the last 2 hours because this will increase BP and skew the results.) Ensure that the client gives verbal consent for the procedure.
4. **SAF** Identify the client using two identifiers.
5. **CCC** Provide privacy. Close the door and pull the curtain.

PROCEDURE

6. **ACC** Review the following:
   - client's level of orientation and ability to follow instructions
   - client's pain level using a consistent facility-approved pain tool.
7. **SAF** Set up an ergonomically safe space. Raise the bed to a comfortable working height and raise the opposite side rail. *Setting up an ergonomically safe space prevents injury to the nurse and client.*
8. **ACC** Have the client rest supine for at least 5 minutes. Remove shoes, socks, and any long-sleeve garments. Provide a blanket if needed.
9. **INF** Perform hand hygiene and apply gloves if there is a risk of exposure to body fluids.
10. **ACC** Select the correct-size BP cuff for the arm and ankle and place both. The bladder within the cuff should be wide enough to encircle 80% of the upper arm or ankle and long enough to be fastened securely. The width of the cuff should be 40% of the extremity circumference.
11. **ACC** Measure the BP in the right arm. (Note: You will complete one side at a time.)
12. **ACC** Apply ultrasound gel to the area you located as the pedal pulse. Next, take the BP in the right ankle using the handheld Doppler angled about 60 degrees toward the client's head. (Note: Determine ahead of time if the posterior tibial pulse or the dorsalis pedis pulse is best.)

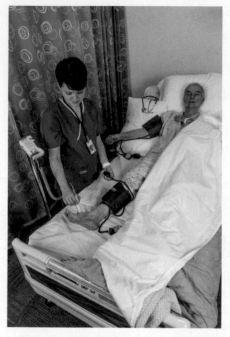

STEPS 11 AND 12 Measure the BP in the right arm. Next, take the BP in the right ankle using a handheld Doppler.

13. **ACC** Calculate the ABI as ankle pressure divided by arm pressure.
14. **ACC** Perform BP measurements in the left arm and ankle.

FINISHING THE SKILL

15. **SAF** Reposition client and bedding. If the bed was raised, return the bed to the lowest position and lower the side rail. *These safety measures reduce the risk of falls.*
16. **INF** Remove gloves, if used, and perform hand hygiene.
17. **EVAL** Evaluate outcomes, including how the client tolerated the procedure and client's understanding of the procedure.
18. **CCC** Answer any client questions.
19. **SAF** Ensure client safety and comfort, and ensure the client can identify and reach the nurse call system, if applicable. *These safety measures reduce the risk of falls.*
18. **COM** Document ABI results and individual BP readings, how the client tolerated the procedure, and pain or other observations in the legal healthcare record. (Note: How to interpret the results is discussed in Box 16.6.)
20. **COM** Notify the authorized healthcare provider if significant findings are noted.

■ CASE STUDY

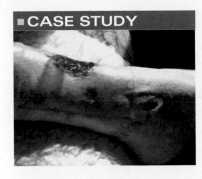

Mr. Adam Beck is a thin, frail, 75-year-old male who lives in his own home with his wife, Bernice, and dog, Sammy. He is just starting home health services for physical therapy. As a part of Mr. Beck's intake, you begin his physical assessment.

Adam has chronic obstructive pulmonary disease (COPD) and had a coronary artery bypass graft (CABG) surgery about 8 years ago. He also had a left hip replacement 2 years ago and has had type 2 diabetes mellitus (DM) for 47 years. In the past 8 years, his DM has not been well controlled. His HgA1c was 10.8 at his emergency room (ER) visit and subsequent authorized healthcare provider visit last week after a fall. When you ask him about his medication, he says he always takes it, but Bernice tells you he has become forgetful and has not been taking his medication or checking his blood glucose levels daily. When questioned further, he admits he is tired of doing the finger-pricks and says, "Why should an old guy like me care anyway!"

Adam tells you he is always tired and prefers to stay in bed. He is unsteady on his feet and fell last week on the way to the bathroom. He went to the ER but had no broken bones, just a bruise on his left leg where he hit the chair edge. Mr. Beck eats small meals. He and his wife both receive Meals on Wheels daily. However, besides toast in the morning, that is all they have during the day.

Case Study Questions

You work for a home health agency, and on your first assessment of Mr. Beck, you find that this *(photo)* is what his leg looks like. Inspect his wound, and then answer the following questions:

1. What should you assess in his home to make it safer?
2. How many wounds do you see on his leg?
3. Why are these most likely vascular wounds?
4. What additional medical tests should he have?
5. Name two ways to treat this wound.
6. **Application of QSEN Competencies:** One of the Quality and Safety Education for Nurses (QSEN) skill competencies for Patient-Centered Care (which we call client-centered care) is to "Elicit expectations of patient and family for relief of pain, discomfort, or suffering" (Cronenwett et al., 2007). How does Mr. Beck's expectation of pain, discomfort, or suffering impact his treatment decisions? An attitude competency is to "Recognize personally held values and beliefs about the management of pain or suffering." How do your expectations of an older man's pain and suffering compare to what Mr. Beck is experiencing?
7. What outcomes do you expect and why?
8. What are Mr. Beck's additional care needs and potential consultations?

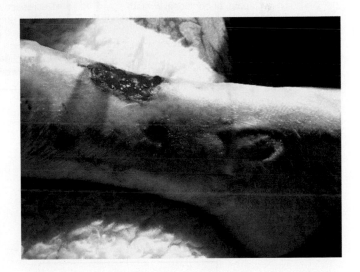

■CONCEPT MAP

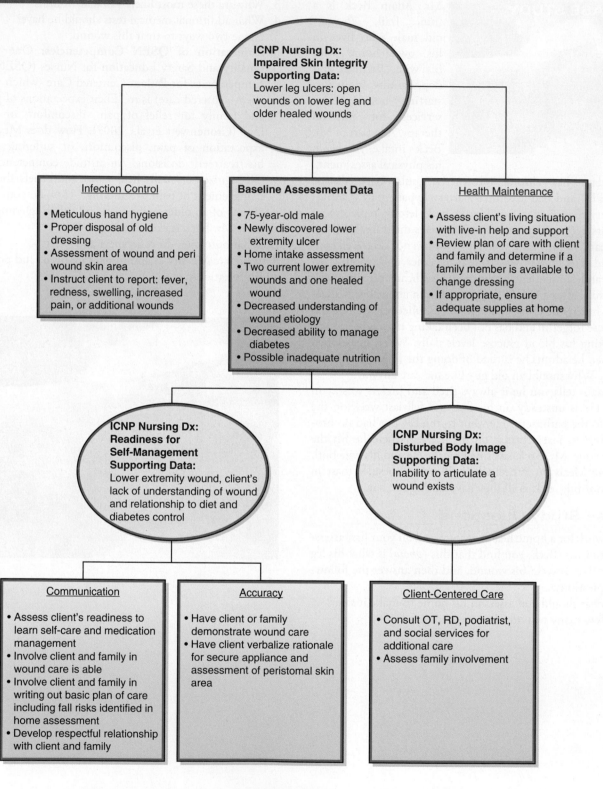

ICNP Nursing Dx: Impaired Skin Integrity Supporting Data: Lower leg ulcers: open wounds on lower leg and older healed wounds

Infection Control
- Meticulous hand hygiene
- Proper disposal of old dressing
- Assessment of wound and peri wound skin area
- Instruct client to report: fever, redness, swelling, increased pain, or additional wounds

Baseline Assessment Data
- 75-year-old male
- Newly discovered lower extremity ulcer
- Home intake assessment
- Two current lower extremity wounds and one healed wound
- Decreased understanding of wound etiology
- Decreased ability to manage diabetes
- Possible inadequate nutrition

Health Maintenance
- Assess client's living situation with live-in help and support
- Review plan of care with client and family and determine if a family member is available to change dressing
- If appropriate, ensure adequate supplies at home

ICNP Nursing Dx: Readiness for Self-Management Supporting Data: Lower extremity wound, client's lack of understanding of wound and relationship to diet and diabetes control

ICNP Nursing Dx: Disturbed Body Image Supporting Data: Inability to articulate a wound exists

Communication
- Assess client's readiness to learn self-care and medication management
- Involve client and family in wound care is able
- Involve client and family in writing out basic plan of care including fall risks identified in home assessment
- Develop respectful relationship with client and family

Accuracy
- Have client or family demonstrate wound care
- Have client verbalize rationale for secure appliance and assessment of peristomal skin area

Client-Centered Care
- Consult OT, RD, podiatrist, and social services for additional care
- Assess family involvement

References

Agency for Healthcare Research and Quality (AHRQ). (2011). Are we ready for this change? In *Preventing pressure ulcers in hospitals: A toolkit for improving quality of care*. Retrieved from https://www.ahrq.gov/professionals/systems/hospital/pressureulcertoolkit/putool1.html.

Avdin, C., Donaldson, N., & Stotts, N. A. (2015). Modeling hospital-acquired pressure ulcer prevalence on medical-surgical units: Nurse workload, expertise, and clinical processes of care. *Health Services Research, 50*(2), 351–373.

Ayello, E. A., Sibbald, R., Ostrow, B., & Smart, H. (2012). Teaching healthcare professionals in resource challenged countries to construct monofilaments for the purpose of diabetic foot screening. *World Council of Enterostomal Therapists Journal, 32*(4), 14.

Ayello, E. A., Zulkowski, K., Capezuti, E., Jicman, W.H., & Sibbald, R.G. (2017). Educating nurses in the United States about pressure injuries.. *Advances in Skin & Wound Care: The Journal for Prevention and Healing, 30*(2), 8394.

Baranoski, S., & Ayello, E. (2015). *Wound care essentials practice principles* (4th ed.). Philadelphia, PA: Springhouse.

Beheshti, A., Shafigh, Y., Parsa, H., & Zangivand, A. (2014). Comparison of high-frequency and MIST ultrasound therapy for the healing of venous leg ulcers. *Advances in Clinical and Experimental Medicine, 23*(6), 969–975.

Boyer, D. (2013). Cultural considerations in advanced wound care. *Advanced Skin Wound Care, 26*(3), 110–111.

Brindle, C. T., & Creehan, S. (2016). Management of surgical wounds. In D. B. Doughty, & L. L. McNichol (Eds.), *Wound, Ostomy and Continence Nurses Society core curriculum: Wound management* (pp. 649–689). Philadelphia, PA: Wolters Kluwer.

Carruthers, K. H., Eisemann, B. S., Lamp, S., & Kocak, E. (2013). Optimizing the closed suction surgical drainage system. *Plastic Surgical Nursing, 33*(1), 38–42.

Centers for Medicare & Medicaid Services. (2017). *Long-term care facility resident assessment instrument 3.0 user's manual version 1.15*. Retrieved from https://downloads.cms.gov/files/mds-30-rai-manual-v115-october-2017.pdf.

Claro, T., Daniels, S., & Humphreys, H. (2014). Detecting *Clostridium difficile* spores from inanimate surfaces of the hospital environment: Which method is best? *Journal of Clinical Microbiology, 52*(9), 3426–3428.

Cronenwett, L., Sherwood, G., Barnsteiner, J., Disch, J., Johnson, J., Mitchell, P., ... Warren, J. (2007). Quality and safety education for nurses. *Nursing Outlook, 55*(3), 122–131. Retrieved from https://qsen.org/competencies/pre-licensure-ksas/.

Fife, C. E., & Carter, M. J. (2012). Wound care outcomes and associated cost among patients treated in US outpatient wound centers: Data from the US wound registry. *Wounds: A Compendium of Clinical Research and Practice, 24*(1), 10–17.

Frank, D. N., Wysocki, A., Specht-Glick, D. D., Rooney, A., Feldman, R. A., St Amand, A. L., & Trent, J. D. (2009). Microbial diversity in chronic open wounds. *Wound Repair and Regeneration, 17*(2), 163–172.

Gehemmo, J., Louvel, A., Nouvellon, M., Caillard, J. F., & Pestel-Caron, M. (2009). Aerial dispersal of methicillin-resistant *Staphylococcus aureus* in hospital rooms by infected or colonized patients. *Journal of Hospital Infection, 71*(3), 256–262.

Grice, E. A., & Segre, J. A. (2011). The skin microbiome. *Nature Reviews Microbiology, 9*(4), 244–253.

Hankin, C. S., Knispel, J., Lopes, M., Bronstone, A., & Maus, E. (2012). Clinical and cost efficacy of advanced wound care matrices for venous ulcers. *Journal of Managed Care Pharmacy, 18*(5), 375–384.

International Classification for Nursing Practice (n.d.). *eHealth & ICNP*. Retrieved from https://www.icn.ch/what-we-do/projects/ehealth-icnp.

James, G. A., Swogger, E., Wolcott, R., Pulcini, E., Secor, P., Sestrich, J., et al., (2008). Biofilms in chronic wounds. *Wound Repair and Regeneration, 16*(1), 37–44.

Kasbekar, A. V., Davies, F., Upile, N., Ho, M. W., & Roland, N. J. (2016). The management of vacuum neck drains in head and neck surgery and the comparison of two different practice protocols for drain removal. *Annals of the Royal College of Surgeons of England, 98*(1), 53–55.

Khanh-Dao Le, L. (2017). *Vacuum drain (surgical): Removal*. [Evidence summary]. Retrieved from The Joanna Briggs Institute EBP Database, JBI@Ovid. JBI551.

National Pressure Injury Advisory Panel (NPIAP). (2016). *Pressure injury stages*. Retrieved from https://npiap.com/page/Pressure InjuryStages.

National Pressure Ulcer Advisory Panel (NPUAP). (2014). European Pressure Ulcer Advisory Panel (EPUAP), and Pan Pacific Pressure Injury Alliance (PPPIA). In E. Haesler (Ed.), *Prevention and treatment of pressure ulcers: Clinical practice guideline*. Osborne Park, Western Australia: Cambridge Media.

Nelson, E. A., & Bell-Syer, S. E. (2014). *Compression for preventing recurrence of venous ulcers*. Cochrane Database of Systematic Reviews. Retrieved from https://doi.org/10.1002/14651858.CD002303.pub3.

Nussbaum, S. R., Carter, M. J., Fife, C. E., DaVanzo, J., Haught, R., Nusgart, M., & Cartwright, D. (2018). An economic evaluation of the impact, cost, and Medicare policy implications of chronic nonhealing wounds. *Value in Health, 21*(1), 27–32.

Piedrahita, C. T., Cadnum, J. L., Jencson, A. L., Shaikh, A. A., Ghannoum, M. A., & Donskey, C. J. (2017). Environmental surfaces in healthcare facilities are a potential source for transmission of *Candida auris* and other *Candida* species. *Infection Control & Hospital Epidemiology, 38*(9), 1107–1109.

Pieper, B., & Zulkowski, K. (2014). The Pieper-Zulkowski pressure ulcer knowledge test. *Advances in Skin and Wound Care, 27*(9), 413–419.

Power, G., Moore, Z., & O'Connor, T. (2017). Measurement of pH, exudate composition and temperature in wound healing: a systematic review. *Journal of Wound Care, 26*(7), 381–397.

Rajpaul, K. (2015). Biofilm in wound care. *British Journal of Community Nursing, 20*(Suppl. 3), S6–S11.

Russo, C., Steiner, C., & Spector, W. (2008). *Hospitalizations related to pressure ulcers among adults 18 years and older, 2006*. HCUP Healthcare Cost and Utilization Project of the Agency for Healthcare Research and Quality. Retrieved from http://www.hcup-us.ahrq.gov/reports/statbriefs/sb64.pdf.

Schmitt, S., Andries, M. K., Ashmore, P. M., Brunette, G., Judge, K., & Bonham, P. A. (2017). WOCN Society position paper: Avoidable versus unavoidable pressure ulcers/injuries. *Journal of Wound, Ostomy and Continence Nursing, 44*(5), 458–468.

Sergent, A. P., Slekovec, C., Pauchot, J., Jeunet, L., Bertrand, X., Hocquet, D., et al., (2012). Bacterial contamination of the hospital environment during wound dressing change. *Orthopaedics & Traumatology: Surgery & Research, 98*(4), 441–445.

Sullivan, N., & Schoelles, K. M. (2013). Preventing in-facility pressure ulcers as a patient safety strategy. *Annals of Internal Medicine, 158*(5, Pt 2), 410–416.

Varnado, M. (2016). Lower extremity neuropathic disease. In D. B. Doughty, & L. L. McNichol (Eds.), *Wound, Ostomy and Continence Nurses Society core curriculum: Wound management* (pp. 475–507). Philadelphia, PA: Wolters Kluwer.

Woo, K. Y., Botros, M., Kuhnke, J., Evans, R., & Alavi, A. (2013). Best practices for the management of foot ulcers in people with Diabetes. *Advances in Skin and Wound Care, 26*(11), 512–524.

Zulkowski, K. (2013). Skin bacteria: Implications for wound care. *Advances in Skin and Wound Care, 26*(5), 231–236..

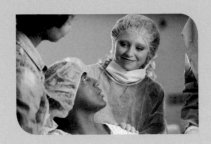

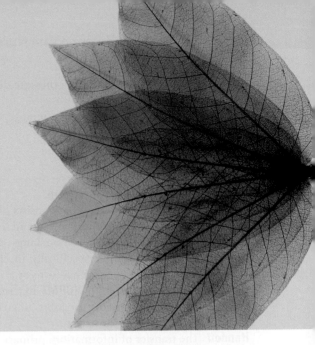

CHAPTER 17

Perioperative Care

"Medicine is the surgery of functions, as surgery proper is that of limbs and organs. Surgery removes the bullet out of the limb, which is an obstruction to cure, but nature heals the wound. What nursing has to do is to put the patient in the best condition for nature to act upon him." | **Florence Nightingale, 1860**

LEARNING OBJECTIVES

By the end of this chapter, the reader will be able to:

1   Identify the three phases of perioperative nursing: preoperative, intraoperative, and postoperative.
2   Discuss the factors that increase surgical risks.
3   Assist in preparing a client for surgery: admission history, assessment, teaching, consent forms, and safety.
4   Provide a client with postoperative instructions for prevention of complications: deep breathing, coughing, positioning, and prevention of deep vein thrombosis.
5   Describe client safety issues during the intraoperative phase, including surgical site verification, positioning,

latex sensitivity, and prevention of surgical site infection.
6   Describe the types of anesthesia and their implications for perioperative nursing care.
7   Discuss complications associated with surgery and anesthesia.
8   Determine key assessments for the client returning from surgery: level of consciousness (LOC), airway, breath sounds, circulation (heart rate and rhythm, blood pressure), urine output, surgical site, and pressure point areas.

703

9 Demonstrate application of a pressure dressing to control bleeding.

10 Demonstrate how to apply and remove antiembolic stockings.

11 Demonstrate the procedure for the use of a sequential compression device.

12 Demonstrate the procedure for the use of a continuous passive motion device.

TERMINOLOGY

Analgesia Loss of ability to feel pain.

Anesthesia A temporary state that consists of unconsciousness, lack of pain, muscle relaxation, and loss of memory.

Antiembolism stockings Elastic stockings worn to prevent emboli or thrombi, specifically in clients who are restricted to bedrest or have had surgery.

Continuous passive motion (CPM) External motorized device to move and stretch the joints of an extremity passively to prevent scar formation.

Handoff The transfer of information, primary responsibility, and authority from one or more nurses to other nurses.

Paralytic ileus Temporary paralysis of the intestine that causes painful abdominal distention, nausea and vomiting, and symptoms of gastrointestinal obstruction.

Sequential compression device (SCD) External motorized device used to intermittently inflate plastic sleeves on the lower extremities to prevent stasis, reducing the risk of thrombi.

Thrombosis The formation of a blood clot inside a blood vessel that obstructs the flow of blood.

Thrombus A clot that forms as a healthy response to a vessel injury.

Venous thromboembolism (VTE) A blood clot that breaks loose and moves to the lungs (pulmonary embolism [PE]) or to the deep veins of the legs (deep vein thrombosis [DVT]).

ACRONYMS

ADLs Activities of daily living
CMP Complete metabolic panel
CPM Continuous passive motion
CTZ Chemoreceptor trigger zone
INR International normalized ratio
IPH Inadvertent postoperative hypothermia
MH Malignant hyperthermia
MHR Maximum heart rate
OR Operating room
OSA Obstructive sleep apnea
PACU Post-anesthesia care unit
PONV Postoperative nausea and vomiting
SCD Sequential compression device
VTE Venous thromboembolism

The perioperative client will transition through three phases: preoperative, intraoperative, and postoperative. The preoperative phase begins when the need or desire for surgery is first identified and ends when the client enters the operating room. The preoperative skills focus on client education. The intraoperative phase includes the surgical procedure and ends with client transfer to the recovery room. The postoperative phase includes care after surgery through the period after discharge home and resolution of the client's postoperative needs. The length of each perioperative phase varies according to the client's condition, type of surgery, and teaching needs. In each phase, nursing care is critical to optimal client outcomes.

In Section 3: Managing Postoperative Care, Skill 17.3, Admitting a Postoperative Client, requires students to incorporate many of the skills from earlier chapters. Although Skills 17.4 to 17.7 are new, student laboratory practice or simulation of a postoperative client is an excellent means to integrate multiple previously learned skills and concepts into complex nursing care.

SECTION 1   Providing Preoperative Education and Care

The focus of nursing care during the preoperative phase is to identify present health concerns, provide information for intraoperative and postoperative needs, and provide client teaching. The client must understand how to prepare for surgery, what to expect during and after the procedure, and the rationale for activities such as progressive mobility that promote healing.

FACTORS AFFECTING SURGICAL RISKS

Assess the client for the following factors, which increase the risk of poor postoperative outcomes:

- Age. The very young and very old are at an increased surgical risk because of an inability to regulate temperature and diminished functionality of the cardiovascular, immune, and metabolic systems (Table 17.1). Older adults may also have preexisting conditions that increase surgical risk.

- Diet. A poor diet, especially low protein status and vitamin and mineral deficiencies, can impair healing after surgery.
- Blood glucose level. A high blood glucose level can slow the healing process.
- Fluid intake. Adequate hydration promotes circulation, which facilitates healing. Fluid also promotes elimination, thins pulmonary secretions, and reduces the risk for thrombosis.
- Medications. Many medications can cause an increased risk during the intraoperative and postoperative phases.
- Obesity. Increased weight impairs lung expansion and thereby increases the risk for atelectasis or pneumonia. In addition, obese clients often experience obstructive sleep apnea (OSA), cardiovascular disease, and type 2 diabetes mellitus. These factors increase the risk for surgical complications and may slow recovery.
- Physical activity. Increased physical activity, such as early ambulation and progressive mobility, prevents the complications of pneumonia, constipation, and thrombosis.
- Preexisting conditions. Cardiovascular disease decreases effective tissue perfusion. Chronic respiratory disease and smoking may prevent full lung expansion and adequate oxygenation of tissues. Coagulation disorders increase the risk of clot formation and bleeding. Diabetes increases the risk of infection and delays wound healing. Liver disease increases bleeding risks and limits detoxification and metabolism, thereby increasing the risk for drug toxicities. Renal disease may reduce the body's ability to regulate fluid balance, blood pressure, and excretion of toxins and medications.
- Substance use. Tobacco use results in impaired circulation and delayed healing. Alcohol and drug use can result in liver damage and cause an increased risk for bleeding and limit detoxification and metabolism, thus increasing the risk for drug toxicities.
- Family history. A family history of muscular dystrophies, clotting abnormalities, or malignant hyperthermia (discussed shortly) increases the client's risk for complications related to the surgery itself and to anesthesia.

NURSING HISTORY AND PHYSICAL EXAMINATION

The preoperative nursing history is an important tool to determine the client's physiologic, cognitive, and psychological preparation for surgery. Information from the client, family members, and previous medical records can help identify health concerns or needs that should be communicated to the healthcare team. The nursing history and physical assessment should include past and current health problems; mental status; physical status; current medications; history of drug, alcohol, and tobacco use; allergies; current vital signs; respiratory and cardiac status; and height and weight. Refer to Table 17.2 for a more extensive list and rationales for obtaining this information before surgery.

TABLE 17.1 Changes With Age That Increase Risk for Surgical Complications

System Change	Nursing Interventions
Cardiovascular: increased risk for decreased cardiac output, altered perfusion, vital sign fluctuations, and clot formation due to: • structural changes in myocardium and valves • decreased sympathetic and parasympathetic innervation to heart • increased calcium and cholesterol deposits, leading to thickened and more rigid vessels	Assess for vital sign changes, presence of dysrhythmias, increased restlessness, or change in level of consciousness. Maintain fluid and electrolyte balance. Encourage ambulation, frequent turning, range-of-motion (ROM) exercises, and use of elastic stockings and intermittent compression devices (ICDs). Provide anticoagulant therapy with education related to mechanism of action, side effects, and interactions.
Respiratory: increased risk for impaired gas exchange and tissue oxygenation due to: • stiffened lung tissue, increased residual capacity, decreased diaphragmatic expansion, and decreased respiratory muscle strength • decreased red blood cells and hemoglobin	Assess respiratory rate and depth, SpO_2. Maintain elevated head of bed (30 degrees or more). Encourage to cough, deep breathe, and use incentive spirometer. Administer packed red blood cells (RBCs) and iron supplements as necessary. Monitor hemoglobin (Hgb), hematocrit (Hct), and RBC levels.
Gastrointestinal: increased risk for gastroesophageal reflux, indigestion, and aspiration due to delayed gastric emptying and decreased sphincter tone	Maintain elevated head of bed (30 degrees or more). Offer small, frequent feedings in lieu of large meals.
Renal: increased risk for fluid and electrolyte imbalances, heart failure, renal failure, urinary tract infections, incontinence, drug toxicity, and sepsis due to: • decreased renal blood flow • decreased glomerular filtration rate • decreased bladder tone and capacity	Determine baseline urine function (blood urea nitrogen [BUN]/creatinine/glomerular filtration rate [GFR]). Monitor closely for adverse drug effects and toxicities. Establish routine voiding schedule (every 2 hours or more if needed). Keep bedside commode, bedpan, and call light within easy reach.
Neurologic: increased risk for injury and infection due to: • sensory losses, decreased tactile sensation, and increased pain tolerance • slowed reaction time • diminished febrile response to infection	Continuously assess pressure points and bony prominences for injury. Institute fall-risk precautions; allow time for processing information and response. Monitor temperature and for other signs of infection (tachycardia, elevated white blood cell [WBC] count, purulent drainage, tissue redness).
Integumentary: increased risk for injury and altered skin integrity (pressure ulcers/skin tears) due to: • thin, fragile skin with loss of subcutaneous tissue	Assess skin every 4 hours; turn and change position every 2 hours. Provide padding for bony prominences.

Adapted from Colloca, Santoro, & Gambassi, 2010.

TABLE 17.2 Preoperative Nursing History and Physical Assessment and Rationale

Nursing History and Physical Assessment	Rationale
Health history	To identify any current or past medical conditions. Previous and current health issues may alert the healthcare team to possible complications.
Mental status	To provide baseline information. Is the client oriented to person, place, time, and situation?
Physical status	To provide baseline information. What is the client's normal level of physical activity?
Medications	To identify current medications and alert the healthcare team to any complications. Include any medications that the client may take, even occasionally. It is also important to ask about any over-the-counter medications and dietary supplements.
Drug and alcohol use	To identify increased risk for complications. Recreational use of drugs or alcohol can interfere with anesthesia or alter bleeding times.
Smoking history	To identify increased risk for complications. Smoking can increase the risk of breathing complications during the intraoperative and postoperative phases.
Allergies	To identify any allergies and possible reactions
Current respiratory and cardiac status	To assess safety of anesthesia and medication administration
Vital signs	To provide a baseline assessment and identify abnormalities

Be sure to include all medications, even those taken occasionally, to identify medications that may increase surgical risk. Some medications, such as warfarin and aspirin, can alter coagulation and increase the risk of bleeding. Antiplatelet medications can inhibit platelet aggregation and also increase the risk of bleeding. Diuretics may alter fluid and electrolyte balance. It is also important to ask about any over-the-counter medications and dietary supplements.

CULTURAL CONSIDERATIONS

Nurses must understand the dynamic and complex concept of culture to provide competent care to a diverse population. Culture is defined as the values, beliefs, and practices shared by a group, which are influenced by internal and external factors such as generational traditions and social position, as well as the cognitive, emotional, behavioral, environmental, and spiritual dimensions of a person (Wong, Sancha, & Gimenez, 2017). Cultural considerations include preferred language, ethnic identity, religious practices, family roles, and social support. When providing care to clients, nurses need to identify any cultural factors that may alter routine procedures. Thus, it

BOX 17.1 Cultural Considerations: Cultural Differences in Postoperative Behaviors

The cultural context and perspective of health, wellness, and illness may significantly affect one's healthcare experience and response to surgery. Galanti (2014) discusses the need for nurses to give careful attention to both verbal and nonverbal cues when assessing postoperative pain in individuals across varying cultures. Similarly, differences in self-care postoperative behaviors exist among various cultures. In a study of three cultural groups (Indian, Chinese, and Caucasian), researchers documented statistically significant differences in incentive spirometer use, deep breathing, coughing, and postoperative activity at 1 week following discharge after coronary artery bypass graft surgery (Gbiri, Ajepe, & Akinbo, 2016). Indian and Chinese immigrants engaged in more activities related to respiratory function (use of incentive spirometer, coughing, and deep breathing) than did their white counterparts. The non-white participants were less likely than Caucasian clients to rest and minimize their level of activity. The Indian and Chinese subjects returned to work at a faster rate and engaged in more heavy lifting, pushing, and pulling of objects than advised. These findings suggest the need for postoperative teaching that is less generic and call for consideration of the socioeconomic variables and learning needs of specific cultural groups. Finally, each person should be approached as an individual first and not as a representative of a particular culture.

is important to respect the client's personal values and beliefs and to individualize care. Box 17.1 identifies cultural differences that might affect perioperative care and discharge teaching.

INFORMED CONSENT

There are four basic elements of the informed consent process that perioperative nurses should understand: capacity, competency, control, and disclosure (Cook, 2016; Simmons, 2016).

- Capacity: To provide informed consent, a client must be an adult or emancipated minor who is mentally competent, alert and oriented, and free from the effects of medications that may alter decisions. The client must have the ability to understand the treatment options and evaluate the risks and benefits of the surgery.
- Competency: The purpose of informed consent is to verify client understanding of the surgical procedure, benefits, possible risks, and alternative approaches.
- Control: Consent is the explicit right of the client. The client has the right to decide who will do what procedure. The client has the right to refuse consent and treatment without coercion or judgment.
- Disclosure: Informed consent protects individual autonomy (the client has the right to be informed and make

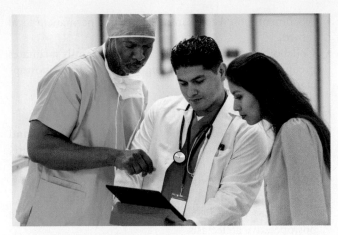

FIG. 17.1 Call the authorized healthcare provider to clarify any uncertainties.

decisions independently) and avoids fraud. A client may claim a lack of informed consent when consent is given for the intervention itself but the disclosure of risks or treatment alternatives is insufficient. Informed consent also provides legal, written documentation (the client must sign to give consent in the United States) (Koch, 2015).

The authorized healthcare provider is responsible for providing information about the procedure, benefits, risks, type of anesthesia, and alternative treatment options. The nurse must verify with the client that the authorized healthcare provider explained the procedure and risks by asking what the client was told about the procedure. This is often done as part of a checklist before surgery. It is the nurses' responsibility to advocate for the client if there are any further questions and call the authorized healthcare provider to clarify any uncertainties (Fig. 17.1).

PREOPERATIVE TEACHING

Preoperative teaching plays an important role in preparing the client for surgery and often relieves anxiety in both the pre- and postoperative phases. Teaching preoperatively is more effective because in the initial postoperative phase, clients are usually sedated, medicated, or in pain and, therefore, less likely to learn.

Preoperative instruction should include a description of the procedure, intended anesthesia, anticipated hospital length of stay, anticipated discharge needs, and physical limitations after surgery. In addition, clients need to know what to expect immediately after their surgery; for example, whether they will require a blood transfusion, experience pain, and need to participate in certain activities and exercise to decrease postoperative complications. With the consent of the client, family members should be included as much as possible during teaching sessions. Clients' preferences and individual learning needs must also be considered. Assess for vision, hearing, and cognitive limitations; the ability to read; and language

barriers. Obtain an interpreter if a language barrier exists. Information can be provided in multiple ways to enhance understanding. Written instructions, video presentation, and face-to-face discussions are the most common ways of providing information.

APPLICATION OF THE NURSING PROCESS

Examples of Related International Classification for Nursing Practice (ICNP) Nursing Diagnoses, Expected Client Outcomes, and Nursing Interventions:

Nursing Diagnosis: Lack of knowledge of treatment regime

Supporting Data: Client scheduled for surgery.

Expected Client Outcomes: Client will exhibit understanding of preoperative teaching by verbalizing or demonstrating postoperative exercises and expectations, such as deep breathing and coughing and the use of the incentive spirometer.

Nursing Intervention Example: Assess knowledge and provide preoperative teaching.

Reference: International Classification for Nursing Practice. (n.d.). *eHealth & ICNP.* Retrieved from https://www.icn.ch/what-we-do/projects/ehealth-icnp.

CRITICAL CONCEPTS
Preoperative Care

Accuracy (ACC)

Accuracy when providing preoperative care is subject to the following variables:
- assessment of client, including vital signs, mobility, skin integrity, lung sounds, circulation, and level of anxiety
- assessment of client's understanding of the informed consent, including procedure and risks
- technique used for processing and carrying out orders, monitoring the client, and providing follow-up care
- number of repetitions and prescribed time of muscle contraction
- proper client positioning.

Client-Centered Care (CCC)

Respect for the client when providing preoperative care is demonstrated by:
- promoting client autonomy and the client's right to make decisions related to life-sustaining treatment
- providing privacy
- ensuring comfort and promoting relaxation
- honoring cultural preferences
- initiating teaching tailored to client's needs
- obtaining an interpreter if the client/family requires
- involving family in history taking and preoperative teaching
- advocating for the client and family.

Infection Control (INF)

When providing preoperative care, healthcare-associated infection associated with the perioperative client is prevented by:

- reducing the transfer and number of microorganisms, primarily through hand hygiene.

Safety (SAF)

When providing preoperative care, implementing safety measures provides a safe care environment and prevents harm, including:

- ensuring verification and documentation of correct client, surgical site, and procedure
- maintaining an environment to support the client's body temperature
- precautions taken to prevent injury during all perioperative phases.

Communication (COM)

- Communication allows for exchanges of information (oral, written, nonverbal, or electronic) between two or more people.

- Documentation records information in a permanent legal record.
- Collaboration with the client and client's family facilitates preoperative care, and teaching ensures optimal postoperative outcomes.

Health Maintenance (HLTH)

Nursing is dedicated to the promotion of health and self-care abilities related to providing preoperative care, including:

- maintaining the health and integrity of the skin
- maintaining the health and integrity of the bladder
- maintaining open alveoli and secretion mobility to reduce postoperative atelectasis
- maintaining circulation and promoting venous return
- maintaining fluid and electrolyte balance.

Evaluation (EVAL)

When providing preoperative care, evaluation of outcomes enables the nurse to determine the efficacy and safety of the care provided, including:

- the client's understanding of preoperative teaching.

■ SKILL 17.1 Preparing a Client for Surgery

EQUIPMENT

Clean gloves
Stethoscope
Blood pressure cuff
Pulse oximetry
Thermometer
Incentive spirometer
Pillow
Folded blanket
Tissues

BEGINNING THE SKILL

1. **SAF** Review the order.
2. **INF** Perform hand hygiene.
3. **CCC** Introduce yourself to the client and family and explain the procedure and the purpose of the preoperative teaching.
4. **SAF** Identify the client using two identifiers.
5. **ACC** Review the nursing history and physical examination. *To establish a baseline assessment.*
6. **CCC** Provide privacy: close the door and pull the curtain.
7. **SAF** Apply name band and allergy band if indicated. *To ensure the safety of the client and confirm any allergies.*

8. **CCC** Determine the emotional needs of the client and the family related to the surgery. *To establish a therapeutic relationship.*

PROCEDURE

9. **ACC** Determine that the client has an informed consent that is signed and dated by the client and the surgeon. *The nurse is responsible for clarifying that the client understands the procedure.*
10. **CCC** Determine if the client has an advance directive. *To understand the client's decisions related to life-sustaining treatments.*
11. **SAF** Determine nothing-by-mouth (NPO) status. Verify the authorized healthcare provider's order of NPO status for 8 to 12 hours prior to surgery.
12. **ACC** Perform preoperative assessment. *To establish baseline criteria and observe for abnormalities to report to the authorized healthcare provider.* Refer to Table 17.2.
13. **SAF** Insert intravenous (IV) line. Verify facility policy; many require an 18- or 20-gauge IV catheter. Use Standard Precautions for IV insertion (see Skill 12.3.).
14. **SAF** Verify preoperative diagnostic screening and alert authorized healthcare provider of any abnormal find-

ings. *To prevent harm to the client from abnormal values.* Refer to Table 17.3.

15. **HLTH** Provide teaching regarding splinting, deep breathing, and coughing. Refer to Chapter 9. *To prepare the client for postoperative deep-breathing and coughing protocol that maintains open alveoli and secretion mobility, thus reducing postoperative atelectasis.*

16. **HLTH** Provide teaching regarding incentive spirometer. Refer to Skill 9.2. *To prepare the client for postoperative care protocol that maintains open alveoli and secretion mobility, thus reducing postoperative atelectasis.*

17. **CCC** Provide teaching regarding pain management.

18. **SAF** Instruct the client to remove dentures or any oral devices; jewelry, including body piercings; artificial nails; wigs; hair clips; makeup; and lotions. *Removable devices and jewelry can cause injury during surgery; makeup and artificial nails can impede assessment.*

19. **HLTH** Apply antiembolism stockings as ordered. Refer to Skill 17.5.

20. **HLTH** Insert indwelling catheter if indicated or assist the client to void before surgery. *To prevent bladder distention or incontinence.* Refer to Chapter 15.

21. **ACC** Administer preoperative medications as ordered.

FINISHING THE SKILL

22. **EVAL** Evaluate outcomes. Is the client ready for surgery? Does the client have an understanding of the postoperative expectations?

23. **CCC** Provide comfort. Assist the client with positioning.

24. **SAF** Ensure client safety. Ensure that the bed is in the lowest position. Ensure that the client can identify and reach the nurse call system. *These safety measures reduce the risk of injury from falls.*

25. **INF** Perform hand hygiene.

26. **COM** Document date, time, assessment findings, client response to teaching, and how the client tolerated the procedures in the legal healthcare record.

TABLE 17.3 Common Preoperative Screenings and Rationales

Diagnostic Test	Rationale
Blood type and crossmatch	To identify blood type for possible blood transfusion
Coagulation studies (prothrombin time [PT], partial thromboplastin time [PTT], international normalized ratio [INR])	To identify bleeding risk
Complete blood count (CBC)	To identify abnormalities in hemoglobin and hematocrit
Comprehensive metabolic panel (CMP)	To identify abnormal levels of electrolytes (potassium, sodium, and magnesium), glucose, liver function tests (alanine aminotransferase [ALT], aspartate aminotransferase [AST]), and renal function tests (blood urea nitrogen [BUN] and creatinine)
Chest x-ray	To identify underlying pulmonary disease; to reveal heart size as an indicator of cardiac function
Electrocardiogram (ECG)	To identify cardiac dysrhythmias
Urinalysis	To identify urinary tract infection or presence of glucose or protein in the urine

■ SKILL 17.2 Instructing Client on Thrombosis Prevention

EQUIPMENT

Clean gloves, if there is risk of exposure to body fluids

BEGINNING THE SKILL

1. **SAF** Review the order.
2. **CCC** Introduce yourself to the client and family.
3. **COM** Explain the procedure and purpose of thrombosis prevention to the client and any family present.
4. **INF** Perform hand hygiene. Apply clean gloves if there is a risk of contact with body fluids.
5. **SAF** Identify the client using two identifiers.
6. **CCC** Provide privacy: close the door and pull the curtain.

Leg Exercises

7. **SAF** Set up an ergonomically safe space. Raise the bed to a comfortable working height. Raise one side rail. *Setting up an ergonomically safe space prevents injury to the nurse and client.*
8. **SAF** Set up a workspace according to your hand dominance (e.g., right-handed on the client's right side).
9. **ACC** Instruct the client to use the great toe to imagine drawing a complete circle while rotating each ankle 360 degrees. Repeat five times. *Maintains joint mobility and promotes venous return.*

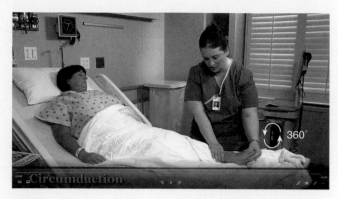

STEP 9 Instruct the client to draw a complete circle.

10. **ACC** Instruct the client to alternate dorsiflexion and plantar flexion of both feet. Repeat five times. (Note: This exercise may be called heel or ankle pumps.) *Promotes venous return.*

11. **ACC** For the quadriceps, instruct the client to tighten the thigh and press the knee against the mattress surface while keeping the leg straight. Relax and then repeat five times. *Promotes venous return.*

12. **ACC** Instruct the client to keep the left leg straight and raise from the mattress, then bend the leg at the hip and knee. Alternate and repeat with the right leg. Perform the exercise five times with each leg. *Promotes venous return and maintains joint mobility.*

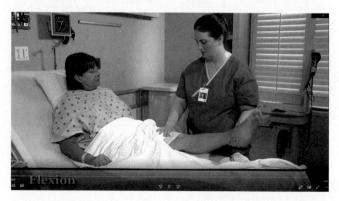

STEP 12 Instruct the client to perform leg exercises.

Turning in Bed

13. **COM** Explain that turning is recommended every 2 hours. *To reduce the risk of postoperative complications.*

14. **CCC** Instruct the client to splint the incision with a pillow (if abdominal). *Splinting the incision minimizes pain.*

15. **COM** To turn to the right side: Instruct the client to raise the left knee and reach across the body, grasping the bedrail on the right side of the bed. *Alternate for turning to the left side.*

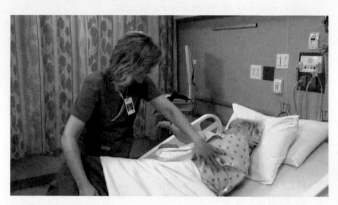

STEP 15 Assist the client with turning.

16. **COM** Instruct the client to push with the bent leg and pull on the handrail to assist in turning. *The client's specific procedure may limit turning ability.*

17. **CCC** Place a pillow to the client's back and between the knees for comfort and alignment. *Supporting the leg and hip in alignment with a pillow prevents internal rotation.*

FINISHING THE SKILL

18. **EVAL** Evaluate outcomes. Does the client have an understanding of the postoperative expectations for thrombosis prevention?

19. **CCC** Provide comfort. Assist the client with positioning.

20. **SAF** Ensure client safety. Place the bed in the lowest position. Ensure that the client can identify and reach the nurse call system. *These safety measures reduce the risk of injury from falls.*

21. **INF** Remove gloves, if used. Perform hand hygiene.

22. **COM** Document date, time, and how the client tolerated the procedure in the legal healthcare record.

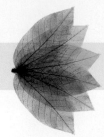

ROLES OF THE SURGICAL TEAM

All operating room personnel must follow the mandates of the U.S. Occupational Safety and Health Administration (OSHA) and wear a sterile gown, disposable shoe covers, mask, head cover, protective eyewear, and gloves to prevent splash exposure from blood. During the intraoperative period, the scrub person and circulating nurse work to maintain a safe and aseptic environment, prevent injury, and provide ongoing assessment of the client during anesthesia.

- The scrub person prepares the surgical table, then anticipates and makes available to the surgeon necessary instruments, drains, sponges, and other equipment. This work allows the surgical procedure to move forward in a timely manner, minimizes anesthesia time, and helps prevent complications. To fulfill the scrub person role, a strong knowledge base and an ability to make quick decisions in an emergency situation are required.
- The circulating nurse works to keep the client free from harm and maintain an efficient, well-coordinated surgical suite. Responsibilities include control of room temperature, humidity, lighting, and asepsis. In addition, the circulating nurse monitors other personnel activities and aseptic practices, all to ensure the protection of clients' rights and well-being.

At the end of the surgical procedure, both the scrub person and circulating nurse account for all instruments and sponges prior to incision closure.

SURGICAL VERIFICATION

When a client enters the surgical suite, all surgical team members must follow Universal Protocol or surgical verification prior to the start of any procedure (The Joint Commission, 2019). This involves a pause in all activity to verify the correct site, correct procedure, and correct client in order to prevent errors and promote clear communication among perioperative team members. The Universal Protocol includes:

- Accurate surgical client identification with two different identifiers
- Review of informed consent with verification that the client understands and verbalizes the pending surgical procedure
- Review of preoperative checklist, laboratory tests, and diagnostic data for consistency and fit with surgical procedure
- Marking of identified surgical cite (e.g., left vs. right distinction; level of spine; digits) with indelible ink and in accordance with client's expectations
- Identification of any present client implants
- Verification of required surgical instruments and necessary equipment

Final "time-out" by all perioperative team members for consensus regarding correct client in the surgical suite and agreed-upon surgical site and procedure prior to incision.

CLIENT POSITIONING

After anesthesia administration, the surgical team positions the relaxed client to provide optimal access to the surgical site, maintain the airway, and ensure ongoing assessment. Care must be taken to maintain correct body alignment and prevent pressure wounds or other skin, nerve, and muscular injuries. Anesthetic medications often compromise perfusion to organs and extremities, which increases the risk of tissue injury. In addition, anesthetized clients lose normal defense mechanisms that signal muscle strain, joint damage, or trauma. Therefore, the circulating nurse and other team members must perform continual assessments of the skin and body position to ensure adequate circulation to body parts. The use of foam padding will protect joints and bony prominences, limiting excessive pressure on the surrounding skin.

Fig. 17.2 identifies the most common client positions during surgery. For most abdominal surgeries, clients lie flat on the back in the dorsal recumbent position. One arm is extended on a side table to allow for administration of IV fluids, blood, and medications. The Trendelenburg position lowers the client's head and upper torso, displaces intestinal organs into the upper abdomen, and allows optimal access for lower abdominal and pelvic procedures. The Sims' position, often used for kidney surgery, places the client on the nonoperative side with a pillow under the groin to elevate the surgical site. For perineal, vaginal, and rectal surgeries, clients lie on their backs, with legs and thighs flexed and the feet placed in stirrups. This is the lithotomy position.

MAINTAINING SAFETY: LATEX SENSITIVITY/ALLERGY

Clients at risk for a latex allergy response include those who have experienced numerous surgeries or frequent urinary catheterizations; have a history of spina bifida or asthma; work in professions with repeated latex exposure; or are allergic to avocados, bananas, chestnuts, kiwi, or raw potato. Reactions vary in severity but may include mild dermatitis characterized by urticaria and redness; a type IV hypersensitivity reaction with hives, localized swelling, itching, rhinorrhea, and coughing; or a life-threatening type I hypersensitivity reaction with generalized edema, wheezing, laryngeal swelling, difficulty breathing, hypotension, dysrhythmias, and cardiac or respiratory arrest. Given the prevalence of latex sensitivity, members of the surgical team must carefully screen clients and follow the Guideline for a Safe Environment of Care

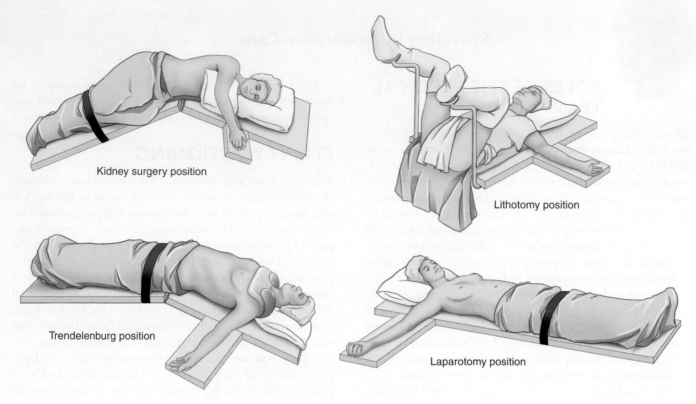

Kidney surgery position

Lithotomy position

Trendelenburg position

Laparotomy position

FIG. 17.2 Positions on the operating table.

from the American Operating Room Nurses (AORN) listed in Box 17.2.

TYPES OF ANESTHESIA

Anesthesia, administered by an anesthesiologist or a certified registered nurse anesthetist (CRNA), provides pain control (analgesia), relaxes or paralyzes muscles, and allows for memory loss (amnesia) during surgery. The four types are conscious sedation and local, regional, and general anesthesia.

Conscious Sedation

When anesthetists administer a combination of medications to relax and block pain without inducing complete unconsciousness, they use conscious sedation. This form of anesthesia is often employed for minor surgical or diagnostic procedures, such as endoscopy or cosmetic surgery. Clients experience drowsiness but maintain the airway independently, respond to touch, and even follow commands if needed. The short-acting sedatives used, such as midazolam (Versed) or propofol (Diprivan), produce an amnesic effect; thus, clients often do not recall events during the procedure. Although conscious sedation helps to control pain and anxiety without great risk of respiratory failure, nurses must still carefully monitor the respiratory rate, oxygen saturation, heart rate, and blood pressure. Prior to the use of conscious

sedation, resuscitation and airway management equipment must be close at hand.

Local Anesthesia

Surgeons typically use local anesthesia to block pain sensation when they perform minor procedures that require sutures for skin lacerations or the removal of a growth. At the conclusion of a major surgery, the surgeon may inject local anesthetics around the surgical site for the relief of postoperative pain. Topical medications such as lidocaine (Xylocaine) or benzocaine (EMLA cream) may be applied to induce surface anesthesia. These medications are absorbed rapidly through the skin and/or mucous membranes.

Regional Anesthesia

Regional anesthesia blocks pain sensations to a larger area, such as an extremity or the upper half of the body. The client remains conscious, although often sedated, but loses feeling as the anesthetic interrupts sensory, motor, and/or sympathetic nerve impulses to and from the surgical site. The anesthetist may perform a peripheral nerve block by injecting an anesthetic into and around specific nerves or nerve groups (e.g., brachial plexus). The Bier block is an IV peripheral technique in which the anesthetist places a tourniquet on the extremity where the surgical procedure will occur and then injects an IV anesthetic below it. The

BOX 17.2 Care of Clients With Latex Allergy

PREOPERATIVE CARE

Notify the surgical team of the latex-sensitive client.

Identify the client with a sensitivity or allergy to latex with a bracelet or wristband and on the medical record.

CARE IN THE SURGICAL SUITE

Develop and implement a protocol to deliver a latex-safe care environment.

Purchase products made from alternatives to natural rubber latex.

Maintain a list of supplies that contain natural rubber latex and alternatives that are latex free.

Implement latex precautions for all clients with latex sensitivity or allergy.

Post signs stating "latex allergy" on all entrances to the operating room.

Schedule latex-sensitive clients as the first cases of the morning, allowing the ventilation system to remove the previous day's latex dust overnight.

Remove all latex products from the surgical suite.

Use latex-free gloves and tourniquets.

Ensure latex-sensitivity is identified in all hand-off communications for the latex sensitive client.

After surgery, transfer the client to a latex-safe care environment, if available.

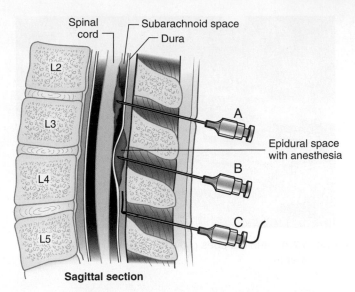

FIG. 17.3 Location of needle point and injected anesthetic relative to dura. **A,** Epidural catheter. **B,** Single-injection epidural. **C,** Spinal anesthesia into the epidural space

tourniquet exerts enough pressure to retain the anesthetic within the extremity without systemic absorption, blocks pain sensation, and limits venous blood return while maintaining arterial circulation. As a result, the Bier block allows rapid anesthesia, decreased bleeding during surgery, and a quick recovery.

Central or spinal anesthesia, often used for abdominal, pelvic, and lower limb surgery, occurs when anesthetists inject an anesthetic into the cerebrospinal fluid or the subarachnoid space, usually below the second lumbar vertebral body. Clients lose sensation and movement below the level of injection but can remain conscious and have less risk of respiratory depression. Still, the spinal anesthetic agent may sometimes travel upward and result in decreased respirations such that clients require mechanical ventilation. Elevation of the client's upper body may limit respiratory paralysis and compromise. Anesthetics also block sympathetic nerve impulses, promote peripheral vascular vasodilation, and cause hypotension, requiring additional fluid support and medication. Headache, nausea, vomiting, and urinary retention are other common adverse effects associated with spinal anesthesia. The circulating nurse monitors the client for all of these complications throughout the surgery. Finally, clients, although unaware, may experience a traumatic or burn injury to the anesthetized area. Nurses in the surgery suite therefore need to assess skin condition and extremity position thoroughly.

Epidural Anesthesia

With epidural anesthesia, the anesthetist inserts a thin indwelling catheter into the epidural space (anywhere within the vertebral column) and injects a larger dose of anesthetic than used with spinal analgesia. Epidural administration typically provides a safer form of anesthesia because medication does not enter the subarachnoid space; however, if the anesthetist inadvertently injects the anesthetic into the subarachnoid space, clients can experience a drop in blood pressure and respiratory failure requiring mechanical ventilation (Fig. 17.3). The circulating nurse monitors the client's vital signs closely. Epidural access not only provides surgical anesthesia but also allows for postoperative analgesia. Epidural analgesia may be provided after surgery to control pain, as described in Chapter 7.

General Anesthesia

The anesthetist provides general anesthesia via the IV and inhalation routes to produce a loss of consciousness and sensation. As a result, the client becomes immobile and does not recall unpleasant or painful aspects of the surgical procedure. If complications occur, general anesthesia allows for adjustments in dosage and can be continued for an extended time frame if needed. During induction, the anesthetist performs endotracheal intubation for airway maintenance and ventilation and administers medications, including muscle relaxants, narcotics, barbiturates, and/or paralytics. In the maintenance phase, anesthesia

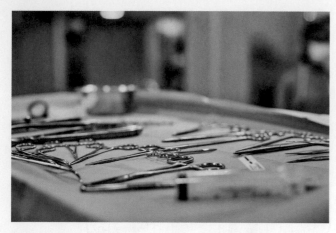

FIG. 17.4 Sterile drapes provide a sterile field for sterile instruments.

continues as the surgical team positions the client, performs skin preparation for incision, and conducts the surgical procedure. In the emergence phase, anesthetics are gradually reduced, and the client begins to waken. Because general anesthesia clients experience respiratory and circulatory depression, they are at greater risk postoperatively for pneumonia, thrombosis, myocardial infarction, stroke, and malignant hyperthermia (discussed shortly). Clients also complain of sore throat after intubation, nausea and vomiting (due to gastrointestinal relaxation), headache, and shivering.

PREPARING THE CLIENT'S SKIN

Surgical site infections have substantial human and financial cost. Many surgical site infections may be preventable (Berrios-Torres et al., 2017). For these reasons, healthcare providers give major attention to the client's skin preparation and SSI prevention prior to surgery. Recommendations call for clients to shower and scrub the surgical site the night before and the morning of surgery with soap or an antibacterial agent. Although evidence indicates that antiseptic showers decrease bacterial colonization, very little data suggest which antibacterial solution (e.g., Betadine, 4% chlorhexidine gluconate) is most effective (Edmiston & Leaper, 2017). Additional skin preparation and hair removal, if needed, occurs before the client enters the surgical suite. Because hair removal with a razor often nicks the skin and results in bacterial invasion, evidence-based practice calls for the use of clippers just prior to the surgical procedure (Kurien, Sansho, Nath, & Varghese (2018). Finally, the administration of prophylactic antibiotics, usually within 1 hour of incision, results in a decrease in

surgical wound infection rates (Rafati, Shiva, Ahmadi, & Habibi, 2014).

All instruments and materials that come in contact with the surgical site must be sterile. Sterile drapes cover body parts, keep the surgical site visible, and provide a field upon which to place sterile instruments (Fig. 17.4). Drapes used in surgery are impervious to moisture. Any item that drops to the side or underneath a draped table is considered unsterile. The front of the surgical teams' gowns from waist up is considered sterile, as are the sleeves from 5 cm (2 inches) above the elbow to the cuff; however, any unscrubbed personnel should remain at least 30 cm (12 inches) away from the sterile field.

CLOSING THE WOUND

At the end of the surgical procedure, scrub nurses may assist with wound closure. Sutures are either absorbable (e.g., chromic, catgut) or nonabsorbable (e.g., silk, synthetic nylon). Nonabsorbable sutures must be removed after the incision heals, whereas absorbable sutures dissolve or are absorbed into the tissue and do not require removal. Surgeon preference, the size and location of the incision, and the type of surgical wound all determine what type of suture is used. The goal is to expose the client to the least amount of foreign suture material as necessary and prevent infection or abscess. One effective method for incision closure is the use of skin staples. These flat, stainless-steel staples can be applied with a staple gun faster and closer to the incision than sutures. Surgeons may also insert and sometimes suture into place drains near the surgical wound. These drains allow removal of excess blood and serous fluid that might otherwise create an environment for bacterial growth and infection. Refer to Chapter 16 for further discussion of wound drainage.

APPLICATION OF THE NURSING PROCESS

Examples of Related ICNP Nursing Diagnoses, Expected
    Client Outcomes, and Nursing Interventions:
Nursing Diagnosis: Risk for latex allergy
Expected Client Outcomes: Client will not experience a latex allergy during the perioperative phase
Nursing Intervention Example: Assess for allergies and communicate any allergies to all members of the healthcare team. Use nonlatex products.
Reference: International Classification for Nursing Practice. (n.d.). *eHealth & ICNP.* Retrieved from https://www.icn.ch/what-we-do/projects/ehealth-icnp.

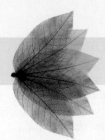

POSTOPERATIVE NURSING CARE

The first stage of recovery from surgery is often referred to as the post-anesthesia or immediate postoperative phase. The surgical team transfers the client from the operating table to a stretcher; then, the anesthetist and circulating nurse (sometimes accompanied by the surgeon) travel with the client to the post-anesthesia care unit (PACU), an open unit located close to the operating room (OR). In the PACU, specialty-trained nurses provide care through the anesthesia recovery period. During transport from surgery to the PACU, the client is at high risk for respiratory and cardiac complications; thus, great care is taken to maintain the airway, monitor vital signs, and ensure optimal circulation. Upon arrival to the PACU, "handoff" communication between the surgical team and the PACU nurse occurs. Through this interactive communication, caregivers address the client's condition, goals, required care, medications, recent or anticipated problems, and safety measures, as listed in Box 17.3.

The second stage of surgical recovery begins in the PACU and continues when the client moves to a postoperative unit. In the PACU, the nurse performs frequent assessments and focuses interventions on airway management; maintenance of respiratory, circulatory, and neurologic function; and pain control. For over two decades, PACU nurses have used the Aldrete or post-anesthesia recovery score (PARS) (Aldrete & Kroulik, 1998) to determine when clients are ready to be discharged from the PACU. The PARS criteria provide a basis for evaluation of the client's level of consciousness, oxygen saturation level, respiratory status, and blood pressure. Scoring occurs on admission to the PACU; again at 5 minutes; then at 15, 30, 45, and 60 minutes; and finally, at the time of discharge. The client must achieve a combined score of 8 to 10 before transfer to a postoperative unit. If scores remain less than 8, clients stay in the PACU or transfer to an intensive care unit. With stable vital signs and the ability to breathe independently, the client transfers to a postoperative unit, where nurses continue to promote healing and prevent postsurgical complications. Outcomes indicative of surgical recovery are identified in Table 17.4.

POSTOPERATIVE ASSESSMENT

Airway/Respiration

Certain types of anesthesia can cause respiratory depression. Therefore, it is essential during the postoperative phase to assess airway patency, respiratory rate and rhythm, depth of ventilation, breath sounds, and pulse oximetry. The normal pulse oximetry ranges between 92% and 100%. Restlessness, tachycardia, and confusion are a few common signs of hypoxia. (See Chapter 3 for more information on respiratory assessment.) Nurses monitor the ability to cough effectively and determine the need for suctioning by listening for crackles and rhonchi. Nurses encourage deep breathing and coughing and the use of incentive spirometry to promote lung expansion and decrease the risk of hypoventilation, atelectasis, and pneumonia. (Review Skills 9.1 and 9.2.)

One of the greatest concerns in the postoperative phase is the risk of airway obstruction as a result of the weak pharyngeal and laryngeal muscle tone after anesthetics, secretions in the pharynx or trachea, or laryngeal edema. Obstructive sleep apnea (OSA) increases the risk of airway obstruction. Clients with OSA require close monitoring and a continuous oxygen saturation monitor. (Refer to Chapters 9 and 18 for more information on airway obstruction and managing OSA.)

Circulation

The postoperative client is at risk for adverse cardiovascular events that occur with fluid-volume deficit, side effects of anesthesia, electrolyte imbalances, and ischemia. Assess the client's blood pressure, heart rate, and rhythm and compare the findings to preoperative baseline assessments. Other signs to assess include alertness; orientation to time, place, and person; warm and pink mucous membranes, quick capillary refill (<3 seconds), strong peripheral pulses, and urinary output of 5 to 10 mL per kilogram. These indicate adequate tissue perfusion. If the blood pressure drops, clients may sense a feeling of impending doom, the heart rate may become irregular, bradycardia or tachycardia may develop, or the client may have chest pain or shortness of breath. For any of these symptoms, the nurse should notify the surgeon.

BOX 17.3 Information Discussed in Postoperative Handoff Communication

Type and duration of surgical procedure
Type and duration of anesthesia
Client allergies
Preoperative status: skin condition, mobility, sensory/perception capacity
Postoperative vital signs, pulse oximetry values
Estimated blood loss
Fluid intake and output
Lab value alterations
Complications during surgery
Existing intravenous catheters, monitoring devices, tubes, drains, catheters
Postoperative orders
Medications administered during surgery
Information related to family dynamics and communication

TABLE 17.4 Evidence of Surgical Recovery

Respiratory stability	The client deep breathes independently and coughs and clears secretions.
Sensory/perception stability	The client is conscious, is aware of surroundings, and reorients easily.
Hemodynamic stability	Vital signs are within baseline range. Blood pressure (BP) may vary across the client's surgical experience. Preoperatively, BP is often increased due to anxiety, pain, or withholding of antihypertensive medications.
Musculoskeletal stability	The client can move all extremities voluntarily or on command to the extent of preoperative status. Movement and sensation are regained after spinal and epidural anesthesia.
Fluid balance	The client voids at minimum 0.5 mL/kg/hr, within intake relatively equal to output. When determining fluid balance, consider the amount of blood loss, emesis, wound and gastric drainage, and urine output.
Surgical wound stability	The client exhibits no excessive blood or fluid loss from the surgical site. Dressings are dry and intact. Drainage is suitable and in line with surgical procedure.

Fluid-volume deficit caused by bleeding or hemorrhage can lead to decreased circulating volume, altered tissue perfusion, and a decrease in the delivery of oxygen and nutrients to cells. Hemorrhage may be either internal (into a body cavity or space) or external (from an incision site or into a drain). Clients with fluid-volume deficit may exhibit a decreased level of consciousness, hypotension, tachycardia, sluggish capillary refill (>3 seconds), or thready pulses, and become pale, with cold and clammy skin. Notify the surgeon if these signs are present.

Nurses maintain the IV infusion to replace fluid volume, apply oxygen therapy, and anticipate orders for possible blood replacement. Expect the authorized healthcare provider to order follow up evaluations of hemoglobin, hematocrit, prothrombin time (PT), partial thromboplastin time (PTT), and international normalized ratio (INR). For external hemorrhage, a pressure dressing may be needed to control the bleeding (see Skill 17.4). Refer to Chapter 12 for more information on administering blood products.

Formation of a blood clot is another concern after surgery. Immobilization increases the risk of blood clots; therefore, early ambulation is important to prevent pulmonary embolism, deep vein thrombosis, and venous thromboembolism. If the client is unable to ambulate, frequent turning (at least every 2 hours) is necessary.

The surgeon may prescribe the use of antiembolism stockings, sequential compression devices (SCDs), or a continuous passive motion (CPM) machine to decrease the risk of the formation of blood clots.

- Antiembolism stockings promote return flow of the venous circulation and prevent venous stasis. The nurse removes the stockings every 8 hours to inspect the client's skin.
- SCDs promote return flow of the venous circulation and prevent venous stasis.
- CPM is most commonly used after knee surgery to help mobilize the joint and thereby reduce the risk of pulmonary embolism, deep vein thrombosis, venous thromboembolism, and formation of scar tissue. (Ekim et al., 2016; Liao et al., 2016)

In addition, clients need to avoid sitting or lying with their feet crossed, raising the bed's knee gatch, or keeping a pillow under their knees because these activities will decrease venous return. Prior to getting clients out of bed for the first time, nurses need to verify activity orders and allow the client to sit on the side of the bed for a few minutes. The positioning of the client before ambulation is described in Chapter 1. Sitting up before ambulating may also prevent orthostatic hypotension, which is described in Chapter 3.

As the client begins to ambulate, the nurse should walk alongside, providing physical support and reassurance (see Chapter 6). Care should be taken not to overly tire the client. Evaluation may include calculating the client's maximum heart rate (MHR). To determine MHR, subtract the client's age from 220. If the client's heart rate exceeds the MHR, return the client to bed immediately, document, and inform the surgeon.

Temperature Control/Malignant Hyperthermia

Surgery and the effects of anesthesia may interfere with normal body temperature maintenance or thermoregulation, and older adults and the very young are at greatest risk. Hypothermia can occur with exposure of the body's surface area, the use of cooling skin preparation agents, decreased surgical suite temperature, IV fluid administration, and blood loss. As a result, clients experience discomfort and an increased risk of SSIs (Billeter et al., 2014) and myocardial ischemia (Sessler, 2016). Shivering, which may indicate hypothermia, also occurs as a side effect of certain anesthetics, and for this reason, the surgeon or anesthetist may prescribe small dosages of clonidine (Catapres). Throughout the perioperative course, nurses must be vigilant to maintain clients' core temperature.

To maintain the safety and comfort of surgical clients, nurses must prevent inadvertent postoperative hypothermia (IPH), which occurs when the core temperature decreases to 36°C or lower. IPH develops as a result of the effects of general or regional anesthesia and body exposure to a cold operating room environment. Clients with IPH are at increased risk for various problems, including shivering, prolonged bleeding, infection, and cardiac dysrhythmias that may result in cardiac arrest or death. Up to 70% of surgical clients experience IPH, and with associated complications, treatment costs and hospital stays increase (Giuliano & Hendricks, 2017).

The treatment of IPH involves active and passive warming methods (Watson, 2018). Active methods deliver heat to a client and can include forced-air warming systems, electric blankets, administration of warm IV fluids, radiant warming systems, and circulating water mattresses. Passive warming methods decrease heat loss by maintaining warm room temperatures between 20°C and 23.8°C (68°F and 75°F) and covering clients with warm blankets or surgical drapes. Research findings indicate that active warming methods are more effective than passive methods in establishing and regulating normal core temperatures, decreasing shivering, and increasing client comfort; however, exact protocols and methods to prevent other complications require further investigation (Watson, 2018).

Active warming methods include forced-air warming devices, which blow warm, filtered air through a hose and are attached to either a blanket or a gown. The warming device is initiated preoperatively, is used to regulate the client's temperature intraoperatively, and is used again postoperatively to warm clients and aid recovery. Forced-air systems have been scrutinized to determine any possible increased risk of SSI, and none has been found (U.S. Food and Drug Administration [FDA], 2017). The concern that forced-air warming devices could change the airflow in the operating room and increase the risk of contamination prompted an airflow study. The study found that the downward laminar airflow from the ceiling counteracted the airflow caused by the forced-air warming device, thereby preventing airflow contamination. Maintaining the client's temperature improves surgical site healing and reduces the rate of SSI (Shirozu, Kai, Setoguchi, Ayagaki, & Hoka, 2018). Refer to the discussion of thermoregulation in Chapter 3 for more information on warming the client.

Malignant hyperthermia (MH) is a potentially life-threatening complication associated with the use of anesthetics and muscle relaxants like succinylcholine. Susceptible individuals include those with a positive family history or preexisting genetic muscular disorders ("Malignant Hyperthermia," 2017). Observe for allergic responses and signs of MH in adult and pediatric clients who have not received anesthesia previously. Suspect MH and notify the qualified healthcare professional when a client exhibits unexpected tachycardia, dysrhythmias, tachypnea, increased carbon dioxide levels, hyperkalemia, and muscle stiffness or rigidity. Temperature elevation occurs as a late sign. To slow the client's rapid metabolic rate and relax the muscles, the nurse may receive orders to increase oxygen levels and administer IV dantrolene sodium (Rosenberg, Pollock, Schiemann, Bulger, & Stowell, 2015). After the client stabilizes, monitor renal function and potassium levels closely for signs of acute kidney injury. Because clients now rotate quickly through PACUs, nurses on postoperative units must also be alert to the signs of and treatment for MH.

Fluid and Electrolyte Balance

Monitoring fluid and electrolyte balance in the postoperative client is essential. Fluid and/or blood loss during the surgery can cause hypovolemia, hypotension, shock, and electrolyte imbalances. PACU nurses should communicate the balance of intake and output during surgery and recovery. It is the nurse's responsibility to assess the client for a history of cardiovascular or renal disease; monitor the client's IV line for patency and the IV site for phlebitis or infiltration. The nurse will assess fluid intake and urine output, including any output from surgical drains and gastric tubes; and monitor for diaphoresis, also considering loss of fluid through the skin and lungs (called insensible fluid loss). For the first several days, the nurse should weigh the client daily and compare to the preoperative weight. Evaluate the client's electrolyte status by comparing postoperative values with the preoperative baseline values.

Neurologic Function

The client is often drowsy because of the anesthetic agent given in the operating room. As the anesthetic begins to metabolize, neurologic functions begin to return. Assess the client's level of consciousness, pupils, gag reflex, hand grips, and movement of extremities. If the client had a surgery that involved the nervous system, a more extensive neurologic assessment may be necessary. For example, assessment of the upper-extremity strength and sensation is required for the client who undergoes cervical spine surgery. It is always important to compare postoperative findings to the client's preoperative baseline assessment. (See Chapter 20 for advanced neurologic assessment information.)

Skin Integrity and Wound Healing

During the recovery and the acute postoperative phase, assess the condition of the skin, identifying any rashes, petechiae, burns, and pressure areas and abrasions. A rash may indicate an allergic reaction or drug sensitivity. Small (1–2 mm) red or purple spots may occur on the skin, called petechiae, caused by minor bleeding from broken capillaries or a clotting disorder. Burns may result from inappropriate placement of electrical cautery devices used to cut, coagulate, and dissect tissue during the surgical procedure. Pressure areas and abrasions may be due to incorrect positioning during surgery. Turn the postoperative area every 2 hours to relieve pressure over bony prominences. Also determine the client's ability to turn and move the extremities. If clients cannot turn on their own, establish and implement a turning protocol to prevent the development of pressure injury.

Dressings are assessed frequently to ensure that they are clean, dry, and intact. Observe the amount, color, consistency, and odor of drainage on the dressing or the drainage collection site. It is common to see a small amount of serosanguineous drainage on the dressings immediately postoperatively. Draw a mark on the dressing along the outer perimeter of the drainage to monitor the amount of drainage. If the drainage is moderate or leaking through the dressing, notify the authorized healthcare provider. Excessive drainage may indicate hemorrhage, and a pressure dressing may be indicated. The nurse may apply more gauze to the surgical site if necessary to reinforce the dressing (refer to Skill 17.4). Many surgeons prefer to change the first postoperative dressing to inspect the incision. When removing the dressing, do not put pressure on the wound. Loosen the edges of the dressing and peel the ends toward the wound while holding the skin with the other hand. During the dressing change, assess for redness, drainage, bleeding, and whether wound edges are approximated.

Urinary Function

Eight to 12 hours before surgery, most clients receive no oral fluids or food (NPO status) to decrease the risk of aspiration during the procedure. This preventative measure, however, can result in decreased urine production. For this reason, clients receive IV fluids and may have an indwelling urinary catheter placed before surgery to monitor urinary output and prevent bladder distention during and after the operation. An empty bladder prevents injury and allows better access to abdominal organs during surgery. Circulating nurses monitor urine production continuously throughout the surgical procedure. A urine output of 1 mL/kg/hour indicates sufficient intravascular volume, adequate renal function, and perfusion.

Postoperatively, the nurse continues to monitor urine production. Document hourly urine output for amount, color, and odor. Dark, concentrated, and decreased urine production (0.5 mL/kg/hr for 2 consecutive hours) in the postoperative phase can indicate hypovolemia, electrolyte imbalance, blood loss, hypoxia, or compromised circulation. If this level of decreased urine output occurs, the authorized healthcare provided should be notified (Baird, 2016). For the prevention of hospital-associated infections, the CDC recommends that caregivers remove indwelling catheters within 24 hours of surgery unless there are important indications for continued use (CDC, 2015). Because of anesthesia, pain, or decreased level of consciousness, some clients do not fully regain bladder function for 6 to 8 hours after surgery, nor can they sense a full bladder. Therefore, nurses may need to palpate right above the symphysis pubis or perform a bladder scan to detect bladder distention. Clients who do not have an indwelling catheter should void within 8 to 12 hours of the surgical procedure. If a bladder scan reveals a urine volume of more than 150 to 200 mL, clients may have urinary retention that requires straight catheterization. Refer to Chapter 15 for information and skills related to performing a bladder scan and a straight catheterization.

Gastrointestinal Function

Postoperative nausea and vomiting (PONV) continue to be the most common postoperative complications, particularly for surgical clients who undergo general anesthesia (Odom-Forren, 2018). These responses are not only unpleasant and uncomfortable but also can lead to aspiration, fluid and electrolyte imbalance, surgical wound dehiscence, esophageal tears, hypertension, and increased intracranial pressure. Individuals react differently to anesthetic agents and experience different thresholds for nausea and vomiting, but both symptoms are under control of the central nervous system's vomiting center in the medulla oblongata and the chemoreceptor trigger zone (CTZ) located in the brain's fourth ventricle (Koyuncu et al., 2017).

Many aspects of the perioperative experience increase the risk for PONV. The most common risk factors related to PONV include the use of volatile anesthetics, surgical organ manipulation, immobility with consequential blood pooling and vestibular disequilibrium, administration of opioids for pain management, hypovolemia, and release of cytokines (Odom-Forren, 2018). In addition, the presence of any pharyngeal tubes or suctioning can lead to mechanical irritation of pharyngeal and vagal nerves, which, in turn, can stimulate nausea and vomiting. Likewise, stomach and duodenal distention, changes in intracranial pressure, and position changes serve as triggers for postoperative nausea and vomiting. In addition, females experience nausea and vomiting twice as often as males, and nonsmokers tend to metabolize anesthetics at a slower rate, thus becoming nauseated more so than smokers. Other predictors for a high risk of PONV include a history of motion sickness, gastroparesis, the use of birth control pills, and anesthesia with nitrous oxide.

When possible, discussion with clients and their family members related to treatment preferences for PONV should take place prior to surgery. American Society of PeriAnesthesia Nurses (ASPAN) guidelines call for prophylactic treatment for clients with moderate and high PONV risks. As prophylactic measures, corticosteroids (dexamethasone), nonsteroidal antiinflammatory drugs, 5HT3 receptor antagonists (ondansetron), or droperidol may be prescribed. The nurse will need to give these medications as ordered. The nurse should also maintain clients' hydration. These interventions should decrease the incidence of PONV (Frandsen & Smith Pennington, 2014). Aromatherapy with inhaled isopropyl alcohol (O'Malley, 2016) and stimulation of acupressure point P6 at three fingers' width from client's wrist (Hofmann, Murray, Beck, & Homann, 2016) have also proven effective when administered before surgery and during the postoperative period. Nurses need to assess clients for PONV risks; determine what antiemetic prophylaxis has been used and proven effective; maintain a quiet, restful environment; position the client with the head of the bed elevated; and finally, continue to assess for nausea and vomiting every time the client is assessed for pain.

Postoperative or Paralytic Ileus

Preoperatively, clients are prescribed NPO status and may even receive laxatives or enemas in order to clear the gut of fecal matter. These measures prevent the release of bowel contents into the peritoneal cavity and decrease the risk for peritonitis (inflamed peritoneum) and sepsis (bloodstream infection). Such preparation, in addition to anesthesia and postoperative opioid pain medication, slows intestinal peristalsis (bowel activity). As a result, some clients experience postoperative or paralytic ileus, a temporary paralysis of the intestine that causes painful abdominal distention, nausea and vomiting, and symptoms of gastrointestinal obstruction (Vather, O'Grady, Bissett, & Dinning, 2014).

Supportive interventions for the prevention of postoperative ileus include sitting in a chair on the first postoperative day and early ambulation. Chewing gum has been found to increase the gastrin plasma concentration and pancreatic polypeptide and increases the duodenal alkali discharge, and it can be effective in the reduction of paralytic ileus

(Pilevarzadeh, 2016). Rocking-chair motion also promotes the early resolution of existing paralytic ileus (Massey, 2010). Reliable indicators of recovery from postoperative ileus include passage of flatus; first bowel movement; tolerance of diet; and resolution of nausea, vomiting, and abdominal distention (Vather et al., 2014).

Progression of Diet for Adequate Nutrition

In the PACU, clients begin taking sips of fluid and ice chips when fully awake. If tolerated, progression to a clear liquid meal of broth, apple juice, and/or tea usually follows. As flatus, peristalsis, and bowel movements return, clients generally progress to a regular diet. A regular diet is encouraged because a clear liquid diet has little nutritional value. In the first postoperative days, offer small amounts of fluids and food every 3 to 4 hours to prevent abdominal distention and vomiting. Encourage foods high in protein and vitamin C to promote tissue and wound repair. Continue to help clients maintain adequate fluid intake, which will soften fecal material, preventing straining and constipation.

Pain

The client's degree of pain varies considerably with the type of surgery. As discussed in Chapter 7, pain should be assessed using a consistent facility-approved tool that is culturally sensitive and age appropriate. See Chapter 7 for more information on pain assessment and management.

POSTOPERATIVE TEACHING

Teaching is important to improve client outcomes and prevent postoperative complications. Postoperative teaching should reinforce preoperative teaching and promote self-care. In addition, teaching should include the following:

- postoperative treatment regimen (e.g., care of the incision, dressing change, prescribed medications)
- prescribed activity
- signs and symptoms of complications and when to notify the authorized healthcare provider
- follow-up appointment schedule
- available community resources.

Throughout the discussion of perioperative care, complications related to surgery have been addressed. Table 17.5 provides a summary of complications, causal factors, and measures for prevention.

APPLICATION OF THE NURSING PROCESS

Examples of Related ICNP Nursing Diagnoses, Expected Client Outcomes, and Nursing Interventions:

Nursing Diagnosis: Risk for infection

Supporting Data: Surgery places individuals at risk for SSI and atelectasis, which could progress to pneumonia. Use of an indwelling Foley catheter during surgery increases the client's risk of a catheter-associated urinary tract infection (CAUTI).

Expected Client Outcomes: The client will remain free from a postoperative infection while in the healthcare setting.

Nursing Intervention Examples: Provide postoperative care, including the following:

- Encourage the client to demonstrate effective coughing and deep breathing.
- Encourage the client to demonstrate proper use of incentive spirometry.
- Encourage and assist with progressive and early ambulation.
- Promote early removal of an indwelling Foley catheter.
- Provide aseptic incisional care per authorized provider orders.

Nursing Diagnosis: Bleeding

Supporting Data: Client oozing blood from the surgical site.

Expected Client Outcomes: The client will not experience significant blood loss from bleeding.

Nursing Intervention Examples: Apply direct pressure. Apply a pressure dressing. Monitor client's skin color and condition, blood pressure, pulse, and level of consciousness.

Reference: International Classification for Nursing Practice. (n.d.). *eHealth & ICNP*. Retrieved from https://www.icn.ch/what-we-do/projects/ehealth-icnp.

CRITICAL CONCEPTS
Providing Postoperative Care

Accuracy (ACC)

Accuracy when providing postoperative care is subject to the following variables:

- assessment of client, including vital signs, mobility, level of discomfort, skin integrity, assessment of incision, lung sounds, circulation, and bleeding
- measurement for antiembolism stocking size and the distance between the gluteal crease and the popliteal area and between the knee and the end of the machine
- proper client positioning.

Client-Centered Care (CCC)

Respect for the client when providing postoperative care is demonstrated through:

- promoting client autonomy and the client's right to make decisions related to life-sustaining treatment
- providing privacy
- ensuring comfort and promoting relaxation
- honoring cultural preferences
- initiating teaching tailored to the client's needs
- obtaining interpreter if client/family requires
- involving family in history taking and perioperative teaching
- advocating for the client and family.

TABLE 17.5 Complications Related to Surgery

Complications	Causal Factors	Preventative Measures/Interventions
Hypoxemia: Decreased oxygen concentration in blood. Symptoms include restlessness, confusion, dyspnea, vital sign changes, diaphoresis, and cyanosis.	Anesthetic agents and pain medication decrease respirations. Pain and poor positioning prohibit adequate lung expansion. History of obstructive sleep apnea.	Monitor level of consciousness, SpO$_2$, respiratory rate, and breath sounds. Obtain order for oxygen supplementation. Maintain airway.
Atelectasis: Collapsed alveoli with increased mucus retention. Symptoms include crackles or diminished breath sounds, increased respiratory rate, dyspnea, and productive cough.	Anesthetic agents, pain, and decreased mobility prevent lung expansion.	Turn, cough, deep breathe, and encourage use of incentive spirometer as ordered while awake. Ensure administration of prescribed breathing treatments.
Pneumonia: Infection and inflammation in alveoli; can be in one or more lobes of the lung. Symptoms include fever, chills, dyspnea, purulent mucus production, and chest pain.	Exposure to bacteria, aspiration and retention of secretions or gastric contents, decreased lung expansion	In addition to previously described measures, treat with prescribed scheduled antimicrobials.
Hemorrhage: Blood loss over a short period of time. Symptoms include restlessness, tachycardia, thready pulse, hypotension, diminished urine output, and cool and clammy skin.	Dislodged clot, ruptured suture at incision line, history of clotting disorder	For external bleed, apply pressure with sterile gauze and notify provider. For internal bleed symptoms, ensure airway, oxygenation, and access for intravenous (IV) fluid administration. Institute rapid response and notify provider.
Hypovolemia: Decreased circulation and perfusion to tissues due to lack of circulating blood volume. Symptoms same as for hemorrhage.	Hemorrhage most likely cause in surgical client; can also be related to vomiting, increased nasogastric drainage, or inadequate fluid resuscitation.	Suspect hemorrhage, look for source of bleeding and treat as noted previously. Increase fluid administration, Plasmanate, or blood products as prescribed.
Thrombus: Clot formation within wall of blood vessel that can occlude distal blood flow. Symptoms include redness, tenderness, swelling in affected extremity, decreased pulse below occlusion site. An **embolus** occurs when a piece of clot breaks loose, travels, and becomes lodged in another organ (e.g., brain, lung, heart).	Trauma to vessel wall, increased blood coagulability, use of birth control pills, venous stasis related to prolonged immobility and dehydration; common after abdominal, pelvic, joint, and extremity surgeries	Early ambulation after surgery; use of prescribed low-molecular-weight heparin, compression stockings, intermittent pneumatic compression devices, and range of motion exercises
Paralytic ileus: Temporary paralysis or interrupted peristalsis of the intestine leading to painful abdominal distention, nausea and vomiting, and symptoms of gastrointestinal obstruction.	Nothing-by-mouth (NPO) status prior to surgery, surgical manipulation of bowel and abdominal organs, influx of air/gas to visualize organs, anesthetic agents and postoperative use of narcotics, immobility	Ambulation on first postoperative day, sitting in chair, rocking in chair. Gradual progression in intake of oral fluids and diet as passage of flatus and bowel movement occur.
Urinary retention: Inability to void within 8 to 10 hours of surgery due to involuntary accumulation of urine in bladder. Symptoms include uncomfortable pressure, distended bladder.	Loss of bladder tone related to use of anesthetics, manipulation, or increased pain medication.	Monitor hourly urinary outputs for 0.5 mL/kg/hr to 1 mL/kg/hr. Confirm bladder distention with scan. Consider straight catheterization for more than 150 to 200 mL.
Urinary tract infection: Infection due to bacterial or yeast invasion of urinary tract. Symptoms include possible fever, chills, dysuria, scant urine output with presence of white blood cells (WBCs) or casts, cloudy urine, frequent urge to void.	Bacterial exposure during catheterization; prolonged use of bladder catheter	Strict sterile technique during catheter insertion; removal of catheter within in 24 hours after surgery
Wound infection/dehiscence: Invasion of bacteria or fungi in wound tissue. Symptoms include redness, tenderness, and purulent drainage at incision; fever, chills, and elevated WBC count; positive cultures; separation of wound at suture line.	Poor aseptic technique during or after surgical procedure; contaminated site prior to surgical intervention (bowel perforation from large intestine contamination); obesity, malnutrition, or decreased perfusion to tissues	Observe wound for symptoms of infection. Wash hands prior to any assessment or dressing application. Maintain aseptic/sterile technique when changing dressings. Encourage diet high in protein and vitamin C. Splint incision with pillow when coughing to prevent strain on suture line.

Infection Control (INF)

When providing postoperative care, healthcare-associated infections associated with the perioperative client are prevented by:

- containment of microorganisms
- reducing the number of microorganisms
- preventing an environment conducive to microbial growth.

Safety (SAF)

When providing postoperative care, implementing safety measures provides a safe care environment and prevents harm, including:

- maintaining an environment to support the client's body temperature
- protecting the client from injury and reducing the risk of falls

- avoiding immobilization for extended periods.

Communication (COM)

- Communication allows for exchanges of information (oral, written, electronic, or nonverbal) between two or more people.
- Documentation records information in a permanent legal record.

Health Maintenance (HLTH)

Nursing is dedicated to the promotion of health and self-care abilities related to providing postoperative care, including:

- maintaining the health and integrity of the skin

- maintaining the health and integrity of the bladder
- maintaining open alveoli and secretion mobility
- maintaining circulation and promoting venous return
- maintaining fluid and electrolyte balance
- reducing the incidence of postoperative atelectasis.

Evaluation (EVAL)

When providing postoperative care, evaluation of outcomes enables the nurse to determine the efficacy and safety of the care provided, including:

- the client's response to the surgical procedure.
- the client's level of pain and response to pain-relief interventions.

■ SKILL 17.3 Admitting a Postoperative Client

EQUIPMENT

Stethoscope
Blood pressure cuff
Pulse oximetry
Thermometer
Clean gloves
Pillow
Folded blanket
Tissues

BEGINNING THE SKILL

1. **SAF** Review the order.
2. **INF** Perform hand hygiene.
3. **INF** Apply clean gloves.
4. **CCC** Introduce yourself to the client and family.
5. **SAF** Identify the client using two identifiers.
6. **CCC** Provide privacy: close the door and pull the curtain.

PROCEDURE

7. **SAF** Set up an ergonomically safe space. Place the head of the bed in the semi-Fowler's position. *To relieve pressure on the abdomen and allow for increased lung expansion.* Raise the bed to a comfortable working height. Raise one side rail. *Setting up an ergonomically safe space prevents injury to the nurse and client.*
8. **SAF** Set up a workspace according to your hand dominance (e.g., right-handed on the client's right side).
9. **ACC** Assess the client's airway; respiratory rate, rhythm, and depth; breath sounds; and oxygenation saturation. *To measure adequate ventilation.*
10. **ACC** Assess heart rate and rhythm, peripheral pulses, blood pressure, skin color, and capillary refill. *To measure adequate circulation and cardiac output.*
11. **ACC** Assess level of consciousness, orientation, gag reflex, and ability to move extremities. *To measure neurovascular response.*

12. **ACC** Assess fluid status. Review status of IV infusions (type of fluid, rate, patency of fluid, and condition of IV site). *To measure adequate hydration status and prevent fluid overload.*
13. **ACC** Assess patency and any drainage from tubes or drains. Assess urinary output. *To monitor bleeding and risk of dehydration or fluid overload.*
14. **ACC** Assess operative site, status of dressing, and drainage (amount, type, and color).
15. **ACC** Assess pain level (scale of 0–10) and nausea and vomiting. Medicate for pain per order.
16. **HLTH** Instruct the client in thrombosis prevention. (Refer to Skill 17.2.)
17. **HLTH** Apply antiembolism stockings as ordered. (Refer to Skill 17.5.)

FINISHING THE SKILL

18. **CCC** Provide comfort. Assist the client with positioning.
19. **SAF** Ensure client safety. Place the bed in the lowest position. Ensure that the client can identify and reach the nurse call system. *These safety measures reduce the risk of injury from falls.*
20. **INF** Remove gloves and perform hand hygiene.
21. **EVAL** Evaluate outcomes:
    What was the client's response to the pain-relief intervention?
    How did the client tolerate the thorough assessment and thrombosis prevention?
22. **COM** Document date, time, postoperative assessment status, care given, and outcomes in the legal healthcare record.
23. **EVAL** Provide follow-up care by frequently monitoring client status according to client needs and facility protocols.

■ SKILL 17.4 Applying Pressure Dressings to Control Bleeding

EQUIPMENT

Clean gloves
Protective gown and mask (as indicated to protect from blood spatter)
Sterile gauze
Gauze bandage
Roller gauze
Adhesive tape
Sandbags
Equipment for vital signs measurement

BEGINNING THE SKILL

1. **ACC** Identify client hemorrhage. *The client may have increased drainage on dressing, drop in blood pressure, and decreased level of consciousness.*
2. **ACC** Quickly locate the external bleeding site.
3. **ACC** Quickly assess the type of bleeding. Arterial bleeding is bright red and gushes in pulsations; it is difficult to control. Venous bleeding is dark red, and the flow is smooth; it will clot more readily than arterial bleeding. Capillary bleeding is dark red, and the flow oozes from the site.
4. **INF** Perform hand hygiene and apply clean gloves (quickly). *To maintain asepsis.*
5. **ACC** Apply direct pressure. *To stop the bleeding.*
6. **SAF** Call for assistance. The bandage must be applied quickly. Do not leave the client.
7. **ACC** Assess the client's skin color and condition, blood pressure, pulse, and level of consciousness. *To compare to baseline assessment. Diaphoresis, hypotension, tachycardia, and altered level of consciousness indicate hypovolemic shock.* Continue to reassess every 5 to 15 minutes.

PROCEDURE

8. **CCC** When assistance arrives, have the second person verify client identification and provide privacy.
9. **SAF** The second person can assist with setting up an ergonomically safe space. Raise the bed to a comfortable working height. Raise one side rail. *Setting up an ergonomically safe space prevents injury to the nurse and client.*
10. **ACC** The first person continues to hold direct pressure while the second person prepares the bandage. *Hold steady, uninterrupted pressure for at least 5 minutes to promote clotting.*
11. **ACC** The second person cuts three to five pieces of adhesive tape and places them within reach, opens sterile

gauze, and unwraps roller bandage. *The bandage must be applied quickly without relieving pressure.*
12. **ACC** The first person applies more sterile gauze to the bleeding site and continues to hold pressure.
13. **ACC** The second person secures gauze with tape on both sides of the dressing, *while pressure is still being applied,* applying even pressure.
14. **ACC** In simultaneous coordination: The first person removes pressure to the bleeding site while the second person quickly covers the center of the dressing with tape. *The bandage must be applied quickly without relieving pressure.*
15. **ACC** The second person continues reinforcing with tape and applying pressure. *To promote clotting.*
16. **SAF** The second person wraps the dressing with the roller gauze, applying two circular turns firmly on both sides of the fingers that are applying pressure. Continue wrapping the roller bandage for four to six more turns. *To apply even pressure over the bleeding site.*

FINISHING THE SKILL

17. **EVAL** Continue to monitor the client's skin color and condition, blood pressure, pulse, and level of consciousness. *To monitor for signs of hypovolemic shock.*
18. **INF** Remove gloves and perform hand hygiene.
19. **CCC** Provide comfort. Assist the client with positioning.
20. **CCC** Ensure client safety. Place the bed in the lowest position. Ensure the client can identify and reach the nurse call system. *These safety measures reduce the risk of injury from falls.*
21. **INF** Perform hand hygiene.
22. **EVAL** Evaluate outcomes:
    What was the client's response to the application of the pressure dressing?
    How did the client tolerate the bleeding and the application of the pressure dressing?
23. **COM** Notify the authorized healthcare provider immediately of your assessment information, care given, and the client's current status.
24. **COM** Document date, time of application of pressure dressing, and how the client tolerated the procedure in the legal healthcare record.
25. **EVAL** Monitor the client for any further evidence of bleeding or hemodynamic changes due to blood loss.

■ SKILL 17.5 Applying and Removing Antiembolism Stockings

EQUIPMENT

Tape measure
Antiembolism stockings
Clean gloves, if there is a risk of exposure to body fluids

BEGINNING THE SKILL

1. **SAF** Review the order.
2. **INF** Perform hand hygiene.
3. **INF** Apply clean gloves, if there is a risk of exposure to body fluids.
4. **CCC** Introduce yourself to the client and family and explain the procedure and the purpose of the antiembolism stockings. Ensure that the client consents to the application of antiembolism stockings.
5. **SAF** Identify the client using two identifiers.
6. **CCC** Provide privacy: close the door and pull the curtain.

PROCEDURE

7. **SAF** Set up an ergonomically safe space. Raise the bed to a comfortable working height. Raise one side rail. *Setting up an ergonomically safe space prevents injury to the nurse and client.*
8. **SAF** Set up a workspace according to your hand dominance (e.g., right-handed on the client's right side).
9. **ACC** Place the client in a supine position for at least 15 minutes before applying stockings. *To prevent pooling of blood in the extremities.*

Applying Antiembolism Stockings

10. **ACC** Assess the client's skin condition and circulation to the legs, including pulses, skin color, temperature, and edema. *To establish a baseline assessment.*
11. **ACC** Use a tape measure to determine the appropriate stocking size.

12. **ACC** Place one hand into the stocking, grasping the heel, and turn inside out to the level of the heel.

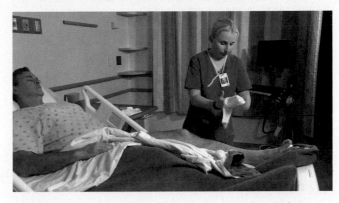

STEP 12 Turn the stocking inside out to the level of the heel.

13. **ACC** Encourage the client to point the toes. Place the stocking over the toes and ease the stocking over the toes and onto the foot. Ensure that the stocking is smooth. *To prevent areas of constriction.*
14. **ACC** Center the client's heel in the heel of the stocking. *To ensure anatomical fit.*
15. **ACC** Pull the stocking over the client's calf until the stocking is fully extended and smooth. *To prevent interference with circulation.* Fit knee-length stockings 2.5 to 5 cm (1–2 inches) below the patella; fit thigh-length stockings 2.5 to 5 cm (1–2 inches) below the gluteal fold.

Removing Antiembolism Stockings

16. **ACC** To remove the stockings, grasp the top of the stocking with your thumb and fingers and gently pull down to the ankle. Then support the foot and ease the stocking over the foot.

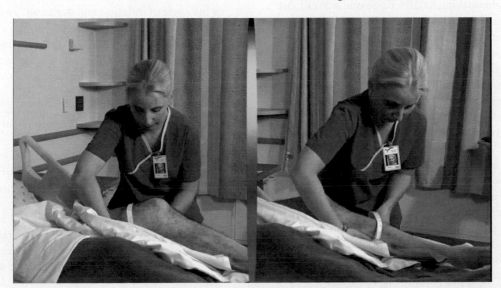

STEP 11 Use a tape measure to determine the appropriate stocking size.

17. **ACC** Stockings should be removed daily or according to facility policy. *To allow for inspecting the skin and bathing the legs.* (Note: After bathing the client's legs, make sure the legs are completely dry before reapplying stockings. Also, stockings should be laundered twice weekly or if visibly soiled and according to facility policy. They should be dried on a flat surface to prevent shrinkage or stretching.)

FINISHING THE SKILL

18. **CCC** Provide comfort. Assist the client with positioning.

19. **SAF** Ensure client safety. Place the bed in the lowest position. Ensure the client can identify and reach the nurse call system. *These safety measures reduce the risk of injury from falls.*
20. **INF** Remove gloves if worn and perform hand hygiene.
21. **EVAL** Evaluate outcomes.
22. **COM** Document date, time of application and/or removal of stockings, and how the client tolerated the procedure in the legal healthcare record.

■ SKILL 17.6 Managing Sequential Compression Devices

EQUIPMENT

Inflation pump
Connection tubing
Clean gloves
Compression sleeves

BEGINNING THE SKILL

1. **SAF** Review the order.
2. **INF** Perform hand hygiene.
3. **INF** Apply clean gloves, if there is a risk of exposure to body fluids.
4. **CCC** Introduce yourself to the client and family and explain the procedure and purpose of the SCD. Ensure that the client consents to the application of SCD.
5. **SAF** Identify the client using two identifiers.
6. **CCC** Provide privacy: close the door and pull the curtain.

PROCEDURE

7. **SAF** Set up an ergonomically safe space. Raise the bed to a comfortable working height. Raise one side rail. *Setting up an ergonomically safe space prevents injury to the nurse and client.*
8. **SAF** Set up a workspace according to your hand dominance (e.g., right-handed on the client's right side).
9. **ACC** Assess the client's skin condition and circulation to the legs, including pulses, skin color, temperature, and edema. *To establish a baseline assessment.*
10. **ACC** Apply antiembolism stockings first if ordered. (See Skill 17.5.)
11. **ACC** Unfold compression sleeve and place on the bed with the cotton lining facing up. *The cotton lining will be against the client's skin and prevent skin irritation.*
12. **SAF** Place the sleeve under the client's leg. For a thigh-length sleeve, place the opening at the popliteal space. *To prevent pressure.* For a knee-length sleeve, place the sleeve above the ankle. *Proper placement of the sleeve prevents injury with inflation of the device.*
13. **ACC** Secure the sleeve around the client's leg with Velcro fasteners. Allow two fingers to fit between the sleeve and the leg. *To allow an appropriate amount of compression.*

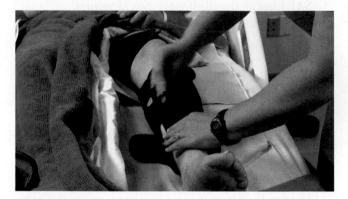

STEP 13 Secure sleeve around the client's leg with Velcro fasteners.

14. **ACC** Connect sleeve to the tubing.
15. **ACC** Set the inflation pump to the ordered pressure amount. Connect the pump to the electrical outlet and turn on the device.
16. **SAF** Monitor the sequential compression device through a full cycle of inflation and deflation. *To ensure proper inflation and deflation to prevent injury.*
17. **SAF** Assess the client's skin condition and circulation to the legs, including pulses, skin color, temperature, and edema. *To ensure proper circulation.*

FINISHING THE SKILL

18. **CCC** Provide comfort. Assist the client with positioning.
19. **SAF** Ensure client safety. Place the bed in the lowest position. Ensure that the client can identify and reach the nurse call system. *These safety measures reduce the risk of injury from falls.*
20. **INF** Remove gloves and perform hand hygiene.
21. **COM** Document date, time of application and/or removal of sequential compression devices, and how the client tolerated the procedure in the legal healthcare record.

■ SKILL 17.7 Managing Continuous Passive Motion

EQUIPMENT

Clean gloves, if there is a risk of exposure to body fluids
Continuous passive motion (CPM) device
Padding for the CPM
Tape measure

BEGINNING THE SKILL

1. **SAF** Review the order.
2. **INF** Perform hand hygiene.
3. **INF** Apply clean gloves if there is a risk of exposure to body fluids.
4. **CCC** Introduce yourself to the client and family and explain the procedure and purpose of the CPM. Ensure that the client consents to the use of CPM.
5. **SAF** Identify the client using two identifiers.
6. **CCC** Provide privacy: close the door and pull the curtain.

PROCEDURE

7. **SAF** Set up an ergonomically safe space. Raise the bed to a comfortable working height. Raise one side rail. *Setting up an ergonomically safe space prevents injury to the nurse and client.*
8. **SAF** Set up a workspace according to your hand dominance (e.g., right-handed on the client's right side).
9. **ACC** Measure the distance between the gluteal crease and the popliteal. *To adjust the length of the CPM and allow for correct placement of the joint.*
10. **ACC** Measure the distance from the knee to the end of the machine. *To adjust the footplate and maintain a neutral position.*
11. **SAF** Set up the device and test it prior to placing the client on the device. *To ensure client safety.*
12. **CCC** Assess the client's pain level using a facility-approved tool before and during the use of the device. The client may require pain medication prior to use. Encourage pain control to ensure compliance with the use of the device to promote healing of the joint and prevent the formation of scar tissue.
13. **CCC** Place appropriate padding on the device. *To prevent skin breakdown and promote comfort.*
14. **ACC** Position the client supine in the middle of the bed. *To ensure proper alignment.*
15. **ACC** Place the device on the bed next to the client.
16. **ACC** Place the affected extremity on the device, making sure the joint is at the joint of the CPM, and ensure a

neutral position. *To allow proper flexion of the knee with movement of the device.*

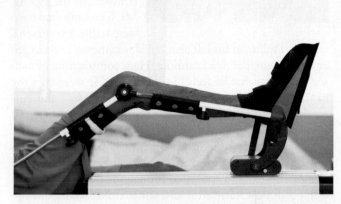

STEP 16 The knee is aligned at the hinge of the CPM.

17. **ACC** Apply the straps on the device around the client's leg, with two fingers fitting between the strap and the leg. *To allow space for the extremity to move and bend with the device.*
18. **ACC** Set the controls at the prescribed levels of flexion and extension. Adjust the controls per authorized healthcare provider order or facility protocol.
19. **EVAL** Turn the device on and monitor the client through the first flexion and extension cycle. *To ensure client safety and comfort.*
20. **CCC** Explain the start and stop button on the remote for the device. *Allow the client to keep the remote to stop the device if needed.*
21. **EVAL** Monitor the device per facility protocol.

FINISHING THE SKILL

22. **CCC** Provide comfort. Assist the client with positioning.
23. **SAF** Ensure client safety. Place the bed in the lowest position. Ensure that the client can identify and reach the nurse call system. *These safety measures reduce the risk of injury from falls.*
24. **INF** Remove gloves (if worn) and perform hand hygiene.
25. **COM** Document date, time of use of CPM, and how the client tolerated the procedure in the legal healthcare record.

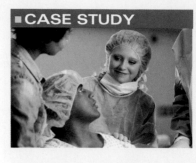

■ CASE STUDY

Mr. Johnson, a 52-year-old African-American male, presents to your medical-surgical unit from the PACU after a bowel resection (colectomy) for tumor removal. In the PACU, Mr. Johnson's vital signs were stable. He presents with an IV line in his left arm, a Foley catheter, and oxygen at 4 L/minute per nasal cannula. He is complaining of nausea and states that he feels like vomiting. He received 4 mg of morphine sulfate intravenously in the PACU and currently receives IV morphine via patient-controlled analgesia (PCA) with a demand dose of 1 mg every 15 minutes. Mr. Johnson's history, obtained preoperatively, reveals that he is a two-pack-per-day smoker. Prior to surgery, Mr. Johnson was prescribed and took two bronchodilators: a combination product of fluticasone and salmeterol (Advair) and albuterol as needed. Upon assessment, Mr. Johnson arouses when his name is called but dozes off easily. He is hesitant to turn, take deep breaths, or cough and reports that his pain is 6 on a 10-point scale. His respirations are 12 to14 breaths per minute, his heart rate is 82 beats per minute, and his blood pressure is 150/88. His skin is cool, and he has good capillary refill in all extremities. Mr. Johnson's oxygen saturation is 94%.

Case Study Questions

1. What priority nursing action will you take for Mr. Johnson immediately?
2. How can you address Mr. Johnson's complaint of nausea? What risk factors does he have for postoperative nausea and vomiting?
3. What other key nursing interventions will be important to implement over the next 24 hours of Mr. Johnson's care?
4. Why might Mr. Johnson arouse to his name but doze off easily?
5. As a result of Mr. Johnson's need for major abdominal surgery, he is at high risk for venous thromboembolism (VTE). What nursing interventions can you employ to prevent the occurrence of a VTE?
6. As Mr. Johnson recovers, what priority points will you include in his teaching plan?
7. **Application of QSEN Competencies:** One of the Quality and Safety Education for Nurses (QSEN) skills for Teamwork and Collaboration is to "Integrate the contributions of others who play a role in helping patient/family achieve health goals" (Cronenwett et al., 2007). How can the nurse facilitate the integration of other members of the healthcare team who may help Mr. Johnson achieve an improved health status?

■CONCEPT MAP

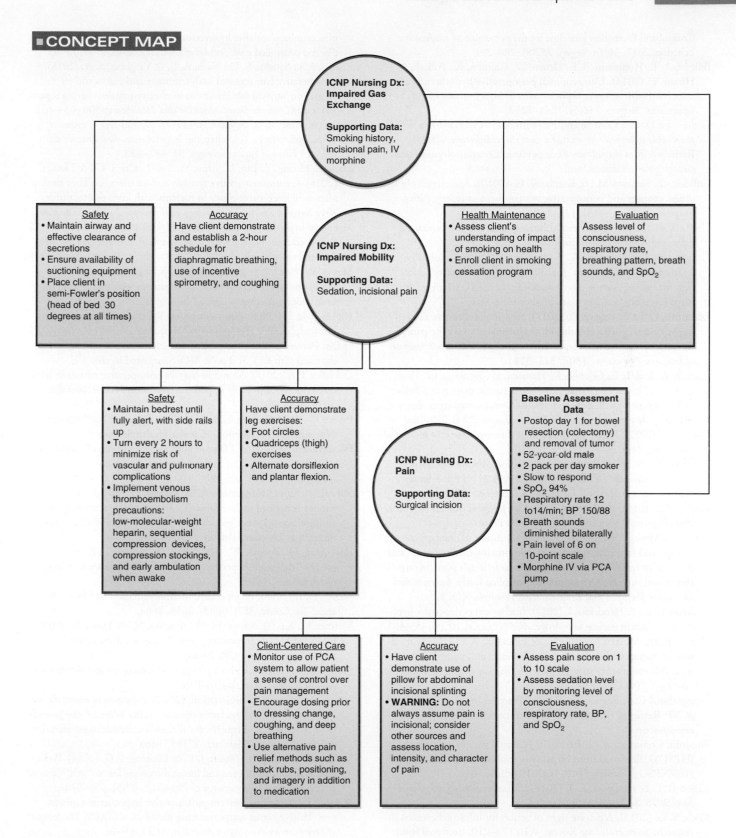

ICNP Nursing Dx: Impaired Gas Exchange

Supporting Data:
Smoking history, incisional pain, IV morphine

ICNP Nursing Dx: Impaired Mobility

Supporting Data:
Sedation, incisional pain

ICNP Nursing Dx: Pain

Supporting Data:
Surgical incision

Safety
- Maintain airway and effective clearance of secretions
- Ensure availability of suctioning equipment
- Place client in semi-Fowler's position (head of bed 30 degrees at all times)

Accuracy
Have client demonstrate and establish a 2-hour schedule for diaphragmatic breathing, use of incentive spirometry, and coughing

Health Maintenance
- Assess client's understanding of impact of smoking on health
- Enroll client in smoking cessation program

Evaluation
Assess level of consciousness, respiratory rate, breathing pattern, breath sounds, and SpO₂

Safety
- Maintain bedrest until fully alert, with side rails up
- Turn every 2 hours to minimize risk of vascular and pulmonary complications
- Implement venous thromboembolism precautions: low-molecular-weight heparin, sequential compression devices, compression stockings, and early ambulation when awake

Accuracy
Have client demonstrate leg exercises:
- Foot circles
- Quadriceps (thigh) exercises
- Alternate dorsiflexion and plantar flexion.

Baseline Assessment Data
- Postop day 1 for bowel resection (colectomy) and removal of tumor
- 52-year-old male
- 2 pack per day smoker
- Slow to respond
- SpO₂ 94%
- Respiratory rate 12 to14/min; BP 150/88
- Breath sounds diminished bilaterally
- Pain level of 6 on 10-point scale
- Morphine IV via PCA pump

Client-Centered Care
- Monitor use of PCA system to allow patient a sense of control over pain management
- Encourage dosing prior to dressing change, coughing, and deep breathing
- Use alternative pain relief methods such as back rubs, positioning, and imagery in addition to medication

Accuracy
- Have client demonstrate use of pillow for abdominal incisional splinting
- **WARNING:** Do not always assume pain is incisional; consider other sources and assess location, intensity, and character of pain

Evaluation
- Assess pain score on 1 to 10 scale
- Assess sedation level by monitoring level of consciousness, respiratory rate, BP, and SpO₂

References

Aldrete, J., & Kroulik, D. (1998). A post-anesthetic recovery score. *Anesthesia and Analgesia, 49*(6), 924–934.

Association of periOperative Registered Nurses (AORN). (2019a). *Guidelines for a safe environment of care. AORN guidelines for perioperative practice 2019.* Denver, CO: AORN, Inc.

Association of periOperative Registered Nurses (AORN). (2019b). *Guideline for prevention of venous thromboembolism: AORN guidelines for perioperative practice 2019.* Denver, CO: AORN, Inc.

Baird, M. S. (2016). *Manual of critical care nursing: Nursing interventions and collaborative management* (7th ed.). St. Louis, MO: Elsevier.

Berrios-Torres, S.I., Umscheid, C.A., Bratzler, D.W., Leas, B., Stone, E.C., Kelz, R.R., …. Schecter, W.P. (2017). Centers for Disease

Control and Prevention guideline for the prevention of surgical site infection, 2017. *JAMA Surgery, 152*(8), 784–791.

Billeter, A. T., Hohmann, S. F., Druen, D., Cannon, R., Polk, J., & Hiram, C. (2014). Unintentional perioperative hypothermia is associated with severe complications and high mortality in elective operations. *Surgery, 156*(5), 1245–1252.

Centers for Disease Control and Prevention. (2015). *Guideline for prevention of catheter-associated urinary tract infections (2009).* Retrieved from https://www.cdc.gov/infectioncontrol/guidelines/cauti/recommendations.html.

Colloca, G., Santoro, M., & Gambassi, G. (2010). Age-related physiologic changes and perioperative management of elderly patients. *Surgical Oncology, 19*(3), 124–130.

Cook, W. E. (2016). "Sign here:" Nursing value and the process of informed consent. *Plastic Surgical Nursing, 36*(4), 182.

Cronenwett, L., Sherwood, G., Barnsteiner, J., Disch, J., Johnson, J., Mitchell, P., … Warren, J. (2007). Quality and safety education for nurses. *Nursing Outlook, 55*(3), 122–131. Retrieved from http://qsen.org/competencies/pre-licensure-ksas/.

Edmiston, C. E., & Leaper, D. (2017). Should preoperative showering or cleansing with chlorhexidine gluconate (CHG) be part of the surgical care bundle to prevent surgical site infection? *Journal of Infection Prevention, 18*(6), 311–314.

Ekim, A. A., İnal, E. E., Gönüllü, E., Hamarat, H., Yorulmaz, G., Mumcu, G., … Orhan, H. (2016). Continuous passive motion in adhesive capsulitis patients with diabetes mellitus: A randomized controlled trial. *Journal of Back and Musculoskeletal Rehabilitation, 29*(4), 779–786.

Flowers, L. (2017). Nicotine replacement therapy. *American Journal of Psychiatry, 11*(6), 4–7.

Frandsen, G., & Smith Pennington, S. (2014). *Abrams' clinical drug therapy: Rationales for nursing practice* (10th ed.). Philadelphia: Wolters Kluwer Health/Lippincott Williams & Wilkins.

Galanti, G. (2014). *Caring for patients from different cultures* (4th ed.). Philadelphia: University of Pennsylvania Press.

Gbiri, C., Ajepe, T., & Akinbo, S. (2016). Efficacy of chest-physiotherapy and incentive-spirometry in improving cardiovascular and pulmonary functional performances in individuals post-thoraco-abdominal surgery: A randomised controlled study. *International Journal of Therapies and Rehabilitation Research, 5*(2), 1.

Giuliano, K. K., & Hendricks, J. (2017). Inadvertent perioperative hypothermia: Current nursing knowledge. *AORN Journal, 105*(5), 453–463.

Hofmann, D., Murray, C., Beck, J., & Homann, R. (2016). Acupressure in management of postoperative nausea and vomiting in high-risk ambulatory surgical patients. *Journal of PeriAnesthesia Nursing, 32*(4), 271–278.

International Classification for Nursing Practice. (n.d.). *eHealth & ICNP.* Retrieved from https://www.icn.ch/what-we-do/projects/ehealth-icnp.

The Joint Commission. (2019). 2019 National patient safety goals (NPSGS). Retrieved from https://www.jointcommission.org/assets/1/6/NPSG_Chapter_HAP_Jan2019.pdf.

Kizior, R. J., & Hodgson, K. J. (2018). *Saunders nursing drug handbook 2018.* St. Louis, MO: Elsevier.

Koch, V. G. (2015). A private right of action for informed consent in research. *Seton Hall Law Review, 4*(1), 174–210. Retrieved from http://scholarship.shu.edu/shlr/vol45/iss1/4.

Koyuncu, O., Leung, S., You, J., Oksar, M., Turhanoglu, S., Akkurt, C., & Turan, A. (2017). The effect of ondansetron on analgesic efficacy of acetaminophen after hysterectomy: A randomized double blinded placebo controlled trial. *Journal of Clinical Anesthesia, 40*, 78–83.

Kurien, J. S., Sansho, E. U., Nath, A. I., & Varghese, S. A. (2018). Pre-operative hair removal with trimmers and razors and its impact on surgical site infections in elective inguinal hernia repair. *Journal of Evidence Based Medicine and Healthcare, 5*(8), 654–658.

Lavand'homme, P., & Steyaert, A. (2017). Opioid-free anesthesia opioid side effects: Tolerance and hyperalgesia. *Best Practice & Research Clinical Anaesthesiology, 31*, 487–498.

Liao, C., Huang, Y., Lin, L., Chiu, Y., Tsai, J., Chen, C., & Liou, T. (2016). Continuous passive motion and its effects on knee flexion after total knee arthroplasty in patients with knee osteoarthritis. *Knee Surgery, Sports Traumatology, Arthroscopy, 24*(8), 2578–2586.

Malignant hyperthermia. (2017). *Harvard medical school health topics A-Z.* Retrieved from https://www.health.harvard.edu/a-toz/malignant-hyperthermia-a-to-z.

Massey, R. (2010). A randomized trial of rocking-chair motion on the effect of postoperative ileus duration in patients with cancer recovering from abdominal surgery. *Applied Nursing Research, 23*(2), 59–64.

Nightingale, F. (1992). *Notes on nursing: What it is and what it is not.* Philadelphia, PA: JB Lippincott Company.

Odom-Forren, J. (2018). *Drain's perianesthesia nursing: A critical care approach* (7th ed.). St. Louis, MO: Saunders Elsevier.

O'Malley, P. A. (2016). Aromatherapy for postoperative nausea in acute care-evidence and future opportunities. *Clinical Nurse Specialist, 30*(6), 318–320.

Pasero, C., & McCaffery, M. (2011). *Pain assessment and pharmacologic management* (E-book). Elsevier Health Sciences.

Pilevarzadeh, M. (2016). Effect of gum chewing in the reduction of paralytic ileus following cholecystectomy. *Biomedical & Pharmacology Journal, 9*(1), 405–409.

Rafati, M., Shiva, A., Ahmadi, A., & Habibi, O. (2014). Adherence to American society of health-system pharmacists surgical antibiotic prophylaxis guidelines in a teaching hospital. *Journal of Research in Pharmacy Practice, 3*(2), 62–66.

Rosenberg, H., Pollock, N., Schiemann, A., Bulger, T., & Stowell, K. (2015). Malignant hyperthermia: A review. *Orphanet Journal of Rare Diseases, 10*, 93.

Sessler, D. I. (2016). Perioperative thermoregulation and heat balance. *The Lancet, 387*(10038), 2655–2664.

Shirozu, K., Kai, T., Setoguchi, H., Ayagaki, N., & Hoka, S. (2018). Effects of forced air warming on airflow around the operating table. *Anesthesiology, 128*, 79–84.

Simmons, K. (2016). Authority to give informed consent for minors. *AORN Journal, 104*(2), P18–P19.

U.S. Food & Drug Administration. (2017). *Information about the use of forced air thermal regulating systems—Letter to health care providers.* Retrieved from https://www.fda.gov/medicaldevices/safety/letterstohealthcareproviders/ucm573837.htm.

Vather, R., O'Grady, G., Bissett, I. P., & Dinning, P. G. (2014). Postoperative ileus: mechanisms and future directions for research. *Clinical & Experimental Pharmacology & Physiology, 41*(5), 358–370.

Watson, J. (2018). Inadvertent postoperative hypothermia prevention: Passive versus active warming methods. *ACORN: The Journal of Perioperative Nursing in Australia, 31*(1), 43–46.

Wong, C., Sancha, C., & Gimenez, T. (2017). A national culture perspective in the efficacy of supply chain integration practices. *International Journal of Production Economics, 193*, 554–565.

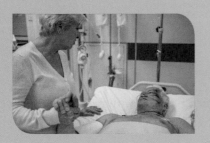

CHAPTER **18**

Advanced Respiratory Management

"Sometimes just breathing is enough." | **Marty Rubin, Author of *The Boiled Frog Syndrome***

SECTION 1 **Caring for a Client With Invasive Mechanical Ventilation**

- **SKILL 18.1** Caring for a Client Receiving Mechanical Ventilation

SECTION 2 **Caring for a Client Who Requires Arterial Blood Gas Sampling**

- **SKILL 18.2** Obtaining Arterial Blood Gases From a Peripheral Arterial Line
- **SKILL 18.3** Obtaining Arterial Blood Gases From the Radial Artery

SECTION 3 **Caring for a Client With a Chest Tube**

- **SKILL 18.4** Assisting With Chest Tube Insertion
- **SKILL 18.5** Maintaining a Chest Tube System and Performing an Occlusive Dressing Change
- **SKILL 18.6** Assisting With Removal of a Chest Tube

LEARNING OBJECTIVES

By the end of this chapter, the reader will be able to:

1. Identify measures to secure and maintain a patent airway when clients are receiving mechanical ventilation.
2. Describe the unique nursing needs of clients receiving mechanical ventilation.
3. Explain the commonly monitored ventilator settings.
4. Describe the nursing interventions for major complications of mechanical ventilation.
5. Demonstrate collecting an arterial blood gas sample from an arterial catheter.
6. Perform arterial puncture to obtain blood gas samples.
7. Identify components of arterial blood gas samples.
8. Identify client conditions that may require the placement of a chest tube.

9. Describe the impact of a pneumothorax on the respiratory system.
10. Identify and describe the three chambers contained in a chest drainage device.
11. Identify key elements of care when maintaining a closed chest tube drainage system.
12. Perform an occlusive dressing change at the chest tube insertion site.
13. Describe the role of the nurse assisting with the insertion of a chest tube.
14. Describe the role of the nurse assisting with the removal of a chest tube.
15. Describe critical factors when changing out a chest tube drainage system.

TERMINOLOGY

Acidosis A blood serum pH below 7.35.

Alkalosis A blood serum pH above 7.45.

Arterial waveform The form of an arterial pressure pulse or displacement wave.

Assist control A ventilator mode in which the client can trigger additional breaths.

Atelectasis An abnormal condition characterized by the collapse of alveoli, preventing the respiratory exchange of carbon dioxide and oxygen in a part of the lungs.

Bronchospasm An abnormal narrowing with partial obstruction of the lumen of the bronchi due to spasm of the peri-bronchial smooth muscle.

Continuous positive airway pressure Mechanical ventilation mode that does not administer any set tidal volume or respiratory rate. A minimum amount of air pressure (5 cm H_2O) provides resistance when the client is exhaling to prevent complete exhalation and collapse of the alveoli.

Controlled mechanical ventilation A ventilator mode in which minute ventilation is determined entirely by set respiratory rate and tidal volume. Does not require any work by the client.

Extubation. The process of withdrawing a tube from an orifice or cavity of the body.

Intermittent mandatory ventilation A ventilator mode in which the client is able to increase the breaths-per-minute ventilation by spontaneous breathing rather than client-initiated ventilator breaths.

Intubation Passage of a tube into a body aperture; specifically, the insertion of a breathing tube through the mouth or nose into the trachea to ensure a patent airway.

Synchronized intermittent mandatory ventilation Ventilator breaths are synchronized with the client's inspiratory effort.

Tidal volume The volume of air in a breath, either inspiration or expiration.

Trochar A sharply pointed surgical instrument contained in a cannula; used for aspiration or removal of fluids from cavities.

Pressure-support ventilation Low limited ventilation that delivers inspiratory pressure until inspiratory flow decreases to a predetermined percentage of peak value.

Ventilator-associated pneumonia A type of nosocomial pneumonia seen in clients on mechanical ventilation, caused by aspiration of secretions or stomach contents.

ACRONYMS

ABG Arterial blood gas

AC Assist control

BPS Behavioral Pain Scale

CMV Continuous mandatory ventilation

CCPOT Critical-Care Pain Observation Tool

CPAP Continuous positive airway pressure

EtCO$_2$ End tidal carbon dioxide concentration

ETT Endotracheal tube

ICUAW Intensive care unit–acquired weakness

IMV Intermittent mandatory ventilation

MDRPI Medical device–related pressure injury

NTT Nasotracheal tube

PEEP Peak end-expiratory pressure

PIP Peak inspiratory pressure

PSV Pressure support ventilation

PUD Peptic ulcer disease

SaO$_2$ Oxygen saturation

SIMV Synchronized intermittent mandatory ventilation

VAE Ventilator-associated event

VAP Ventilator-associated pneumonia

Inadequate oxygenation and gas exchange can be a life-threatening emergency (as discussed in Chapter 9). To supplement oxygenation, supplemental oxygen can be provided via nasal cannula, mask, or continuous positive airway pressure (CPAP); however, the client provides the ventilation.

When a client is not able to provide adequate ventilation despite supplemental oxygen or noninvasive ventilation using an orofacial/naso-facial mask and the positive airway pressure of CPAP, then the next level of support is invasive mechanical ventilation.

SECTION 1 Caring for a Client With Invasive Mechanical Ventilation

Mechanical ventilation is the process of using a ventilator to provide breaths that facilitate the transport of oxygen and carbon dioxide to and from the alveoli for the purpose of pulmonary gas exchange. Mechanical ventilation may either assist clients with breathing or replace spontaneous breathing. Clients require mechanical ventilation to protect the airway; improve pulmonary gas exchange; relieve respiratory distress; assist with healing of the airway, lungs, brain, or spinal cord; in surgery; or in drug-overdose situations (Baird, 2016). It can also decrease systemic or myocardial oxygen consumption and reduce intracranial pressure. Mechanical ventilation is typically delivered by an endotracheal tube or nasotracheal tube or via tracheostomy.

THE AIRWAY: ENDOTRACHEAL TUBES

Endotracheal tubes (ETTs) are flexible artificial airways used for short-term airway management. ETTs and nasotracheal tubes (NTTs) come in a variety of sizes based on the inner diameter of the tubing and may be cuffed or uncuffed (Fig. 18.1). ETTs range in size from 2 mm for a neonate to 9 mm for a large adult. The average ETT sizes for a woman are 7 to 7.5 mm, and those for a man are 8 to 9 mm. Cuffed ETTs are typically used for adults and children but not typically for neonates.

ETTs are inserted by authorized healthcare providers. Intubation is not within the scope of a registered nurse without special certification. Nurses assist with intubation and monitor the client during the procedure. Typically, an ETT is inserted orally using a laryngoscope, and then an oropharyngeal airway may also be inserted to prevent biting on the tube. Fig. 18.2 identifies the equipment to insert an ETT. Sometimes medical or anatomical situations may warrant an NTT, but it has a greater incidence of sinusitis (Baird, 2016). Intubation attempts should take only 15 to 20 seconds (American Association of Critical-Care Nurses [AACN], 2017). The nurse assists with client positioning and monitors the oxygenation status of the client. Pulse oximetry should be continuously monitored. Intubation is a frightening and stressful experience for the client. The nurse assesses the anxiety level and pain of the client, administers prescribed medications, and monitors the client's response.

Ensuring Placement

As soon as the ETT is placed, the nurse evaluates placement by listening for equal air movement bilaterally, observes for equal chest expansion with each breath, and monitors the client's oxygen saturation via pulse oximetry. In addition, the use of a colorimetric end-tidal CO_2 (EtCO$_2$) monitor allows for the measurement of carbon dioxide to further confirm ETT placement in the trachea (Fig. 18.3).

Confirmation of accurate ETT placement is made with an x-ray ordered by the authorized healthcare provider. The distal tip of the ETT should rest approximately 2 to 4 cm (0.75–1.5 inches) above the carina for adults (AACN, 2017). ETTs have radiopaque markers along the length of the tube to provide the clinician with depth measurements. Once the correct placement of the ETT has been confirmed by x-ray, the nurse should secure the tube and note the position of the tube marking relative to the client's teeth or gums. The entrance to the naris is used for an NTT (e.g., 30 cm at entrance to right naris). The size of the ETT or NTT should also be documented. The nurse continues to monitor the placement of the ETT as long the client is intubated. Unintended extubation is a risk, and the nurse takes safety measures to reduce that risk, especially during ETT securement and client positioning.

Securing and Stabilizing the Endotracheal Tube

There are a number of devices and methods for securing an ETT, which include commercial tube holders or the more traditional use of twill tape or standard adhesive tape. Fig. 18.4 shows a commercial securement device and the traditional use of tape to secure an ETT. Nurses sometimes use foam dressing or hydrocolloid membrane on clients' cheeks to help prevent skin breakdown. Commercial tube holders are generally more comfortable for clients and more secure if the tube requires manipulation (AACN, 2017). However, commercial devices are also a potential source of pressure

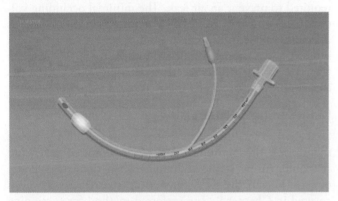

FIG. 18.1 Cuffed endotracheal tube.

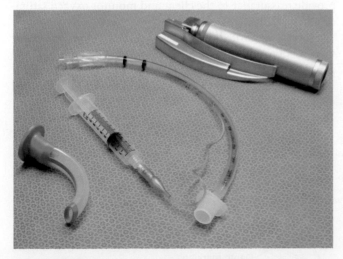

FIG. 18.2 Equipment to insert an endotracheal tube (ETT). *Left* to *right:* oropharyngeal airway (bite block), 10-mL syringe to inflate the cuff, cuffed ETT, and laryngoscope.

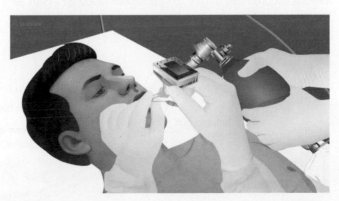

FIG. 18.3 Use of a colorimetric end-tidal CO_2 monitor further confirms endotracheal tube (ETT) placement in the trachea.

injury. Medical device–related pressure injuries (MDRPIs) are localized injuries to the skin or mucous membranes as a result of pressure from a device. Critically ill clients in the intensive care unit (ICU) have several risk factors for pressure injury, including altered level of consciousness, impaired sensation, nutritional compromise, diminished tissue perfusion, and potential use of vasoactive medications (Hampson et al., 2018). Studies have found that ETTs and their means of securement are a significant source of MDRPIs (Hanonu & Karadag, 2016). A strategy to reduce the risk of the ETT causing an MDRPI is to change the ETT position at least every 2 hours (Hollister Education, n.d.). Healthcare facilities may have protocols related to how many and which level of providers are required to reposition the ETT using a commercial tube holder or retape the ETT using a traditional tape method. One risk related to frequent repositioning is the possibility of accidental extubation. The critical element

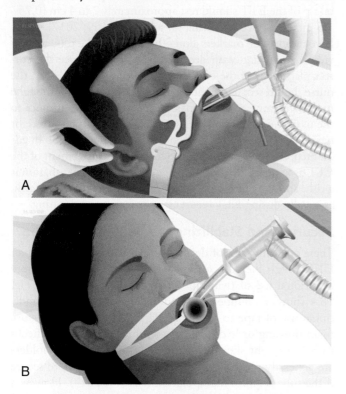

FIG. 18.4 A, Endotracheal tube (ETT) secured with a commercial securement device. B, Traditional taped ETT with an oral airway serving as a bite block.

is protecting the client's airway. Nurses should frequently assess the lips and skin underneath mechanical devices, particularly on the cheeks and back of the neck, to determine if skin breakdown is present (Hampson et al., 2018).

Cuffed Endotracheal Tubes

The distal end of a cuffed tube has an inflatable balloon, or cuff, surrounding the outer cannula. The ETT cuff seals the airway to prevent the gases injected by mechanical ventilation from escaping and to prevent secretions from entering the trachea. Once the ETT is inserted, the cuff is inflated by attaching an air-filled 10-mL syringe to the distal end of the inflating tube at the pilot balloon and instilling the air. Fig. 18.5 identifies the components of the cuffed ETT. The cuff pressure is measured using a cuff manometer (Fig. 18.6). Cuff pressures are generally maintained between 20 and 25 cm H_2O mm Hg but are dependent on the outer diameter of the ETT and the size of the client's airway. Cuff pressures are measured on a routine basis. Frequent monitoring of cuff inflation should occur because overinflation of the cuff can cause damage to the tracheal mucosa. Underinflation allows an audible air leak around the cuff. Two different but similar techniques are used to determine the minimum cuff pressure required to prevent an air leak. The minimal occluding volume (MOV) is determined by listening over the trachea as the cuff is inflated and stopping at the point when no air leak is heard. If the trachea is sealed, the client is not able to speak (Fig. 18.7). The minimal leak technique (MLT) decreases the cuff pressure until a faint leak is heard (Mondor, 2017a).

Maintaining a Patent Airway

Strategies to maintain the patency of the ETT include monitoring the humidification of the inspired gases and suctioning using sterile technique when there is evidence of secretions in the ETT. Suctioning an artificial airway is covered in Chapter 9. The preferred method for suctioning when the client is on mechanical ventilation is the closed method (see Skill 9.13). During the suctioning procedure, provide reassurance to the client and monitor oxygen saturation before, during, and after the procedure.

Nurses, authorized healthcare providers, and respiratory therapists provide collaborative care to maintain a secure and patent airway in the management of clients with an ETT. Unexpected extubation or compromise of the ETT tube caused

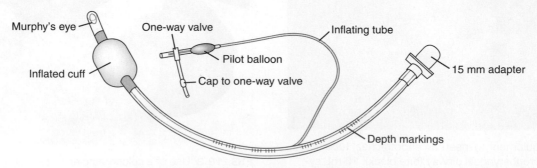

FIG. 18.5 Cuffed endotracheal tube with adapter, inflating tube and pilot balloon, depth markings, inflated cuff, and Murphy eye.

by a client's condition can lead to airway trauma, hypoxia, and death (Lizarondo, 2017). Vigilance by nurses and other healthcare providers requires a team approach, as Box 18.1 illustrates.

PROVIDING MECHANICAL VENTILATION

There are essentially two ways that mechanical ventilators can give a breath. One gives a breath measured by the volume of air in each breath, called volume-controlled (VC) mechanical ventilation. The other gives a breath based on the pressure of airflow; this is called pressure-controlled (PC) ventilation. In years past, adults were usually placed on VC mechanical ventilation, whereas children and infants were placed on PC mechanical ventilation. Today, PC is increasingly used for both adult and pediatric populations (Rittayamai et al., 2015). In

addition, ventilators can be set for different levels of ventilator support. The maximum level of support is controlled mandatory ventilation (CMV), which provides a set number of breaths per minute and requires no respiratory effort from the client. The assist-control (AC) mode provides a set number of breaths and also supports breaths that are triggered by the client. The intermittent mandatory ventilation mode (IMV) provides a minimum number of breaths per minute and allows the client to increase the number of breaths per minute by spontaneous breathing rather than client-initiated ventilator breaths (Rittayamai et al., 2015). A much lower level of support is synchronized intermittent mandatory ventilation (SIMV), in which ventilator breaths are synchronized with client inspiratory effort (Seckel & Bucher, 2017). Both PC and VC ventilators can give breaths that are client initiated or timed. The selected mode is determined by the authorized healthcare provider and is initiated based on the client's needs and the ventilators and protocols available within a clinical setting.

Mechanical Ventilation Settings

Mechanical ventilators, regardless of whether they are PC or VC, will have some of the same settings. Settings include the following:

- Respiratory rate—number of breaths per minute delivered by the ventilator
- Fraction of inspired oxygen (FiO_2)—may range from 21% (room air) to 100%
- Sensitivity—determines the amount of effort the client must generate to initiate a ventilator breath
- Pressure support (PS)—positive-pressure setting used to assist the client's inspiratory pressure

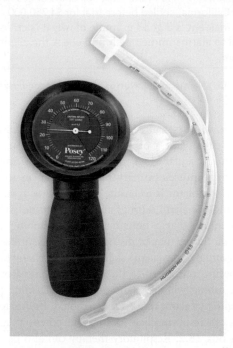

FIG. 18.6 Handheld cuff manometer to measure cuff pressure.

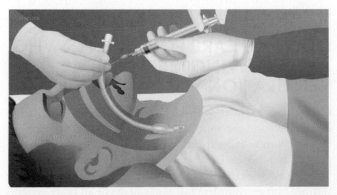

FIG. 18.7 The cuff is inflated, stopping at the point when no air leak is heard. This is the minimal occluding volume (MOV).

BOX 18.1 Lessons From Experience: Emergency Airway Management During Seizure

Ms. Crain is a 38-year-old female with a history of multiple sclerosis admitted to a critical care unit secondary to a decreased level of consciousness (LOC). She is intubated and on mechanical ventilation, and she is being treated for electrolyte imbalances. The nurse is providing oral care when Ms. Crain begins having a seizure in which she clenches her teeth on the endotracheal tube and is unable to be oxygenated via the ventilator. The seizure lasts for approximately 3½ minutes and requires the nurse and respiratory therapist to work together to oxygenate the client. The respiratory therapist deflates the endotracheal cuff and provides ventilation using a bag-mask device to oxygenate the client. A second nurse works to secure the bite block and insert an oral airway in order to allow the client to be reattached to the ventilator. Ms. Cain's oxygenation status remains above 90% during the seizure, and there are no apparent problems related to hypoxia. The rapid response by the respiratory therapist in deflating the cuff and providing oxygen via the bag-mask device allowed the client to receive sufficient oxygen to prevent an anoxic injury. The collaborative and timely efforts between the nurses and the respiratory therapist prevented more serious problems from occurring for Ms. Cain.

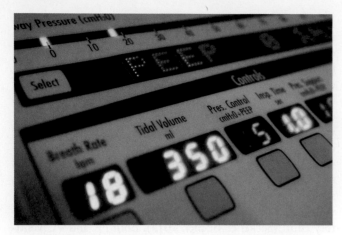

FIG. 18.8 Control panel on a mechanical ventilator.

- High-pressure limit—regulates the maximum pressure the ventilator can generate to deliver the tidal volume

For both PC and VC ventilators, time is an important factor when giving mechanical breaths. The inspiratory time (T_i) is the time it takes to give the breath, and the expiratory time (T_e) is the time allotted for expiration. The i:e ratio is a fraction that reflects the inspiratory time/expiratory time. This is very important at fast respiratory rates. There must be enough time for the air to exhale, or the air pressure will increase, like blowing up a balloon. Both VC and PC ventilators have high-pressure alarms (Baird, 2016).

For PC ventilators, there are three important pressures for the nurse to monitor:
- Mean airway pressure (MAP)
- Peak inspiratory pressure (PIP)—maximum pressure during inspiration, set on the ventilator
- Positive end-expiratory pressure (PEEP)—positive pressure applied at the end of expiration of ventilator breaths
VC ventilators give a preset volume for each breath. For VC ventilators, airway pressure is a dependent variable, and the settings to monitor include the following:
- Inspiratory flow rate—speed at which the tidal volume is delivered
- Tidal volume (V_t)—volume of gas delivered to client during each ventilator breath
- Peak inspiratory flow rate

These settings are individualized to the client's needs, and the authorized healthcare provider makes changes related to the current blood gas analysis and response to current ventilator settings. A written order for ventilator settings is required (Fig. 18.8).

Capnography

Capnography is an additional setting that may be monitored. It is the $EtCO_2$ concentration measured at the end of expiration. The waveform, or capnogram, shows the levels of CO_2 during the respiratory cycle. Clients who may need this type of monitoring include those who have acute airway obstruction or apnea, hypercapnia, or hyperthermia. Capnography monitoring may also be indicated for clients who are receiving opioids or other types of narcotics that increase the risk of sedation and respiratory depression (see Chapter 7). The

---

BOX 18.2 Lessons From the Courtroom: Alarms Sound in the ICU, Nurse Does Not Respond, Hypoxic Brain Injury Results

A 22-year-old client experienced a traumatic brain injury as a result of a fall from a moving vehicle. He had become somewhat responsive but was on a ventilator, with both arms and hands in restraints. The family was asked to leave the room during shift report. They were not allowed back into the room when the new nurse's shift began. The nurse assigned to the client was busy in another nearby room for a considerable amount of time. The 22-year-old client's airway became obstructed, and an alarm sounded when his oxygen saturation dropped. The cardiac monitor showed bradycardia and eventually asystole, which sounded additional alarms. When the situation was noticed, a code was called, and the client was resuscitated. However, he had already experienced significant, permanent, hypoxic brain damage. The lawsuit, filed in the Superior Court of Los Angeles County, California, settled before trial for $4,750,000.

This incident is a good example of why it is critical to respond to alarms immediately and check the client without delay.

Reference: ICU: Alarms Sound, Nurse Does Not Respond, Hypoxic Brain Injury Results, 2009.

$EtCO_2$ allows nurses and other healthcare professionals to assess the effectiveness of mechanical ventilation interventions, neuromuscular blockades, and prone positioning.

One of the nurse's primary responsibilities in managing a mechanical ventilator is to ensure the ventilator is functioning properly and the alarm settings are on at all times. The alarms signal the nurse that a potentially life-threatening condition exists; circuit tubing may be disconnected, the ventilator may be malfunctioning, or the client's status may have changed. A rapid, system-specific assessment of the client, the ventilator, and the ventilator tubing will allow the nurse to determine the problem. A ventilator alarm must not be ignored. Failure to respond to alarms can result in client deaths and potential lawsuits, as shown in Box 18.2. Respiratory therapy can also be alerted to assist in the identification of the problem that is causing the alarm. If the problem persists and the cause cannot be immediately identified, the client may need to be disconnected from the ventilator and given breaths with a manual resuscitation bag. For a list of complications that trigger alarms, see Box 18.3.

NURSING CARE FOR CLIENTS WHO ARE RECEIVING MECHANICAL VENTILATION

Caring for a client who requires mechanical ventilation extends beyond the ventilator, its circuitry, and the artificial airway. Nurses expand care to think holistically about the person and his or her family, including emotional needs. Nurses provide client-centered care even in the critical care setting. Nurses complete full assessments of all body systems with an understanding of the impact of mechanical ventilation, manage additional equipment the client requires, and

BOX 18.3 Ventilator Alarms

LOW-PRESSURE ALARMS
- Ventilator tubing disconnected from endotracheal tube
  - Intervention: Reconnect tubing to endotracheal tube.
- Endotracheal tube displaced or extubated
  - Intervention: Check tube placement. Replace if appropriate.
  - Intervention: Manually ventilate client with Ambu bag if extubated.
  - Intervention: Contact healthcare provider immediately.
- Underinflated or damaged cuff
  - Intervention: Attempt to reinflate. Use manometer to determine appropriate inflation pressure.
  - Intervention: If unable to inflate, contact the authorized healthcare provider immediately because the client may require reintubation.
- Leak in ventilator circuitry
  - Intervention: Reconnect loose circuitry. Assess for holes or malfunction.
- Ventilator malfunction
  - Intervention: Manually ventilate client with Ambu bag.
  - Intervention: Secure another ventilator.

HIGH-PRESSURE ALARMS
- Increased airway pressure, decreased lung compliance, chest wall resistance
  - Intervention: Assess lung sounds, pain, and position.
  - Intervention: Administer analgesics if appropriate.
  - Intervention: Reposition and reassess lung sounds.
  - Intervention: Call the authorized healthcare provider if no improvement.
- Secretions in airway; potential for mucus plug
  - Intervention: Suction if appropriate. Encourage the client to cough if appropriate.
  - Intervention: Call the authorized healthcare provider if unable to remove secretions.
- Condensation in circuitry
  - Intervention: Remove fluid from tubing.
- Client biting endotracheal tube, coughing, gagging, or agitated
  - Intervention: Insert bite block if needed.
  - Intervention: Check patency and accuracy of position of endotracheal tube.
  - Intervention: Provide education to the client if anxious. Administer prescribed medication if indicated.
- Bronchospasm
  - Intervention: Assess the client for cause. Contact the authorized healthcare provider. Provide treatment as ordered.

Adapted from Baird, 2016; Mora Carpio & Mora, 2018.

implement protocols to reduce the risk for serious complications from mechanical ventilation.

Impaired Communication

Clients who are intubated cannot verbally communicate their needs. Furthermore, many clients are sedated when receiving mechanical ventilation. The trend today is less and lighter sedation, which allows the nurse more opportunities for communication. Developing alternative communication strategies can help alleviate some of the client's and family's fears, reduce feelings of frustration, and allow the client to participate in his or her care. However, fatigue, physical strength, and cognitive impairment, such as delirium, have a profound impact on the client's ability to communicate as well (Holm & Dreyer, 2018). Frequently used tools to assist with communication include providing a communication board (Fig. 18.9), providing pencil and paper for written communication, or running through a list of likely issues phrased as yes-or-no questions with a predetermined means of response (e.g., thumbs-up or thumbs-down, one blink or two, or simple head nods). A study with nonsedated clients emphasized that continuous information about the ETT, the temporary nature of their voicelessness, and the purpose of mechanical ventilation was essential to reduce anxiety and enhance a sense of security. Despite the lack of sedation, these clients are very ill and may have poor memory and/or comprehension of what they were told. Communication in the ICU requires the nurse to be alert to the changing needs and communication abilities of the client (Holm & Dreyer, 2018).

The goal of nursing care for the client who requires mechanical ventilation is to monitor the client's response to ventilator support and reduce the risk of complications. Physiologic and psychosocial nursing care interventions are imperative for clients who are ventilated. The Society of Critical Care Medicine published 2018 clinical practice guidelines for the prevention and management of pain, agitation/sedation, delirium, immobility, and sleep disruption in adult clients, referred to as the PADIS guidelines (Devlin et al., 2018). For each of these, communication with the client and family and collaboration with the healthcare team is critical for improving client outcomes.

Pain

Typically, critically ill adults on mechanical ventilation do experience pain, both during rest and during procedures. Pain management is complicated by difficulties with self-report. Validated behavioral pain scales, including the Behavioral Pain Scale (BPS) and the Critical-Care Pain Observation Tool (CCPOT), are recommended for their validity and reliability. Opioids, nonopioid analgesics (including acetaminophen, ketamine, and nonsteroidal antiinflammatory drugs [NSAIDs]), local anesthetics, and nonpharmacologic strategies may all be applied in a "multimodal analgesia" approach to bring pain relief (Devlin et al., 2018). For more information about pain management and nonpharmacologic comfort strategies, refer to Chapter 7.

Agitation/Sedation

Nurses monitor the degree of sedation when caring for a client on mechanical ventilation. Light levels of sedation facilitate spontaneous breathing and early mobilization and are therefore associated with improved outcomes. Nurse-targeted sedation is when nurses at the bedside implement an established sedation protocol and titrate medication to

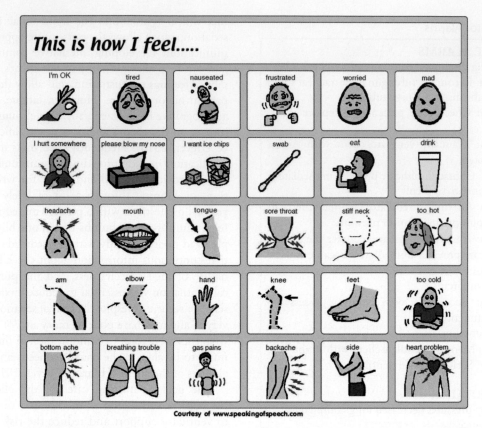

FIG. 18.9 Example of a communication board for clients in the intensive care unit (ICU).

achieve targeted sedation scores on an established sedation assessment tool. Nonbenzodiazepine sedatives are preferable to benzodiazepine sedatives (Devlin et al., 2018).

Delirium

Delirium is defined as an acute change in consciousness that is accompanied by inattention and either a change in cognition or perceptual disturbance. There may be hyperactive delirium, which is marked by agitation, attempting to remove invasive equipment, and/or emotional lability. There may also be the other end of the spectrum: hypoactive delirium, which is marked by withdrawal, apathy, and/or decreased responsiveness. It is a common problem in the ICU, affecting up to 80% of ICU residents. It is associated with increased length of stay and poor clinical outcomes. Assessment for delirium using a valid tool should be a part of ICU care. (Devlin et al., 2018). Nurses can intervene to minimize clients' risk of delirium by utilizing delirium assessment tools adopted by ICUs, such as the Intensive Care Delirium Screening Checklist (ICDSC). Nurses review the client's medications for those that may cause delirium, such as benzodiazepines. Box 18.4 relates the unexpected actions of a client at risk for delirium.

Implementing daily awakening trials and encouraging early progressive mobility and exercise decrease the risk of delirium. Multi-intervention approaches, such as the ABCDEF Bundle of care described in Box 18.5, have been

BOX 18.4 Expect the Unexpected: Unplanned Extubation

Mr. Talbott is a 76-year-old male with a history of emphysema and chronic obstructive pulmonary disease (COPD) who had a small bowel resection secondary to a paralytic ileus 2 days ago. He is intubated with a 7.0 endotracheal tube (ETT) taped at his left lip at a depth of 25 cm. His wife has been at his side all day, but she has gone home to rest. He has been calm and cooperative while she was present. He has not required sedation or restraints but is receiving pain medication every 4 hours. It is now 9:00 PM, and the nurse caring for Mr. Talbott assessed him at 8:00 PM. She is preparing 9:00 PM medications. She hears a ventilator alarm and asks a fellow nurse to check because she has removed narcotics and cannot leave them unattended. The nurse in Mr. Talbott's room immediately calls for assistance, and his assigned nurse responds. Mr. Talbott has his hands tightly on his ETT and is about to extubate himself. Both nurses work together to keep the ETT in place and talk to Mr. Talbott calmly and quietly in an effort to reorient him to the environment and explain his situation. They recognize that the use of pain medications, the potential for delirium, and the anxiety of being intubated on a ventilator all contribute to the potential for extubation. The nurses' quick response to a ventilator alarm and calm presence in a potentially dangerous situation prevent a serious complication of unplanned extubation.

BOX 18.5 ABCDEF Bundle

Use the ABCDEF Bundle developed at Vanderbilt University Medical Center:

A is for assess, prevent, and manage pain.
B is for both spontaneous awakening trial and spontaneous breathing trial.
C is for choice of analgesia and sedation.
D is for delirium monitoring and management.
E is for early progressive mobilization and ambulation.
F is for family engagement and empowerment.

Reference: Marra, Lay, Pandharipande, & Patel, 2017.

shown to result in significantly less delirium (Devlin et al., 2018). If delirium is identified, the nurse's primary responsibility is to keep the client safe.

Immobility

Implementing rehabilitation and early mobilization of critically ill adults is recommended. Prolonged bedrest and mechanical ventilation commonly result in weakness, to the extent that the term *intensive care unit–acquired weakness* (ICUAW) has been identified. Studies have found that survivors of critical illnesses may continue to have functional, physical, cognitive, and/or psychological disabilities that persist for years after discharge (Arias-Fernandez, Romero-Martin, Gomez-Salgado, & Fernandez-Garcia, 2018). ICUAW is associated with many problems, including the development of pressure injuries, pneumonia and atelectasis, joint contractures, and thromboembolism. These complications lead to longer lengths of stay and the potential for poor outcomes related to deconditioning, weight loss, and significant functional limitations (Arias-Fernandez et al., 2018). Early mobilization and rehabilitation are strategies to prevent ICUAW, and they have the additional benefit of reducing delirium (Delvin et al., 2018). Rehabilitation and early mobilization are a new area of evidence research, and the body of evidence is evolving rapidly; nevertheless, the evidence supports the positive increase in strength, mobility, and quality of life; less time on mechanical ventilation; and a higher probability of discharge to home. Getting critically ill clients moving requires a multidisciplinary team of physical therapists, respiratory therapists, and nurses to manage the client's needs.

Sleep

Sleep is the final factor identified in the new guidelines. Sleep disruption is very common in the ICU and is thought to contribute to ICU delirium, longer duration of mechanical ventilation, impaired immune function, and neurocognitive dysfunction. Studies suggest a relationship between the quantity of rapid eye movement (REM) sleep and delirium (Delvin et al., 2018). When clients are mechanically ventilated, their sleep duration is lower than normal, and sleep fragmentation is higher. Several studies identify the relationship between sleep deprivation and mental status changes, including delirium; what remains unknown is if poor sleep is a cause for delirium (Delvin et al., 2018).

REDUCING THE RISK OF COMPLICATIONS OF MECHANICAL VENTILATION

Nurses have the potential to reduce complications by using evidence-based, facility-approved protocols. Mechanical ventilation has several potential complications, including:

- aspiration
- ventilator-associated pneumonia (VAP)
- peptic ulcer disease (PUD)
- gastrointestinal bleeding
- venous thromboembolic events
- difficulty managing secretions.

Reducing the Risk of Aspiration

Aspiration is a risk when a client has an ETT and is receiving mechanical ventilation, even with a cuffed endotracheal tube. The presence of an oral ETT increases salivation. The ETT passes through the epiglottis, preventing it from closing and forming an effective seal. Aspiration can occur from an accumulation of pooled secretions above the ETT cuff. Deflation or manipulation of the cuff may allow these pooled secretions to enter the trachea. Sometimes called a microaspiration, these sections are full of microorganisms and may result in pneumonia. Strategies to prevent aspiration include using an ETT with a means of suctioning secretions just above the cuff and suctioning prior to deflating the cuff or repositioning the ETT (McBeth, Montes, Powne, North, & Natale, 2018).

Clients who are critically ill have an increased risk not only for microaspiration but also for aspiration of regurgitated gastric contents. This presents a dilemma because nutrition is essential for healing, yet those who are receiving enteral feedings are at greater risk. Nurses monitor enteral feeding tube placement per facility protocols in an effort to reduce this risk. Evidence suggests that the following interventions can reduce the risk for aspiration in clients who are mechanically ventilated:

- Maintain the head of the bed (HOB) at 30 to 45 degrees unless medically contraindicated.
- For clients at high risk of aspiration, use a continuous feeding method.
- Consider postpyloric placement of a feeding tube.
- Monitor physical symptoms of difficulty with tolerating feedings or digestion, such as distension or passing of stool or gas.
- Ask about the use of prokinetic agents to reduce opiate-induced changes in motility (Baird, 2016).

For more on reducing the risk of aspiration, see the discussion of gastrointestinal therapy in Chapter 5.

Ventilator-Associated Pneumonia

When clients contract pneumonia after receiving mechanical ventilation for a minimum of 48 hours, it is identified as

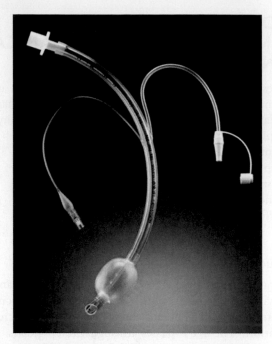

FIG. 18.10 Endotracheal (ETT) tube with subglottic secretion drainage port.

ventilator-associated pneumonia (VAP). Specific equipment and nursing care strategies can significantly reduce the risk of VAP. As discussed previously, microaspiration of the endogenous flora of oropharyngeal secretions around the endotracheal tube cuff increases the risk for VAP. Evidence suggests that the use of ETTs with subglottic secretion drainage ports when clients are likely to be intubated for more than 48 to 72 hours can reduce the incidence of VAP (Klompas et al., 2014). Fig. 18.10 shows an ETT with subglottic secretion drainage. Mortality due to VAP is estimated to be between 9% and 13% (Health Research & Educational Trust [HRET], 2017). Elevating the HOB 30 to 45 degrees decreases the risk of aspiration. Oral hygiene with 0.12% oral chlorhexidine is also an intervention in the prevention of VAP (Institute for Healthcare Improvement [IHI], 2017). Although the evidence is mixed, the logic is sound that the use of a toothbrush and providing good oral care along with careful oral suctioning reduces the bacteria in the oral cavity (AACN, 2017).

When healthcare facilities implement care bundles, like the one described later in this chapter for ventilated clients, the reduction in VAP and improved client outcomes surpass the individual percentage of improvement expected from the evidence related to each individual care item. It is surmised that the coordinated, team-centered approach has positive synergistic impacts on care.

Peptic Ulcer Disease Prophylaxis

Clients receiving mechanical ventilation are at an increased risk for stress ulcers and, as a result, subsequent gastrointestinal bleeding. Medications such as histamine 2 blockers and proton-pump inhibitors are frequently prescribed. Including pharmacy and making PUD prophylactic medication routine are suggested best practices for preventing this complication.

Bundles

The IHI (2017) recommends five interventions to improve the care of ventilated clients and prevent ventilator-associated events (VAEs).

1. Elevate the HOB between 30 and 45 degrees. Elevating the HOB may reduce the potential for microaspiration of gastric contents.
2. Provide PUD prophylaxis if not contraindicated. Although the use of peptic ulcer prophylaxis may increase the incidence of nosocomial pneumonia, the potential for a gastrointestinal bleed may be far more serious.
3. Provide deep venous thrombosis prophylaxis. Clients on ventilators have multiple risk factors for deep vein thrombosis, including immobility and sedation. Sequential compression devices (SCDs), antiembolic stockings, and compression boots can be used if medications cannot be utilized. Application of SCDs and antiembolism stockings is described in Chapter 17.
4. Provide daily sedative interruption and daily assessment of readiness to extubate. Interruption of sedation has demonstrated decreased mechanical ventilation days, decreased complications, and a decreased number of days in critical care.
5. Provide daily oral care. Use an oral chlorhexidine gluconate (0.12%) rinse twice daily. Moisturizer can be applied to the oral mucosa and lips every 2 to 4 hours. Good oral hygiene serves to reduce oral mucosa flora that could result in upper respiratory tract bacterial colonization.

APPLICATION OF THE NURSING PROCESS

Examples of Related International Classification for Nursing Practice (ICNP) Nursing Diagnoses, Expected Client Outcomes, and Nursing Interventions:

Nursing Diagnosis: Impaired breathing
Supporting Data: Client requires mechanical ventilation.
Expected Client Outcomes: Client will:
- maintain arterial blood gases within established parameters
- remain free of dyspnea or restlessness
- effectively maintain a patent airway
- effectively mobilize secretions
- maintain a respiratory rate within established parameters and ventilator settings.
Nursing Intervention Example: Ensure the ventilator is functioning properly and the alarm settings are on at all times.

Nursing Diagnosis: Risk for delirium
Expected Client Outcomes: Client will:
- be free of injury throughout hospitalization
- be able to demonstrate orientation to person, time, place, and situation.
Nursing Intervention Example: Assess for delirium each shift.
Reference: International Classification for Nursing Practice. (n.d.). *eHealth & ICNP.* Retrieved from https://www.icn.ch/what-we-do/projects/ehealth-icnp.

CRITICAL CONCEPTS
Caring for a Client With Invasive Mechanical Ventilation

Accuracy (ACC)

Accuracy when caring for a client with an ETT on mechanical ventilation is affected by the following variables:

Client-Related Factors
- Ability to communicate with the healthcare team
- Level of anxiety, level of consciousness, sedation, or delirium

Nurse-Related Factors
- Maintaining and securing client's airway in the appropriate position
- Maintaining appropriate depth of endotracheal tube
- Appropriate cuff inflation
- Proper assessment of lungs sounds and the need for suctioning client

Equipment-Related Factors
- Ventilator and alarm settings per written orders
- Proper calibration of equipment
- Maintaining ventilator circuit tubing

Client-Centered Care (CCC)

When caring for a client receiving mechanical ventilation, respect for the client includes:
- obtaining consent for procedures and promoting autonomy
- explaining the procedure and arranging for an interpreter if needed
- providing privacy and ensuring comfort
- answering questions that the client or family may have
- advocating for the client and family.

Infection Control (INF)

Healthcare-associated infection can be prevented when caring for a client with an ETT on mechanical ventilation by:

- containment of microorganisms
- preventing and reducing the transfer of microorganisms
- reducing the number of microorganisms.

Safety (SAF)

Safety measures for clients with an ETT or NTT on mechanical ventilation prevent harm and provide a safe care environment by:
- verifying that the ventilator alarms are on at all times
- ensuring that airway devices are patent and secured at all times.

Communication (COM)

- Communication exchanges information (oral, written, nonverbal, electronic) between two or more people.
- Documentation records information in a permanent legal record.
- Collaborating with the client and other healthcare professionals is essential when caring for the client receiving mechanical ventilation.

Health Maintenance (HLTH)

Nursing is dedicated to the promotion of health when caring for a client with an ETT on mechanical ventilation by:
- protecting the client's oral mucosa during and after suctioning
- protecting the client's skin and mucous membranes from ETT securement devices and ventilator tubing
- protecting the client's sleep from interruption.

Evaluation (EVAL)

Evaluation of the outcomes allows the nurse to determine the efficacy of the care provided when caring for clients receiving mechanical ventilation.

■ SKILL 18.1 Caring for a Client Receiving Mechanical Ventilation

EQUIPMENT

Clean gloves
Communication board
Materials for communication in writing
10-mL syringe for endotracheal cuff
Cuff manometer
Twill tape
Adhesive remover
Oral care products: soft toothbrush, nonfoaming toothpaste
Chlorhexidine gluconate (0.12%) oral rinse
Yankauer suction catheter
Stethoscope
Noise- and light-reduction sleep aides

BEGINNING THE SKILL

1. **CCC** Introduce yourself to the client and family.
2. **SAF** Identify the client using two identifiers.

PROCEDURE

3. **INF** Perform hand hygiene. Apply clean gloves *each* time you are exposed to body fluids. Then remove gloves and perform hand hygiene.
4. **CCC** Provide privacy. *Providing privacy in layers enhances client-centered care.*

Assessment of the Client on Mechanical Ventilation

5. **ACC** Assess the client's level of consciousness (LOC). Use the Glasgow Coma Scale to assess LOC if needed (see Chapter 20). Obtain vital sign measurements.

6. **ACC** If a sedative is prescribed, assess the client's level of sedation using a facility-approved sedation tool. Determine when the daily interruption of sedation will occur. *Interruption of sedation has demonstrated decreased mechanical ventilation days, decreased complications, and a decreased number of days in critical care. Interruption in sedation can concur with early mobilization.*

7. **CCC** Assess the client and family's ability to understand assessments and procedures, and address any distress that might be present.

8. **CCC** Identify special needs related to communication barriers due to level of health literacy, language, or hearing impairment. Secure professional interpreters if available.

9. **CCC** Develop a strategy for communicating with the client (e.g., using a writing tablet, letter board, or communication board.) *This reduces anxiety and increases the client's cooperation.*

10. **CCC** Orient the client frequently to self, location, date and year, time of day, the reason for hospitalization/treatment, the presence of the ETT, temporary nature of voicelessness, and the location of the nurse's call system.

11. **COM** Explain all assessments and procedures to the client and family.

12. **CCC** Assess the client for pain using a facility-approved pain scale (e.g., BPS, CCPOT). *The Society for Critical Care Medicine recommends the use of an established pain assessment tool for clients on mechanical ventilation.*

13. **ACC** Assess the client for delirium using a facility-approved delirium assessment tool. Review the client's medication list for medications that increase the risk for delirium, such as benzodiazepines. *Delirium is associated with increased length of stay, increased time on mechanical ventilation, increased mortality, and even permanent cognitive impairment (Baird, 2016).*

Assessment of ETT Placement, Stabilization, and Client Ventilation

14. **SAF** Apply gloves and inspect the position of the ETT. Note the position of the tube marking relative to the client's teeth or gums. Compare the current position to the position at the time of x-ray for placement verification.

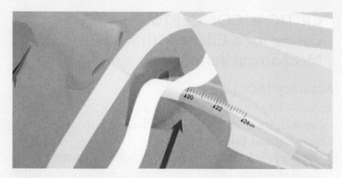

STEP 14 Inspect the position of the tube marking relative to the client's teeth or gums.

15. **HLTH** Inspect the client's lips, cheeks, back of the neck, and all other areas at risk for skin breakdown secondary to intubation.

16. **SAF** Reposition the ETT if using a commercial securement device. If the ETT is taped into position, remove the tape, reposition, and change the tape. If cuff deflation is needed, perform deep oral suctioning first. Reposition bite block, if used. *The presence of an ETT is the primary risk factor for an MDRPI.* **WARNING:** If the securement device or tape on an ETT is changed, ensure that a second nurse is present to hold the tube in place and prevent accidental extubation.

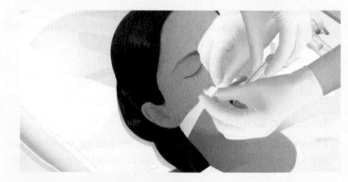

STEP 16 If the ETT is taped into position, remove the tape, reposition, and change the tape.

17. **ACC** Measure cuff inflation using a manometer and make adjustments if necessary.

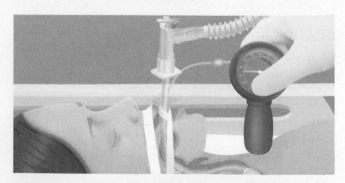

STEP 17 Measure cuff inflation using a manometer.

18. **ACC** Verify ventilator mode, pressure support, tidal volume, PEEP, oxygen concentration (FiO$_2$), flow rate (40–60 L/min), and programmed respiratory rate (e.g., 12–14 breaths/min) against the authorized healthcare provider's orders. Inspect circuitry attachments and ensure connections are secure.

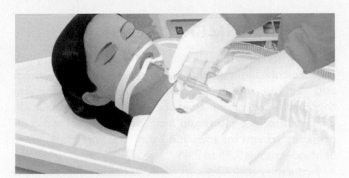

STEP 18 Inspect circuitry attachments and ensure connections are secure.

19. **SAF** Set and confirm the accuracy of alarms, delays, and thresholds on ventilator settings. **WARNING:** Ensure that the client's ventilator alarms are ON at all times. Do not silence.
20. **ACC** Assess the client's response to mechanical ventilation by assessing oxygenation status via pulse oximetry (SPO$_2$) and capnography (EtCO$_2$). Assess for equal chest wall movement.
21. **ACC** Assess the client's respiratory system by auscultating lung sounds and assessing for any audible secretions. Suction the ETT only if secretions are present (see Chapter 9).
22. **ACC** Verify the accuracy of electronic vital sign monitor readings by obtaining vital sign measurements.

Preventing Complications of Mechanical Ventilation

23. **HLTH** Elevate the HOB between 30 and 45 degrees. *The semirecumbent position may reduce the potential for microaspiration of oral and/or gastric contents.*
24. **INF** Provide oral care: (1) Brush teeth with a soft toothbrush, (2) suction oropharyngeal secretions, and (3) use an oral rinse of chlorhexidine gluconate (0.12%). Apply a mouth moisturizer to lips and oral mucosa every 2 to 4 hours. *Providing oral care reduces the risk of VAP.* (Note: Apply gloves for this procedure; then remove gloves and perform hand hygiene after the procedure.)

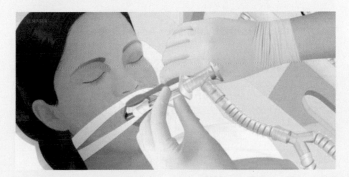

STEP 24 Provide oral care.

25. **HLTH** Check medications to ensure the client is receiving PUD prophylaxis. Contact the authorized healthcare provider if the order is not found. *PUD prophylaxis is best practice to prevent stress ulcers and potential gastrointestinal bleeding.*
26. **HLTH** Check for SCDs and antiembolism stockings on the client's legs. Check medications to determine if the client is also receiving pharmacologic thrombosis prophylaxis.
27. **COM** Collaborate with physical therapy and family members to determine the best time for range-of-motion exercises and/or early mobilization. These need to be at a time when sedation is interrupted. (Note: As identified in the 2018 PADIS guidelines, rehabilitation/mobilization beginning within a few days of mechanical ventilation is safe, feasible, and beneficial [Balas et al., 2018].)
28. **CCC** Administer analgesia and possibly light sedation as indicated by assessment findings. *Clients receiving mechanical ventilatory assistance may have pain.* (Note: PADIS guidelines advocate that analgesia take priority over sedation [Balas et al., 2018].)
29. **CCC** Collaborate with respiratory therapy and family member to plan and prepare for time periods of uninterrupted sleep. (Note: Breathing changes when one is asleep; assist-control [AC] ventilation is recommended from improving sleep vs. pressure-support ventilation.) Nighttime sleep is preferable to (and perhaps more feasible than) daytime. Use noise- and light-reduction measures, such as the use of earplugs and an eye mask. Multicomponent strategies within individualization have the most likelihood of success. Clustering care to minimize interruptions is a universal approach. *Sleep habits are highly individual; strategies to promote healthy sleep should be individualized. For example, some individuals may feel cold and want sleep socks, and others may feel too warm and want a small fan.* (Delvin et al., 2018).

FINISHING THE SKILL

30. **SAF** Ensure client safety. Ensure the bed is in the lowest position. Ensure the client can identify and reach the nurse call system. *These safety measures reduce the risk of injury from falls.*
31. **CCC** Ensure client comfort. Provide reassurance and emotional support.
32. **EVAL** Evaluate the outcomes. Verify the client's status and safety before leaving the bedside.
33. **INF** Remove gloves and perform hand hygiene.
34. **COM** Document assessment findings, care given, and outcomes in the legal healthcare record, including the following:
    - assessment findings for LOC, sedation, pain, and delirium
    - size and depth of ETT or NTT
    - any changes of ETT position or with the securement device

- skin assessment under securement device
- ETT cuff pressure
- condition of the lips, mouth, and tongue
- oral care, oral suctioning, and application of moisturizer, as provided

- respiration rate and other vital signs
- ventilator settings
- medications administered
- SCD and/or antiembolism stocking present
- how the client tolerated the procedure.

ARTERIAL BLOOD GASES

Arterial blood gas (ABG) sampling is the gold standard for assessment and management of ventilated clients or those who require long-term oxygen therapy (AACN, 2017). In addition to measuring gas exchange and acid–base balance, ABGs are used to assess respiratory and nonrespiratory components of the blood and to help determine the effectiveness of therapy for the client. Therefore, clients who are receiving mechanical ventilation require ABG monitoring. Nurses may receive special training to perform an arterial puncture in order to collect an ABG. Nurses collect and analyze arterial blood samples to provide accurate results to facilitate appropriate treatment and interventions. Nurses collaborate with respiratory therapists and other members of the healthcare team to obtain and interpret ABGs in emergency departments, surgical areas, and ICUs.

ABGs are generally analyzed in a clinical laboratory or using a handheld ABG blood gas analyzer within a hospital unit (also called a point-of-care device) (Fig. 18.11). The components of blood gases include SaO_2, PaO_2, $PaCO_2$, pH (acidity or alkalinity), and bicarbonate (HCO_3). There is a very narrow range for each of the components of an ABG. Normal values for ABGs are provided in Table 18.1. Altered ABGs and acid–base imbalances can affect all body systems and could eventually lead to tissue hypoxia and cell destruction and death.

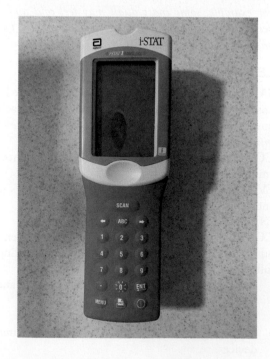

FIG. 18.11 Handheld arterial blood gas (ABG) blood analyzer.

ACID–BASE IMBALANCES

Clients with critical illnesses often have an acid–base imbalance, described as a disturbance in the equilibrium between acid and base substances within the body. The significant concepts to understand about acid–base imbalance are acids, bases, and the respiratory and metabolic regulatory and compensatory systems for acids and bases. The normal pH range of blood serum is 7.35 to 7.45.

Respiratory acidosis occurs when ventilation does not expel sufficient CO_2. The result is an increase in CO_2 in the blood. The CO_2 combines with H_2O to form carbonic acid, resulting in more acidic blood. Some causes of respiratory acidosis include problems in primary lung function (e.g., emphysema, chronic obstructive pulmonary disease [COPD]), changes in the lungs from secondary problems (e.g., lung cancer), and any condition that obstructs the airway (e.g., mucus plug) or depresses respiratory effort (e.g., brain trauma).

Respiratory alkalosis occurs when too much CO_2 is expelled. The result is an insufficient amount of carbonic acid (H_2CO_3) in the blood, resulting in more alkaline blood. Hyperventilation results in respiratory alkalosis. The most common cause is hypoxia. The compensatory response to hypoxia is breathing faster; the client breathes faster to try to get more oxygen and blows off CO_2, resulting in respiratory alkalosis. Additional conditions that may cause hyperventilation resulting in respiratory alkalosis include fever, pain, anxiety, and brain injury.

Metabolic acidosis occurs when acids accumulate in the body and overwhelm the body's compensatory mechanisms. There are several types of metabolic acidosis with differing etiologies. Lactic acidosis results from a buildup of lactic acid. In healthy individuals, this occurs with extensive exercise, but with the very ill, it occurs from lack of oxygen. This is most often the cause in hospitalized clients requiring oxygen and mechanical ventilation. Other causes include diabetic acidosis that results from the buildup of ketone bodies, resulting in diabetic ketoacidosis, and hyperchloremic acidosis that results from excessive loss of sodium bicarbonate, such as can occur with severe diarrhea. The compensatory mechanism is to convert the acids

TABLE 18.1 Normal Values for Acid–Base and Serum Chemistries

Arterial Blood Gases	Arterial
pH	7.35–7.45
PaO_2	80–100 mm Hg
$PaCO_2$	35–45 mm Hg
HCO_3	24–28 mEq/L
SaO_2	>95%

Reference: Pagana & Pagana, 2013.

and eliminate the carbon dioxide via the lungs. The sign of this compensatory mechanism is primarily an increase in the depth of respirations, hyperpnea, or long, deep breaths. The result is that CO_2 is eliminated from the lungs.

Metabolic alkalosis is the presence of too much bicarbonate or the loss of acid in the blood and may be caused by a loss of stomach acid, either from excessive vomiting or from gastrointestinal suctioning. Diuretics, massive transfusions of whole blood in which citrate is metabolized to bicarbonate, and ingestion of sodium bicarbonate (baking soda) are other causes of metabolic alkalosis. The respiratory compensation

for this acid–base disturbance is that the respiratory rate and depth decrease, and CO_2 is retained in the lungs.

In summary, understanding gas exchange and acid–base imbalances is clinically important because it helps the nurse and other members of the healthcare team gain insight into the client's condition. In addition, proper monitoring can help determine the need for and response to mechanical ventilation and oxygen therapy. Working as a team, nurses and other healthcare professionals can predict complications and provide appropriate treatment and care.

SECTION 2 Caring for a Client Who Requires Arterial Blood Gas Sampling

ABGs are obtained either by using a peripheral arterial line or by performing an arterial puncture, usually of the radial artery. Obtaining an accurate ABG sample is dependent on several accuracy-related variables. The nurse is responsible for many aspects of care and skill performance that affect the results of the ABG, including the timing of ventilator changes relative to the ABG, the technique used to obtain the sample, and time between sample collection and analysis. Safe, accurate, and timely performance of this skill can make a difference in the accuracy of the results and therefore the initiation of appropriate treatment.

INDWELLING ARTERIAL CATHETER SAMPLING

Arterial catheters may be inserted into adults and children by an authorized healthcare provider. The radial artery is the preferred site. The brachial artery is a potential site, but it is

the primary blood supply to the arm and does not have collateral circulation. The femoral artery is also a potential site but has a greater risk for infection due to the proximity to the groin. Ultrasound guidance is recommended when available (AACN, 2017). In newborns, the umbilical artery is initially accessed. The indications for arterial catheters include to the need to monitor invasive arterial blood pressure; the need for frequent blood sampling, including ABGs; and the need to monitor the effects of vasoactive drugs (AACN, 2017).

The arterial catheter is attached to a transducer system that includes pressure tubing, a three-way transducer stopcock, and a bag of sterile intravenous (IV) fluid within a pressurized sleeve (Fig. 18.12). The pressurized sleeve exerts a sustained pressure of 300 mm Hg on the IV fluid in order to allow infusion of approximately 3 mL per hour into the catheter to maintain patency and prevent backflow of arterial blood into the tubing. Keep in mind that arterial blood is under pressure, the pressure of the client's blood pressure. Therefore, fluid connected to arterial blood must be pressurized to prevent backflow.

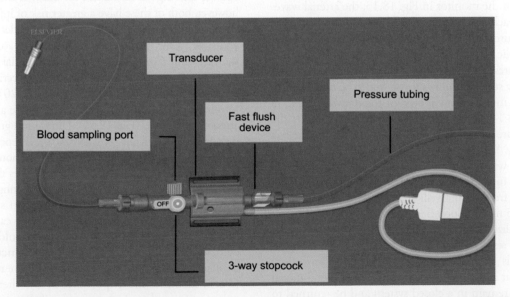

FIG. 18.12 Transducer system with blood sampling port, transducer, fast flush device, pressure tubing, and cable.

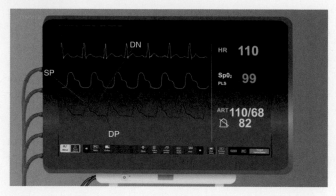

FIG. 18.13 The bottom waveform on the monitor shows the arterial blood pressure waveform. Each wave represents a pulse. The peak of the waveform represents the systolic pressure (SP), and the lowest point of the waveform represents the diastolic pressure (DP). The dicrotic notch (DN) represents the closing of the aortic valve.

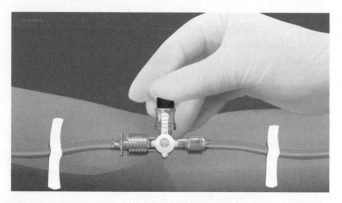

FIG. 18.14 A three-way stopcock for drawing arterial blood samples from catheter in the closed position.

The transducer system provides an electrical interface between the arterial catheter and a cardiac monitor. This is what allows continuous monitoring of the client's blood pressure. The transducer converts pressure signals within the client's vasculature to electrical responses that can be visualized as a waveform. As you can see on the monitor in Fig. 18.13, the arterial waveform represents each pulse. The peak of the waveform represents the systolic pressure, and the lowest point of the waveform represents the diastolic pressure. The waveform may show a dicrotic notch, which represents the closing of the aortic valve.

The three-way stopcock allows the device to be turned off to the client or the monitor and allows for the drawing of blood samples (Fig. 18.14). An inline flushing system controls the amount of pressure within the flush, thereby decreasing the risk for arterial injury. When drawing a blood sample in some systems, the initial withdrawal of fluid is wasted because this is a mixture of the infusing normal saline and the client's blood. Often, sampling from an indwelling arterial catheter requires a waste of at least 5 mL of blood that can contribute to anemia if a client is hospitalized long term. However, the waste is required because accurate results cannot be obtained from blood that is mixed with fluids from the continuous infusion. Devices are now available that allow the initial withdrawal of blood mixed with IV fluid to remain in a closed system and be returned to

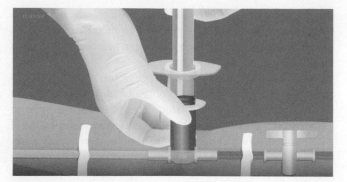

FIG. 18.15 Blood conservation devices have a reservoir for the mixed blood and IVF that eliminates the need to discard blood when drawing blood samples.

the client once a sample is drawn. (Fig. 18.15) This is termed a *blood conservation strategy* and has resulted in a decrease in phlebotomy blood loss. Blood conservation is important because it is reported that 90% of ICU patients become anemic by the third day (Jones, Spangler, Keiser, & Turkelson, 2019). Hospital-acquired anemia has an increased risk of mortality and length of hospital stay (Jones et al., 2019). The volume of blood loss may be reduced by up to 70 mL/day through the use of a blood conservation sampling device. This in turn decreases the risk of anemia and the potential accompanying risk for a blood transfusion. Blood conservation devices are useful in decreasing client blood loss and staff blood exposure and have the potential for long-term client benefits (Page, Retter, & Wyncoll, 2013). Diligent nursing care will prevent complications.

ARTERIAL PUNCTURE SAMPLING

In the adult and pediatric populations, arterial puncture involves palpating an artery and performing a percutaneous puncture. In many facilities, nurses must be specially trained and have certification in order to perform this procedure. Typically, the radial artery is the preferred site. This site is easy to access, and the artery is superficial and easier to stabilize (AACN, 2017). Additional sites for drawing ABGs include the brachial and femoral arteries; however, both of these have a greater risk of injury. The brachial artery is larger than the radial artery but lies deep within the arm and close to the median nerve. This makes accessing this vessel more difficult. Complications related to arterial puncture include pain, vasospasm, hematoma formation, infection, hemorrhage, and neurovascular compromise (AACN, 2017). Nurses performing this skill should carefully review the anatomy of veins, arteries, and nerves (Fig. 18.16). Ultrasound guidance is recommended when available (AACN, 2017). If repeated samples will be needed, an indwelling arterial catheter should be considered because repeated puncture of a site increases the risk of hematoma, scarring, or laceration of the artery (Hong Chu, 2017).

Client cooperation assists the nurse in successfully performing any skill, but arterial punctures can be very painful, and clients may find it difficult to hold still. This may contribute to the need for a repeated puncture, which can damage the artery as well as surrounding nerves. The AACN (2017) identifies the importance of anesthetizing the puncture site. Several options are a possibility, including EMLA

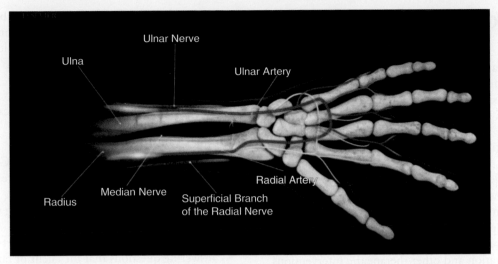

FIG. 18.16 Arteries and nerves in the hand and wrist.

BOX 18.6 Modified Allen Test

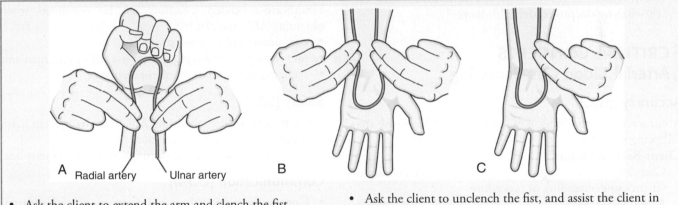

A Radial artery   Ulnar artery   B   C

- Ask the client to extend the arm and clench the fist.
- Compress the radial and ulnar artery with your index and middle finger.

- Ask the client to unclench the fist, and assist the client in relaxing the arm.
- Remove compression from the ulnar artery only.
- Color should return to the client's palm within 6 seconds.

cream, lidocaine ointment, or an injection of 0.2 to 0.3 mL of 1% lidocaine prior to performing an arterial puncture.

To further reduce the risk of complications from arterial punctures, the client's selected extremity/hand should be assessed for warmth, circulation, and sensation. In addition, the modified Allen test should be done according to facility policy in order to assess the patency of the radial and ulnar arteries. The modified Allen test checks to see if the circulation to the hand from the ulnar artery is sufficient to provide perfusion to the hand. Refer to Box 18.6 for the steps to the modified Allen test. If the modified Allen test shows that ulnar perfusion is not sufficient, then it may be necessary to identify alternative sites for arterial blood draws. Placing an arterial line in the radial artery without adequate ulnar artery perfusion could result in tissue necrosis.

Two additional complications can be prevented or minimized. Arterial punctures have the potential to introduce bacteria into an artery. To prevent infection, strict application of the critical concept of infection control is required. In addition, applying safety measures will minimize the potential for bleeding, bruising, or injury to the blood vessel. Apply pressure to the site for up to 5 minutes when clients are receiving anticoagulant

therapy. Clients with slow clotting times may need pressure held for longer, depending on their medical history and condition.

Accurate client assessment, proper client positioning, and client-centered education are essential components of performing arterial punctures. Observing the client's respirations and monitoring oxygenation via pulse oximetry or capillary refill (see Chapter 9) are key assessments. Client teaching includes explaining the procedure and how the results assist the authorized healthcare provider in determining appropriate interventions. Education for clients and families also includes information regarding the primary reason for arterial punctures. This education can allay fears and is an aspect of client-centered care.

In summary, the goal of obtaining a specimen for ABG analysis is to provide diagnostic information to help healthcare providers to determine if the client is experiencing a respiratory or metabolic disorder. It also guides changes to mechanical ventilation parameters and settings to help correct the problem. Nurses can work collaboratively with other professionals to assess the client's respiratory status and to provide safe and effective care when obtaining ABGs. Specialized training may be indicated for these skills.

APPLICATION OF THE NURSING PROCESS

Examples of Related ICNP Nursing Diagnoses, Expected Client Outcomes, and Nursing Interventions:

Nursing Diagnosis: Impaired gas exchange

Supporting Data: Client is on mechanical ventilation.

Expected Client Outcomes: The client will demonstrate improved ventilation and adequate oxygenation, as demonstrated by:

- clear lung fields
- respiration rate and depth within established parameters
- oxygenation and other components of ABGs within established parameters
- verbalized or acknowledged understanding of oxygen supplementation and other therapeutic interventions.

Nursing Intervention Example: Monitor ABGs per order.

Reference: International Classification for Nursing Practice. (n.d.). *eHealth & ICNP.* Retrieved from https://www.icn.ch/what-we-do/projects/ehealth-icnp.

CRITICAL CONCEPTS
Arterial Blood Gas Sampling

Accuracy (ACC)

Accuracy when obtaining ABG samples is affected by the following variables:

Client-Related Factors

- Client's age, medical history, vascular volume, cardiac output
- Client's understanding of procedure
- Activity level
- Temperature

Nurse-Related Factors

- Positioning of client
- Preparation and technique used to obtain direct ABGs
- Correct identification of anatomical landmarks used to locate puncture site
- Angle of needle insertion for direct ABGs
- Preparation and technique used to obtain ABGs by arterial line
- Technique used to store and transport ABG samples

- Time between sample collection and lab analysis
- Recent changes in mechanical ventilator settings
- Documentation of inaccurate mechanical ventilator settings or percentage of oxygen delivered

Equipment-Related Factors

- Proper calibration of equipment
- Correct location of indwelling arterial catheter

Client-Centered Care (CCC)

Respect for the client when obtaining ABGs includes:

- obtaining verbal consent for procedures and promoting autonomy
- explaining the procedure and arranging for an interpreter if needed
- providing privacy and ensuring comfort
- answering questions that the client or family may have
- advocating for the client and family.

Infection Control (INF)

Healthcare-associated infection can be prevented when obtaining ABG samples by:

- containment of microorganisms
- preventing and reducing the transfer of microorganisms
- reducing the number of microorganisms.

Safety (SAF)

Safety measures when obtaining ABG samples prevent harm and provide a safe care environment by:

- preventing blood loss and clotting within the catheter line.

Communication (COM)

- Communication exchanges information (oral, written, nonverbal, or electronic) between two or more people.
- Documentation records information in a permanent legal record.
- Collaboration with the client and other healthcare professionals is essential when obtaining arterial blood gas samples.

Evaluation (EVAL)

Evaluation of the outcomes allows the nurse to determine the efficacy and accuracy of the care provided.

■ SKILL 18.2 Obtaining Arterial Blood Gases From a Peripheral Arterial Line

EQUIPMENT

Clean gloves

Sterile 4 × 4 gauze pads,

Antiseptic solution

3-mL heparinized, vented syringe

Appropriate blood specimen tubes (or ABG kit)

Labels with the client's name and appropriate identifying data

Laboratory form and specimen labels

Goggles or fluid shield face mask

Needleless blood sampling access device and cannula (for closed arterial sampling system)

Extra blood specimen tube (for discard)

Sterile, nonvented cap or needleless cap

BEGINNING THE SKILL

1. **CCC** Introduce yourself to the client and family.
2. **SAF** Identify the client using two identifiers.
3. **CCC** Provide privacy. *Providing privacy in layers enhances client-centered care.*
4. **INF** Perform hand hygiene.

PROCEDURE

5. **CCC** Assess the client's/family's ability to understand the procedure, and address any distress that might be present.

6. **CCC** Identify special needs related to communication barriers due to illiteracy, language, or hearing difficulties. Secure professional interpreters if available. *Reduces anxiety and increases the client's cooperation.*
7. **CCC** Explain the procedure.
8. **CCC** Obtain verbal consent when possible.
9. **ACC** Assess the following:
   a. client's activity level
   b. recent changes in supplemental oxygen
   c. recent changes to mechanical ventilator settings.
   Blood gases need to reflect the client's sustained response to intervention. If changes in oxygen have been implemented, the information from blood gases will not be accurate.
10. **ACC** Record temperature. *pH increases, and PaO_2 and $PaCO_2$ decrease, as temperature decreases.*
11. **SAF** Set up an ergonomically safe space. Raise the bed to a comfortable working height. Raise one side rail. *Setting up an ergonomically safe space prevents injury to the nurse and client.*
12. **INF** Apply gloves and other personal protective equipment (PPE) as needed.
13. **ACC** Place client in reclining position with the HOB elevated 45 degrees. *This position facilitates breathing and is usually comfortable for the client.*
14. **ACC** Position the client's arm to provide access to arterial line stopcock port located proximal to the client.

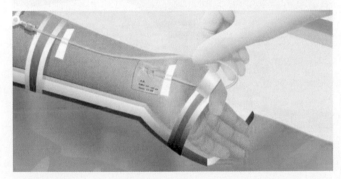

STEP 14 Position client's arm to provide access to arterial line's stopcock.

15. **ACC** Assess the patency of the arterial catheter.
    a. Observe the waveform on the monitor (see Fig. 18.12). A clear waveform indicates that the arterial line is patent.
    b. Ensure catheter and dressing are dry and intact, without signs of leaking.
16. **ACC** Prepare ABG syringe by expelling air and excess heparin with plunger.
17. **SAF** Turn the three-way stopcock so that it is off to the access port.
18. **ACC** Remove the nonvented cap from the access port.
19. **INF** Place the cap upside down on a flat surface to minimize contamination (if reusing cap).
20. **INF** Scrub access port with antiseptic for 15 seconds.
21. **ACC If using a needleless syringe:**
    a. Attach a needleless syringe to the stopcock:
    b. Turn the stopcock away from client's access site to allow blood flow into the syringe.

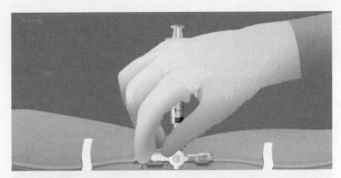

STEP 21B Turn the stopcock away from the client's access site.

c. Draw waste (discard volume) slowly per protocol. If using a blood conservation device, draw back on the plunger to fill the blood reservoir.

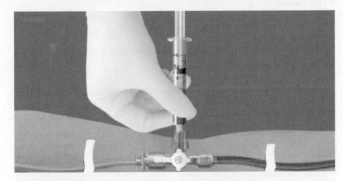

STEP 21C Draw waste slowly per protocol.

d. Turn the stopcock off to the client's access site. **WARNING:** If the stopcock is not turned to the off position, blood will continue to flow from the port, causing unnecessary blood loss.

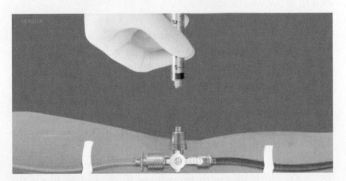

STEP 21D Turn stopcock off to the client's access site.

e. Remove the syringe.
f. Discard the waste and the syringe in appropriate container (Steps e and f are not performed if using a blood conservation device.)
g. Attach heparinized syringe for sample. *Heparin serves as an anticoagulant but can decrease the pH as well as $PaCO_2$.*
h. Obtain sample. Turn stopcock away from client's access site and gently draw or allow appropriate amount of arterial blood to flow into heparinized syringe. Arterial blood should flow into the syringe easily. *Gentle technique prevents hemolysis.*

i. Turn stopcock to off position. Remove syringe.

j. If using a blood conservation device, return the blood in the blood reservoir to the client.

22. **ACC If using a blood-sampling device or vacutainer:**

    a. Attach blood-sampling device to the stopcock port.

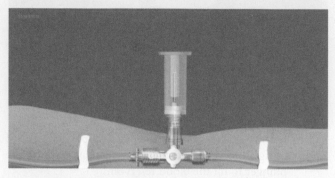

STEP 22A Attach blood-sampling device to port.

    b. Turn stopcock away from client access site.

    c. Attach appropriate tube to blood-sampling device to draw waste volume.

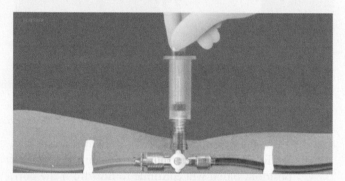

STEP 22C Attach appropriate tube to blood-sampling device to draw waste volume.

    d. Turn stopcock to off position.

    e. Remove the tube and sampling device.

    f. Discard in appropriate container.

    g. Attach heparinized syringe for sample. *Heparin serves as an anticoagulant but can decrease the pH as well as $PaCO_2$.*

    h. Draw appropriate amount of arterial blood into the heparinized syringe.

    i. Turn stopcock to off position. Remove syringe.

23. **SAF** Flush line with transducer flush device. Flush the port with transducer flush device. Flush the port using a syringe or blood specimen tube if using a blood-sam-

pling device. Ensure that arterial catheter tubing and port are free of blood. *Prevents clotting of catheter.*

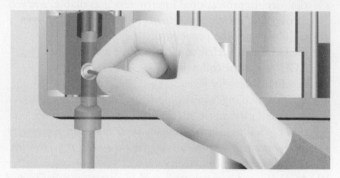

STEP 23 Flush the line with the transducer flush device.

24. **ACC** Gently expel air bubbles from ABG syringe sample, and place sterile cap on sample. *Air bubbles can change the sample and cause a falsely high PaO_2 and falsely low $PaCO_2$.*

25. **INF** Place a new, sterile, nonvented cap on the access port of the stopcock or replace with previous cap. *Prevents contamination of arterial catheter and transducer system.*

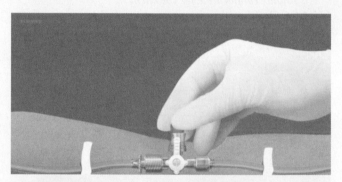

STEP 25 Place a new, sterile, nonvented cap on the access port of the stopcock.

26. **COM** Attach client label to syringe with date and time arterial sample was drawn. Ensure the specimen label contains two client identifiers. Label the specimen in the presence of the client. *National safety guidelines recommend labeling specimens in the presence of the client.*

27. **ACC** Perform blood gas analysis with point-of-care device, or transport to the lab promptly. (Note: Some facilities require that the sample be placed in an ice slurry, particularly if there will be a delay in analysis. Blood gas analysis should be performed within 30 minutes of collection to ensure accuracy [AACN, 2017].)

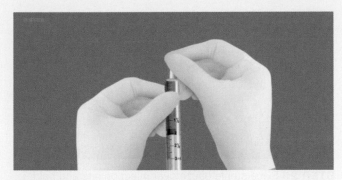

STEP 27 Perform analysis or transport sample promptly to ensure accuracy.

28. **INF** Remove gloves and perform hand hygiene.

FINISHING THE SKILL

29. **SAF** Ensure client safety. Place the bed in the lowest position. Ensure that the client can identify and reach the nurse call system. *These safety measures reduce the risk of injury from falls.*

30. **CCC** Ensure client comfort. Provide reassurance and emotional support.
31. **SAF** Ensure alarms are on and arterial waveform returns.
32. **EVAL** Evaluate the outcomes. Verify the client's oxygenation status before leaving the bedside.
33. **INF** Perform hand hygiene.
34. **COM** Document assessment findings, care given, and outcomes in the legal healthcare record, including the following:
    - client's ability to tolerate procedure
    - changes in oxygen saturation
    - patency of arterial line
    - results of arterial blood gas analysis (The results may be automatically uploaded to the client's electronic health record.)
    - changes in ventilator settings based on the authorized healthcare provider's orders.

■ SKILL 18.3 Obtaining Arterial Blood Gases From the Radial Artery

EQUIPMENT

Gloves
PPE
Sterile gauze
>0.5% chlorhexidine gluconate solution
Tape or adhesive bandage
3-mL heparinized, vented syringe
20- to 25-gauge and 25-mm (1-inch) needle with needle cover/needle guard
Client identification label and laboratory paperwork
Biohazard bag (if not point of care)
Thermometer
Small towel or washcloth

BEGINNING THE SKILL

1. **CCC** Introduce yourself to the client and family.
2. **SAF** Identify the client using two identifiers.
3. **CCC** Provide privacy. *Providing privacy in layers enhances client-centered care.*
4. **INF** Perform hand hygiene.

PROCEDURE

5. **CCC** Assess the client's/family's ability to understand the procedure, and address any distress that might be present.
6. **CCC** Identify special needs related to communication barriers due to illiteracy, language, or hearing difficulties. Secure professional interpreters if available. *Reduces anxiety and increases the client's cooperation.*

7. **CCC** Explain the procedure.
8. **CCC** Obtain verbal consent from the client when possible.
9. **ACC** Assess the client for the following:
    - oxygenation status over last 30 minutes
    - activity level
    - recent changes in supplemental oxygen
    - recent changes in mechanical ventilator settings

    Blood gases need to reflect the client's sustained response to intervention. If changes in oxygen have been implemented, the information from blood gases will not be accurate.

10. **ACC** Record the client's temperature. *When a client's temperature decreases, pH increases, and PaO_2 and $PaCO_2$ decrease.*
11. **SAF** Set up an ergonomically safe space. Raise the bed to a comfortable working height. Raise one side rail. *Setting up an ergonomically safe space prevents injury to the nurse and client.*
12. **INF** Apply clean gloves and other PPE as needed.
13. **ACC** Place the client in a reclining position with the HOB elevated 45 degrees. *This position facilitates breathing and is usually comfortable for the client.*
14. **ACC** Select site on client for direct arterial puncture.
15. **SAF** Perform modified Allen's test to assess for circulation (see Box 18.6).
16. **ACC** Support the client's arm and hyperextend the selected wrist. Use a small, rolled washcloth or towel for support.

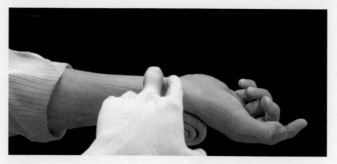

STEP 16 Support arm and hyperextend the wrist.

17. **ACC** Pull the plunger of the heparinized syringe to approximately the 1- to 1.5-mL mark per facility protocol. *Pulling the plunger allows the syringe to fill automatically when the artery is punctured. All air must be expelled from the syringe before analysis of the blood.*

18. **INF** Position the sterile gauze and adhesive within reach.

19. **ACC** Use your nondominant hand to palpate, and locate the radial artery with your index and middle finger.

20. **SAF** Stabilize the radial artery at the site proximal to the puncture site.

21. **INF** Use a facility-approved antiseptic to clean the injection site. Allow the site to air dry. (Note: Skin preparation with >0.5% chlorhexidine preparation with alcohol is the CDC guideline [CDC, 2015].)

22. **INF** Cleanse the site according to facility protocol.

23. **CCC** Use distraction/relaxation methods or provide local anesthesia per facility policy (see Chapter 7). *Most clients report paint during this procedure. The use of an anesthetic agent reduces pain. Distraction may decrease the client's anxiety.*

24. **ACC** Hold the needle at a 30- to 45-degree angle. Use one fluid motion to insert the needle bevel up into the pulsation site.

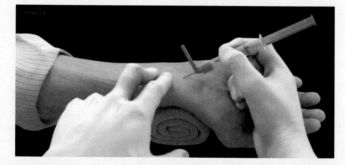

STEP 24 Enter the artery at a 30- to 45-degree angle.

25. **ACC** Observe the syringe for backflow of blood. Advance the needle slowly if you do not immediately observe blood return.

26. **ACC** Do not advance the needle once you see blood return.

27. **ACC** Allow the syringe to fill completely. *Arterial blood should flow into the syringe easily. Using a gentle technique and allowing the sample to flow will prevent hemolysis.*

28. **SAF** Once the syringe is filled, withdraw the needle using one continuous motion.

29. **SAF** Place sterile gauze over injection site and hold pressure for at least 5 to 10 minutes.

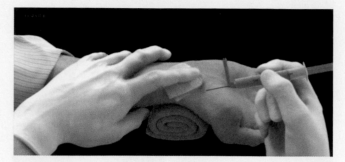

STEP 29 Place sterile gauze over injection site and hold pressure for 5 to 10 minutes.

30. **SAF** Stabilize the plunger to avoid air aspiration. Engage the needle safety device.

31. **ACC** While continuing to hold pressure over the injection site, gently mix the blood in the syringe.

32. **ACC** Expel any air bubbles from the sample. *Air from the environment can cause errors in blood gas analysis.*

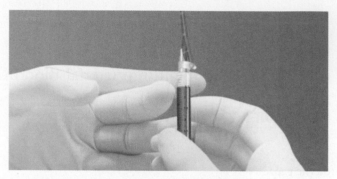

STEP 32 Expel air bubbles from sample.

33. **SAF** Remove the needle from the syringe and discard per agency protocol.

34. **SAF** Cap with safety cap. *Prevents blood spillage.*

35. **ACC** Attach client label to syringe with date and time of arterial puncture. Ensure specimen label contains two client identifiers. Label specimen in the presence of the client. *National safety guidelines recommend labeling specimens in the presence of the client.*

36. **ACC** Perform blood gas analysis with point-of-care device, or transport for analysis as soon as possible per facility policy. (Note: Some facilities require that the sample be placed in an ice slurry, particularly if there will be a delay in analysis. Check facility policy.)

37. **SAF** Dispose of equipment.

38. **INF** Remove gloves and perform hand hygiene.

FINISHING THE SKILL

39. **SAF** Ensure client safety. Place the bed in the lowest position. Ensure the client can identify and reach the nurse call system. *These safety measures reduce the risk of injury from falls.*

40. **CCC** Ensure client comfort. Provide reassurance and emotional support.

41. **EVAL** Evaluate the outcomes. Ensure that the client is not in respiratory distress before leaving the bedside.

42. **INF** Perform hand hygiene.
43. **COM** Document assessment findings, care given, and outcomes in the legal healthcare record, including the following:
    - date, time, and puncture site
    - results of modified Allen's test
    - administration of local anesthetic if used
    - client assessment

- site assessment: pre- and post-arterial puncture
- temperature
- oxygen saturation (SaO_2)
- oxygen therapy and ventilator settings
- results of ABG analysis (results may be automatically uploaded to the client's electronic health record)
- client response and how the client tolerated the procedure.

SECTION 3 Caring for a Client With a Chest Tube

Chest tubes, or thoracic catheters, may be placed in the intrapleural space, the parietal pleura, or the mediastinal space to drain air, fluid, or both from the chest. The intrapleural space is the potential space between the visceral pleura, a thin serous membrane covering the lungs and inner chest wall (Fig. 18.17). The parietal pleura is a thin, serous membrane lining the chest walls and diaphragm. The mediastinal space contains the organs and tissues separating the lungs, including the heart, large vessels, trachea, esophagus, thymus, lymph nodes, and connective tissue. The semiflexible, transparent chest tube cannula allows blood, fluid, transudate, or air to drain from the intrapleural, parietal, or mediastinal space. Chest tube therapy also prevents fluid and air return to the pleural space and restores negative pressure to allow the lung to expand if placed in the pleural or parietal space.

Inhalation and exhalation are the result of pressure changes within the thoracic cavity. When fluid or air enters the pleural space, the pressure gradient in the thoracic cavity is affected, impairing lung expansion. If the pleural space continues to fill, the lung will eventually collapse (Mondor, 2017b). *Hemothorax* is the term used to describe when blood fills the lung space due to an injury, such as fractured ribs, or surgical intervention. When fluid fills the lung space, it is called a pleural effusion, and when pus fills the lung space due to infection, it is called empyema (Li, 2017). A pneumothorax occurs when air enters the space surrounding the lungs through either damaged lung tissue leaking air or a hole in the chest wall (Fig. 18.18). A spontaneous pneumothorax occurs when a bleb, or air-filled sac on the lung surface, ruptures, allowing air to leak into the pleural space (Mondor, 2017b). Blebs can occur and rupture due to lung disease but may also be seen in healthy, young people (Mondor, 2017b). A tension pneumothorax describes a condition in which the air building up in a pneumothorax has no way to escape the pleural space, causing not only the collapse of the lung but compression of the heart and a mediastinal shift (Mondor, 2017b). The mediastinal

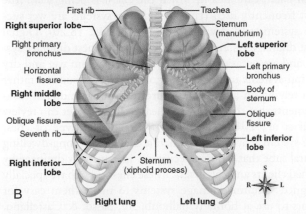

FIG. 18.17 The lung tissue is surrounded by the pleural space and the pleural lining.

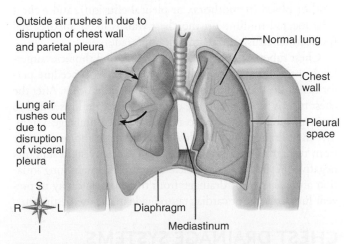

FIG. 18.18 A pneumothorax occurs when air enters the space surrounding the lungs through either damaged lung tissue leaking air or a hole in the chest wall.

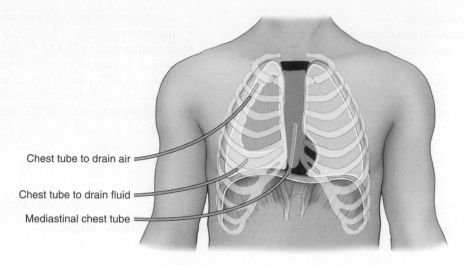

FIG. 18.19 A chest tube on the upper chest wall typically removes air; a chest tube on the lower chest wall drains fluid or blood, and a midline tube is likely a mediastinal tube.

shift causes compression of the lung that has not collapsed, further compromising the respiratory system. When there is a combination of both air and blood filling the lung space, it is known as a hemopneumothorax (Mondor, 2017b). Chest tubes located in the pleural space allow for drainage of air, blood, and/or other fluids, allowing the lung to expand properly and reducing tension in the thoracic cavity.

As previously mentioned, chest tubes can also be placed in the mediastinal space. This is often seen following cardiothoracic surgery to drain fluids to prevent surgical complications such as pericardial effusion or cardiac tamponade (Mondor, 2017b). However, chest tubes are also used as treatment rather than prevention for pericardial effusion or cardiac tamponade when an indwelling catheter is determined to be appropriate. As identified in Fig. 18.19, the location of the chest tube's insertion site on the chest wall can be a clue to its purpose. For example, a chest tube found on the upper chest wall is typically used to remove air (pneumothorax), a chest tube located on the lower chest wall is used to drain fluid or blood (hemothorax or pleural effusion), and a chest tube located midline on the chest wall is likely mediastinal (pericardial effusion or cardiac tamponade).

Chest tubes are inserted during cardiac and thoracic surgeries, in procedural areas of the hospital, or in a procedure performed at the bedside when emergent situations occur. After the chest tube is inserted into the client, the distal end is secured to drainage tubing connected to a water seal chest drainage system. The chest drainage system allows fluid drainage and prevents air from reentering the pleural cavity. The closed system supports negative pressure in the thoracic cavity to maintain lung inflation and assists with drainage from the thoracic cavity to prevent lung collapse or cardiac tamponade in the mediastinum.

CHEST DRAINAGE SYSTEMS

There are many varieties of chest drainage systems available for use with chest tubes. The system used will depend on

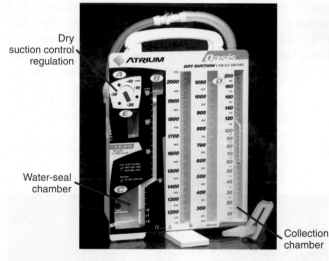

FIG. 18.20 Example of closed chest drainage system—dry suction.

the client's condition, the authorized healthcare provider's preferences, and the availability of the system in the facility or client care area in which the client is being seen. The most frequently used types of drainage systems are wet suction systems and dry suction systems (Fig. 18.20). Digital chest drainage systems are another type of chest drainage system and are occasionally used. They differ from wet and dry suction systems in that they create their own suction rather than relying on an external source and provide digital measurements that the authorized healthcare provider can review (Arai et al., 2018) (Fig.18.21). Yet another type of chest tube system may be used when a client has a long-dwelling pleural tube that requires recurrent, intermittent drainage by trained clients and caregivers. These chest tubes have specially designed vacuum drainage systems to make them easy for clients to use at home (Chalhoub, Ali, Sasso, & Castellano, 2016). This section focuses on the management of wet and dry suction systems because they are the most widely used.

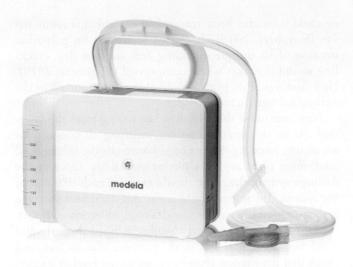

FIG. 18.21 Example of a digital chest drainage system.

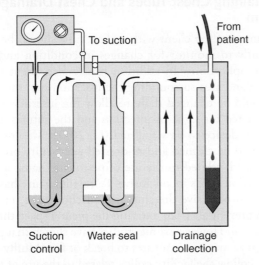

FIG. 18.22 Three chambers in a chest drainage device: drainage collection, water seal, and suction control.

Types of Chambers

Both wet suction and dry suction chest drainage systems include the three chambers: drainage collection chamber, water seal chamber, and suction control chamber (Fig. 18.22).

Drainage Collection Chamber

The drainage collection chamber is connected to extension tubing, and the extension tubing is connected directly to the chest tube. The chamber's graduated markings allow the nurse to determine the quantity of output during each shift, as well as the total output for the duration of the client's treatment with the chest tube. Sudden changes in the amount of output (e.g., quantities greater than 100 mL/hr after the initial drainage has tapered) or changes in the character of the output (e.g., from serosanguinous to bright red blood) could indicate a complication such as a hemorrhage. Notify an authorized healthcare provider of unusual or excessive drainage per written parameters and facility policy.

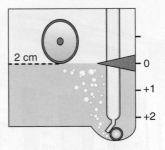

FIG. 18.23 Bubbling in the water seal provides the nurse information about the pleural space and/or chest tube drainage system.

Water Seal Chamber

The water seal chamber allows air to leave the chest but prevents air from reentering the chest from the drain. When the chest tube is in the pleural space (not the mediastinal space), the activity in the water seal gives the nurse information about the status of the pleural space. Bubbling when the client breaths in indicates the evacuation of air from the pleural space, sometimes referred to as an air leak. Finding an air leak on assessment may be anticipated, as would be the case in a chest tube placed to evacuate air in a pneumothorax (Fig. 18.23). The water seal chamber may also assist healthcare providers in identifying leaks. A new air leak could indicate a change in the client's condition or a leak somewhere in the chest tube or drainage system. Tidaling (an up-and-down movement of the water in the water seal chamber) reflects the rise and fall of pressure within the pleural space. Tidaling will typically gradually decrease as the lung expands to fill the pleural space (Mondor, 2017b). If tidaling stops suddenly, the chest tube or drainage line could be occluded and should be inspected (Mondor, 2017b).

Suction Control Chamber

The suction control chamber can be either wet or dry. Negative pressure is applied to the pleural or mediastinal space to assist in the evacuation of fluid or air. The suction control chamber is filled with water in wet suction systems and connected to an external suction source, typically wall suction (Mondor, 2017b). The water in the chamber regulates the wall suction to control the amount of suction actually applied to the chest tube (Mondor, 2017). In a dry suction system, the suction chamber contains an internal regulatory mechanism to maintain pressure so that no water is necessary (Mondor, 2017b). The negative pressure in dry systems is typically set at -20 cm H_2O but can be manually adjusted to what is prescribed (Fig. 18.24).

CARING FOR THE CLIENT WITH A CHEST TUBE AND CHEST DRAINAGE SYSTEM

The nurse's responsibilities in caring for a client with a chest tube and chest drainage system include assisting with setting up and connecting the chest tube to the drainage system,

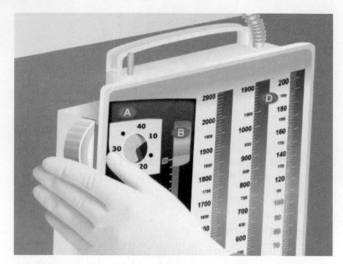

FIG. 18.24 Suction in dry systems is typically set at −20 cm H₂O.

assessing the client, monitoring equipment, performing routine care, documenting characteristics and quantity of output throughout the shift, and educating the client. The nurse may also be responsible for assisting the authorized healthcare provider with the removal of the chest tube. In addition, it is also important to have basic skills in troubleshooting chest tubes (discussed shortly).

Assisting With Chest Tube Insertion

Inserting a chest tube is a sterile, invasive procedure that can be very painful. If the chest tube is not placed under general anesthesia, the nurse's role is to provide emotional support, administer analgesia as prescribed, and provide education prior to and during the procedure. In addition, the nurse usually sets up the chest tube drainage system, secures the connections, and adjusts the external suction as prescribed. Cardiac and pulmonary assessments are performed following the procedure in order to evaluate the immediate response and check for complications. The authorized healthcare provider typically orders a chest x-ray to confirm correct placement of the chest tube.

Assessing the Client With a Chest Tube

When assessing a client with a chest tube, a good rule is to begin at the client and work toward the drainage system. The nurse should begin with a thorough cardiac and pulmonary assessment, noting any abnormalities. The nurse should consider that some abnormal findings can be anticipated based on why the chest tube was placed. For example, decreased lung sounds on the right side could be reasonably anticipated if a chest tube was recently placed for a right hemothorax or pneumothorax but not if the client had a mediastinal chest tube placed. Assessment of the insertion site should include an inspection of the dressing to ensure it is clean, dry, and intact. The area around the insertion site should also be examined for signs of infection and palpated for crepitus. Crepitus, or subcutaneous emphysema, is air that has escaped from the lung space

or chest tube and been trapped in the subcutaneous tissue (Sommers, 2019). It can be identified on palpation because of its unique crackling feel and the dry, crackling sound it makes when compressed (Sommers, 2019). New findings of crepitus should always be reported to the authorized healthcare provider.

Next, the nurse should follow the tubing from the insertion site to the drainage system, ensuring all connections are secure, assessing the drainage present in the tubing, and confirming there are no kinks or occlusions. Once at the drainage system, the nurse should examine each chamber of the system. The nurse should assess and document the type and amount of drainage in the drainage collection chamber, confirm that the water seal chamber is filled properly and check for bubbling indicating the presence of an air leak, and check that the suction chamber is set to the level of suction prescribed.

Maintaining Chest Tubes and Chest Drainage System

Assessment of the client with a chest tube should be done frequently to monitor for changes in condition and possible complications. In addition to the assessment of the dressing and area surrounding the insertion site, the dressing should be changed daily to allow the insertion site to be inspected for signs of infection and the sutures or stabilization device to be visualized (Li, 2017). The insertion site should be cleaned and re-dressed per facility protocol. The research related to the use of petroleum gauze around the insertion site is inconclusive. Petroleum gauze has been used as an occlusive dressing around chest tube insertion sites to prevent air from entering the pleural space through the incision. However, some studies have shown that petroleum gauze may cause sutures to break or fail (Muffly et al., 2012). Follow the facility policy related to the use of petroleum gauze.

After the dressing change, the nurse should confirm that the extension tubing is securely connected to both the chest tube and the drainage system to allow the system to function properly and prevent inadvertent disconnection. The extension tubing is looped on the bed to prevent dependent loops that would allow the drainage to block the tubing, thereby changing the desired negative pressure in the pleural space. Looping the tubing on the bed also allows slack in the tubing to prevent dislodgement as the client moves in bed. The extension tubing should never be stripped or milked to remove a clot because this can cause extreme levels of negative pressure to build up in the tubing (Flynn Makic, Rauen, Jones, & Fisk, 2015). If stripping or milking is performed, the high negative pressure created will reach the end of the chest tube once the clot is dislodged and can injure tissue. The appropriate placement for a chest drainage system is below the client's chest to promote drainage and secured to the bed frame. The placement of the system, the status of the water seal chamber, the amount of suction, and the amount and characteristics of the chest tube drainage should be monitored frequently.

Replacing a Chest Tube Drainage System

The chest drainage system is disposable. Once the collection chamber is full, the drainage system can be replaced with a new system. A new chest drainage system is set up using sterile technique. This is done prior to disconnecting the old one to minimize the time the chest tube is clamped during the exchange of the two drainage systems. Clamp the chest tube during a chest tube drainage system change by using two padded hemostats, clamped opposite of each other. Remove the clamps as soon as the new system is set up and connected appropriately. Clamping a chest tube for extended periods of time could result in tension pneumothorax or other complications (Li, 2017). The old chest drainage system should be secured in a biohazard bag and placed in a large biohazard disposal container.

Assisting With Chest Tube Removal

Assisting with the removal of a chest tube includes educating and supporting the client during the process; appropriate disposal of used equipment; and postprocedural assessments, including vital signs, oxygen saturation, and pain, using a facility-approved pain assessment tool. Immediate concerns include diminished breath sounds; changes in heart rate, rhythm, or heart sounds; labored respirations; chest pain; and decreased oxygen saturation. Prior to the removal of a chest tube, the suction is often discontinued by the authorized healthcare provider to eliminate a possible air leak (Muzzy & Butler, 2015).

Prior to removal of the chest tube, clean the insertion site with a facility approved antiseptic solution per facility policy. Assess the site for redness, swelling, or discharge. Administer analgesia 30 minutes prior to chest tube removal, if ordered, and assess the client's pain pre- and postprocedure. The sutures used to secure the chest tube are clipped with sterile scissors, and the suture material is removed with sterile tweezers. Clean gloves can be used for this procedure if sterile technique is used.

Just before the chest tube is removed, instruct the client to take a big breath and exhale as the tube is pulled out. This prevents air from entering the pleural space until the insertion site is covered. After the chest tube is removed, cover the insertion site with petroleum gauze per facility policy if a pleural site. Mediastinal sites may have sutures or Steri-strips applied to close the site. Both sites are then covered with an occlusive dressing. Once the chest tube is removed and the dressing is applied, the client can resume normal breathing. The chest tube and drainage system should be secured in a biohazard bag and placed in a large biohazard disposal container.

TROUBLESHOOTING THE CHEST TUBE AND DRAINAGE SYSTEM

Nurses also assess for possible complications related to potential air leaks or equipment malfunctions. Indications of leaks in the system or problems with equipment can manifest as changes in the client's respiratory assessment or cardiovascular assessment as well as changes in the drainage system. If assessment findings indicate a new or worsening air leak seen in the water seal chamber of the drainage system, the nurse should first try to identify the source of the leak (Muzzy & Butler, 2015). The nurse should check that all connections are secure, and if the air leak persists, the nurse may briefly clamp the chest tube as close as possible to the client if facility policy allows (Muzzy & Butler, 2015). If the air leak stops after clamping, the source of the leak is either internal or at the insertion site; if it continues, the source is in the tubing or system, and a change of equipment may be necessary (Muzzy & Butler, 2015). If air has entered the pleural space, symptoms could include increasing respiratory distress and asymmetrical chest movement. Remember that one of the most serious complications of chest tubes is a tension pneumothorax, which can be indicated by tracheal deviation, a shift of the trachea to one side.

If a chest tube is ever disconnected from the extension tubing or drainage system unexpectedly, air can fill the pleural space. The priority is to prevent the occurrence or reoccurrence of a pneumothorax. Facility policy may dictate the nurse's actions in this instance; however, options include cleansing the connections with facility-approved antiseptic and reconnecting as soon as possible, submersing the chest tube in *sterile* saline until a new drainage system can be set up, or quickly setting up and connecting a new drainage system if one is readily available. Clamping the chest tube if disconnected is no longer advised due to the risk of tension pneumothorax (Mondor, 2017).

When a chest tube is inadvertently dislodged from the client, the potential for a pneumothorax also exists. Immediately place a gloved hand over the insertion site and request assistance (Muzzy & Butler, 2015). An extra petroleum gauze should be kept at the bedside for this type of situation. Place the petroleum gauze over the site and cover with a gauze and tape dressing, taping only three sides to allow any air in the pleural space an escape route (Muzzy & Butler, 2015). Contact the authorized healthcare provider for further instructions. For more information on troubleshooting, see Table 18.2.

APPLICATION OF THE NURSING PROCESS

Examples of Related ICNP Nursing Diagnoses, Expected Client Outcomes, and Nursing Interventions:
Nursing Diagnosis: Impaired breathing, as seen by the following:
- decreased lung expansion
- asymmetrical chest expansion and breath sounds.

Supporting Data: Client has a pneumothorax and chest tube.
Expected Client Outcome: The client will have no signs of impaired breathing, as demonstrated by the following:
- Client's respiratory rate will return to baseline.
- Client will have symmetrical chest expansion and breath sounds

TABLE 18.2 Troubleshooting for Chest Tubes and Chest Drainage Systems

Problem	Possible Causes	Immediate Interventions
Chest tube inadvertently removed from client's thorax	Tension on chest tube (dependent loops, turning client without sufficient slack) Confused client removes tube independently Degradation of sutures, with subsequent migration of chest tube	Cover insertion site with gloved hand. Call for assistance. Place petroleum gauze over site and cover with a gauze dressing, taping only three sides to allow air an escape route. Contact authorized healthcare provider.
Sudden absence of tidaling	Clots, kinks in tubing, or dependent loops	Remove clots by gently squeezing or twisting tubing, if facility policy allows. Remove kinks. Reposition tubing to eliminate dependent loops.
New onset or worsening of constant, vigorous bubbling in water seal chamber	Indicates an air leak	Verify that chest tube has not migrated or been dislodged. Check that all connections are secured. Use padded hemostats, proximal to distal, to determine if leaks exist in tubing. When bubbling stops, the leak is between the hemostat and client. Replace chest drainage system if necessary.
New or worsening crepitus around the chest tube insertion site	Air leaking into the subcutaneous tissue Possible blockage in drainage system Wound at insertion site needs to be sealed	Notify authorized healthcare provider.
Chest tube becomes disconnected from chest drainage system	Connection not taped securely Tubing may have been pulled during ambulation or turning	Wipe the connections with facility-approved antiseptic. Immediately reconnect tubes. Insert chest tube into a bottle of *sterile* saline. Connect to new drainage system if readily available. Ask client to cough.
Chest drainage system tips over	Not secured to bed frame Tipped over during ambulation or movement	Return unit to upright position. Assess fluid levels in water seal and suction chambers and replace as needed. Mark collection chambers at current levels of output. Calculate output. It may be necessary to change the chest drainage device to determine output or if suction and water seal chambers cannot be replaced properly.

Nursing Intervention Example: Maintain drainage and negative pressure by positioning the tubing that is attached to the chest tube on the bed and preventing dependent loops.

Reference: International Classification for Nursing Practice. (n.d.). *eHealth & ICNP*. Retrieved from https://www.icn.ch/what-we-do/projects/ehealth-icnp.

CRITICAL CONCEPTS
Caring for a Client With a Chest Tube

Accuracy (ACC)

Accuracy when caring for a client with a chest tube is affected by the following variables:

Nurse-Related Factors
- Positioning and preparation of client for insertion
- Positioning the tubing to prevent negative pressure
- Proper assessment of the client's respiratory status
- Proper monitoring of client and chest tubes
- Precise measurement of output each shift
- Troubleshooting techniques

Equipment-Related Factors
- Proper functioning and setting of the suction regulator
- Functioning of the chest tube drainage system
- Integrity of extension tubing and absence of holes or defects

Client-Centered Care (CCC)

When caring for a client with a chest tube, respect for the client is demonstrated by:
- ensuring that written consent is obtained for an invasive procedure and verbal consent is given for noninvasive procedures
- explaining the procedure and arranging for an interpreter if needed
- providing privacy and ensuring comfort
- answering questions that the client or family may have
- advocating for the client and family
- providing culturally sensitive explanations.

Infection Control (INF)

Healthcare-associated infection when caring for a client with a chest tube is prevented by:
- containment of microorganisms
- preventing and reducing the transfer of microorganisms
- reducing the number of microorganisms
- preventing an environment conducive to microbial growth.

Safety (SAF)

Safety in caring for a client with a chest tube is accomplished by implementing safety measures and providing a safe care environment by:

- maintaining secure, connected chest drainage tubes and a secure chest tube drainage system
- effectively troubleshooting for leaks and other complications

Communication (COM)

- Communication exchanges information (oral, written, nonverbal, or electronic) between two or more people.
- Documentation records information in a permanent healthcare record.
- Collaboration with the client and other healthcare professionals is essential when caring for a client with a chest tube.

Health Maintenance (HLTH)

Nursing is dedicated to promotion of health when using chest tubes by:
- protecting the client's skin at the insertion site
- caring for the client's skin after the chest tube is removed.

Evaluation (EVAL)

Evaluation of outcomes enables the nurse to determine the efficacy of the care provided when caring for a client with a chest tube.

▪ SKILL 18.4 Assisting With Chest Tube Insertion

EQUIPMENT

PPE
Disposable absorbent pad
Facility-approved pain assessment tool
Wet or dry suction closed chest tube drainage system
Sterile water (if wet suction)
Suction canister and tubing
Suction regulator
Connector (e.g., 5-in-1 tubing connector or "Y" connector, if more than one chest tube is to be connected to the chest tube drainage system)
Adhesive tape (~2.5 cm/ [1 inch] in width), to secure tube connections and to anchor chest tube to client
Sterile gloves
Occlusive dressing materials:
Petroleum gauze (7.6 cm × 91.4 cm [3 inches × 36 inches])
Split 4 × 4 gauze dressings/drain sponges (2)
4 × 4 gauze pads (3–4)
Occlusive (nonporous) tape
Sterile supplies and equipment required by the authorized healthcare provider to insert a chest tube, as follows:
Chest tube of appropriate size
Facility-approved antiseptic solution (2% chlorhexidine or povidone-iodine) and gauze or antiseptic swabs
Needle holder
Sterile gown, mask, and cap, eye protection
Sterile thoracotomy procedure tray

BEGINNING THE SKILL

1. **INF** Perform hand hygiene and apply PPE if indicated.
2. **INF** Apply clean gloves.
3. **CCC** Introduce yourself to the client and family. Check that consent was obtained. Ensure that the client understands the reason for the procedure and the steps of the procedure.
4. **SAF** Identify the client using two identifiers.
5. **CCC** Provide privacy. *Providing privacy in layers enhances client-centered care.*

PROCEDURE

6. **CCC** Place a disposable absorbent pad under the client to protect linens.
7. **ACC** Position the client for privacy, comfort, and accessibility for the procedure. Elevate the HOB 30- to 60-degrees and position the arm above the head. *This allows access for the authorized healthcare provider.*

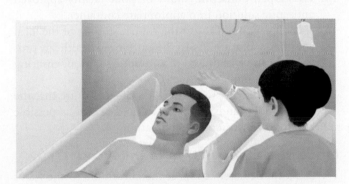

STEP 7 Elevate the head of bed to a 30- to 60-degree angle and position the client's arm above the head.

8. **SAF** Raise the bed to an ergonomically safe working height. Raise one side rail. *Setting up an ergonomically safe space prevents injury to the nurse and client.*
9. **ACC** Assess the client's respiratory, cardiovascular, and pain status, including:
   - vital signs
   - respiratory rate, depth, effort, and chest excursion
   - breath sounds, noting asymmetry
   - pulse oximetry values and capillary refill time
   - pain, using a facility-approved tool
   This will provide a baseline assessment to evaluate the changes after the insertion of the chest tube.
10. **ACC** Administer oxygen as ordered. Monitor the client's response to the supplemental oxygen with a pulse oximeter or capnography. *Presence of a hemothorax or pneumothorax impairs gaseous exchange. Supplemental oxygen may be necessary to maintain oxygenation.*

11. **CCC** Administer the prescribed sedative, analgesia, or emergency medication as ordered. *Analgesia and sedation may require time to take effect. If the need for the chest tube does not allow waiting, local analgesia will be administered at the insertion site.*

12. **ACC** Prepare the closed chest drainage system per manufacturer's instructions.

13. **INF** Use sterile technique to open the thoracotomy tray. Drop any additional sterile items onto the inner packaging using sterile technique.

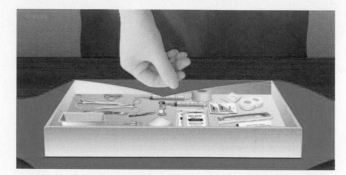

STEP 13 Use sterile technique to open the thoracotomy tray.

14. **INF** Open antiseptic swabs or pour facility-approved antiseptic solution into appropriate container.

15. **INF** Open and disinfect the rubber stopper of the local anesthetic solution. Assist the authorized healthcare provider during withdrawal of antiseptic solution, ensuring aseptic technique.

16. **CCC** Provide reassurance to the client. Ensure that the client understands the need to hold as still as possible and follow instructions on breathing.

Once the Chest Tube Is Inserted

17. **ACC** Immediately connect the chest tube to the water seal chest drainage system.

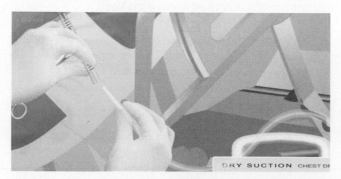

STEP 17 Immediately connect the chest tube to the water seal chest drainage system.

18. **ACC** Observe for bubbling or tidaling in the water seal chamber with a pleural chest tube. *The water seal acts as a one-way valve, and the tidaling reflects the rise and fall of respirations.* (Note: The water level increases during inspiration and decreases during expiration for a client who is not ventilated. The opposite is true for a mechanically ventilated client.)

19. **ACC** Initiate the prescribed amount of suction.

20. **ACC** Position the chest tube drainage system so that it is below the level of chest tube insertion, secured to the bed frame, and in an upright position. If the client has a pleural chest tube, ensure that the chest drainage system is on the same side as the tube. *Promotes drainage and prevents tension and displacement of tube.*

21. **ACC** Position the extension tubing on the client's bed. Prevent dependent loops. *Dependent loops can prevent drainage and cause positive pressure.*

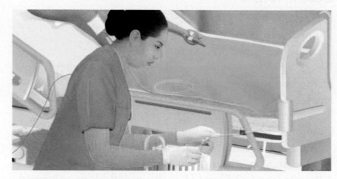

STEP 21 Position the extension tubing on the client's bed.

22. **INF** Dress the insertion site with occlusive dressing per order and facility policy. (See Skill 18.5.)

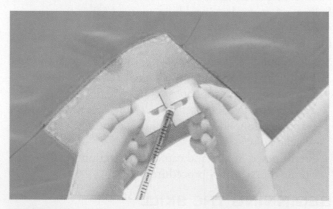

STEP 22 Dress the insertion site with occlusive dressing per order.

23. **SAF** Secure the connection of the distal end of the chest tube to the chest drainage system per manufacturer's recommendations. *Securing the tubing prevents disruptions in the flow of drainage and contamination.* (Note: The tape should not obscure view of the drainage.)

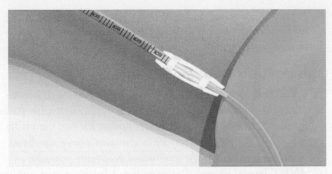

STEP 23 Secure the connection of the distal end of the chest tube to the chest drainage system.

24. **EVAL** Monitor for bubbling or tidaling in the water seal chamber. *Intermittent bubbling with inspiration may be an expected finding in a client with a pneumothorax. However, persistent bubbling may indicate an air leak in the connections.*
25. **EVAL** Confirm proper functioning of the suction control. *Proper functioning of the suction control facilitates evacuation of the pleural or mediastinal space.*
26. **EVAL** Evaluate the client's respiratory, cardiovascular, and pain status, including:
    - vital signs
    - respiratory rate, depth, effort, and chest excursion
    - breath sounds, noting asymmetry
    - pulse oximetry values and capillary refill time
    - pain, using a consistent facility-approved tool
    Identify any changes following the insertion of the chest tube that indicate the client's response to the chest tube therapy.
27. **ACC** Assess the amount, color, and consistency of the drainage in the collection chamber.

28. **SAF** Dispose of sharps in appropriate container.
29. **INF** Dispose of soiled materials and equipment.

FINISHING THE SKILL

30. **INF** Remove gloves and perform hand hygiene.
31. **CCC** Ensure client comfort. Provide reassurance and emotional support.
32. **SAF** Ensure client safety. Place the bed in the lowest position. Ensure that the client can identify and reach the nurse call system. *These safety measures reduce the risk of injury from falls.*
33. **EVAL** Evaluate the outcomes. Verify client's respiratory, cardiovascular, and pain status before leaving the bedside.
34. **INF** Perform hand hygiene.
35. **SAF** Check order with the authorized healthcare provider for a chest x-ray to confirm correct chest tube placement.
36. **COM** Document assessment findings, care given, and outcomes in the legal healthcare record, including the following:
    - vital signs
    - respiratory rate, depth, effort, and chest excursion
    - bilateral breath sounds, noting any asymmetry
    - pulse oximetry values and capillary refill time
    - pain or discomfort using a facility-approved pain assessment tool before and after the procedure
    - how the client tolerated the procedure
    - amount, color, and consistency of chest drainage
    - description of insertion site and dressing
    - assessment of the water seal bubbling and amount of suction
37. **EVAL** Provide follow-up care by continuing to monitor the client's respiratory, cardiovascular, and pain status as well as the chest tube placement and drainage. *Continuous monitoring helps ensure that the chest tube will function properly and remain intact.*

■ SKILL 18.5 Maintaining a Chest Tube System and Performing an Occlusive Dressing Change

EQUIPMENT

Clean gloves
PPE, to protect you and/or your uniform from exposure to body fluids
Sterile gloves
Facility-approved pain assessment tool
Facility-approved antiseptic solution (e.g., chlorhexidine gluconate) and gauze or antiseptic swabs
Sterile water (if wet suction)
Sterile cleansing solution
Cotton-tipped applicators
Adhesive tape to secure tube connections and to anchor chest tube to client
Occlusive dressing materials:
    Petroleum gauze (7.6 cm × 91.4 cm [3 inches × 36 inches])

Split 4 × 4 gauze dressings/drain sponges (2)
4 × 4 gauze pads (3–4)
Occlusive (nonporous) tape

BEGINNING THE SKILL

1. **INF** Perform hand hygiene and apply PPE if the client has transmission precautions ordered or to protect you and/or your uniform from exposure to body fluids.
2. **INF** Apply clean gloves.
3. **CCC** Introduce yourself to the client and family and explain the procedure. Ensure verbal consent for the dressing change.
4. **SAF** Identify the client using two identifiers.
5. **CCC** Provide privacy. *Providing privacy in layers enhances client-centered care.*

PROCEDURE

Assessment of the Client and Chest Tube Drainage System

6. **SAF** Set up an ergonomically safe space. Raise the bed to a comfortable working height. Raise one side rail. *Setting up an ergonomically safe space prevents injury to the nurse and client.*

7. **ACC** Begin with the client and work your way to the chest tube drainage system. Assess the client's respiratory and pain status, including:
   - vital signs
   - respiratory rate, depth, effort, and chest excursion
   - breath sounds, noting any asymmetry
   - pulse oximetry values and capillary refill time
   - pain, using a facility-approved tool

   This assessment is to evaluate respiratory and pain level changes after the insertion of the chest tube.

8. **SAF** Position the extension tubing on the client's bed. *Promotes drainage and prevents tension and displacement of the tube.* If the client has a pleural chest tube, ensure that the chest drainage system is below the level of the chest on the same side as the tube. *Dependent loops prevent drainage and can cause positive pressure.*

9. **ACC** Assess the amount, color, and consistency of the fluid inside the chest drain tubing. *The drainage in the chest drain device is collected over a period of time, and the color may change.*

10. **SAF** Check for the secure connection of the chest tube to the chest drain device tubing.

11. **SAF** Ensure the connections are wrapped with strong tape or manufacturer-recommended securement ties to help maintain the connection.

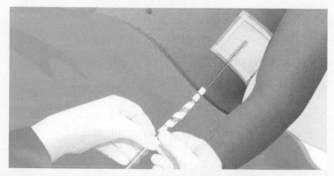

STEP 11 Ensure the connections are wrapped with strong tape to help maintain the connection.

12. **SAF** Confirm the position and security of the chest tube drainage system.

13. **ACC** Assess for bubbling or tidaling in the water seal chamber. *Intermittent bubbling with inspiration may be an expected finding in a client with a pneumothorax. However, persistent bubbling may indicate an air leak in the connections.*

14. **ACC** Assess the proper functioning of the suction control. If using a wet suction chest tube drainage system, sterile water may need to be added because evaporation causes the level to decrease over time. *Proper functioning of the suction control facilitates evacuation of the pleural or mediastinal space.*

Chest Tube Dressing Change

15. **CCC** Position the client for privacy, comfort, and accessibility for the procedure. Place an absorbent disposable pad under the affected side to protect linens. Elevate the HOB 30 to 60 degrees and position the arm above the head. *This allows access for the authorized healthcare provider.*

16. **INF** Change gloves. Perform hand hygiene and apply clean gloves.

17. **INF** Remove the tape, existing gauze pads, drain sponges, and petroleum gauze. Discard soiled materials.

18. **ACC** Assess the skin at the chest tube insertion site. Identify skin irritation, inflammation, or exudate as signs of infection.

19. **SAF** Confirm that the sutures anchoring the chest tube are intact.

20. **ACC** Palpate the skin surrounding the insertion site for evidence of subcutaneous emphysema (e.g., crepitus). *Crepitus may indicate an air leak.*

21. **INF** Remove gloves and perform hand hygiene.

22. **INF** Prepare sterile field:
    a. Open the packages of drain sponges and petroleum gauze pads using sterile technique.
    b. Pour prescribed sterile solution into a sterile basin to clean the site.
    c. Place cotton-tipped applicators into the sterile solution.

22. **INF** Apply sterile gloves.

23. **INF** Clean the skin at the insertion site with facility-approved solution and according to facility protocol.

24. **INF** Clean the chest tube per facility protocol.

25. **ACC** Wrap the petroleum gauze around the chest tube at the insertion site to establish an airtight seal if this is the facility policy. *To seal the insertion site from air entry.*

26. **ACC** Place the drain sponges around the tube in opposite directions.

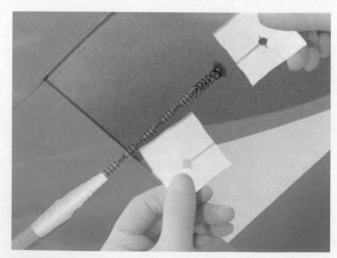

STEP 26 Place the drain sponges around the tube in opposite directions.

27. **ACC** Place two gauze pads over the drain sponges. Cover the gauze pads with an occlusive dressing.
28. **COM** Label the dressing with the date, time, and your initials, per facility policy.
29. **SAF** Confirm the chest tube is secured to the client's skin below the dressing. *This prevents movement of the tube at the insertion site.*

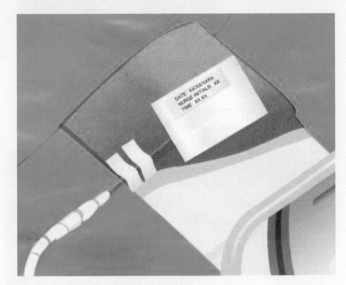

STEP 29 Confirm the chest tube is secured to the client's skin below the dressing.

30. **SAF** Loop the tubing that is attached to the chest tube on to the bed. *Dependent loops can exert positive pressure.*

31. **INF** Dispose of soiled materials.
32. **INF** Remove gloves and perform hand hygiene.

FINISHING THE SKILL

33. **CCC** Ensure client comfort. Provide reassurance and emotional support.
34. **SAF** Ensure client safety. Place the bed is in the lowest position. Ensure that the client can identify and reach the nurse call system. *These safety measures reduce the risk of injury from falls.*
35. **EVAL** Evaluate the outcomes. Verify the client's respiratory status before leaving the bedside.
36. **INF** Perform hand hygiene.
37. **COM** Document assessment findings, care given, and outcomes in the legal healthcare record, including the following:
    - vital signs
    - respiratory rate, depth, effort and chest excursion
    - breath sounds, noting any asymmetry
    - pulse oximetry values and capillary refill time
    - pain level using a facility-approved pain assessment tool
    - amount, color, and consistency of chest drainage
    - assessment of the water seal bubbling and amount of suction
    - chest tube insertion site assessment, including if sutures are intact
    - assessment of the dressing that was removed and the new dressing
    - how the client tolerated the dressing change procedure
    - medication administered.

■ SKILL 18.6 Assisting With Removal of a Chest Tube

EQUIPMENT

Analgesia, if ordered
Absorbent pad to protect linens (disposable)
Sterile and clean gloves
Surgical mask
PPE, to protect you and/or your uniform from exposure to body fluids
Facility-approved antiseptic solution and gauze or antiseptic swabs
Occlusive dressing materials:
Sterile petroleum gauze
Two to four 4 × 4 gauze pads for chest tube insertion site
Occlusive (nonporous) tape
Sterile suture removal tray, which usually includes the following:
    Scissors and small gauze
    Biohazard waste bag

BEGINNING THE SKILL

1. **INF** Perform hand hygiene and apply PPE to protect you and/or your uniform from exposure to body fluids.
2. **CCC** Introduce yourself to client and family and explain the procedure. Ensure that the client gives verbal consent. *Explanation decreases anxiety, and consent promotes autonomy.*
3. **SAF** Identify the client using two identifiers.
4. **CCC** Provide privacy. *Providing privacy in layers enhances client-centered care.*

PROCEDURE

5. **ACC** Assess the client's respiratory and cardiovascular status, including:
    - vital signs
    - respiratory rate, depth, effort, and chest excursion
    - breath sounds, noting symmetry
    - pulse oximetry values and capillary refill time

This will provide a baseline assessment to determine if there are any changes after removal of the chest tube.

6. **CCC** Assess the client's pain status, using a facility-approved pain assessment tool. Provide comfort measures as ordered. Administer analgesia if ordered and wait an appropriate time. An alternative is for the healthcare provider to administer local analgesia at the insertion site. Application of cold packs has also been shown to decrease discomfort with chest tube removal (AACN, 2017). *Decreasing pain and anxiety increases client cooperation.*

7. **SAF** Set up an ergonomically safe space. Raise the bed to a comfortable working height. Raise one side rail. *Setting up an ergonomically safe space prevents injury to the nurse and client.*

8. **ACC** Raise the HOB 30 to 45 degrees and position the disposable absorbent pad under the affected side to protect linens. *Raising the HOB facilitates respiratory effort.*

9. **CCC** Position the client for privacy, comfort, and accessibility for the procedure. Position the arm above the head. *This allows access for the authorized healthcare provider.*

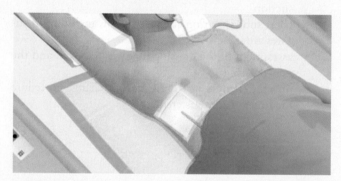

STEP 9 Position the client for privacy, comfort, and accessibility for the procedure.

10. **INF** Using sterile technique, open the following items:
    - suture removal tray
    - sterile petroleum gauze for pleural insertion site
    - two to four sterile 4 × 4 gauze sponges
11. **INF** Open packages of antiseptic swabs and drop onto sterile tray without touching contents.
12. **INF** Perform hand hygiene and apply clean gloves.
13. **INF** Remove the existing dressing.
14. **ACC** Assess the site for redness, swelling, or discharge.
15. **INF** Dispose of soiled dressing and clean gloves; perform hand hygiene.
16. **INF** Apply sterile gloves. Apply sterile mask and gown as indicated.
17. **INF** Using sterile technique, clean the skin at the insertion site with facility-approved antiseptic solution in the facility-prescribed manner. Allow to air dry.

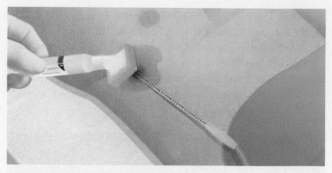

STEP 17 Clean the skin at the insertion site with facility-approved antiseptic solution.

18. **ACC** Clip sutures to release chest tube.
19. **ACC** Remove silk sutures with tweezers.

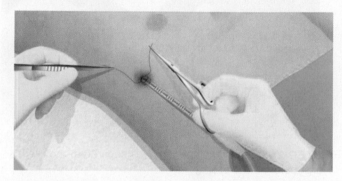

STEP 19 Remove silk sutures with tweezers.

20. **ACC** Instruct the client to perform a Valsalva maneuver (i.e., take a deep breath and hold it). *This prevents the client from gasping or sucking in air during chest tube removal.*

21. **SAF WARNING:** Immediately after advanced healthcare provider has removed chest tube: Cover pleural insertion site with petroleum gauze or mediastinal insertion site with Steri-strips or several 4 × 4 gauze sponges. Cover the gauze sponges with foam tape or other occlusive nonporous tape. *The occlusive dressing prevents air from reentering the pleural space.*

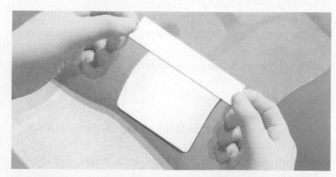

STEP 21 Cover pleural insertion site with petroleum gauze and several gauze sponges, and them cover with foam tape.

22. **INF** Discard chest tube and closed chest tube drainage system in a biohazard bag.
23. **INF** Remove sterile gloves and perform hand hygiene.
24. **EVAL** Evaluate the client's respiratory, cardiovascular, and pain status after chest tube removal, including:
    - vital signs
    - respiratory rate, depth, effort, and chest excursion
    - breath sounds, noting symmetry
    - pulse oximetry values and capillary refill time
    - pain status, using a facility-approved pain assessment tool. *The expected outcome is that the client has no changes in respiratory or cardiovascular status and that pain resulting from the chest tube removal resolves.*

FINISHING THE SKILL

25. **CCC** Ensure client comfort. Provide reassurance and emotional support.
26. **SAF** Ensure client safety. Place the bed in the lowest position. Ensure that the client can identify and reach the nurse call system. *These safety measures reduce the risk of injury from falls.*
27. **EVAL** Evaluate the outcomes. Verify the client's respiratory status before leaving the bedside.
28. **INF** Perform hand hygiene.
29. **COM** Document assessment findings, care given, and outcomes in the legal healthcare record, including:
    - vital signs
    - respiratory rate, depth, effort, and chest excursion
    - breath sounds, noting symmetry
    - pulse oximetry values and capillary refill time
    - insertion site appearance
    - how the client tolerated the procedure
    - any pain or discomfort using a facility-approved pain tool
    - medications administered.
30. **EVAL** Monitor the client's respiratory status and pain level following chest tube removal.

■ CASE STUDY

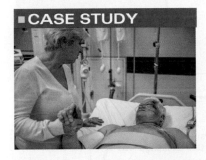

Mr. Bill Lockhart is a 74-year-old male with a 50-year, 1.5-pack-per-day smoking history. He was diagnosed with chronic obstructive pulmonary disease (COPD) 7 years ago. He and his wife come to the emergency room after Mr. Lockhart experiences a fall in their garage. He reports he has lost 15 pounds in the past 6 months and generally feels weak. He has difficulty sleeping and has been using three pillows under his head at night to help him breathe more easily.

At the time of admission, Bill is having progressive dyspnea and a productive but weak cough, with copious, thick yellow sputum. His heart rate is 110 beats per minute, respiratory rate is 30 breaths per minute, and blood pressure is 135/85. His temperature is slightly elevated at 37.2°C, and his oxygen saturation is 88%. He has bilateral expiratory wheezes, and diminished breath sounds in the lung bases are noted. He has bilateral pitting edema of his lower extremities. He is admitted with a diagnosis of pneumonia.

He is initially placed on orofacial CPAP at 45% O_2. However, within a few hours Mr. Lockhart becomes increasingly dyspneic, with more apparent use of accessory muscles. Capnography shows increasing CO_2 concentration. An arterial puncture for ABGs is obtained, as follows:
- pH is 7.25.
- PaO_2 is 60 mm Hg.
- $PaCO_2$ is 55 mm Hg.
- HCO_3^- is 28.

Because Mr. Lockhart is acidotic with increasing CO_2, he is intubated by the authorized healthcare provider with an 8.0 ETT taped at a 26-cm depth at the left lip. The mechanical ventilator is set for assist-control (AC) ventilation at a rate of 16, tidal volume of 550, and FiO_2 at 35%. After Mr. Lockhart is placed on the ventilator, he has a frightened look on his face, and he begins to bite and chew on his ETT. He begins to exhibit increasing agitation and restlessness. Mrs. Lockhart is asking, "What can I do to help him?"

Case Study Questions

1. Considering Mr. Lockhart's physical status and the signs and symptoms on admission, what are the priority nursing diagnoses regarding his care?
2. Based on the ABG values provided, what acid–base imbalance is Mr. Lockhart experiencing?
3. Mr. Lockhart will require ABG sampling to monitor his response to ventilator therapy. Which method of ABG sampling will have the least risk? What test will the nurse perform prior to the sampling?
4. The ICU where Mr. Lockhart is admitted implements the ABCDEF Bundle. Mr. Lockhart appears frightened and agitated and is chewing on the ETT. What aspects of care can the nurse address to assist this client?
5. How might the nurse caring for Mr. Lockhart explain the role of family to Mrs. Lockhart?
6. How can the nurse facilitate communication with Mr. Lockhart and decrease his anxiety?
7. **Application of QSEN Competencies:** One of the Quality and Safety Education for Nurses (QSEN) skill competencies for Evidence-Based Practice is to "Participate in structuring the work environment to facilitate integration of new evidence into standards of practice" (Cronenwett et al, 2007). How can the nurse structure the ICU environment to integrate the PADIS guidelines? What about integrating the ABCDEF Bundle?

■ CONCEPT MAP

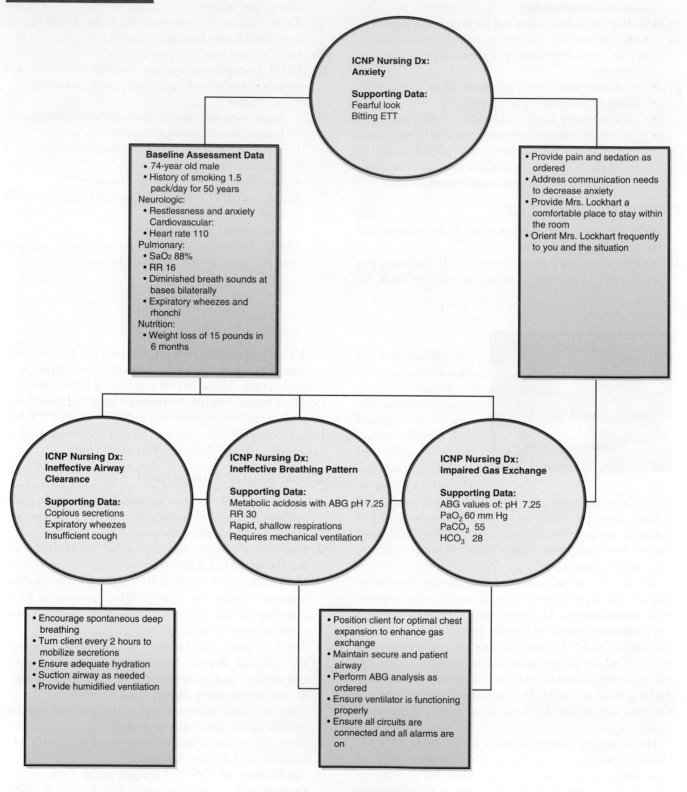

ICNP Nursing Dx:
Anxiety

Supporting Data:
Fearful look
Bitting ETT

Baseline Assessment Data
- 74-year old male
- History of smoking 1.5
  pack/day for 50 years
Neurologic:
- Restlessness and anxiety
  Cardiovascular:
- Heart rate 110
Pulmonary:
- SaO_2 88%
- RR 16
- Diminished breath sounds at
  bases bilaterally
- Expiratory wheezes and
  rhonchi
Nutrition:
- Weight loss of 15 pounds in
  6 months

- Provide pain and sedation as
  ordered
- Address communication needs
  to decrease anxiety
- Provide Mrs. Lockhart a
  comfortable place to stay within
  the room
- Orient Mrs. Lockhart frequently
  to you and the situation

ICNP Nursing Dx:
Ineffective Airway
Clearance

Supporting Data:
Copious secretions
Expiratory wheezes
Insufficient cough

ICNP Nursing Dx:
Ineffective Breathing Pattern

Supporting Data:
Metabolic acidosis with ABG pH 7.25
RR 30
Rapid, shallow respirations
Requires mechanical ventilation

ICNP Nursing Dx:
Impaired Gas Exchange

Supporting Data:
ABG values of: pH 7.25
PaO_2 60 mm Hg
$PaCO_2$ 55
HCO_3 28

- Encourage spontaneous deep
  breathing
- Turn client every 2 hours to
  mobilize secretions
- Ensure adequate hydration
- Suction airway as needed
- Provide humidified ventilation

- Position client for optimal chest
  expansion to enhance gas
  exchange
- Maintain secure and patient
  airway
- Perform ABG analysis as
  ordered
- Ensure ventilator is functioning
  properly
- Ensure all circuits are
  connected and all alarms are
  on

References

American Association of Critical-Care Nurses. (2017). In D. L. Weigand (Ed.), *AACN Procedure manual for high acuity, progressive, and critical care* (7th ed.). St. Louis, MO: Elsevier.

Arai, H., Tajiri, M., Kameda, Y., Shiino, K., Ando, K., Okudela, K., & Masuda, M. (2018). Evaluation of a digital drainage system (Thopaz) in over 250 cases at a single site: A retrospective case-control study. *Clinical Respiratory Journal, 12*(4), 1454–1459.

Arias-Fernandez, P., Romero-Martin, M., Gomez-Salgado, J., & Fernandez-Garcia, D. (2018). Rehabilitation and early mobilization in the critical patient: Systematic review. *Journal of Physical Therapy Science, 30,* 1193–1201.

Baird, M. S. (2016). *Manual of critical care nursing: Nursing interventions and collaborative management* (7th ed.). St. Louis, MO: Elsevier.

Balas, M. C., Weinhouse, G. L., Denehy, L., Changques, G., Rochwerg, B., Misak, C., & Fraser, G. L. (2018). Interpreting and implementing the 2018 pain, agitation/sedation, delirium, immobility, and sleep disruption clinical practice guideline. *Critical Care Medicine, 46,* 1464–1470.

Centers for Disease Control and Prevention. (2015). *Guidelines for the prevention of intravascular catheter-related infections (2011).* Retrieved from https://www.cdc.gov/infectioncontrol/guidelines/bsi/recommendations.html.

Chalhoub, M., Ali, Z., Sasso, L., & Castellano, M. (2016). Experience with indwelling pleural catheters in the treatment of recurrent pleural effusions. *Therapeutic Advances in Respiratory Disease, 10*(6), 566–572.

Cronenwett, L., Sherwood, G., Barnsteiner J., Disch, J., Johnson, J., Mitchell, P., ... & Warren, J. (2007). Quality and safety education for nurses. *Nursing Outlook, 55*(3), 122–131. Retrieved from http://qsen.org/competencies/pre-licensure-ksas/.

Devlin, J. W., Skrobik, Y., Gélinas, C., Needham, D. M., Slooter, A. J. C., Pandharipande, P. P., & Alhazzani, W. (2018). Clinical practice guidelines for the prevention and management of pain, agitation/sedation, delirium, immobility, and sleep disruption in adult patients in the ICU. *Critical Care Medicine, 46*(9), e825–e873.

Flynn Makic, M. B., Rauen, C., Jones, K., & Fisk, A. C. (2015). Continuing to challenge practice to be evidence based. *Critical Care Nurse, 35*(2), 39–50.

Hampson, J., Green, C., Stewart, J., Armitstead, L., Degan, G., Aubrey, A., Paul, E., & Tiruvoipati, R. (2018). Impact of the introduction of an endotracheal tube attachment device on the incidence and severity of oral pressure injuries in the intensive care unit: A retrospective observational study. *BMC Nursing, 17*(4), 1–8.

Hanonu, S., & Karadag, A. (2016). A prospective, descriptive study to determine the rate and characteristics of and risk factors for the development of medical device-related pressure ulcers in intensive care units. *Ostomy Wound Management, 62*(2), 12–22.

Health Research & Educational Trust. (2017). *Preventing ventilator-associated events (VAE) change package: 2017 Update.* Chicago, IL: Health Research & Educational Trust. Retrieved from http://www.hret-hiin.org/topics/ventilator-associated-event.shtml.

Hollister Education. (n.d.). *eLearning course: AnchorFast oral endotracheal tube fastener.* Retrieved from https://www.hollister.com/eLearning/Hollister/AnchorFast/story_html5.html.

Holm, A., & Dreyer, P. (2018). Nurse-patient communication within the context of non-sedated mechanical ventilation: A hermeneutic-phenomenological study. *British Association of Critical Care Nurses, 23*(2), 88–94.

Hong Chu, W. (2017). *Arterial blood gases: Clinician information.* [Evidence summary]. Retrieved from The Joanna Briggs Institute EBP Database, JBI@Ovid. JBI177.

ICU: Alarms sound, nurse does not respond, hypoxic brain injury results. (2009). *Legal Eagle Eye Newsletter for the Nursing Profession, 17*(3). Retrieved from http://www.nursinglaw.com.

Institute for Healthcare Improvement. (2017). *How-to guide: Prevent ventilator-associated pneumonia.* Cambridge, MA: Institute for Healthcare Improvement. Retrieved from http://www.ihi.org/resources/Pages/Tools/HowtoGuidePreventVAP.aspx.

International Classification for Nursing Practice. (n.d.). *eHealth & ICNP.* Retrieved from https://www.icn.ch/what-we-do/projects/ehealth-icnp.

Jones, S., Spangler, P., Keiser, M., & Turkelson, C. (2019). Impact of nursing education of phlebotomy blood loss and hospital-acquired anemia. *Dimensions of Critical Care Nursing, 38*(1), 13–19.

Klompas, M., Branson, R., Eichenwald, R., Greene, L. R., Howell, M. D., Lee, G., & Berenholtz, S. M. (2014). Strategies to prevent ventilator-associated pneumonia in acute care hospitals: 2014 Update. *Infection Control and Hospital Epidemiology, 35*(8), 915–936.

Li, Y. (2017). *Chest drains: Maintenance.* [Evidence summary]. Retrieved from The Joanna Briggs Institute EBP Database, JBI@Ovid. JBI1634.

Lizarondo, L. (2017). *Endotracheal tube placement verification: Ultrasound.* [Evidence summary]. Retrieved from The Joanna Briggs Institute EBP Database , JBI@Ovid. JBI1319.

Marra, A., Lay, E. W., Pandharipande, P. P., & Patel, M. B. (2017). The ABCDEF Bundle in critical care. *Critical Care Clinics, 33*(2), 225–243.

McBeth, C. L., Montes, R. S., Powne, A., North, S. E., & Natale, J. E. (2018). Interprofessional approach to the sustained reduction in ventilator-associated pneumonia in a pediatric intensive care unit. *Critical Care Nurse, 38*(6), 36–46.

Mondor, E. E. (2017a). Upper respiratory problems. In S. L. Lewis, L. Bucher, M. M. Heitkemper, & M. M. Harding (Eds.), *Medical-surgical nursing: Assessment and management of clinical problems* (10th ed.) (pp. 475–497). St. Louis, MO: Elsevier.

Mondor, E. E. (2017b). Lower respiratory problems. In S. L. Lewis, L. Bucher, M. M. Heitkemper, & M. M. Harding (Eds.), *Medical-surgical nursing: Assessment and management of clinical problems* (10th ed.) (pp. 499–537). St. Louis, MO: Elsevier.

Mora Carpio, A. L., & Mora, J. I. (2018). Ventilator management. *StatPearls.* Retrieved from https://www.ncbi.nlm.nih.gov/books/NBK448186/.

Muffly, T. M., Couri, B., Edwards, A., Kow, N., Bonham, A. J., & Paraíso, M. F. R. (2012). Effect of petroleum gauze packing on the mechanical properties of suture materials. *Journal of Surgical Education, 69*(1), 37–40.

Muzzy, A. C., & Butler, A. K. (2015). Managing chest tubes: Air leaks and unplanned tube removal. *American Nurse Today, 10*(5), 10–13.

Pagana, K., & Pagana, T. (2013). *Mosby's diagnostic and laboratory test reference* (11th ed.). St. Louis, MO: Mosby.

Page, C., Retter, A., & Wyncoll, D. (2013). Blood conservation devices in critical care: A narrative review. *Annals of Intensive Care.* Retrieved from http://www.annalsofintensivecare.com/content/3/1/14.

Rittayamai, N., Katsios, C. M., Beloncle, F., Friedrich, J. O., Mancebo, J., & Brochard, L. (2015). Pressure controlled vs volume controlled ventilation in acute respiratory failure: A physiology-based narrative and systemic review. *CHEST, 148*(2), 340–355.

Seckel, M. A., & Bucher, L. (2017). Critical care. In S. L. Lewis, L. Bucher, M. M. Heitkemper, & M. M. Harding (Eds.), *Medical-surgical nursing: Assessment and management of clinical problems* (10th ed.) (pp. 1554–1585). St. Louis, MO: Elsevier.

Sommers, M. S. (2019). Pneumothorax. In *Davis's diseases and disorders: a nursing therapeutics manual* (6th ed.). Philadelphia: FA Davis Company.

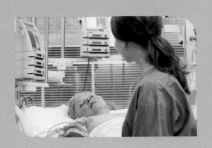

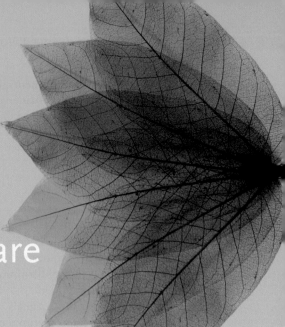

CHAPTER 19

Advanced Cardiovascular Care

"It is only with the heart that one can see rightly; what is essential is invisible to the eye." | **Antoine de Saint Exupéry (*The Little Prince*, 1943)**

LEARNING OBJECTIVES

By the end of this chapter, the reader will be able to:

1 Provide a brief overview of the normal anatomy and physiology of the heart.
2 Discuss the concept of perfusion and how it relates to normal cardiovascular processes.
3 Identify examples of alterations in cardiovascular processes and decreased perfusion.
4 Discuss principles related to cardiac conduction and electrocardiogram (ECG) monitoring.

5 Place the client on continuous ECG (hardwire or telemetry) cardiac monitoring.
6 Perform a 12-lead ECG.
7 Discuss dysrhythmias and alterations of cardiac conduction.
8 Perform or assist with elective synchronized cardioversion.

9 Demonstrate the critical elements of caring for a client who has a temporary or permanent pacemaker.

10 Discuss cardiac emergencies and links in the cardiac chain of survival.

11 Analyze the clinical cues for a client who develops acute ischemic chest pain.

12 Demonstrate the critical elements of caring for a client after an emergency cardiac catheterization.

13 Perform emergency (asynchronous) defibrillation on a client.

14 Prioritize the care for a client in cardiac arrest.

TERMINOLOGY

Acute coronary syndrome (ACS) General term that refers to a group of symptoms or conditions (ischemic chest pain, angina, etc.) that is associated with coronary artery obstruction resulting in the disruption of blood flow to the myocardium (heart muscle).

Artifact Extraneous electronic signals caused by outside interference. Artifact can sometimes cause distortions on an ECG tracing and may inadvertently be mistaken for dysrhythmias.

Biphasic Energy waveforms that travel in two directions, as with biphasic defibrillators.

Cardiac output (CO) Volume of blood, measured in liters (L), pumped per minute by the heart. The formula for calculating cardiac output is CO = HR (heart rate) × SV (stroke volume).

Defibrillator An electronic device that delivers an electric shock (measured in joules) to the client's heart to terminate dysrhythmias and allow the intrinsic pacemaker (or SA node) to reestablish normal sinus rhythm.

Depolarization Electrical activity that occurs as a wave when there is movement of ions across a cell membrane. On the ECG, depolarization is represented by the P wave (corresponds with atrial contraction) and the QRS complex (corresponds with ventricular contraction).

Dysrhythmia Refers to abnormal or disordered rhythm of the electrical activity of the heart

Electrocardiogram (ECG) Graphic representation, display, or record of the electrical (not muscle) activity of the heart. An ECG may also be referred to as an EKG.

Impedance Amount of resistance to the current or flow of energy during defibrillation. This can be affected by variables such as body mass, diaphoresis, and quality of contact with paddles.

Implantable cardioverter-defibrillator (ICD) Battery-powered device, usually implanted under the client's skin. It can detect dysrhythmias and deliver a shock to restore normal rhythm.

Intrinsic Inherent or occurring naturally within the body (e.g., client's own intrinsic heart rate)

Ischemia Inadequate or reduced blood flow to the heart or other organs of the body.

Isoelectric Refers to absence of electrical activity or baseline on an ECG. Waveforms below the line have a negative (downward) deflection, and those above the line have a positive deflection.

Joules Amount of energy (or current) selected for defibrillation or cardioversion.

Left ventricular ejection fraction (LVEF) Measurement of amount of blood ejected by the client's left ventricle with each heartbeat. The normal LVEF may range between 55% and 70%.

Repolarization Recovery or return of the cells to their resting state. This electrical activity is represented by the T wave on the ECG and corresponds to myocardial relaxation.

ACRONYMS

ACS Acute coronary syndrome
AHA American Heart Association
ARC American Red Cross
AV Atrioventricular
ECG Electrocardiogram
ICS Intercostal space
MI Myocardial infarction
NSTEMI Non–ST-segment elevation myocardial infarction
RRT Rapid response team
SA Sinoatrial
STEMI ST-segment elevation myocardial infarction
VF Ventricular fibrillation
VT Ventricular tachycardia

Cardiac disease is a leading cause of death in the United States and worldwide (Centers for Disease Control and Prevention [CDC], 2017). In addition to early recognition and prevention, nurses have a critical role in helping clients recover from cardiac alterations and restoring them to health. Nurses also have an important role with respect to helping clients maintain optimal cardiovascular perfusion. This chapter discusses concepts and skills related to advanced cardiovascular care. It is not intended to replace an advanced critical care textbook. Skills related to peripheral vascular care, such as the use of compression devices, are discussed in Chapter 17.

CARDIOVASCULAR SYSTEM

The cardiovascular system (also known as the circulatory system) includes the heart, lungs, blood vessels (arteries, veins, capillaries, arterioles, venules), and lymphatics. At the center of this intricate network is the heart, a muscular organ located within the mediastinum beneath the sternum. There are four chambers in the heart: the right and left atria (upper chambers) and the right and left ventricles (lower chambers). These chambers are separated by valves to prevent backflow. The main function of the heart is to pump blood, which contains oxygen, nutrients, and other vital substances, to provide nourishment to the cells within the body.

The Concept of Perfusion

The concept of perfusion refers to central perfusion (cardiac output or amount of blood pumped by the heart per minute) as well as tissue perfusion (Wilson, 2017). In order for adequate perfusion and oxygenation of the tissues to occur, the heart, blood vessels, and lungs must work in harmony. An adequate circulating blood volume must also be maintained. As shown in Fig 19.1, oxygen-poor or deoxygenated blood enters the right atrium through the superior vena cava (which receives blood from the head, neck, and upper thorax) and the inferior vena cava (which receives blood from the structures inferior to or below the upper thorax). The blood is then pumped from the right atrium into the right ventricle. From the right ventricle, the blood is pumped into the pulmonary artery, which branches into the right and left pulmonary arteries that go to the right and left lungs, respectively.

Once the deoxygenated blood is in the lungs, it enters into the pulmonary capillary network, where gas exchange takes place. Oxygenated blood then leaves the lungs via the right and left pulmonary veins, which drain into the left atrium. After this occurs, the oxygenated blood enters the left ventricle. The left ventricle is the primary pumping chamber of the heart, and it is normally thicker and larger than the right ventricle. The left ventricle pumps the oxygenated blood into the aorta, which then carries this blood (via the ascending and descending aortic branches) to the organs and the upper and lower extremities of the body.

As blood is pumped out of the left ventricle, some of the oxygenated blood flows from the aorta into the coronary artery network, which is near the surface of the heart. The coronary arteries supply oxygen to all areas of the heart. As with other organs of the body, the coronary arteries require adequate circulating blood volume and adequate perfusion in order for oxygenation of the tissues to occur. The major coronary arteries are shown in Fig. 19.2.

Cardiovascular Alterations and Disruptions in Perfusion

Various conditions can cause disruptions in perfusion and cardiovascular function. One example of a condition that can cause a disruption in perfusion is a blockage of one or more of the coronary arteries, leading to acute coronary syndrome (ACS) and cardiac ischemia (see Section 4 of this chapter).

Other examples of alterations include an inability of the heart to work effectively as a pump (heart failure) or an insufficient amount of volume in the pump (hypovolemia). Reduced intravascular volume can be caused by internal or external blood loss, or it could be caused by a shifting of fluids out of the intravascular space to other areas of the body. In contrast, a client may exhibit heart failure when the heart is weak or pumping inefficiently. In this situation, the heart may have a low left ventricular ejection fraction (LVEF) and is not able to compensate by ejecting or pumping enough blood to meet the oxygen and metabolic demands of the body. Finally, increased intravascular volume or fluid overload may cause the left ventricle to decompensate and lead to heart failure as well. Heart failure is caused by damage to the heart muscle (as with myocardial infarction), or it can be related to other conditions, such as cardiomyopathy. Left-sided or left ventricular heart failure results from the inability of the left ventricle to contract efficiently, which leads to lower LVEF and, eventually, an overload of blood in the left atrium, resulting in an increased backpressure, which may lead to pulmonary congestion. Left-sided heart failure may lead to right-sided heart failure because of the inability of the right ventricle to pump blood effectively against the increasing back pressure within the lungs, which can further cause volume overload and peripheral edema. In severe cases, a client can develop stages of cardiogenic shock, resulting in reduced cardiac output and impaired tissue perfusion. Clinical manifestations may include, but not be limited to, the following:

- Decreased blood pressure (significantly below baseline)
- Low urine output (less than 0.5 mL/kg per hour over 2 hours)

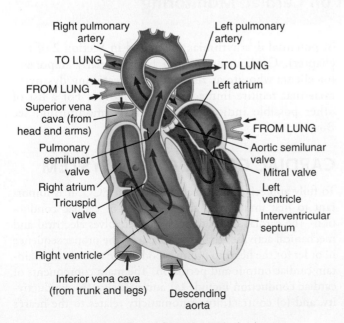

FIG. 19.1 Blood flow through the heart.

Right pulmonary artery
TO LUNG
FROM LUNG
Superior vena cava (from head and arms)
Pulmonary semilunar valve
Right atrium
Tricuspid valve
Right ventricle
Inferior vena cava (from trunk and legs)
Left pulmonary artery
TO LUNG
Left atrium
FROM LUNG
Aortic semilunar valve
Mitral valve
Left ventricle
Interventricular septum
Descending aorta

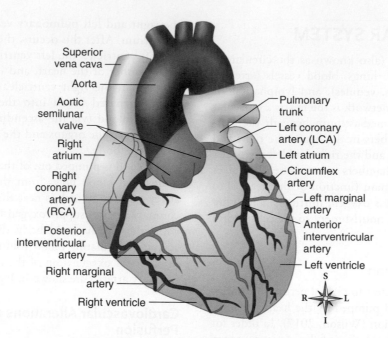

Fig. 19.2 Coronary arteries of the heart.

- Cool, clammy skin (particularly extremities)
- Weak, thready pulses in extremities
- Changes in mental status, restlessness, or confusion
- Rapid, shallow respirations and alterations in oxygen (O₂) saturation
- Activity intolerance or inability to perform normal activities.

Clients who have alterations of the cardiovascular system may require care in a variety of settings. Common skills nurses may need to perform include, but are not limited to, electrocardiogram (ECG) monitoring, providing care for clients who require cardioversion or cardiac pacemakers, and providing care for clients who have various cardiac emergencies.

SECTION 1 Caring for a Client on Cardiac Monitoring

One of the most common procedures performed for clients is cardiac monitoring. An electrocardiogram (ECG), also sometimes referred to as EKG, is a noninvasive procedure and graphic record of the electrical activity of the heart. The primary purpose of the ECG is to detect the transmission of cardiac impulses and obtain information about the heart rate, rhythm, and other characteristics. However, the ECG does not replace assessment by the nurse at the bedside, nor does it detect all cardiac pathology.

The indications for cardiac monitoring vary, depending on the client's condition. Some clients, such as those who are critically ill, may require continuous cardiac monitoring, whereas other clients may be monitored intermittently as a precautionary measure during certain procedures. One of the most common indications for cardiac monitoring is for clients who have existing

or potential dysrhythmias (discussed in Section 2 of this chapter). Cardiac monitoring is particularly important for clients who are at risk for life-threatening dysrhythmias that require immediate defibrillation. For a list of other possible indications for cardiac monitoring, see Box 19.1.

CARDIAC CONDUCTION SYSTEM

To fully appreciate the mechanism of an ECG, it is important to first understand the principles of cardiac conduction. The cardiac conduction system involves electrical and mechanical activities that must occur in the proper sequence in order for the heart to pump blood to the tissues and maintain cardiac output and perfusion. The main components of cardiac conduction include (a) automaticity, (b) conductivity, and (c) contractility. Automaticity relates to the heart's ability to produce an electrical impulse from a stimulus. Conductivity is the heart's ability to conduct an electrical impulse from one cell to the next. Contractility is the ability of the muscle fibers in the heart to shorten after receiving an impulse, resulting in contraction. These events must occur in the proper sequence with the correct timing.

As illustrated in Fig. 19.3, the electrical impulse travels through the heart in an organized fashion with each heartbeat. Normally, the sinoatrial (SA) node, known as the heart's "pacemaker," discharges approximately 60 to 100

times per minute. The impulse from the SA node spreads through both atria and results in depolarization and contraction of the atrial muscles; it then travels through internodal pathways to the atrioventricular (AV) node. When the impulse reaches the AV node, the conduction velocity slows slightly in order to allow complete emptying of the circulating blood volume from the atria into the ventricles. This "slight delay" function of the AV node is critical because incomplete filling of the client's ventricles could ultimately result in reduced stroke volume and cardiac output.

After the impulse passes through the AV node, it continues through the AV bundle of His and down the right/left bundle branches into the Purkinje network of both ventricles. The conduction through the Purkinje fibers (which look like thousands of tiny branches) results in ventricular depolarization. This "wave" of depolarization produces contraction. However, the electrical activity, not myocardial contraction, is what is seen on the client's ECG (Jacobson, 2019a).

THE ECG TRACING

To ensure that the ECG tracing is adequate, the nurse will observe the electronic tracing on the monitor as well as the rhythm strip on graph paper that may be printed out and posted. It is important for the nurse to be able to recognize the normal ECG waveforms and components. A tracing of good quality will be clear and free from extraneous artifact, and the primary ECG components (P, QRS, T, and the PR interval, ST segment or interval, QT interval) should be easy

BOX 19.1 Possible Indications for Cardiac Monitoring

- Chest pain and/or associated symptoms
- Acute coronary syndrome (ACS) (suspected or confirmed)
- Acute heart failure (right or left ventricular failure)
- Electrolyte disturbances (e.g., low or high potassium or magnesium levels)
- Palpitations, syncope (fainting), dizziness, or irregular pulse that deviates from baseline
- History of cardiac ischemia, dysrhythmias, or conduction disorders
- High-risk procedures or surgery that could cause cardiac disturbances
- Sudden or unusual change in physiological status or post-resuscitation
- Overdose of medications that are a high risk for cardiac toxicity

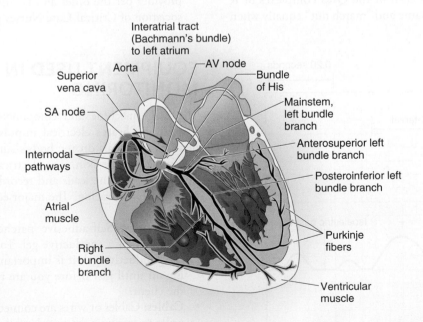

FIG. 19.3 Cardiac conduction pathway.

to identify. In addition to the ECG components, the boxes on the graph paper should also be clear. The grid on the graph paper consists of vertical and horizontal boxes that measure time (horizontal boxes) and amplitude or voltage (vertical boxes). Each small box on the horizontal axis is equal to 0.04 seconds, and each large box is 0.20 seconds. On the vertical axis, each small box measures 1 mm (0.1 mV), and each large box measures 5 mm (0.5 mV). For an illustration of the major ECG components and the ECG measurement intervals, see Fig 19.4.

Depending on the setting, nurses may also be required to measure and evaluate some of the ECG components (e.g., PR, QRS, and QT intervals; ST segment) in order to monitor the client for any changes. A description of basic ECG elements is as follows (Jacobson, 2019a):

- **P wave:** This small deflection (usually 2.5 mm or less in height) represents atrial muscle depolarization or contraction. The P wave should precede every QRS wave.
- **QRS complex:** The QRS complex represents ventricular depolarization. As shown in Fig 19.4, the Q wave is the initial downward deflection below the isolectric baseline, followed by the R wave. The R wave is a taller complex that has an upward or opposite deflection from the Q and S waves. The S wave (second downward deflection) follows the R wave. The normal width of the QRS complex is 0.04 to 0.10 in an adult (Jacobson, 2019a), and it should always precede the T wave. However, the width of the QRS may vary slightly depending on the client. Notify the authorized healthcare provider if the width is outside the established parameters for the client per the order and facility policy. If the heart rate is regular, the distance between each of the QRS complexes or R waves should be the same and "march out" equally when measured.

- **T wave:** Represents repolarization (recovery) of the ventricles. The T wave should normally follow and deflect in the same direction as the QRS complex.
- **U wave:** Small wave that sometimes follows the T wave. It may be enlarged when repolarization is prolonged. This may be caused by the presence of certain medications or by conditions such as electrolyte disorders (e.g., low potassium, magnesium, or calcium).
- **PR interval:** This interval is normally 0.12 to 0.20 seconds, and it is measured from the beginning of the P wave to the beginning of the QRS complex. The PR interval may be prolonged in clients who have certain conduction alterations such as AV block.
- **ST segment:** This is measured from the end of the QRS complex to the beginning of the T wave. Normally, this segment is isoelectric (at baseline). If the ST segment is elevated or depressed more than 1 to 2 mm, the client may be having cardiac ischemia as part of ACS (see Section 4 of this chapter). For examples of ST-segment and T-wave alterations, see Fig 19.5.
- **QT interval:** This will vary depending on age, gender, and heart rate. It is measured from the beginning of the QRS complex to the end of the T wave. Generally, it should not measure more than 0.45 in men and 0.46 in women (Jacobson, 2019a). The length of the QT interval may be affected by the client's heart rate. Thus, the QT interval is usually corrected for heart rate using a facility-approved formula. A prolonged QT interval can be induced by certain medications and may lead to life-threatening dysrhythmias. If a client has a prolonged QT interval above established parameters or greater than 0.50 (corrected for heart rate), notify the authorized healthcare provider per the order and facility policy (American Association of Critical-Care Nurses [AACN], 2016).

EQUIPMENT USED IN ECG MONITORING

The ECG machine and components help to detect and amplify the heart's electrical impulses. These impulses are detected as signals on the body's surface by electrodes that are applied to the skin. The electrical signals are then conducted through the leads and recorded on the graph paper to produce the tracing. The major equipment for the ECG is as follows:

- **Electrodes:** Self-adhesive patches that are disposable and contain a conductive gel. To avoid "drying out" of the conductive gel, it is important to not peel the backing off until just before you are ready to place them on the client.
- **Cables:** Cables or wires are connected to the electrodes in order to transmit the signals to the ECG machine. These are usually labeled or color-coded.
- **ECG machine:** Transmits the signal to a screen (or oscilloscope) for viewing. The machine also records the ECG tracing on the calibrated ECG graph paper.

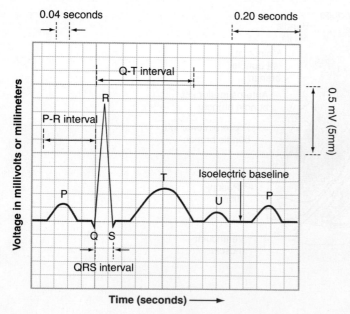

FIG. 19.4 Electrocardiogram (ECG) components and intervals.

ECG alterations associated with ischemia

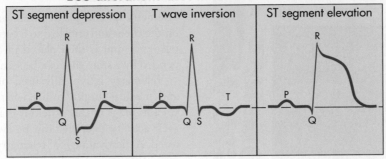

FIG. 19.5 Examples of ST-segment and T-wave alterations.

LEAD PLACEMENT FOR ECG MONITORING

A lead is a tracing or a "view" of the electrical activity of the heart from different angles or vectors across the body. These angles are obtained by a group or pairs of electrodes on the client (Randazzo, 2016; Wung, 2017). A lead also refers to the cables or wires that are used to connect the monitor or ECG machine to the client's electrodes.

To understand how leads work, think about how electricity flows. Usually, the flow of electricity or vector is from negative to positive. In this context, the word *vector* relates to the electrical activity, emanating from the heart, that has both magnitude and direction. If electrical currents flow from the negative to positive electrodes, upright or positive deflections will be produced. If electrical currents flow away from the positive electrodes, a negative deflection will appear (Pelter, Kozik, & Carey, 2017).

The client's lead connections may be labeled as positive or negative, and they may be color-coded. The decision about which lead to select for ECG monitoring is determined by the needs of the client. The three-lead system is simple and easy to use. However, a disadvantage of the three-lead system is that it

does not allow for monitoring precordial/chest leads. Thus, a five-lead system, which does allow for precordial views, is usually preferred and more commonly used. A five-lead system consists of four limb leads and one precordial lead. Examples of a three-lead system and a five-lead system are illustrated in Fig. 19.6. For labeling purposes, the limb leads are referred to as right arm (RA), left arm (LA), or left leg (LL) leads. For the five-lead system, the labels *V* (precordial vector) or *C* (chest lead) may be used (Pelter et al. 2017). As shown in the figure, the precordial/chest lead V1 is located at the fourth intercostal space at the right sternal border. An alternative precordial/chest lead is V6 (not shown), which is located at the client's left midaxillary line at the fifth intercostal space. However, V1 is usually the preferred precordial lead for monitoring dysrhythmias (AACN, 2016; Jacobson 2019a).

Depending on the client's needs and the manufacturer recommendations, a six-lead system may be used that allows the two precordial/chest leads (V1 and V6) to be viewed at the same time. For some clients, such as those with ACS or myocardial injury, continuous 12-lead or ST-segment monitoring may be indicated (see Section 4 of this chapter).

When performing ECG monitoring, the critical concept of accuracy is paramount. Accurate identification of

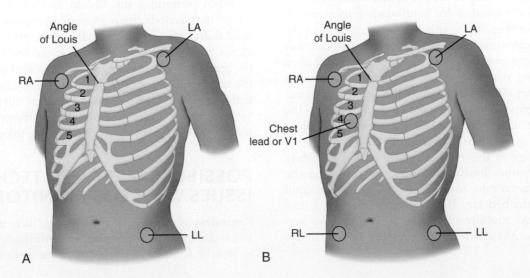

FIG. 19.6 Examples of a three-lead and a five-lead system. **A,** Three-lead system. **B,** Five-lead system.

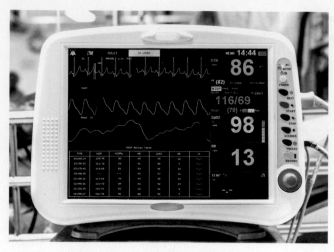

FIG. 19.7 Example of a bedside cardiac monitor.

landmarks and placement of electrodes and leads are essential for an accurate ECG tracing. Misplacement of an electrode by just one intercostal space can affect the morphology of the ECG components, which can result in misdiagnosis (AACN, 2016).

TYPES OF ECG MONITORING

The type of monitoring used will vary depending on the client's condition and the setting where he or she is receiving care. In the acute care setting, continuous bedside monitoring (hardwire and telemetry) is typically used. In outpatient or home settings, long-term ambulatory ECG monitoring may be indicated.

Continuous (Hardwire) Bedside Monitoring

With continuous (hardwire) ECG monitoring, the lead wires are attached directly to the client, and the impulses are transmitted to the monitor for continuous display on the bedside monitor (Fig. 19.7). This is most often used for clients in critical care areas (e.g., intensive or coronary care, surgery, recovery and emergency room). These clients will often have monitoring systems that can simultaneously monitor and display other vital functions as well, such as oxygen saturation, capnography, blood pressure, and respirations. The ECG tracing is usually transmitted to a central monitoring (CM) station for 24-hour observation.

The advantage of this type of system is that it enables the nurse and other healthcare providers to observe the client's ECG, heart rate, and rhythm at a glance for rapid assessment at the bedside. The disadvantage is that it may limit the client's mobility. When using this type of system, ensure that the alarms are set properly and are always turned on.

Using Telemetry

Telemetry systems use electrodes and lead wires that are placed on the client and attached to a battery pack. The battery pack/telemetry unit is then placed in a device or pouch and suspended by a strap that can be secured and worn by the client.

Telemetry is typically used on cardiac step-down units and medical-surgical units where monitoring is provided. An advantage of this system is that clients can ambulate, and their activity tolerance can be evaluated while being monitored. A disadvantage of telemetry is that the client's activity may cause artifact and distort the quality of the tracing. Like the hardwire ECG, telemetry systems can provide 24-hour observation by the CM station.

PERFORMING A 12-LEAD ECG

A 12-lead ECG is a test that evaluates the heart from 12 different angles or perspectives. This is accomplished by using 10 electrodes that view the heart from two perpendicular planes, the frontal and horizontal planes. This is similar to taking a picture from different positions. The frontal leads (leads I–III; AVR, AVL, and AVF) view the heart from a vertical or frontal plane, and the transverse precordial/chest leads (V1–V6) view the heart from a horizontal plane (Fig. 19.8) (Randazzo, 2016; Wung, 2017). To improve understanding and enhance accuracy, it is also important to consider anatomical reference points such as the midclavicular, anterior axillary, and midaxillary lines. The precise placement of the 12-lead ECG electrodes is described in Skill 19.2.

Because more leads are used at different angles, the 12-lead ECG typically provides a more in-depth diagnostic analysis of the heart than a five-lead or six-lead ECG monitoring system. The 12-lead ECG is also the gold standard for the initial evaluation of clients who have ACS and suspected myocardial ischemia or infarction (Caple & Heering, 2018). Additionally, the 12-lead ECG may be used as a screening tool before certain high-risk medical or surgical procedures. An example of a 12-lead ECG is provided in Fig. 19.9.

When performing the 12-lead ECG, it is important to ensure the electrodes/leads are placed properly and maintain good skin contact. The limb leads must be placed on the limbs in the same place bilaterally, *not* on the torso. In addition, the precordial or chest leads should be placed on the chest in the appropriate intercostal spaces, as previously discussed. It is also important for the client to remain as still and relaxed as possible, with the legs uncrossed, during the procedure. This reduces the chance of artifact from outside interference.

POSSIBLE SAFETY AND TECHNICAL ISSUES WITH ECG MONITORING

Regardless of the type of monitoring, there are key safety and technical issues that must be considered. As described in Box 19.2, alarm safety is one of the most serious safety

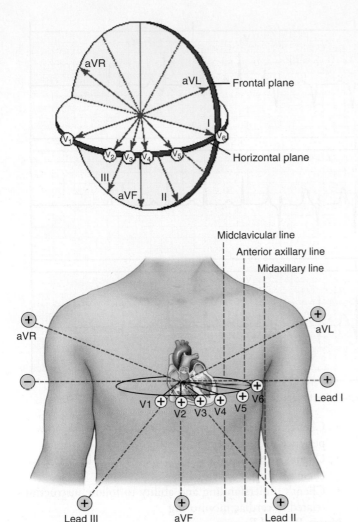

FIG. 19.8 Frontal and horizontal planes of a 12-lead electrocardiogram (ECG). (Note: In this image, V1 to V6 represent the horizontal plane, not electrode placement.)

technical problems with ECGs, as well as troubleshooting tips, see Box 19.3. An important concept to remember is that your first priority is the client. If a technical problem does arise with the ECG, assess your client's level of consciousness first to ensure the client is not having any distress, and then troubleshoot for technical problems with the ECG. If there is not a technical problem and the client has a possible dysrhythmia, assess your client further (e.g., obtain a palpated pulse and blood pressure) and provide the appropriate interventions as described in Section 2 of this chapter.

SUMMARY

When caring for a client who requires cardiac monitoring, accuracy and communication are two of the most important critical concepts to consider. This is particularly true if the client is at risk for impaired cardiac function. Consistent technique, proper identification of electrode sites, and communication with other members of the healthcare team will enhance accuracy and early identification of changes in the client's status. However, it is important to note that cardiac monitoring is only one tool and is not used in isolation. Additional assessment parameters such as the client's physical exam and subjective signs and symptoms must also be considered.

Collaboration and Teamwork

When performing cardiac monitoring, there may be several members of the healthcare team involved. Thus, collaboration and teamwork are essential. For example, an ECG technician may assist with performing a 12-lead ECG, and CM technicians assist with monitoring the client in the CM station. However, the registered nurse (RN) is responsible for reviewing and analyzing the rhythm strips, measuring the ECG components, and contacting the authorized healthcare provider per facility policy. The RN is also responsible for proper documentation in the client's record.

issues. Client fatalities have occurred because of alarm incidents, including alarms being inadvertently left off, high/low alarms not being reset, alarms not being configured properly, or monitoring systems never being turned on when placed on the client at the time of admission. The National Patient Safety Goals by The Joint Commission have identified the need to ensure that alarms on medical equipment, including the ECG, are heard and responded to in a timely manner.

Some technical problems that can occur with ECG monitoring include poor tracings, artifact and interference from outside activity (Fig. 19.10), poor skin contact with electrodes, and difficulty keeping the electrodes in place. Electrodes can also cause skin breakdown, particularly for clients who have to wear them long term. Proper skin preparation and follow-up monitoring of the client's skin can avert these complications. For additional examples of

APPLICATION OF THE NURSING PROCESS

Examples of Related International Classification for Nursing Practice (ICNP) Nursing Diagnoses, Expected Client Outcomes, and Nursing Interventions:

Nursing Diagnosis: Risk for impaired cardiac function

Supporting Data: Client has history of heart failure and alterations in ECG findings.

Expected Client Outcomes: Client will have no evidence of impaired cardiac function, as seen by:
- vital signs and ECG results within established parameters
- absence of signs and symptoms of heart failure (see narrative discussion)

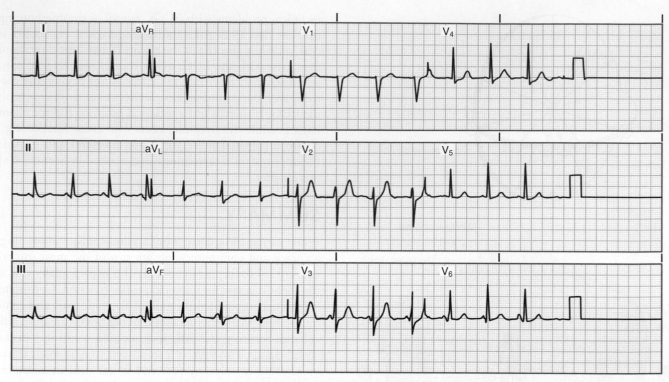

FIG. 19.9 Example of a 12-lead electrocardiogram (ECG).

- skin warm and dry
- ability to tolerate activities of daily living.

Nursing Intervention Examples: Monitor client's vital signs and other parameters of cardiac function, and ensure accuracy when performing cardiac monitoring.

Nursing Diagnosis: Risk for impaired skin integrity
Supporting Data: Client has redness and irritation where ECG electrodes are located.

Expected Client Outcomes: Client will have no evidence of impaired skin integrity, as seen by:
- absence of skin breakdown or excoriation at electrode sites
- absence of pain, discomfort, or redness at electrode sites.

Nursing Intervention Example: Monitor the client's skin integrity where electrodes are placed.

Reference: International Classification for Nursing Practice. (n.d.). *eHealth & ICNP*. Retrieved from https://www.icn.ch/what-we-do/projects/ehealth-icnp.

CRITICAL CONCEPTS
Caring for a Client on Cardiac Monitoring

Accuracy (ACC)

When caring for a client on cardiac monitoring, accuracy is affected by the following variables:

Client-Related Factors
- Client's assessment, including age, level of consciousness, and orientation

- Client's medical history, including history of previous experience with cardiac monitoring
- Client's skin integrity where electrodes will be placed and client's history of allergies
- Client's understanding and ability to follow instructions related to cardiac monitoring

Nurse-Related Factors
- Proper technique regarding lead selection and preparation and placement of skin electrodes
- Proper identification of anatomical landmarks used for electrode placement
- Proper technique for troubleshooting and documenting cardiac monitoring
- Preparation of client and instructions regarding cardiac monitoring
- Adherence to standards and guidelines related to monitoring (e.g., AACN)

Equipment-Related Factors
- Proper functioning of cardiac monitoring equipment (e.g., ECG machine, cables)
- Proper functioning of battery-operated devices (e.g., telemetry monitoring)

Client-Centered Care (CCC)

When caring for a client on cardiac monitoring, respect for the client is demonstrated by:
- explaining the procedure and the need for cardiac monitoring
- providing culturally sensitive explanations
- answering questions, arranging for an interpreter if needed, and promoting autonomy
- ensuring privacy and comfort when positioning the client for the ECG

BOX 19.2 Lessons From Experience: Cardiac Monitors: An "Alarming" Scenario

Mr. Snow, a 69-year-old client with a history of coronary artery disease (CAD) and dysrhythmias, has been admitted to the unit following cardiac surgery. Since admission, his vital signs, oxygen saturation, and heart rhythm have remained stable, and his incisional pain has been controlled with medication.

After 24 hours, Mr. Snow begins to increase his activity while also remaining on the electrocardiogram (ECG) monitor. His wife has remained with him at the bedside. One evening, after Mr. Snow has been moving around more, his monitor alarm begins to go off with increasing frequency (at 10:40 PM, 11:15 PM, and 12:30 AM). After the nurse troubleshoots, she realizes the technical problems with the ECG are related to artifact, increased movement, and discomfort. The nurse checks the ECG leads and medicates Mr. Snow for pain. The nurse also provides comfort measures such as enhancing the client's environment and providing gentle massage (see Chapter 7). As the nurse leaves the room, Mrs. Snow remarks, "Can you please do something about that alarm? My husband hasn't been able to sleep for days!"

At approximately 6:30 AM, Mr. Snow's alarm goes off again. However, this time when the nurse checks on Mr. Snow, he is seizing. The nurse immediately checks the monitor and sees that Mr. Snow has a rapid ventricular tachycardia (VT). There is no discernable pulse. The nurse immediately defibrillates Mr. Snow (who is successfully converted to sinus rhythm) and calls the emergency team.

What is your take-away from this case study? This is a good example of why it is critical for alarms to remain on at a volume that can be heard at all times. Because numerous alarms go off in acute/critical care areas, "alarm fatigue" can occur, not only for staff but for family members and clients as well. The Joint Commission, American Association of Critical-Care Nurses (AACN), and other entities have developed strategies to prevent alarm fatigue. For example, proper electrode skin preparation and changing electrodes every 24 hours may help to prevent loss of adherence and contact of the electrodes. Additional strategies include individualizing alarm parameters for the needs of the client and checking alarm settings during handoff communication and whenever there is a change in the client's condition or caregiver (AACN, 2018).

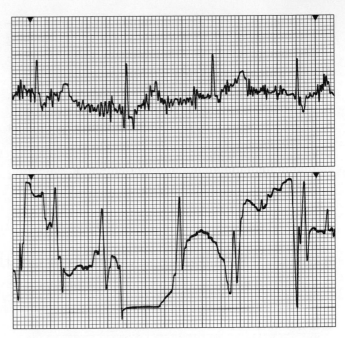

FIG. 19.10 Examples of electrocardiogram (ECG) artifact.

BOX 19.3 Possible Technical Problems With ECGs and Troubleshooting

- **Possible Technical Problems With ECGs**
  - Artifact (waveform interference) or 60-cycle interference
  - Intermittent/absent electrocardiogram (ECG) trace or low-amplitude complexes
  - Baseline drift, wandering, or irregular ECG baseline
  - Excessive triggering of monitor alarms
- **Troubleshooting Tips**
  - Are the ECG cables and leads intact and properly inserted into the monitor?
  - Is the electrode contact poor due to client diaphoresis or other problem? Was the skin prepped properly for the electrodes? Is the electrode gel still moist?
  - Is the appropriate lead selector on the monitor turned on?
  - Does the gain (sensitivity) need to be adjusted? Is the gain too high or low?
  - Is the client restless, or is there excessive cable movement?
  - Does the client have muscle tremors or excessive shivering?
  - Are there electrical devices (e.g., heating pads, radios) near the client that could cause interference? Are the devices in compliance with medical facility standards?
- **Possible Interventions**
  - Check leads, cables, and electrodes. Adjust sensitivity/gain on the monitor.
  - Change electrodes and ensure that electrodes are moist (not dry). If the client has excessive diaphoresis, use 4 × 4 gauze or other methods to dry off the chest.
  - Stabilize cables and leads. Tape electrodes with hypoallergenic tape if needed. Use comfort measures to help client's restlessness and anxiety.
  - Set high/low alarms based on the needs of the client. Do *not* turn alarms off.

- advocating for the client and family and explaining the procedure.

Infection Control (INF)

When caring for a client on cardiac monitoring, healthcare-associated infection is prevented by:
- preventing and reducing the transfer of microorganisms
- reducing the number of microorganisms
- proper cleaning of ECG equipment.

Safety (SAF)

When caring for a client on cardiac monitoring, safety measures prevent harm and maintain a safe care environment by:

- ensuring that cardiac alarms are turned on at all times, assessing for allergies to latex and other substances, and ensuring that the cardiac monitor safety guidelines are always followed.

Communication (COM)

- Communication exchanges information (oral, written, nonverbal, or electronic) between two or more people.
- Documentation records information in a permanent healthcare record.
- Collaboration with the healthcare team and client enhances safe and effective care, and ensures that the client remains on the monitor with the alarms properly set.

Health Maintenance (HLTH)

Nursing is dedicated to the promotion of health when caring for a client on cardiac monitoring, including:
- protecting and caring for the client's skin where electrodes have been placed.

Evaluation (EVAL)

Evaluation of outcomes when caring for a client on cardiac monitoring enables the nurse to determine the efficacy of the care provided.

■ SKILL 19.1 Placing a Client on a Continuous ECG Monitor (Hardwire or Telemetry)

EQUIPMENT

Disposable pre-gelled electrodes
Electrode skin-prep pads
Adhesive-remover pads for electrode removal (if needed)
Hypoallergenic tape (if needed to secure electrodes)
Gauze pads (if needed to dry client's chest)
Bedside cardiac (ECG) monitor (for hardwire monitoring)
Battery pack (for telemetry monitoring)
Cable for leads (must be compatible with ECG monitor and leads)
Clean gloves and personal protective equipment (PPE) (only if exposure to body fluids is expected)
Clippers (if needed for chest hair)
Marker pen (for writing date/time on electrodes)
Washcloth and soap (if needed for cleaning area for electrodes)
Pouch or carrying case for battery pack (telemetry only)

BEGINNING THE SKILL

1. **ACC** Review the order for continuous ECG monitoring:
   - type of continuous ECG monitoring (e.g., hardwire monitor or telemetry)
   - type of lead (e.g., 5, 6, or 12 lead).
2. **ACC** Review the client's medical/surgical history and history of cardiac monitoring.
3. **INF** Perform hand hygiene.
4. **CCC** Introduce yourself to the client and family.
5. **SAF** Identify the client using two identifiers.
6. **CCC** Provide privacy and explain the procedure. *Providing privacy in layers enhances client-centered care.*
7. **CCC** Obtain verbal consent for the procedure. *Promotes autonomy.*

PROCEDURE

8. **ACC** Assess the client for the following:
   - **SAF** allergies to adhesive gel, latex, or any other substance
   - level of consciousness and orientation to person, time, place, and situation

   - integrity of skin where ECG electrodes are likely to be placed
   - any complaints of chest pain, palpitations, or other symptoms.
9. **INF** Apply gloves and/or PPE if exposure to body fluids is likely.
10. **SAF** Elevate the client's bed to an ergonomically safe working height. (Note: After the procedure, return the bed to the lowest position to reduce the risk of falls.)

Preparing the Equipment

11. **ACC** **If the client is being placed on a hardwire continuous bedside monitor:**
    a. Check the monitor and ensure that it is calibrated and working properly.
    b. **SAF** Check the cable and ensure it is compatible with the bedside monitor.
    c. **SAF** Inspect lead wires and ensure they are not damaged (e.g., fraying, broken wires).
    d. Ensure that lead wires are inserted into the cable securely. *Securing cables and lead wires reduces the risk of artifact and interference in the ECG tracing.*
    e. Ensure that the client cable is inserted properly into the bedside monitor.

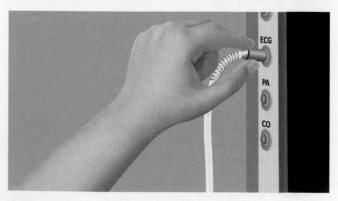

STEP 11E Insert the cable into the monitor.

12. **ACC If the client is being placed on a telemetry monitor:**
    a. Insert new battery pack securely into telemetry unit per manufacturer instructions, and ensure polarity markings are matched up properly on the transmitter.
    b. Ensure that telemetry cables and leads in the telemetry unit are secure and intact.

Preparing the Client

13. a. **ACC** Position the client supine or with the head of the bed elevated slightly if tolerated. *Facilitates application of electrodes in correct position.*
    b. **CCC** Drape client appropriately and expose only the area of the body where the electrodes will be placed. *Protects the client's dignity and prevents the client from getting chilled.*
    c. **HLTH** If there is excessive hair on the chest, clip hair with facility approved clippers. *Excessive hair could interfere with skin contact/conduction.* (Note: Avoid shaving because it could cause microscopic tears in the skin, which could create an entry point for microorganisms [Caple & Karakashian, 2018].)

14. **ACC** Identify sites for placing electrodes on client per facility policy and guidelines.
    a. Avoid selecting electrode sites around bony areas, joints, areas of redness, or lesions. *Placing electrodes in these areas could cause irritations and extraneous artifact.*
    b. Use anatomical landmarks to find optimal sites and palpate intercostal spaces.
    c. Identify client's sternal notch (angle of Louis). Palpate the upper part of the sternum or suprasternal notch. Then move your fingers to palpate each of the intercostal spaces (ICSs) within the appropriate reference lines (Pelter et al., 2017). (Note: For more information about anatomical landmarks and lines of reference, such as the midclavicular line, midaxillary line, and anterior axillary line, see Chapter 4.)

15. **ACC** Cleanse sites for electrode placement with warm water. Remove any lotion or oils from the skin. Allow skin to dry completely. *Excessive oils or lotions interfere with conductivity.* (Note: Some facilities may require specific solutions to remove dead skin cells.)

16. **ACC** Gently abrade electrode sites with an ECG prep, dry gauze, or washcloth according to facility policy. *This procedure may help to remove dead skin cells and residue.*

17. **ACC** Open electrode packaging and remove electrodes from package. Do *not* peel off electrode backing until ready to apply. *Electrode gel can dry out quickly if exposed to air.*

18. **ACC** If the leads/cables are "snap style," attach (or snap) the lead wires onto the electrodes *before* removing the backing and placing the electrodes on the client. *Snapping the cables onto the electrodes after they are placed on the client could be uncomfortable (Pelter et al., 2017).*

19. **COM** Write the time/date on each electrode pad with a marker if required by facility policy. *Enhances communication with other healthcare providers as to when electrodes need to be changed to protect the client's skin.*

20. **ACC** Carefully peel the backing off of the electrodes and ensure that the center of the pad is moist with the conductive gel. (Note: Avoid touching the adhesive back of electrode.) *Touching the adhesive backing with your fingers can decrease the adherence of the electrode.*

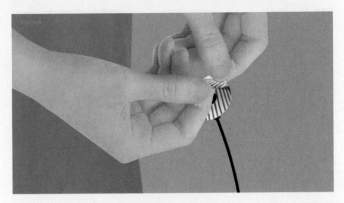

STEP 20 Prepare electrodes.

Applying the Electrodes/Leads

(Note: Apply electrodes per facility policy and manufacturer guidelines. The lead selection is based on the client's needs and other factors such as chest wall space [Jacobson, 2019a].)

21. **ACC Using a five-lead system:** (Pelter et al., 2017)

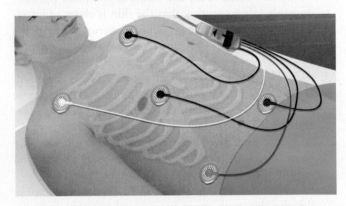

STEP 21 Five-lead system.

   a. Place right-arm (RA) electrode in the infraclavicular fossa near the right shoulder just below the client's right clavicle.
   b. Place (LA) left-arm electrode in the infraclavicular fossa near the left shoulder just below the client's left clavicle.
   c. Place right-leg (RL) electrode below the client's right rib cage or hip.
   d. Place left-leg (LL) electrode below the client's left rib cage or hip. (Note: Some facilities prefer the leg electrodes to be placed at or below the level of the umbilicus.)
   e. Place precordial chest lead electrode at fourth ICS at right sternal border for viewing V1 lead *or* at fifth ICS, at midaxillary line, for viewing V6. (Note: V1 is the preferred lead for viewing dysrhythmias [AACN, 2016; Jacobson, 2019a].) (Note: Depend-

ing on the manufacturer, the leads may be labeled using a color-coded system such as white [RA], black [LA], green [RL], red [LL], and brown [V1 or V6].

22. **ACC Using a six-lead system:**

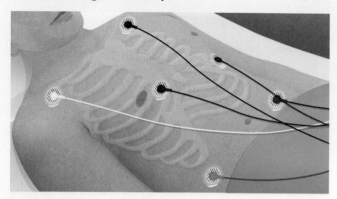

STEP 22 Six-lead system.

   a. Place limb electrodes as described in Steps 21a through 21d.
   b. Place both precordial chest leads V1 and V6 as described in step 21e.
   c. Ensure that the V6 electrode is placed under, not over, the breast. If the client has pendulous breasts, ask the client to lift the breast as you place the electrode (after ensuring that the skin is clean and dry). (Note: If the client cannot lift the breast, apply gloves and assist the client, then remove gloves and perform hand hygiene [Caple & Heering, 2018].)

23. **ACC** Select appropriate lead selectors. V1 is preferred. (Note: Whenever possible, select at least two leads to be displayed.) *This facilitates accuracy (AACN, 2016; Pelter et al., 2017).*

24. **ACC** For each electrode, ensure that the adhesive side of the electrode is on the client's skin with a secure seal around the perimeter of the electrode.

25. **ACC** If the client is diaphoretic or has profuse sweating, dry the skin with gauze before applying the electrode. *Clean and dry skin facilitates adherence and prevents irritation.*

26. **ACC** If the client has a pacemaker, an alternate site for chest electrodes may have to be used, such as the upper shoulders or back. *Placing the electrodes directly over a pacemaker could interfere with the tracing.*

27. **ACC** Verify that the appropriate lead wires/cables or clips are attached to ECG electrodes and ensure they are secure. *Loose cables/leads can interfere with ECG conduction.*

28. **COM** Tape down electrodes (and a small loop of lead) with hypoallergenic tape if necessary. *Securing the electrodes in place prevents displacement and loss of ECG tracing.*

29. **SAF** Position cable with adequate slack to minimize tension.

30. **ACC** If the client is on telemetry, place the unit in a pouch or gown pocket and ensure that the ties are secure. (Note: If the telemetry unit has a transmitter, instruct the client to push the button and notify the nurse for any unusual symptoms.)

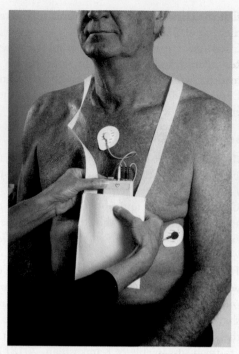

STEP 30 Secure telemetry.

31. **ACC** Confirm the ECG tracing and ensure that all of the components and waveforms can be visualized without artifact/interference. Obtain the client's apical and/or peripheral pulse rate, and ensure that the client's manual heart rate matches the heart rate displayed on the bedside monitor. (Note: If the client is on telemetry, check the tracing at the CM station.)

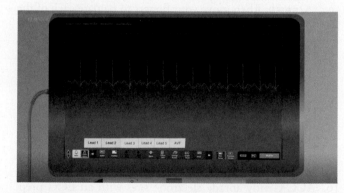

STEP 31 Confirm the ECG tracing.

32. **ACC** If the ECG tracing is not visible or is of poor quality (e.g., baseline drift, artifact), check the cables, lead wires, and electrodes, and troubleshoot accordingly (see Box 19.3).

33. **SAF** Set monitor alarm limits according to policy or order. **WARNING:** Ensure that alarms are turned *on* and that high/low parameters have been set accordingly.

34. **COM** Notify CM station about the client being placed on bedside monitor or telemetry and ensure the CM technicians can see the client's tracing. Give CM the following information:
   • client's name, electronic ID number, date of birth, age, and gender

- client's diagnosis and purpose of cardiac monitoring
- client's lead placement and alarm parameters (high/low).

35. **ACC** Print the ECG rhythm strip as required by facility policy. Record time, date, client name, and other pertinent information, such as vital signs or client symptoms, as indicated.

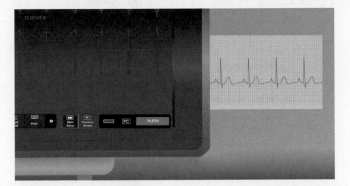

STEP 35 Obtain a rhythm strip.

36. **SAF** Provide client/family teaching about the monitor and instruct them that certain activities and movements may trigger alarms. **WARNING**: Instruct client and family *not* to turn off alarms.
37. **ACC** Instruct the client and family to avoid electric blankets or other electrical devices near the client. *Electrical devices such as electric blankets can cause artifact and disrupt the tracing.*
38. **EVAL** Continue to monitor the client and ensure that the electrodes remain intact, with good skin contact. If electrodes become wet or loose, replace as needed. *Facilitates ECG tracing.*
39. **EVAL** Evaluate quality of ECG tracing at regular intervals. Document other parameters, such as QT interval, PR interval, ST-segment elevation, and so forth, based on policy and order. **WARNING:** Notify the authorized healthcare provider if the QT interval is prolonged and not within established parameters or of any other unexpected finding in the ECG components.

40. **SAF** Monitor the alarms at frequent intervals and ensure they are turned on.

FINISHING THE SKILL

41. **INF** Remove gloves and PPE (if worn).
42. **INF** Perform hand hygiene.
43. **SAF** Ensure client safety and comfort. Ensure that the bed is in the lowest position, and verify that the client can identify and reach the nurse call system. *These safety measures reduce the risk of falls.*
44. **EVAL** Evaluate the outcomes. Is the client's ECG tracing clear and without artifact?
45. **COM** Document assessment findings, care provided related to cardiac monitoring, and outcomes in the legal healthcare record, including the following:
    - date and time the monitoring was initiated and type of lead used
    - quality of ECG tracing at initiation and rhythm strip printout at regular intervals
    - alarm settings, high/low parameters, and other alarm parameters (e.g., vital signs)
    - frequency of electrode changes and the condition of skin under the electrode sites
    - time and date that CM station is informed of client information
    - signature of the nurse initiating the monitoring. (Note: An electronic signature may be required.)
46. **HLTH** Provide follow-up care: Replace electrodes every 24 hours and rotate sites according to facility policy. Assess electrode sites for irritation or blistering, and clean residue off the client's skin before applying new pads. *Changing pads daily protects the client's skin integrity and reduces the chance of loss of electrode adherence.* (Note: If previous pad sites are irritated, ensure that skin is clean/dry, and apply new pads a few inches from old pad sites.)
47. **SAF** If the client is on telemetry, change batteries when electrodes are changed per facility policy.

■ SKILL 19.2 Performing a Diagnostic 12-Lead ECG

EQUIPMENT

Facility approved 12-lead ECG machine
Disposable pre-gelled electrodes
Electrode skin prep pads
Gauze pads (if needed to dry client's chest)
Adhesive remover pads for electrode removal (if needed)
Hypoallergenic tape (if needed to secure electrodes)
12-lead ECG machine, cables, and graph paper
Clean gloves, PPE (only if exposure to body fluids is expected)
Clippers (if needed for chest hair)
Washcloth and soap (if needed for cleaning area for electrodes)

BEGINNING THE SKILL

1. **ACC** Review the order for 12-lead ECG.
2. **ACC** Review the client's medical/surgical history and history of 12-lead ECGs.
3. **INF** Perform hand hygiene.
4. **CCC** Introduce yourself to the client and family.
5. **SAF** Identify the client using two identifiers.
6. **CCC** Provide privacy and explain the procedure. *Providing privacy in layers enhances client-centered care.*
7. **CCC** Obtain verbal consent for the procedure. *Promotes autonomy.*

PROCEDURE

8. **ACC** Assess the client for the following:

- **SAF** allergies to adhesive gel, latex, or any other substance
- level of consciousness and orientation to person, time, place, and situation
- integrity of skin where ECG electrodes are likely to be placed
- any complaints of chest pain, palpitations, or other symptoms.

9. **ACC** Determine if the client has had any previous 12-lead ECGs for comparison.

Preparing the 12-Lead ECG Machine

10. a. **ACC** Ensure that the 12-lead ECG machine is in working order and properly calibrated.
    b. **ACC** Verify that there is adequate ECG graph paper in the ECG machine.
    c. **SAF** Confirm that correct cable is connected to the ECG machine. Inspect the lead wires and ensure they are intact and not damaged (e.g., fraying, broken wires).

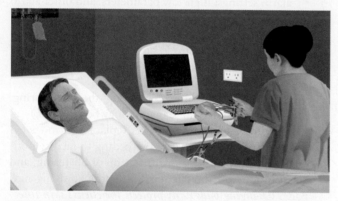

STEP 10C Check the lead wires.

    d. **SAF** Connect the ECG machine to a power source. Confirm that the machine meets medical facility requirements and that the third prong of the outlet is intact (Caple & Heering, 2018).

11. **ACC** Enter input and client information into ECG machine (e.g., medical record number, name, date of birth, gender, diagnosis, and any report of symptoms such as chest pain).

12. **INF** Apply gloves and/or PPE if exposure to body fluids is likely.

Preparing the Client

13. a. **SAF** Elevate the client's bed to an ergonomically safe working height. (Note: After the procedure, return the bed to the lowest position to reduce the risk of falls.)
    b. **ACC** Position the client supine or with the head of the bed elevated slightly if tolerated. *This facilitates application of electrodes in the correct position.*
    c. **CCC** Drape the client appropriately and expose only the area of the body where the electrodes will be placed. *Protects the client's dignity and prevents the client from getting chilled.*
    d. **HLTH** If there is excessive hair on the chest, clip hair with facility-approved clippers. *Excessive hair could*

interfere with skin contact/conduction to electrodes. (Note: Avoid shaving because it could cause microscopic tears in the client's skin, which could create an entry point for microorganisms [Caple & Karakashian, 2018].)

14. **ACC** Identify sites for placing the electrodes for a 12-lead ECG and mark with an indelible marker per facility policy. *This facilitates accuracy and consistency if there are repeated ECGs.*
    a. Avoid selecting electrode sites around bony areas, joints, areas of redness, or lesions. *Placing electrodes in these areas could cause irritation and extraneous artifact.*
    b. Use anatomical landmarks to find optimal sites and palpate intercostal spaces (ICSs).
    c. Identify client's sternal notch (angle of Louis). Palpate the upper part of the sternum or suprasternal notch. Then move your fingers down to palpate the ICSs within the appropriate reference lines. *(For more information about anatomical landmarks and lines of reference [e.g., midclavicular line, midaxillary line, anterior axillary lines], see Chapter 4.)*
    d. For precordial leads, avoid using the nipple as a reference point. *The nipple location can vary, and it may not provide an accurate landmark (Randazzo, 2016).*

15. **ACC** Cleanse sites for electrode placement with warm water. Remove any lotion or oils from the skin. Allow the skin to completely dry. *Excessive oils or lotions interfere with conductivity.* (Note: Some facilities may require specific solutions to remove dead skin cells.)

16. **ACC** Gently abrade electrode sites with an ECG prep, dry gauze, or washcloth according to facility policy. *This procedure may help to remove dead skin cells and residue.*

17. **ACC** Open electrode packaging and remove electrodes from package. Do *not* peel off electrode backing until ready to apply. *Electrode gel can dry out quickly if exposed to air.*

18. **ACC** If the lead/cables are "snap style," attach (or snap) the lead wires onto the electrodes *before* removing the backing and placing the electrodes on the client. *Snapping the cables onto the electrodes after they are placed on the client could be uncomfortable (Pelter et al., 2017).*

19. **ACC** Carefully peel the backing off the electrodes and ensure that the center of the pad is moist with the conductive gel. (Note: Avoid touching the adhesive back of electrode.) *Touching the adhesive backing with your fingers can decrease the adherence of the electrode.*

Applying the Electrodes and Lead Wires on Client

(Note: Apply electrodes/leads per facility policy and guidelines. If the electrode placement has to be altered due to wounds, dressings, pads, and so forth, note the alternative sites clearly on the 12-lead ECG recording [Wung, 2017].)

20. **ACC** Apply limb electrodes. Place electrodes just proximal to wrists and ankles per facility policy and guidelines, and ensure they are placed in the same location bilaterally.

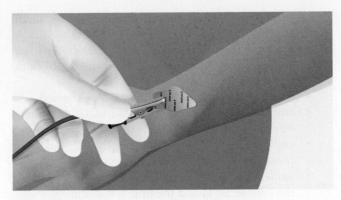

STEP 20 Applying limb electrodes and leads.

a. Place RA electrode on the client's right arm just proximal (or above) the right wrist.
b. Place LA electrode on the client's left arm just proximal to the left wrist.
c. Place RL electrode on the client's right leg just proximal (or above) the right ankle.
d. Place LL electrode on the client's left leg just proximal to the left ankle.
21. **ACC** Apply precordial or chest electrodes (V leads 1–6).

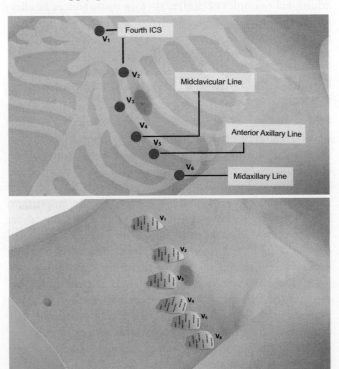

STEP 21 Identify sites and apply precordial electrodes.

a. Place V1 electrode at fourth ICS just to the right of the sternum (right sternal border).
b. Place V2 electrode at fourth ICS just to the left of the sternum (left sternal border).
c. Place V3 electrode midway between V2 and V4.
d. Place V4 at the fifth ICS left midclavicular line.
e. Place V5 at the anterior axillary line at the same level as V4 (fifth ICS).

f. Place V6 at the midaxillary line at the same level as V4 and V5 (fifth ICS).
22. **ACC** For each electrode, ensure that the adhesive side of the electrode is on the client's skin with a secure seal on the electrode. (Note: If the client is diaphoretic or has profuse sweating, dry the client's skin with gauze pad before applying electrode to facilitate adherence.)
23. **ACC** If the client has pendulous breasts, ask the client to lift the breast as you place the electrodes (V3–V6) under the breast (after ensuring the client's skin is clean and dry). (Note: If the client cannot lift the breast, apply gloves and assist the client, then remove gloves and perform hand hygiene [Caple & Heering, 2018].)
24. **ACC** Attach appropriate lead wires/cables or clips to electrodes (if not already done), and ensure they are secure. *Loose cables/leads can interfere with ECG conduction.*

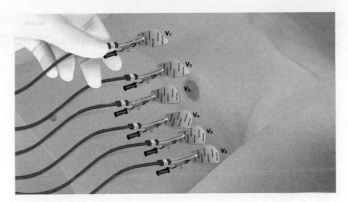

STEP 24 Attach lead wires.

25. **ACC** Instruct the client to place the arms at side and to relax and remain as still as possible; ensure that the client's legs are not crossed or pressing against the bed. *Facilitates an accurate ECG tracing.*
26. **ACC** Move electronic devices such as cell phones, electric heating blankets, or other devices away from the client. *These devices can interfere with ECG tracing.*
27. **ACC** Press start button to run 12-lead ECG. Verify that ECG tracing can be visualized without artifact. *Determines if troubleshooting is needed during procedure.*
28. **ACC** If tracing is not visible or is of poor quality (artifact, etc.), check client movement, cables, lead wires, and electrodes. Repeat ECG after troubleshooting (see Box 19.3).
29. **EVAL** Continue to monitor client. Ensure that electrodes remain intact, with good skin contact, during the procedure (usually about 5–10 minutes). *Facilitates proper tracing.*
30. **ACC** After ECG is complete, remove cables from electrodes; turn off machine.
31. **HLTH** Remove electrodes and clean conductive gel from the skin. If there is any difficulty with removal, use adhesive remover pads. *Protects skin and promotes comfort.*
32. **EVAL** Compare 12-lead ECG with previous 12-lead ECGs to check for any significant changes, and forward the ECG and other information to the authorized healthcare provider.

FINISHING THE SKILL

33. **INF** Dispose of electrodes and clean ECG machine/cables with disinfectant per policy.
34. **INF** Remove gloves and PPE (if worn).
35. **INF** Perform hand hygiene.
36. **SAF** Ensure client safety and comfort. Ensure that the bed is in the lowest position and verify that the client can identify and reach the nurse call system. *These safety measures reduce the risk of falls.*
37. **EVAL** Evaluate the outcomes. Did the client tolerate the procedure? Is this 12-lead ECG tracing adequate? Can all of the ECG waveforms and components be identified?
38. **COM** Document assessment findings, cardiac medication administration, and outcomes in the legal healthcare record:
    - date and time the 12-lead ECG was performed
    - trends and comparison of 12-lead ECGs with previous 12-lead ECGs
    - any symptoms reported during the 12-lead ECG procedure (e.g., chest pain, palpitations)
    - name of the authorized healthcare provider receiving the 12-lead ECG and the time it was sent.

SECTION 2 Caring for a Client With a Dysrhythmia or Altered Cardiac Conduction

Have you ever wondered what it means when your client has an irregular pulse or an unusually slow or rapid pulse? It may be related to a dysrhythmia, an alteration in the client's cardiac conduction. These alterations could involve dysrhythmias (abnormal rhythms of the heart) or conduction disorders such as heart block. The treatment varies, depending on the client. Many clients who have dysrhythmias or conduction disorders remain hemodynamically stable and only need close monitoring, whereas other clients may require additional interventions.

DYSRHYTHMIAS AND CONDUCTION DISORDERS

When discussing dysrhythmias and conduction disorders, it is helpful to clarify the terms. The term *arrhythmia* means "without rhythm." *Dysrhythmia* means "disturbed rhythm." For the purposes of this section, the term *dysrhythmia* will be used. It is important to note that not all dysrhythmias are conduction disorders, although some dysrhythmias may develop from conduction disorders (AHA, 2016b).

As discussed in Section 1 of this chapter, the electrical impulses in the heart normally begin in the SA node and then travel through the atria and ventricles in an organized manner. On an ECG, this would be manifested as normal sinus rhythm (NSR). However, when a dysrhythmia occurs, the impulse may begin outside of the SA node, which may then create ectopic (or irregular) heartbeats. This "ectopy" may arise from the atria, the AV junction, or the ventricles. In general, dysrhythmias that originate in the ventricles tend to be more dangerous than those that originate in the atria.

If a client has a conduction disorder, there may be a problem with the *progression* of conduction. For example, when a client has a bundle-branch block, the electrical impulse must find an alternate route of travel, which could slow down the contraction of one of the ventricles for a fraction of a second.

This pathology may or may not cause symptoms, although it would likely be seen on an ECG (AHA, 2016b). For a list of additional examples of cardiac rhythm disturbances or alterations that may be seen, see Box 19.4. For more in-depth information on the interpretation of specific dysrhythmias, refer to an ECG analysis text.

Clinical Implications of Dysrhythmias and Conduction Disorders

From a practical standpoint, the seriousness of a dysrhythmia or conduction disorder depends on the etiology or cause. For example, if a client has cardiac ischemia (see Section 4 of this chapter), a dysrhythmia could indicate the heart has increased "irritability" that could potentially get worse. The nature or clinical manifestations of the disorder are also important. Some clients may have isolated ectopic beats or very short runs of ectopy, whereas other clients may develop sustained dysrhythmias. The longer or more frequently a dysrhythmia occurs, the greater is the risk of the client developing inefficient and decreased ventricular filling and a decreased cardiac output. The client may also develop vital sign changes. For example, a decrease in the client's cardiac output may result in a drop in blood pressure and/or a compensatory increase in the client's heart rate. Additional manifestations may include, but not be limited to, the following:
- anxiety and sense of fear or panic
- cold, clammy skin and decreased perfusion to the extremities
- dizziness or lightheadedness
- fluttering sensations or sense of palpitations in the chest or neck
- syncope (fainting) or feelings of near-syncope
- fatigue and feeling overly tired or "drained"
- shortness of breath and/or difficulty breathing
- chest pain or "tightness" in the chest or other area of the body.

CRITICAL CONCEPTS

BOX 19.4 Examples of Cardiac Rhythm Disturbances

- **Disturbances That Involve the Sinoatrial (SA) Node**
  - Sinus bradycardia (SB) (rate below 60 beats/minute)
  - Sinus tachycardia (ST) (rate above 100 beats/minute)
  - Sinus dysrhythmia or sinus arrest (pauses)
- **Dysrhythmias That Involve in the Atria**
  - Premature atrial contractions (PACs)
  - Premature atrial tachycardia (PAT)
  - Atrial fibrillation (A-fib)
  - Atrial flutter (A-flutter)
- **Disturbances That Involve the Atrioventricular (AV) Node, Bundle Branches, or Other Areas of Conduction**
  - First-degree AV block
  - Second-degree AV block (Mobitz I or Wenckebach or Mobitz II)
  - Third-degree (complete) AV block
  - Bundle-branch block (BBB)
- **Dysrhythmias That Involve Ventricles**
  - Premature ventricular contractions (PVCs)
  - Ventricular tachycardia (VT)
  - Ventricular fibrillation (VF)
  - Ventricular asystole

Reference: Jacobson, 2019a.

Assessment and Care for a Client With a Dysrhythmia

A key component of excellent nursing is astute assessment. A client can develop a dysrhythmia in any setting. When you enter the client's room, immediately check the client's level of consciousness and vital signs, and determine if the client is hemodynamically stable. If the client is *not* hemodynamically stable, call the rapid response team (RRT) and authorized healthcare provider immediately. After first checking your client, check the leads, cables, electrodes, and ECG monitor if applicable, and make sure there is not a technical problem with the ECG (see Box 19.3). In some cases, artifact could be mistaken as a dysrhythmia.

During the dysrhythmia, perform a rapid head-to-toe bedside assessment and assess your client for any symptoms he or she may be experiencing. For example, is your client having palpitations (fluttering sensations in the chest)? Does the client feel lightheaded, as if he or she is about to pass out? Is the client having chest pain? Is the client having trouble breathing, or does the client feel short of breath? How is the client's oxygen saturation? If the client is on an ECG monitor, check the client's pulse and compare it with the heart rate on the monitor to assess if there is a discrepancy. This helps determine if the client is "perfusing" during the dysrhythmia. In addition, document the onset of the dysrhythmia as well as when it resolved (AACN, 2016).

If the client remains in a sustained dysrhythmia or exhibits symptoms that are different from baseline, remain with the client and monitor the client's vital signs and level of consciousness. Ensure that emergency equipment, such as the automated external defibrillator (AED) or defibrillator is nearby. Clients with dysrhythmias may deteriorate quickly. The authorized healthcare provider must be notified, and if the client is in distress, the RRT or emergency team must be summoned (see Section 4 of this chapter). Check the client's lab work (if ordered) because some electrolyte disorders, such as low potassium or magnesium levels, may cause dysrhythmias.

USING SYNCHRONIZED CARDIOVERSION

When a client has a rapid dysrhythmia that does not respond to medications or resolve spontaneously, additional procedures may be required. If the client has an altered level of consciousness and the dysrhythmia is life threatening, emergency defibrillation is required without delay (see Section 4 of this chapter). However, if the dysrhythmia is hemodynamically stable and the client is awake and alert, elective cardioversion may be indicated. Cardioversion is a procedure that is done by using a defibrillator synchronized with the client's QRS complex. This is used for dysrhythmias that originate *above* the ventricles, such as atrial fibrillation (AF) or supraventricular tachycardia (SVT), and do not respond to medical therapy. Synchronization with the QRS complex or R wave is crucial so that the shock does not occur on the T wave during repolarization. If a shock is delivered during this vulnerable recovery phase, it could destabilize the client's conduction pathway and cause dangerous ventricular dysrhythmias (Jacobson, 2019a).

If the client has an elective cardioversion, preparation often begins days or weeks before the procedure. The reason for this is that clients who have chronic atrial dysrhythmias (e.g., atrial fibrillation) may be at increased risk for clot formation in the left atrium. The clot could then be dislodged as a thrombus and enter the circulatory system after conversion to sinus rhythm. Thus, the client may be placed on anticoagulants to prevent clot formations before the cardioversion. In addition, clients who are on certain medications, such as digoxin or potassium, may need to have blood levels monitored to ensure they do not have any drug toxicity before the procedure.

Performing or Assisting With Elective Synchronized Cardioversion

Depending on the facility, the nurse may be responsible for performing and/or assisting with the procedure. Before the procedure, confirm that the equipment is working and that emergency equipment (e.g., suction, crash cart) is nearby. The defibrillator should be facility approved; capable of synchronization mode; and equipped with a built-in oscilloscope, ECG monitor, and calibrated graph paper.

Accuracy is one of the most important critical concepts when preparing for and performing synchronized cardioversion. In order to increase the chance for successful cardioversion, the adhesive pads must be placed accurately based on anatomical landmarks and the manufacturer recommendations. Because elective cardioversion is often indicated for atrial dysrhythmias, placement of the pads may be slightly different than for ventricular dysrhythmias. For more details on pad placement, see Skill 19.3. For more information on different types of defibrillators and remote, "hands-free" defibrillation, see Section 4 later in the chapter.

Providing client-centered care and comfort is also important. Because cardioversion is uncomfortable, the client must receive sedation or anesthesia such as propofol from an authorized healthcare provider. To ensure the client's safety, monitoring the client's oxygen saturation, along with vital signs, will be necessary. Before the cardioversion, ensure that the client has a patent intravenous (IV) access device in order to administer IV medications for an immediate effect.

During the cardioversion, confirm that the synchronization on the defibrillator is in the proper synchronization mode and that it is accurately recognizing the client's QRS complexes. Usually, there will be a bright-colored marker on the QRS complexes and not on the tall T waves. The machine should *not* discharge until it recognizes the QRS complex. If more than one shock is required, the synchronization may have to be reset (Hambach, 2017a; Jacobson, 2019a).

SUMMARY

In summary, a client who develops dysrhythmias or conduction disorders may be at risk for decreased perfusion and impaired cardiac output. Therefore, the nurse must continue to monitor the client closely for changes in vital signs and other changes in the client's clinical status, such as decreased level of consciousness and/or decreased urine output. The nurse must also maintain a calm presence and provide reassurance as needed for the client and family.

APPLICATION OF THE NURSING PROCESS

Examples of Related ICNP Nursing Diagnoses, Expected Client Outcomes, and Nursing Interventions:

Nursing Diagnosis: Impaired cardiac output

Supporting Data: Recurrent dysrhythmias; client has been feeling lightheaded.

Expected Client Outcomes: The client will have improved cardiac output, as seen by:

- blood pressure and pulse at baseline and within established parameters
- LVEF measurement within established parameters
- extremities warm to the touch
- urine output of at least 0.5 mL/kg per hour over 2 hours

Nursing Intervention Examples: Monitor vital signs (e.g., blood pressure, pulse) and client's level of consciousness. Monitor urine output and warmth of extremities.

Reference: International Classification for Nursing Practice. (n.d.). *eHealth & ICNP.* Retrieved from https://www.icn.ch/what-we-do/projects/ehealth-icnp.

CRITICAL CONCEPTS
Caring for a Client With a Dysrhythmia or Altered Cardiac Conduction

Accuracy (ACC)

When caring for a client who has a dysrhythmia or altered cardiac conduction, accuracy is affected by the following variables:

Client-Related Factors

- Client's assessment, including age, level of consciousness, and orientation
- Client's medical history; history of dysrhythmias or conduction disorders
- Client's history of previous cardioversion or defibrillation procedures
- Client's clinical status and presence of recent damage to the heart or heart failure
- Client's electrolyte status or lab results (e.g., potassium or magnesium levels)

Nurse-Related Factors

- Knowledge of anatomy/physiology related to altered cardiac conduction
- Proper identification of landmarks used for placement of pads and/or paddles
- Adherence to facility policy and guidelines related to using cardioversion
- Properly setting up synchronized mode for cardioversion

Equipment-Related Factors

- Proper functioning of cardioversion equipment (e.g., synchronized mode)

Client-Centered Care (CCC)

When caring for a client who has a dysrhythmia or altered cardiac conduction, respect for the client is demonstrated by:

- explaining the procedure, answering questions, and encouraging follow-up questions about cardioversion
- promoting autonomy by ensuring that informed consent has been obtained before cardioversion
- providing privacy and culturally sensitive explanations, and arranging for an interpreter if needed
- ensuring comfort by providing appropriate sedation and/or pain medication during elective cardioversion and advocating for the client and family.

Infection Control (INF)

When caring for a client who has a dysrhythmia or altered cardiac conduction, healthcare-associated infection is prevented by:

- preventing and reducing the transfer of microorganisms
- reducing the number of microorganisms.

Safety (SAF)

When caring for a client who has a dysrhythmia or altered cardiac conduction, safety measures prevent harm and maintain a safe care environment by:

- ensuring that cardiac alarms are turned on and ensuring that the synchronized mode and safety guidelines are used for cardioversion
- assessing for allergies to latex and other substances, including medications.

Communication (COM)

- Communication exchanges information (oral, written, nonverbal, or electronic) between two or more people.
- Documentation records information in a permanent healthcare record.
- Collaborating with other healthcare professionals, including staff in the CM unit, facilitates accurate identification and interpretation of dysrhythmias.

Health Maintenance (HLTH)

Nursing is dedicated to the promotion of health when caring for a client who has a dysrhythmia or altered cardiac conduction, including the following:

- prevention of burns and proper care of skin during elective cardioversion.

Evaluation (EVAL)

Evaluation of outcomes enables the nurse to determine the efficacy, accuracy, and safety of the care provided.

■ SKILL 19.3 Performing or Assisting With Elective Cardioversion

EQUIPMENT

Defibrillator adhesive pads if needed (pre-gelled or adhesive)

Defibrillator/monitor with synchronization abilities, ECG oscilloscope, and recorder

ECG calibrated graph paper (for defibrillator)

IV devices and equipment (e.g., IV pole, fluid)

IV sedatives and other medications as prescribed

ECG cables and monitoring equipment (bedside or portable)

Emergency equipment on standby (e.g., crash cart, suction)

Stethoscope and blood pressure cuff

Oxygen saturation monitor and supplemental oxygen (if needed)

BEGINNING THE SKILL

1. **ACC** Review order.
2. **ACC** Review the following:
   - client's dysrhythmia diagnosis (e.g., atrial fibrillation, atrial flutter, SVT)
   - history of previous cardioversions or other cardiac procedures
   - lab work such as digoxin or potassium to ensure levels are not toxic.
3. **INF** Perform hand hygiene.
4. **CCC** Introduce yourself to the client and family.
5. **SAF** Identify the client using at least two identifiers.
6. **CCC** Provide privacy and explain the procedure. *Providing privacy in layers enhances client-centered care.*
7. **CCC** Obtain verbal and written consent for the procedure. *Promotes autonomy.*
8. **SAF** Assess the client for allergies, including any medications or sedatives that may be used for the procedure.
9. **ACC** Assess the client for the following:
   - level of consciousness and orientation to person, time, place, and situation
   - medications client has taken in the last 36 to 48 hours
   - any complaints of chest pain, palpitations, or other symptoms.

10. **SAF** If the client has transdermal medication, remove the patch and clean residual from the skin. *Transdermal patches could cause burns and interfere with energy transfer (Hambach, 2017a).*
11. **SAF** Confirm that the client has had nothing by mouth (NPO) for the designated amount of time. *Reduces risk of aspiration if the client has an emergency and has to be intubated.* (Note: The client may be allowed to take medications and sips of water when they are on NPO status.)
12. **SAF** Confirm that the client has a patent IV device, without any signs of infiltration. *The IV device may be needed for sedatives or medications that may be given.*
13. **SAF** Ensure that emergency equipment (e.g., crash cart, suction, oxygen, bag-mask device, intubation equipment) is nearby. *Facilitates preparation for any emergencies.*

Preparing the Equipment for the Procedure

14. a. **ACC** Use facility-approved defibrillator (suitable for cardioversion and synchronization) that is also equipped with ECG oscilloscope screen and monitor.
    b. Ensure that machine is plugged in and working properly.
    c. Confirm that machine has ECG graph paper loaded.
15. **INF** Apply gloves and PPE if there is a risk of exposure to body fluids.

Preparing the Client

16. a. **SAF** Raise the bed to an ergonomically safe working height. (Note: After the cardioversion procedure, return the bed to the lowest position to reduce the risk of falls.)
    b. Position the client supine or with the head of the bed elevated slightly if tolerated.
    c. Assess the presence of any pacemakers, implantable defibrillators, or other devices. *Defibrillating over these devices could disrupt their function.*
    d. Assess the integrity of the client's skin where the electrodes and pads will be placed. Ensure that the skin is dry and intact. *Skin must be dry and not wet to avoid*

contact burns. (Note: Avoid areas of skin with breakdown, redness, or burns.)

   e. Prepare the client's skin and attach the monitor electrodes and leads on the defibrillator per manufacturer instructions and facility policy (see Skill 19.1).

17. **CCC WARNING:** Verify that the client is adequately sedated per orders. *This procedure can be painful.* (Note: Conscious sedation or anesthesia such as propofol may also be used by an authorized health care provider.)

18. **ACC** Verify that the client's rhythm can be visualized on the defibrillator monitor.

19. **ACC** Use a monitor lead that shows a tall QRS complex or R wave. *This will facilitate proper synchronization.*

20. **SAF** Place the defibrillator in synchronization mode. Ensure that the QRS complex or R wave has a marker to identify the correct synchronization of the defibrillator with the client's rhythm. *This helps the defibrillator sense the QRS complex and synchronize properly.*

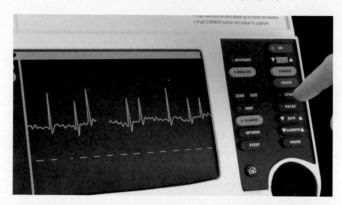

STEP 20 Press synchronization mode.

21. **SAF** Observe for visual flashing , such as the presence of red arrows, and an audible beep with each QRS complex or R wave. *This will indicate that the QRS complex is consistently being sensed properly by the machine.* (Note: If each QRS is not being sensed, adjust the gain on the monitor until the marker appears on each R wave [Hambach, 2017a].)

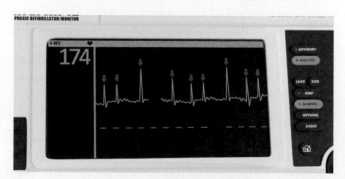

STEP 21 Verify consistent synchronization with each R wave.

22. **ACC** Print a rhythm strip and label per policy before the procedure. *Documents precardioversion rhythm for comparison and will verify synchronization mode markers.*

Placing the Defibrillator Pads (for Cardioversion) on the Client

23. **ACC** Apply conductive gel pads (for paddles) or self-adhesive pads for "hands-free" remote defibrillation/cardioversion per manufacturer instructions or policy.

   a. **Anterior/posterior (A/P) placement:** Place anterior pad *(top image)* immediately adjacent and right lateral to sternum, under the right clavicle. The center, or midline, of the anterior pad should be at the fourth ICS. Place the posterior pad *(bottom image)* below the scapula and left lateral to the spine. The center of the posterior pad should be placed at the level of the T7 vertebra. (Note: The A/P position is recommended for cardioversion procedures to enhance current flow through the client's atria [Zoll Medical Corporation, 2017].)

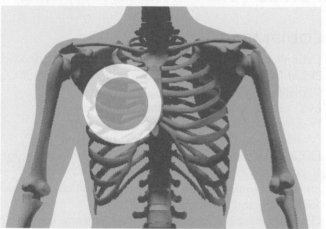

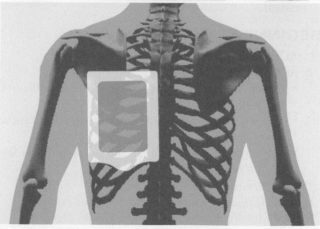

Step 23A Anterior/posterior (AP) placement. (Note: The anterior pad is top image and the posterior pad is bottom image.)

   b. **Anterior/anterior (A/A) or sternal/apex placement:** The sternal pad is in the same position as or slightly higher than the A/P position. It is also below the clavicle. The center of the apex pad should be placed in the left midaxillary line at the fifth ICS.

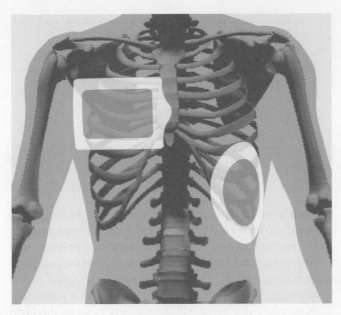

STEP 23B Sternal/apex placement.

   c. Avoid using alcohol-soaked pads. *Alcohol is combustible with electrical currents.*
   d. Avoid placing pads over breast tissue. *Breast tissue can increase resistance.*
   e. Avoid placing pads over an implantable cardioverter-defibrillator (ICD) or pacemaker. If the client has a pacemaker, place the pads at least 2.5 cm (1 inch) from the pulse generator and lead wires (Hambach, 2017a; Zoll Medical Corporation, 2017).
24. **ACC** Set defibrillator monitor to run a continuous tracing during the procedure.
25. **ACC** Charge the defibrillator at the amount of energy (*joules*) according to order or policy. (Note: The amount of joules used will vary according to the type of dysrhythmia the client has. The lowest amount of energy necessary to convert the client's rhythm is the standard of care.)
26. **SAF** Recheck the synchronization on the defibrillator and ensure that it is working properly and that markers can consistently be seen on each QRS complex.
27. **SAF WARNING:** When the defibrillator is charged, verbally state "ALL CLEAR" and count down three times while checking to ensure everyone is clear from the bed, client, and equipment.

28. **SAF** Press "shock" on the discharge button on the defibrillator machine or on each paddle while checking again to ensure everyone is still clear. Hold the discharge button until the current has been fully discharged. *There may be a slight delay in synchronization mode because the machine is sensing and synchronizing with the client's QRS complex (Hambach, 2017a).* (Note: If using paddles, place the paddles on the conduction pads on client's chest and apply equal firm pressure on each paddle. Press the "shock" buttons on the paddles simultaneously.)
29. **ACC** Check the monitor to determine whether the client has converted to an organized rhythm (see the image below). If the dysrhythmia persists, increase the joules and repeat the procedure per order and facility policy.
30. **EVAL** After the procedure, monitor the client's vital signs, level of consciousness, and oxygen saturation as the client comes out of sedation or anesthesia. Reorient the client to surroundings if needed, and assess if there is a change from the client's baseline.
31. **ACC** Print ECG strip or check a 12-lead ECG if ordered (see Skills 19.1 and 19.2).
32. **HLTH** Remove defibrillator pads and/or clean conductive gel off client's skin if used.
33. **HLTH** Assess the client's skin and ensure there are no burns or signs of breakdown.
34. **SAF** Provide follow-up care. **WARNING:** Ensure that monitor alarms on ECG monitor remain turned on and that the high and low alarms are set appropriately per order.

FINISHING THE SKILL

35. **INF** If paddles were used, clean them between clients per facility policy with appropriate solution.
36. **INF** Remove gloves and PPE (if used) and perform hand hygiene.
37. **SAF** Ensure client safety and comfort. Ensure that the bed is in the lowest position, and verify that the client can identify and reach the nurse call system. *These safety measures reduce the risk of falls.*
38. **EVAL** Evaluate the outcomes. Did the client convert to sinus rhythm as expected?
39. **COM** Document assessment findings, care given related to the dysrhythmia, and outcomes in the legal healthcare record, including the following:

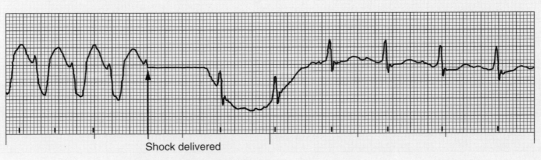

Shock delivered

STEP 29 Confirm an organized rhythm.

- time and date of elective cardioversion and amount of joules used
- outcome of cardioversion; rhythm before and after cardioversion
- amount and type of sedation or anesthesia used
- vital signs and oxygen saturation during and after cardioversion
- condition of client's skin after cardioversion
- client's tolerance of the procedure.

SECTION 3 Caring for a Client With a Cardiac Pacemaker

CARDIAC PACEMAKERS

Clients who have disorders that result in a decreased cardiac output and decreased perfusion may be candidates for an artificial pacemaker. A pacemaker is a device that delivers electrical stimulation to the heart in order to initiate depolarization and contraction. Pacemakers may be indicated when the client's heart rate is too slow (severe bradycardia) or for conduction disorders such as symptomatic heart blocks and SA or AV nodal dysfunctions. They may also be indicated for some rapid dysrhythmias, such as SVT, not responsive to other treatment (Jacobson, 2019a).

HOW A PACEMAKER WORKS: MAJOR FUNCTIONS AND COMPONENTS

A pacemaker simulates the role of the client's SA node or natural pacemaker. For conduction to occur, a closed-loop circuit must exist. With cardiac pacing, this circuit consists of the pulse generator, the conducting lead, and the client's myocardium. The pulse generator is the power source, and the leads (thin, insulated wires) transfer the electrical current to the myocardium (Jacobson, 2019a). The basic functions of pacemakers include the following:

- **Sensing:** Pacemaker's ability to "sense" (or monitor) intrinsic (or natural) electrical activity. Thus, when a pacemaker senses the client's heartbeat, it will not deliver a paced beat. This is a critical function because if the pacemaker does not sense the client's intrinsic beats, it could fire randomly and create a random stimulus.

- **Pacing or pulse generation:** Ability of pacemaker to "pace" or send an electrical impulse to the heart through the pacing lead when the client's intrinsic rate is too slow (or too fast, or irregular, depending on how the pacemaker is programmed). This will be seen as a "spike" at the appropriate place on the client's ECG. For a ventricular pacemaker, this spike will appear just prior to the QRS complex.

- **Capture:** Successful stimulation by pacemaker impulse that results in depolarization or contraction. An indication that this is working properly is a visible pacemaker spike/stimulus followed by either an atrial or ventricular "paced beat" or a paced rhythm (Fig. 19.11). The ability of the heart to "capture" is affected by certain variables, including the strength of the stimulus and the condition of the myocardial tissue (Spotts, 2017).

TYPES OF PACEMAKERS

The type of pacemaker used is determined by the severity and nature of the client's condition, the client's hemodynamic stability, and the anticipated length of time the client may need the pacemaker. The two main categories of pacemakers are temporary and permanent. A temporary pacemaker is usually indicated for short-term use, whereas a permanent pacemaker is placed for more long-term use. A temporary pacemaker may also be used while clients are stabilizing and waiting to receive a permanent pacemaker.

Another device a client may need is the biventricular pacemaker. Biventricular pacing, also known as cardiac resynchronization therapy (CRT), is used to improve cardiac function and treat heart failure. CRT is accomplished

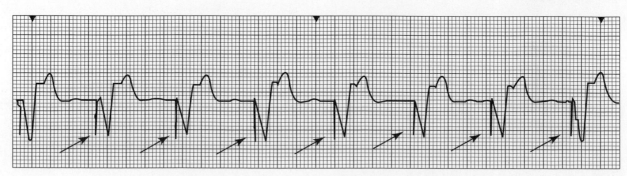

FIG. 19.11 Example of paced rhythm. Note the pacer spike before each paced beat.

by placing a third lead in the left ventricle (via the lateral or posterior left ventricular vein), in addition to placing leads in the right atrium and right ventricle. This is done to stimulate both ventricles to contract simultaneously. The goal is to help the client's heart pump efficiently and improve cardiac output (Jacobson, 2019b).

TEMPORARY PACEMAKERS

Temporary pacemakers are usually placed in a hospital critical care setting. They may be indicated when a client suddenly develops acute conditions such as severe bradycardia (heart rate less than 40 beats per minute), SA node disruptions, high-grade heart block, and other disorders associated with an acute decrease in the client's cardiac output.

One of the distinguishing features of temporary (as opposed to permanent) pacemakers is that the pacemaker pulse generator is external and accessible outside of the client and thus can be adjusted by the nurse and other providers. To protect the settings, the pulse generator usually has a clear shield or cover (Fig. 19.12). The settings on the pulse generator are ordered by the authorized healthcare provider and may include the following (Jaffe & Balderrama, 2017):

- **Pacing rate:** Number of impulses sent by the pulse generator to the client's myocardium (usually 60–80/minute). To avoid increased oxygen consumption, the rate should be set as low as possible while also maintaining an optimal cardiac output.
- **Energy output:** Level of electrical output measured in milliamperes (also referred to as the "mA"). The mA will vary (depending on the type of pacemaker the client

has), and it is usually adjusted until adequate "capture" is achieved. With a temporary pacemaker, capture is assessed by observing the appearance of the client's ECG (electrical ECG) and by palpating the client's pulse (mechanical capture).

- **Mode:** When a fixed rate (or asynchronous mode) is used, the pacemaker delivers a preset stimulus, regardless of the client's intrinsic myocardial activity. In the "demand" (or synchronous) mode, the pacemaker can "sense" the client's intrinsic activity and thus only delivers a stimulus when needed. The demand mode is often preferred so that the pacemaker does not compete with the client's rhythm.
- **Sensitivity:** Ability of the pulse generator to detect or sense the client's intrinsic activity, more specifically, the client's R wave. Some external temporary devices, such as transcutaneous pacemakers, may not have a separate setting for this function. To assess sensitivity, observe the client's ECG for the presence of pacer spikes, followed by successfully captured beats (Jaffe & Balderrama, 2017).

The type of temporary pacemaker used for a client depends on the client's needs and clinical status. Two of the most common types of temporary pacemakers include transcutaneous and transvenous devices. A transcutaneous pacemaker is an external, noninvasive device, whereas a transvenous pacemaker is invasive. A more detailed description of these devices follows.

Temporary Transcutaneous Pacemakers

Temporary transcutaneous pacemakers (TCPs) require external pacemaker pads (which may also be called *pacing electrodes*), as opposed to internal pacing wires, and they are usually only used in an emergency until a temporary or permanent transvenous pacemaker can be inserted. Many of these systems have built-in ECG monitoring, and some models also have the ability to defibrillate the client if needed (see Section 4 of this chapter). Because it is relatively easy to apply, the TCP may be preferred for clients who cannot wait for a transvenous pacemaker.

Depending on the facility, the nurse may be responsible for placing the pacemaker pads/electrodes as well as properly operating the TCP. Before the application of the TCP, the skin must be properly cleaned and prepared in order to facilitate the most optimal conduction. The pacing electrodes are placed on the client's chest (usually in an anterior/posterior position) and attached to the external pulse generator. The external pulse generator can then be adjusted according to the client's needs/orders.

When caring for clients with TCPs, ensure that the device is capturing properly. With a TCP, a captured beat should appear as a very wide (usually greater than 0.12 second) QRS complex preceded by a pacer spike. Because this type of pacemaker is external, the energy output (mA) requirements are higher than for other types of pacemakers. As a result, the client may have more discomfort and require sedation. The

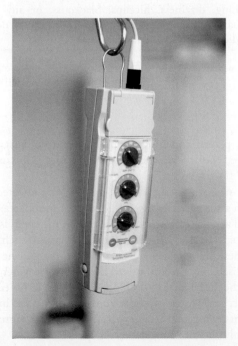

FIG. 19.12 Pulse generator for an external temporary pacemaker.

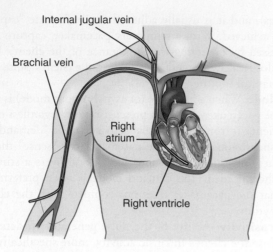

FIG. 19.13 Transvenous pacemaker (TVP) sites.

client's risk for burns may also be higher. Check the client's skin for impaired skin integrity, and follow the manufacturer instructions closely.

Temporary Transvenous Pacemakers

Temporary transvenous pacemakers (TVPs) are inserted and guided transvenously (most often through the right internal jugular or subclavian vein) by the cardiologist into the myocardium (Fig. 19.13). They may be indicated for clients who do not respond to the TCP and/or clients who are waiting for a permanent pacemaker. As with all pacemakers, observe the client's rhythm and ensure the pacemaker activity is consistent with parameters (Jacobson, 2019a).

When using a TVP, check the battery on a regular basis and ensure that it is not low. It is also important to secure the device and ensure that the lead wires do not migrate or become dislodged. In addition, the external pulse generator must be protected. As previously identified in Fig. 19.12, pulse generators often have clear plastic covers that can protect the settings.

Because the TVP is invasive, the insertion site must be monitored closely for any signs of bleeding or infection, such as purulent drainage, redness, or edema. Change the dressing if it is damp or loose, and report signs of infection to the authorized healthcare provider.

PERMANENT PACEMAKERS

If the client's disorder has not resolved, the client may have a surgical placement of a permanent pacemaker. Depending on the client's disorder, the leads are usually placed transvenously in the appropriate chamber of the heart (right atrium, right ventricle, or both). The pulse generator for the pacemaker is usually placed in a surgically created pocket subcutaneously under the client's clavicle. Once the pacemaker is

BOX 19.5 Home Care Considerations: Permanent Pacemakers

A new pacemaker can cause anxiety. Before discharge, ensure that the client and family have postprocedure instruction sheets and contact numbers for any questions or concerns. Key teaching strategies for the client may include, but are not limited to, the following:

- **Reinforce activity instructions.** It may take at least 6 to 8 weeks for complete healing to occur and for the pacemaker to settle into place. The client should wear the arm immobilizer as instructed and avoid sudden, jerky movements that would cause abduction (the arm to pull away from the body). The client should also avoid raising the arms above the head for at least 5 days (or as ordered) and avoid carrying heavy objects (usually anything over 3 lb).
- **Teach the client to keep track of his or her heart rate.** Confirm that the client knows the programmed upper and lower rate. Teach the client to count the pulse for a full minute and record it. Instruct the client to contact the healthcare provider if his or her pulse drops below the set rate or is above the acceptable rate limit guide.
- **Reinforce teaching regarding pacemaker maintenance.** Instruct the client to avoid causing pressure over the area where the pacemaker is located. If the client is female, encourage her to wear a soft pad on the pacemaker incision to protect it from a bra.
- **Encourage the client to carry his or her pacemaker ID card.** This is important in case of an emergency or if the client has to go through a metal detector (e.g., airport security).
- **Encourage the client to contact the healthcare provider for unusual symptoms.** Clients should contact their healthcare provider if they experience swelling, trouble breathing, dizziness, hiccups, blackouts, or any other unusual symptom. These symptoms may (or may not be) an indication of pacemaker failure.

Reference: American Heart Association, 2016c.

properly placed and programmed, the cardiologist or other authorized healthcare provider can make adjustments as needed.

After placement, the client's arm on the affected side is placed in a sling for the first 24 hours for immobilization, and overhead activity is restricted. In addition, the client is assessed closely for indicators of adequate cardiac output, such as warm extremities, stable vital signs, and adequate urine output. Before discharge, the authorized health care provider will verify that the pacemaker is working within programmed parameters. Discharge teaching and follow-up care are also important for clients with permanent pacemakers. For more information on home care considerations, see Box 19.5.

TABLE 19.1 Examples of Cardiac Pacemaker Complications

Complication	Characteristics and Possible Interventions
Sensing problems: • Undersensing • Oversensing	• Undersensing or "failure to sense" can occur if pacemaker does not sense client's own intrinsic beats. May result in inappropriate "firing" or random pacemaker spikes. • Oversensing can occur if pacemaker senses outside or extraneous signals. This could inhibit function of pacer. • Sensitivity on pacemaker may need to be adjusted. Check battery.
• Failure to capture:	• Pacemaker delivers a stimulus but is not able to initiate depolarization and contraction of the myocardium. • Pacer spikes are visualized but are not followed by paced or "captured" beats (e.g., absence of P wave for atrial pacing and/or absence of QRS complex for ventricular pacing). • Check all connections and leads. Ensure battery is not low.
• Failure of pulse generator or "failure to pace"	• Pacemaker does not deliver a pacemaker stimulus as programmed. • Absence of pacemaker spikes and absence of paced beats. • Check all connections and leads. Battery may need to be changed.
• Myocardial irritability • Diaphragmatic irritability	• Pacemaker leads could migrate after placement and cause irritability at the site of the catheter tip. • Myocardial irritability could be manifested as "ectopic beats" or ventricular dysrhythmias (in the case of ventricular pacer). • Diaphragmatic irritability or pacing could be manifested by "hiccups" or muscle twitching. • Pacemaker leads may need to be repositioned and stabilized. Be alert for other serious complications (e.g., perforation).
• Infection or phlebitis	• Monitor insertion site for redness, swelling, or drainage. • Secure leads to minimize movement and prevent irritation.

References: Jacobson, 2019b; Jaffe & Balderrama, 2017; Spotts, 2017.

POSSIBLE COMPLICATIONS/SAFETY ISSUES WITH PACEMAKERS

Although pacemakers can provide lifesaving benefits, there are potential complications. In particular, issues related to temporary pacemakers in the acute care setting may require troubleshooting. For a list of complications and possible interventions, see Table 19.1. In addition to possible complications, there are safety issues to consider when working with pacemakers. Pacemaker devices work by using electrical currents. Thus, unsafe electrical devices could affect function. Some key safety tips for pacemakers are as follows (AHA, 2016d):

• Be aware of your client's environment and any possible hazards. Are there any loose or frayed lead wires exposed on a temporary pacemaker? If so, ensure these are covered properly.
• Avoid placing defibrillator paddles (if used) directly over the client's pacemaker. If a defibrillator or AED is used, check the pacemaker to ensure it is working properly.
• Use caution when using a transcutaneous electrical stimulator (TENS) unit. These devices may affect certain types of pacemakers with unipolar programming.
• If the client must receive therapeutic radiation treatments, shield the pacemaker as much as possible if it lies directly within the radiation field.
• Avoid exposure to magnetic resonance imaging (MRI). Although there are conditional MRI pacemakers, many clients have pacemakers that can be damaged by the magnetic field created by an MRI. Regardless of the type of pacemaker your client has, follow safety precautions, and provide client and family teaching to reduce the risk of complications.

APPLICATION OF THE NURSING PROCESS

Examples of Related ICNP Nursing Diagnoses, Expected Client Outcomes, and Nursing Interventions:
Nursing Diagnosis: Risk for bradycardia
Supporting Data: Client has episodes of second-degree heart block.
Expected Client Outcomes: The client will remain in normal sinus rhythm (NSR), as seen by:
• heart rate above 60 beats per minute
• absence of bradycardic or syncopal (fainting) episodes
• extremities warm to touch bilaterally
• peripheral pulses at client's baseline and equal bilaterally.
Nursing Intervention Example: Monitor client's vital signs and heart rhythm.
Reference: International Classification for Nursing Practice. (n.d.). *eHealth & ICNP*. Retrieved from https://www.icn.ch/what-we-do/projects/ehealth-icnp.

CRITICAL CONCEPTS
Caring for a Client With a Pacemaker

Accuracy (ACC)

When caring for a client who has a pacemaker, accuracy is affected by the following variables:

Client-Related Factors

- Client's assessment, including age, level of consciousness, and orientation
- Client's medical history; client's history of previous pacemaker insertions
- Client's condition and presence of recent damage to the heart or heart failure
- Client's electrolyte status or lab results (e.g., potassium, magnesium levels)

Nurse-Related Factors

- Preparation of client and instructions regarding client's pacemaker device
- Adherence to guidelines related to temporary and permanent pacemakers

Equipment-Related Factors

- Proper functioning of pacemaker and pacemaker pulse generator

Client-Centered Care (CCC)

When caring for a client with a pacemaker, respect for the client is demonstrated by:

- explaining the procedure, answering questions, and encouraging follow-up questions about pacemaker procedure and care
- promoting autonomy by obtaining informed consent before pacemaker procedure
- advocating for the client and family by providing culturally sensitive explanations and arranging for an interpreter if necessary
- ensuring comfort by providing appropriate sedation and/or pain medication during and after pacemaker procedure.

Infection Control (INF)

When caring for a client with a pacemaker, healthcare-associated infection is prevented by:

- preventing and reducing the transfer of microorganisms
- reducing the number of microorganisms
- preventing an environment conducive to bacterial growth

Safety (SAF)

When caring for a client who has a pacemaker, safety measures prevent harm and maintain a safe care environment by:

- ensuring that safety guidelines are followed at all times and ensuring that wires and pulse generator box for pacemaker are intact and protected
- assessing for allergies to latex and other substances, including medications.

Communication (COM)

- Communication exchanges information (oral, written, nonverbal, or electronic) between two or more people.
- Documentation records information in a permanent healthcare record.
- Documentation of pacemaker function and capture on the ECG strip enhances communication and client care.

Health Maintenance (HLTH)

Nursing is dedicated to the promotion of health when caring for a client with a pacemaker, including the following:

- care of skin under electrodes for temporary subcutaneous pacing
- prevention of burns when using subcutaneous pacing
- securing TVP wires to minimize movement.

Evaluation (EVAL)

- Evaluation of outcomes enables the nurse to determine the efficacy and safety of the care provided.

■ SKILL 19.4 Caring for a Client With a Transcutaneous Pacemaker (TCP)

EQUIPMENT

Transcutaneous pacing device (TCP)
Pacing pads/electrodes (for TCP)
Defibrillator (for standby)
IV sedatives and other medications as prescribed
Emergency equipment on standby (e.g., crash cart, suction)
Stethoscope and blood pressure cuff
Oxygen saturation monitor
Supplemental oxygen (if needed)

BEGINNING THE SKILL

1. **ACC** Review order for temporary TCP, including:
   - TCP settings (pacer rate, mA, mode).
2. **ACC** Review the following:

- medical and surgical history (past and present), including history of past placement of pacemaker devices (temporary or permanent), and conduction disorder diagnosis
- lab work that could affect paced rhythms (e.g., electrolytes, potassium, magnesium).

3. **INF** Perform hand hygiene.
4. **CCC** Introduce yourself to the client and family.
5. **SAF** Identify the client using two identifiers.
6. **CCC** Provide privacy and explain the procedure. *Providing privacy in layers enhances client centered care.*
7. **CCC** Ensure that consent is obtained for the TCP procedure.
8. **SAF** Assess the client for allergies, including any medications or sedatives that may be used for the procedure.

9. **ACC** Assess the client for the following:
   - level of consciousness and orientation to person, time, place, and situation
   - any complaints of shortness of breath, palpitations, or other symptoms
   - level of pain or discomfort using a facility-approved pain scale.
10. **INF** Apply gloves and PPE if risk of exposure to body fluids.
11. **SAF** Obtain vital signs and oxygen saturation. Compare to baseline.
12. **CCC** If the client is having pain, medicate the client according to orders and facility policy. *Transcutaneous pacing can be a very uncomfortable procedure for the client.*
13. **SAF** If the client is on sedation medication, assess the level of sedation using a facility approved scale. *Clients with TCPs are frequently on sedation and/or pain medication.*
14. **SAF** Confirm that the client has a patent IV device, without any signs of infiltration. *This may be needed for sedatives or medications that may be given.*
15. **SAF** Ensure that emergency equipment (e.g., crash cart, suction, oxygen, bag-mask device, intubation equipment) is nearby. *Facilitates preparation for any emergencies.*
16. **SAF** Verify that the client's room is environmentally safe:
    a. Ensure that electrical equipment is in compliance with medical facility standards.
    b. Inspect cables being used and ensure they are intact without any frayed edges or loose wires. *Frayed wires can cause an electrical hazard.*
17. **ACC** Determine the type of pacemaker the client has and whether or not ECG monitoring is in place, and ensure cables are attached. (Note: Some temporary pacers have built-in ECG systems. If not, ensure that the client is on continuous cardiac bedside monitoring with alarms set.)
18. **SAF** Raise the bed to an ergonomically safe working height and position the client at a 20- to 30-degree angle if tolerated and not contraindicated. (Note: After the procedure, return the height of the bed to the lowest position to reduce the risk of falls.)
19. **CCC** Drape the client to expose only the chest while protecting privacy.

Checking Placement and Condition of Site for Transcutaneous Pacemaker

20. **ACC** Check pacemaker pads/electrodes and ensure that they are secure. Ensure that anterior pad/electrode is positioned left of the sternum at the left fourth ICS at the left midclavicular line. The posterior pacing pad/electrode should be on the back between the left scapula and the spinal column at the level of the

heart (Spotts, 2017). *The AHA recommends the A/P position for this procedure (Caple & Karakashian, 2018).*

21. **HLTH** Inspect the skin around pads/electrodes. Ensure there are no burns or skin breakdown. *Transcutaneous pacemakers can cause burns due to the high energy output.*
22. **ACC** Replace pacing pads/electrodes if they are loose, or if they have been on the client longer than the manufacturer recommends (Note: Pacemaker pads/electrodes cannot be repositioned. If they are loose, they must be replaced [Caple & Karakashian, 2018].)
    a. Remove old pads and dispose. Clean any gel residue from the skin. Inspect for burns. If present, report to the authorized healthcare provider.
    b. Prepare skin for new pads and ensure that it is clean and dry. Avoid alcohol or benzoin. *These substances are combustible in the presence of electrical currents.*
    c. If the client has excessive hair, clip hair. Do *not* shave hair. *Shaving could cause microscopic tears of the skin, which could cause infection or irritation.*
    d. Prepare new pads. Remove protective liners from each pad.
    e. Roll each pad (one at a time) onto skin at the identified sites. *Rolling the pad reduces the potential for air trapping and improves contact and conduction.*
    f. Avoid placing pads over bony areas, and avoid any areas of skin breakdown.
    g. Gently press down the pad and ensure that the entire pad (including edges) is in place. Avoid cutting the pad. *Good contact of the entire pad with the skin helps conduction.*

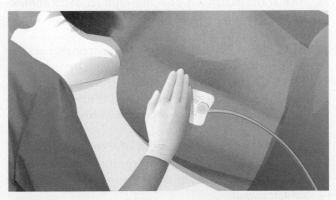

STEP 22G Ensure that the anterior TCP pad and the posterior TCP pad are secure.

Checking the Pulse Generator and Settings for Transcutaneous Pacemaker

23. a. **ACC.** Ensure that the pulse generator/monitor is intact and attached securely to the cables.
    b. Check the pacing rate (usually 60–80).

c. Check the mA (energy output; usually 40–80 mA). (Note: Energy requirements are higher for TCPs because conduction has to go through skin.)

d. Check mode (synchronous/demand or asynchronous). (Note: The synchronous/demand mode is usually preferred. Some machines are automatically synchronous when ECG electrodes are connected to the client [Caple & Karakashian, 2018].)

Verifying the Proper Function of Transcutaneous Pacemaker

24. **ACC** Confirm that pacemaker ECG lead shows an adequate QRS complex or R wave. *This helps the pacemaker sense the QRS complex and synchronize properly.*

25. **ACC** Verify "electrical capture" by observing the client's ECG each time the pacemaker fires (as evidenced by pacemaker spikes). Electrical capture should appear as a wide QRS (ventricular complex) with a T wave in the opposite deflection. (Note: Capture on a TCP may be much wider and difficult to visualize because of interference.)

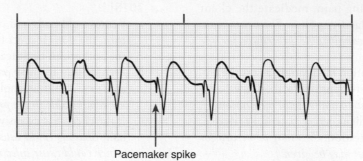

Pacemaker spike

STEP 25 Verify capture.

26. **SAF** Ensure that pacemaker spike is in front of each "paced" QRS complex (for ventricular pacemakers) and that there are not random pacer spikes. *Random pacer spikes could indicate that the pacemaker is failing to sense, which could lead to life-threatening dysrhythmias.*

27. **ACC** Verify "mechanical capture" by palpating the client's femoral *or* peripheral pulses.

28. **SAF** If the pacemaker does not capture, check connections, leads, and pacing pads/electrodes (in the case of TCP) (see Table 19.1).

29. **ACC** Print a rhythm strip to verify pacemaker activity per policy.

30. **EVAL** Continue to monitor the client's rhythm to ensure the pacemaker is working, and continue to monitor vital signs and oxygen saturation frequently as indicated.

31. **EVAL** Monitor pulses, level of consciousness, and warmth in extremities at frequent intervals, and monitor client's urine output. *These are indicators of adequate cardiac output.*

32. **EVAL** Continue to monitor the client for any pain or discomfort and monitor sedation level. *Transcutaneous pacing can be a very uncomfortable procedure for the client.*

33. **SAF WARNING:** Ensure that the cardiac monitor alarms on the ECG monitor remain turned on and that the high and low alarms are set appropriately per order.

FINISHING THE SKILL

34. **INF** Remove gloves and PPE (if used) and perform hand hygiene.

35. **SAF** Ensure client safety and comfort. Ensure that the bed is in the lowest position, and verify that the client can identify and reach the nurse call system. *These safety measures reduce the risk of falls.*

36. **EVAL** Evaluate the outcomes. Is the client's heart rate at or above 60 beats per minute? Is the client's skin intact under the pacing electrodes/pads without signs of redness or irritation?

37. **COM** Document assessment findings, care given related to the temporary pacemaker (TCP), and outcomes in the legal healthcare record, including the following:
   - settings: rate, mA (energy output), and mode (demand or asynchronous)
   - appearance of captured beats and grading of pulses bilaterally
   - level of pain using a facility-approved scale; pain medication given
   - condition of client's skin where TCP pads or electrodes were placed.
   - Hemodynamic response (e.g., blood pressure)

■ SKILL 19.5 Caring for a Client With a Transvenous Pacemaker (TVP)

EQUIPMENT

Transvenous temporary pacemaker device (TVP)
Pulse generator (for TVP)
9-V battery for TVP
Defibrillator (for standby in case of emergency)
Dressing change supplies and chlorhexidine swabs (if needed for TVP)
Emergency equipment on standby (e.g., crash cart, suction)
Stethoscope and blood pressure cuff
Oxygen saturation monitor
Supplemental oxygen (if needed)

BEGINNING THE SKILL

1. **ACC** Review order for temporary TVP, including the following:
   - TVP pacemaker settings (pacer rate, mA, mode).
2. **ACC** Review the following:
   - medical and surgical history (past and present), including history of past placement of pacemaker devices (temporary or permanent) and conduction disorder diagnosis
   - lab work that could affect paced rhythms (e.g., electrolytes, potassium, magnesium).
3. **INF** Perform hand hygiene.
4. **CCC** Introduce yourself to the client and family.
5. **SAF** Identify the client using two identifiers.
6. **CCC** Provide privacy and explain the procedure. *Providing privacy in layers enhances client-centered care.*
7. **CCC** Ensure that consent is obtained for the TVP procedure.
8. **SAF** Assess the client for allergies, including any medications or solutions that may be used for the procedure. (Note: Some solutions, such as betadine or prep pads, contain iodine.)
9. **ACC** Assess the client for the following:
   - level of consciousness and orientation to person, time, place, and situation
   - any complaints of shortness of breath, palpitations, or other symptoms
   - any complaints of persistent hiccups. *Hiccups could be an indication of irritability caused by the temporary pacer (TVP) wire on the myocardium (see Table 19.1).*
10. **INF** Apply gloves and PPE if there is a risk of exposure to body fluids.
11. **SAF** Obtain vital signs and oxygen saturation. Compare to baseline.
12. **SAF** Confirm that the client has a patent IV device, without any signs of infiltration. *This may be needed for sedatives or medications that may be given.*
13. **SAF** Ensure that emergency equipment (e.g., crash cart, suction, oxygen, bag-mask device, intubation equipment) is nearby. Facilitates preparation for any emergencies.
14. **SAF** Verify that the client's room is environmentally safe:

a. Ensure that all electrical equipment is in compliance with the medical facility standards.
b. Inspect cables being used and ensure they are intact, without any frayed edges or loose wires. *Frayed wires can cause an electrical hazard.*
15. **SAF** Raise bed to an ergonomically safe working height and position the client at a 20- to 30-degree angle if tolerated and not contraindicated. (Note: After the procedure, return the height of the bed to the lowest position to reduce the risk of falls.)
16. **CCC** Drape the client to expose only the chest while protecting privacy.

Checking Placement and Condition of Site for Transvenous Pacemaker

17. **ACC** Inspect pacemaker leads for the TVP. Ensure that they are intact and attached securely to the pulse generator, without signs of frayed or broken edges.
18. **INF** Inspect insertion site for the TVP. Ensure that there is no redness, edema, purulent drainage, or bleeding at site. *TVPs are invasive. Observe for infection.*
19. **INF** If dressing is wet or loose, clean site with chlorhexidine swabs or facility-approved solution, and change according to facility policy. (see Skill 13.3.)

Checking the Pulse Generator and Settings on the Transvenous Pacemaker

20. a. **ACC** Ensure that the pulse generator is intact and attached securely to the cables. (Note: Usually a TVP pulse generator will have a plastic cover to lock in place.)
    b. Secure the pulse generator near the client. Avoid hanging on IV pole. *Hanging the generator on an IV pole can cause tension and dislodgement of pacing wires.*
    c. Check the TVP pacing rate (usually 60–80).
    d. Check the mA (energy output; usually 2–3 mA). (Note: Energy requirements are lower for TVPs than TCPs because the pacing wire with TVPs has contact with the myocardium.)
    e. Check mode (synchronous/demand or asynchronous). (Note: Some machines are automatically synchronous when ECG electrodes are connected.)
    f. Ensure that sensitivity is set according to orders (Jaffe & Balderrama, 2017).

Verifying the Proper Function of the Transvenous Pacemaker

21. **ACC** Confirm that pacemaker ECG lead shows an adequate QRS complex or R wave. *This helps the pacemaker sense the QRS complex and synchronize properly.*
22. **ACC** Verify electrical capture by observing client's ECG each time the pacemaker fires (as evidenced by pacemaker spikes). Electrical capture should appear as a wide QRS (ventricular complex) with a T wave in the opposite deflection.

23. **SAF** Ensure that the pacemaker spike is in front of each "paced" QRS complex (for ventricular pacemakers) and that there are not random pacer spikes. *Random pacer spikes could indicate that the pacemaker is failing to sense, which could lead to life-threatening dysrhythmias.*

24. **ACC** Verify mechanical capture by palpating the client's femoral or peripheral pulses.

25. **SAF** If the pacemaker does not capture, check connections and transvenous pacing leads (see Table 19.1).

26. **ACC** Print a rhythm strip to verify TVP activity per facility policy.

27. **EVAL** Continue to monitor the client's rhythm to ensure the pacemaker is working, and continue to monitor vital signs and oxygen saturation frequently as indicated.

28. **EVAL** Monitor pulses, level of consciousness, and warmth in extremities at frequent intervals, and monitor client's urine output. *These are indicators of adequate cardiac output.*

29. **SAF** Provide follow-up care and monitoring. **WARNING:** Ensure that monitor alarms on ECG monitor remain turned on and that the high and low alarms are set appropriately per order.

30. **SAF** Recheck batteries in pulse generator box and replace if low. (Note: Some facilities require that batteries be changed every 24 hours for temporary pacemakers.)

FINISHING THE SKILL

31. **INF** Remove gloves and PPE (if worn) and perform hand hygiene.

32. **SAF** Ensure client safety and comfort. Ensure that the bed is in the lowest position, and verify that the client can identify and reach the nurse call system. *These safety measures reduce the risk of falls.*

33. **EVAL** Evaluate the outcomes. Is the client's pacemaker capturing properly? How is the client's hemodynamic response? Is the client's blood pressure within established parameters?

34. **COM** Document assessment findings, care given related to the temporary pacemaker (TVP), and outcomes in the legal healthcare record, including the following:
    - location and condition of insertion site for TVP
    - condition of TVP insertion site (e.g., any irritation, redness, or drainage)
    - presence, condition, and type of dressing on TVP site
    - settings: rate, mA (energy output), and mode (demand or asynchronous)
    - appearance of captured beats and grading of pulses bilaterally
    - Hemodynamic response (e.g., blood pressure)

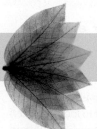

SECTION 4 Caring for a Client With a Cardiac Emergency

Cardiac emergencies can occur at any time in any setting. Providing rapid assessment, timely interventions, and follow-up care can minimize injury and prevent the loss of life. The key is to be prepared and respond as quickly as possible while also remaining calm and providing emotional support and care to the client and family. The critical concepts of client-centered care, accuracy, and communication are essential. Teamwork and collaboration are also important.

CARING FOR A CLIENT WITH ISCHEMIC CHEST PAIN

Ischemic chest pain (also called angina) is a potentially life-threatening emergency. Angina is a warning signal, and it is considered to be unstable if it is a new symptom, if it occurs with rest or low activity, or if it increases in duration or intensity (Leeper, 2019). The cause of unstable angina is myocardial (cardiac) ischemia or a lack of blood flow and oxygen to the heart, and it is part of a broad spectrum of clinical presentations known as acute coronary syndrome (ACS). ACS may be caused by a complete or partial blockage of a coronary artery, and most people recognize this as

a myocardial infarction (MI) or heart attack. ST-segment changes on the client's ECG are also important to consider. These findings may be classified as (non–ST-segment elevation myocardial infarction (NSTEMI) or ST-segment elevation myocardial infarction (STEMI). As discussed in Section 1, clients with ACS may require continuous ST-segment monitoring to detect subtle changes (see previously identified Fig. 19.5).

If left untreated, unstable angina and ACS can progress to MI, life-threatening dysrhythmias, heart failure, and death. Nurses are held to a high standard with respect to providing care for these clients. Thus, assessment and early recognition of ischemic chest pain are essential.

A list of warning signs of ischemic chest pain is provided in Box 19.6. Some clients, such as women and clients with diabetes and/or vascular disorders, may not have classic symptoms of chest pain (AHA, 2016a). Therefore, it is important to ask the client about other signs and symptoms (Fig. 19. 14). The critical assessment parameters of ischemic chest pain can be measured using the PQRST scale (**P**rovoking factors, **Q**uality, **R**adiating, **S**everity, **T**ime) (see Skill 19.6) (Leeper, 2019). Many clients who have chest pain are in denial, or they may say something like "Oh, this is probably just indigestion or a touch of the flu." or "I'm just

BOX 19.6 Possible "Warning Signs" of Cardiac Ischemia

- Denial that there is anything wrong
- Substernal discomfort in middle of chest that may feel dull, heavy, or achy and may radiate to the back, neck, jaw, stomach, or arms
- Tight-feeling chest that may be described as "indigestion"
- Shortness of breath or dyspnea (with or without chest pain)
- Feelings of nausea and/or extreme fatigue
- Diaphoresis (or sweating); client may describe as a "cold sweat"
- Feelings of lightheadedness and/or dizziness
- Pallor (due to less oxygenation and perfusion)
- Sense of anxiety or feelings of "impending doom"

References: American Heart Association, 2016a; Chu. 2017.

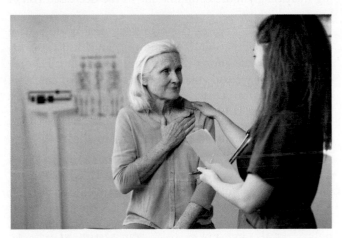

FIG. 19.14 Assess for associated symptoms of cardiac ischemia.

tired right now." Some people may perceive their pain as a discomfort or an annoyance as opposed to pain.

If a client is compromised or unable to communicate verbally, additional assessment parameters will have to be used, such as nonverbal indicators. For example, is the client diaphoretic (sweaty) or cold and clammy? Is the client grimacing, or does the client appear distressed? Manifestations of chest pain can vary, depending on the individual.

Immediate Interventions for Clients With Ischemic Chest Pain

When caring for a client with ischemic chest pain (or associated symptoms), it is critical to intervene as quickly as possible. The goal is 100% relief in order to prevent further myocardial damage. In addition to obtaining a 12-lead ECG, interventions may include immediate bedrest, supplemental oxygen, and administration of nitroglycerin (NTG) or other medications (e.g., IV morphine) as ordered by the authorized healthcare provider. The goal of these interventions is to improve the client's coronary blood flow and oxygenation.

To help the cardiologist definitively diagnose the presence and/or extent of myocardial damage, biomarkers such as serum troponin levels may be ordered along with other possible diagnostic tests. Nursing care for clients with ischemic chest pain must focus on providing an environment that is as calm and noise-free as possible and reducing the client's anxiety.

EMERGENCY CARDIAC CATHETERIZATION

If the cardiologist determines that the client's ischemic chest pain is related to a partial or complete blockage of a coronary artery, then a reperfusion procedure such as an emergency cardiac catheterization may be indicated. This procedure can prevent or minimize myocardial damage from cardiac ischemia. During the procedure, a cardiologist will access the client's radial or femoral artery to introduce a catheter that will be advanced to the client's heart, which will allow the cardiologist to locate and open the blocked coronary artery. In most cases, the cardiologist will use a small inflatable balloon to press plaque buildup against the walls of the coronary artery. Once blood flow has been restored to damaged myocardium, the cardiologist will place a stent, which is a small mesh metal tube or cylinder, in the area of the plaque buildup to keep the artery open. To prevent the stent from clotting, anticoagulants are usually ordered (Leeper, 2019).

Caring for Clients After Emergency Cardiac Catheterization

After receiving an emergency cardiac catheterization, clients may develop complications, such as retroperitoneal bleeding, hematoma, chest pain, or dysrhythmias. Thus, it is important for nurses to continuously monitor for these complications and educate clients about ways to prevent complications from occurring. Specific interventions, such as prescribed bedrest and postprocedure IV fluids and medications, are ordered by the authorized healthcare provider. Bedrest and immobilization of the extremity near the cardiac catheter insertion site can prevent the disruption and irritation of the insertion site, either in the groin or the wrist, and prevent bleeding from occurring. In addition, a compression bandage is usually in place on the insertion site. IV fluids after the cardiac catheterization help flush out the contrast dye that was used during the procedure, which is potentially harmful to the client's kidney function if not excreted.

After the client returns to the unit, continue to monitor the client closely for bleeding and bruising at the insertion site. This is particularly important if the client has been receiving anticoagulants. In most cases, the client will remain on ECG monitoring after the procedure, and the client's vital signs and catheter insertion site will be checked at frequent intervals. The client's peripheral pulses distal to the insertion site must also be frequently checked.

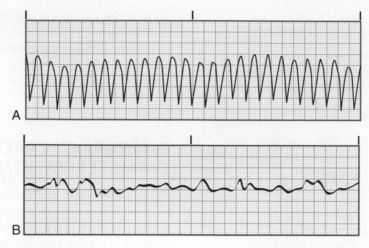

FIG. 19.15 Examples of life-threatening dysrhythmias. **A**, Ventricular tachycardia (VT). **B**, Ventricular fibrillation (VF).

PROVIDING EMERGENCY DEFIBRILLATION

When a life-threatening dysrhythmia such as pulseless rapid ventricular tachycardia (VT) or ventricular fibrillation (VF) occurs (Fig. 19.15), quick and early emergency defibrillation is required. Theoretically, the electrical current that is provided with defibrillation depolarizes the myocardium and terminates the abnormal electrical activity, which then allows the client's own intrinsic pacemaker (SA node) to kick in and reestablish normal sinus rhythm (Hambach, 2017b). Defibrillation is only used for "shockable" dysrhythmias that have some type of electrical activity, such as VT or VF.

Synchronization Versus Asynchronization

As discussed earlier in Section 3, clients who have hemodynamically stable dysrhythmias with an organized QRS complex may be candidates for medical interventions or synchronized elective cardioversion (see Skill 19.3). Emergency cardioversion (for clients with a QRS complex) is indicated if the client is *not* hemodynamically stable. However, when a client has a dysrhythmia with no QRS complex, the synchronization mode should *not* be selected. This is an important distinction because the synchronization mode will not fire in the absence of the QRS complex (such as with VF), and the defibrillator will not discharge (Hambach, 2017b).

Types of Defibrillators

The type of defibrillator will vary, depending on the setting. In most facilities, manual biphasic (as opposed to monophasic) defibrillators are used, whereby the energy waveforms travel through the heart in two directions (positive and then negative), thus requiring lower amounts of energy to defibrillate the client (Hambach, 2017b). As with cardioversion (see Section 3 of this chapter), the machine must be equipped with an ECG monitor/oscilloscope and graph paper that allows for a continuous printout during the procedure. Many defibrillators also have a "quick look" feature that allows visualization of the client's rhythm when the paddles are in place. Although paddles may be used, self-adhesive

pads/electrodes for "hands-free" defibrillation are becoming increasingly more common due to the decreased risk of burns and injury.

Some of the newer, state-of-the-art defibrillators have unique features that allow monitoring and display of O_2 saturation as well as other vital functions. Additionally, some defibrillators have code management systems that can store data for review at a later point in time. An example of a biphasic manual defibrillator is shown in Fig. 19.16.

Using an Automated External Defibrillator

An AED is a system that can be used in any setting in which it is available and by anyone who is trained. This device incorporates a rhythm analysis and voice-command feature that guides the responder/operator through a sequence of steps. It also advises the responder when a shock is recommended. Because of the critical importance of early defibrillation, the AHA has advised that AEDs be available in areas where there are large numbers of people and where access to care may not be accessible, such as schools, airports, and other areas (Jacobson, 2019a). In addition, AEDs are increasingly used in some facilities to provide rapid access to defibrillation outside of the critical care units. As with all defibrillators, there are important safety guidelines to consider. For more information on AEDs, refer to current AHA or American Red Cross (ARC) guidelines. For special considerations regarding pediatric defibrillation, see Box 19.7.

CARING FOR A CLIENT WHO IS IN CARDIAC ARREST

When a cardiac arrest occurs, every second counts. For every minute there is a delay in care, the client's chance of survival can decrease by as much as 10% (ARC, 2016). As a result, the AHA has developed the "Cardiac Chain of Survival." The links in this chain are as follows:

- Immediate recognition and activation of emergency response
- Early cardiopulmonary resuscitation (CPR), with an emphasis on high-quality chest compressions

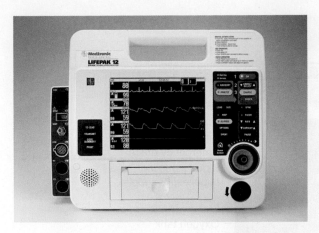

FIG. 19.16 Biphasic manual defibrillator.

- Rapid defibrillation (without delay for VF or pulseless VT)
- Effective advanced life support
- Integrated post–cardiac arrest care

Responding in a Cardiac Arrest

In the acute care setting, a rapid response team (RRT) or a "code" team will usually be summoned to manage the emergency. However, the client's nurse and other members of the healthcare team who initially respond also have a vital role in the emergency.

The nurse who is initially at the scene will assess the client and determine if the client is unresponsive and pulseless, call for help (or have an assistant call for help), and initiate CPR per AHA guidelines until a defibrillator or AED is available. The nurse must remain with the client and must *not* leave the room. Ideally, a backboard or other type of hard surface should be placed under the client (if available) to facilitate effective chest compressions.

A second responding nurse or other healthcare provider should ensure the emergency team has been called and that an AED or defibrillator, a manual resuscitation bag and mask, and a crash cart are rapidly brought to the scene (if they are not already there). The crash cart (Fig. 19.17) will have airway and intubation supplies (top drawer), a *full* oxygen tank, emergency medications, and other items that will be needed. Wall regulators for oxygen, suction, nasogastric (NG) sump tubes, and so forth should be set up and ready. If the backboard is not in the room, it will usually be on the side/back of the crash cart. It is a good idea to become familiar with the location and contents of the crash cart on the unit *before* an emergency occurs.

Regarding the sequence of CPR and defibrillation, follow AHA guidelines and facility policy. The evidence is conflicting as to whether or not CPR should *always* be performed first before defibrillation. For clients who are receiving ECG monitoring, immediate defibrillation (without delay) is indicated for VF and pulseless VT. However, if defibrillation is not readily available or

successful, cycles of CPR should be continued per AHA guidelines.

When performing CPR, position yourself directly over the client, and ensure that the chest compressions are effective in order to facilitate myocardial blood flow. As discussed in Box 19.8, the AHA guidelines reconfirm the importance of minimizing interruptions in chest compressions and improving the quality of CPR. As noted, these guidelines are evidence based and supported by ongoing research.

Post-Resuscitation

If the client is successfully resuscitated, continue to monitor the client closely. Care of the client will vary depending on how long the client was in cardiac arrest and the client's metabolic condition. When feasible, perform a head-to-toe assessment, including a neurologic assessment, and compare the results to the client's baseline. If the client is awake and responsive, the client may need to be reoriented to the surroundings. The client and family will need emotional support as well. Collaborate and consult with other members of the healthcare team as needed.

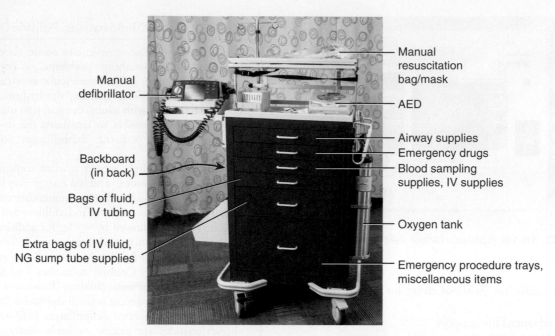

Manual resuscitation bag/mask

Manual defibrillator

AED

Airway supplies

Emergency drugs

Blood sampling supplies, IV supplies

Backboard (in back)

Bags of fluid, IV tubing

Extra bags of IV fluid, NG sump tube supplies

Oxygen tank

Emergency procedure trays, miscellaneous items

FIG. 19.17 Example of a crash cart.

APPLICATION OF THE NURSING PROCESS

Examples of Related ICNP Nursing Diagnoses, Expected Client Outcomes, and Nursing Interventions:

Nursing Diagnosis: Risk for ineffective tissue perfusion

Supporting Data: Client has a history of ACS and unstable angina.

Expected Client Outcomes: The client will have increased tissue perfusion, as seen by:

- absence of chest pain or other symptoms of tissue ischemia
- vital signs and oxygen saturation within established parameters
- extremities warm to touch, without signs of shock or pallor.

Nursing Intervention Examples: Monitor the client's vital signs and other parameters of tissue perfusion. Provide oxygen as ordered and indicated.

Reference: International Classification for Nursing Practice. (n.d.). *eHealth & ICNP*. Retrieved from https://www.icn.ch/what-we-do/projects/ehealth-icnp.

CRITICAL CONCEPTS
Caring for a Client With a Cardiac Emergency

Accuracy (ACC)

When caring for a client with a cardiac emergency, accuracy is affected by the following variables:

BOX 19.8 Lessons From the Evidence: American Heart Association (AHA) Evidence-Based Guidelines: Quality of Chest Compressions and CPR

Based on research data and evidence-based systematic reviews of the International Liaison Committee on Resuscitation (ILCOR), the AHA guidelines continue to emphasize the importance of high-quality chest compressions and CPR. Some of the key features of these guidelines are as follows:

- **Ensure that chest compressions are done at an adequate rate (100–120/minute):** Although chest compressions need to be quick (at least 100/minute), they must also be effective. The updated guidelines include the upper limit based on a study indicating that a too-rapid rate (>120) may result in decreased compression depth.
- **Ensure that the chest is compressed an adequate depth (5 cm [2 inches]):** For adults, the compression depth should be at least 5 cm (2 inches). The updated guidelines also note that the depth should not be more than 6 cm (2.4 inches) due to the risk of possible injury.
- **Allow full recoil, and avoid leaning on the client during CPR:** Full chest recoil is facilitated by allowing the chest to return to its neutral state during the decompression phase of CPR. Leaning on the client (which would prevent chest recoil) may result in decreased venous return and reduced myocardial blood flow.
- **Minimize the interruption of chest compressions.** This remains a key point. The goal is to have a compression fraction (or time that compressions are performed during cardiac arrest) as high as possible. Interruptions should be minimized and limited to less than 10 seconds when doing pulse checks and when using automated external defibrillators (AEDs).

Reference: Kleinman et al., 2015.

Client-Related Factors
- Client's assessment, including level of consciousness and orientation
- Client's age, gender, past and present medical history; history of cardiac disorder
- Client's condition, presence of recent damage to the heart or heart failure
- Client's ability to report symptoms (e.g., chest pain, shortness of breath)
- Client's metabolic/electrolyte status (e.g., potassium, magnesium levels, etc.)

Nurse-Related Factors
- Knowledge and proper implementation of the links in the cardiac chain of survival
- Anticipation, preparation, assessment, and proper identification of unstable angina, dysrhythmias, and other possible cardiac emergencies
- Adherence to and understanding of approved guidelines

Equipment-Related Factors
- Proper functioning of wall outlets for oxygen and suction and proper functioning of any other emergency equipment
- Availability of crash cart, full oxygen tank, and other emergency equipment.

Client-Centered Care (CCC)

When caring for a client with a cardiac emergency, respect for the client is demonstrated by:
- explaining the procedures that may occur during cardiac emergencies
- providing culturally sensitive explanations and arranging for an interpreter if necessary

- answering questions for the client and family
- ensuring comfort during and after cardiac emergencies
- providing privacy and advocating for the client and family.

Infection Control (INF)

When caring for a client with a cardiac emergency, healthcare-associated infection is prevented by:
- preventing and reducing the transfer of microorganisms
- reducing the number of microorganisms.

Safety (SAF)

When caring for a client with a cardiac emergency, safety measures prevent harm and maintain a safe care environment by:
- ensuring that alarms are turned on at all times and emergency equipment is used per manufacturer guidelines.
- assessing for allergies and ensuring that measures are taken to minimize any injuries to the client during emergencies.

Communication (COM)

- Communication exchanges information (oral, written, nonverbal, or electronic) between two or more people.
- Collaboration, interdisciplinary cooperation, and teamwork with other healthcare professionals will facilitate positive client outcomes during cardiac emergencies.
- Documentation records information in a permanent healthcare record.

Evaluation (EVAL)

Evaluation of outcomes enables the nurse to determine the efficacy of the care provided.

■ SKILL 19.6 Caring for a Client With Acute Ischemic Chest Pain

EQUIPMENT

Clean gloves and PPE, if there is a risk of exposure to body fluids
Stethoscope and blood pressure cuff
ECG monitoring equipment (bedside or portable)
Emergency equipment on standby
Defibrillator and crash cart on standby
Oxygen saturation monitor
Supplemental oxygen (if needed)
Medications (e.g., acetylsalicylic acid [ASA], NTG, morphine) (if ordered)
NTG infusion (glass bottle) and special nonabsorbing tubing (if ordered)

BEGINNING THE SKILL

1. **ACC** Review the following:
   - medical history and current diagnosis such as Acute Coronary Syndrome (ACS)

- relevant lab results, such as cardiac enzymes or biomarkers (e.g., troponin levels). *Elevated serum troponin levels could indicate the client has had an acute MI.*
2. **INF** Perform hand hygiene.
3. **CCC** Introduce yourself to the client and family.
4. **SAF** Identify the client using at least two identifiers.
5. **CCC** Provide privacy and explain the procedure. *Providing privacy in layers enhances-client centered care.*

PROCEDURE

6. **ACC** Perform rapid bedside assessment. Assess level of consciousness and presence of chest pain or associated symptoms. If the client is in immediate distress, summon the RRT per facility policy. (Note: The authorized healthcare provider must be notified at the onset of ischemic chest pain.)
7. **ACC** Obtain the client's vital signs (particularly pulse, blood pressure, and respirations) and oxygen saturation; perform a cardiac assessment (see Chapter 4). Note if

there is a change from the client's baseline before chest pain. *Vital signs may be affected by ischemic chest pain.*

8. **SAF** Assess the client for allergies. Look at the client's armband, and ask client verbally about allergies. Note allergies to any medications or allergies to latex or other substances that may be used. *This is an important safety measure.*

9. **ACC** Assess the nature of the client's chest pain and other symptoms.
   - **P** (Provoking): What aggravates the pain? Is it at rest or brought on by activity?
   - **Q** (Quality): Where is the pain located (e.g., center of chest, substernal, or epigastric area)? How does the pain feel (e.g., dull, heavy, pressure, tightness)? Are there any associated symptoms (e.g., shortness of breath, nausea/vomiting, or "cold sweat")?
   - **R** (Radiating): Is the pain radiating to the client's left or right arm, jaw, neck, back, or anywhere else?
   - **S** (Severity): What is the level of the client's pain on a scale of 1 (least) to 10 (worst)?
   - **T** (Time): When did the pain start or how long did it last (in minutes)?

10. **ACC** Obtain a stat 12-lead ECG (if not already done), and place the client on continuous bedside ECG monitoring. Compare 12-lead ECG with previous to see if there are any changes from baseline, and ensure that results are sent to the authorized healthcare provider. (Note: Continuous 12-lead monitoring may be required, depending on the client's condition.)

11. **ACC** Assess the client for dysrhythmias and note if there is a deviation from baseline. *Dysrhythmias can cause chest pain due to decreased blood flow and oxygen to the myocardium. Dysrhythmias can also increase the client's myocardial oxygen demand and compromise coronary artery blood flow by reducing the heart's diastolic filling time.*

12. **SAF** Ensure that emergency equipment, oxygen, and the defibrillator are nearby and ready to use. *Clients who develop acute ischemic chest pain can sometimes deteriorate quickly.*

13. **SAF** If the client has shortness of breath, ensure that the head of the bed is elevated at least 30 to 45 degrees. *Elevating the head of the bed can help with diaphragmatic expansion and oxygenation.*

14. **INF** Apply gloves and PPE (if needed).

15. **ACC** Place the client on supplemental oxygen as indicated and per order to keep oxygen saturations within established parameters. *Helps provide oxygenation to the myocardium.*

16. **ACC** Insert an IV access device (if the client doesn't already have one), and ensure that there is no indication of infiltration (see Chapter 12). *An IV device may be needed for emergency medications.*

17. **ACC** Give emergency medications as ordered, such as nitroglycerin (either sublingual [SL] spray tablets, or IV), or other medications as ordered (see Chapters 11 and 12). *These medications may be used to improve blood flow (by vasodilatation) to the myocardium or to reduce preload (in the case of morphine) to reduce myocardial oxygen consumption.*

18. **ACC** Continue to administer sublingual NTG as ordered, or titrate IV NTG per order, until chest pain is relieved. Monitor blood pressure and pulse. *Cardiac medications such as NTG can affect blood pressure and pulse.* (Note: The goal with ischemic chest pain is 100% relief.)

19. **ACC** Prepare the client for emergency cardiac catheterization as indicated and ordered (see Skill 19.6).

20. **EVAL** Continue to monitor the client's vital signs and other vital functions.

21. **CCC** Provide a quiet environment and provide emotional support to the client and family. *A quiet environment will help reduce stress and anxiety during ischemic pain.*

22. **SAF** Provide follow-up care as needed. If chest pain is relieved, continue to monitor the client on a regular basis. **WARNING:** Ensure that ECG alarms are turned on before you leave the room.

FINISHING THE SKILL

23. **SAF** Ensure client safety and comfort. Ensure that the bed is in the lowest position, and verify that the client can identify and reach the nurse call system. *These safety measures reduce the risk of falls.*

24. **EVAL** Evaluate the outcomes. Is the client's chest pain relieved? Are the client's vital signs within established parameters? Is the client's 12-lead ECG within established parameters?

25. **COM** Document assessment findings, care given related to the client's ischemic chest pain, and outcomes in the legal healthcare record, including the following:
   - client's ischemic chest pain assessment (based on PQRST model)
   - presence of other symptoms, such as shortness of breath or palpitations
   - onset of chest pain and time that authorized healthcare provider notified
   - time that 12-lead ECG obtained and authorized healthcare provider who received it
   - use of continuous 12-lead or ST-segment monitoring during chest pain
   - oxygen saturation and vital signs during ischemic chest pain episode.

■ SKILL 19.7 Caring for a Client After an Emergency Cardiac Catheterization

EQUIPMENT

Stethoscope and blood pressure cuff

Clean gloves and PPE, if there is a risk of exposure to body fluids

Gauze pads (if needed to change insertion site dressing)

Transparent dressing (if needed to change insertion site dressing)

ECG monitoring equipment (bedside or portable)

IV access devices and equipment (e.g., IV pole, fluid)

Oxygen saturation monitor

Supplemental oxygen (if needed)

Emergency equipment on standby (e.g., crash cart, suction)

BEGINNING THE SKILL

1. **ACC** Review orders for the following:
   - bedrest instructions
   - postprocedure IV fluids
   - postprocedure position (supine or head elevated no more than 30 degrees)
2. **ACC** Review the following:
   - medical and surgical history (past and present), including previous MIs cardiac catheterizations, and/or cardiac stent placement
   - lab work that could affect rhythms (e.g., electrolytes, potassium, magnesium)
   - history of anticoagulant use and time/day client last took anticoagulants.
3. **INF** Perform hand hygiene.
4. **CCC** Introduce yourself to the client and family.
5. **SAF** Identify the client using at least two identifiers.
6. **CCC** Provide privacy. *Providing privacy in layers enhances client-centered care.*

PROCEDURE

7. **ACC** Assess the client for the following:
   - **SAF** allergies to medications, latex, or other substances that may be used after cardiac catheterization
   - level of consciousness and orientation to person, time, place, and situation
   - any complaints of shortness of breath, palpitations, or other symptoms
   - **CCC** any pain/discomfort at cardiac catheterization insertion site.
8. **INF** Apply gloves and PPE if there is a risk of exposure to body fluids.
9. **SAF** Obtain vital signs and oxygen saturation, and ensure that the client is connected to the ECG monitor (see Skill 19.1). Compare to the client's baseline. (Note: If needed, raise the client's bed to an ergonomically safe working height, then return the bed to the lowest position after care is provided.)
10. **SAF** Confirm that the client has a patent IV access device, without any signs of infiltration. *This may be needed for IV fluids or medications that may be given.*

11. **ACC** Assess the cardiac catheter insertion site for any sign of bleeding or hematoma, and assess the compression bandage (if present) to ensure that it is secure and intact.
    - If the cardiac catheterization used a radial approach, the catheter insertion site will be located on the right wrist.
    - If the cardiac catheterization used a femoral approach, the catheter insertion site will be located on either the right or left groin.
12. **SAF WARNING:** If bleeding is present, apply gloves and then apply pressure directly on and proximal to the insertion site per facility policy. Contact the authorized healthcare provider.
13. **ACC** If indicated and allowed by policy, reinforce or change the catheter insertion site dressing using gauze pads and transparent dressing if needed and ordered. (Note: If Step 12 or Step 13 were performed, remove gloves and perform hand hygiene before continuing care.)
14. **ACC** Assess the client for other complications, such as bruising or retroperitoneal bleeding (e.g., unilateral back or flank pain, decreased blood pressure, increased heart rate). If this occurs, notify the authorized healthcare provider immediately.
15. **ACC** Perform a system-specific cardiac physical assessment, including auscultation of heart tones (see Chapter 4). *This serves as a baseline for future assessments.*
16. **ACC** Assess pulses distal to the insertion site. Mark pulses with an indelible marker if difficult to locate. Note the color and warmth of extremities. *Assessment of pulses and warmth in extremities distal to the insertion site ensures that circulation has not been compromised by a thrombus or other complication (see Chapters 3 and 4 for assessment of pulses).* **WARNING:** If the distal pulses are not palpable or heard with a Doppler and/or this assessment deviates from the client's baseline, notify the authorized healthcare provider.
17. **ACC** Start IV fluids if ordered by the authorized healthcare provider. *Supplemental hydration after a cardiac catheterization helps to clear the contrast agent and reduces the risk of nephrotoxicity.*
18. **SAF** Instruct client to avoid manipulating, flexing, or moving the joint nearest to the cardiac catheter insertion site. *Manipulation of the joint can irritate the site and cause a hematoma.*
19. **ACC** Assess the cardiac catheter insertion site per order or facility policy. (Note: The site is usually monitored every 15 minutes the first hour after the client's arrival to the unit, followed by every 30 minutes for the next 2 hours, then every hour for the next 12 hours.)
20. **EVAL** Continue to monitor the client's vital signs and oxygen saturation for the remainder of the time the client is on the unit.

21. **CCC** Maintain a quiet, calm environment and provide support to the client and family. *A quiet environment will help reduce stress and anxiety during ischemic pain.*

FINISHING THE SKILL

22. **SAF** Ensure client safety and comfort. Ensure that the bed is in the lowest position, and verify that the client can identify and reach the nurse call system. *These safety measures reduce the risk of falls.*
23. **EVAL** Evaluate the outcomes. The client will have no evidence of bleeding or hematoma near the insertion site. The client's extremities will be warm with intact distal pulses.
24. **COM** Document assessment findings, care provided after receiving cardiac catheterization, and outcomes in the legal healthcare record, including the following:
    * assessment of the cardiac catheter insertion site and condition of compression dressing
    * assessment of client's pulses distal to the catheter insertion site and grading bilaterally
    * date and time if additional pressure was used to control bleeding and who was notified.

■ SKILL 19.8 Providing Emergency (Asynchronous) Manual Defibrillation

EQUIPMENT

Facility-approved defibrillator/monitor with ECG oscilloscope and recorder
"Hands-free" defibrillator pads or electrodes if used (pregelled or adhesive)
Conductive gel pads (if needed for paddle use)
ECG calibrated graph paper (for defibrillator)
Emergency equipment on standby (e.g., crash cart, suction)
Manual resuscitation bag and mask (if needed)
Clean gloves and PPE, if there is a risk of exposure to body fluids
Oxygen saturation monitor, supplemental oxygen (if needed)

BEGINNING THE SKILL

1. **INF** Perform hand hygiene.
2. **CCC** Introduce yourself to the family (if they are in the room). (Note: Depending on facility policy, the client's family/significant others may have permission to remain in the room.)
3. **SAF** Identify the client using at least two identifiers.
4. **CCC** Provide privacy. *Providing privacy in layers enhances client-centered care.*

PROCEDURE

5. **ACC** Perform a rapid assessment and check the client's level of consciousness. Assess the client's rhythm and pulse. If the client has a lethal dysrhythmia (e.g., VF or a pulseless, nonperfusing VT) and/or if the client is quickly deteriorating, summon the RRT or emergency team and retrieve the defibrillator or AED. (Note: Emergency defibrillation without sedation is only indicated if the client is seizing, pulseless, unresponsive, or in cardiac arrest.)
6. **SAF** If a defibrillator is not immediately available and the client is in cardiac arrest, perform CPR (with minimal interruptions in chest compressions) per AHA guidelines.
7. **SAF** Ensure that a second responding nurse retrieves emergency equipment (e.g., crash cart, suction, oxygen, bag-mask device, intubation equipment) to be on standby.
8. **INF** Apply gloves and PPE if there is a risk of exposure to body fluids.
9. **ACC** If the client is not on a continuous bedside monitor, attach the defibrillator monitor. (Note: Some defibrillators also have a "quick look" feature" that allows visualization of the client's rhythm when the paddles are placed on the chest.)
10. **ACC** If the client has any metallic objects or transdermal nitropaste on the skin, remove and clean off any residue. *Metallic objects and transdermal patches can interfere with conduction.*
11. **SAF** Ensure that the client is in a dry environment and that the client's chest is dry. *Because water is a conductor of electricity, it could cause the nurse responder to receive a shock and burn the client. It could also interfere with energy conduction to the heart (Hambach, 2017b).*
12. **ACC** Apply conductive gel pads (for paddles) or self-adhesive pads for "hands-free," remote defibrillation per manufacturer or facility policy.
    a. **Sternum-apex location:** Place one pad at apex, left midaxillary line, and the other pad just below the right clavicle on the right side of sternum.

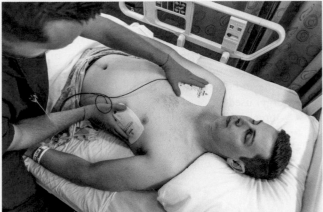

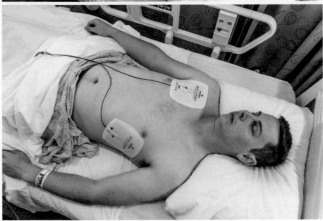

STEP 12A Position defibrillator pads (sternum-apex location shown).

   b. **Anterior/posterior location (self-adhesive pads):** Place one pad in anterior left precordial area or below left clavicle; place posterior pad below scapula.

   c. Avoid using alcohol-soaked pads. *Alcohol is combustible with electrical currents.*

   d. Avoid placing pads over breast tissue. *Breast tissue can increase resistance.*

   e. Avoid placing pads over an ICD or pacemaker. If the client has a pacemaker, place at least 2.5 cm (1 inch) from the pulse generator and lead wires (Hambach, 2017b).

13. **ACC** Set defibrillator/monitor to run a continuous tracing during the procedure.

14. **ACC** Charge the defibrillator at the amount of energy (*joules*) according to order or policy. (Note: The amount of joules used may range from 100 to 360 joules and will vary according to the dysrhythmia and the type of defibrillator used. Biphasic defibrillators use less energy than monophasic defibrillators. Use the lowest amount of energy necessary to convert the rhythm.)

15. **SAF WARNING:** If the client has a dysrhythmia (e.g., VF) with no QRS, do *not* use the synchronization mode. *The defibrillator won't discharge if it doesn't sense the R wave.*

16. **SAF** If using paddles, place them on the conductive pads in the proper location. Apply equal, firm pressure on each paddle (about 25 lb each) (Jacobson, 2019b)

17. **SAF** Quickly recheck the client and the rhythm on the monitor. *Prevents unnecessary shock.*

18. **SAF WARNING:** Announce "ALL CLEAR" and count down three times while checking to ensure everyone is clear from the bed, client, and equipment. *These safety measures help ensure that other responders at the scene are not inadvertently shocked.*

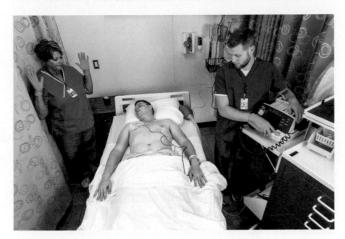

STEP 18 Ensure "all clear" before the shock.

19. **ACC** Press the "shock" button on the remote defibrillator machine or on each paddle. If using paddles, press the "shock" button on each paddle at same time with equal pressure.

20. **SAF** Check the client and check the monitor to determine if the client has converted to sinus rhythm. If dysrhythmia persists and the client is still unresponsive and pulseless, immediately resume CPR and cardiac arrest procedure per AHA guidelines. (Note: If the first shock is not successful, the joules are usually increased according to order or facility protocol.)

21. **ACC** If the client has stable rhythm, check vital signs, level of consciousness, neurologic status, and oxygen saturation. Assess if there is a change from the client's baseline.

22. **CCC** Reorient the client to surroundings if necessary. *Dysrhythmias, particularly if they result in a loss of consciousness and hemodynamic changes, can cause disorientation.*

23. **SAF** Ensure that IV line is established. *Prepares for emergency drugs if needed.*

24. **ACC** Print an ECG strip or check a 12-lead ECG if ordered (see Section 2).

25. **CCC** Remove conductive pads or adhesive pads, and clean skin if needed. Assess the client's skin and ensure there are no burns or injury. (Note: Depending on the manufacturer, adhesive defibrillator pads may remain on the client for reuse if they are not damaged or crimped.)

26. **SAF** Provide follow-up care and ensure that the monitor alarms on ECG monitor remain turned on and that the high and low alarms are set appropriately per order.

FINISHING THE SKILL

27. **INF** If paddles were used, clean per facility policy with appropriate solution.
28. **INF** Remove gloves and PPE (if used) and perform hand hygiene.
29. **SAF** Ensure safety and comfort. Remain with the client until the RRT and authorized healthcare provider arrive per facility policy.
30. **EVAL** Evaluate the outcomes. Was the client successfully defibrillated into sinus rhythm? Are the client's vital signs and level of consciousness within established parameters?
31. **COM** Document assessment findings, care given related to emergency defibrillation, and outcomes in the legal healthcare record, including the following:
    - time and date of defibrillation, amount of joules (energy) used
    - outcome of defibrillation, rhythm before and after defibrillation
    - length of time before first defibrillation (e.g., ≤2 minutes).

■ SKILL 19.9 Responding to a Client (Adult) in Cardiac Arrest

This skill is not intended to replace your basic life support [BLS]/advanced cardiac life support [ACLS] provider course for CPR on an adult client. For more information on adult CPR, as well as pediatric CPR (for infants and children), refer to current AHA guidelines.

EQUIPMENT

Backboard (for CPR)
Clean gloves and PPE, if there is a risk of exposure to body fluids
Manual resuscitation bag and mask
Emergency equipment and crash cart (fully stocked)
Defibrillator adhesive pads (if "hands-free" paddles are used)
Conductive gel pads (if paddles used)
Facility approved defibrillator/monitor with ECG oscilloscope, recorder, and graph paper
Stethoscope and blood pressure cuff, oxygen saturation monitor
Oxygen equipment and portable oxygen tank (usually on crash cart)

BEGINNING THE SKILL

1. **INF** Perform hand hygiene.
2. **CCC** Introduce yourself to the family (if they are in the room). (Note: Depending on facility policy, the client's family/significant others may have permission to remain in the room.)
3. **SAF** Identify the client and provide privacy. *Providing privacy in layers enhances client-centered care.*
4. **INF** Apply gloves and PPE if there is a risk of exposure to body fluids.

PROCEDURE

5. **SAF** Determine if the client is unresponsive and without signs of life (no breathing or pulse). If the client is in cardiac arrest, call the RRT and remain with the client. (Note: Ask an assistant or unit clerk to summon the emergency team and retrieve an AED or defibrillator if possible. If you are alone, follow current AHA guidelines and facility policy.)
6. **ACC** If the client is receiving ECG monitoring, assess the rhythm. If the client has a pulseless dysrhythmia (e.g., VF), immediately proceed to emergency defibrillation (see Skill 19.8).
7. **SAF** If the client is not receiving ECG monitoring or if a defibrillator is not available, place the client in the supine position and immediately initiate BLS per the current AHA guidelines. (Note: A manual resuscitation bag and mask should be used for rescue breaths, and a hard surface or backboard should be placed under client to facilitate effective chest compressions.)
8. **ACC** While doing chest compressions, ensure that you have proper alignment and are positioned directly over the client. Place the client's bed in the lowest position and/or get a footstool if needed. *This allows you to be positioned over the client to facilitate effective chest compressions.* (Note: While doing CPR, avoid a rocking motion, and avoid leaning on the client. Allow the chest to recoil and return to its natural position to facilitate venous return.)
9. **SAF WARNING:** Continue to remain with the client. There must always be at least one nurse in the room with the client, if possible, during a cardiac arrest.
10. **SAF** Ensure that a second responding nurse (if available) retrieves an AED or defibrillator with an ECG monitor (if not already in the room), a crash cart, oxygen, and other equipment. (Note: The second responding nurse should assist with the manual resuscitation bag and mask and help maintain a complete seal on the mask. If you are alone, administer compressions and rescue breaths per AHA guidelines while minimizing interruptions in chest compressions.)
11. **SAF** Continue cycles of CPR and AED per AHA guidelines and facility policy until the RRT arrives. (Note: The RRT usually manages the arrest once they arrive.)
12. **SAF** Ensure that wall suction and oxygen flow meters are set up and working, and assist team with securing an IV line, setting up emergency pacer, or other procedures as needed.

13. **COM** Confirm that someone is recording the events of the cardiac arrest. *Provides documentation.* (Note: This task will often be assigned by the emergency team.)

14. **COM** Collaborate with the the RRT or other healthcare providers as needed with sending emergency lab work, communicating with family, calling chaplain, or other tasks as needed.

15. **ACC** If the client is successfully resuscitated, provide post-resuscitation care and prepare to transfer to critical care if indicated. Maintain the client in the appropriate recovery position as ordered (e.g., side-lying position).

16. **ACC** Check vital signs and do a head-to-toe assessment (particularly the client's level of consciousness and neurologic status). Note if there is a change from baseline. *Clients who have been in cardiac arrest may need to be reoriented to the immediate surroundings.*

17. **CCC** Assess the client for pain or discomfort and assess for possible bruising around the sternum or rib cage. *Chest compressions can sometimes cause tenderness, bruising, or injury.*

18. **CCC** Provide follow-up care with the family and provide support as needed.

FINISHING THE SKILL

19. **INF** If defibrillator paddles were used, clean per facility policy with appropriate solution.

20. **INF** Remove gloves and PPE (if used) and perform hand hygiene.

21. **SAF** Ensure client safety and comfort. Remain with the client until the client is stabilized and transferred to the critical care unit if indicated.

22. **EVAL** Evaluate the outcomes. Was the client successfully resuscitated? Is the client's hemodynamic and neurologic status at the pre-arrest baseline? Is the client oriented?

23. **COM** Document assessment findings, care given, and outcomes in the legal healthcare record, including the following:
    - time of cardiac arrest, time emergency team notified, and time team arrived
    - sequence of events and list of personnel who were present and assignments
    - length of time before first compressions and defibrillation were started
    - notification of the family and support provided (e.g., chaplain care).

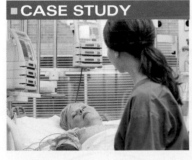

■ CASE STUDY Ms. Rice is a 58-year-old female who has been admitted to the medical-surgical unit following a cholecystectomy. She has a long history of diabetes, as well as coronary artery disease (CAD). Since admission, she has been comfortable with stable vital signs.

One afternoon after ambulating to her bathroom, Ms. Rice calls the nurse into her room and states, "I feel sick to my stomach." After further assessment, the nurse notes that Ms. Rice is short of breath and has a dull ache on the left side of her neck and jaw area. Her blood pressure is elevated, and her oxygen (O_2) saturation is 88%, which is significantly different from her baseline assessment, and her pulse feels irregular and weak. After placing Ms. Rice on bedrest, the nurse calls the authorized healthcare provider who orders a 12-lead ECG, cardiac monitoring, and lab tests (e.g., troponin level). Nitroglycerin (SL) and supplemental oxygen are also ordered.

After evaluating Ms. Rice's test results, the cardiology team decides to do an emergency cardiac catheterization for reperfusion and place a stent in Ms. Rice using a femoral approach in her right groin. After the procedure, Ms. Rice is admitted to the critical care unit for continued care and monitoring. Her vital signs and O_2 saturation are stable, she is pain-free, and her dressing is dry and intact. The post-procedure orders include bedrest, IV fluids, anticoagulants, vital signs, and pulse checks. She also remains on ECG monitoring. The nurse notifies CM about Ms. Rice's status and communicates with the staff about the high/low alarm parameters.

Later that night, Ms. Rice becomes increasingly restless and states that she is having some trouble sleeping. Although Ms. Rice has no pain or other symptoms, the critical care nurse notes that she has a small amount of bleeding on her right groin dressing. After applying pressure to the site (with gloves) and checking Ms. Rice's vital signs, the nurse contacts the authorized healthcare provider. She also uses comfort measures such as controlling noise to help Ms. Rice relax. The nurse reports all of this information to the oncoming nurse as part of handoff communication.

Case Study Questions

1. After Ms. Rice was initially admitted to the medical-surgical unit, her condition changed. Considering her medical history and signs and symptoms, what was the top priority regarding her care, and why? How did the medical-surgical nurse in this scenario recognize and analyze cues and demonstrate clinical judgment and reasoning?

2. What methods and strategies can be used to assess ischemic chest pain? Considering Ms. Rice's gender, history, and other factors, what are the challenges regarding the assessment?

3. After the 12-lead ECG and other tests, the cardiology team performs an emergency cardiac catheterization for reperfusion and stent placement. What are some possible complications?

4. Later in the evening after the catheterization, Ms. Rice becomes increasingly restless. What are the possible hazards of increased restlessness or movement by Ms. Rice? How can the critical care nurse ensure safety as well as client-centered care in this situation?

5. **Application of QSEN Competencies:** Two of the Quality and Safety Education for Nurses (QSEN) Teamwork and Collaboration attitudes are to "appreciate the risks associated with handoffs among providers and across transitions in care" and to "value teamwork and the relationships upon which it is based" (Cronenwett et al., 2007). How did the critical care nurse in this scenario demonstrate these competencies when communicating with the CM staff and the oncoming nurse? What are additional ways the nurse could enhance handoff communication and safety for Ms. Rice?

■CONCEPT MAP

ICNP Nursing Dx:
Risk for Impaired
Cardiac Function
Supporting Data:
Initial vital sign changes
Weak, thready irregular pulse
Oxygen (O_2) saturation changes

- Continue to assess BP and pulse
- Monitor O_2 saturation
- Ensure that vital signs are within established parameters.
- Monitor extremity pulses bilaterally

Baseline Assessment Data
- 58 years old
- History of CAD and diabetes
- C/O feeling "sick at my stomach" after ambulating
- C/O dull ache on left side of neck and jaw area
- Vital signs/O_2 sat. changes
- 12-lead ECG changes
- Cardiac catheterization and stent placement
- Increased restlessness

ICNP Nursing Dx:
Risk for Ineffective
Tissue Perfusion
Supporting Data:
History of CAD
Cardiac ischemia signs/symptoms

ICNP Nursing Dx:
Anxiety
Supporting Data:
Sleep difficulty
Restlessness

- Maintain client on bedrest during ischemic symptoms
- Place client on O_2 per orders/policy
- Administer medication such as nitroglycerin as ordered
- Obtain 12-lead ECG per order/policy
- Provide post-cardiac catheterization care

- Maintain calm, "noise-free" environment
- Provide explanations
- Use non-jargon language
- Enhance client's environment
- Provide comfort measures

References

American Association of Critical-Care Nurses. (2016). *AACN practice alert: Accurate dysrhythmia monitoring in adults*. Retrieved from https://www.aacn.org/newsroom/aacn-updates-cardiac-monitoring-practice-alerts.

American Association of Critical-Care Nurses. (2018). *AACN practice alert. Managing alarms in acute care across the life span. Electrocardiography and pulse oximetry*. Retrieved from https://www.aacn.org/clinical-resources/practice-alerts/managing-alarms-in-acute-care-across-the-life-span.

American Heart Association. (2016a). *Warning signs of a heart attack*. Retrieved from http://www.heart.org/HEARTORG/Conditions/-HeartAttack/WarningSignsofaHeartAttack/Warning-Signs-of-a-Heart-Attack_UCM_002039_Article.jsp.

American Heart Association. (2016b). *Conduction disorders*. Retrieved from http://www.heart.org/HEARTORG/Conditions/Arrhythmia/AboutArrhythmia/Conduction-Disorders_UCM_302046_Article.jsp.

American Heart Association. (2016c). *Living with your pacemaker*. Retrieved from http://www.heart.org/HEARTORG/Conditions/Arrhythmia/PreventionTreatmentofArrhythmia/Living-With-Your-Pacemaker_UCM_305290_Article.jsp#.VimutqJlfO4.

American Heart Association. (2016d). *Devices that may interfere with your pacemaker*. Retrieved from http://www.heart.org/HEARTORG/Conditions/Arrhythmia/PreventionTreatmentofArrhythmia/Devices-that-may-Interfere-with-Pacemakers_UCM_302013_Article.jsp.

American Red Cross, (2016). First aid/CPR/AED. In *Participant's manual*. Yardley, PA: StayWell Publishing.

Caple, C., & Heering, H. (2018). Electrocardiogram: Performing—An overview. In *Nursing practice & skill*. Ipswich, MA: EBSCO Publishing. Retrieved from Cinahl Information Systems.

Caple, C., & Karakashian, A. L. (2018). Transcutaneous cardiac pacing: Monitoring. In *Nursing practice & skill*. Ipswich, MA: EBSCO Publishing. Retrieved from Cinahl Information Systems.

Centers for Disease Control. (2017). *Heart disease fact sheet*. Retrieved from http://www.cdc.gov/dhdsp/data_statistics/fact_sheets/fs_heart_disease.htm.

Chu, W. H. (2017). *Acute chest pain: Myocardial ischemia*. Retrieved from The Joanna Briggs Institute EBD Database, JBI@Ovid. JBI1669.

Cronenwett, L., Sherwood, G., Barnsteiner, J., Disch, J., Johnson, J., Mitchell, P., ... Warren, J. (2007). Quality and safety education for nurses. *Nursing Outlook, 55*(3), 122–131. Retrieved from http://qsen.org/competencies/pre-licensure-ksas/.

Hambach, C. (2017a). Cardioversion. In D. L. Wiegand (Ed.), *AACN procedure manual for high acuity, progressive, and critical care* (7th ed.) (pp. 293–301). St. Louis, MO: Saunders Elsevier.

Hambach, C. (2017b). Defibrillation (external). In D. L. Wiegand (Ed.), *AACN procedure manual for high acuity, progressive, and critical care* (7th ed.) (pp. 302–308). St. Louis, MO: Saunders Elsevier.

International Classification for Nursing Practice. (n.d.). *eHealth & ICNP*. Retrieved from https://www.icn.ch/what-we-do/projects/ehealth-icnp.

Jacobson, C. (2019a). Interpretation and management of basic cardiac rhythms. In S. M. Burns, & S. A. Delgado (Eds.), *AACN essentials of critical care nursing* (4th ed.) (pp. 37–70). New York, NY: McGraw Hill.

Jacobson, C. (2019b). Advanced ECG concepts. In S. M. Burns, & S. A. Delgado (Eds.), *AACN essentials of critical care nursing* (4th ed.) (pp. 459–500). New York, NY: McGraw Hill.

Jaffe, S. E., & Balderrama, D. (2017). Transvenous pacing: Monitoring. In *Nursing practice & skill*. Ipswich, MA: EBSCO Publishing. Retrieved from Cinahl Information Systems.

Kleinman, M. E., Brennan, E. E., Goldberger, Z. D., Swor, R. A., Terry, M., Bobrow, B. J., & Rea, T. (2015). Part 5: Adult basic life support and cardiopulmonary resuscitation quality: 2015 American Heart Association Guidelines update for cardiopulmonary resuscitation and emergency cardiovascular care. *Circulation, 132*(Suppl 2), S414–S435. Retrieved from http://circ.ahajournals.org/content/132/18_suppl_2/S414.full.pdf+html.

Leeper, B. (2019). Cardiovascular system. In S. M. Burns, & S. A. Delgado (Eds.), *AACN essentials of critical care nursing* (4th ed.) (pp. 245–274). New York, NY: McGraw Hill.

Pelter, M. M., Kozik, T. M., & Carey, M. G. (2017). Cardiac monitoring and electrocardiographic leads. In D. L. Wiegand (Ed.), *AACN procedure manual for high acuity, progressive, and critical care* (7th ed.) (pp. 467–476). St. Louis, MO: Saunders Elsevier.

Randazzo, A. (2016). *Prime medical training: Guide to 12-lead ECG placement*. Retrieved from https://www.primemedicaltraining.com/12-lead-ecg-placement/.

Rossano, J. W., Jones, W. E., Lerakis, S., Millin, M. G., Nemeth, I., Cassan, P., & Bradley, R. N. (2015). The use of automated external defibrillators in infants: A report from the American Red Cross Scientific Advisory Council. *Pediatric Emergency Care, 31*(7), 526–530.

Spotts, C. (2017). Permanent pacemaker (assessing function). In D. L. Wiegand (Ed.), *AACN procedure manual for high acuity, progressive, and critical care* (7th ed.) (pp. 388–398). St. Louis, MO: Saunders Elsevier.

Stephenson, E. A., & Berul, C. I. (2015). Pediatric ventricular fibrillation treatment and management. *Medscape*. Retrieved from http://emedicine.medscape.com/article/892748-treatment.

Wilson, S. (2017). Perfusion. In J. F. Giddons (Ed.), *Concepts for nursing practice* (3rd ed.) (pp. 167–188). St. Louis, MO: Elsevier.

Wung, S. (2017). Twelve-lead electrocardiogram. In D. L. Wiegand (Ed.), *AACN procedure manual for high acuity, progressive, and critical care* (7th ed.) (pp. 494–500). St. Louis, MO: Saunders Elsevier.

Zoll Medical Corporation. (2017). *Keys to successful cardioversion*. Retrieved from https://www.zoll.com/medical-technology/cardioversion/.

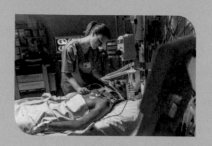

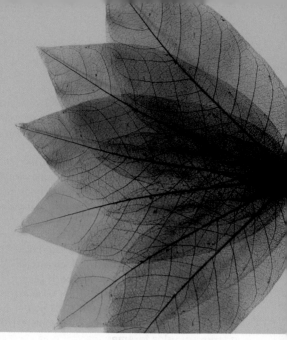

CHAPTER 20

Advanced Neurologic Care

"The human brain is a most unusual instrument of elegant and as yet unknown capacity" | **Attributed to Stuart Seaton, Author**

LEARNING OBJECTIVES

By the end of this chapter, the reader will be able to:

1. Identify the pathophysiologic changes associated with an acute neurologic injury.
2. Perform an advanced neurologic assessment on a critically ill client.
3. Use a pupillometer device.
4. Identify the indications and contraindications for a lumbar puncture (LP).
5. Demonstrate the critical elements of caring for a client who is receiving an LP.
6. Identify signs and symptoms of increased intracranial pressure (ICP).

7. Demonstrate the critical elements of caring for a client with an external ventricular drain (EVD) and ICP monitoring.
8. Obtain ICP readings.
9. Discuss selected neurologic emergencies.
10. Provide care for a client who requires seizure precautions.
11. Discuss screening tools that may be used for recognizing an acute stroke.
12. Assess a client who may be having an acute stroke.

TERMINOLOGY

Aphasia Inability to understand or express language.

Cerebrospinal fluid A serum-like fluid that continuously circulates around the ventricles of the brain, the spinal cord, and the subarachnoid space to allow for buoyancy of the brain inside the skull and to provide appropriate nutrition to the brain.

Cranial nerves Peripheral nerves (12 pairs) that arise from the brain and have motor or sensory function. These nerves are often tested during a neurologic exam.

Glasgow coma scale A commonly used summative scoring system of eye, verbal, and motor responses to describe level of consciousness (LOC). The scores can range from 3 (lowest) to 15 (highest). A lower score is associated with a more impaired LOC.

Interventricular foramen (foramen of Monro) A small interventricular opening on both the right and left ventricles of the brain that connects the third ventricle at the midline of the brain.

Intracranial pressure (ICP) Pressure or force exerted by the brain, cerebrospinal fluid, and cerebral blood flow inside the skull.

Intracranial pressure waveforms (P1, P2, P3) Three distinct monitor waveforms that can demonstrate pathologic changes in intracranial pressure over the cardiac cycle.

Level of consciousness The extent of alertness, awareness, orientation, and responsiveness to the environment experienced by an individual at a given time.

Monro–Kellie doctrine Observation that the cranial cavity is a closed space and that the sum of brain tissue, cerebrospinal fluid, and cerebral blood flow is constant, and therefore, a change in one component necessitates a change in the other.

Motor function Precise, purposeful movement of small and large muscle groups.

Neurological Pupil index (NPi) An algorithm to convey the reactivity of the pupil to a light source or a pupillometer to determine early pupillary changes related to changes within the brain.

Reflex An involuntary movement that does not require conscious thought.

Sensory function The ability to detect information from our senses, including sight, smell, pain, touch, temperature, hearing, and taste.

Tragus A small, fleshy prominence at the external auditory canal opening.

ACRONYMS

CBF Cerebral blood flow
CN Cranial nerve
CPP Cerebral perfusion pressure
CSF Cerebrospinal fluid
DTR Deep tendon reflexes
EVD External ventricular drain
FAST Face, arm, speech, time
GCS Glasgow Coma Scale
ICP Intracranial pressure
LOC Level of consciousness
LP Lumbar puncture
MEND Miami Emergency Neurologic Deficit
NIHSS National Institutes of Health Stroke Scale
NINDS National Institute of Neurological Disorders and Stroke
NPi Neurological Pupil index
PERRLA Pupils equal, round, regular, and reactive to light and accommodation
TBI Traumatic brain injury

The human neurologic system is highly complex. The nervous system has two major components, the brain and the spinal cord, which must communicate and coordinate together seamlessly to maintain vital functions of the autonomic, sensory, and motor processes of the body. The vital functions of the cerebral cortex, cerebellum, hypothalamus/thalamus, brainstem, limbic system, basal ganglia, midbrain, and cranial nerves must also be maintained. Effective neurologic functioning requires timely transmission of nerve impulses across synapses, adequate levels of neurotransmitters, and maintenance of the brain tissue, myelin sheath, and other structures. If any of these elements or processes are disrupted, the client may experience an alteration in his or her neurologic function. Thus, the nurse's expertise in this area is essential.

The primary focus of this chapter is skills related to alterations of the brain and intracranial processes. Cervical immobilization procedures related to alterations of the client's spinal cord, such as halo traction and the application of cervical collars, are discussed in Chapter 6. Logrolling a client and safe client transfers are discussed in Chapter 1.

INTRACRANIAL PROCESSES

Intracranium and *intracranial* are all-encompassing terms that describe the components within the skull. Between the skull and the brain, there are multiple layers of tissue that function to protect the brain. These layers, from outermost to innermost, include the dura mater, subdural space, arachnoid mater, subarachnoid space, and pia mater, which lies directly on the surface of the brain (Fig. 20.1). The dura mater, arachnoid mater, and pia mater are layers of protective tissue. The subarachnoid space (between the pia mater and arachnoid mater) contains cerebrospinal fluid (CSF), which allows the space to act as a "shock absorber" to cushion and protect the brain.

The three main regions of the brain are the cerebrum, the cerebellum, and the brainstem. These regions and other anatomical structures of the brain and central nervous system are illustrated in Fig. 20.2. As shown in Fig. 20.3, the lobes of the cerebrum include the right and left frontal lobes, the right and left parietal lobes, the right and left temporal lobes, and the occipital lobe.

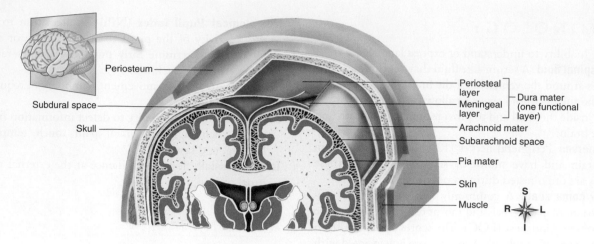

FIG. 20.1 Outer layers of the brain.

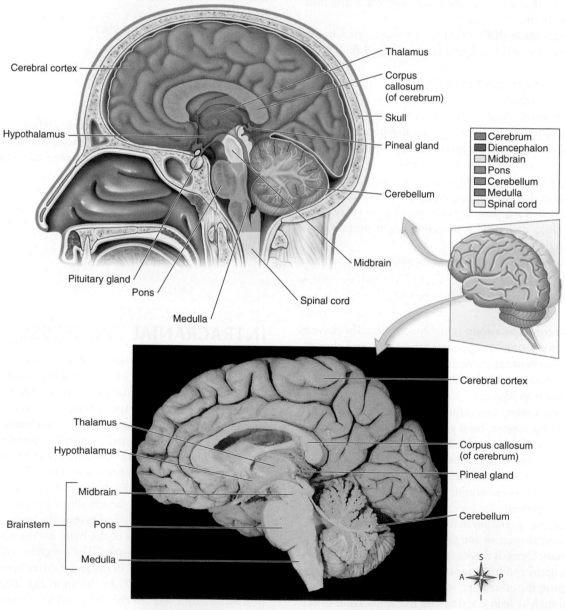

FIG. 20.2 Regions and structures of the brain.

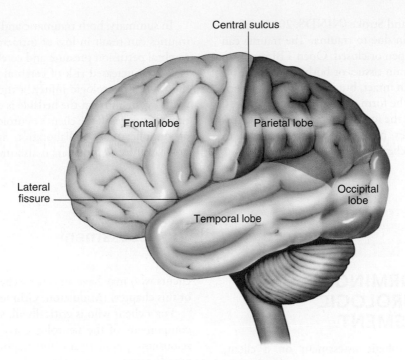

FIG. 20.3 Lobes of the brain.

Maintenance of Intracranial Homeostasis

The cranium is a closed space that does not leave much room for alterations. The Monro–Kellie doctrine recognizes that in order to maintain homeostasis, there must be a constant in three main components. These components include the client's brain tissue, which encompasses approximately 80% of the intracranial volume; the cerebral blood flow volume, which comprises approximately 10% of the intracranial volume; and the cerebrospinal fluid, which makes up another 10% of the intracranial volume (Weerakkody & Goel, 2018).

The brain allows for some compliance to abnormalities such as intracerebral hemorrhage or a brain tumor by adjusting the percentages of the three components. However, given the limited amount of space in the cranium, there can only be so much accommodation before brain damage occurs. This damage usually occurs in the form of a midline shift of the brain but can ultimately lead to cerebral herniation. Herniation is the downward shift of the brain into the spinal column—the only opening into the cranium—which results in loss of cerebral blood flow. Once herniation affects the brainstem, the client's respiratory centers are adversely affected. The client may also have signs of increased intracranial pressure (ICP) (discussed in Section 2 of this chapter).

Cerebral Blood Flow and Cerebral Perfusion Pressure

To maintain the health of the three main components previously discussed, the brain must receive blood from the heart. Considering the Monro–Kellie doctrine, the brain must only receive a certain amount of blood at a certain amount of pressure from the heart to maintain homeostasis. The pressure at which the brain receives blood from the heart is called *cerebral perfusion pressure* (CPP). CPP is calculated by subtracting the client's measured intracranial pressure (ICP) from the mean arterial pressure (MAP). The formula is CPP = MAP – ICP. The MAP refers to the blood pressure created by the heart, and the ICP refers to the pressure within the skull (see Section 2 of this chapter.). A well-perfused brain has a CPP of 50 to 70 mm Hg (Urden, Stacy, & Lough, 2016). The term *cerebral blood flow* (CBF) refers to the blood that circulates through the brain. The goal for the client is to maintain optimal CBF and CPP and to avoid cerebral herniation.

MAJOR NEUROLOGIC INJURIES: TRAUMATIC AND NONTRAUMATIC

In the acute care or critical care setting, a client may have various neurologic injuries that can be traumatic or non-traumatic. Examples of neurologic injuries include intracerebral hemorrhage, subdural hematoma, subarachnoid hemorrhage, acute stroke, or a mass such as a brain tumor. The causes of these neurologic injuries that result in bleeding within the cranium may be due to trauma. However, nontraumatic causes of these injuries include hemorrhages related to high blood pressure, hemorrhages in the setting of anticoagulant usage, or even spontaneous hemorrhages without a definitive cause. Other alterations within the brain can include lesions that take up space within the cranium and cause a shift within the cranium. These lesions can include brain tumors, arterial-venous malformations, and atrial venous fistulae, which are both abnormal connections of arteries and veins within the cranium and/or spinal cord.

One of the most serious neurologic injuries related to trauma is traumatic brain injury (TBI). The National Institute of Neurological Disorders and Stroke (NINDS, 2018) defines TBI as damage to the brain due to trauma. The trauma can result in the injury being open or closed. Open TBI results in penetration of the skull, brain tissue, or both. In closed TBI, the cerebral contents remain intact, but the client may experience injury to the skull in the form of nondisplaced fractures, injury to the brain tissue in the form of hematomas or hemorrhage, or concussive injuries. Both open and closed TBI can occur with or without the client's loss of consciousness.

In summary, both traumatic and nontraumatic neurologic injuries can result in loss of intracranial homeostasis, altered cerebral perfusion pressure and cerebral blood flow, increased ICP, and increased risk of cerebral herniation. Regardless of the client's neurologic injury, a thorough neurologic assessment by the nurse at the bedside is essential for early recognition of changes in the client's neurologic status and prevention of complications. Collaboration and communication with other healthcare providers is also imperative.

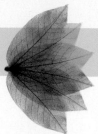

SECTION 1 Advanced Neurologic Assessment

PERFORMING A NEUROLOGIC ASSESSMENT

When performing a neurologic assessment on a client, accuracy is one of the most important critical concepts. Neurologic changes can be subtle; therefore, an accurate examination at the beginning of a shift is important to determine the client's baseline neurologic status for comparison with subsequent assessments. The neurologic assessment also allows the healthcare team to monitor the client's response to treatment and evaluate outcomes. Various scales exist to quantify the findings of a neurologic assessment, including the National Institutes of Health Stroke Scale (NIHSS) and the Miami Emergency Neurologic Deficit (MEND) exam (discussed in Section 3 of this chapter). One of the most widely recognized tools is the Glasgow Coma Scale (GCS), which measures three components: eye opening, verbal response, and motor response (Table 20.1). However, most experts do not recommend using the GCS alone for

clients who may have an acute ischemic stroke (see Section 3 of this chapter) (Middleton, Grimley, & Alexandrov, 2015).

For a client who is critically ill, six of the most important components of the neurologic assessment are level of consciousness, pupillary size and response, motor function, sensory function, deep tendon reflexes, and a neurologic score using the GCS or another approved scale. The assessment will vary according to whether the client is conscious or unconscious. The assessments should also focus on airway, breathing, and circulation because TBIs or other neurologic injuries can affect autonomic functions, such as breathing and blood pressure. Thus, it is also important to obtain the client's vital signs and pulse oximetry readings (see Chapter 3).

ASSESSMENT OF LEVEL OF CONSCIOUSNESS

Assessment of the level of consciousness (LOC) begins the moment you enter the room and observe the client. During the neurologic assessment, the nurse can gather valuable information by sitting down at eye level and interacting with the client, while also observing the client's alertness and ability to respond (Fig. 20.4). For example, do the client's eyes open spontaneously, or is some level of stimulation required? Is the client able to make eye contact and maintain alertness, or does he or she become inattentive and drowsy after a few minutes? The

TABLE 20.1 Glasgow Coma Scale

Glasgow Coma Scale (GCS)	Response	Score
Best eye response	4—Spontaneously 3—To verbal command 2—To painful stimuli 1—Eyes do not open	_____
Best verbal response	5—Oriented 4—Confused 3—Inappropriate words 2—Incomprehensible words 1—Nonverbal	_____
Best motor response	6—Obeys commands 5—Localized to painful stimuli 4—Withdraw from painful stimuli 3—Flexion to painful stimuli 2—Extension to painful stimuli 1—No motor response	_____
		Total: _____

Note: The highest GCS score possible is 15. The higher the number, the better the GCS score.

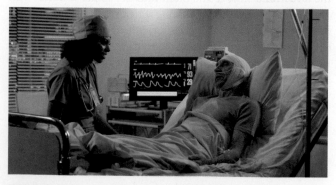

FIG. 20.4 Assess neurologic parameters, including LOC, during your interactions with the client.

TABLE 20.2 Assessment of Level of Consciousness (LOC)

Alert	Client is fully awake and completely interactive upon initial interaction
Drowsy	Client is less alert but will communicate and concentrate with very little stimulation
Somnolent	Client requires more stimulation and will drift back to sleep quickly without stimulation
Lethargic	Client may require noxious stimulation to induce very limited interaction
Obtunded	Client with most arousable state of lethargy if stimulated
Stupor	Client definitely requires noxious stimulation and may only respond with a groan
Coma	Client without response to persistent noxious stimulation and without sleep and wake cycles
Vegetative state	Client without perception of environment but with sleep and wake cycles, including eyes open

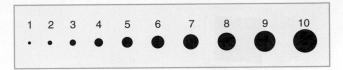

FIG. 20.5 Pupil size chart.

amount of stimulation needed, if any, can help to determine the client's LOC. See Table 20.2 for a comparison of the various descriptions of LOC. A client may arouse with verbal stimuli or may require light tactile or noxious stimuli. Evaluation of the client's LOC, including the client's participation, attention, and concentration, will continue throughout the exam.

It is important to remember that a client's LOC is, of course, influenced by client sedation. Thus, for a more accurate assessment, the authorized healthcare provider may order that sedation be decreased or stopped prior to the exam, which is sometimes referred to as a "sedation vacation."

ASSESSMENT OF PUPILLARY RESPONSE AND FUNCTION

In a neurologic assessment, the pupillary response is the primary cranial nerve examination (see Chapter 4). The client's pupil reactivity to light and the quality and equality of that reactivity bilaterally are important assessment parameters that should be included in the documentation. The acronym PERRLA is often used to document pupillary response and refers to pupils equal, round, regular, and reactive to light and accommodation. Accommodation refers to the ability of the pupils to focus on objects close up and far away. The three basic elements of a pupillary exam are as follows:

- **Shape of each pupil**—The expected findings are round pupils bilaterally, unless the client has a known anomaly at baseline, such as a cataract defect.
- **Reaction to light**—An expected finding is brisk constriction of the pupil to light bilaterally. There should also be a constriction reaction in the opposite pupil called *consensual pupillary reflex*. A slower constriction response of pupils to light is referred to as "sluggish" pupils, and no pupillary response to light is referred to as "fixed" pupils.
- **Size of the pupil**—Pupils are usually measured in millimeters (mm). An expected finding is equal pupil size bilaterally. There are resources available to help determine the size of pupils; for example, many penlights display

pictures of pupillary sizes measured in millimeters. See Fig. 20.5 for an illustration of varying pupil sizes in mm.

Continuous monitoring for pupillary changes is a critical component of a complete neurologic assessment, and it is important to obtain a baseline pupillary exam in order to detect subtle changes. Pupillary changes are an early sign of worsening neurologic injury, including increased ICP. An increase in ICP can also cause pressure on the third cranial nerve, the oculomotor nerve, causing the pupil to become sluggish or nonreactive. Any change or unexpected finding in the client's pupillary response must be reported to the authorized healthcare provider immediately. For more information regarding the cranial nerves, see Chapter 4.

USING A PUPILLOMETER DEVICE FOR ASSESSMENT OF PUPILS

If the client is going to need repeated pupillary assessments or if additional information is needed, a pupillometer might be indicated. A pupillometer is a handheld device used by nursing per facility policy or as ordered by the authorized healthcare provider. The use of this device has become more common in recent years (Anderson, Elmer, Shutter, Puccio, & Alexander, 2018). With this relatively new technology, nurses can detect subtle changes in the client's ongoing pupillary exams.

When using the pupillometer, follow the manufacturer recommendations closely. The device delivers a flash of light, examines the pupillary response, then gives objective data regarding the pupillary response. The pupillometer has an attachment device that is dedicated to a specific client, and it will only be disposed of once the client no longer requires exams. This attachment will store the client's individual pupillary exam history in order to view trends over time. An example of a pupillometer is shown in Fig. 20.6A, and an attachment device for the pupillometer is shown in Fig. 20.6B.

Pupillometer Data Points

The two important objective data points the pupillometer will display are the size of each pupil and the Neurological Pupil index (NPi) of each pupil (Fig 20.7). The NPi is an algorithm created to standardize the description of how a pupil responds to light. The naked eye of the examiner can only subjectively distinguish between brisk, sluggish, or nonreactive. The NPi is displayed in the form of a value ranging from 1 to 5. An NPi value that is greater than or equal to 3 is considered to be a normal, brisk pupillary response. Any number less than 3 is considered to be an abnormal, sluggish reaction (Box 20.1). When comparing the pupils bilaterally, a difference in size of greater than 0.7 mm or other abnormal

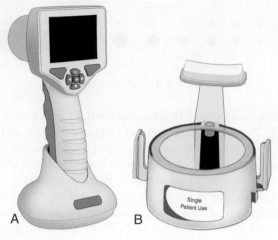

FIG. 20.6 A, Example of a pupillometer in a docking station. **B,** Example of an attachment device for a pupillometer.

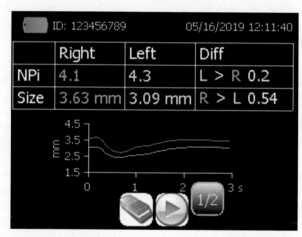

FIG. 20.7 Example of data points on a pupillometer screen.

BOX 20.1 Expected Parameters for Pupillometer Measurements (NPi Scale)

- A Neurological Pupil index (NPi) score of 3.0 to 4.9 is considered to be a normal/"brisk" pupil assessment, per the NPi algorithm.
- An NPi score of less than 3 is considered an abnormal/ "sluggish" pupil assessment, per the NPi algorithm.
- The difference in size between the left and right pupil should not be greater than 0.7 mm. If it is, this is considered an abnormal finding.
- **Nonresponsive pupil:** An NPi of zero is considered to be a nonreactive pupil. This is an abnormal finding.

Reference: NeurOptics, 2018.

finding must be reported to the authorized healthcare provider immediately because this could indicate an increase in the client's ICP. For more information related to critical pupillometer findings, see the NeurOptic instructions at https://neuroptics.com/wp-content/uploads/2018/09/NPi-200-Quick-Start-Guide.pdf.

TABLE 20.3 Speech Centers

Aphasia Type	Disability	Location
Expressive aphasia	Inability to speak or read written language	Broca's area, located in the left inferior frontal lobe
Receptive aphasia	Inability to understand speech or written language	Wernicke's area, located in the left posterior temporal lobe

ASSESSMENT OF VERBAL RESPONSE AND FUNCTION

Language is another important part of a thorough neurologic exam. It is necessary to assess the client's ability to speak clearly and to communicate verbally. To accurately assess these functions, you must first understand the major alterations of speech. *Dysarthria* is impaired articulation of the muscles used to speak, which can be secondary to damage to certain areas of the brain. Dysarthria may also be related to a mechanical dysfunction (e.g., a problem with the client's tongue control, palate, or lips), which may be caused by trauma, illness, or disease. For example, a client with dysarthria may have slurred speech.

Another alteration of speech is *aphasia*, which is the inability to understand or express language. Aphasia can occur when specific areas of the brain are damaged. As described in Table 20.3, there are two types of aphasia: receptive and expressive. *Receptive aphasia* affects the client's ability to *understand* language. *Expressive aphasia* is the inability of the client to *express* language. As you can imagine, the inability to communicate can be very frustrating for a client, particularly when his or her cognitive function is intact. The client may understand what he or she *wants to say* but may not be able to say it correctly or at all.

ASSESSMENT OF MOTOR AND SENSORY FUNCTION

The motor exam evaluates muscle tone and strength. The strength scale ranges from 0 to 5, with 0 being flaccid or complete paralysis and 5 being normal (Table 20.4). When evaluating motor function, the nurse compares muscle tone and strength bilaterally.

For a client with a decreased LOC, noxious stimuli may be required to assess motor function. Because a noxious stimulus sufficient to produce a motor response will usually cause pain, the motor exam helps indirectly evaluate the client's sensory function, which can be displayed as withdrawal from pain, localization, a verbal response, or a grimace. *Localization* can be defined as attempting to stop the noxious stimulation by using the unaffected extremity, crossing midline toward the weak extremity where the noxious stimulus is applied, and trying to remove the stimulus. Use the least amount of stimulus possible. In an unconscious client with a neurologic injury, the trapezius squeeze or sternal rub technique may be used to assess the central pain response. To assess the client's motor or sensory function in an extremity, apply firm pressure to one of the digits in that particular extremity. For example, if you are trying to elicit a response of the right arm, apply pressure to the cuticle nailbed of one of the digits of the right hand.

It is important to note that the client's elicited responses to pain stimuli should be considered in the context of the entire clinical picture. In other words, the responses may be due to a reflex and may not reliably indicate consciousness or motor response.

A final component of the motor exam is assessing for signs of neurologic posturing. Decorticate posturing and decerebrate posturing can occur on one or both sides of the body and may indicate that the client has severe brain damage. As shown in Fig. 20.8A, decorticate posturing is characterized by flexion in the arms, wrists, and fingers. In addition, the elbows are flexed and held toward the core or chest, the legs are extended and may have internal rotation, and the feet may be plantar-flexed with internal rotation.

TABLE 20.4 Motor Strength Exam Grading

Grade Scale	Description of Response
5	Normal strength—Movement against gravity with resistance
4	Decreased strength—Movement against gravity with some resistance
3	Decreased strength—Movement against gravity
2	Decreased strength—Movement possible if gravity eliminated
1	Decreased strength—Palpable or visible flicker of muscle contraction
0	No strength—No contraction; total paralysis

With decerebrate posturing (Fig. 20.8B), the arms are extended and held close to the body; the legs are extended and held together, with the toes pointed down; the head and neck are extended; and the back may be arched.

ASSESSMENT OF DEEP TENDON REFLEXES

Eliciting deep tendon reflexes (DTRs) is another component of an advanced neurologic assessment. DTR is graded 0 (absent) to 4+ (hyperactive). (See Chapter 4.) DTR assessment can provide information about the client's ability to localize nerve innervations and corresponding motor response. Primitive reflexes such as the Babinski reflex reflect the client's central nervous system function. The Babinski reflex is described in Skill 20.1, step 22 of this chapter.

LIFESPAN CONSIDERATIONS

When completing an advanced neurologic assessment of an older adult, it is important to understand the client's baseline level of functioning. Clients of advanced age are at risk for cognitive changes and may require assistance with activities of living. Without knowing this baseline, it is difficult to know what findings to expect and what findings to accept as baseline function. For example, it would be unfair to expect a client to know the date when he or she is unable to keep up with this information at home and does not have a neurologic injury. This information can be obtained by discussing the client's baseline function with his or her loved ones. This is also a good example of why the critical concept of communication is important.

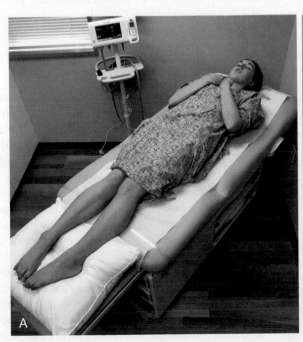
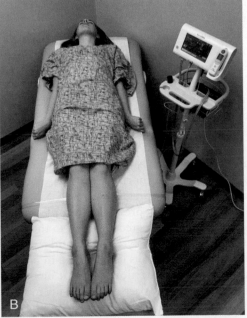

FIG. 20.8 Types of abnormal posturing. **A,** Decorticate posturing. **B,** Decerebrate posturing.

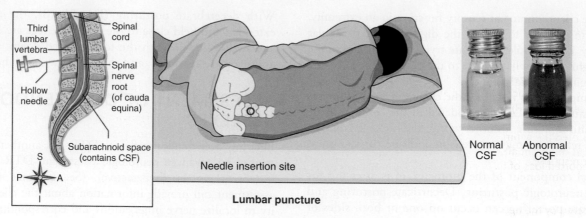

Lumbar puncture

FIG. 20.9 Location and positioning for lumbar puncture.

DIAGNOSTIC PROCEDURES

As part of the advanced neurologic assessment, diagnostic procedures are often performed. One of the most common diagnostic procedures used is a lumbar puncture (LP). The LP (also called a spinal tap) is used to collect CSF cerebrospinal fluid (CSF) for analysis, measurement of the opening pressure of CSF, or injection of medications and/or dye into the CSF space. Prior to the LP, a computed tomography (CT) scan may be completed to determine if there is abnormal swelling of the brain or increased ICP, which would be contraindications for an LP. In addition, this can place patient at a higher risk for cerebral herniation. After it is determined that there are no contraindications and informed consent is obtained, the client may be prepared for the LP.

Assisting With the Lumbar Puncture Procedure

When assisting with an LP procedure, help the client into a lateral recumbent "C-shaped" or fetal position—chin to chest, knees to abdomen (Fig. 20.9). The client is often positioned on the left side during an LP. However, the client may be positioned on either side, depending on physical limitations, preference of the authorized healthcare provider, or client comfort. During an LP, the authorized healthcare provider injects a local anesthetic into the lower lumber space around L3 and L4. A spinal needle is then inserted between vertebrae L3 and L4 through the dura mater and into the subarachnoid space. Once the needle is in place, the authorized healthcare provider may determine the opening pressure of the CSF using a manometer. After the opening pressure is recorded, a sample or samples of CSF are collected and sent to the lab for further evaluation. The needle is removed, and a dressing is placed over the site. Pressure is usually held in place for a few minutes to ensure no additional CSF or blood leaks out of the puncture site. As part of follow-up monitoring, the nurse must observe the client for complications (discussed shortly).

Lifespan Considerations: Positioning Clients During a Lumbar Puncture

For geriatric clients, positioning for an LP may be difficult due to musculoskeletal changes and other changes associated with the normal aging process. For example, older adults who have arthritis or immobility will need additional assistance to stay immobile during the procedure. While the client is lying on his or her side, provide joint support and facilitate alignment of the spine by placing a pillow between the client's knees. Older adult clients may also have a decreased spatial awareness, which could increase their fall risk. Stay close to the client at all times during the LP, and never leave the client unattended on the bed or procedure table while the side rail is down.

Pediatric clients may require conscious or unconscious sedation during an LP. In addition, positioning may need to be varied based on the age of the child. Developmental consideration and preparation are needed for toddlers, preschoolers, and early-school-age children. Consider utilizing a facility-approved child-life specialist to assist during the procedure if available.

Contraindications and Potential Complications of Lumbar Puncture

Overstimulation from an LP can cause cerebral herniation and possible brain death. Thus, an LP should never be performed on any client who is experiencing increased ICP or who is at high risk for sudden increases in ICP (Chioffi, 2017). Another contraindication for performing an LP is a bleeding or clotting disorder. The LP procedure utilizes a needle to puncture through the skin and into the subarachnoid space; therefore, a client who is at high risk for bleeding/clotting problems can bleed into and out of the space. As noted in Box 20.2, the nurse must also be alert for certain medications such as anticoagulants that can cause bleeding and alert the authorized healthcare provider regarding these contraindications.

A potential complication of an LP is a decrease in the movement and sensation of the lower extremities. Other possible complications include, but may not be limited to, a spinal hematoma or infection. Clients may also experience a headache or back pain, particularly if there is a CSF leak.

BOX 20.2 Lesson From the Courtroom: Complications of a Lumbar Puncture

In a case filed in the Texas Court of Appeals, a client presented to the emergency room (ER) with a stiff neck and headache. The physician ordered aspirin and Lovenox. A lumbar puncture (LP) was ordered, which was performed by a neurologist. The nurses involved with the client's care administered the aspirin and Lovenox at noon, before the LP, and at midnight after the procedure. The next day, the client reported loss of feeling in his legs, back pain, and an inability to urinate, all consistent with a spinal hematoma. Although stat magnetic resonance imaging (MRI) was ordered by the neurologist at 6:00 AM, it was not done until 3:00 PM the next day. Despite a surgical intervention at another hospital, the client was unable to recover from the spinal hematoma, and he became a paraplegic.

Although the jury in the case found the physicians to be primarily liable, the court ruled that the nurses were also negligent and partly responsible for the client's outcome. In addition, the court noted that the nurses should have recognized that anticoagulant medications are contraindicated when an LP is performed due to the high risk of bleeding and spinal hematoma formation. In addition, the court asserted that the nurses failed to appreciate the urgency for the ordered MRI even though the client was having signs of complications. As a side note, the nurses settled with the client as individuals out of court prior to the trial (Lumbar puncture: Patient given contraindicated drugs, nurses ruled partly responsible, 2012). This case demonstrates the importance of understanding the precautions and contraindications of the procedures the client is receiving, such as an LP, and whether the client is taking medications that increase risk. In addition, this case underscores the importance of recognizing signs and symptoms of possible complications and the need for immediate interventions without delays. Finally, this case illustrates the need for adequate and timely communication and follow-up with other members of the healthcare team.

If the client has any of these signs and symptoms, or if there is a change in the client's neurologic assessment or status, contact the authorized healthcare provider immediately. It is also important to follow post-procedure orders and facility policy regarding positioning. For example, some clients may be required to remain on bedrest or remain flat for a certain amount of time (if tolerated) after an LP. This must be ordered by the authorized healthcare provider.

SUMMARY

As identified below, the critical concepts of accuracy, client-centered care, infection control, safety, communication, and evaluation are imperative when performing an advanced neurologic assessment and providing advanced neurologic care. In particular, accuracy is important in order to monitor trends and detect subtle changes and to prevent complications. The goal is for the client to establish neurologic homeostasis and maintain an effective neurologic status.

APPLICATION OF THE NURSING PROCESS

Examples of Related International Classification for Nursing Practice (ICNP) Nursing Diagnoses, Expected Client Outcomes, and Nursing Assessment:

Nursing Diagnosis: Effective neurologic status

Supporting Data: Client's previous neurologic exams have been within established parameters.

Expected Client Outcomes: The client will continue to demonstrate an effective neurologic status, as seen by the following parameters:
- neurologic exam scores (e.g., NIHSS, MEND exam, GCS) at the client's baseline and/or within established parameters
- awake and alert, responsive, and oriented to person, place, time, and situation
- pupillary response briskly reactive and equal bilaterally
- appropriate deep tendon reflexes within established parameters bilaterally
- absence of decerebrate or decorticate posturing.

Nursing Assessment Example: Assess the client's LOC, pupillary response, verbal response, motor and sensory function, and DTRs, at specified intervals.

Reference: International Classification for Nursing Practice. (n.d.). *eHealth & ICNP*. Retrieved from https://www.icn.ch/what-we-do/projects/ehealth-icnp.

CRITICAL CONCEPTS
Advanced Neurologic Assessment

Accuracy (ACC)

Accuracy related to advanced neurologic assessment is sensitive to the following variables:

Client-Related Factors
- Client's age, culture, and language
- Client's LOC and ability to follow commands
- Mobility and ability to be positioned for assessment and LP
- Neurologic history and diagnosis, and medical status
- Neurologic exam scores (e.g., NIHSS, MEND exam, GCS)
- Level of pain, discomfort, or emotional distress
- Presence of any disabilities (e.g., vision or hearing impairment)
- Environment (e.g., noise, temperature, distractions)

Nurse-Related Factors
- Technique used for performing neurologic assessments
- Proper positioning of client for assessment and LP
- Proper calibration and positioning of pupillometer device
- Proper identification of appropriate landmarks for assessment and LP
- Personal bias or assumptions during neurologic assessment
- Ability to verify findings and perform further assessment, as needed

Equipment-Related Factors
- Properly functioning and fully charged pupillometer

Client-Centered Care (CCC)

When performing an advanced neurologic assessment, respect for the client is demonstrated by:
- promoting autonomy and ensuring that a consent form is signed for LP or other procedures
- arranging for an interpreter if necessary
- providing privacy during procedure and assessment and only exposing what is necessary during neurologic assessment and LP
- ensuring comfort and reducing environmental stimuli
- honoring cultural preferences during neurologic procedure and LP
- advocating for the client and family by explaining procedures.

Infection Control (INF)

When performing an advanced neurologic assessment, healthcare-associated infection is prevented by:
- preventing and reducing the transfer of microorganisms
- reducing the number of microorganisms.

Safety (SAF)

When performing an advanced neurologic assessment, safety measures prevent harm to the client by maintaining a safe care environment, including:
- safe positioning and fall prevention during procedures
- verifying the absence of contraindications for procedures.

Communication (COM)

- Communication exchanges information (oral, written, nonverbal, or electronic) between two or more people.
- Documentation of the neurologic assessment records information in a permanent legal record.

Evaluation (EVAL)

When performing an advanced neurologic assessment, evaluation of outcomes enables the nurse to determine the accuracy of the assessment and the efficacy of the care provided, including:
- monitoring for trends and changes in diagnostic information, outcomes, and assessment findings.

■ SKILL 20.1 Performing a Neurologic Assessment

EQUIPMENT

Clean gloves and personal protective equipment (PPE), if there is a risk of exposure to body fluids
Penlight
Blood pressure cuff and stethoscope
Reflex hammer
Stethoscope
Pulse oximeter

BEGINNING THE SKILL

1. **SAF** Review the client's medical and surgical history, and determine if there are contraindications to any procedures used for the neurologic exam.
2. **INF** Perform hand hygiene.
3. **CCC** Introduce yourself to client and family.
4. **SAF** Identify the client using two identifiers.
5. **CCC** Provide privacy and explain the procedure. *Providing privacy in layers enhances client-centered care.* Obtain verbal consent if possible.
6. **INF** Apply clean gloves and PPE, if there is a risk of exposure to body fluids.

PROCEDURE

Assess the Client's Mental Status (Level of Consciousness and Orientation)

7. **ACC** Assess the client's LOC (see Table 20.2). *This will determine how to proceed with the neurologic assessment and pro-*

vide a baseline assessment of the client. (Note: A client's level of consciousness can range from awake and alert to comatose.)

8. **ACC** Assess the client's orientation (if the client is verbalizing). (Note: If the client is awake but unable to verbalize, use alternative methods of communication, such as writing and hand gestures.)
   a. Person—"What is your full name?"
   b. Place—"Where are you right now?"
   c. Time—"What is today's date?" or "What year is it?"
   d. Situation—"Why are you here today?"

9. **CCC** If the client is unresponsive or comatose, interact with the client, even if you are not sure if the client can hear you. *Clients with neurologic injuries may hear you even if they cannot respond.*
   a. Call the client by his or her full name.
   b. Apply light touch, such as a gentle shoulder shake.
   c. Apply a noxious stimulus, such as pressure on the nailbed.

10. **ACC** Assess client's vital signs and oxygen saturation levels (see Chapter 3). *The client's vital signs and oxygen saturation can alter, as well as be altered by neurologic injuries.*

Assess the Client's Pupillary Response to Light

11. **ACC** Ensure that the lights in the room are dimmed if necessary. *Dimming the room lights may help illuminate and visualize the pupils, particularly for manual pupillary checks.*

12. **ACC** Use a pupillometer if available and check the pupils bilaterally (see Skill 20.2).

13. **ACC** If using a penlight to manually check the pupils bilaterally, see Skill 4.4, step 29 in Chapter 4. (Note: The pupillary response in the illuminated eye and opposite [nonilluminated] eye should be constriction. This is a consensual pupillary reflex.)

14. **ACC** Compare the client's pupillary response to the client's baseline exam. If the client has changes, notify the authorized healthcare provider. (Note: The expected finding is that both pupils should be equal, round, regular, and reactive to light and accommodation [PER-RLA].) *Pupillary changes such as unequal sizes, irregularly shaped pupils, or pupils that are sluggishly reactive may indicate that the client has altered intracranial pressure or another issue (see Fig. 20.5 for varying pupil sizes).*

Assess the Client's Verbal Response

15. **ACC** Assess language (if verbal) by assessing for aphasia (see Table 20.3 and the narrative text). *This helps to assess which area of the brain may be affected.*
    a. Ask the client to name a simple object, such as a pen. (Note: If the client does not appear to be aware of what is being asked, this could be an example of receptive aphasia.)
    b. Ask the client a simple question, such as, "What is your name?" (Note: If the client tries to answer but uses the wrong word or the answer is incomprehensible, this could be an example of expressive aphasia. This is especially true if the client appears to be frustrated because the client knows the correct answer but is unable to express the correct words.)
    c. Ask the client to repeat a simple phrase, such as, "No ifs, ands, or buts." (Note: If the client is unable to do so, it could be an example of expressive and/or receptive aphasia, or it could be a mechanical issue or dysarthria, as described in the narrative text.)

Assess the Client's Motor Strength

16. **ACC** Assess the client's upper extremity strength (if the client can follow commands).
    a. Ask the client to hold both arms straight out in front and close his or her eyes for 10 seconds. Watch for one arm to drift downward, revealing weakness.
    b. Ask the client to grip your crossed middle and index fingers.
    c. While attempting to pull your fingers from the client's grasp, assess whether or not the strength of the client's grip is bilaterally symmetric (see Skill 4.8, step 31 in Chapter 4).

17. **ACC** Assess the strength of the legs and ankles (if the client can follow commands).
    a. Ask the client to hold each leg individually straight out in front of them for 5 seconds. Watch for downward drift, revealing weakness.
    b. Ask the client to plantar-flex and dorsal-flex ankles. Compare mobility bilaterally.
    c. Ask the client to press the sole of each foot against your hand as if "pressing the gas pedal" (see Skill 4.8, step 37 in Chapter 4).
    d. Compare ankle/foot strength bilaterally and note if the client's strength is equal in both ankles/feet. *Weakness on one side of the body can provide information about the location of the injury within the brain.* (Note: Strength can be scored on a 1-to-5 scale [see Table 20.4].)

18. **ACC** If the client has a decreased LOC, assess motor strength and sensory function simultaneously:
    a. Deliver noxious stimulus (e.g. applying pressure to the end of the client's nailbed).
    b. Evaluate client response. (Note: Depending on the severity of the neurologic injury, there will be varying motor responses.) Responses may include the following:
    - localizing (see the narrative text)
    - withdrawal of extremities
    - decorticate posturing
    - decerebrate posturing
    - no motor response.

Assess the Client's Sensation

19. **ACC** If the client is able to communicate verbally or with gestures, lightly touch each extremity while asking the client if the sensation feels the same bilaterally (see Chapter 4).

20. **ACC** If the client is unconscious or unable to feel light touch:
    a. Deliver noxious stimuli as described in step 18.
    b. Record findings as "Client sensitive to light touch" or "Client responds to noxious stimuli." *This will facilitate communication with other healthcare providers.*

Assess the Client's Deep Tendon Reflexes

21. **ACC** Assess the patellar and triceps reflex (see Skill 4.5, steps 46 and 47).

22. **ACC** Assess the plantar reflex (Babinski reflex). Stroke the client's heel upward to just below the little toe, then across the ball of the foot toward the great toe with the rounded end of a reflex hammer handle or other tool. (Note: The expected finding for an adult, or any client over 2 years of age, is plantar flexion of all of the toes and inversion or turning in of the foot, also known as a negative Babinski sign. An abnormal, positive Babinski sign, is dorsiflexion, or upgoing, of the great toe and fanning of the other toes [Jarvis, 2016].)

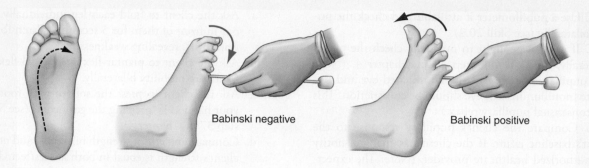

STEP 22 Babinski reflex.

Evaluate Neurologic Assessment Score

23. **EVAL** Determine the GCS (see Table 20.1) or score from another facility-approved scale, such as the NIHSS or MEND exam. Use information obtained from the client's neurologic assessment. (Note: For clients who may have an acute ischemic stroke, the NIHSS is often recommended instead of the GCS score [Middleton et al., 2015] [see Section 3 of this chapter].)

FINISHING THE SKILL

24. **INF** Remove gloves and PPE if used and perform hand hygiene.
25. **SAF** Ensure safety and comfort. Ensure that the bed is in the lowest position, and verify that the client can iden-

tify and reach the nurse call system. *These safety measures reduce the risk of falls.*

26. **EVAL** Evaluate the outcomes. Is the client's neurologic exam within established parameters for the client? Did the client tolerate the neurologic exam?
27. **COM** Document assessment findings, care given, and outcomes in the legal healthcare record, including the following:
    * time the neurologic assessment was completed
    * neurologic assessment findings
    * NIHSS, MEND exam, or GCS score
    * any change from the baseline assessment (if this is a subsequent assessment)
    * information reported to the authorized healthcare provider (as applicable).

■ SKILL 20.2 Using a Pupillometer

EQUIPMENT

Clean gloves
Pupillometer device (exact models may differ depending on the facility)
Programmable guard attachment for pupillometer (for single client use)
Antiseptic wipe
Gauze pad (if needed to assist in opening client's eye)
Pupillometer docking station

BEGINNING THE SKILL

1. **ACC** Review order for pupillometer procedure. (Note: Some facilities have standing orders for the pupillometer and allow the nurse's discretion to determine if there is an indication for this procedure based on the client's risk for pupillary changes.)
2. **ACC** Review the client's medical and surgical history.
3. **SAF** Review the following:
   * risk factors for pupillary changes, including brain hemorrhage, cerebral herniation, brainstem or spinal

cord lesion, or compression of cranial nerve III (Portran, Cour, Hernu, de la Salle, & Argaud, 2017)
   * any contraindication for a pupillometer procedure, including broken skin, swelling, infection, or fracture around the orbit of the eye
   * any allergies to latex, plastic, tape, or other devices.
4. **INF** Perform hand hygiene.
5. **CCC** Introduce yourself to the client and family.
6. **SAF** Identify the client using two identifiers.
7. **CCC** Provide privacy and explain the procedure. *Providing privacy in layers enhances client-centered care.* Obtain verbal consent if possible.
8. **SAF** Ask the client verbally about any known allergies.

PROCEDURE

9. **ACC** Perform a neurologic assessment (see Skill 20.1). (Note: If the client's neurologic status has declined from baseline, notify the authorized healthcare provider immediately.)
10. **ACC** Assess client for the following:
    * baseline pupillary assessment

- ability to follow commands and understand instructions.

11. **ACC** Obtain pupillometer from docking station and ensure that it is fully charged.

12. **INF** Obtain a new guard attachment for single client use. *Prevents cross-contamination.* (Note: New guard attachments are usually only necessary upon the first pupillary exam because they are programmed individually and dedicated to the client for continued use while in the facility.)

13. **INF** Apply clean gloves.

14. **SAF** Position the client or the client's bed at an ergonomically safe working height. *Facilitates accurate assessment of pupils without injury to the nurse or client.*

15. **SAF** Carefully inspect each eye. **WARNING:** Do not use the pupillometer device if there is a visible skin injury around eye, known orbital bone injury, or signs of swelling.

16. **SAF** Enter the client's personal identifier information (e.g., last four digits of client's medical account number) into the pupillometer per facility policy.

17. **ACC** Attach the client's guard attachment to the pupillometer. Ensure that it is securely in place by hearing the "click." *Prevents attachment from inadvertently becoming dislodged.*

18. **ACC** Ask the client to look ahead. *Facilitates eye opening and visualization of the pupil.*

19. **ACC** While holding the pupillometer securely with your dominant hand, place the pupillometer guard attachment on the client's orbital bone (gently but with steady pressure) at a 90-degree angle. Do not tilt the pupillometer. *This angle facilitates visualization of the pupil and accurate assessment.* (Note: The pupillometer exam may start with either eye; both the right and left pupil will be assessed.)

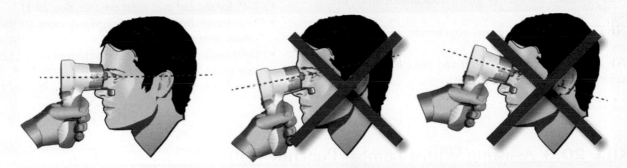

STEP 19 Position pupillometer at the correct angle.

20. **ACC** If the client is unconscious or unable to cooperate, gently use a gauze pad with the help of an assistant or with your nondominant hand (thumb and forefinger) to help keep the client's eye open. *Eye must be open fully to properly visualize the entire pupil.*

21. **ACC** Confirm that the entire circumference of the pupil (left or right) is seen within the screen. *Facilitates accurate visualization and measurement of the pupil.*

22. **ACC** Once visualization is confirmed, press and hold either the "left" or "right" button until the pupillometer locates the pupil by surrounding the pupil with a circle. (Note: This may take approximately 3 seconds and can vary depending on the manufacturer.)

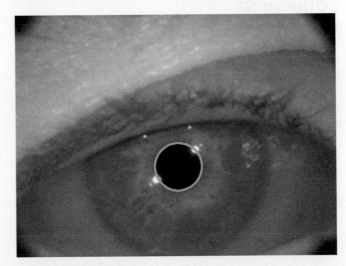

STEP 22 Confirm pupil capture.

23. **COM** Warn the client that there will be a flash of light, and ask the client not to blink. *Avoiding blinking facilitates accuracy and prevents a "tracking problem" during the procedure.*

24. **ACC** Release the button and hold the pupillometer steady as it delivers the flash of light and records the pupillary reaction to light. Ensure that the reading was

measured properly. *This ensures an accurate reading.* (Note: If there is a message on the screen to "repeat" or "rescan," an error may have occurred. Repeat the procedure if necessary in order to obtain an accurate result.)

25. **ACC** Reposition the client as needed and repeat steps 18 to 24 on the opposite eye. (Note: The touchscreen can be used to display the results. Select the video icon to view the video playback of the readings if needed [NeurOptics, 2018])

26. **SAF** Place the client's bed back to the lowest position after the procedure. *Prevents injury to the client.*

27. **EVAL** Compare new findings to baseline pupillary exam and notify the authorized healthcare provider of any changes. *This facilitates timely interventions for the client in order to prevent further deterioration in the client's neurologic status.*

28. **ACC** Separate the client's guard attachment from the pupillometer.

29. **INF** Clean the client's guard attachment and store per facility policy.

30. **INF** Disinfect the pupillometer and place back in charger or docking station per policy.

FINISHING THE SKILL

31. **INF** Remove gloves and PPE if used and perform hand hygiene.

32. **SAF** Ensure safety and comfort. Ensure that the bed is in the lowest position, and verify that the client can identify and reach the nurse call system. *These safety measures reduce the risk of falls.*

33. **EVAL** Evaluate the outcomes. Did the client tolerate the procedure? Were you able to visualize the client's pupils adequately? How do the results compare to previous results?

34. **COM** Document assessment findings, care given, and outcomes in the legal healthcare record, including the following:
    - time the assessment was completed
    - pupil size in millimeters (mm) for the left and right eye
    - NPi for the left and right eye (see Box 20.1)
    - any change from baseline pupillary exam (if this is a subsequent assessment)
    - information communicated to the authorized healthcare provider (as applicable).

■ SKILL 20.3 Assisting With a Lumbar Puncture (LP)

EQUIPMENT

PPE (sterile gowns, sterile gloves, face masks with eye shields, and caps)
Bedside table
Linens/towels for client positioning
Sterile lumbar puncture kit
Laboratory/specimen labels
Glucometer/blood draw supplies for simultaneous serum blood glucose level
Preservative-free antiseptic solution
Bandage

BEGINNING THE SKILL

1. **ACC** Review and verify orders.
2. **SAF** Identify any contraindications, such as bleeding or clotting disorder, anticoagulant use, increased ICP, or risk for herniation. *A client who is at risk for bleeding or clotting problems can potentially bleed into and out of the CSF space. A sudden increase in ICP due to overstimulation from the procedure can cause further elevation in ICP (Chioffi, 2017).*
3. **INF** Perform hand hygiene.
4. **CCC** Introduce yourself to the client and family.
5. **SAF** Identify the client using two identifiers.
6. **CCC** Provide privacy and explain the procedure. *Providing privacy in layers enhances client-centered care.*
7. **CCC** Ensure that informed consent has been obtained.
8. **SAF** Check the client's armband and ask the client verbally if he or she has any allergies, including an allergy to antiseptic solution. (Note: Antiseptic must be preservative-free.)

9. **ACC** Encourage the client to empty his or her bladder, and make sure there is no bladder distention. *A full bladder can prevent the client from maintaining an accurate position during the procedure and cause physiologic changes during the procedure due to the discomfort.*

10. **ACC** Obtain baseline vital signs. *Allows comparison with post-procedure vital signs.*

11. **ACC** Perform a neurologic assessment, including mental status, motor exam, and sensation, paying close attention to the lower extremities (see Skill 20.1). *This will be compared to the post-procedure assessment to ensure the client has not suffered an adverse event.*

12. **ACC** Assess the client for structural problems such as congenital/developmental deformities, kyphosis, and scoliosis. *These issues may hinder the client's ability to maintain proper positioning.* (Note: This assessment can be done by positioning the client in a flexed position of the neck and spine, as with the "fetal position.")

PROCEDURE

13. **INF** Perform hand hygiene again and apply gloves.

14. **INF** Set up sterile tray or open supplies as needed to ensure they are accessible to the authorized healthcare provider performing the LP.

15. **SAF WARNING:** Ensure that a preservative-free antiseptic solution is used. *A preservative-free antiseptic solution is used to prevent the neurotoxicity that could be caused by preservatives. Allergies to the solution or a history of shellfish allergy should be identified prior to the procedure.*

16. **SAF WARNING:** Ensure that there is a "time-out" verification to confirm that this is the correct client, correct site, and correct procedure (The Joint Commission, 2015). *Prevents wrong-client, wrong-site, and wrong-procedure errors.*

17. **SAF** Raise the client's bed to an ergonomically safe height. (Note: Be sure to lower the client's bed back to the lowest position after the procedure.) **WARNING:** Do not walk away from the client while the bed is raised and the siderail is down. *Reduces the risk of falls.*

18. **ACC** Assist the client into a lateral recumbent position (left or right side) with the head and neck flexed (chin should touch the chest) and knees pulled up to the chest (ask the client to "hug" his or her knees once the knees are pulled up). *This allows the spaces between the vertebrae to open for proper needle placement.*

19. **CCC** Assist the client to maintain position during the procedure. Support the client with one hand on his or her shoulder and one on the hip. Remind the client to remain as still as possible. *The client can become fatigued or anxious or may have physical challenges that affect mobility and adherence to the position.* (Note: To provide privacy and to protect the client's dignity, only expose what is necessary for the exam.)

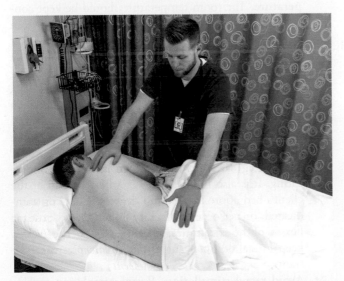

STEP 19 Hold the client's position and only expose what is neccesary.

20. **CCC** Reassure and calm the client as needed. *Reduces client anxiety during the procedure.*

21. **EVAL** Monitor the client's respiratory status, vital signs, and complaints of pain and discomfort. *Diaphragm expansion is limited in the procedure due to the positioning, which can affect respiratory effort. Pain can indicate incorrect placement of needle at insertion site or neurologic compromise.*

22. **ACC** If the authorized healthcare provider will be measuring the CSF opening pressure:
    a. Note and record the opening pressure value.
    b. Observe and record characteristics of the CSF (e.g., color, clarity). (Note: CSF should be clear and colorless.)

23. **SAF** Label CSF specimens with the client's name and other identifying information and label according to the order in which they were collected. Ensure that the spec-imens are labeled in the presence of the client per facility policy. *Labeling specimens in the presence of the client is a best-practice safety recommendation.* (Note: The laboratory tests may include, but not be limited to, glucose, protein, cell count, gram stain, cultures, and cytology.)

24. **SAF** Assist the authorized healthcare provider to hold pressure at the aspiration site if needed. *Minimizes bleeding at insertion site.*

25. **SAF** Discard needles and syringes into appropriate biohazard sharps container.

26. **EVAL** Obtain the client's serum glucose level per order. Label the specimen in the presence of the client and send it to the laboratory per facility policy. *This will be used to compare with the CSF glucose level to determine if CSF appears to be infected. A normal CSF glucose level is two-thirds of the serum glucose level. Lower CSF glucose levels suggest bacterial infection.*

FINISHING THE SKILL

27. **SAF** Send the labeled CSF specimens (after reverifying the labels for accuracy) to the laboratory as ordered by the authorized healthcare provider.

28. **EVAL** Monitor the client for LOC, vital signs, and oxygen saturation. *Monitoring allows for early detection of complications.*

29. **EVAL** Inspect dressing over the LP insertion site for excess bleeding or clear drainage.

30. **INF** Remove gloves and PPE if used and perform hand hygiene.

31. **SAF** Ensure safety and comfort. Ensure that the bed is in the lowest position, and verify that the client can identify and reach the nurse call system. *These safety measures reduce the risk of falls.* (Note: Follow post-procedure orders regarding client positioning after an LP.)

32. **EVAL** Evaluate the outcomes. Did the client tolerate the procedure? Is the client having a post-procedure headache or any other signs and symptoms after the LP?

33. **COM** Document assessment findings, care given, and outcomes in the legal healthcare record:
    • date and time of the LP procedure
    • outcomes of the procedure
    • client's response and how client tolerated the procedure
    • condition and appearance of the LP insertion site
    • serum glucose level.

34. **EVAL** Provide follow-up monitoring, including the following: (Note: If any of these signs and symptoms occur, notify the authorized healthcare provider immediately.)
    a. Continue to monitor the client for changes in vital signs, decreased LOC, headache, stiff neck, and photophobia. *Suggestive of new subarachnoid hemorrhage.*
    b. Monitor the LP insertion site for hematoma or bleeding.
    c. Monitor the client for an inability to void independently. *Indicates possible LP complication or inappropriate spinal needle placement.*
    d. Monitor for decreased motor strength/sensation in the lower extremities. *Indicates possible LP complication or inappropriate spinal needle placement.*

As discussed in the chapter introduction, intracranial pressure (ICP) is the force exerted by the brain, CSF, and cerebral blood flow (CBF) inside the skull, which is expressed by the Monro–Kellie doctrine. An elevated ICP can occur due to neurologic trauma such as TBIs, brain tumors, infections, and hemorrhages. A sudden increase in ICP or a sustained elevation in ICP over a period of time can result in secondary brain injury such as cerebral herniation. Some of the possible signs and symptoms of increased ICP are listed in Box 20.3. Caring for clients at risk for increased ICP focuses on maintenance of physiologic integrity of the brain tissue, CBF, and CSF, as well as management of interventions that affect these factors. For clients with established increased ICP, the focus is on reducing the ICP and then maintaining the ICP within the parameters ordered by an authorized healthcare provider.

The expected parameters of an ICP value vary depending on the client's age, body build, positioning, anatomy, and neurologic status. It is important to look at trends for the individual client. An ICP that is elevated for one client may not be unusual for another client. However, a widely accepted range of a benign ICP is 0 to 15 mm Hg (Cox, 2017). An ICP value of greater than 14 or 15 mm Hg may be considered elevated. The authorized healthcare provider will set parameters and determine when an elevated ICP requires notification and possible interventions.

INTERVENTIONS FOR CLIENTS WITH INCREASED ICP

Interventions that may decrease the client's ICP include regulation of blood pressure and body temperature; fluid balance; administration of steroids or hypertonic saline; and maintenance of effective respiratory function, including

BOX 20.3 Signs and Symptoms of Increased Intracranial Pressure (ICP)

- Headache
- Blurred vision
- Decreased level of consciousness
- Vomiting (may be projectile)
- Weakness or difficulty speaking
- Cushing's triad (bradycardia, alteration in rate and character of respirations, and alteration in blood pressure [e.g., widened pulse pressure])
- Pupillary changes
- Changes in respirations
- Loss of brainstem reflexes
- High-pitched cry and poor feeding (infants)

induced hyperventilation in an intubated client. Lower levels of carbon dioxide (CO_2) in the blood may temporarily decrease an elevated ICP. Monitoring the client's oxygen saturation using pulse oximetry and monitoring end-tidal carbon dioxide ($EtCO_2$) using capnography may also be helpful (see Chapter 18). The following interventions are additional examples of measures that may decrease or help prevent increased ICP in clients:

- **Provide a calm environment.** A noisy environment can increase the client's ICP. The client's LOC may be altered but his or her hearing may remain intact. Thus, the client's environment should be quiet, with efforts to cluster nursing care. Regardless of whether the client is conscious or unconscious, use a calm voice to explain each intervention. Use of restraints can also increase a client's ICP. Although safety is paramount, avoid restraints whenever possible in order to decrease stimulation and prevent increased ICP.
- **Control the client's temperature and the room temperature.** The room temperature should be kept consistent to keep the client's body temperature within established parameters. If ordered, a cooling blanket for thermoregulation may be used. (Note: For more information on thermoregulation and using a cooling blanket, see Chapter 3.)
- **Provide proper positioning of the client.** Provide midline positioning and alignment of the head and neck by ensuring the client's head is not leaning to one side. In addition to decreasing the client's ICP, proper positioning can enhance the accuracy of ICP monitoring. It is also important to elevate the head of the client's bed approximately 30 degrees if not contraindicated, or per order or facility policy. Avoid extreme flexion of the extremities, at the waist, or of the neck to keep intraabdominal and intrathoracic pressure constant.
- **Avoid rectal stimulation.** Rectal stimulation can increase ICP. Avoid using rectal thermometers. In addition, medication administration should be limited to oral, enteral, or intravenous routes, with avoidance of rectal medication administration.

CARING FOR A CLIENT WITH AN EXTERNAL VENTRICULAR DRAIN AND PERFORMING ICP MONITORING

Intracranial pressure can be monitored in two ways: (1) indirect clinical evaluation and monitoring of the client's LOC, pupillary response, and other parameters (see Skill 20.1), and (2) direct invasive monitoring, as through an external ventricular drain (EVD). An EVD can be used to temporarily control ICP by draining excess CSF or blood from the ventricles of the brain. The CSF is accessed and/or drained by the placement of a catheter into the ventricular system of the brain; the catheter is then attached to an external drainage system that is a component of the EVD (see Fig. 20.10).

CSF drainage through an EVD is ordered as continuous or intermittent. As shown in Fig. 20.11, the burette is the chamber that the CSF flows into, and it contains and measures the amount of CSF that is drained over a certain amount of time. Depending on the manufacturer, the burette may also be called a drip chamber. The volume or rate of CSF flow is controlled by adjusting the level or height of the burette relative to the interventricular foramen.

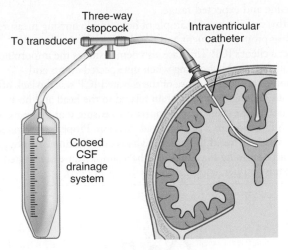

FIG. 20.10 Intracranial components and placement of an external ventricular drain (EVD).

In addition to draining CSF, the EVD may also be attached to a transducer and monitor, which can provide information in the form of ICP waveforms and ICP pressure values similar to those provided by an arterial pressure-monitoring system. ICP monitoring not only allows for direct measurement of the client's ICP but also provides information about the adaptive capacity of the client's intracranial dynamics from the waveform assessment (discussed shortly).

When caring for clients with an EVD and ICP monitoring, it is essential that all devices be calibrated correctly and that various lines are free of kinks. In addition, the systems must be kept sterile. It is also important to maintain the insertion site and any dressings to prevent infection.

Positioning the client with an ICP monitor follows the same recommendations identified for a client with elevated ICP. As noted previously, the client's head needs to remain in midline (not be turned to the side) to avoid jugular venous compression, which would affect CBF and CSF drainage and subsequently increase the ICP. In addition, the head of the bed needs to be elevated to approximately 30 degrees if not contraindicated or ordered otherwise by the authorized healthcare provider. As illustrated in Box 20.4, nursing measures such as client positioning and alignment may have a dramatic impact on a client's ICP.

Ensuring Accuracy With ICP Monitoring

Prior to obtaining an ICP reading, it may be necessary to zero the transducer. The exact procedure will depend on the manufacturer instructions and facility policy. To ensure accuracy, zero the transducer at atmospheric pressure before each reading and each time that the client changes positions. As Fig. 20.11 illustrates, the fluid-filled transducer is zeroed using a laser level device or laser pointer while in line with the tragus of the client's ear. The tragus is an anatomical

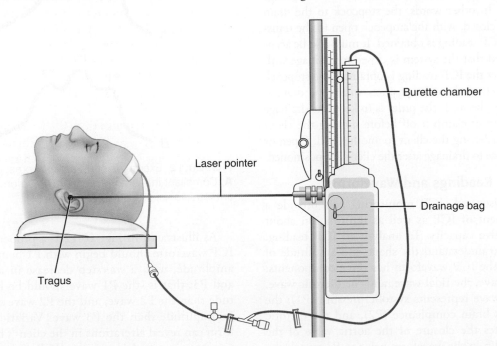

FIG. 20.11 Example of an external ventricular drain (EVD) setup with a laser pointer. The tragus of the ear is an anatomical landmark that represents the location of the interventricular foramen.

BOX 20.4 Lessons From Experience: Troubleshooting for ICP Elevation

Ms. Fitzgerald, a 55-year-old female, was admitted to the critical care unit for a right hemispheric intracerebral hemorrhage (blood within the brain tissue) with intraventricular hemorrhage (blood within the ventricles of the brain). She was intubated upon arrival to the emergency room (ER) due to her decreased level of consciousness and inability to protect her airway. She also had an external ventricular drain (EVD) placed due to early cerebral herniation related to cerebral edema and hydrocephalus, an enlargement of the ventricle of the brain due to blood within the ventricles. After several days, Ms. Fitzgerald required a craniectomy to relieve the swelling. For the first 3 days after surgery, Ms. Fitzgerald's intracranial pressure (ICP) remained within established parameters (15 mm Hg or less). Although her ICP was occasionally elevated, it generally responded well to treatment and nursing measures.

On post-craniectomy day 4, after being repositioned for her bath, the nurse noticed that Ms. Fitzgerald's ICP had increased to 29 mm Hg. Realizing that the stimulation of the bath and other activities might have elevated the client's ICP, the nurse ensured that Ms. Fitzgerald's bed was elevated 30 degrees and allowed her to rest before measuring the ICP again. The nurse also opened the EVD to allow cerebrospinal fluid (CSF) to drain as needed and performed additional troubleshooting measures, such as checking for any kinks or disruptions in the system. In addition, the nurse re-zeroed the transducer and ensured that it was at the level of the tragus (see Fig. 20.11).

After waiting at least 5 minutes, the nurse rechecked the ICP reading again and found it to now be even worse: 32 mm Hg. At this time, the nurse obtained vital signs (which were within normal range), performed a neurologic assessment, and contacted the authorized healthcare provider, who ordered mannitol to be administered. Mannitol is a powerful diuretic that is often used for clients with neurologic injuries. Although mannitol and other measures had worked in the past, Ms. Fitzgerald's ICP remained elevated at 30 mm Hg after the interventions.

The client's nurse then asked another experienced neurocritical care nurse to assess the situation. This nurse assessed Ms. Fitzgerald's positioning and realized the pillow placed behind the neck for comfort was causing her head to protrude forward. The nurse removed the pillow and rechecked the ICP. Slowly, the client's ICP decreased to her baseline and expected range.

This case is a good example of how simple nursing measures such as proper alignment and positioning can significantly affect a client's ICP. This case also demonstrates the importance of diligent troubleshooting when unexpected events and responses occur. The cause of the elevated ICP was the lack of venous drainage from the brain related to the head and neck position of the client. It is important to ensure that a client with an EVD maintains a neutral head position. Proper positioning may also help avoid the use of high-risk medications. Although client positioning may appear to be a simple cause of elevated ICP, it is an intervention that may be overlooked.

landmark associated with the interventricular foramen where CSF is generated. This provides a benchmark for accuracy of the baseline ICP and subsequent readings.

ICP measurements are more accurate when the drainage system is closed. In other words, the stopcock to the drain should be off, or closed, with the stopcock open to the transducer when the ICP reading is obtained. It must also be accurately documented that the system is closed to drainage with each reading. After the ICP reading is obtained, the stopcock should then be returned to the position where the drain is open, if ordered to be so. If the order is to keep the drainage system open, close or clamp it off before moving the client in the bed or transferring the client to another bed. Open or unclamp the device to drainage after the client is repositioned.

Analyzing ICP Readings and Waveforms

As previously discussed, ICP monitoring can provide a direct measurement of ICP as well as information about the brain's adaptive capacity. To analyze an ICP reading, it is important to understand the shape and amplitude of the waveforms. The ICP waveform has three components: the percussion wave, the tidal wave, and the dicrotic wave. The percussion wave represents systolic pressure (P1), the tidal wave shows brain compliance (P2), and the dicrotic wave demonstrates the closure of the aortic valve of the heart (P3). The dip in the waveform prior to P3 reveals the dicrotic notch, which is a low point in pressure just before the aortic valve closes.

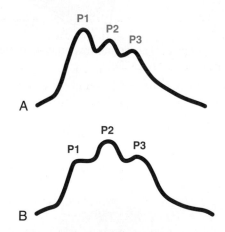

FIG. 20.12 Examples of intracranial pressure waveforms. **A,** Compliant intracranial pressure waveform. **B,** Noncompliant intracranial pressure waveform.

As illustrated in Fig. 20.12A, a proper or "compliant" ICP waveform should begin with P1 being the highest in amplitude, with a stairstep decrease in amplitude in P2 and P3; that is, the P1 wave should be higher in amplitude than the P2 wave, and the P2 wave should be higher in amplitude than the P3 wave. Variations in the waveform can reveal alterations in the client's brain. Generally, prior to an actual increase in ICP, the amplitude of the waveforms will start to increase. Ultimately, if the P2 wave becomes greater in amplitude compared with the P1 wave, the client may have decreased brain compliance. An example of a "noncompliant" ICP waveform is illustrated in Fig. 20.12B.

SUMMARY

In summary, ICP can be monitored by indirect methods such as neurologic evaluation and monitoring of the client's signs and symptoms. ICP can also be measured by direct methods using an EVD and ICP monitoring system. Regardless of the methods used, the critical concepts of accuracy and communication are imperative. These critical concepts are also interrelated. For example, to facilitate accurate ICP readings, there must be effective communication and consistent technique used for ICP monitoring among nurses and other healthcare providers. This is essential to provide the appropriate interventions for a client with increased ICP.

APPLICATION OF THE NURSING PROCESS

Examples of Related ICNP Nursing Diagnoses, Expected Client Outcomes, and Nursing Interventions:

Nursing Diagnosis: Increased intracranial pressure
Supporting Data: The client has experienced recent neurologic trauma and has an increased ICP reading.
Expected Client Outcomes: The client will have decreased ICP, as demonstrated by:
- absence of signs and symptoms of increased ICP (see Box 20.3)
- ICP readings within the established parameters for the client (e.g., 15 mm Hg or less)
- neurologic exam within established parameters.

Expected Client Outcomes: The client will remain within established parameters for regulation of temperature, heart rate, respiratory rate, blood pressure, oxygen saturation, and $EtCO_2$.
Nursing Intervention Examples: Monitor vital signs. Provide measures that will decrease the client's ICP (e.g., elevate the head of bed 30 degrees, maintain midline head alignment).
Reference: International Classification for Nursing Practice. (n.d.). *eHealth & ICNP.* Retrieved from https://www.icn.ch/what-we-do/projects/ehealth-icnp.

CRITICAL CONCEPTS
Caring for a Client With Increased Intracranial Pressure

Accuracy (ACC)

Caring for a client with increased ICP is subject to the following variables:
Client-Related Factors
- Client's age and medical status
- Client's LOC, vital signs, oxygen saturation, and $EtCO_2$

- Neurologic history and diagnosis, as well as diagnostic and procedural evaluations
- Neurologic exam scores (e.g., NIHSS, MEND exam, GCS)
- Level of pain, discomfort, or emotional distress
- Environment (e.g., noise, temperature, distractions)

Nurse-Related Factors
- Technique used for performing ICP monitoring and neurologic assessments
- Recognition of signs and symptoms of increased ICP
- Positioning of client and proper identification of landmarks for ICP monitoring
- Calibration and positioning of ICP monitoring devices
- Observation and analysis of ICP waveforms
- Proper maintenance and monitoring of EVD

Equipment-Related Factors
- Proper functioning of ICP monitoring devices

Client-Centered Care (CCC)

When caring for a client with increased ICP, respect for the client is demonstrated by:
- promoting autonomy and ensuring that consent is obtained for EVD placement
- providing privacy
- ensuring comfort and reducing environmental stimuli
- honoring cultural preferences and arranging an interpreter if necessary
- advocating for the client and family during ICP monitoring.

Infection Control (INF)

When caring for a client with increased ICP, healthcare-associated infection is prevented by:
- preventing and reducing the transfer of microorganisms
- reducing the number of microorganisms.

Safety (SAF)

When caring for a client with increased ICP, safety measures prevent harm and maintain a safe care environment, including:
- providing safe management of monitoring devices and drains during client positioning.

Communication (COM)

- Communication exchanges information (oral, written, nonverbal, or electronic) between two or more people.
- Documentation records information in a permanent legal record.
- Communication between the nurse and other healthcare providers enhances the accuracy of the ICP readings and improves client care.

Evaluation (EVAL)

When caring for a client with increased ICP, evaluation of outcomes enables the nurse to determine the efficacy of the care provided, including the following:
- monitoring and comparing ICP values, trends, and neurologic assessment findings.

▪ SKILL 20.4 Caring for a Client With an External Ventricular Drain (EVD) and Obtaining Intracranial Pressure (ICP) Readings

EQUIPMENT

Clean gloves and PPE, if there is a risk of exposure to body fluids
Penlight
Level or laser pointer

BEGINNING THE SKILL

1. **ACC** Review and verify the order for height of drain, how often to drain CSF, and how often to measure the ICP.
2. **COM** Review documentation of previous-shift assessment findings. *This facilitates communication and allows comparison of new findings with previous findings.*
3. **INF** Perform hand hygiene.
4. **CCC** Introduce yourself to the client and family.
5. **SAF** Identify the client using two client identifiers.
6. **CCC** Explain to the family and the conscious or unconscious client what is being done. *An unconscious client may still have intact hearing.*
7. **CCC** Provide privacy. *Providing privacy in layers enhances client-centered care.*

PROCEDURE

8. **INF** Apply clean gloves if there is a risk of exposure to body fluids.
9. **ACC** Perform advanced neurologic assessments hourly or as ordered (see Skill 20.1).
10. **ACC** Assess for signs and symptoms of elevated ICP, which can include, but may not be limited to, the following (see previously identified Box 20.3):
    - change in pupillary exam including size, shape, and contraction
    - decreased level of consciousness
    - changes in vital signs (e.g., bradycardia, widened pulse pressure, changes in rate and character of respirations)
    - elevated ICP reading.
11. **ACC** Verify proper client position:
    a. Ensure the client's head is in midline position. *This allows for proper venous drainage of blood from the brain in order to not contribute to elevated ICP.*
    b. Ensure the head of the bed is at 30 degrees or per order.
12. **ACC** Verify that the transducer is at the level of the tragus (interventricular foramen in the brain) using either a level device or laser pointer (see Fig. 20.11).
13. **ACC** Assess the drainage system for any problems and alert the authorized healthcare provider as necessary:
    a. Assess insertion site for signs of infection or drainage.
    b. Assess system tubing for kinks or leaks at insertion site or at any connection sites along the drainage tubing.
    c. Assess for air in drainage tubing.
    d. Assess for clots along drainage tubing.

    e. Assess if system is open or closed to drainage and verify this with the order.
14. **SAF** Verify that alarm limits are set to the correct "high" and "low" range as ordered. **WARNING:** Do *not* turn alarms off. *Setting the alarm limits follows safety guidelines.*
15. **ACC** Zero the transducer per manufacturer instructions, institution policy, and the order. *This allows the transducer to read the ICP at atmospheric pressure in order to give the most accurate reading.* The general process is as follows:
    a. Turn the stopcock toward the drainage system.
    b. Assess the height of the drain and ensure the transducer is at the level of the tragus.
    c. Remove the cap covering the lumen to the transducer.
    d. Press "zero" on the monitor and allow the monitor to recalibrate.
    e. Recap the transducer lumen.
    f. Turn the stopcock toward the pressure tubing to allow the transducer to read the ICP.
    g. Watch for the ICP number on the monitor to remain constant; accept this number as the client's ICP value.
    h. Turn the stopcock toward the transducer to allow for drainage of CSF per the order or facility policy.
16. **EVAL** Evaluate the ICP waveforms. *The ICP waveforms can give insight into the compliance of the brain and whether the drain is in the proper position (see Fig. 20.12).*
17. **EVAL** Monitor the ICP value and record hourly or as ordered in conjunction with the neurologic assessment. (Note: The specifics on obtaining the ICP number will be dependent on the exact monitoring system at each individual institution. However, most systems are similar in the fact that if the drain is open to drain CSF, then it is not accurately reading the ICP. The drain must be temporarily clamped or closed to drainage to read an accurate ICP.)
18. **EVAL** Monitor the CSF drainage for color, clarity, and amount. If there is a change in the characteristics of the CSF or if it becomes darker or blood-tinged, notify the authorized healthcare provider immediately. *The expected finding is that the CSF is clear. Blood-tinged drainage or excessive drainage could indicate rebleeding in the brain.*
19. **COM** Calculate and document the client's CPP if indicated or ordered. (Note: The formula for calculating cerebral perfusion pressure is CPP = MAP – ICP.)

FINISHING THE SKILL

20. **INF** Remove gloves and PPE if used and perform hand hygiene.
21. **SAF** Ensure safety and comfort. Ensure that the bed is in the lowest position, and verify that the client can identify and reach the nurse call system. *These safety measures reduce the risk of falls.*

22. **EVAL** Evaluate the outcomes. Did the client tolerate the procedure? Is the EVD intact and free from any signs of infection? Are the client's ICP readings improving or remaining within established parameters? How do the current ICP readings compare to previous readings?
23. **COM** Document findings and compare to past trends in assessment findings.
24. **SAF** Alert the authorized healthcare provider if the following occurs:

a. The ICP reading is not within written or established parameters for the client.
b. There are significant changes in the appearance or amount of CSF.
c. There are changes in the client's neurologic assessment.
d. There are any other abnormal or unexpected findings.

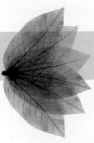

SECTION 3 Caring for a Client With a Neurologic Emergency

Clients who have a neurologic injury (traumatic or nontraumatic) can develop complications at any time. When caring for these clients, the focus must be on early recognition and assessment, ongoing monitoring, timely interventions, and prevention of further complications. For the purpose of this section, two common neurologic emergencies will be discussed: seizures and strokes. These emergencies may be seen in a variety of different settings and clinical areas.

CARING FOR A CLIENT WHO IS HAVING A SEIZURE

A seizure is an abnormal firing of electrical charges within the brain. The intensities of these charges can vary, making the presentation of seizures vary as well. The neurologic disorder known as epilepsy can be defined as at least two unprovoked seizures with a return to baseline between them. *Unprovoked seizure* means there is not another explanation for why the client may be having seizures. Possible causes of provoked seizures can include neurologic injuries, such as brain tumors, TBI, stroke, and subdural hematomas. Metabolic disturbances may include hypercalcemia, hyponatremia, hypoglycemia, and drug overdose or withdrawal.

There are multiple types of seizures, which can be further broken down into subtypes. The main seizure presentations are partial seizures and generalized seizures. Partial seizures only involve one part of the brain, and therefore usually only one area of the body is affected. These can present as a tremor in one part of the body. In generalized seizures, the entire brain is involved, causing the full body to be affected and producing tonic-clonic movements that may be accompanied by a loss of consciousness. During a partial seizure, a client may or may not have a change in LOC. If the client does not have a change in LOC, this is referred to as a simple-partial seizure. If there is a change in the client's LOC, it is referred to as a complex-partial seizure. A subtype of generalized seizure is called an absence (pronounced absonz) seizure, which is described as a staring spell in which

the client has no recollection of the episode. This condition can be difficult to diagnose, and it may be mistaken for an individual who is daydreaming.

Reducing the Risk of Seizures

For clients at risk of having a seizure, prevention is a top priority. There are many medications, called antiepileptics, to assist in reducing the risk of seizures that clients with known epilepsy can take regularly as seizure prophylaxis. There are also emergency medications that can be given to stop a seizure while it is happening, such as benzodiazepines (e.g., diazepam, lorazepam). In some cases, the client may have to be sedated by the authorized healthcare provider. Administer medications as prescribed and continue to monitor the client closely.

In addition to medications, clients who are at risk for seizures are also placed on seizure precautions. This is important in many settings, including the acute care environment. Seizure precautions reduce the risk of client injury during a seizure. Precautions prior to a seizure may include, but are not be limited to, padding the bedrails of the client's bed, putting up all bed rails to prevent rolling out of bed, and removing sharp objects from the environment.

During a seizure, steps that promote safety include turning the client to his or her side, removing any constricting clothing or ties, and detaching restraints. Restraints can cause muscle strains if the client is seizing against them. The nurse's calm demeanor and ability to provide a safe care environment can reduce the client and family's anxiety during a seizure.

CARING FOR A CLIENT WHO MAY BE HAVING AN ACUTE STROKE

The English word *stroke* comes from the Greek word *apoplexia,* meaning "struck down by violence." This descriptive name originated because of the sudden onset of a stroke. Although a stroke often affects clients suddenly, the consequences may be lifelong.

There are two major types of stroke, ischemic stroke and hemorrhagic stroke. An ischemic stroke is caused by a blockage of an artery inside the brain, leading to a loss of blood flow

BOX 20.5 Risk Factors for Ischemic Stroke

- Hyperlipidemia
- Hypertension
- Diabetes mellitus
- Cardiac dysrhythmias (e.g., atrial fibrillation, atrial flutter)
- Known carotid stenosis
- Cigarette smoking
- Obesity
- Family history of stroke

BOX 20.6 Signs and Symptoms of an Acute Stroke

- Sudden difficulty with vision in one or both eyes, diplopia (double vision)
- Sudden loss of balance or coordination or sudden dizziness
- Sudden numbness or weakness or drooping of features on one side of the face
- Sudden numbness or weakness of the leg or arm, particularly on one side of the body
- Sudden confusion or change in mental status
- Drooling from mouth and/or dysphagia (difficulty swallowing)
- Difficulty with speech and language; speech may be slurred
- Loss of consciousness or change in level of consciousness

Reference: American Stroke Association, 2018.

and resulting in damage to a specific area within the brain. A hemorrhagic stroke is caused by the rupture of a vessel inside the brain, leading to bleeding into the brain tissue. Ischemic strokes are much more common than hemorrhagic strokes, comprising over 85% of all strokes. However, with both types of stroke combined, stroke is the fifth-leading cause of death in the United States (American Stroke Association, 2018). Some risk factors for ischemic stroke are listed in Box 20.5. Sadly, of the clients who survive a stroke, many will have lasting deficits.

It is important to quickly recognize the signs and symptoms (Box 20.6) of a stroke in order for a client to obtain treatment promptly to decrease the amount of brain injury. Sometimes the first sign of a stroke *is* the stroke. Depending on the type of stroke, the treatments can vary. Among other interventions, possible treatments for an ischemic stroke can include a thrombolytic agent called a tissue-type plasminogen activator (tPA) or a procedure called a mechanical thrombectomy to remove the clot. Possible treatments for a hemorrhagic stroke may include correction of any coagulopathy as well as evacuation of the hemorrhage or other surgical interventions.

Basic Nursing Care and Screening for Clients Who May Be Having a Stroke

As part of a multidisciplinary team, nurses have a crucial role with respect to rapid assessment, triage, and timely interventions for clients who may be having an acute stroke. In addition to helping clients navigate through the healthcare system, the nurse can facilitate treatments and transfer to the intensive care or specialized stroke units (Middleton et al., 2015).

BOX 20.7 Lessons From the Evidence: Effectiveness of the FAST and BE-FAST Exams

In a study conducted by Aroor, Singh, and Goldstein (2017), the records of 736 clients who had been admitted to a stroke unit were analyzed over a 12-month time frame. The objective of the study was to determine if the clients had any signs and symptoms that would be captured by using the FAST screening. In addition, a revised mnemonic BE-FAST that includes evaluation of gait balance (B) and eye or vision symptoms (E) was evaluated. As part of the inclusion criteria, all of the subjects were determined to have a diagnosis of acute ischemic stroke.

According to the authors, 14.1% of the subjects did not have signs and symptoms that would have been identified by the FAST exam. However, a sensitivity analysis revealed that with the addition of balance and gait assessment (B) and eye and vision assessment (E), there was an increase in the recognition of strokes, and the proportion of clients with strokes who would not have been identified was reduced to 2.6%. The authors acknowledged that more research and prospective studies are needed in different settings to validate these findings (Aroor et al., 2017).

The client is particularly vulnerable during the first 72 hours after a stroke. Some key interventions for these clients include (1) early recognition of symptoms and complications; (2) oxygen saturation monitoring; (3) vital sign monitoring, particularly of the client's blood pressure; (4) cardiac monitoring (see Chapter 19); (5) blood glucose monitoring; and (6) screening for dysphasia and aspiration risk (Middleton et al., 2015). It is also important to remain with the client and provide close monitoring until the rapid response team (RRT) arrives per facility policy.

Examples of Tools Used for Stroke Assessment

An acute stroke can happen anywhere at any time. The choice of the appropriate screening tool can make a tremendous difference. One tool that is well known and easy to use is the "FAST" exam. (American Stroke Association, 2019) The acronym correlates with *face, arm, speech, time.* One advantage of this tool is that it is simple to use and can be taught to anyone, including family members and individuals in the community. However, one study found that the FAST exam may not identify certain clients who are having an acute ischemic stroke. Thus, the consideration of additional clinical parameters, such as balance and vision changes, may be warranted (Box 20.7).

National Institute of Health Stroke Scale (NIHSS)

The National Institute of Health Stroke Scale (NIHSS) is a tool used in many facilities and is recommended and supported by current practice and evidence-based guidelines. In addition, this tool has demonstrated validity and reliability, and it measures stroke disability as well as possible long-term outcomes (Know Stroke, n.d.; Middleton et al., 2015). However, it should be noted that the NIHSS exam is fairly complex and may require training and certification of the examiner. The basic components of the NIHSS calculator include the client's **LOC** and ability to answer two questions correctly and follow two simple commands; **best gaze** (horizontal eye movement); **visual fields** (vision in all four quadrants); **facial palsy** (symmetry in the smile and ability to raise eyebrows and close eyes equally); **motor function** (unexpected drift in upper and lower extremities); **limb ataxia** (ability to perform a finger-nose-finger test and heel-shin test bilaterally); **sensory** (differentiation of sharp or dull stimuli); **best language** (ability to identify or describe images on the NIHSS naming sheet and the ability to read a list of sentences); **dysarthria** (presence of slurred speech); and **extinction and inattention** (lack of awareness of right or left side). For a more detailed graphic version of the NIHSS that includes images and detailed instructions, see the NINDS website at https://www.stroke.nih.gov/documents/NIH_Stroke_Scale_Booklet_508C.pdf. The text version of the NIHSS is available at https://www.stroke.nih.gov/documents/NIH_Stroke_Scale_508C.pdf.

When using the NIHSS, score what the client actually does, not what you think the client should do. It is also important not to coach the client or tell them how they should respond. Variables that may affect the test include preexisting disabilities, such as weakness or visual deficits, and clients who are intubated and have language impairments. To enhance accuracy, record the results as the test is being administered and use consistent assessment techniques for each exam (KnowStroke, n.d.).

Miami Emergency Neurologic Deficit (MEND) Exam

Another tool that is often used and has demonstrated validity is the Miami Emergency Neurologic Deficit (MEND) exam (Fig. 20.13). This exam is a quick, concise evaluation of a client who is believed or confirmed to have suffered an ischemic stroke. The advantage of the MEND exam is that it can be easily mastered and is less time consuming to use than the NIHSS. The MEND exam also enhances communication between nurses and other members of the healthcare team in different settings. For example, it can initially be used to obtain a baseline assessment in the pre-hospital setting and then used again for re-evaluations in the acute care facility (Advanced Stroke Life Support [ASLS], 2018). The main components of the MEND exam are:

- **Mental status** (e.g., assessment of the client's LOC, speech, and ability to answer questions, such as what month or year it is, as well as the ability to follow commands)
- **Cranial nerves** (e.g., assessment of facial droop, visual fields, and horizontal gaze)
- **Limbs** (e.g., assessment of arm or leg drift; sensory and motor function of the arms and legs; arm and leg coordination such as the finger-nose test or heel-shin test).

Regardless of the setting, a consistent and reliable screening tool must be used in order for accurate comparisons to be made between different facilities and different shifts. This will help nurses and other members of the healthcare team collaborate and provide excellent and timely care for these clients.

SUMMARY

The critical concepts of accuracy, safety, client-centered care, infection control, communication, and evaluation are all relevant when caring for a client who is having a neurologic emergency. In particular, maintaining safety, providing timely care, and preventing injury are important when caring for a client who is having a stroke or seizure. In addition, effective teamwork and collaboration between nurses and other healthcare providers are essential in order to facilitate optimal outcomes for the client and prevent complications during a neurologic emergency.

APPLICATION OF THE NURSING PROCESS

Examples of Related ICNP Nursing Diagnoses, Expected Client Outcomes, and Nursing Interventions:

Nursing Diagnosis: Risk for injury
Supporting Data: Client has a history of seizures.
Expected Client Outcomes: The client will have no injuries from seizure activity, as seen by:
- absence of visible injuries after seizures
- absence of reported injuries by client
- neurologic exam within established parameters.

Nursing Intervention Examples: Implement seizure precautions. Keep bed in lowest position. Remain with the client and contact the RRT per facility policy.

Reference: International Classification for Nursing Practice. (n.d.). *eHealth & ICNP.* Retrieved from https://www.icn.ch/what-we-do/projects/ehealth-icnp.

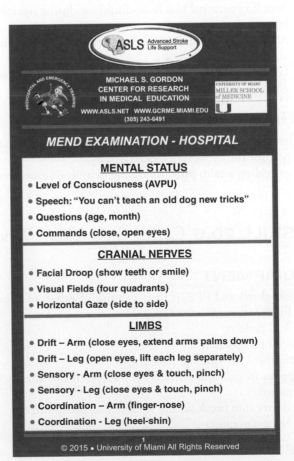

FIG. 20.13 Miami Emergency Neurologic Deficit (MEND) exam.

CRITICAL CONCEPTS
Caring for a Client With a Neurologic Emergency

Accuracy (ACC)

Caring for a client with a neurologic emergency is subject to the following variables:

Client-Related Factors

- Client's age and medical status, as well as neurologic history and diagnosis
- Client's vital signs (blood pressure, pulse, temperature, respirations)
- History of seizures or risk factors for seizures
- History of stroke or risk factors for stroke
- Neurologic assessment and exam score (e.g., NIHSS, MEND exam)
- Level of pain, discomfort, or emotional distress
- Vision, hearing, or any disabilities
- Environment (e.g., noise, temperature, distractions)

Nurse-Related and System-Related Factors

- Rapid assessments and interventions to improve client outcomes
- Technique and screening tool used for assessing the client for stroke
- Adherence to stroke protocols and seizure precautions used in the facility
- Avoiding personal bias or assumptions during neurologic emergencies
- Ability to verify findings and perform further assessment, as needed
- Follow-up monitoring and care following a neurologic emergency

Client-Centered Care (CCC)

When caring for a client with a neurologic emergency, respect for the client is demonstrated by:

- providing a calm presence during neurologic emergencies
- providing privacy and protecting the client's dignity
- ensuring comfort and reducing environmental stimuli
- honoring cultural preferences and arranging for an interpreter if necessary
- advocating for the client and family and providing updates about the client's condition.

Infection Control (INF)

When caring for a client with a neurologic emergency, healthcare-associated infection is prevented by:

- preventing and reducing the transfer of microorganisms
- reducing the number of microorganisms.

Safety (SAF)

When caring for a client with a neurologic emergency, safety measures prevent harm and maintain a safe care environment, including:

- ensuring that the environment is free from hazards or obstacles that could harm the client
- following evidence-based stroke and seizure protocols.

Communication (COM)

- Communication exchanges information (oral, written, nonverbal, or electronic) between two or more people.
- Collaboration with other healthcare providers will facilitate rapid care and reduce complications for clients who are having neurologic emergencies.
- Documentation records information in a permanent legal record.

Evaluation (EVAL)

When caring for a client with a neurologic emergency, evaluation of outcomes enables the nurse to determine the efficacy of the care provided.

■ SKILL 20.5 Caring for a Client Who Requires Seizure Precautions

EQUIPMENT

Clean gloves and PPE, if there is a risk of exposure to body fluids
Bedrail padding
Clock or stopwatch
Equipment for vital sign assessment
Supplies to gain intravenous (IV) access, if not already obtained
Medication to break seizure if needed as prescribed (e.g., IV benzodiazepine)

BEGINNING THE SKILL

1. **ACC** Review the client's history and assess the client's risk factors for having seizures, including the following: brain tumor, brain hemorrhage, central nervous system infection, electrolyte imbalance, metabolic abnormality, or known epilepsy. *Knowledge of the client's risk for seizures will facilitate safety and early preparation for seizure management.*
2. **INF** Perform hand hygiene.
3. **CCC** Introduce yourself to the client and family.
4. **SAF** Identify the client using two identifiers.
5. **CCC** Provide privacy. *Providing privacy in layers enhances client-centered care.*

PROCEDURE

6. **INF** Apply gloves and PPE if there is a risk of exposure to body fluids.

7. **SAF** Obtain or ensure the client has IV access per facility protocol. *IV access is important for possible emergency administration of ordered medications for seizure activity.*

Implementing Seizure Precautions

8. **SAF** Ensure client's environment is safe and free from hazards. *Prevents injuries.*
   - Lower the client's bed to the lowest position.
   - Put up the bed railing.
   - Place padding on bedrails; blankets are sufficient if custom padding is not available.
   - Decreased stimulation in the room, such as television or extended visitation.
   - Remove sharp objects within immediate reach.
   - Remove any electrical hazards or glass near the client, such as lamps.

Providing Immediate Care for the Client Who Is Seizing

9. **SAF** Implement safety measures for the seizing client:
   - Turn the client to his or her side. *Prevents aspiration of emesis into the lungs.*
   - Remove any constricting clothing or ties. *Prevents airway obstruction or injuries.*
   - Detach restraints if in place. *Restraints can cause muscle strains and possible injury if the client is seizing against them.*
   - Protect the client's head. Use a pillow or soft padding under the client's head if not contraindicated.
   - If the client is standing up when the seizure begins, help lower the client gently to the floor to prevent the client from falling.
10. **SAF** Ensure safety of self and others if the client has severe agitation. *Clients may be disoriented and confused following a seizure.* **WARNING:** Do not leave the client alone during a seizure.
11. **COM** Alert the authorized healthcare provider and emergency RRT as required by facility policy. *Collaboration enhances client care.*
12. **ACC** Administer seizure-breaking medication as ordered by the authorized healthcare provider and observe the effect of the medication after administration
13. **ACC** Time the duration of the seizure. *Timing helps identify the risk to the client and the type of seizure.*
14. **ACC** Examine the nature of the seizure (e.g., Does the client have a blank stare? Is the client having tremors or tonic-clonic movements?). (Note: There are many types of seizures, and the presentation of the seizure will need to be described to the authorized healthcare provider.)
15. **ACC** Obtain a complete set of vital signs and assess LOC. *Clients may have a change in clinical status or decreased LOC following seizure activity.*
16. **ACC** Notify the authorized healthcare provider of the seizure. Report the following:
   - onset of seizure
   - duration of seizure
   - presentation of seizure
   - client's current neurologic status after seizure and if emergency response team alerted
   - vital signs and any medications that are administered
   - client behavior prior to the seizure. *There may be precipitating behavior prior to seizures that can alert the client or healthcare provider that a seizure may be coming.*
17. **CCC** Explain recent events related to the seizure and provide emotional support to the client and family. *Seizures can be scary, confusing, and unsettling to the client and family.*

FINISHING THE SKILL

18. **INF** Remove PPE and gloves if used and perform hand hygiene.
19. **SAF** Ensure safety and comfort. Ensure that the bed is in the lowest position, and verify that the client can identify and reach the nurse call system. *These safety measures reduce the risk of falls.*
20. **EVAL** Evaluate the outcomes. Is the client's neurologic status normal and within expected parameters after the seizure? Is the client free from injuries after the seizure?
21. **COM** Document findings.
   - Onset, duration, presentation, and characteristics of the seizure
   - Client's vital signs after the seizure
   - Client's neurologic status, including LOC, before and after seizure
   - Conversation with authorized healthcare provider
   - Conversation with the client and/or client's family
   - Name and dosage of any medications that were administered and the client's response.
22. **ACC** Prepare to carry out new orders from the authorized healthcare provider (e.g., seizure-breaking medications).
23. **EVAL** Provide follow-up monitoring for any further seizure activity.

■ **SKILL 20.6** Assessing a Client Who May Be Having an Acute Stroke

EQUIPMENT

Clean gloves and PPE, if there is a risk of exposure to body fluids

BEGINNING THE SKILL

1. **ACC** Review the client's history and risk factors for having a stroke (see Box 20.5).
2. **INF** Perform hand hygiene.
3. **CCC** Introduce yourself to the client and family.
4. **SAF** Identify the client using two identifiers.
5. **CCC** Provide privacy and explain the procedure. *Providing privacy in layers enhances client-centered care.* Obtain verbal consent.

PROCEDURE

6. **INF** Apply gloves and PPE if there is a risk of exposure to body fluids.
7. **ACC** Identify the change in the client's exam requiring the need to perform a rapid assessment.
8. **ACC** Assess the client's LOC and other neurologic parameters (see Skill 20.1). If the client is in immediate distress, notify the authorized health care provider and RRT immediately per facility policy.
9. **ACC** Obtain vital signs and compare to the client's baseline vital signs. *The client's vital signs (particularly blood pressure and pulse) are important parameters to consider with a possible stroke.*

Perform a Stroke Screening Exam Using a Facility-Approved Tool

10. **ACC** If using NIHSS or MEND exam, see Fig. 20.13 or the narrative text.
11. **ACC** If using the FAST or BE-FAST exams, perform the following:
    a. **Balance:** Assess the client's balance and gait and any difficulty with ambulation.
    b. **Eyes:** Assess the client for vision changes (e.g., blurred vision, diplopia [double vision]).
    c. **Face:** Instruct the client to smile. Observe closely and compare one side of the client's face to the other while assessing for droop on one side.

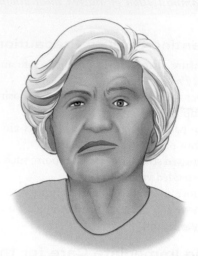

STEP 11C Assess the client's facial characteristics.

d. **Arms:** Ask the client to hold both arms straight out in front of the body. Do *not* allow the client to rest the elbows on the trunk. Observe for inability to raise one arm. If able to raise both arms, instruct the client to close his or her eyes and watch for subtle drift of one arm compared with the other. (Note: The expected finding is that there is no drift.)

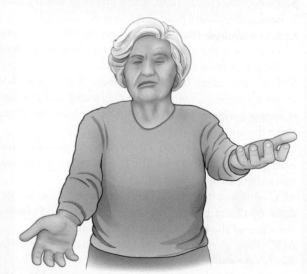

STEP 11D Assess the client's arm drift.

e. **Speech:** Ask the client to state a simple phrase, such as, "Today is a sunny day" or "No ifs, ands, or buts." Note if the client has difficulty forming words or has incomprehensible speech, inappropriate response, or slurred speech. (Note: The expected finding is that the client's speech will be clear, with no deficits.)

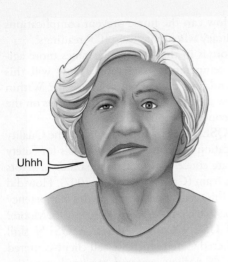

Uhhh

STEP 11E Assess the client's speech patterns.

f. **TIME:** Note the time of onset and get emergency help immediately. *"Time is brain"—the more time that passes without getting care, the more permanent damage can be done.*

12. **ACC** Consider additional signs of stroke, including sudden-onset numbness, dizziness, light-headedness, confusion, drooling, sudden headache, and so forth (see Box 20.6).

13. **ACC** Assess the client's pupils for size, symmetry, and response to light (see Skill 20.1). *Pupillary changes such as pupils of differing sizes bilaterally, sluggishly reactive pupils, or nonreactive pupils can be a sign of increased ICP or other adverse neurologic change.*

14. **EVAL** Determine if there is a change from the client's baseline exam. *A change in the client's neurologic status could determine whether this is an acute event or not.*

15. **COM** Notify the authorized healthcare provider with new information immediately if needed. *Collaboration with other health care providers enhances client care. Any delay in notifying the authorized healthcare provider could delay treatment for the client.*

16. **SAF** Remain with the client until the authorized healthcare provider or RRT arrives. *This facilitates safe care until additional interventions or transfer to intensive care can occur.*

17. **ACC** Prepare for any new orders from the authorized healthcare provider, such as stat medications (e.g., tPA, other medications), stat laboratory work, or scans.

FINISHING THE SKILL

18. **INF** Remove gloves and PPE if used and perform hand hygiene.

19. **SAF** Ensure safety and comfort. Ensure that the bed is in the lowest position, and verify that the client can identify and reach the nurse call system. *These safety measures reduce the risk of falls.*

20. **EVAL** Evaluate the outcomes. Did the client receive timely care? *The standard is for the client to receive care as rapidly as possible after the onset of stroke symptoms.*

21. **COM** Document the findings, including the following:
   - results of stroke screening (e.g., NIHSS; MEND, FAST, or BE-FAST exam)
   - notification of the authorized healthcare provider and RRT
   - time of onset of the client's symptoms
   - time the RRT arrived.

■ CASE STUDY

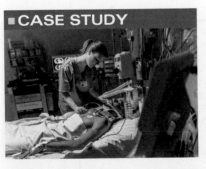

Mr. Moore, a 38-year-old male with a past medical history of seizures and hypertension, arrives at the emergency room (ER) via ambulance following a motor vehicle accident (MVA). He was driving his motorcycle on the highway when a truck side-swiped his tire and his motorcycle spun off the road and into an embankment. Mr. Moore, who was not wearing a helmet, was thrown off the motorcycle and to the ground. He has been conscious, but drowsy since the first responders arrived on the scene. Visible injuries include contusions and lacerations to his head, including the forehead and left orbital area, and along his forearms and shoulders.

Upon arrival at the ER, Mr. Moore's vital signs and neurologic exam are stable. Although drowsy, he awakens to verbal stimuli. He is intubated and on ventilatory support (see Chapter 18), and he has a cervical collar in place as a precaution (see Chapter 6). He is also on continuous ECG monitoring (see Chapter 19). During the assessment, the nurse notes that Mr. Moore has a history of epileptic seizures.

While in the ER, Mr. Moore complains to the nurse of a headache. In addition, he has become increasingly drowsy and difficult to arouse, and he has pupillary changes. The nurse reviews the orders and notes that an LP is ordered. Before gathering the equipment, the nurse alerts the healthcare team about Mr. Moore's symptoms and her concern about the LP. The LP is canceled by the authorized healthcare provider until magnetic resonance imaging (MRI) and further tests can be obtained. The nurse ensures that the head of Mr. Moore's bed remains elevated to 30 degrees and awaits further orders. The nurse also continues to address Mr. Moore by name, and she provides explanations about procedures even though she is not sure he can hear her.

The imaging results confirm that Mr. Moore has a subarachnoid hemorrhage (SAH). The neurosurgeon plans for placement of an external ventricular drain (EVD) to monitor intracranial pressure (ICP) and drain additional cerebrospinal fluid (CSF) as needed. In addition, Mr. Moore is admitted to the intensive care unit (ICU), and he will continue to receive intracranial pressure (ICP) monitoring. The ICU nurses keep Mr. Moore's family updated as much as possible, and they allow visitation per facility policy and client preference. The nurses also provide explanations and emotional support to Mr. Moore and his family. While in the ICU, Mr. Moore becomes increasingly restless and agitated, and his temperature is elevated above established parameters.

Case Study Questions

1. Considering Mr. Moore's injuries sustained in the MVA, what are the highest priorities of care after he is admitted to the ER?

2. Considering Mr. Moore's history of seizures, what additional monitoring and safety measures should the nurse implement?

3. Mr. Moore experiences new symptoms after arrival to the ER. What is the significance of these symptoms? What interventions are important to implement, including positioning?

4. Why was it critical for the nurse to alert the authorized healthcare provider about these symptoms as well as her concerns regarding the LP?

5. After Mr. Moore's EVD is placed, he is transferred to intensive care. What are key assessments and care related

to the EVD? How can the nurse prevent complications and ensure accuracy when obtaining ICP readings?

6. While Mr. Moore is in the ICU, he becomes more agitated, and his temperature is elevated. How will this affect his ICP, and how can the nurse intervene? Within this context, how are the ICNP nursing diagnoses on the accompanying concept map interrelated?

7. **Application of QSEN Competencies:** One of the Quality and Safety Education for Nurses (QSEN) skills for Safety is to communicate concerns of potential hazards or errors to the healthcare team (Cronenwett et al., 2007). How did the ER nurse in this scenario demonstrate this competency and prevent a possible hazard or safety issue for Mr. Moore?

8. **Application of QSEN Competencies:** A QSEN skill for Patient-Centered Care (which we call client-centered care) is to provide patient-centered care with sensitivity and respect for the diversity of human experience (Cronenwett et al., 2007). How did the nurses demonstrate this competency? How did they show respect and sensitivity for Mr. Moore ?

■ CONCEPT MAP

ICNP Nursing Dx: Decreased Intracranial Adaptive Capacity

Supporting Data:
Subarachnoid hemorrhage
Symptoms of increased ICP

Baseline Assessment Data
- 38-year-old male
- Motor vehicle accident
- Head injury
- Symptoms of increased intracranial pressure
- Subarachnoid hemorrhage
- EVD placement
- ICP monitoring
- Increased temperature
- Increased agitation in ICU

ICNP Nursing Dx: Increased Intracranial Pressure

Supporting Data:
Symptoms of increased ICP
Increased agitation

- Monitor Mr. Moore's vital signs and neurologic status
- Ensure that EVD is intact and patent without kinks
- Maintain head in midline with proper alignment
- Keep head elevated 30 degrees per order

- Monitor for signs and symptoms of increased ICP
- Maintain calm environment
- Avoid rectal temperatures
- Use comfort measures for Mr. Moore

ICNP Nursing Dx: Impaired Thermoregulation

Supporting Data:
Head injury
Elevated temperature

- Maintain normothermic body temperature
- Control room temperature
- Use cooling blanket per order

References

Advanced Stroke Life Support. (2018). *Miami emergency neurologic deficit.* Retrieved from http://www.asls.net/mend_about.php.

American Stroke Association. (2018). *Impact of stroke (stroke statistics).* Retrieved from https://www.strokeassociation.org/STROKEORG/AboutStroke/Impact-of-Stroke-Stroke-statistics_UCM_310728_Article.jsp.

American Stroke Association. (2019). *F.A.S.T.* Infographic. Accessed at https://www.stroke.org/en/about-stroke/stroke-symptoms/learn-more-stroke-warning-signs-and-symptoms.

Anderson, M., Elmer, J., Shutter, L., Puccio, A., & Alexander, S. (2018). Integrating quantitative pupillometry into regular care in a neurotrauma intensive care unit. *Journal of Neuroscience Nursing, 50*(1), 30–36.

Aroor, S., Singh, R., & Goldstein, L. B. (2017). BE-FAST (Balance, Eyes, Face, Arm, Speech, Time): Reducing the proportion of strokes missed using the FAST mnemonic. *Stroke, 48*(2), 479–481.

Chioffi, S. (2017). Lumbar puncture (assist). In L. Wiegand (Ed.), *AACN procedure manual for high acuity, progressive, and critical care* (7th ed.) (pp. 873–879). St. Louis: Elsevier.

Cox, S. (2017). Intraventricular catheter with external transducer for cerebrospinal fluid drainage and intracranial pressure monitoring. In L. Wiegand (Ed.), *AACN procedure manual for high acuity, progressive, and critical care* (7th ed.) (pp. 842–855). St. Louis: Elsevier.

Cronenwett, L., Sherwood, G., Barnsteiner, J., Disch, J., Johnson, J., Mitchell, P., ... Warren, J. (2007). Quality and safety education for nurses. *Nursing Outlook, 55*(3), 122–131. Retrieved from http://qsen.org/competencies/pre-licensure-ksas/.

International Classification for Nursing Practice. (n.d.). *eHealth & ICNP.* Retrieved from https://www.icn.ch/what-we-do/projects/ehealth-icnp.

Jarvis, C. (2016). *Physical examination and health assessment.* [e-book]. St. Louis: Elsevier.

The Joint Commission Universal Protocol. (2015). Retrieved from https://www.jointcommission.org/standards/universal-protocol/.

Know Stroke. (n.d.). National Institutes of Health Stroke Scale. National Institute of Neurologic Disorders and Stroke. Retrieved from https://www.stroke.nih.gov/resources/scale.htm.

Lumbar puncture: Patient given contraindicated drugs, nurses ruled partly responsible. (2012). *Legal Eagle Eye Newsletter for the Nursing Profession.* Retrieved from http://www.nursinglaw.com/lumbar-puncture-nurses.pdf.

Middleton, S., Grimley, R., & Alexandrov, A. W. (2015). Triage, treatment, and transfer: Evidence-based clinical practice recommendations and models of nursing care for the first 72 hours of admission to hospital for acute stroke. *Stroke, 46,* e18–e25.

National Institute of Neurological Disorders and Stroke. (2018). *Traumatic brain injury information page.* Retrieved from https://www.ninds.nih.gov/Disorders/All-Disorders/Traumatic-Brain-Injury-Information-Page.

NeurOptics. (2018). *NPi-200 pupillometer system quick start guide.* Retrieved from https://neuroptics.com/wp-content/uploads/2018/09/NPi-200-Quick-Start-Guide.pdf.

Portran, P., Cour, M., Hernu, R., de la Salle, S., & Argaud, L. (2017). Pupillary abnormalities in non-selected critically ill patients: An observational study. *Journal of Thoracic Disease, 9*(8), 2528–2533.

Urden, L., Stacy, K., & Lough, M. (2016). *Priorities in critical care nursing.* St. Louis: Elsevier.

Weerakkody, Y., & Goel, A. (2018). Monro-Kellie hypothesis. *Radiopaedia.* Retrieved from https://radiopaedia.org/articles/monro-kellie-hypothesis.

Adapted from *VHA Safe Patient Handling and Mobility Algorithms* 2014 and 2016: Fig 1.2; Fig 1.3; Fig 1.4

Aehlert B: *ECGs Made Easy,* ed 6, St Louis, 2013, Mosby: Fig 19.3; Skill 19.3, Step 29

Ball J et al.: *Seidel's Guide to Physical Examination,* ed 8, St Louis, 2015, Mosby: Fig 4.8; Skill 4.4, Step 30, part B; Skill 4.9, Step 26; Skill 4.9, Step 30

Bonewit-West K: *Clinical Procedures for Medical Assistants,* ed 9, St. Louis, 2015, Saunders. In Aehlert B: *ECGs Made Easy,* ed 6, St Louis, 2013, Mosby: Skill 19.1, Step 30

Canale ST, Beaty JH: *Campbell's Operative Orthopaedics,* ed 12, Philadelphia, 2013, Mosby. In Lewis S et al: *Medical-Surgical Nursing: Assessment and Management of Clinical Problems,* ed 10, St. Louis, 2017, Mosby: Fig 6.7B

Cdc.gov: Fig 2.5; Skill 2.15, Step 7 (both photos)

Clinical Skills Videos: Specialty Collections: Critical Care Collection, ed 1: Skill 3.4, Step 11B; Skill 3.4, Step 11C; Skill 5.10, Step 15; Fig 13.3A; Fig 13.3B; Fig 13.4; Skill 13.3, Step 10; Skill 13.3, Step 11; Skill 13.3, Step 18; Skill 13.3, Step 21; Skill 13.5, Step 14; Skill 13.5, Step 16; Skill 13.5, Step 17; Skill 13.5, Step 19; Skill 13.5, Step 20; Skill 13.6, Step 19; Skill 13.5, Step 34; Skill 13.7, Step 23; Skill 13.7, Step 25; Skill 13.7, Step 26; Skill 13.8, Step 22; Skill 13.8, Step 23; Skill 13.9, Step 2; Skill 13.9, Step 25; Skill 14.2, Step 16; Skill 14.3, Step 15; Skill 14.3, Step 16; Skill 14.3, Step 18; Skill 14.4, Step 13c; Skill 14.4, Step 13d; Skill 14.4, Step 13e; Skill 14.4, Step 13g; Skill 14.4, Step 16; Skill 14.5, Step 13; Skill 14.5, Step 14; Skill 14.5, Step 18; Skill 14.5, Step 19; Skill 14.6, Step 13; Skill 14.6, Step 16; Skill 14.6, Step 17; Skill 14.8, Step 16; Skill 14.8, Step 17; Skill 14.8, Step 18; Skill 14.8, Step 19; Skill 14.9, Step 12; Skill 14.9, Step 13; Skill 14.9, Step 17; Skill 14.9, Step 20; Skill 14.9, Step 21; Skill 14.9, Step 22; Skill 14.9, Step 27; Skill 14.9, Step 28; Fig 18.12; Fig 18.13; Fig 18.14; Fig 18.15; Fig 18.16; Skill 18.2, Step 14; Skill 18.2, Step 21B; Skill 18.2, Step 21C; Skill 18.2, Step 21D; Skill 18.2, Step 22A; Skill 18.2, Step 22C; Skill 18.2, Step 23; Skill 18.2, Step 25; Skill 18.2, Step 27; Skill 18.3, Step 16; Skill 18.3, Step 24; Skill 18.3, Step 29; Skill 18.3, Step 32; Fig 18.17, part A; Fig 18.24; Skill 18.4, Step 7; Skill 18.4, Step 13; Skill 18.4, Step 17; Skill 18.4, Step 21; Skill 18.4, Step 22; Skill 18.4, Step 23; Skill 18.5, Step 11; Skill 18.5, Step 26; Skill 18.5, Step 29; Skill 18.6, Step 9; Skill 18.6, Step 17; Skill 18.6, Step 19; Skill 18.6, Step 21; Skill 19.1, Step 11E; Skill 19.1, Step 20; Skill 19.1, Step 21; Skill 19.1, Step 22; Skill 19.1, Step 31; Skill 19.1, Step 35; Skill 19.2, Step 10C; Skill 19.2, Step 20; Skill 19.2, Step 21 (both images); Skill 19.2, Step 24

Clinical Skills Videos: Specialty Collections: Maternal Newborn Collection, ed 1: Skill 7.15, Step 15; Skill 7.16, Step 14

Clinical Skills Videos: Specialty Collections: Neonatal Collection, ed 1: Skill 3.5, Step 3; Skill 3.5, Step 4; Skill 3.5, Step 9; Skill 5.10, Step 15

Clinical Skills Videos: Specialty Collections: Pediatrics Collection, ed 1: Skill 6.9, Step 9A; Skill 6.10, Step 15; Skill 6.11, Step 13; Skill 6.11, Step 15; Skill 7.12, Step 12A, part A; Skill 7.12, Step 12A, part B; Skill 7.12, Step 19; Skill, 7.12, Step 30; Skill, 7.12, Step 32; Skill 7.15, Step 19 (both images); Skill 7.16, Step 12, part A; Skill 9.11, Step 17; Skill 9.11, Step 23; Skill 9.12, Step 20; Skill 9.12, Step 24A; Skill 9.12, Step 25; Skill 9.12, Step 48; Skill 9.13, Step 14; Skill 9.13, Step 17

Clinical Skills Videos: Specialty Collections: Respiratory Care Collection, ed 1: Fig 9.3; Fig 9.16; Fig 9.17; Skill 9.10, Step 11A; Skill 9.10, Step 12; Skill 9.10, Step 16; Skill 11.6, Step 17D; Skill 11.6, Step 21; Fig 18.1; Fig 18.3; Fig 18.4; Fig 18.7; Skill 18.1, Step 14; Skill 18.1, Step 16; Skill 18.1, Step 17; Skill 18.1, Step 18; Skill 18.1, Step 24

Clinical Skills Videos: Essentials Collection: Essentials Collection, ed 1: Skill 1.13, Step 8B; Skill 1.13, Step 9C; Skill 1.13, Step 10A; Skill 2.8, Step 12; Skill 3.3, Step 7; Skill 3.3, Step 8; Skill 3.3, Step 9; Skill 3.10, Step 9; Skill 3.11, Step 9; Skill 3.11, Step 10; Skill 3.18, Step 10; Skill 3.18, Step 14; Skill 3.18, Step 17; Skill 3.18, Step 18; Skill 5.5, Step 22; Skill 5.5, Step 29; Skill 5.5, Step 30; Skill 5.5, Step 33; Skill 5.5, Step 40; Skill 5.7, Step 11; Skill 5.11, Step 22A; Skill 5.11, Step 22E; Skill 5.11, Step 22F; Skill 9.1, Step 9; Skill 9.1, Step 13; Skill 9.2, Step 9; Fig 9.7; Fig 9.11; Fig 9.12; Skill 9.6, Step 11; Skill 9.7, Step 7E; Skill 9.7, Step 9E; Skill 9.7, Step 10F; Skill 9.14, Step 10A; Skill 9.14, Step 10B; Skill 9.14, Step 14; Skill 9.14, Step 17; Skill 9.14, Step 22; Skill 9.14, Step 23; Skill 9.14, Step 28; Skill 9.14, Step 29; Skill 9.14, Step 30; Skill 9.14, Step 31; Skill 11.7, Step 22; Fig 16.1; Fig 16.2; Skill16.1, Step 12; Skill16.1, Step 15; Skill16.1, Step 17D; Skill16.1, Step 17E; Skill 16.2, Step 12; Skill 16.4, Step 8; Skill 16.4, Step 15; Skill 16.4, Step 18; Skill 16.4, Step 19; Fig 16.5; Skill 16.6, Step 11; Skill 16.6, Step 12; Skill 16.6, Step 14' Skill 16.6, Step 18; Skill 16.6, Step 20; Skill 16.6, Step 23; Skill 16.7, Step 12; Skill 16.7, Step 15; Skill 16.7, Step 17; Skill 16.7, Step 18; Skill 16.7,

Step 21; Skill 17.2, Step 9; Skill 17.2, Step 12; Skill 17.2, Step 15; Skill 17.5, Step 11 (both images); Skill 17.5, Step 12; Skill 17.5, Step 13

Clinical Skills Videos: Skills for Nursing Collection: Perioperative Collection, ed 1: Skill 10.4, Step 14 ; Fig 10.1; Skill 10.6, Step 4; Skill 10.6, Step 8; Skill 10.6, Step 9; Skill 10.7, Step 10; Skill 10.7, Step 14; Skill 10.7, Step 16; Skill 10.7, Step 17; Skill 10.8, Step 7; Skill 10.8, Step 9; Skill 10.8, Step 11; Skill 10.8, Step 14; Skill 10.9, Step 6; Skill 10.9, Steps 8 and 9; Skill 10.9, Step 10; Skill 10.9, Steps 13 and 14; Skill 10.9, Step 15

Clinical Skills Videos: Skills for Nursing Collection: Emergency Collection, ed 1: Skill 6.6, Step 11; Skill 6.6, Step 12; Skill 9.9, Step 12; Skill 15.2, Step 14; Skill 15.2, Step 15; Skill 15.2, Step 16; Skill 15.2, Step 17; Skill 15.3, Step 8; Skill 15.3, Step 10; Skill 15.3, Step 13; Skill 15.3, Step 17; Skill 19.3, Step 20; Skill 19.3, Step 21

Clinical Skills Videos: Skills for Nursing Collection: Essentials Collection, ed 1: Skill 2.1, Step 12; Skill 2.1, Step 14; Skill 2.2, Step 8; Skill 2.2, Step 9; Skill 2.3, Step 57G; Skill 2.4, Step, Step 10; Skill 2.5, Step 13; Skill 2.5, Step 16; Skill 2.6, Step 10; Skill 2.8, Step 12; Skill 2.8, Step 13; Skill 2.10, Step 8; Skill 2.10, Step 11; Skill 2.10, Step 15; Skill 2.11, Step 8; Skill 2.11, Step 17; Skill 2.12, Step 21; Skill 2.12, Step 23; Skill 2.13, Step 10; Skill 2.14, Step 11; Skill 2.14, Step 12; Skill 2.16, Step 8; Skill 2.16, Step 11; Fig 2.9; Skill 2.20, Step 12; Skill 2.21, Step 12A; Skill 2.21, Step 13C; Skill 2.21, Step 13D; Skill 2.21, Step 16; Skill 2.21, Step 17; Fig 2.14; Skill 2.23, Step 13; Skill 2.23, Step 20; Skill 2.23, Step 28C (both photos); Skill 2.23, Step 36; Skill 2.23, Step 37; Skill 2.23, Step 39; Skill 2.23, Step 41; Skill 2.24, Step 14; Skill 2.24, Step 16; Skill 2.25, Step 14; Skill 2.25, Step 16; Skill 2.25, Step 17; Skill 2.25, Step 19; Skill 2.25, Step 25; Skill 2.25, Step 29; Skill 2.25, Step 33; Skill 2.25, Step 40; Fig 4.3; Fig 4.4; Fig 4.5; Skill 4.3, Step 12D; Skill 4.4, Step 16; Skill 4.4, Step 26; Skill 4.4, Step 30, part A; Skill 4.4, Step 34; Skill 4.5, Step 25; Skill 4.5, Step 26B; Skill 4.5, Step 26D; Skill 4.5, Step 46; Skill 4.6, Step 30; Skill 4.6, Step 35H; Skill 4.7, Step 13; Skill 4.7, Step 14; Skill 4.7, Step 15; Skill 4.7, Step 19A; Skill 4.7, Step 19B; Skill 4.8, Step 19; Skill 5.2, Step 13; Skill 5.2, Step 18; Skill 5.4, Step 24; Skill 7.5, Step 19; Skill 7.5, Step 25; Skill 11.3, Step 22B; Skill 11.5, Step 25; Skill 11.5, Step 26B; Skill 11.5, Step 35; Skill 11.10, Step 21E; Skill 11.10, Step 22D; Skill 11.12, Step 17H; Skill 11.19, Step 18; Fig 12.8; Skill 12.3, Step 14; Skill 12.3, Step 17 (both images); Skill 12.3, Step 18; Skill 12.3, Step 19; Skill 12.3, Step 22; Skill 12.3, Step 23; Skill 12.3, Step 24; Skill 12.3, Step 28; Skill 12.3, Step 30; Skill 12.6, Step 14; Skill 12.6, Step 16; Skill 12.9, Step 9; Skill 12.9, Step 11; Skill 12.9, Step 17; Skill 12.9, Step 23A; Skill 12.9, Step 25; Skill 12.10, Step 6; Skill 12.10, Step 16; Skill 12.10, Step 19A; Skill 12.10, Step 21B; Skill 12.11, Step 25; Skill 12.11, Step 31; Skill 12.11, Step 33; Skill 12.11, Step 39; Skill 14.2, Step 14; Skill 15.7, Step 15; Skill 15.7, Step 22; Skill 15.7, Step 27; Skill 15.7, Step 22; Skill 15.7, Step 32; Skill 15.7, Step 34; Skill 15.8, Step 26; Skill 15.8, Step 32; Skill 15.8, Step 35; Skill 15.9, Step 14; Skill 15.9, Step 21; Skill 15.9, Step 26; Skill 15.9, Step 32; Skill 15.9, Step 43; Skill 15.10, Step 16; Skill 15.10, Step 21; Skill 15.10, Step 36; Skill 15.10, Step 39; Skill 15.10, Step 40; Skill 15.10, Step 45; Skill 15.11, Step 16 (both images); Skill 15.11, Step 19 (both images); Skill 15.12, Step 11; Skill 15.13, Step 11; Skill 15.13, Step 20; Skill 15.13, Step 23; Skill 15.14, Step 20; Skill 15.14, Step 21; Skill 15.14, Step 25; Skill 15.14, Step 35; Skill 15.15, Step 12; Skill 15.15, Step 13; Skill 15.16, Step 14; Skill 15.16, Step 19; Skill 15.16, Step 23; Skill 15.16, Step 22; Skill 15.16, Step 26; Skill 15.16, Step 27; Skill 15.16, Step 30

Copyright Hill-Rom Services, Inc. Reprinted with permission. All rights reserved: Fig 2.11; Fig 2.13

Copyright The International Dysphagia Diet Standardisation Initiative 2016. Retrieved from https://iddsi.org/ framework: Fig 5.2

Copyright Zulkowski, 2015: Chapter 16 opening photo; Chapter 16 case study photo; Table 16.1 photos; Box 16.4

Courtesy Atrium Medical Corporation, Hudson, NH. In Lewis S et al: *Medical-Surgical Nursing: Assessment and Management of Clinical Problems,* ed 10, St. Louis, 2017, Mosby: Fig 18.20

Courtesy B. Braun Medical Inc., Bethlehem, PA: Skill 7.16, Step 12, part B

Courtesy Brandis Goodman and the Tube Feeding Awareness Foundation: Fig 5.8

Courtesy Dale Medical Products, Inc., Plainville, MA. In Perry A et al: *Fundamentals of Nursing,* ed 8, St. Louis, 2013, Mosby: Fig 9.22

Courtesy Dr. Charles Hollen: Fig 4.2; Fig 7.6

Courtesy Dr. Christopher Hollen: Fig 8.3; Fig 8.5

Courtesy Gentherm, Cincinnati, OH: Fig 3.2; Skill 3.4, Step 16

Courtesy Howmedica, Inc, Allendale, PA. In Lewis S et al: *Medical-Surgical Nursing: Assessment and Management of Clinical Problems,* ed 10, St. Louis, 2017, Mosby: Fig 6.7A

Courtesy ICU Medical, San Clemente, CA: Fig 7.7; Fig 7.8

Courtesy Medela Healthcare, Switzerland: Fig 18.9

Courtesy NeurOptics, Laguna Hills, CA: Fig 20.7; Skill 20.2, Step 19; Skill 20.2, Step 22

Courtesy Össur® Americas, Foothill Ranch, CA: Fig 6.10, part A

Courtesy Philips Healthcare, Andover, MA. In Wiegand DL: *AACN Procedure Manual for High Acuity, Progressive, and Critical Care,* ed 7, 2017, St. Louis, Elsevier: Fig 19.7

Courtesy Shannon Davis: Fig 8.11

Courtesy Zoll Medical Corporation, Chelmsford, MA: Skill 19.3, Step 23A (both images); Skill 19.3, Step 23B

Description column data from Kirton C: Assessing edema, *Nursing 96* 26(7):54, 1996. Illustration from Seidel H et al: *Mosby's Guide to Physical Examination,* ed 7, St Louis, 2011, Mosby: Fig 4.7

Goldman L, Schafer AI: *Goldman's Cecil Medicine,* ed 24, Philadelphia, 2012, Saunders. In Lewis S et al: *Medical-Surgical Nursing: Assessment and Management of Clinical Problems,* ed 10, St. Louis, 2017, Mosby: Fig 9.15

Harkreader H et al: *Fundamentals of Nursing: Caring and Clinical Judgment,* ed 3, St. Louis, 2007, Elsevier. In Wilson, SF, Giddens JF: *Health Assessment for Nursing Practice,* ed 6, St. Louis, 2017, Mosby: Skill 4.6, Step 19

Hockenberry M et al: *Wong's Essentials of Pediatric Nursing,* ed 10, St. Louis, 2017, Mosby: Fig 8.9; Skill 11.18, Step 24

istock.com: Chapter 1 opening photo; Chapter 1 case study photo; Chapter 2 opening photo; Fig 2.7; Fig 2.12; Chapter 2 case study photo; Chapter 3 opening photo; Chapter 3 case study photo; Chapter 4 opening photo; Box 4.4 photo; Chapter 5 opening photo; Chapter 5 case study photo; Chapter 6 opening photo; Fig 6.1; Chapter 6 case study photo; Chapter 7 opening photo; Fig 7.2; Chapter 7 case study photo; Chapter 8 opening photo; Fig 8.4; Fig 8.6; Fig 8.7; Fig 8.10; Chapter 8 case study photo; Chapter 9 opening photo; Fig 9.13; Fig 9.14; Chapter 9 case study photo; Skill 9.6, Step 10; Skill 9.8, Step 16; Chapter 10 opening photo; Chapter 10 case study photo; Chapter 10 opening photo; Chapter 10 case study photo; Chapter 11 opening photo; Chapter 11 case study photo; Fig 11.4; Fig 11.11; Chapter 12 opening photo; Fig 12.12; Fig 12.13; Chapter 12 case study photo; Chapter 13 opening photo; Chapter 13 case study photo; Chapter 14 opening photo; Chapter 14 case study photo; Chapter 15 opening photo; Chapter 15 case study photo; Fig 15.2; Fig 15.3; Chapter 17 opening photo; Fig 17.1; Fig 17.4; Skill 17.7, Step 16; Chapter 17 case study photo; Chapter 18 opening photo; Fig 18.2; Fig 18.8; Chapter 18 case study photo; Chapter 19 opening photo; Chapter 19 case study photo; Fig 19.12; Fig 19.14; Chapter 20 opening photo; ; Chapter 20 case study photo; Fig 20.4

Kamal A, Brocklehurst JC: *Color Atlas of Geriatric Medicine,* London, 1991, Wolfe. In Wilson, SF, Giddens JF: *Health Assessment for Nursing Practice,* ed 6, St. Louis, 2017, Mosby: Skill 4.3, Step 14

Knit-Rite 4-Way Shrinker. Photo credit: Knit-Rite, Inc. Copyright 2019: Skill 6.14, Step 18

Lewis S et al: *Medical-Surgical Nursing: Assessment and Management of Clinical Problems,* ed 10, St. Louis, 2017, Mosby: Fig 13.1; Fig 17.3

Lewis S et al: *Medical-Surgical Nursing: Assessment and Management of Clinical Problems,* ed 9, St. Louis, 2014, Mosby: Fig 8.7; Fig 19.13; Skill 19.4, Step 22G; Skill 19.4, Step 25; Fig 19.15; Fig 19.16; Fig 20.10

Lowdermilk DL, Perry SE: *Maternity and Women's Health Care,* ed 9, St. Louis, 2007. In Ball J et al.: *Seidel's Guide to Physical Examination,* ed 8, St Louis, 2015, Mosby: Skill 4.9, Step 18

McCance K et al: *Pathophysiology: The Biologic Basis for Disease in Adults and Children,* ed 7, St Louis, 2014, Mosby: Fig 19.1; Fig 19.5

Modified from Seidel H et al: *Mosby's Guide to Physical Examination,* ed 7, Mosby, 2011. In Wilson SF, Giddens JF: *Health Assessment for Nursing Practice,* ed 5, St. Louis, 2013, Mosby: Skill 4.6, Step 19

Modified from Swartz MH: *Textbook of Physical Diagnosis: History and Examination,* ed 6, Philadelphia, 2010. In Wilson SF, Giddens JF: *Health Assessment for Nursing Practice,* ed 5, St. Louis, 2013, Mosby: Skill 4.4, Step 14

Patton KT et al: *Essentials of Anatomy & Physiology,* St. Louis, 2012, Mosby: Fig 14.2; Fig 18.17; Fig 18.18

Patton KT, Thibodeau GA: *The Human Body in Health and Disease,* ed 7, St. Louis, 2018, Mosby: Fig 19.2; Fig 20.9

Patton, KT, Thibodeau, GA: *The Human Body in Health and Disease,* ed 6, St. Louis, 2014, Mosby: Fig 2.2; Fig 9.1; Fig 14.1; Fig 15.1

Patton KT, Thibodeau GA: *Structure and Function of the Body,* ed 15, St. Louis, 2014, Elsevier: Fig 20.2; Fig 20.3

Patton, KT, Thibodeau, GA: *Anatomy & Physiology,* ed 10, St. Louis, 2019, Mosby: Fig 20.1

Patton, KT, Thibodeau, GA: *Anatomy & Physiology,* ed 8, St. Louis, 2013, Mosby: Fig 4.6

Patton KT, Thibodeau GA: *Anthony's Textbook of Anatomy & Physiology,* ed 20, St. Louis, 2013, Mosby: Fig 12.1

Perry A et al: *Clinical Nursing Skills & Techniques,* ed 8, St. Louis, 2014, Mosby: Fig 6.8; Fig 6.9; Fig 6.10B; Skill 6.12, Step 8 (Image courtesy Össur Americas. All rights reserved.); Fig 11.10

Perry A et al: *Fundamentals of Nursing,* ed 8, St. Louis, 2013, Mosby: Skill 2.18, Step 9; Skill 2.18, Step 10; Skill 5.3, Step 18B; Skill 7.12, Step 14

Reprinted with permission of Nellcor Puritan Bennett Inc., Pleasanton, CA: Fig 18.10

Rumack C et al: *Diagnostic Ultrasound,* ed 4, Philadelphia, 2011, Mosby: Fig 13.2

Sorrentino SA, Remmert L: *Mosby's Textbook for Nursing Assistants,* ed 8, St. Louis, 2012, Mosby. In Yoost BL, Crawford LR: *Fundamentals of Nursing: Active Learning for Collaborative Practice,* 2e, St. Louis, 2020, Elsevier: Fig 6.4

United States Department of Agriculture (USDA): Fig 5.1

Wesley K: *Huszar's ECG and 12-Lead Interpretation,* ed 5, St. Louis, 2017, Elsevier: Fig 19.8 (first image); Fig 19.9; Fig 19.10; Fig 19.11

Wiegand DL: *AACN Procedure Manual for High Acuity, Progressive, and Critical Care,* ed 7, 2017, St. Louis, Elsevier: Box 18.6

Williams P: *de Wit's Fundamental Concepts and Skills for Nursing,* ed 5, St. Louis, 2018, Mosby: Skill 14.1, Step 19

Wilson SF, Giddens JF: *Health Assessment for Nursing Practice,* ed 6, St. Louis, 2017, Mosby: Skill 4.6, Step 28; Skill 4.8, Step 36

Yoost BL, Crawford LR: *Fundamentals of Nursing: Active Learning for Collaborative Practice,* ed 2, St. Louis, 2020, Elsevier: Fig 7.1; Fig 8.1; Skill 11.3, Step 21B; Fig 11.15; Skill 11.18, Step 25; Skill 11.18, Step 26

INDEX

Page numbers followed by *f, t,* or *b* indicate figures, tables, or boxes, respectively.